Practical General Practice

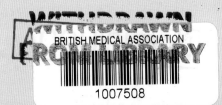

Practical General Practice
Guidelines for Effective Clinical Management

SEVENTH EDITION

Adam Staten, MA (Cantab), MBBS, MRCP (UK), DRCOG, DMCC, PGCertCE, MRCGP

General Practitioner
Milton Keynes, UK

Paul Staten, MBBS, MA (Cantab), DRCOG, MRCGP

General Practitioner
Milton Keynes, UK

For additional online content visit
ExpertConsult.com

ELSEVIER
Edinburgh   London   New York   Oxford   Philadelphia   St Louis   Sydney   2019

ELSEVIER

First edition 1988
Second edition 1992
Third edition 1999
Fourth edition 2003
Fifth edition 2006
Sixth edition 2011
Seventh edition 2020

Notices

Practitioners and researchers must always rely on their own experience and knowledge in evaluating and using any information, methods, compounds or experiments described herein. Because of rapid advances in the medical sciences, in particular, independent verification of diagnoses and drug dosages should be made. To the fullest extent of the law, no responsibility is assumed by Elsevier, authors, editors or contributors for any injury and/or damage to persons or property as a matter of products liability, negligence or otherwise, or from any use or operation of any methods, products, instructions, or ideas contained in the material herein.

ISBN: 9780702055522

Senior Content Strategist: Pauline Graham
Content Development Specialist: Carole McMurray
Content Coordinator: Susan Jansons
Project Manager: Radjan Lourde Selvanadin
Design: Brian Salisbury
Illustration Manager: Narayanan Ramakrishnan
Illustrator: Graphic World
Marketing Manager: Deborah Watkins

Printed in China

Last digit is the print number: 9 8 7 6 5 4 3 2 1

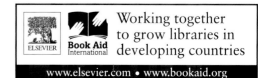

Contents

Preface

It is 30 years since the publication of the first edition of this textbook and since then, a time during which five further editions of the book have been published, a wealth of research and numerous guidelines have been produced as part of the worldwide crusade to practise the evidence-based medicine, for which this book was in some ways a forerunner.

This is the first edition not to be edited by Alex Khot and Andrew Polmear, whose vision and passion for producing straightforward, evidence-based, and above all practical guidelines for general practitioners working at the coal face of primary care originally brought this textbook into being. We hope this edition follows those principles and remains a reliable desktop companion for GPs.

Producing a guidelines-based book like this is much like the endless work of Sisyphus pushing his boulder up a hill in Tartarus for all eternity, only to watch it roll back down before reaching the summit. The pace of change in medicine, the rate at which guidelines are produced, and at which consensus opinion changes, makes it almost inevitable that a book such as this is at risk of being out of date before the ink is dry on the page. However, guidelines tend to change by evolution rather than revolution and the content of this book, produced by experts working in the real world of daily practice, is likely to differ only by nuance in the coming years from the guidance produced by the various esteemed medical institutions.

As ever, this book should be seen as a guide and a template from which general practitioners can derive their own ways of working based on a logical, structured approach. The chapters of this book are designed to mirror the mental processes of the doctor during the general practice consultation and so help that doctor to synthesise rational and safe treatment plans for his or her patients.

Whilst keeping pace with the changes in guidance has made the production of this book a challenge, the wealth and breadth of research and guidance currently available has also enabled our contributors to produce more robust guidance than has ever previously been possible.

In recognition of the fact that previous editions of this book have attracted a readership outside of the United Kingdom, this edition has deliberately been designed to be less UK focused with guidance based on guidelines and opinion from around the globe. Where possible the details of patient support groups, relevant to specific diseases in different countries, have also been included to reflect the more global outlook of this edition.

Adam Staten
Paul Staten

The Structure of the Book

Bullets

Different coloured bullet points have been used to provide emphasis for different types of comment:

- Black bullets are for general information or explanation e.g. 'Treatment can be expected to….'
- Pink bullets are instructions for questions that should be asked, examinations that should be performed, or investigations and treatments that should be undertaken e.g. 'Ask the patient x, y and z', 'Examine for a, b and c'.
- Grey bullets are used where there is a subdivision of another heading.

Lists

Where we present a list in no particular order we use:

(a) chest pain; or
(b) hypotension; or
(c) heart failure.

Where the order is important we number the list:

1. Sit the patient up.
2. Give oxygen.
3. Give diamorphine …

Boxes

These are used to highlight information that might otherwise get lost in the text: guidelines, a list of tests as a 'work-up' for a patient with a particular condition, or patient organisations for example.

References

Our aim is to reference every statement of fact. Where such a statement is not accompanied by a reference, the reader can assume it is taken from the reference in a box at the start of that section.

Acknowledgements

Firstly we would like to thank Alex Khot and Andrew Polmear whose vision led to the production of the first six editions of this text book; we hope that this current edition lives up to the high standards they have set. We would, of course, like to thank all our contributors who have worked to ever tightening deadlines, to produce a set of great chapters, frequently swimming against the tide of new guidance and research to keep this edition up to date as we have moved through production. We would particularly like to thank Mr Iain Wilson, Mr Robert Hone, and Dr Naema Alam who all stepped in at the last moment with invaluable advice and contributions to help get this book to press.

An enormous thank you must go to the team at Elsevier, in particular, Carole McMurray, Pauline Graham, and Radjan Lourde Selvanadin for whom the last few months and years must have felt like something of a cat herding exercise.

Adam would like to thank his wife Shiva and his daughters Rose and Grace who have had to tolerate a husband and father who has spent many vacant hours tapping slowly at his laptop. Paul would like to thank his partner Erica for her help and support.

List of Contributors

The editor(s) would like to acknowledge and offer grateful thanks for the input of all previous editions' contributors, without whom this new edition would not have been possible.

Annemieke Bikker, MSc
Teaching Fellow
University of Edinburgh
Usher Institute of Population Health Sciences and
    Informatics
College of Medicine and Veterinary Medicine
Edinburgh, Scotland

Ruth Margaret Bland, BSc, MBChB, MD, FRCPCH
Consultant General Paediatrics
Royal Hospital for Children and Honorary Associate
    Clinical Professor
Institute of Health and Wellbeing
University of Glasgow
Glasgow

David Nicholas Blane, BSc, MBChB, MPH
Clinical Academic Fellow
General Practice and Primary Care
University of Glasgow
Glasgow

Christopher Burton, MD, FRCGP
Professor of Primary Medical Care University of Sheffield
Sheffield

David Carty, MBChB, PhD, FRCP
Consultant Endocrinologist
Department of Diabetes, Endocrinology and Clinical
    Pharmacology
Glasgow Royal Infirmary
Glasgow

Jane Colgan, MBChB, DTH&H, MRCP
Specialty Doctor
Monklands Hosptial
Lanarkshire
Airdrie, Scotland

Lynsay Crawford, MBChB
Clinical University Teacher
School of Medicine, University of Glasgow
Deputy Director of Vocational Studies
School of Medicine, University of Glasgow
GP Partner
Balmore Surgery
Possilpark Health and Care Centre
Glasgow

Ben Dietsch, MBChB
Lead Specialty Doctor
Willen Hospice
Milton Keynes

**Kieran Dinwoodie, MBChB, MRCGP, DRCOG, DTM&H,
Dip Derm**
General Practitioner Principal
Calderside Medical Practice
Blantyre

Al Dowie, PhD
General Practice and Primary Care
University of Glasgow
Glasgow

Russell Drummond, MBChB
Honorary Clinical Associate Professor
School of Medicine, Dentistry and Nursing
University of Glasgow
Glasgow

Suzannah Drummond, MBBS, FRCOphth
Consultant in Ophthalmic Surgery
Ophthalmology
Tennent Institute of Ophthalmology
Glasgow

Anchal Goyal, MBBS, nMRCGP, DRCOG, DPD, GPwSI
Dermatology
NHS Lanarkshire
Monklands District General Hospital, Airdrie

Kate Hughes, MBChB PhD MRCP (Diabetes and Endocrinology)
Consultant Physician and Diabetologist and
    Endocrinologist
Honorary Senior Lecturer
School of Medicine, Dentistry and Nursing
University of Glasgow
Glasgow

Heather Lafferty, MBChB, MRCP
Consultant Physician and Gastroenterologist
Queen Elizabeth University Hospital
Glasgow

Lynn A. Legg, PhD, MPH
Research Fellow
Scottish Centre for Excellence in Rehabilitation Research
University of Strathclyde
Glasgow

Sharon Mackin, MBChB (Hons), MRCP
Specialty Registrar Diabetes and Endocrinology
Department of Diabetes and Endocrinology
Glasgow Royal Infirmary
Glasgow

John MacLean, MBChB, MRCGP, FRCPS (Glas), FFSEM, DRCOG
General Practitioner
Maryhill Health and Care Centre and
    Sport and Exercise Medicine Doctor
Hampden Sports Clinic and Scottish FA and
    Honorary Clinical Associate Professor
University of Glasgow
Glasgow

Frances McManus, MBChB, BMedSci, PhD, MRCP (Diabetes and Endocrinology)
Consultant Physician
Department of Diabetes
Endocrinology and Clinical Pharmacology
Glasgow Royal Infirmary
Glasgow

Stewart W. Mercer, MD, PhD, FRCGP, FFPHM, FRCPE
Professor of Primary Care Research
University of Glasgow
Director of the Scottish School of Primary Care
Glasgow

Catriona Nisbett, MBChB, MRCGP, MRCP, DRCOG, Dip Dermatology
General Practitioner
The Murray Surgery, East Kilbride

Declan Nugent, MB BCh, BAO, MRCGP
General Practitioner
Glasgow

Hilary Pinnock, MBChB, MD, MRCGP
Reader
Allergy and Respiratory Research Group, Centre for
    Population Health Sciences
University of Edinburgh
Edinburgh, Scotland
General Practitioner
Whitstable Medical Practice
Whitstable

Hilary Lockhart Pearce, MBChB, MRCPCH
Consultant General Paediatrics
Royal Hospital for Children
Glasgow

Lindsey Pope, MBChB, MRCGP, PGCertMedEd, FHEA
Clinical Senior University Teacher
General Practice and Primary Care
University of Glasgow
Glasgow

Ian Reeves, BSc, BM
Department of Medicine for the Elderly
Southern General Hospital
Glasgow

Neil Ritchie, MBChB, PhD, MRCP(UK) (Infectious Diseases)
Clinical Lecturer in Infectious Diseases
Institute of Infection, Immunity and Inflammation
University of Glasgow
Glasgow

John Paul Seenan, MBChB, MD, MRCP
Consultant
Department of Gastroenterology
Queen Elizabeth University Hospital
Glasgow

Aziz Sheikh, BSc, MBBS, MSc, MD
Chair of Primary Care Research and Development
University of Edinburgh
Usher Institute of Population Health Sciences and
    Informatics
College of Medicine and Veterinary Medicine
Edinburgh

Dominique Thompson, MBChB, MRCGP (Dist)
GP and Director
Buzz Consulting
Bristol

Jane Tracy, MBBS, DRACOG, GCHE
Director
Centre for Developmental Disability Health Victoria
Monash University
Melbourne, Victoria, Australia

Harry Hao-Xiang Wang, PhD
Associate Professor
School of Public Health
Sun Yat-Sen University
PR China
Honorary Senior Lecturer
General Practice and Primary Care
University of Glasgow
Glasgow

Iain Wilson, MBBS, BSc, MRCS
Surgical Trainee
Queen Alexandra Hospital
Portsmouth

1

Principles and Practice of Primary Care

ADAM STATEN

CHAPTER CONTENTS

OBJECTIVES

- Primary care can be defined as any care that is delivered in the community as opposed to the inpatient setting. In wealthier countries primary care is usually considered to be the first level of care provision, whereas in poorer countries it may be seen as a systemwide strategy to providing access to healthcare (World Health Organization [WHO], 2003).
- It is widely recognised that building health services around high-quality primary care results in better public health, fewer inequalities in healthcare by socioeconomic class, and lower rates of unnecessary hospital admissions (Kringos, Boerma, van der Zee, & Groenewegen, 2013).
- The structure of primary care varies widely from country to country but there are key similarities to treating patients in the community that are true in all countries, and all healthcare systems, including the interaction between healthcare, social care, and third sector organisations, a

holistic approach to patient care, and an approach to patient care that is proactive rather than reactive.
- The WHO (2003) recognises the core principles of primary care to be:
  1. universal access to care and coverage based on need;
  2. commitment to health equity as part of development oriented to social justice;
  3. community participation in defining and implementing health agenda;
  4. intersectoral approaches to health.
- These principles are underpinned by the declaration of Alma-Ata, made in 1978 (WHO 1978) in which primary care was defined as "essential health care based on practical, scientifically sound and socially acceptable methods and technology made universally accessible."

Challenges of Primary Care

Population Challenges

- The provision of holistic care is at the heart of primary care and providing this care is increasingly challenging with a global population that is increasing in size, age, and multimorbidity.
- The increasing capability to diagnose and treat disease leads to increasing patient demand and increasing resource cost both in terms of time and finance.
- Particularly in developed nations, the rise of illnesses related to lifestyle factors such as smoking, alcohol consumption, and obesity create a burden to the healthcare system and are a complicating factor to many other illnesses. Globally, infectious diseases such human immunodeficiency virus/acquired immunodeficiency syndrome (HIV/AIDS) contribute to the increasing burden on primary healthcare (and the wider healthcare system).
- An increasing emphasis in maintaining wellness rather than simply treating ill health has put primary care at the forefront of screening programmes, education programmes, and primary preventative treatment.
- The increasing capabilities of modern medicine, the emphasis on keeping people well, and wider public access to healthcare information (via the internet, for example) all contribute to rising patient expectations and managing these expectations in a resource limited environment can prove very challenging. In the United Kingdom the General Medical Council (GMC) found that this rise in expectations was a key contributing factor to the 100% increase in complaints made against doctors between 2007 and 2012 (GMC, 2014). Rising patient expectations is also frequently cited as a reason for doctors leaving their role in primary care (Leese, Young, & Sibbald, 2002).

The Challenge of External Factors

- Healthcare is expensive and funding for primary care is not always adequate to meet the needs of the population it serves. For example, in many developing countries funding is diverted away from the provision of comprehensive primary care in favour of providing vertical care programmes targeting specific issues such as HIV/AIDS or childhood immunisations (Maeseneer et al., 2008).
- The provision of healthcare can become highly politicised and interference in healthcare from politicians for political purposes, rather than to improve patient care, can be a source of real frustration and dissatisfaction for doctors.
- Doctors now practice in the full glare of the media (and social media) spotlight. Not only can this be intimidating and exposing, but doctors working in general practice are often left to undo the damage done by inaccurate messages promulgated by the media.
- A worldwide tendency to increasing litigation and, in some circumstances, the criminalisation of medical error

add to the pressures of working within primary care and medicine in general.

The Evolving Primary Care Team

- Whilst general practitioners (GPs) are usually considered to be central to the provision of primary care services, the primary care team includes all those professionals who contribute to the health and well-being of patients in the community.
- With the increasing complexity of healthcare provision, and the increasing complexity of the patients who receive treatment in the community, any attempt for GPs to practice in isolation without recourse to the wider primary healthcare team is likely to result in frustration for the GP and poor-quality, possibly dangerous care for patients.
- The roles and responsibilities of the primary care team are to some extent limitless. It is characteristic of primary care that practitioners working in the community are expected to deal to a greater or lesser extent with every problem that a patient may present. Often these problems are not simply medical and they may be complicated by, or indeed may primarily be, psychological or social problems.
- Many tasks in primary care are as well, and often better, performed by members of the primary care team other than GPs.
- The structure of primary care teams varies from country to country—for example, in the United Kingdom dentists usually work separately from GPs, but in other European countries it is common for doctors and dentists to be colocated. Similarly, professionals such as social workers and mental health nurses are located alongside GPs in many countries.
- As coordinating patient care becomes ever more complex it is vital that the extended primary care team works coherently to avoid patient neglect or duplication of effort to deliver effective, rational care to patients.
- Workforce problems in primary care in many countries have led to the innovation of new roles for established healthcare professionals within primary care and the creation of entirely new types of healthcare professionals.
- The primary care team in any community should be tailored to suit the healthcare needs of the local population and it is therefore essential for anyone involved with workforce planning to be familiar with the variety of professionals that can contribute to providing primary healthcare.
- To deal with the demands of modern healthcare, doctors should see themselves as having a key role in driving healthcare policy toward establishing the most effective primary care teams for their particular populations.

Nurse Practitioners

- Nurse practitioners, or advanced nurse practitioners, are trained beyond the usual competences of registered nurses so that they are able to practice autonomously and assess and diagnose undifferentiated problems, to synthesise treatment plans (Royal College of Nursing, 2012). Key to this is their ability to prescribe independently.

- Nurse practitioners work in many different areas of healthcare but within primary care they provide care both for acute illness (usually by providing consultations for minor illness) and chronic disease (such as performing routine reviews in respiratory illness or diabetes).
- They are well established in Anglophone countries where they are seen as a key resource in helping to manage patient demand, but they are less well recognised in other parts of the world.
- Training to become an advanced nurse practitioner varies from country to country and depends on the area of healthcare in which the nurse is working, but in the United Kingdom the Royal College of Nursing provides accredited training courses to upskill nurses and prepare them for an advanced role.
- Evidence suggests that nurse practitioners provide good levels of patient satisfaction and good patient outcomes, but the evidence of cost effectiveness remains equivocal (Martin-Misener et al., 2015).

Physiotherapists

- Up to 30% of primary care consultations relate to musculoskeletal problems, many of which are best dealt with by physiotherapists. However, direct access to physiotherapists for patients is not necessarily the norm within primary care.
- Direct access is usually available to patients in Australia, absent in the United States, and patchy throughout the European Union. This variability in access is despite the fact that the majority of countries, particularly within Europe, have the requisite legislation and train their physiotherapists to have the requisite competencies to practice independently. Often the barriers to enabling direct access come from within the medical profession itself, despite the potential reduction in workload that physiotherapists can provide (Chartered Society of Physiotherapists, 2013). Where direct access is not available patients must usually come via their primary care physician to get access to physiotherapy.
- The provision of direct access physiotherapy has been shown to be both clinically and cost effective (Mallet et al., 2014).

Clinical Pharmacists

- Clinical pharmacists have an extended role that involves direct patient-facing activity with particular respect to medicine management. Their key roles are in optimising medication and dosage regimes, de-conflicting medications that may interact, and ensuring the cost effectiveness of medications. Many are also involved in the management of minor ailments and chronic disease.
- As polypharmacy in an ageing population becomes more common, expertise in medicine management will be increasingly important and an increasing workload burden for general practitioners.
- The role is perhaps best established in the United States where clinical pharmacists have been working and evolving their role over a period of decades. In 1997 the WHO published policy statements that envisaged an expanded future role for pharmacists that would benefit patients in healthcare systems globally. Since then the role has become increasingly recognised in the Anglosphere and across Europe. Clinical pharmacists are also invaluable in bolstering the primary care teams in countries where doctor numbers are low.

Physician Assistants/Associates

- To train as a physician assistant (also known as a *physician associate*) the trainee must already have a degree in a life or healthcare science subject. Physician assistants then undergo an intense period of training in the medical model to enable them to interview, examine, and diagnose patients; order and interpret tests; and perform procedures according to competency. They may work in a variety of settings from surgery to emergency medicine, but many work in primary care.
- The physician assistant is a dependent medical practitioner who works under the supervision of a physician. The ability to prescribe is variable depending on the country (or US state) in which the individual works.
- The physician assistant is a US invention; the role was established there over 50 years ago. Currently there are around 100,000 physician assistants practicing. They have been shown to be cost effective and acceptable to patients, and in recent years several countries have shown interest in developing training programmes to produce physician assistants to alleviate pressure on primary care doctors (Legler, Cawley, & Fenn, 2007).

Mental Health Professionals

- Mental health problems are an enormous part of primary care, either as the presenting problem or as a complicating factor for other problems. Up to one third of all general practice appointments are thought to involve a mental health component.
- Given this workload and the economic burden of mental health in primary care, the WHO has produced policy emphasising the importance of providing good-quality primary mental healthcare. However, it remains unusual for mental health nurses, or other mental health professionals who are capable of delivering psychologic treatments, to be embedded within the primary care team.
- Since 2014 in the Netherlands there has been a deliberate shift in the provision of mental healthcare from secondary to primary care. This has been largely facilitated by increasing the number of mental health nurses working

alongside GPs such that between 2010 and 2014 the proportion of practices in the Netherlands with a mental health nurse increased from 20% to over 80%. This has not reduced GP workload but has increased the number of long appointments available in the community to patients with mental health problems (Magnée et al., 2016).

- A Cochrane review of the effectiveness of counselling provided within primary care found that it was clinically more effective in the short term than usual care (although not in the long term) and associated with similar costs to usual care (Bower et al., 2011).

Medical Assistants

- Medical assistants primarily work within primary care teams in the United States. They are allied health professionals who work in both administrative and clinical roles. Their duties may include scheduling appointments, handling correspondence, updating patient notes, as well as performing clinical procedures such as ECGs and blood draws, assisting the physician during procedures, or preparing patients for examination.
- It is suggested that they are a key means by which doctors can relieve themselves of their administrative workload and so enable themselves to focus more on direct patient care (Sinsky et al., 2013).

Use of Technology

The use of technology within medicine has the potential to improve patient care and make the working life of primary healthcare professionals easier and less stressful. As technologies develop it is important that those working within primary care stay alert to new ways in which this technology can be applied to their own working environments.

Electronic Medical Records
(Davies et al., 2016)

- The use of electronic medical records (EMRs) is common but not ubiquitous. In New Zealand, Scandinavia, and the United Kingdom the use of medical records is almost universal, but this is not the case in other developed nations; for example, in Canada rates are below 80% and in Switzerland they are below 60%.
- Even where EMRs are used the capabilities of different systems vary enormously with the most advanced allowing the review of results, correspondence, production of patient summaries, transfer of electronic prescriptions to pharmacies, and prompts and alerts for patient review. This allows for more seamless care, reduction in duplication of work, and the setting up of efficient and reliable patient recall systems for patient review and monitoring.
- Higher levels of doctor satisfaction with their EMRs have been shown to correlate with overall higher job satisfaction.

Telemedicine

- Telemedicine (or telehealth) relates to the remote monitoring of patients and the transfer of biometric data from the patients' home to their doctor. It has perhaps been most utilised when dealing with cardiovascular or respiratory disease to enable early detection of decompensation of the monitored illness and proactive, early management.
- As technology advances and equipment such as blood pressure monitors and oxygen saturation probes become cheaper it is likely that this will be seen as a convenient and cost-effective means of managing patients. It has the added advantage of engaging patients with their own care and empowering them to take responsibility for managing their illness.
- The cost effectiveness of telemedicine remains uncertain (Henderson, 2013), but it is likely that increasing amounts of remote monitoring will become part and parcel of future general practice; and as its use becomes more common its cost effectiveness will improve.

Communications Technology

- We have more ways to communicate with one another than ever before—via telephone, email, text message, or video phone. These technologies present the possibility of interacting with our patients and our colleagues more efficiently and more flexibly.
- Younger patients in particular are comfortable with communicating electronically. For example, the use of virtual clinics that employ email and text messaging to communicate with young diabetic patients has dramatically improved attendance rates (Mayor, 2016).
- Video phone applications (such as Skype) have been used in a variety of settings: providing remote care for refugees, orthopaedic follow-up, and psychiatric consultation. GPs in the United Kingdom have experimented with using Skype™ to review patients in nursing homes.
- There are numerous email or phone-based systems that can be employed to enable GPs to access specialist advice rapidly, which may obviate the need for an acute admission or a referral for specialist advice.

Models of Care

- As the burden of caring for enlarging and ageing populations increases, the way in which patients are seen in primary care will need to be adapted to increase capacity within the system.
- GPs need to adapt the ways in which they see their patients to suit their particular patient populations. Some of these varied models of seeing patients will be reliant on the technologies discussed earlier in the chapter; others require a fresh approach to the traditional medical consultation.

Telephone Triage

- Telephone triage is a means by which patient demand and flow can be managed. It has become popular, particularly in the United Kingdom, as a way to reduce the number of patients that need to be seen face to face and involves patients speaking to a health professional (usually a doctor or a nurse) by phone to assess the need for a face-to-face review before the patient is offered an appointment.
- Some who advocate the system estimate that up to 60% of primary care problems can be resolved over the phone and there is evidence suggesting that patients find this means of interacting with their GP satisfactory.
- However, the ESTEEM trial was a large-scale trial of telephone triage which found that, although clinician contact time on the day of the appointment request was reduced, overall clinician contact time was no different to usual care, which to some extent undermines its purpose (Holt et al., 2016).

Shared Medical Appointments

- Shared medical appointments are part medical consultation, part education session. Groups of patients with the same condition are seen together for an extended appointment and educated about their condition and how it can be managed. This saves overall clinician time whilst increasing the contact time the patient has with the clinician. Other benefits include empowering patients to self-manage and the creation of a peer support network for patients.
- They have been used in a range of settings including diabetes, maternity, physiotherapy, and liver disease. Patients report higher levels of satisfaction with shared medical appointment care than with usual care (Heyworth et al., 2014).

The General Practitioner Consultant

- This is a model of care that relies on the GP having a team of varied allied health professionals at hand.
- This model of care relies on central triage which directs patients toward the relevant professional (e.g., physiotherapist, mental health nurse, physician associate). The GP is not directly involved in the initial patient contact but is called in to consult on cases that are beyond the capability of the allied health professional.
- Theoretically this frees up the GP to dedicate time to those most complex patients who require the most skilled input albeit at the expense of the regular and recurrent patient contacts that many would argue provide job satisfaction in primary care.

The Virtual Ward

- The virtual ward is a concept designed to manage patients, often housebound patients, who require intense, proactive, and multidisciplinary input. It is an elaboration on the concept of the multidisciplinary team and may or may not make use of telehealth data.
- Versions of the virtual ward that have been trialled usually involve a team consisting of community nurses, GPs, geriatricians, and possibly representatives from social services. This team meets at regular intervals to discuss a case load of complex patients.
- By meeting regularly and having input from a number of disciplines this approach aims to improve proactive care and so reduce the risk of an acute decompensation in illness requiring hospital admission. It should also reduce duplication of effort by improving communication between all those involved in the patient's care.

Caring for the Doctor

The Burnout Syndrome

- The world of general practice is without doubt stressful and continues to become more so as a result of the challenges detailed already in this chapter. A 2015 Commonwealth Fund survey of primary care in 10 developed nations found that significant proportions of doctors in all 10 countries found their work in general practice either very stressful or extremely stressful (Davies et al., 2016).
- The phenomenon of physician burnout is well recognised but often not well handled. The three key features of burnout are usually described as:
  1. emotional exhaustion;
  2. depersonalisation;
  3. an absent sense of personal accomplishment.
- The burnout syndrome overlaps with, and is complicated by, anxiety and depression and shares key features with those issues such as social withdrawal, absenteeism from work, and problems with drug and alcohol abuse.
- Doctors are at high risk of burnout as they are selected based on personality traits such as perfectionism, high achievement, a sense of responsibility, and competitiveness, which all put them at higher risk of burning out.
- Work within medicine exposes people to extended periods of extreme emotional stress (both their own and that of other people), which contributes to burnout.
- A perceived stigma to mental illness amongst doctors also means that doctors tend to seek help late by which point the damage may well be significant, including suicidality.

Finding Help and Treatment

- It is important that those working within general practice recognise the signs of stress and burnout both in themselves and in their colleagues and feel able to seek help or suggest that their colleagues seek help.

- Treatment for the burnout syndrome, or for depression or substance misuse problems in general, is along standard lines and includes cognitive behavioural therapy (CBT), medication, and counselling. These can be sought via the doctors' own GP although many are reluctant to seek help in this way for themselves. Alternatively, many countries have mental health programmes specifically for medical professionals that can operate on an anonymous basis.
- Self-help techniques such as mindfulness also have a good evidence base amongst doctors working in primary care and many simple mindfulness techniques can be learnt via online apps.
- GPs also have the opportunity to tackle the source of their distress either by changing the way in which they work or by changing the type of work that they do within the varied world of primary care.

Further Reading

Staten, A., & Lawson, E. (2017). *GP wellbeing: Combatting burnout in general practice*. London: CRC Press.

References

Bower, P., Knowles, S., Coventry, P. A., et al. (2011). Counselling for mental health and psychosocial problems in primary care. *Cochrane Database of Systematic Reviews*, (9), CD001025.

Chartered Society of Physiotherapists. (2013). Direct access and patient/client self-referral to physiotherapy: A review of contemporary practice within the European Union. *Physiotherapy, 99*, 285–291.

Davies, E., et al. (2016). *Under pressure: What the Commonwealth Fund's 2015 international survey of general practitioners means for the UK*. Retrieved from http://www.health.org.uk/publication/under-pressure#sthash.3qqLghqH.dpuf.

General Medical Council. (2014). *What's behind the rise in complaints about doctors from members of the public*. Retrieved from https://gmcuk.wordpress.com/2014/07/21/whats-behind-the-rise-in-complaints-about-doctors-from-members-of-the-public/.

Henderson, C. (2013). Cost effectiveness of telehealth for patients with long term conditions (Whole Systems Demonstrator telehealth questionnaire study): Nested economic evaluation in a pragmatic, cluster randomised controlled trial. *British Medical Journal (Clinical Research Ed.), 346*. doi:https://doi.org/10.1136/bmj.f1035.

Heyworth, L., et al. (2014). Influence of shared medical appointments on patient satisfaction: A retrospective 3-year study. *Annals of Family Medicine, 12*, 324–330.

Holt, T., et al. (2016). Telephone triage systems in UK general practice: Analysis of consultation duration during the index day in a pragmatic randomised controlled trial. *The British Journal of General Practice, 66*, e214–e218.

Kringos, D. S., Boerma, W., van der Zee, J., & Groenewegen, P. (2013). Europe's strong primary care systems are linked to better population health but also to higher health spending. *Health Affairs, 32*, 686–694. doi:10.1377/hlthaff.2012.1242.

Leese, B., Young, R., & Sibbald, B. (2002). GP principals leaving practice in the UK. *The European Journal of General Practice, 8*, 62–68.

Legler, C. F., Cawley, J. F., & Fenn, W. H. (2007). Physician assistants: Education, practice and global interest. *Medical Teacher, 29*, e22–e25.

Maeseneer, J., van Weel, C., Egilman, D., et al. (2008). Funding for primary health care in developing countries. *BMJ (Clinical Research Ed.), 336*, 518–519.

Magnée, T., de Beurs, D. P., de Bakker, D. H., et al. (2016). Consultations in general practices with and without mental health nurses: An observational study from 2010 to 2014. *BMJ Open, 6*, e011579.

Mallett, R., et al. (2014). Is physiotherapy self-referral with telephone triage viable, cost-effective and beneficial to musculoskeletal outpatients in a primary care setting? *Musculoskeletal Care, 12*, 251–260.

Martin-Misener, R., et al. (2015). Cost effectiveness of nurse practitioners. *British Medical Journal Open, 5*, e007167.

Mayor, S. (2016). Use texts, apps, and Skype to keep young people with diabetes engaged with services, says guidance. *British Medical Journal (Clinical Research Ed.), 352*, i394.

Royal College of Nursing. (2012). *Advanced Nurse Practitioners: An RCN Guide to advanced nursing practice, advanced nurse practitioners and programme accreditation*.

Sinsky, C., et al. (2013). In search of joy in practice: A report of 23 high-functioning primary care practices. *Annals of Family Medicine, 11*, 272–278.

World Health Organisation. (1978). *Declaration of International Conference on Primary Health Care*, Alma-Ata, USSR, 6–12 September.

World Health Organisation. (2003). *The World Health Report: Shaping the future*. Geneva: WHO Publishing.

2

Long-Term Conditions

STEWART W. MERCER, HARRY HAO-XIANG WANG

CHAPTER CONTENTS

OBJECTIVES

- A long-term condition (LTC) is commonly defined as *a condition that requires ongoing medical care, limits what one can do, and is likely to last for a year or more.*
- Common long-term conditions include diseases such as coronary heart disease, diabetes, asthma, and stroke. Patients with such conditions are commonly seen and managed in primary care in the long term. Less common chronic conditions seen in general practice include multiple sclerosis, Parkinson disease, and muscular dystrophy.
- Conditions once considered terminal are now commonly seen, and regarded as long-term conditions, due to improved survival rates from treatments, and this includes many cancers and infectious diseases such as human immunodeficiency virus (HIV) and acquired immunodeficiency syndrome (AIDS).

Prevalence of Long-Term Conditions

- Prevalence rates of individual long-term conditions vary considerably between different countries and populations, though in most countries, including developing countries, long-term conditions are increasing rapidly in the population. This is true in all age groups, although certain conditions affect certain age groups more than others.
- It should be borne in mind that all prevalence estimates of long-term conditions are based on data collection methods that have some flaws. Thus prevalence estimates will vary according to how the condition is defined and measured.

Comorbidity and Multimorbidity

- International studies have demonstrated that many people living with chronic disorders have multiple chronic health problems simultaneously. The co-occurrence of one or more additional long-term conditions to a person with an index condition (a condition of primary concern) is termed *comorbidity*. For example, a patient with diabetes and asthma, being cared for by a diabetologist, may be considered by the specialist physician as a diabetic with comorbidity. It is a term mainly used by specialists reflecting their own area of expertise.
- In general practice, patients commonly have two or more long-term conditions without one being clearly an index condition, and indeed the extent to which different conditions affect patients often varies over time. Thus in primary care the term *multimorbidity* (MM) is preferred to comorbidity.

Prevalence of MM

- Multimorbidity is common and has been rising in prevalence over recent years. For example, a Canadian study of 21 family practices in Quebec reported a multimorbidity prevalence of 69% in 18- to 44-year-olds, 93% in 45- to 64-year-olds, and 98% in those over age 65, with the number of chronic conditions varying from 2.8 in the youngest to 6.4 in the oldest (Fortin et al., 2005). In the United Kingdom, a large, nationally representative study in Scotland found that over 40% of the whole population (all ages included) had at least one long-term condition, and almost 25% of the entire population had multimorbidity (Barnett et al., 2012).

- The prevalence of multimorbidity increases substantially with age and is present in most people aged 65 years or older. However, the Scottish study also found that the absolute number of people with multimorbidity was higher in those younger than 65 years than those over 65 years, thus long-term conditions and multimorbidity should not be considered simply a problem of old age.

Global Burden

- Over recent decades, life expectancy has improved dramatically and currently exceeds the age of 75 on average, in nearly 60 countries. This is due to improved living circumstances, greater access to universal education, and rapid advances in clinical medicine and public health.
- The ageing of the global population is regarded as the most crucial driver of increases in the burden of chronic diseases. It is particularly evident in wealthier countries where many people are living much longer now than ever, though not necessarily healthier in their extra years. It is estimated that by 2020, the incidence of long-term conditions will increase by approximately 30% to 40% as the population ages.

Deprivation Effects

- Health is seldom distributed evenly across populations and in most (if not all) countries of the world, the poorest health is found in those living in situations of poverty. This is also true of multimorbidity, which tends to be worse in those of the lowest socioeconomic status. The study in Scotland (discussed earlier) revealed an astonishingly precise relationship between multimorbidity and deprivation. Multimorbidity in those living in the most deprived areas also develops some 10 to 15 years younger than in the least deprived decile of the population.
- Many (though not all) studies have found that multimorbidity is more common in women than in men.

Effects of MM

- Many LTCs are associated with increased mortality and/ or morbidity, and this is exacerbated by increasing levels of multimorbidity. There is a clear linear relationship between levels of multimorbidity and death rate.
- Multimorbidity also increases hospital admission rates, even for potentially avoidable admissions and has a major negative impact on quality of life.

Healthcare Utilisation

- Patients with LTCs and multimorbidity may have higher overall vulnerability to diseases and less resistance to acute health threats (e.g., higher susceptibility to influenza). These interacting influences lead to a complex pattern in the demand and utilisation of health services.
- Multimorbidity leads to an increased likelihood of referrals between different providers of healthcare (often in a vertical manner—i.e., general practitioner [GP] to several specialists, but also between specialists, especially in centres of excellence). Excessive use of specialist care leads to a rapid rise in healthcare expenditure. Multimorbidity has become one of the most salient influences on cost of healthcare due to the heavy burden on the healthcare utilisation.

Mental and Physical

- LTCs span both mental and physical conditions, and commonly patients have both. This relationship is bidirectional in that patients with mental health problems commonly go on to develop physical health problems, and patients with a wide range of LTCs are more likely to go on to develop mental health problems than the general population.

Polypharmacy

- A common problem in patients with LTCs is polypharmacy, which is usually defined as *being on five or more regular medications*. In patients with multimorbidity, polypharmacy is even more common. This has serious implications for iatrogenesis. Indeed, a common reason for hospital admission, especially in the elderly, is medication side effects and interactions. Not only is this harmful to patients, but it also infers a huge financial drain on healthcare systems.
- A second problem with polypharmacy is adherence to medication regimens. Research has shown that once patients get to five or more medications per day their adherence begins to decline. That's not to say that patients stop taking all their tablets, but they do tend to be creative in developing their own regimens, especially skipping tablets that have effects that they don't like such as loop diuretics.
- Patients often have strong perceptions of which tablets may be giving them side effects (even if this is unlikely to be the case), which can be influenced by a whole host of things such as pill size, colour, and taste. It has been suggested that polypills (combination pills with several ingredients—e.g., for cardiovascular disease) may enhance adherence by reducing the number of tablets required each day, though at present there is little evidence to support this.

Clinical Guidelines

- A likely major driver of polypharmacy is guidelines. The development of clinical guidelines based on evidence collated from randomised controlled trials has been one of the major advances in the delivery of evidence-based medicine over the last 20 years. However, guidelines are invariably single-disease focused. They give good advice on when to start medications in single LTCs, though seldom give advice on when to stop them. This, combined with the fact that most patients with LTCs have multimorbidity, means that most patients rapidly accumulate new prescriptions and thus polypharmacy.

Evidence-Based General Practice

- The rise of evidence-based medicine (EBM) has been one of the greatest achievements in medical research and the implementation of EBM into general practice has resulted in huge improvements in the management of LTCs. Statin prescribing for hypercholesterolaemia, antihypertensive prescribing for hypertension, achievement of glycaemic control in diabetes through insulin, or drug interventions are a few examples of EBM. The gold standard research method that underpins EBM is the randomised controlled trial (RCT).
- It is such evidence of benefit from RCTs that underpins clinical guidelines. However, there is a danger of overextrapolating findings from RCTs on specific populations (e.g., men <65 years) to a much wider population (e.g., both sexes, elderly). It is also important to realise that most RCTs on LTCs are on patients with single conditions, and most trials actively exclude patients with comorbidity or multimorbidity from taking part in such trials. A recent Cochrane review of interventions specifically for patients with multimorbidity found only a handful of RCTs published worldwide.
- Care must thus be taken not to blindly apply guidelines to all multimorbid patients without consideration of the individual patient's needs, circumstances, and priorities. Clinical judgment and shared decision making based on informed choice are vital tools in the management of patients with LTCs, alongside clinical guidelines.

Management

- The management of patients with LTCs is a large and important part of the work of general practice and primary care. In the United Kingdom, about 80% of patients who consult their GP or practice nurse have an LTC, and as we have seen, most of these patients are likely to have more than one LTC.
- The majority of care for most patients with LTCs can safely be undertaken in primary care, especially once any acute phase has been dealt with by secondary care (e.g., myocardial infarction in patients with congenital heart defect [CHD], initiation of insulin in newly diagnosed type 1 diabetic) and the diagnosis is confirmed.
- In the United Kingdom practice nurses are increasingly involved in the routine care of patients with LTCs (e.g., in conducting annual reviews of patients with hypertension, asthma). These nurses require suitable training and supervision and it is important to emphasise that they are not working autonomously but in partnership with the GPs, who remain the key clinicians in dealing with patients with complex LTCs.

Organisational

- The effective management of patients with LTCs in primary care depends on a well-organised and strong primary care system. The work of the late Barbara Starfield, a preeminent primary care clinical researcher, has shown that countries with strong primary care systems deliver higher quality of care and are more cost effective.
- Thus a well-funded and well-developed primary care system is a basic requisite for the cost-effective management of the vast numbers of patients with LTCs.
- Many models exist with regard to how the management of patients with LTCs is best organised, but one of the best known and most widely used is the chronic care model developed by Wagner and colleagues in the United States. The chronic care model defines a range of important factors, which they suggest need to be addressed to promote effective management of chronic disease. These factors include:
  a. clinical information systems (e.g., disease registers so that patients with known LTCs can be identified and recalled);
  b. delivery system design (e.g., annual review at a planned visit, with members of the primary care team working in a coordinated and complementary way);
  c. decision support (e.g., evidence-based practice guidelines, access to specialist advice);
  d. self-management support (e.g., by giving information, coaching, and motivation to support patients to manage their own conditions better).
- These four factors are thought to work together to improve patient's functional and clinical outcomes as a result of prepared and proactive primary care staff having productive interactions with informed and activated patients.
- Although the chronic care model is intuitively appealing and gives a comprehensive overview of how best care may be achieved, it should be noted that evidence for its effectiveness outside the United States is limited and achieving certain aspects of it can be very difficult in practice.
- The model envisages self-management support as being not just a function of the healthcare system but also a collaborative function of communities. Although this makes good sense in theory, as primary care is imbedded within communities, and communities often have a range of assets that could help people with LTCs (e.g., charitable organisations, faith groups, lunch clubs, exercise facilities), effective linkages between primary healthcare providers and local community resources are hard to achieve in practice.

Inverse Care Law

- An important issue compounding the effective management of patients with LTCs in primary care is the continuing existence of the *inverse care law* in many (if not all) countries around the world. The term was first introduced in the 1970s by Julian Tudor Hart, a GP working in a socioeconomically deprived population in Wales. The inverse care law states that the availability of good medical care tends to vary inversely with the need for it in the population served. In general terms, this means that the poorest patients have the worst healthcare.

- This is of course abundantly clear within healthcare systems that are largely privately run. However, it is sadly also true of systems that have a national health service, such as the United Kingdom. The reason for this is that within the United Kingdom, primary care services (and the number of GPs in an area) are not distributed according to health need but according to population size.
- Although health need rises two- to threefold from the most affluent to the most deprived patients, the distribution of GPs is flat across deprivation deciles. In practice, this means that patients who live in poorer areas have worse access to high-quality care (longer waiting times to see a GP, shorter consultation length) with primary care practitioners in deprived areas being more stressed due to the greater need, demand, and clinical complexity of the patients.
- The inverse care law is of course not a law as such; it is a situation brought about by policy decisions through governments as the funders of healthcare. Such policies could be changed, and doctors themselves can advocate for such change. In Scotland, for example, the GPs working in the 100 most deprived areas of the country formed an informal group, GPs at the Deep End, which has been active in vocalising the problems they and their patients face.

What Do Patients With LTCs Need From General Practice?

(a) Practice Organisation. Practices need to be well organised in caring for patients with LTCs, with effective means of identifying patients (i.e., electronic disease registers) and arranging proactive anticipatory care rather than simply reacting to problems that patients present with in an unplanned way. The best way to organise such anticipatory care will depend on the practice resources and the patient population. For example, in more affluent areas, patients with LTCs are more likely to be proactive in their self-management by attending booked reviews, etc. Patients in deprived areas more commonly have additional social and psychologic problems and thus may fail to attend booked appointments for reviews and so more anticipatory care may need to be done within the reactive consultation. This of course has implications for consultation length, but some practices in deprived areas are able to give longer consultations (e.g., 15–20 minutes) when it is needed, by having spare time slots within booked sessions which can be moved so that a 10-minute slot can be changed immediately into a 20-minute slot.

(b) Empathic, Person-Centred Care. The encounter between doctor and patient should never be reduced to a dry tick box exercise where the GP blandly follows protocol. General practice defines itself as a discipline that provides holistic, generalist medicine. Holism means taking a biopsychosocial (and at times spiritual) approach to care. General practice is community based and community facing. Nowhere else in medicine is whole-person care so possible on a population level and so needed. We have the opportunity to get to know our patients and their families over time, and thus provide much needed continuity of care. Our care is comprehensive and coordinated; delivered with compassion and caring. Empathy is important in all therapeutic relationships and empathic care is supported by values of altruism. Empathy is especially valued by patients with multimorbidity. Empathy leads to higher patient and practitioner satisfaction, and better outcomes; research has shown that patients never feel enabled in consultations without GP empathy. Empathy has also been linked to better adherence with treatment regimens, reduction in symptom severity, and improved well-being. The effects of empathy can be direct and immediate or indirect and longer term.

(c) Generalism. GPs need to be expert generalists, which not only requires excellent technical clinical skills and knowledge and effective communication skills, but also to be skilled in interpretive medicine, integrating multiple sources of knowledge (including biomedical, biographical, and professional) in a dynamic exploration and interpretation of the individual illness experience. Practicing interpretive medicine leads to decisions about what is wrong, and what is needed to intervene, which supports an outcome of health as a resource for living, with the patient as an active partner in coproducing health.

Conclusions

- As the population ages, the dramatic rise in the prevalence of LTCs is the major challenge facing the world and most of its countries. It is also the major challenge facing general practice and primary care.
- Multimorbidity is the norm not the exception, yet guidelines and EBM are largely derived from research which excludes patients with multimorbidity.
- In managing patients with single or multiple LTCs, general practice and primary care teams need to be well organised to care for such patients and to be proactive and anticipatory rather than simply reactive. This requires a strong primary care system with adequate resources.
- Patients with multiple complex needs, must be at the centre of care, not the round pegs in the square holes of single disease–focused approaches. Holism lies at the heart of good management, and empathic, patient-centred care is a key requirement of the two facets of high-quality primary care for patients with LTCs—generalism and interpretive medicine.

References

Barnett, B., Mercer, S. W., Norbury, M., Watt, G., Wyke, S., & Guthrie, B. (2012). The epidemiology of multimorbidity—authors reply. *Lancet, 380,* 1383–1384.

Fortin, M., Bravo, G., Hudon, C., Vanasse, A., & Lapointe, L. (2005). Prevalence of multimorbidity among adults seen in family practice. *Annals of Family Medicine, 3,* 223–228.

3

Communication Skills

ANNEMIEKE BIKKER, LYNSAY CRAWFORD

CHAPTER CONTENTS

OBJECTIVES

- Good communication skills are central to general practice; without them you cannot be an effective clinician. However extensive your clinical knowledge, the inability to communicate that information, or interact and engage with patients, renders that knowledge ineffective. The consequences of ineffective or poor communication are unsatisfactory consultations (patients' concerns not elicited or hidden agendas not revealed); poor concordance with advice or medication and therefore poorer outcomes; less patient satisfaction; less patient enablement; and increased incidence of complaints.
- Good communication is crucial not just with patients but with all other colleagues (nurses, receptions staff, relatives, pharmacist, secondary care, etc.).

Professional Requirement

- The professional requirements related to communication skills are outlined in the General Medical Council's (GMC, 2013) Good Medical Practice as:
  a. treat patients as individuals and respect their dignity;
  b. treat patients politely and considerately;
  c. respect patients' rights to confidentiality;
  d. work in partnership with patients;
  e. listen to, and respond to, their concerns and preferences;
  f. give patients the information they want or need in a way they can understand;
  g. respect patients' right to reach decisions with you about their treatment and care;
  h. support patients in caring for themselves to improve and maintain their health;
  i. work with colleagues in the ways that best serve patients' interests.

- The Royal College of General Practitioners (RCGP, 2016) curriculum statement states that general practitioners (GPs) should display:
  a. an understanding of the wider context in which the consultation takes place;
  b. an understanding of the structure of the consultation;
  c. commitment to an ethical and reflective attitude.

Communication Skills

Verbal Communication

- During consultations it is important to use a mixture of question types:
  a. Open questions
  b. Closed questions
  c. Focused questions
  d. Indirect questions
- Question types to avoid:
  a. Leading questions
  b. Compound/double questions
- As well as questions, language is used for other purposes:
  a. Social exchanges ("Good morning" or comments on the weather)
  b. Facilitations ("Go on" or "uh uh")
  c. Repetition/restatement (repeating back what has just been said)
  d. Confrontation (confronting with an observation: "You look worried/sad/angry")
  e. Clarification/interpretation (clarifying what the patient has said: "So the tiredness started after your sleep pattern was disturbed?")
  f. Judgmental statements (responses that state the value judgment of the doctor: "Anyone who smokes cigarettes is foolish")
  g. Reassurance, explanation, instruction, or advice

Nonverbal Communication

- This includes:
  a. dress and appearance;
  b. facial expression;
  c. gaze and eye contact;
  d. gestures;
  e. posture;
  f. proximity—comfort zones;
  g. body contact and touch;
  h. mirroring;
  i. pacing.

Paralinguistics

- This is the term given to those aspects of vocalization, such as the speed, loudness, and pitch of the voice. These may convey information about emotions, attitudes, or personality (e.g., a soft, slow hesitant voice is associated with depression while a more rapid, loud voice suggests anger or excitement).

Rapport

- One of the most common mistakes in communication is to talk too much and listen too little. In listening to patients it is important to really listen and to let patients know that you are listening to them. This establishes trust and rapport.
- Rapport can be established and maintained at four levels:

  Level 1: Nonverbal level—by matching body language; posture, gestures, facial expressions, and eye contact
  Level 2: Paralinguistics/voice level—by matching breathing rate, tone, pitch, tempo
  Level 3: Language level—by matching or using another's words
  Level 4: Values level—by connecting with shared beliefs and values

- Sensitivity to patient's cues (Silverman et al., 2013):
  1. Be alert to patient's verbal cues (prompts, throw-away comments) and nonverbal cues (body language, facial expression, vocal cues) to elicit emotional content of the illness, ideas, effect on daily living, and expectations.
  2. Clarify the emotions that the patient is hinting at (e.g., by repeating or checking out a verbal cue: "You said that the cough worries you, especially at night. What theories do you have about what it might be?" or a nonverbal cue: "Am I right in thinking that you are puzzled by the information that I gave you?").
  3. Explicitly acknowledge cues as appropriate.
- Demonstrating empathy to help develop rapport involves (Derksen et al., 2013):
  1. understanding (or reconstruct and imagine) the patient's situation, perspective, and feelings;
  2. verbally communicating that understanding to check its accuracy (e.g., "I can see that you are very worried about the test results");
  3. acting on that understanding in a helpful therapeutic way.
- Empathy does not require you to have experienced the same problem as the patient or to like the patient. Research shows that patients consider empathy to be a key component of quality of care and that empathy is linked to patient enablement (Derksen et al., 2013; Mercer et al., 2012).

Ideas, Concerns, Effect, and Expectations

- This includes obtaining an understanding of how the patient sees the situation and experiences the illness, as well as exploring the disease. Enquire about (Stewart et al., 2014):
  a. feelings that reflect the emotional content of the illness (e.g., "Do you have any concerns about…?");

b. ideas about what the patient thinks is the cause (e.g., "What do you think is causing it?");

c. effect on the patient's daily life (e.g., how illness limits daily activities and impairs their capacity to fulfil certain responsibilities);

d. expectation of the consultation (e.g., "What were you expecting from seeing me today?").

- By taking other factors into account (age, culture, the physical environment, or people affected by the illness), the patient's experience of the illness is put into the context of the person's life (e.g., "Who is at home with you?").

- This can be summarized as the ICEE framework, in which the doctor explores:

a. patient's ideas (I) about what is wrong;

b. patient's feelings/concerns (C) about the illness;

c. impact/effect (E) of the patient's problems;

d. patient's expectations (E) about what should be done.

Sharing Information

- The GMC states that you must "give patients the information they want or need to know in a way they can understand."

- Tailor the explanation to the patient by taking into account the patient's needs and beliefs (e.g., "You mentioned depression and tiredness. I think tiredness is more likely because…").

  - Observe the patient's reactions to check if the explanation needs refinement.

  - Find out what and how much the patient wants to know to match the amount and type of information to the patient's needs and preferences (e.g., the diagnosis, coping techniques or support available, the causes of the illness, or side effects of treatment).

  - Check what the patient already knows (e.g., "I don't know how much you know about high blood pressure, can you tell me?").

  - Avoid jargon or check the patient's understanding of the technical term used.

  - Back up verbal information with written information, if appropriate, and ensure this is in the relevant language.

  - Check the patient's understanding.

Depending on the patient, Thistlethwaite and Morris (2006) suggest that the explanation is based on three domains (Table 3.1).

Shared Decision Making

- "Shared decision making is an approach where clinicians and patients make decisions together using the best available evidence" (Elwyn et al., 2010).

- The shared decision-making process includes (Thistlethwaite & Morris, 2006):

a. giving information to the patient on treatment options, possible risks, and benefits in a way that the patient understands;

TABLE 3.1   Sharing Information

Type of Explanation	Type of Questions	Purpose
Interpretive	What *What is diabetes?*	To interpret or clarify
Descriptive	How *How do my kidneys work?*	To describe a concept or process
Giving reasons	Why *Why did this happen to me?*	To give reason based on principle, motives, or values

b. helping the patient to balance the risks and benefits and make sure that their choice is based on fact rather than misconception.

Informed Consent

- The GMC (2013) states that it is the responsibility of the person providing treatment or undertaking an investigation to obtain consent: *Expressions of consent* (from GMC General Medical Council [available at www.gmc-uk.org/gmp]).

- According to the GMC (2013), you must give patients the information they want or need about:

a. the diagnosis and prognosis;

b. any uncertainties, including options for further investigations;

c. options for treating and managing the condition, including the option not to treat;

d. the purpose of proposed treatments and what these will involve;

e. the potentials risks, burdens, and likelihood of success of each option;

f. whether a proposed investigation or treatment is experimental (part of research or innovative);

g. who is responsible for the treatment, the roles of those involved, the involvement of students;

h. their right to refuse to take part in research or teaching;

i. their right to seek a second opinion;

j. any bills they will have to pay;

k. any conflicts of interest that you may have;

l. information on any treatments with potential greater benefit than the ones offered by you or your organization.

- Before accepting patients' consent, you must consider whether they have been given the information they want or need, and how well they understand the details and implications of what is proposed. This is more important than how their consent is expressed or recorded.

- Patients can give consent orally or in writing, or they may imply consent by complying with the proposed examination or treatment (e.g., by rolling up their sleeve to have their blood pressure taken).
- In the case of minor or routine investigations or treatments, if you are satisfied that the patient understands what you propose to do and why, it is usually enough to have oral or implied consent.
- In cases that involve higher risk, it is important that you get the patient's written consent. This is so that everyone involved understands what was explained and agreed.
- By law you must get written consent for certain treatments, such as fertility treatment. You must follow the laws and codes of practice that govern these situations.

Confidentiality

- The GMC, in Confidentiality (2009), states the principles of confidentiality and respect for patients' privacy. This includes:
  a. making sure that any personal information about patients that you hold or control is effectively protected at all times against improper disclosure;
  b. instances when personal information can be disclosed, including if it is required by law, patients consent to this disclosure (either implicitly for the sake of their own care or expressly for other purposes), or if it justified in the public interest.

Working With Interpreters

- The GMC states you should make sure that arrangements are made, wherever possible, to meet patients' language and communication needs.
- Ask that the interpretation be in the first person without omissions, editing, polishing, or outside conversations.
- Ask the interpreter to clarify (in his or her own words) any misunderstandings that occur due to cultural differences.
- Position yourself so that you face and speak directly to the patient rather than the interpreter.
- Talk with the patient in the first person (using "I").
- Maintain direct eye contact with the patient.
- Do not direct your questions or inquiries to the interpreter.
- Ask the patient to repeat any instructions and explanations given to ensure that they are understood.
- Issues to be aware of (Lloyd & Bor, 2004):
  - Meanings can be altered in the translation process.
  - The patient can be embarrassed by the presence of an interpreter due to the sensitive nature of the problem, especially when the interpreter is of the same nationality.
  - The patient's ideas can be reinterpreted by interpreter or translated in a shortened version.

Adherence and Compliance

- Tate (2010) states several reasons why patients follow or do not follow the treatment:
  a. Some patients adhere because they are told by the doctor to do so.
  b. If the patient understands and believes the explanation given by the doctor then the patient is more likely to adhere to treatment.
  c. If the patient's own understanding matches that of the doctor and the agenda is shared, then the patient is most likely to adhere.
  d. Shared decision making and linking the management plan with the patient's beliefs are key to ensuring adherence and compliance.

Physical Arrangement of the Room

- The physical arrangement of the room can facilitate or hinder communication (Lloyd & Bor, 2004).
- Arrangement of seats
  - Turning away and facing a computer can indicate disinterest, so the patient may not give information critical to the consultation.
  - Arrangements such as sitting sideways or facing each other without a desk in the middle, and being at the same eye level, will facilitate communication.
  - Usually the patient's chair is stable with four legs and the doctor's chair is often a swivel seat on wheels, which helps to complete the various tasks and to face the patient and the computer at different times.
- Use of computer. Communication guides (Silverman et al., 2013) suggest:
  a. waiting until patients have finished their opening statement before looking at the computer;
  b. turning your attention back to patients if they start to speak whilst you are looking at the computer;
  c. explaining to patients what you are doing so they understand the process.

The Structure of the Consultation

The ability to select from different consultation styles and skills to navigate through the consultation facilitates the need to meet patients with different expectations and preferences.

The Consultation

- Pendleton et al. (1984) defined seven tasks performed by doctors, which form the aims for each consultation. It is not suggested that all tasks should be completed in every consultation, though they argue that continued omission of one or more tasks will negatively impact on consultation outcome. Tasks 1 to 5 identify what the doctor needs to achieve. Tasks 6 and 7 relate to the entire consultation and highlight the use of time and resources, and the development of an effective doctor–patient relationship.

- The seven tasks:
  a. To define the reason for the patient's attendance, including:
     1. the nature and history of the problem(s);
     2. the aetiology (or cause) of the problem (i.e., the interaction of the physical, psychologic, and social factors);
     3. the patient's ideas, concerns, and expectations;
     4. the effects of the problems (on daily living).
  b. To consider other problems that are present but not presented by the patient, that is:
     1. continuing problems (e.g., previous problems discussed at earlier consultations or social conditions relevant to the current problem);
     2. modifiable risk factors (health promotion).
  c. To choose with the patient an appropriate action for each problem.
  d. To achieve a shared understanding of the problems with the patient (including giving explanations that relate to patient's ideas about the problem).
  e. To involve the patient in the management and encourage him or her to accept appropriate responsibility. The level of involvement that is appropriate will vary from patient to patient and from problem to problem.
  f. To use time and resources appropriately:
     1. in the consultation;
     2. in the long term.
  g. To establish or maintain a relationship with the patient that helps to achieve the other tasks (e.g., the doctor–patient relationship encourages the sharing of decisions).

The Inner Consultation

- Neighbour (1987) uses five checkpoints (subgoals) in the consultation alongside an awareness of minimal cues (verbal and nonverbal) to help discover the unspoken agenda. He emphasizes the importance of the start of the consultation in which the patient conveys more information then often is realized. Ideally, a checkpoint is reached before moving to the next.
- The five-stage model:
  a. Connecting—with the patient and developing rapport
  b. Summarizing—your understanding of the problem (events and emotional content)
  c. Handing over—the management plan that is understood, accepted, and agreed with the patient. Strategies for handing over include:
     1. negotiating;
     2. influencing;
     3. gift wrapping.
  d. Safety netting—and planning for the unexpected to manage uncertainty (e.g., using a specific time frame such as, "Come back in 2 weeks if it doesn't get better"). Neighbour points to three safety netting questions:
     1. If I am right, what do I expect to happen?
     2. How will I know if I am wrong?
     3. What would I do then?

  e. Housekeeping and taking care of yourself through stress prevention. Various options are given on what to do about job stress during and outside the consultation.

The Calgary Cambridge Method

- The Calgary Cambridge Method (Kurtz et al., 2003) integrates the tasks of the consultation and skills for communication.
- Silverman et al. (2013) analysed 71 communication skills, grouped under six headings. The skills needed depend on the context and the outcomes that the doctor and patient want to achieve.
- These skills include:
  a. initiating the session
     - Establishing initial rapport
     - Identifying reason(s) for attendance
  b. gathering information
     - Exploration of patient's problems
     - Additional skills for understanding the patient's perspective
  c. providing structure to the consultation
     - Making organization overt
     - Attending to flow
  d. building the relationship
     - Using appropriate nonverbal behaviour
     - Developing the rapport
     - Involving the patient
  e. explaining and planning
     - Providing the right amount and type of information
     - Aiding accurate recall and understanding
     - Achieving a shared understanding: incorporating the patient's perspective
     - Planning: shared decision making
  f. closing the session
     - Forward planning
     - Ensuring appropriate point of closure

The CARE Approach

- The CARE Approach (Bikker et al., 2014) aims to foster the achievement of empathic, patient-centred communication in health care encounters and is based on the Consultation and Relational Empathy (CARE) measure, a patient-rated experience measure. It is a broad set of guiding principles to be applied flexibly depending on the situation and circumstance.
- It consists of four interacting components that form an integrated cyclical process:
  a. Connecting: Actively engaging with the patient to create or deepen rapport and to facilitate open communication in a safe environment
  b. Assessing: Listening and taking a holistic approach to fully understand the patient's situation, perspective, and feelings (and their attached meanings)
  c. Responding: Communicating your understanding (and checking its accuracy) in a caring and

compassionate way, responding positively with clear explanations if appropriate

d. Empowering: Helping patients to feel more in control according to their abilities, preferences, and values and planning their treatment in partnership with them

Overviews of Consultation Models

http://www.bradfordvts.co.uk/online-resources

http://www.skillscascade.com/models.htm

http://www.gp-training.net/training/communication_skills/consultation/index.htm

How to React to a Complaint

- The General Medical Council (2013) states, "You must respond promptly, fully and honestly to complaints and apologize when appropriate."
- MDDUS recommends to:
  a. ask colleagues for support;
  b. make sure someone else in the practice deals with the complaint if you are subject of the complaint;
  c. keep good contemporaneous notes (this is absolutely critical!);
  d. be open to accepting that something may have gone wrong;
  e. share learning from complaints with the whole practice;
  f. let the complainant know what the practice plans to do to put things right.

Telephone Consultations

- There is a limited but growing body of research with regard to telephone consultations and guidance on how best to use this form of consultation (Bunn et al., 2007; Cochrane, 2009). The review by Car and Sheikh (2003) shows that patient satisfaction with telephone consultations is high.
- McKinstry et al. (2010) found that in comparison to face-to-face consultations, telephone consultations tend to be shorter (4.6 versus 9.7 minutes), deal with fewer problems, and typically contain less information gathering, counselling/advice, and rapport building. They also found that telephone consultations were less likely to include sufficient information to exclude important serious illnesses. They suggest that telephone consultations may be more suited to structured follow-up and management of long-term conditions than for in-hours acute management.
- In an exploratory study, McKinstry et al. (2011) found that the content of the consultations was equally well remembered by patients, irrespective of whether these were conducted by telephone or face-to-face methods. In both cases, recall was poorer in patients presenting multiple problems and with brain injury.

Communication Skills for Telephone Consultations

- Car and Sheikh (2004) suggests using the same skills as in face-to-face consultations, and being systematic in covering the following:
  1. Active listening (including verbal facilitation [e.g., "mm, I see…", "tell me a bit more…"]) and increased questioning/detailed history taking (e.g., "What does the rash look like?") to compensate for lack of visual cues
  2. Frequent clarifying and paraphrasing (to ensure that the messages have been sent and received in both directions)
  3. Picking up verbal (red flag words/warning signs) and nonverbal cues (such as pace, pauses, change in voice intonation [e.g., "I can hear from your voice that you are not sure about…"])
  4. Offering opportunities to ask questions
  5. Offering patient education
  6. Documentation

Confidentiality

- Telephone consulting is considered to have some additional risk with respect to confidentiality with the risk of a conversation being overheard as the area of most concern (McKinstry et al., 2009).
- To minimize and manage breaches in confidentially in telephone consultations and conversations McKinstry et al. (2009) suggests the following:
  - Reception areas should be organized so that telephone calls are taken out of earshot of other patients.
  - Care should be taken not to identify patients in a way other patients can hear (e.g., rather than repeating names ask for date of birth).
  - Doctors should avoid taking calls in reception or other staff areas, particularly in small communities.
- Phone etiquette
  - Check the provided number with the number on the patient's record. If it does not match, additional care might be needed.
  - Always check when phoning patients that they are in an environment where they can speak comfortably and confidentially.
  - Unless you recognize a patient's voice always confirm identity by date of birth, or better still, last consultation reason.
  - Avoid getting involved with third party consultations; always ask to speak directly to the patient if possible.
  - If asking patients to provide details of a problem, receptionists should explain why they are asking (e.g., "so the doctor can prioritize") and explain that patients do not have to give any information if they do not wish to.
  - Practices should have caller identification switched off.

- If messages are left at all on an answering machine they should be confined to confirmation that the clinician called and a request to call back.
- If in doubt, ask to see the patient.

Guidance on Remote Prescribing

- The GMC (2013), in *Good Practice in Prescribing and Managing Medicines and Devices*, states that to prescribe "you must satisfy yourself that you can make an adequate assessment, establish a dialogue and obtain the patient's consent" and that you "may prescribe only when you have adequate knowledge of the patient's health, and are satisfied that the medicines serve the patient's needs."
- Nonsurgical cosmetic medicinal products cannot be prescribed remotely.

Email Consultations

- There is inconclusive evidence on effects of email for clinical communication between patients' health care professionals on quality of care. There is no evidence-based guidance on how email might best be used in clinical practice (Atherton et al., 2012; Atherton et al., 2018).
- There is little consensus about the rules of patient–provider online interactions and the important role that can be played by staff in responding to certain types of messages.
- Based on a systematic review Car and Seikh (2004) concluded that successful communication through emails depends on a shared understanding by doctor and patient on its role, advantages, and limitations. They suggest introducing a standard protocol to inform patients on how emails are dealt with in the practice.

Confidentiality

Topps (2006) suggests the following to increase patient confidentiality:
- Avoid specifics, especially in touchy subject areas.
- Stick to logistic information, such as appointment availability.
- Warn patients that anything they write or say may go astray so they should be careful.
- Warn users of email systems that employers/owners have right of access.
- Warn system users that they cannot assume confidentiality just because they are communicating with a doctor's office.
- Avoid confirming information given by the patient—it may be speculative by another party.
- Never write or say anything that you would not be happy seeing printed on a newspaper front page.

References

Atherton, H., Sawmynaden, P., Sheikh, A., Majeed, A., & Car, J. (2012). Email for clinical communication between patients/ caregivers and healthcare professionals between patients/caregivers and healthcare professionals. *Cochrane Database of Systematic Review*, (11), CD007978.

Atherton, H., Brandt, H., Ziebland, S., Bikker, A., Campbell, J., Gibson, A., et al. (2018). Alternatives to the face-to-face consultation in general practice; focused ethnographic case study. *British Journal of General Practice*, 8(669).

Bikker, A. P., Cotton, P., & Mercer, S. W. (2014). *Embracing Empathy in Healthcare. A universal approach to person-centred, empathic healthcare encounters*. London: Radcliffe.

Bunn, F., Byrne, G., & Kendall, S. (2007). The effects of telephone consultation and triage on healthcare use and patient satisfaction: a systematic review. *British Journal of General Practice*, 57(542), 714–722.

Car, J., & Sheikh, A. (2003). *Telephone consultations. British Medical Journal*, 326, 7396.

Car, J., & Sheikh, A. (2004). Email consultations in health care: 1—scope and effectiveness. *British Medical Journal*, 329, 435.

Derksen, F., Bensing, J., & Lagro-Janssen, A. (2013). Effectiveness of empathy in general practice: a systematic review. British Journal of General Practice, 606, e76–e84.

Elwyn, G., Laitner, S., Coulter, A., Walker, E., Watson, P., Thomson, R., et al. (2010). Implementing shared decision making in the NHS. *BMJ*, 341, c5146.

General Medical Council. (2009) *Confidentiality: good practice in handling patient information*. https://www.gmc-uk.org/ethical-guidance/ethical-guidance-for-doctors/confidentiality. (Accessed 8 August 2018).

General Medical Council. (2013). *Good medical practice*. London, England: GMC. Retrieved from www.gmc-uk.org/gmp.

Kurtz, S. M., Silverman, J. D., Benson, J., & Draper, J. (2003). Marrying Content and Process in Clinical Method Teaching: Enhancing the Calgary-Cambridge Guides. *Academic Medicine*, 78(8), 802–809.

Lloyd, M., & Bor, R. (2004). *Communication skills for medicine* (2nd ed.). London: Harcourt.

McKinstry, B., Watson, P., Pinnock, H., Heaney, D., & Sheikh, A. (2009). Telephone consulting in primary care: a triangulated qualitative study of patients and providers. *British Journal of General Practice*, 59(563), 433–440.

McKinstry, B., Hammersley, V., Burton, C., et al. (2010). The quality, safety and content of telephone and face-to-face consultations: a comparative study. *BMJ Quality and Safety*, 19, 298–303.

Mckinstry, B., Watson, P., Elton, R. A., Pinnock, H., Kidd, G., Meyer, B., et al. (2011). Comparison of the accuracy of patients' recall of the content of telephone and face-to-face consultations: an exploratory study. *Postgraduate Medical Journal*, 87(1028), 394–399.

Mercer, S. W., Jani, B. D., Maxwell, M., Wong, S. Y. S., & Watt, G. C. M. (2012). Patient enablement requires physician empathy: a cross-sectional study of general practice consultations in areas of high and low socioeconomic deprivation in Scotland. *BMC Family Practice*, 13, 6.

Neighbour, R. (1987). *The inner consultation*. Int: Kluwer Academic Publishers.

Pendleton, D., Schofield, T., Tate, P., & Havelock, P. (1984). *The consultation: an approach to learning and teaching*. Oxford: Oxford University Press.

Royal College of General Practitioners. (2016). *The RCGP curriculum: Professional & clinical modules*.

Silverman, J. D., Kurtz, S. M., & Draper, J. (2013). *Skills for Communicating with Patients* (3rd ed.). CRC Press.

Stewart, M., Brown, J. B., Weston, W. W., McWhinney, I. R., McWilliam, C. L., & Freeman, T. R. (2014). *Patient-centered medicine: transforming the clinical method* (3rd ed.). Oxon: Radcliffe Medical Press.

Tate, P. (2010). *The Doctor's Communication Handbook*. Oxon: Radcliffe Publishing.

Thistletwaite, M. (2006). The Patient-doctor Consultation in Primary Care: Theory and Practice. Royal College of General Practitioners.

4

Ethics

AL DOWIE

CHAPTER CONTENTS

OBJECTIVES

- The primary objective of this chapter is to offer general practitioners a practical aid to clinical ethical thinking without feeling they need to be armed with a master's degree in moral philosophy or medical law. While much of the ethics of patient care is centred on the three Cs of capacity, consent, and confidentiality, specific ethical territory that general practitioners commonly have to negotiate include the following:
  a. fit notes;
  b. medical reports;
  c. fitness to drive;
  d. confidentiality and disclosure;
  e. young patients and consent;
  f. parental rights and responsibilities;
  g. child protection;
  h. termination of pregnancy;
  i. compulsory hospital admission and treatment;
  j. adult patients lacking capacity;
  k. power of attorney;
  l. advance decisions/advance directives;
  m. resuscitation decisions;

  n. decisions against treatment to sustain life;
  o. death certification.
- Clearly, then, general practice ethics has its own characteristics due to those features of clinical practice that are particular to it as a specialty (Papanikitas and Spicer, 2018; Rogers and Braunack-Mayer, 2009).
- In medical ethics generally, domains that tend to recur include the following (Stirrat, Johnston, Gillon, & Boyd, 2010):
  a. foundations of medical ethics and law;
  b. professionalism: good medical practice;
  c. patients: their values, narratives, rights, and responsibilities;
  d. informed decision making and valid consent/refusal;
  e. capacity and incapacity;
  f. confidentiality;
  g. justice and public health;
  h. children and young people;
  i. mental health;
  j. beginning of life;
  k. toward the end of life;
  l. medical research and audit.

General Practice Ethics

- Distinctive features of general practice ethics include:
  a. Maintaining trust for longer-term clinical relationships
  b. Accentuated importance of confidentiality in the context of local communities
  c. Professional relationships with multiple patients from the same household
  d. Complexity in care of patients with multimorbidity
  e. Highly interprofessional context
  f. Public health obligations
  g. Rationing decisions in the management of individual patients
  h. Considerations of social responsibility and health inequality

Different Meanings of Ethics

- The moment a patient enters the consulting room, the doctor is already in an ethical context. In that sense ethics

TABLE 4.1	Different Meanings of Ethics	
Shorthand for	**Interpretation**
Philosophical ethics	Abstract, critical discussion of ethical concepts (metaethics)
Ethical theory	Normative discussion of obligation in generalized terms
Ethical analysis	Deliberation on ethical theory in specific circumstances (also known as *applied* or *practical*
Bioethics	ethics)
Biomedical ethics	Ethical analysis and/or governance and protocols with respect to biological and life sciences
Medical ethics	Ethical analysis and/or governance and protocols with respect to scientific medicine
Health care ethics	Ethical analysis and/or governance and protocols with respect to medical practice
Research ethics	Ethical analysis and/or governance and protocols with respect to practice in the health professions
Public health ethics	Governance and protocols with respect to research practices and research ethics committees
	Population-based responsibilities, resource allocation, and policy in relation to health inequalities

Adapted from Dowie, A., & Martin, A. (2011). Ethic and law in the medical curriculum. AMEE Education Guide No. 53. Dundee: Association for Medical Education in Europe.

TABLE 4.2	Normative Domains in Medicine	
Ethical	Criteria for *self-directed practice* that is not derived from the regulator or the state (though the three sets of criteria may or may not coincide), whereby obligation is guided by principles, values, and responsibilities in connection with relevant, ordinate interests.
Legal	Criteria for *state-sanctioned practice*, whereby obligation is within a formal system of entitlements and duties as specified in the law, which is subject to criteria of ethical and sociocultural standards.
Professional	Criteria for *validated practice*, whereby obligation is according to the academic and clinical standards set by accrediting and regulatory authorities (in the United Kingdom, the General Medical Council) as both a prior condition and a continuing requirement for licensed practice through periodic appraisal, and in fulfilment of the supplementary criteria for membership of learned societies and Royal Colleges.

Adapted from Dowie, A., & Martin, A. (2011). Ethic and law in the medical curriculum. AMEE Education Guide No. 53. Dundee: Association for Medical Education in Europe.

in general practice is very much concerned with everyday, ordinary, and routine aspects of patient care, even if the presenting complaint is far from simple one.

- An *issue* is a controversy, and a *dilemma* is a difficult choice between alternatives. Ethical issues and dilemmas are not the substance of most clinical practice, which is not usually controversial and does not often entail awkward ethical alternatives from which to choose. Sometimes the difficulty lies in not yet possessing the relevant knowledge base or a structured approach to ethical reasoning such as those illustrated later in the chapter.
- Because the single word *ethics* is used as a convenient shorthand for widely differing domains, ambiguity surrounding the term frequently leads to misunderstanding wherever it arises. Table 4.1 illustrates a range of various meanings.

Ethics, Law, and Professionalism

- This chapter uses *ethics* as shorthand for yet another category in addition to those listed in Table 4.1, namely the practice of professional ethics. This is a threefold nexus involving ethics, law, and professionalism. These normative domains in clinical practice, while distinct, combine with each other as intertwined

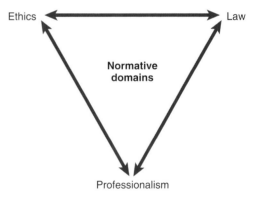

• **Fig. 4.1** Interplay of ethics, law, and professionalism.

strands. Table 4.2 teases out these strands as (1) self-directed practice, (2) state-sanctioned practice, and (3) validated practice.
- Ethical, legal, and professional norms arise from separate discourses with separate histories that nevertheless bear upon each other dynamically, as opposed to being simply static zones with overlapping areas of intersection (Fig. 4.1).
- Ethical norms answer to the requirements of law and to the standards set by the General Medical Council and other

• EXAMPLE 4.1 Referral Request for Termination of Pregnancy

Miss Caitlin Thomas, a 20-year-old student who has recently registered at the practice, attends Dr. Pal's morning surgery to seek referral for an early medical termination of pregnancy (TOP). As a matter of personal conscience, Dr. Pal is unable to participate in TOP referrals.

• EXAMPLE 4.2 Patient Access to Medical Records

Mrs. Kezia Rosen is a retired manager who was discharged from hospital last week following hip replacement surgery and is recovering at home. Her son has come to the practice with a signed letter from his mother requesting access to her medical records, which she wishes him to collect on her behalf.

professional bodies. It is possible for practitioners to take an ethical stance personally that differs from what is sanctioned by the other two sources of norms, for example in matters of conscience. When this is in conflict with the other domains, it is an external standard that prevails, since the individual practitioner is ultimately accountable to the law and to the profession. It can happen, though, that external norms may shift toward personal ethical positions in line with contemporary society.

- Legal norms in medicine are informed by professional codes and ethical reasoning. Standards that are set out in legislation need to be interpreted to particular cases heard in the courts, so that the application of statutes becomes clarified over time to take account of potential injustices. Acts of Parliament are also subject to processes of updating and streamlining, as seen for example in progressive improvements to equality law.

- *Ethical.* In Example 4.1, Dr Pal's ethical commitments inform her clinical practice because they are central to her sensibility as a person and formation as a professional. This is important for every doctor, whatever stance is taken, not only on this but on any area of ethical significance. It may be that the practitioner has thought through a reasoned position on the subject, or equally it could be a tacit view in terms of conscience.

- *Legal.* Miss Thomas is entitled to seek access to abortion services in the United Kingdom under the terms of the Abortion Act 1967, as amended by the Human Fertilisation and Embryology Act 1990, subject to the statutory conditions.

- *Professional.* Professional norms are under-girded by the legal minimum and the imperatives of ethical responsibility, and as a safeguard may also go beyond what is strictly required both ethically and legally. For example, a health authority may apply more stringent data protection measures than are otherwise mandated by law to act as a buffer against preventable breaches of confidential information held on patients in their health records. The General Medical Council recognizes the prerogative of a

doctor not to assist in the arrangements for a TOP, while also requiring Dr. Pal to direct Miss Thomas without delay to another practitioner who can facilitate this if it is her intention to proceed.

- *Ethical.* Example 4.2 is one of the exceptions to the general obligation of confidentiality for medical professionals not to disclose the personal information of patients to other parties. As well as necessary disclosure to other members of the health care team involved in the clinical management of patients, any disclosure can be made for which the patient gives explicit consent. This can include, for example, medical reports for third parties such as employers or, as in this case, disclosure to another person whom the patient has identified. However, there is still the obligation to exercise care in doing so, for example by making appropriate checks and safeguarding against unnecessary disclosure.

- *Legal.* The question of Mrs. Rosen gaining access to her medical records is a legal one. In the United Kingdom, the Data Protection Act 2018 provides for the right of access by persons (called *data subjects*) on whom records are kept, whether paper or electronic, which includes medical records. It also provides for access by others such as Mrs. Rosen's son with her explicit consent. The Act requires appropriate measures to preserve the security and integrity of records, which entails providing copies rather than originals. Prompt response is required, and compliance following receipt of the written subject access request, as in Mrs. Rosen's case, must be within 30 days. This must be provided free of charge, with the exception of requests that are excessive.

- *Professional.* It is essential to maintain Mrs. Rosen's trust in responding to her request, which includes attention both to the duty of confidentiality and to the proper disclosure that is sanctioned by law. Communication skills are central to this, for example in explaining the 30-day compliance period, and the provision of copies rather than the original record. It is also appropriate to clarify the details of Mrs. Rosen's request, to confirm if it is for a part or the whole of her medical records (medical notes, papers, correspondence, imaging, printouts of electronic files), and whether there might be a specific concern that can be addressed directly.

Ethical Reasoning

- "What were your reasons for acting as you did, doctor?" This is a typical question that arises in practical examinations for college membership, or in hearings before a fitness to practice panel, or in litigation before a court when counsel is leading evidence or cross-examining. The implication is that for a practitioner's actions to be defensible there has to be an underlying rationale that is coherent and can stand up to scrutiny. George Bernard Shaw's wry commentary on the professions being "a conspiracy against the laity" is countered by society's insistence on ethical accountability as a safeguard against professional collusion.

- When thinking through our ethical decision making in clinical practice, it is not necessary to be equipped with a working knowledge of theories in philosophical ethics. Instead there are practicable approaches to ethical analysis that, while informed by a theoretical understanding of ethics, are oriented toward making justifiable decisions rather than focusing on technical discussion. None of these is capable of making ethical decisions on our behalf; ultimately they all require the individual to make her or his own judgment.
- Three methods in ethical analysis are illustrated to clarify the process of ethical reasoning, out of which the practitioners can arrive at their own ethical conclusion:
  a. Benefits, Burdens, and Risks
  b. The Four Principles
  c. The Four Topics

Benefits, Burdens, and Risks

- Ethically uncertain situations may sometimes yield straightforwardly to a basic analysis of benefits, burdens, and risks, which can be clarified during the course of the clinical encounter through reflection-in-action (Example 4.3).
- In Example 4.3, we can readily weigh the relative proportions of risks, burdens, and benefits to see the clear lack of ethical justification for screening (Table 4.3). There still remains the matter of responding to the father in an appropriately professional fashion, but the ethical analysis thought through during the course of the consultation will inform that discussion in terms of the father's concern for his daughter's best interests.

The Four Principles

- A merit of the benefits, burdens, and risks approach is that it is highly patient centred, but on its own this can entail the limitation of suspending wider concerns of ethical significance, such as considerations of stewardship, sustainability, and the rights of other stakeholders, including the practitioner's institutional responsibilities in leadership and management.
- The more nuanced framework from which it derives is the classic distillation of ethical theory in health care contexts detailed by Beauchamp and Childress (2013). Their four principles of (1) justice, (2) respect for autonomy, (3) beneficence, and (4) nonmaleficence offer a widely known but easily misunderstood set of ethical criteria that have particular relevance to medical practice (Table 4.4).
- Again, these cannot do our reasoning for us, and indeed ethical principles may so conflict with each other that we have to exercise our judgment to arbitrate between them. For example, there may be a new and more effective drug therapy available for a particular illness, but due to the number of patients potentially involved the additional cost to the practice would be at the expense of other prescribing priorities. Rather, the four principles act as signposts to help us identify the ethically significant aspects of a clinical situation on which to base our actions.
- *Justice.* In Example 4.4, fairness to Mr. Gordon involves taking seriously the persistence of unpleasant symptoms,

---

• EXAMPLE 4.4   Troubling Symptoms yet Normal Test Results

James Gordon is a 55-year-old patient who experiences sudden attacks of nausea, sweating, and headache roughly once a month and sometimes more frequently. He is moderately hypotensive. Following referral to the local general hospital recently, there were no abnormal findings from other investigations. As there has been no improvement in his symptoms, he is desperate for some resolution and is determined to have further investigations including a computed tomography (CT) scan, for which he is willing to pay. He asks for referral to a different consultant at another hospital as a private patient.

• EXAMPLE 4.3   A Father Requests Genetic Testing for His Daughter

Following his wife's death from breast cancer, Mr. Svoboda is anxious about the possibility of a genetic cause that may have been passed on to his daughter, who is now 10 years old. He wants her to be tested for inherited BRCA1 and BRCA2 mutations associated with the disease.

TABLE 4.3   A Father Requests Genetic Testing for His Daughter

Benefits	Burdens	Risks
None to the child, even in the event of an "all-clear," since it is the father who is seeking reassurance here; in the event of an untoward result, there are no risk-reduction strategies relevant to childhood.	Undergoing a screening process that is not clinically indicated at her age. Harmful consequences to the child in the event of an untoward test result; introduction of a damaging anxiety unnecessarily early in her life about the likelihood of future disease.	Unpleasant experience for the daughter attending the clinic to have a sample taken. Distress resulting from the explanation given to the daughter (so as to gain her assent) of why she is undergoing the screening process. Possibility of generating a negative association with medical services that may be harmful to the child's trust and impact on how she relates to health professionals and clinical encounters in the future.

TABLE 4.4 The Four Principles

Interpretation	Examples	Not to Be Confused With
1. Justice		
Fairness	Avoiding statements in patient notes that are pejorative (e.g., poor historian). A patient who is a frequent attender to your practice, and in your view unnecessarily so, insists on a hospital referral. Your letter to the consultant is careful not to suggest disparagingly that the patient needlessly consumes clinical time and resources (e.g., "This patient is never away from my surgery").	Legal justice Retributive justice One-size-fits-all style of equal distribution; blind disregard for significant differences in the needs of patients.
2. Respect for Autonomy		
Respect for self-determination	A patient who presents with chronic obstructive pulmonary disease declines any help with smoking cessation. You focus instead on achieving therapeutic concordance in view of the patient's multimorbidity, and signal that you might come back to the smoking another time. An elderly patient with a stress-related illness is adamant that she will continue to look after her husband at home, despite his advancing dementia and the availability of a place in a local care home. Rather than press the issue you suggest keeping this as an option and arrange a timely follow-up with her.	The idea that anything we want to do is our own concern.
3. Beneficence		
Acting in the patient's best interests	A patient fails to attend an appointment to discuss the results of a blood test, which shows abnormal liver function indicative of harmful alcohol dependency. You then have a letter sent out and ask reception staff to contact the patient by telephone to arrange an urgent appointment. A Muslim patient has recently started a course of medication three times daily, but is greatly concerned as it will not be possible for him to sustain this regimen during Ramadan. You write him up instead for a single daily dose which is not ideal for a steady concentration but will provide him with sufficient cover during the fast.	Doing good Benevolence
4. Nonmaleficence		
Weighing benefits of treatment versus risk of harm	A patient with mild to moderate depressive illness had become dependent on the medication and was stepped down on these leading to complete withdrawal. His symptoms have since returned, and because the previous treatment worked so effectively, he requests the same prescription. You ask him instead to try cognitive behavioural therapy in combination with a safer but less potent drug. A patient is suffering poor quality of life directly as a result of her experience of menopause. She is finding it impossible to fulfil her obligations at work, thus exposing her to loss of income, and is also unable to cope at home, with consequences for relationships with her husband and teenage children. You offer her hormone replacement therapy as the risks in the interim are not disproportionate to the overall improvement she is likely to gain.	Do no harm Nonmalevolence Nonmalfeasance

which interfere with his ability to work and to enjoy social activities. It also involves offering some alternative to the pursuit of more tests as a private patient that either repeat those already done or are not clinically indicated in the absence of abnormal findings. Options might include exploring other approaches in primary care or offering a referral as previously for a second opinion.

- *Respect for autonomy*. It is a matter of Mr. Gordon's self-determination whether he should pursue medical attention as a private patient. If Mr. Gordon insists on going ahead then it is proper to respond with due cooperation. Further, in so doing the ongoing professional relationship of trust and confidence is promoted.
- *Beneficence*. With a view to Mr. Gordon's best interests, it is appropriate to offer guidance on the usefulness of repeating tests that were performed only recently to no avail, and the advisability of incurring the unwarranted personal expense he is contemplating. It is possible that

he is not fully aware of the scientific basis for being hesitant about this and would benefit from an explanation.

- *Nonmaleficence.* Beyond the economic harm of paying for private consultations and unnecessary clinical workup, given Mr. Gordon's impaired ability to work, and the potential burdens of inconvenience and stress, there is also the reality that no investigations are entirely free of risk. With regard to his intention to seek a CT scan, it may be that he does not appreciate the exposure to ionizing radiation entailed. Taken together, all the risks require to be outweighed by the benefits, and this would be an important area in communicating with Mr. Gordon.

The Four Topics

- One of the difficulties with the four principles approach is that its abstraction may not easily be amenable to some clinical situations in real life. As an alternative, Jonsen, Siegler, and Winslade (2015) set out their four-topic approach that is patient centred while also being cognizant of governing obligations and values, thereby combining strengths of the two models discussed earlier. It provides a structure for comprehensive assessment of ethical relevance by considering in sequence:
  1. Medical indications
  2. Patient preferences
  3. Quality of life
  4. Contextual features.
- These assessments, though separate, are kept together to ensure attention to what is ethically salient in the round, and in the light of that to help clarify what would be the most appropriate way to proceed. The order of topics denotes an expanding horizon of attention rather than a hierarchy of ethical importance, and Example 4.5 illustrates how they might be used.

• EXAMPLE 4.5   A Patient Seeking Antibiotics

Ken Porter is a 28-year-old science teacher who has been steadily troubled by unsightly acne over the past 15 months. He comments that even throughout adolescence he never experienced a skin problem so badly. Work is difficult enough without feeling embarrassed in front of his classes, and it also interferes with his personal life. Topical preparations purchased over-the-counter have not proved useful, and this is his first visit to the practice since the onset.

- *Medical indications.* Though not a severe case of acne, neither is it a transient flare-up, and Ken's complexion is obviously a significant and continuing problem. It is likely that the demands of work contribute to this, and health choices may also be a factor in promoting the condition of his skin in the long term.

- *Patient preferences.* Ken is categorical that he would rather not put up with the problem indefinitely and he would like antibiotic therapy to clear it up quickly. That aside, it would be appropriate to alert him to lifestyle options that could help with this, including diet and exercise, and possibly also practical considerations such as hand hygiene in the workplace.

- *Quality of life.* In addition to the normal stress of his job, the chronic unsightly appearance of his skin is substantially affecting his quality of life and the confidence to enjoy social contact. The benefit to Ken of an efficient and effective approach to managing his acne would be significant.

- *Contextual factors.* Antimicrobial stewardship is a responsibility in professional ethics because of the risks of unwarranted prescribing that impact both on the patient concerned and on the wider community. Decisions on a case-by-case basis depend, in part, on the proportionality of likely benefit to the individual. In Ken's situation, an important contextual factor at his stage of adulthood is the opportunity to form relationships with the potential for life partnership and family, which in this instance is preventably limited by his presenting complaint.

Summary: Professional Ethics in General Practice

- This chapter has clarified distinctive qualities of general practice ethics; the nature of professional ethics comprising the three intertwined domains of ethics, law, and professionalism; and some practicable approaches to ethical analysis.
- To conclude, the mnemonic PROFESSIONAL ETHICS can be formed from 18 key terms used in this chapter (Table 4.5).

TABLE 4.5	Professional Ethics in General Practice	
P	Public trust	Upholding the confidence of society in the profession
R	Regulatory framework	Normative criteria of practice in relation to maintaining registration
O	Obligations	Duty of care, responsibilities to colleagues, statutory requirements
F	Formation	Continuing professional development, reflective practice, values, professional identity
E	Ethical framework	Normative criteria of practice in relation to moral reasoning

TABLE 4.5	Professional Ethics in General Practice—cont'd	
S	Standards	Performance benchmarks in clinical practice
S	Social responsibility	Attention to the effects of policy and practice on communities
I	Institutional roles	Leadership, management, participating in organizational structures
O	Outcomes	Attention to the efficacy of practice, clinical audit
N	Non-collusion	Not engaging jointly in pretence against or with patients
A	Appraisal	Accountability to clinical supervision
L	Legal framework	Normative criteria of practice in relation to the State
E	Everyday	Emphasis on the ordinary and routine in clinical situations
T	Thought-through	Ethical reasoning, principles of ethical practice
H	Habits	Character of the practitioner; habits of the head, hands, and heart (knowledge, skills, and attitudes) that characterize the practice of medical professionals
I	Intentions	Attention to the goals of clinical practice in specific situations
C	Consequences	Attention to the scope for unintended outcomes that could result from actions that are being considered
S	Safety	Acting in line with measures to avoid preventable harm

Adapted from Dowie, A., & Martin, A. (2011). *Ethic and law in the medical curriculum*. AMEE Education Guide No. 53. Dundee: Association for Medical Education in Europe.

References

Beauchamp, T. L., & Childress, J. F. (2013). *Principles of biomedical ethics* (7th ed.). Oxford: Oxford University Press.

Dowie, A., & Martin, A. (2011). *Ethics and law in the medical curriculum*. AMEE Education Guide No. 53. Dundee: Association for Medical Education in Europe.

Jonsen, A. R., Siegler, M., & Winslade, W. J. (2015). *Clinical ethics: A practical approach to ethical decisions in clinical medicine* (8th ed.). New York, NY: McGraw Hill.

Papanikitas, A., & Spicer, J. (Eds.), (2018). *Handbook of primary care ethics*. Boca Raton, FL: CRC Press/Taylor & Francis Group.

Rogers, W. A., & Braunack-Mayer, A. J. (2009). *Practical ethics for general practice* (2nd ed.). Oxford: Oxford University Press.

Stirrat, G. M., Johnston, C., Gillon, R., & Boyd, K. (2010). Medical ethics and law for doctors of tomorrow: The 1998 consensus statement updated. *Journal of Medical Ethics, 36*, 55–60.

5

Disability

LYNN LEGG, JANE TRACY

CHAPTER CONTENTS

OBJECTIVES

- A disabled person is a person who has a disability. A person is disabled if he or she has a sensory, physical, mental, or intellectual impairment and the impairment has a substantial adverse effect on his or her ability to carry out daily activities required to maintain health and well-being. (Office for Disability Issues UK, 2010).
- Impairments are not synonymous with underlying pathology, but rather the manifestation of that pathology.
- Disability can result from a wide spectrum of sensory, physical, mental, or intellectual impairments ranging from mild to serious:
  - *Recurring episodic impairments:* mental health conditions (depression, bipolar affective disorders, schizophrenia), asthma, and epilepsy
  - *Progressive impairments:* macular degeneration, chronic obstructive pulmonary disease (COPD), dementia, motor neurone disease, cancer, multiple sclerosis (MS), osteoarthritis, rheumatologic disorders
  - *Permanent impairments:* personality disorder, developmental disabilities, sensory impairment, traumatic brain injury, stroke
  - *Transient or self-limiting impairments:* head and neck pain, frozen shoulder, cellulitis, or flu
  - *Circadian rhythm impairments:* rheumatoid arthritis, morning stiffness and functional disability in the early morning
  - *Seasonal rhythm impairments:* seasonal affective disorder
  - *Impairments following surgical or medical interventions:* recovery from joint replacement surgery, reduced upper limb strength and pain due to breast cancer treatment

Effect of Impairment on Carrying Out Normal Day-to-Day Activities

- Complete or substantial dependence on another.
- Time taken may be significantly longer (e.g., dressing and toileting) (Australian Bureau of Statistics, 2012a).
- May affect a person's ability to sustain an activity for long periods of time or carry out the activity repeatedly. A person may be able to carry out an activity (such as walking) but suffer significant pain in doing so, which in turn may limit the performance of that activity (Australian Bureau of Statistics, 2012a).
- An impairment may not have an adverse effect on a person's ability to carry out a single daily living activity in isolation (such as getting out of bed). However, the effect of an impairment on the person's ability to carry out multiple interconnected activities (such as getting out of bed, toileting, showering, dressing, breakfasting to go to work) may be substantial. (Office for Disability Issues UK, 2010)
- Interruption of normal day-to-day activities such as a frequent need to go to the toilet. (Office for Disability Issues UK, 2010)
- May have a circadian rhythm such as rheumatoid arthritis (i.e., joint pain, morning stiffness, and functional disability in the early morning hours). (Office for Disability Issues UK, 2010)
- May affect a person's ability to estimate or assess danger (e.g., road safety, touching very hot things, or an inability to protect oneself from potential exploitation or violence). (Office for Disability Issues UK, 2010)
- May cause a person to modify a behaviour (e.g., a person with rheumatoid arthritis may limit activities first thing in the morning to avoid pain or to wait for prescribed medications to take effect). Equally, a person may employ an avoidance strategy if there is a risk of considerable embarrassment in social situations such as faecal incontinence or facial disfigurement. (Office for Disability Issues UK, 2010)
- Physical impairments can cause mental effects and vice versa (e.g., a person with fatigue or pain may experience difficulties in remembering or concentrating). Similarly, mental impairments can have physical manifestations (e.g., a person with a mental impairment such as depression may experience difficulty in carrying out physical activities). (Office for Disability Issues UK, 2010)

Prevalence of Disability

Disability is common, and it becomes more so as populations age. Approaches to measuring disability vary but it is estimated that 15% of the world's population have a disability (WHO, 2011). The prevalence is 18.5% in Australia (Australian Bureau of Statistics, 2012b), 18% of the population of England and Wales report limitations in ability to perform day-to-day activities as a consequence of long term health problems or disability. (Reference: Census 2011, UK. Office for National Statistics).

Human Rights and Disability

All people have equal rights to participate in their communities and to access community services, including health services. People with disabilities experience inequalities and social injustice, including rejection, isolation, discrimination, harassment, stigma, segregation, and institutionalisation. They also currently experience barriers in accessing education and employment opportunities, and timely and appropriate health care and services.

Rehabilitation

- The WHO (2011) defines rehabilitation as "a set of measures that assist individuals who experience, or are likely to experience, disability to achieve and maintain optimal functioning in interaction with their environments."
- The term *rehabilitation* is also a process aimed at enabling persons with a disability "to reach and maintain their optimal, physical, sensory intellectual, psychological and social functional levels thus providing them with the tools they need to attain independence and self-determination".
- The aims of rehabilitation are to:
  a. prevent loss of function;
  b. improve or restore function;
  c. compensate for lost function;
  d. halt or slow decline in function;
  e. maintain function. WHO. World report on Disability. 2011

Physical and Rehabilitation Medicine

Physical and rehabilitation medicine doctors (physiatrists) are involved in the diagnosis of health conditions, assessment of functioning, and prescription of medical and technologic interventions that manage health conditions and optimize functional capacity.

Health and Social Care Professionals

Health and social care professionals include occupational therapists, physiotherapists, orthotists and prosthetists, speech and language therapists, rehabilitation nurses, audiologists, psychologists, social workers, and rehabilitation technologists.
- Interventions include:
  - Guided practice (such as practice walking and transferring after knee replacement)
  - Self-management strategies for people with long term health conditions
  - Education and training
  - Exercises
  - Manual therapy
  - Use of specific techniques (such as reminiscence therapy, biofeedback, acupuncture, graded activity)
  - Alternative or compensatory strategies (such as augmentative and alternative communication)

- Environmental modification (internal and external physical adaptations to the home)
- Provision of assistive technologies
- Advice and information
- Work with unpaid carers
- Support and counselling
- Promotion of a healthy lifestyle and physical activity

Assistive Technologies

A product or service designed to enable persons with a disability to achieve and maintain optimal functioning in interaction with their environments.
- Examples of assistive technologies:
  - *For people with mobility impairments:* wheelchairs, prostheses, orthoses, scooters, bath boards and seats, ramps, grab rails, stair lifts
  - *For people with visual impairments:* Braille-based typewriters (braillers) and embossers, access technology such as screen reader programs, high-contrast spectacles, radio for people with visual impairment
  - *For people with hearing impairments:* cochlear implants, amplified telephones and mobiles, vibrating alarm clocks, products to relieve the effect of tinnitus, hearing aids
  - *For people with cognitive impairment:* computer-based technology for recording of information, text to speech apps or programs that assist people with writing and reading difficulties, pictorial-based electronic timetables, GPS devices
  - *For people with speech impairments:* speech synthesizers, communication boards, modified typewriters, text to voice software
  - *Equipment for activities of daily living:* modified eating utensils, dressing aids, adapted personal hygiene equipment, emergency call systems, dosette boxes for medication

Rehabilitation Settings

- Rehabilitation services can be delivered in a variety of settings including hospitals, clinics, GP surgeries, the home, residential or nursing care homes, school, and work (Australian Bureau of Statistics, 2012b).

Evidence-Based Rehabilitation

Examples of systematic reviews in rehabilitation include:
- Occupational therapy for adults with problems in activities of daily living after stroke
- Multidisciplinary rehabilitation for acquired brain injury in adults of working age
- Home-based versus centre-based cardiac rehabilitation
- Physical rehabilitation for older people in long-term care
- Multidisciplinary rehabilitation for older people with hip fractures
- Multidisciplinary rehabilitation for adults with multiple sclerosis

- Multidisciplinary biopsychosocial rehabilitation for neck and shoulder pain among working age adults
- Multidisciplinary biopsychosocial rehabilitation for subacute low back pain among working age adults
- Pulmonary rehabilitation following exacerbations of chronic obstructive pulmonary disease
- Vocational rehabilitation for people with severe mental illness
- Exercise-based cardiac rehabilitation for coronary heart disease
- Cognitive rehabilitation for people with schizophrenia and related conditions

Source: The Cochrane Library (http://www.cochrane.org)

Intellectual Disability/Learning Disability/ Developmental Disability

Terminology

- *Learning disability* is synonymous with *intellectual disability. Intellectual disability* involves impairments of intellectual functioning, acquired during the developmental period, that impact on the persons ability to manage the tasks of daily life in conceptual, social and practical domains. Severity relates to the deficits in adaptive functioning. (American Psychiatric Association, 2013). *Developmental disability* includes motor impairments (cerebral palsy), social impairments (autism spectrum disorders), sensory impairments (vision and hearing), and cognitive impairment (intellectual disability).

- People with intellectual disability have a significantly reduced ability to understand new or complex information and to learn and apply new skills. This results in a reduced ability to cope independently (WHO, 2013).
- It is estimated that around 1% of the population have an intellectual disability (depending on definitions and methods of ascertainment) (McKenzie et al., 2016).

The Importance of Language

Language reflects the attitudes of the speaker, and influences those of others. Inappropriate language can cause hurt and offense to people with disabilities and their families and friends. People with disabilities are people first. Their disability impacts on their life experience, but it does not define them. Using 'person-first' language, such as 'Nick is a man with intellectual disability' focuses attention on the person, rather than the disability.

Health and Learning Disability: The Evidence

- People with learning disabilities experience:
  - higher rates of morbidity and premature death than their non–learning-disabled peers, a significant proportion of which is avoidable (Emerson & Baines, 2010; Heslop et al., 2013; Hollins & Tuffrey-Wijne, 2013; World Health Organisation, 2018; Trollor et al., 2017);
  - chronic and complex health and social needs;
  - barriers to accessing health care;
  - fewer opportunities for preventive health and health promotion interventions;
  - more undiagnosed and un/undertreated health conditions. (Lennox, Bain, & Rey-Conde, 2007; Emerson, et al., 2011; Kavanagh, Krnjacki, & Kelly, 2012; Trollor et al., 2017).
- *Hospital care:* People with intellectual disabilities encounter particular barriers to high quality care while in hospital (Iacono et al., 2014).
- *Standardized health assessments* are effective in the detection of previously unrecognized and/or unmet health needs, including life-threatening conditions, and lead to targeted actions to address health needs (Lennox, Bain, & Rey-Conde, 2007; Robertson, Roberts, Emerson, Turner, & Greig, 2011; Sullivan et al., 2011).
- *Consensus guidelines* in the primary care of adults with developmental disabilities (Sullivan et al., 2011) provide evidence under these headings:

- General Issues in Primary Care for Adults with Developmental Disability
- Physical Health Guidelines for Adults with Developmental Disability
- Behavioural and Mental Health Guidelines for Adults with Developmental Disability
- Care should be delivered to people with disabilities as part of a *collaborative team*.
- The *aetiology of the disability* should be established.
- Be aware of the *communicative role of behaviour* and the behavioural manifestations of illness, pain or discomfort (physical and mental), and environmental stressors.
- *Disease prevention* is essential.
- Avoid the unnecessary or inappropriate use of medications that may cause harm.
- Be aware of the *increased prevalence* in people with disabilities of:
  - vision and hearing impairment;
  - dental disease;
  - cardiac disorders (congenital and acquired);
  - musculoskeletal disorders including spasticity, scoliosis, osteopenia/osteoporosis, osteoarthritis;
  - respiratory disorders, particularly aspiration pneumonia, which are among the most common causes of death for people with developmental disability;
  - epilepsy, as seizures are a prominent cause of death;
  - gastrointestinal disease, particularly reflux and constipation, and the impact of these on quality of life and behaviour (*Helicobacter pylori* is more common in people with developmental disability.);
  - endocrine disorders such as thyroid disease, hypogonadism, and diabetes;
  - mental health, as these disorders can be difficult to identify when people have communication difficulties. Effective treatment depends on accurate diagnosis.

Providing Primary Health Care

- *Person-first approach.* Think first of the person as a man or woman of a particular age, background, and physique. What care would you provide to this person if he or she did not have a disability? Is there any reason to modify that care? If so, why?
- Then *consider the person's disability:*
  - *How does the intellectual disability affect health* and health care? Consider the person's life experiences and opportunities, communication and cognitive abilities, ability to make considered decisions, and ways the person plans and anticipates consequences.
  - *What is the cause of the disability* and does that aetiologic diagnosis inform health care? For example, someone with Down syndrome (DS) is at increased risk, for a lifetime, of thyroid dysfunction, hearing and vision impairment, immune deficiency, and respiratory infection. In the teens, 20s, and 30s, these individuals are at risk of depression and anxiety; and in their 40s and beyond they are at risk of Alzheimer disease.

- *Demonstrate respect:*
  - *Address the person directly* and use a tone of voice consistent with his or her age.
  - *Ask the person's permission* before inviting the accompanier into the consultation or asking questions of the accompanier, and always ensure the focus remains on the person.
- *Support the person to understand.* Many people with intellectual and associated developmental disabilities have communication difficulties:
  - *Address the person by name,* and use eye contact and/or touch to get his or her attention.
  - *Assume competence* when unsure of someone's ability to understand, and then adjust accordingly. A person's ability to understand may be better than his or her ability to express oneself (and vice versa).
  - *Speak slowly, in short clear sentences.*
  - *Explain what will happen* in the consultation to help the person know what to expect.
  - *Ask one question at a time* and provide adequate time for the person to think about your question and formulate a reply. Avoid leading questions and check responses by asking again in a different way.
  - Avoid using abstract concepts such as time, as the person may find them more difficult to understand. Use significant events such as meals, social or sporting events, birthdays or celebrations, rather than hours/days/months when asking questions related to time.
  - *Use visual information* (pictures, diagrams, signs, gestures) to aid comprehension.
  - *Check understanding* by asking the person to demonstrate or repeat what you have said in his or her own words.
  - Some people may have *limited literacy* and thus may have difficulty reading patient information or appointment letters. The person may wish to involve support workers or family members to assist with these tasks.
- *Support the person to express oneself.* Cognitive impairment makes identifying and verbalizing difficult and physical condition may impact on speech.
  - If you do not know, ask the person how he or she communicates (i.e., to indicate yes/no, use communication aids).
  - If the person uses a communication device, ensure he or she has access to it, then read the directions (usually on or in the device or book) and use it together.
  - Use visual cues such as objects, pictures, or diagrams.
- *If you can't understand then ask for help.* There may be times when you do not understand what the person is saying. In this situation, it may be helpful to ask the person:
  - to repeat a response;
  - to say it another way (using different words, for instance);
  - to illustrate his or her method of saying "yes" and "no" and then ask yes/no questions to identify what is being said;
  - if you could ask an accompanier to help you understand.
- *Never pretend to understand when you do not* as this devalues the person's communication. If you can't understand after using the strategies listed, acknowledge the importance of the message by apologizing and expressing regret at not understanding.
- *All people communicate.* People communicate through facial expression, body language, and behaviour. It may be clear that someone finds a sensation unpleasant from a grimace, is cold by shivering, or wants to leave when becoming agitated and looking toward the door. Acknowledging the person's experience and communication demonstrates that you hear, value, and respect his or her wishes.

Reasonable Adjustments

- Reasonable adjustments are those required under the antidiscrimination legislation to ensure services are as accessible and effective for people with disabilities, including intellectual disabilities, as they would be for people without disabilities (Turner & Robinson, 2011).
- Knowing a patient has an intellectual disability provides guidance to the general practitioner (GP) as to the reasonable adjustments to care that may be required to ensure equity. A person may:
  - require more time for a consultation to enable him or her to understand the information presented and have a chance to ask questions;
  - wish to have a family member, paid carer, or advocate present during the consultation;
  - have difficulty reading and writing and may need information presented in easy English or in audio form;
  - find it difficult to wait in a waiting room and it may be more appropriate to wait with his or her carer in comfortable surroundings nearby and be rung a few minutes before the appointment.

Advocacy

People with intellectual disabilities require their doctor to be an advocate in negotiating the health system and making sure their rights to equity in health care are upheld.

Principles of Practice

1. Take a person-centred approach by seeking to understand the perspective, personality, experiences, and strengths of each person.
2. Support empowerment of the person to make as many decisions as possible about his or her own life.
3. Enable choice by providing information about choices and support for the person to choose which suits him or her best.
4. Treat each person with dignity and respect, recognizing the inherent shared humanity in all people.

Legal Issues of Consent and Capacity

- For children, parents generally hold legal power to make decisions on their behalf.

- For adults, it is presumed that they can make their own decisions about health care. If this is in doubt it is up to the health practitioner to establish the person's legal capacity and ability to:
  1. understand the information provided;
  2. believe and retain the information provided;
  3. evaluate the relevant information;
  4. express a choice.
- People who do not have capacity will require someone to assist them or to make the decision on their behalf. Whatever their capacity the person concerned should be as actively involved in decision making as possible.

Comprehensive Health Care

- Holistic health care is that in which the person's physical and mental health are understood and supported in the context of that person's social context and life experiences.
- All doctors should adopt a proactive approach to a person's health care.
- Comprehensive health assessments should always include a systems review, a medication review, and, for those in whom the cause of their intellectual disability is unknown, consideration of an aetiogic review every few years is recommended. Understanding of the genetic causes of disability is growing rapidly, and referral to genetic services could be enlightening.
- Comprehensive care includes a focus on disease prevention (immunization, cancer screening, etc.) and health promotion (adequate exercise, healthy diet, not smoking, etc.).

Mental Health Issues

- People with intellectual disabilities have a higher rate of mental health issues.
- Depression, anxiety, mania, and psychosis all occur in people with intellectual disabilities. When people have cognitive and/or communication impairments they will express their symptoms through changes in their behaviour. Depression may present as social withdrawal, irritability, changes in appetite and sleep; mania as increased activity, vocalization, and sleep disturbance; psychosis as unexplained fear or appearing to respond to visual or auditory hallucinations.
- Treatment of disorders of mental health is the same as in the general population. **Effective treatment depends on accurate diagnosis.** Vigilance by both the GP and family/support staff with respect to response to medication and side effects is vital, as the patient is likely to have difficulty reporting these.
- Principles of medication use:
  1. Effective treatment depends on accurate diagnosis.
  2. Start at a low dosage and increase slowly (start low, go slow).
  3. Always use the lowest effective dose.
  4. Review medications regularly with particular regard to indications and side effects.

HEALTH CARE FOR PEOPLE WITH INTELLECTUAL DISABILITIES

Some Tips for Consultations

	Challenge	One Possible Solution
Prior to appointment	Required appointment may not be made	General practitioner or nurse initiates appointment and reminds patient
	Person/family/staff may not know what information is required	Contact person and/or carer and detail information required at appointment
	Waiting time may be an issue	Minimise waiting time
		Arrange for person to wait nearby in comfortable surroundings (park, coffee shop, car). Ring him or her a few minutes before appointment
At consultation	Person may feel anxious or frightened	Greet warmly and establish rapport by chatting about something of interest to person
	Person may become irritated	Speak to the person concerned. Remember he or she is your patient, not the family member or paid carer
	Person may get bored, become anxious, or want to leave	Include the person in the discussion, both verbally and nonverbally, no matter his or her capacity
	Information given at consultation may not be retained/passed on accurately to those involved in care	Write a summary of outcomes of consultation, the next steps in care, and who is responsible
After consultation	Person may be anxious next time	Discuss with patient/carer what went well, and how to improve for next time
		Record in notes

RESOURCES FOR HEALTH PROFESSIONALS

Understanding Health and Intellectual Disability: www.intellectualdisability.info

Therapeutic Guidelines Ltd. (2012). *Management guidelines: Developmental disability.* Version 3. Melbourne: Therapeutic Guidelines Ltd. https://tgldcdp.tg.org.au/fulltext/quicklinks/management_guideline.pdf

NSW Agency for Clinical Innovation: www.aci.health.nsw.gov.au/resources/intellectual-disability/intellectual_disability_training/id-training-videos

Management Guidelines: Developmental Disability (2012) https://tgldcdp.tg.org.au/fulltext/quicklinks/management_guideline.pdf

The Guide: Accessible Mental Health Services for People with Intellectual Disability. A guide for providers. https://tgldcdp.tg.org.au/fulltext/quicklinks/management_guideline.pdf

Down Syndrome

- People with DS still experience significant barriers to the receipt of high-quality health care, and health outcomes compare unfavourably with those of the general population (Therapeutic Guidelines—Developmental Disability 2012; Tracy 2011; Torr et al., 2010).
- They are at increased risk of a range of physical and mental health conditions, often live with multiple unrecognized health issues, and have limited access to disease prevention and health promotion interventions.

Health Care for Children With Down Syndrome

- *General care.* As for all children, primary care has responsibility for monitoring health and development. Health promotion and disease prevention: diet, exercise, weight management, immunizations.
- *Neonatal examination and investigation* to identify congenital anomalies, including cardiac and gastrointestinal malformations.
- *Nutrition.* Dietitians can also offer information and support (note: calcium, vitamin D for osteoporosis prevention).
- *For families.* Link to services and supports, including early intervention services, dental services, allied health services, and support services such as the Down Syndrome Association.
- *Hearing.* Auditory brainstem evoked response at 0 to 6 months; audiology annually from 1 to 5 years; two yearly from age 5 to 18 years and at any time concern regarding hearing loss is raised by parents, carers, or screening tests.
- *Vision.* Ophthalmologic examination at 0 to 6 months; annually to age 5 years; 2 yearly to age 18 years and at any time concern regarding vision is raised by parents, carers, or screening tests.
- *Endocrine.* Check thyroid function at birth then annually throughout childhood and again if suggestive symptoms or signs are noted. Assess specifically for undescended testes and hypogonadism.

- *Dental/oral health.* Dental review 3 to 6 monthly from first teeth for monitoring development plus prevention and treatment of oral disease.
- *Gastrointestinal.* Monitor diet and weight. Consider gastrooesophageal reflux disease (GORD), *H. pylori*, coeliac disease, and constipation as these are all more common in children with DS.
- *Atlantoaxial instability.* Monitor for signs and symptoms of cord compression.
- *Haematologic/immunologic.* Be alert to increased risk of infections and leukaemia.

Health Care for Adolescents With Down Syndrome

- *Sexuality.* Girls will require education and support to manage periods (see Resources for Carers). Everyone requires additional advice about sex and contraception. Teenagers with DS are more vulnerable to sexual exploitation/abuse. They require education about appropriate behaviours (themselves and others), how to keep themselves safe, and how to get help if needed. For those unable to advocate for themselves, adequate protection and supervision are required to ensure their safety.
- *Skin.* Folliculitis/acne may affect self-esteem and interactions with others. Energetic treatment is required.
- *Mental health.* Biologic, psychologic, and social factors contribute to increased risk of disorders of mental health, especially anxiety and depression.
- *Transition from paediatric to adult services.* Consider all services used by the child and family: recreation, respite services, school and postschool options (employment, education, other), and mental health services. The GP has an important role in providing support and guidance through this time of change. Encourage the adolescent to take an increasingly active role in his or her health management.

Health Care for Adults With Down Syndrome

- *Health monitoring.* Risk factor identification (e.g., cardiovascular disease).
- *Health promotion and disease prevention.* Diet, exercise, weight management, cancer screening (may include smear test, mammography, bowel cancer screening), immunizations.
- *Annual health assessments* underpin proactive health care and enable early detection, health promotion, and disease prevention.
- *Behaviour change.* A change in behaviour is a communication—consider disorder of physical, dental, or mental health, and environmental causes.
- *Dental and oral health.* Dental review 6 monthly.
- *Cardiovascular.* Mitral valve prolapse may develop during adulthood (50% of adults)—regular cardiac examination and/or echocardiography is required.
- *Atlantoaxial instability.* Cervical cord compression (~2% of people with DS). Symptoms/signs include neck pain,

torticollis, limb weakness, increased reflexes, change in gait and/or bladder/bowel function, sensory changes.
- *Hearing*. Audiology 3 yearly and if suspicion of hearing loss raised by carers or screening
- *Vision*. Ophthalmological review at 30 years; every 5 years thereafter and if suspicion of visual loss raised by carers or screening.
- *Thyroid function*. Annually and whenever suggestive symptoms or signs are noted
- *Mental health*. Biologic, psychologic, social factors contribute to increased risk of disorders. Anxiety and depression more common.
- *Alzheimer disease*. Average age of diagnosis early 50s; rare under 45 years; exclude physical/mental cause of functional decline.
- *Gastrointestinal*. Increased risk of GORD, coeliac disease, and chronic constipation.
- *Osteoporosis*. Bone mineral density testing in early adulthood and repeat at menopause in women and ~40 years for hypogonadal men. Discuss and implement prevention strategies: diet and exercise, and calcium and vitamin D supplementation if levels are low or the person is on an anticonvulsant.
- *Medication*. Regular (3 monthly) review. Monitor response and side effects: reevaluate indications and efficacy (cease if ineffective); ensure lowest effective dose; educate patient and carers about expected response and side effects. Consider prepackaging of medication by pharmacy to ensure accurate dosing and safety. Be aware of sensitivity to psychoactive medication ("Start low, go slow") and be vigilant for side effects (behaviour change may be an early symptom).

Health Care for Older People With Down Syndrome

- The increasing lifespan of people with DS means more people experience the conditions of ageing including menopausal symptoms, arthritis, cardiovascular disease, osteoporosis, sensory loss, and dementia.
- Alzheimer disease occurs earlier in people with DS with an average age of diagnosis in the early to mid-50s. Symptoms may be difficult to differentiate from physical disease (e.g., hypothyroidism, anaemia); medication effects (e.g., nausea, confusion, dizziness); mental illness (e.g., depression, psychosis); and sensory deterioration (e.g., hearing and vision).

RESOURCES FOR PARENTS AND PROFESSIONALS

Down Syndrome Association of Australia: http://www
.downsyndrome.org.au
Down Syndrome Association UK; http://www.downs
-syndrome.org.uk
Down Syndrome Association Scotland: www.dsscotland
.org.uk
Down Syndrome Association Ireland: http://downsyndrome
.ie/campaigns-and-projects/person-first-language/

- Proactive assessment and investigation is required to exclude treatable causes of functional decline.

Carers

- In Australia, around 12% identify as carers (Australian Bureau of Statistics, 2012a); 70% of primary carers are women and 83% of carers were caring for someone in their household. Figures are similar in the United Kingdom (Carers Trust UK, 2012).
- When a person comes to his or her medical practitioner accompanied by a carer it is important to:
  a. establish the relationship between the person and carer;
  b. clarify the carers role;
  c. ensure the person's consent for the carer to be present;
  d. speak directly to the person, not to the carer. If the person finds it difficult to express oneself, or if you have trouble understanding the person, ask if you may ask questions of the carer. Always involve and include the person in the consultation through verbal and nonverbal communication.
  e. write down the key outcomes of the consultation, any follow-up tasks that are required (investigations, further information, monitoring for response to treatment and side effects of medication, etc.), and arrangements for review. This information must be given to the person and/or the carer to ensure it is relayed accurately to other carers involved.

Caring for the Carers

- Family members who care for a relative tend to have lower rates of workforce participation, lower incomes, and reduced connection with their social group and communities.
- They may find aspects of care difficult, and struggle to make the time to address their own physical and mental health issues.
- It may therefore be helpful if the GP invites the carer to come for his or her own consultation to discuss ways to acquire assistance with the caring role (services, equipment, therapy, local activity groups for people requiring care, respite, etc.).
- The consultation also provides an opportunity to review the carer's physical and mental health status and needs, and to address current and potential issues.

Resources for Carers

- *Carer organizations* provide advice, peer support, and access to information and resources. Examples:
  - Carers UK: http://www.carersuk.org/newsroom/stats-and-facts
  - Carers Australia: http://www.carersaustralia.com.au
- *Local councils/authorities* provide information about services, resources, support, and activities.
- *Therapy services* include occupational therapists, physiotherapists, and speech therapists.

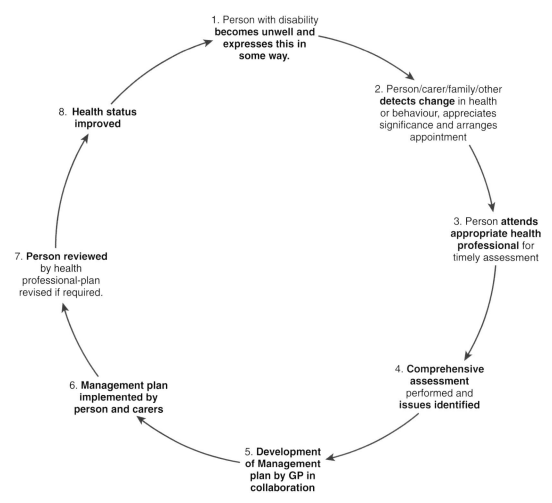

• **Fig. 5.1** Cycle of good health care. *GP,* General practitioner.

Cycle of Good Health Care— A Shared Responsibility

- Optimal health care for someone with a disability requires a cycle (Fig. 5.1) (Tracy, 2013). At each step there is a risk that the next may not occur.
- GPs and support staff/family have a shared responsibility to work collaboratively with the person with the intellectual disability to ensure the steps of the cycle are worked through and completed to ensure the person concerned achieves and maintains optimal health and function.

Further Reading

World Health Organization. (2013). *ICF Online.*

Office for National Statitistics. (2013). *Disability in England and Wales, 2011 and comparison with 2001.*

United Nations. (2006). *Convention on the rights of persons with disabilites and optional protocol.*

Equality and Human Rights Commission. (2013). *The United Nations Convention on the rights of people with disabilites—What does it mean for you? 2010.* Equality and Human Rights Commission.

World Health Organization. (1946). *Preamble to the Constitution of the World Health Organization as adopted by the International Health Conference,* New York, June 1946; signed July 1946 by the representatives of 61 states (Official Records of the World Health Organization, no. 2, p. 100) and entered into force on 7 April 1948.

Turner, S. L., Nair, A., Sedki, I., Disler, P. B., & Wade, D. T. (2005). Multi-disciplinary rehabilitation for acquired brain injury in adults of working age. *Cochrane Database of Systematic Reviews.*

Taylor, R. S., Dalal, H., Jolly, K., Moxham, T., & Zawada, A. (2010). Home-based versus centre-based cardiac rehabilitation. *Cochrane Database of Systematic Reviews.*

Crocker, T., Forster, A., Young, J., Brown, L., Ozer, S., ... Smith, J. (2013). Physical rehabilitation for older people in long-term care. *Cochrane Database of Systematic Reviews.*

Handoll-Helen, H. G., Cameron, I. D., Mak-Jenson, C. S., & Finnegan, T. P. (2009). Multidisciplinary rehabilitation for older people with hip fractures. *Cochrane Database of Systematic Reviews.*

Khan, F., Turner, S. L., Ng, L., Kilpatrick, T., & Amatya, B. (2007). Multidisciplinary rehabilitation for adults with multiple sclerosis. *Cochrane Database of Systematic Reviews.*

Hillier, S. L., & McDonnell, M. (2011). Vestibular rehabilitation for unilateral peripheral vestibular dysfunction. *Cochrane Database of Systematic Reviews.*

Karjalainen, K. A., Malmivaara, A., van-Tulder, M. W., Roine, R., Jauhiainen, M., ... Hurri, H. (2003). Multidisciplinary biopsychosocial rehabilitation for neck and shoulder pain among working age adults. *Cochrane Database of Systematic Reviews.*

Chung-Charlie, S. Y., Pollock, A., Campbell, T., Durward, B. R., & Hagen, S. (2013). Cognitive rehabilitation for executive dysfunction in adults with stroke or other adult non-progressive acquired brain damage. *Cochrane Database of Systematic Review.*

Puhan, M. A., Gimeno, S. E., Scharplatz, M., Troosters, T., Walters, E. H., & Steurer, J. (2011). Pulmonary rehabilitation following exacerbations of chronic obstructive pulmonary disease. *Cochrane Database of Systematic Reviews.*

Khan, F., Ng, L., Gonzalez, S., Hale, T., & Turner, S. L. (2008). Multidisciplinary rehabilitation programmes following joint replacement at the hip and knee in chronic arthropathy. *Cochrane Database of Systematic Reviews.*

Khan, F., Amatya, B., Ng, L., Drummond, K., & Olver, J. (2013). Multidisciplinary rehabilitation after primary brain tumour treatment. *Cochrane Database of Systematic Reviews.*

Thomson, L., Handoll-Helen, H. G., Cunningham, A. A., & Shaw, P. C. (2002). Physiotherapist-led programmes and interventions for rehabilitation of anterior cruciate ligament, medial collateral ligament and meniscal injuries of the knee in adults. *Cochrane Database of Systematic Reviews.*

Crowther, R., Marshall, M., Bond, G. R., & Huxley, P. (2001). Vocational rehabilitation for people with severe mental illness. *Cochrane Database of Systematic Reviews.*

Heran, B. S., Chen-Jenny, M. H., Ebrahim, S., Moxham, T., Oldridge, N., … Rees, K. (2011). Exercise-based cardiac rehabilitation for coronary heart disease. *Cochrane Database of Systematic Reviews.*

McGrath, J., & Hayes, R. L. (2000). Cognitive rehabilitation for people with schizophrenia and related conditions. *Cochrane Database of Systematic Reviews.*

Ostelo-Raymond, W. J. G., Costa-Leonardo, O. P., Maher, C. G., de-Vet-Henrica, C. W., & van-Tulder, M. W. (2008). Rehabilitation after lumbar disc surgery. *Cochrane Database of Systematic Reviews.*

Mehrholz, J., Kugler, J., & Pohl, M. (2012). Locomotor training for walking after spinal cord injury. *Cochrane Database of Systematic Reviews.*

The Cochrane Collaboration. (2013). *The Cochrane Library.*

Bigby, C., Douglas, J., & Iacono, T. (2018). *Enabling mainstream systems to be more inclusive and responsive to people with disabilities: Hospital encounters of adults with cognitive disabilities.* Report for the National Disability Research and Development Agenda. Melbourne: Living with Disability Research Centre, La Trobe University. *Electronic copies* are available from the La Trobe University Research Repository http://hdl.handle.net/1959.9/563533.

References

American Psychiatric Association. (2013). *Diagnostic and statistical manual of mental disorders* (5th ed.). Arlington, VA.

Australian Bureau of Statistics. (2012a). *Carers. Disability Ageing and Carers.* Retrieved from http://www.abs.gov.au/ausstats/abs@.nsf/Lookup/4F768035180A4CD7CA257C21000D8228?open document.

Australian Bureau of Statistics. (2012b). *Disability. Disability Ageing and Carers.* Retrieved from http://www.abs.gov.au/ausstats/abs@.nsf/Lookup/A813E50F4C45A338CA257C21000E4F36?open document.

Carers Trust UK. (2012). http://www.carersuk.org/newsroom/stats-and-facts.

Emerson, E., & Baines, S. (2010). *Health inequalities and people with learning disabilities in the UK: 2010.* Durham: Improving Health & Lives: Learning Disabilities Observatory.

Emerson, E., Madden, R., Graham, H., Llewellyn, G., Hatton, C., & Robertson, J. (2011). The health of disabled people and the social determinants of health. *Public Health*, 125(3), 145–147.

Heslop, P., Blair, P., Fleming, P., Hoghton, M., Marriott, A., & Russ, L. (2013). *Confidential inquiry into premature deaths of people with learning disabilities.* Bristol: Norah Fry Research Centre, University of Bristol.

Hollins, S., & Tuffrey-Wijne, I. (2013). Meeting the needs of patients with learning disabilities. *British Medical Journal*, 346, doi: https://doi.org/10.1136/bmj.f3421.

Iacono, T., Bigby, C., Unsworth, C., Douglas, J., & Fitzpatrick, P. (2014). A systematic review of hospital experiences of people with intellectual disability. *BMC Health Services Research*, 14.

Kavanagh, A., Krnjacki, L., & Kelly, M. (2012). *Disability and Health Inequalities in Australia: Research Summary: Addressing the Social and Economic Determinants of Mental and Physical Health.* Victorian Health Promotion Foundation, Carlton South, Vic. Available at https://www.vichealth.vic.gov.au/media-and-resources/publications/disability-and-health-inequalities-in-australia.

Lennox, N., Bain, C., & Rey-Conde, T. (2007). Effects of a comprehensive health assessment programme for Australian adults with intellectual disability: a cluster randomized trial. *International Journal of Epidemiology*, 36(1), 139–146.

McKenzie, K., Milton, M., Smith, G., et al. *Curr Dev Disord Rep* (2016) 3: 104. https://doi.org/10.1007/s40474-016-0085-7.

Office for Disability Issues UK. (2010). *Equality Act 2010 Guidance.*

Robertson, J., Roberts, H., Emerson, E., Turner, S., & Greig, R. (2011). The impact of health checks for people with intellectual disabilities: A systematic review of evidence. *Journal of Intellectual Disabilities Research*, 55, 1009–1019. doi:10.1111/j.1365-2788.2011.01436.x. [Epub 2011 Jul 5].

Sullivan, W. F., Berg, J., Bradley, E., Cheetham, T., Denton, R., Heng, J., et al. (2011). Primary care of adults with developmental disabilities. Canadian Consensus Guidelines. *Canadian Family Physician*, 57, 541–553.

Therapeutic Guidelines Ltd. (2012). *Management guidelines: Developmental disability.* Version 3. Melbourne: Therepeutic Guidelines Ltd.

Torr, J., Strydom, A., Patti, P., & Jokinen, N. (2010). Aging in down syndrome: Morbidity and mortality. *Journal of Policy and Practice in Intellectual Disabilities*, 7(1), 70–81.

Tracy, J. (2011). Australians with Down syndrome—health matters. *Australian Family Physician*, 40, 202–208.

Tracy, J. (2013). Disability in the mainstream: Improving healthcare provided to people with intellectual disability and the role of mainstream and specialist services. In C. Bigby & C. Fyffe (Eds.), *Making mainstream services accessible and responsive to people with intellectual disability: What is the equivalent of lifts and Labradors? Proceedings of the Seventh Roundtable on Intellectual Disability Policy.* Bundoora: Living with Disability Research Group, Faculty of Health Sciences, La Trobe University.

Trollor, J., Srasuebkul, P., Xu, H., et al. (2017). Cause of death and potentially avoidable deaths in Australian adults with intellectual disability using retrospective linked data. *BMJ Open*, 7, e013489. doi:10.1136/bmjopen-2016-013489.

Turner, S., & Robinson, C. (2011). *Reasonable adjustments for people with learning disabilities—implications and actions for commissioners and providers of healthcare. Learning Disabilities Observatory.* http://

www.improvinghealthandlives.org.uk/uploads/doc/vid_11084_
IHAL%202011%20-01%20Reasonable%20adjustments%20
guidance.pdf.

World Health Organization. (2011). *World report on disability 2011.*
Geneva: WHO.

World Health Organisation. (2013). *Fact sheet 352. Disability
and health.* http://www.who.int/mediacentre/factsheets/fs352/en/
index.html#.

World Health Organisation. (2018) *Fact Sheet: Disability and health.*
www.who.int/news-room/fact-sheets/detail/disability-and-health.

6

Children's Health

RUTH MARGARET BLAND, HILARY LOCKHART PEARCE

CHAPTER CONTENTS

The Child With a Fever

- Fever is one of the most common reasons for seeking medical help. There are many causes of acute fever, and it is important to take a thorough history and examine the child carefully. In most cases the fever is due to a viral illness that will be self-limiting.

- The challenge for the general practitioner (GP) is identifying the child with a potentially serious bacterial infection. If a child is acutely unwell then he or she should be referred to hospital immediately, particularly if there is no obvious source for the fever, in which case the child will require a septic screen. Classic signs of particular infections, such as the stiff neck and headache of meningitis, may not be present in infants who often present with fever, pallor, and irritability, and so a GP needs to maintain a high index of suspicion for underlying serious infection.

What to Ask About the Child

- It is important to ask how long the fever has been present. A fever of more than 8 days duration, with no source, suggests underlying pathology requiring further investigation (see upcoming discussion). A parental history of fever should always be taken seriously, even if a pyrexia is not recorded by the examining doctor, as it is likely that the child has been given paracetamol or a similar medication.
- Ask about how long the fever has been present and whether the child is getting better or worse.
- In all cases of fever ask specifically about a rash—a blanching rash is often present with viral infections but a non-blanching rash may indicate an underlying serious bacterial infection.
- Explore how the child is feeding and whether he or she is refusing feeds or vomiting. Ask specifically about any symptoms that may point to a cause for the fever, including vomiting and diarrhoea (possible gastroenteritis), cough and coryzal symptoms (pneumonia or other respiratory infection), pulling at an ear (possible otitis media). In an older child ask about pain passing urine (possible urinary tract infection [UTI]), painful joint (possible septic arthritis), and seizures (possible meningitis or herpes encephalitis).

Ask if other members of the family have been unwell and whether there has been any recent travel abroad.

What to Look for on Examination
Guideline

National Institute for Health and Care Excellence. (2013). Feverish illness in children. NICE clinical guideline 160. Available from https://www.nice.org.uk/guidance/cg160/resources/support-for-education-and-learning-educational-resource-traffic-light-table-pdf-189985789.

- The National Institute for Health and Care Excellence (NICE) has produced a traffic light system for signs and symptoms that predict the risk of serious illness in children under 5 years of age which will be familiar to most UK general practitioners.

NICE Traffic light system for identifying the risk of serious illness in under 5s

	High Risk: Refer Urgently	Intermediate Risk: Refer	Low Risk: Manage at Home
Colour: skin / lips/tongue	Pale/mottled/ashen/blue	Pallor reported by parent/carer	Normal colour
Activity	No response to social cues Appears ill to health professional Does not wake if roused Weak, high pitched or continuous cry	Not responding normally to social cues No smile Wakes only with prolonged stimulation Decreased activity	Responds normally to social cues Content/smiles Strong normal cry or not crying Stays awake or awakens quickly
Respiratory	Grunting Respiratory rate (RR) >60 breaths/min Moderate/severe chest indrawing	Nasal flaring RR: 6–12 months >50 breaths/min; >12 months >40 breaths/min Oxygen saturation ≤95% Crackles in chest	
Circulation and hydration	Reduced skin turgor	Tachycardia: <12 months: >160 beats/min; 12–24 months: >150 beats/min; 2–5 years: >140 beats/min Capillary return time ≥3 sec Dry mucous membranes Poor feeding in infants Reduced urine output	Normal skin and eyes Moist mucous membranes
Other	≤3 months: temp ≥38°C Non-blanching rash Bulging fontanelle Neck stiffness Status epilepticus Focal neurologic signs Focal seizure	3–6 months: temp ≥39°C Fever ≥5 days Rigors Swelling of limb or joint Non–weight-bearing limb, not using an extremity	None of the amber or red symptoms or signs

- In addition to the clinical findings listed, examine the child for specific signs that could indicate the source of fever, including examining for pus on the tonsils, inflammation of the tympanic membranes, swelling and inflammation of the joints, enlargement of the lymph nodes, and tenderness in the abdomen.

What to Do

- The priority is to decide whether to refer the child for further investigations, and whether this needs to be done urgently (see the NICE guidelines provided earlier).
- In older children who are not acutely unwell and in whom no source of acute fever can be found, the following investigations are useful: urinalysis and urine culture, full blood count (FBC), C-reactive protein (CRP), stool culture.
- A normal white cell count and CRP, and a negative urinalysis, are reassuring; and it is unlikely that there is any serious pathology underlying the fever.
- It is not advisable to prescribe antibiotics to children without a source for the fever. Most children who are not acutely unwell with fever do not have underlying bacteraemia.
- If an unwell child presents with a non-blanching rash and fever, suspect meningococcal disease and give intramuscular (IM) antibiotics before urgent transfer to hospital.

Pyrexia of Unknown Origin

A pyrexia of unknown origin (PUO) is a fever of 8 days or more in a child in whom there is no source of fever after initial investigations have been done. These children should be referred for further investigation. The list of causes is vast, including infectious bacterial diseases (Lyme disease, salmonella); viral illnesses (Epstein-Barr virus); fungal and parasitic diseases; connective tissue diseases; Kawasaki disease and malignancy.

The Child With a Cough

- Cough is a common symptom in children. It can be acute (<3 weeks) or chronic (3–12 weeks). In infants think about pertussis and bronchiolitis. Most acute coughs in older children are caused by viruses, but if the child is unwell with fever and tachypnoea then pneumonia must be excluded.
- Causes of chronic cough include asthma, pertussis, viruses including adenovirus, bacteria including mycoplasma, and postnasal drip

What to Ask About the Child

- Ask about the duration of the cough to find out if it is acute or chronic. Most acute coughs are caused by viruses and will be self-limiting. However, viruses such as adenoviruses can cause coughs that last up to 3 months.

- Ask if there is a pattern to the coughing. Children with pertussis have paroxysmal spells of coughing but are generally well with no respiratory symptoms between the episodes of spasmodic coughing. A child with asthma may have exercise-induced, or nocturnal, cough. An infant with gastro oesophageal reflux (GOR) may experience coughing after feeding or when prone, for example when put into his or her cot to sleep, when the parents might report a nighttime cough.
- Ask about the onset of the cough. If it started suddenly with no prodromal symptoms, then ask about a history of choking and consider the possibility of an inhaled foreign body.
- Ask whether the cough sounds wet or dry. The cough associated with asthma sounds dry, while the cough associated with a respiratory infection sounds wet and may be productive of sputum. A barking cough associated with stridor is typical of croup, while a harsh paroxysmal cough is suggestive of pertussis.
- Check whether there are associated symptoms that might point to the aetiology of the cough (for example, whether the child has fever, nasal discharge, increased work of breathing, reduced exercise tolerance, anorexia, fatigue, or weight loss). If the child has a persistent cough associated with fever and night sweats, ask whether the child has been exposed to tuberculosis (TB).
- For infants and young children, ask whether the caregivers have noted any episodes of apnoea, which may be associated with pertussis, bronchiolitis, and GOR.
- Sinusitis may present with persistent cough and tenderness over the sinuses, and the child may present with facial pain.
- Ask about feeding, appetite, and weight gain. In infants vomiting and cough may suggest a diagnosis of gastrooesophageal reflux.
- In the family history, specifically ask about atopy, asthma, or a TB contact.
- Take a child's immunization status, in particular bacillus Calmette-Guérin (BCG) and pertussis.

What to Look for on Examination

- Assess if the child is acutely unwell (refer to page 39), in particular looking for cyanosis or pallor; signs of respiratory distress include nasal flaring, grunting, chest indrawing, or an increased respiratory rate (>50 breaths/min in children 0–12 months; >40 breaths/min in children >12 months of age). Refer urgently as appropriate if these signs are present.
- In young children, most information will be gained by observation. However, it is useful to auscultate the chest for crackles and wheeze if the child is not distressed and crying. If there are crackles, determine whether they are generalized (e.g., in an infant with bronchiolitis) or localized (e.g., in a child with lobar pneumonia).

- Examine the upper respiratory tract, including the tonsils, ears, and nose.
- Palpate the face over the region of the sinuses, as tenderness over these areas may suggest sinusitis.
- Look for evidence of a chronic respiratory illness including a chest deformity (e.g., sulci, increased anterior-posterior diameter) and finger clubbing.
- Weigh the child and plot this on an appropriate growth chart and compare with previous measurements to assess growth. Failure to thrive associated with a cough needs further investigation.

What to Do

- Have a low threshold for referring infants with a clinical diagnosis of a lower respiratory illness, bronchiolitis, or pertussis to secondary care if they are ex-preterm (as they can deteriorate quickly), have had apnoeic episodes with this illness, or have been admitted to hospital previously with a respiratory illness. For children over 1 year of age with pneumonia, if they are not acutely unwell they may be managed at home with an oral antibiotic and antipyretic.
- A child with a sudden onset of cough and a possible history of choking should be referred urgently for investigation of an inhaled foreign body. These children may also have stridor.
- If a child has a persistent nocturnal cough that you think may be asthma, give a trial of an inhaled steroid. If the child does not respond to this, then refer to secondary care.
- Refer all children with a persistent cough for more than 1 month who are not improving.
- Refer all children with a cough and failure to thrive for further investigations, which may include imaging, assessment of immune function, and bronchoscopy.
- In infants with a possible diagnosis of gastrooesophageal reflux try an antireflux medication.

The Child With Wheeze

- Wheeze within the context of a viral illness is common in pre-school children. One third of children will have at least one episode of wheeze before they are 3 years old. The diagnosis of asthma, in children under the age of 5, is a clinical one. In older children, asthma is diagnosed if more than one of the following symptoms is present: recurrent wheeze, cough, difficulty breathing, and chest tightness. The diagnosis should be supported with spirometry in children old enough to comply with assessment (usually around the age of 5).
- A trial of a β-2 agonist may demonstrate reversibility of bronchospasm, but in children less than 2 years of age the response to bronchodilator therapy is not always consistent. The diagnosis should be considered if there are other features, including nocturnal cough or exercise-induced symptoms. A family, or personal, history of atopy may also be helpful.

What to Ask About the Child

- Ask about the pattern and frequency of episodes of wheeze. Is the wheeze frequent and episodic with definite triggers, such as exercise or cold weather, suggestive of asthma? Or does the wheeze only occur with upper respiratory tract infections and is therefore more likely to be a viral-induced wheeze, particularly in a younger child?
- Ask if the child has associated symptoms, including a dry cough, respiratory symptoms with exercise, disturbed sleep, or snoring. Children with asthma may have a nocturnal or early morning cough. A wet-sounding cough is less likely to be asthma.
- Ask about family history. A diagnosis of asthma is more likely if there is a family or personal history of atopy, including eczema, hay fever, or other allergies.
- Ask if the wheeze has been present since birth; and if so, consider a diagnosis of tracheobronchomalacia.
- Check if the child was born prematurely and if he or she was intubated and ventilated. Such children may be more likely to deteriorate quickly with respiratory illnesses and may need referral to secondary care more promptly than children born at term with no neonatal complications.
- Always ask whether the child is exposed to cigarette smoke and check his or her growth.

What to Look for on Examination

- Assess if the child is acutely unwell, in particular looking for cyanosis or pallor, and signs of respiratory distress.
- In a child with known asthma, look out for the so-called silent chest with no wheeze. This is a dangerous sign as it indicates little air movement.
- Be aware of children who are so breathless that they cannot talk in sentences. This is a dangerous sign indicating severe respiratory distress. Children who are agitated or exhausted should also be referred urgently.
- Auscultate for wheeze. A generalized wheeze is present in asthma and in infants with bronchiolitis. Also check for crackles, which may suggest lower respiratory tract infection.
- If the child is old enough measure a peak expiratory flow and compare this to the reference charts and, if available, to previous measurements of the child.
- Look for evidence of a chronic respiratory condition, including a chest deformity (e.g., sulci) and finger clubbing.
- Weigh the child, plot on an appropriate growth chart, and compare with previous measurements. Failure to thrive associated with a cough or wheeze needs further investigation; also consider referring these children to secondary care.

What to Do

- Management of acute wheeze in a child who is unwell includes oxygen therapy, β-2 agonist via a nebulizer or multidosing with an inhaler through a spacing device, oral steroids, and referral to secondary care if indicated. For longer term management of asthma, refer to guidelines, including the British Guideline on the Management of Asthma, which provides a stepwise approach to the medical management of asthma.
- For children with viral-induced wheeze who are well between episodes, treatment with a β-2 agonist for acute symptoms may be beneficial. However, β-2 agonists are often ineffective for children under the age of 1 year.
- For all children it is useful to provide advice to the families about related triggers, including avoidance of smoke, pollen, and animal dander where appropriate.
- Refer children to secondary care if they have wheeze and are not growing well, have recurrent chest infections, or have a chronic cough.

The Child With Constipation

- Constipation is a very common reason for referral to secondary care. Parents are often concerned that the child has underlying pathology and often come to hospital expecting that investigations, including imaging, will be carried out.
- More than 90% of cases of constipation are idiopathic (i.e., have no underlying anatomical or physiological cause). It is important to provide a clear explanation to the parent and child (where appropriate), implement a management plan, and arrange regular follow-up to ensure that the child responds to treatment.

What to Ask About the Child

- Ask about the frequency and consistency of the stools (use the Bristol stool chart to help children and caregivers to identify the type of stools they are passing). Fewer than three formed stools per week, and stools that are hard or like rabbit droppings, are features of constipation.
- Explore whether the child has abdominal pain while passing stool and between episodes of stooling. Children with constipation often experience regular lower abdominal pain and pain on defecation particularly if the stools are large and hard.
- Ask if there has ever been blood coating the stool, suggesting a fissure caused by constipation.
- Ask about episodes of diarrhoea. Sometimes children with constipation present with diarrhoea, but this is overflow diarrhoea, passed with no sensation and often offensive to smell. Caregivers will often report that the child is lazy and failing to go to the toilet in time, and caregivers are often concerned about treating the child with laxatives (see upcoming discussion), as they feel it will make the

diarrhoea worse. However, overflow diarrhoea will not resolve until any impacted faeces are passed.
- In the past history, ask whether the child passed meconium within the first 48 hours after delivery. Failure to pass meconium, or constipation beginning in the first few weeks of life, may indicate an underlying pathology (e.g., Hirschsprung disease). However, it is important to stress that most cases of constipation are idiopathic and the child will require no investigations.
- As with all children, check that the child is thriving and otherwise well.

What to Look for on Examination

- Assess if the child is acutely unwell. A distended abdomen, especially in a child who is also vomiting, requires urgent referral to secondary care. Palpate the abdomen for faecal masses, which are most often felt above the pelvic rim in children with constipation. Check the child's height and weight and plot on a chart, comparing with previous measurements. A child who is failing to thrive with constipation should be referred to secondary care for exclusion of other disorders, including coeliac disease and hypothyroidism.
- There is no need to perform a rectal examination on a child with constipation in primary care. This will cause distress to the child and not help with the diagnosis. However, it is useful to check the appearance of the anus externally. In a young infant, check that the anus is patent, as in rare cases an imperforate anus may have been missed on neonatal examination. Check if there is an anal fissure which may be the cause of bleeding per rectum, or multiple fissures or a fistula which may be suggestive of other pathology such as Crohn's disease. Bruising around the anus may indicate possible child abuse.
- Neuromuscular causes of constipation are rare, but check that there is no obvious deformity of the spine, to rule out a sacral dimple with no visible base, and that the child does not have abnormal tone, power, gait, or reflexes. In a toddler check for delayed walking that could indicate an underlying neuromuscular problem.

What to Do

- Investigations are not normally required and idiopathic constipation can usually be managed in primary care. The key points of management are reassurance, a clear management plan, and follow-up to check response to treatment.
- It is important to explain that constipation is common and that diet alone is unlikely to solve the problem, particularly in the short term. Explain the importance of starting a laxative to soften the stools, with the goal of passing a soft stool at least once per day. Explain that it is preferable to have stools that are too loose rather than too hard at this stage.

- Explain that if a child is soiling (overflow diarrhoea), this behaviour is not deliberate and should not be punished. It is often a relief to caregivers and children to understand that overflow diarrhoea will stop once the constipation resolves.
- Treatment includes disimpaction if this is required and then regular treatment with appropriate laxatives. Paediatric Movicol (a macrogol) is the laxative of choice for children. Clear guidance on doses for disimpaction and maintenance are given in the British National Formulary for Children and in the NICE guidelines.
- Give clear instructions on how to take the laxative, explaining that it should not be stopped and started, and that some abdominal pain and loose stools will be experienced during the first days of administration. Caregivers often stop giving laxatives as the child passes loose stools, but explain that this is to be expected in the first few days.
- Children are often fearful of sitting on the toilet and attempting to pass stool. Once the stools are soft, encourage the child to sit on the toilet for 5 to 10 minutes after breakfast and evening meal. Giving a child balloons to blow up whilst on the toilet, and providing a foot stool for comfort if unable to reach the floor, are strategies to encourage pushing.
- Arrange follow-up for the child to check on response to treatment and to suggest modifications in laxative doses as required. If the child has faecal impaction then arrange follow-up after 1 week. Check adequate fluid intake.

The Child With Abdominal Pain

- At least 10% of schoolchildren will experience abdominal pain regularly. There are many causes and the challenge is to identify the child with underlying pathology and to avoid unnecessary tests on children with functional abdominal pain who do not require them.

What to Ask About the Child

- Ask at what age the pain started. Take seriously abdominal pain commencing in young children (<5 years), in whom constipation has been excluded.
- Explore about the frequency and pattern of the pain, bearing in mind that children with underlying pathology will experience pain irrespective of play or other activities.
- Ask if the pain wakes the child at night, as functional pain does not tend to cause nocturnal wakening.
- Explore if there is a relationship to eating, as *Helicobacter pylori* disease may be associated with upper abdominal and retrosternal pain on eating.
- Ask if any particular foods aggravate the pain. Pain can occur in coeliac disease after eating gluten.
- Ask if the pain is associated with pallor, nausea, or a family history of migraine. Children can get abdominal migraine that presents with nonspecific abdominal pain but not necessarily headache.

- Ask specifically about vomiting. Bilious vomiting usually has a surgical cause and children should be referred to secondary care. Children with an acute surgical cause for their vomiting are usually unwell (e.g., a child with acute appendicitis will usually present with listlessness and anorexia in addition to abdominal pain).
- Ask about the stools and whether defecation is associated with pain. Diarrhoea, blood, or mucus per rectum *may* indicate underlying pathology (e.g., inflammatory bowel disease). However, constipation with a fissure may also cause blood that coats the stools and is a common cause of abdominal pain.
- Check whether the child has other symptoms that may indicate underlying pathology. For example, mouth ulcers, joint pains, and anal skin tags are associated with Crohn's disease.
- Explore for factors in the social history that may be sources of anxiety, including problems at school, difficulties with parents, parental separation or divorce.
- Ask about dysuria, which may suggest UTI.

What to Look for on Examination

- Examine for an acute abdomen or surgical cause for abdominal pain. Check for acute/rebound tenderness on palpation, a distended abdomen, fever, lethargy, and a furred tongue.
- Functional abdominal pain is nonspecific. Children often vaguely point to their umbilicus when trying to localize the pain and do not usually complain of tenderness when their abdomen is palpated.
- Measure and plot the child's weight and height on a growth chart and compare to previous measurements. A child with abdominal pain associated with weight faltering needs further investigations to rule out conditions such as inflammatory bowel disease and coeliac disease.
- Check the anus externally for skin tags, fissures, fistulae, and ulceration (there is no need to do a PR [rectal] exam). A fissure may be present with constipation. Skin tags, multiple fissures, and fistulae may suggest inflammatory bowel disease, and should be further investigated.
- Finger clubbing in a child with abdominal pain is suggestive of underlying pathology, including inflammatory bowel disease. Similarly, mouth ulcers may indicate Crohn's disease (but may also be an incidental finding).

What to Do

- If you are concerned that there is underlying pathology the following investigations may be helpful in distinguishing between functional and nonfunctional pain:
  - Faecal calprotectin. Levels over 200 μg/g *may* be suggestive of inflammatory bowel disease and these children should be referred.
  - Blood tests: FBC, ferritin, inflammatory markers (CRP, erythrocyte sedimentation rate [ESR]), liver function tests, coeliac antibody screen.

- Faecal *H. pylori* antigen may be helpful in children with upper abdominal/retrosternal pain and pain on eating, or those with a family history of *H. pylori* disease.
  - Urine culture to exclude UTI.
  - Normal investigations are often reassuring to parents.
- If the child is constipated manage appropriately. Drug treatment may be helpful in the following conditions: serotonin antagonists in abdominal migraine and mebeverine in irritable bowel syndrome. For debilitating functional abdominal pain psychology input may be required.

The Child With Diarrhoea

- It is important to distinguish between acute (<2 weeks) and chronic (>2 weeks) diarrhoea.
- Acute diarrhoea is often associated with vomiting and is usually caused by viruses, including rotavirus, adenovirus, and calicivirus. Rarely acute diarrhoea is caused by bacteria (*Salmonella, Shigella, Yersinia, Campylobacter*) or protozoa (*Giardia* and *Cryptosporidium*).

What to Ask About the Child

- Ask about the duration of the diarrhoea and distinguish between acute and chronic diarrhoea.
- Enquire whether the child has vomiting, as gastroenteritis causes acute diarrhoea and vomiting.
- Specifically ask whether the child has blood in the diarrhoea. This is found in infections (also see haemolytic uraemic syndrome [HUS]) and in inflammatory bowel disease if the diarrhoea is chronic.
- Ask about recent travel abroad as this may indicate the aetiology of the diarrhoea (e.g., *Salmonella*).
- Ask if the child lives on a farm or has had contact with animals, and consider whether the child could have *Campylobacter.*
- Ask whether the child has ongoing abdominal pain or other symptoms suggestive of inflammatory bowel disease or coeliac disease. If the child has constipation, consider whether the diarrhoea is overflow diarrhoea.
- Ask about the child's diet, as fruit juices, diluting juice, fizzy drinks, and sugar-free chewing gum may cause osmotic diarrhoea.

What to Look for on Examination

- Assess whether the child is acutely unwell and in need of acute admission for treatment of severe dehydration or severe underlying infection.
- Check for petechiae, which may be present in HUS and sepsis.
- Examine the abdomen for tenderness, masses, and organomegaly.
- Plot the child's current weight and height on a growth chart and compare with previous measurements. (Remember, if the child is dehydrated his or her weight will be lower than normal.)
- Check whether the child has finger clubbing suggestive of underlying chronic pathology.
- Check the anus externally for skin tags, fissures, fistulae, and ulceration (there is no need to do a PR exam), particularly if you are suspecting a chronic underlying cause. A fissure may be present with constipation. Skin tags, multiple fissures, and fistulae may suggest inflammatory bowel disease and should be further investigated.
- Check the mouth for ulcers, which may indicate underlying pathology (e.g., Crohn's disease) but may also be an incidental finding.

What to Do

- Acutely unwell children should be referred.
- If the child can be managed at home, consider sending stools for culture if there is blood in the stool, or the child has travelled abroad recently.
- For children with bloody diarrhoea it is wise to check the blood count, electrolytes, glucose and renal function. Antibiotics may be required in the following specific circumstances to treat diarrhoea:
  - If *Giardia* is isolated from the stool, give metronidazole for 3 days. Asymptomatic patients do not require treatment.
  - If *Campylobacter* is isolated from the stool, give erythromycin if there is systemic upset or persistent blood in the stools, although many cases will resolve without antibiotic treatment (consult with your local microbiologist if in doubt).
  - If *Salmonella* or *Shigella* are isolated from the stool, consider referral to secondary care for treatment and management, particularly if the child is systemically unwell or is under 1 year old.
- If any of the following organisms are cultured from the stool, notify the environmental health department: *Shigella, Salmonella, Giardia, Campylobacter, Cryptosporidium, Escherichia coli 0157.* Discuss children with *E. coli 0157* with secondary care, due to its association with HUS.
- In cases of chronic diarrhoea and failure to thrive or other symptoms, consider further investigations and/or referral. Inflammatory bowel disease and coeliac disease may present with diarrhoea in children.
- If a dietary cause for osmotic diarrhoea has been found, suggest relevant dietary modifications.
- It is important to provide appropriate advice for feeding a child during diarrhoea. Many caregivers may think that it is important to starve the child by providing only water, but this is not helpful. Practical tips about feeding include the following:
  - For breastfed infants, encourage continued breastfeeding which will provide both calories and water.
  - For non-breastfeeding infants, it is rarely necessary to withdraw feeds as this may delay recovery.
  - It is rarely necessary to restrict lactose in the diet.

- Oral rehydration solution (ORS) may be prescribed in moderate dehydration for replacement of fluids during the first 4 hours. After this, recommence normal feeds, with ORS given after each loose stool at a dose of 10 mL/kg body weight. Do not keep children on ORS for prolonged periods of time, as they will become ketotic due to low calorie intake and may then experience abdominal pain and deteriorate clinically.

The Child With a Murmur

- Most murmurs are innocent.
- The majority of pathological heart murmurs are picked up in infancy or have been found on an antenatal scan. As many infants are now discharged from hospital a few hours after birth, they may present to primary care in the first few days of life with either heart failure or cyanosis. These children require urgent referral to hospital for investigation and management.
- Murmurs are often picked up at the routine 6-week baby check. These murmurs should also be referred to secondary care for assessment.
- The key features of an innocent murmur are the seven Ss (Bronzetti & Corzani, 2010):
  1. Sensitive (change with position and respiration)
  2. Short duration
  3. Single (no associated clicks or gallops)
  4. Small (nonradiating)
  5. Soft (low amplitude)
  6. Sweet (not harsh, but musical)
  7. Systolic

What to Ask About the Child

- Ask about cardiac symptoms, including chest pain, syncope, impaired exercise tolerance, colour changes, and cyanosis.
- Ask whether the murmur has ever been noted previously.
- Enquire about the child's feeding, appetite, and growth. All children who are failing to thrive with a murmur should be further investigated.
- Check if there is a family history of cardiac disease. Children have an increased risk of congenital heart disease if they have a first degree relative with a history of congenital heart disease.

What to Look for on Examination

- Assess if the child is acutely unwell.
- Check for cyanosis and pallor and whether there are signs or symptoms that could indicate heart failure, including tachycardia, an enlarged liver, sweating, and difficulties with feeding (particularly in infants).
- Feel for the femoral pulses. Decreased or absent femoral pulses and a short systolic murmur may indicate coarctation of the aorta, a murmur that may not be picked up in early childhood.

- The most common murmur will be an innocent one. On auscultation an innocent murmur will change with the child's position (often being loudest when the child is lying down), have a short duration, will not radiate to the precordium or back, have a soft quality often described as "musical," and be systolic with no associated clicks or gallops.

What to Do

- Refer urgently all children with a murmur who have cyanosis or signs of heart failure (tachycardia, sweating, poor feeding, tachypnoea, enlarged liver, or failure to thrive).
- Also refer urgently all children noted to have a murmur in the first 48 hours of life.
- Refer children whose murmur is not consistent with the findings of an innocent murmur, including a widely radiating or particularly loud murmur.
- Refer those who have cardiac symptoms, including syncope, chest pain, or concerns regarding growth.
- If you think the murmur is an innocent one:
  1. document your findings;
  2. arrange to review the child again to reassess the murmur (if the child is currently unwell, arrange review once the acute illness has resolved);
  3. there is no need to refer to secondary care if the child is well and the murmur has the characteristics of an innocent murmur.

The Child Who Collapses

- Syncope is a temporary loss of consciousness resulting in collapse, caused by reduction in oxygenation to the brain. There are a number of causes, the most common of which are vasovagal episodes (fainting) and reflex anoxic syncope (RAS). RAS is most common in the toddler age group.
- Rare cardiac causes of syncope include arrhythmias (long QT syndrome, Wolff-Parkinson-White syndrome) and cardiac abnormalities (aortic or pulmonary stenosis). As syncope may result in abnormal movements, including stiffening of the body or limbs, convulsive jerking, or drowsiness following the event, syncope may sometimes be confused for epilepsy.
- Breath holding attacks also occur in the toddler age group. During these events the child gets cross, starts to cry, holds his or her breath, turns blue, and collapses. The cyanosis is due to the glottis being held closed. These events are respiratory in origin and an electrocardiogram (ECG) taken at the time would not show asystole.

What to Ask About the Child

- Obtain a detailed history of the event, including what happened before, during, and after the collapse. Try to obtain a history from a witness and, if old enough, the child. In vasovagal episodes the child will often have prodromal features, including sweating, dizziness, and pallor.

- Ask about the frequency of episodes and, if the child has had more than one episode, whether the episodes have similar features. Enquire whether there are specific triggers to the events. Breath-holding attacks occur when a child is crying; RAS occurs in response to a noxious stimulus. Events during exercise or whilst supine are unusual in benign cases of syncope and children with these features should be referred to secondary care.
- Check if there is a history of sudden death in a family member under 30 years of age or a family history of sudden infant death syndrome, and refer children with a positive family history for further assessment.
- If possible, ask the family to capture one of these events on video.

What to Look for on Examination

Usually the child will present with a history of collapse, rather than immediately after the collapse. In most cases the child will have a normal examination. However:
1. examine the cardiovascular system, including blood pressure (take whilst sitting and standing and look for a postural drop in pressure, which may be the cause of a vasovagal episode);
2. examine the neurological system, looking for cranial nerve abnormalities, asymmetry of tone or power, or an abnormal or unstable gait suggestive of an underlying neurologic condition, which would be a rare cause of collapse. In RAS, check the conjunctivae and palmar creases for signs of iron deficiency anemia.

What to Do

- All children with syncope should have an ECG to rule out a rare but potentially fatal cardiac problem. Ideally the ECG should be read by an experienced paediatrician. The exception is classic breath-holding attacks when the child is seen to cry, hold his or her breath, and turn blue. An electroencephalogram (EEG) is not usually required in cases of syncope.
- A clear explanation and reassurance is required for parents and children. Prevention of vasovagal episodes includes the following strategies:
  - Children can learn to recognize the prodromal symptoms and sit with the arms folded and legs crossed to maintain their blood pressure and prevent syncope.
  - Suggest increasing fluids and dietary salt.
- It is difficult to prevent RAS or breath-holding attacks. Sometimes advising the parents to blow gently on the face of a child about to have a breath holding attack may abort the event.

The Child With Chest Pain

- Chest pain is a common reason for 10- to 16-year-olds to attend the emergency department. It can cause significant concern to parents and children but in the majority of cases is noncardiac in origin.

- The most common cause is a musculoskeletal problem; but also consider respiratory causes including asthma and pneumonia, gastrointestinal causes including oesophagitis, and anxiety associated with hyperventilation.

What to Ask About the Child

- Ask about the duration, frequency, location, and description of the pain.
- Enquire whether the pain occurs at rest, on exertion, or during the night.
- Check whether there are associated symptoms, including syncope, pallor, sweating, palpitations, all of which are concerning.
- Ask whether there are respiratory or gastrointestinal symptoms, including asthma or GOR.
- Check whether analgesia helps the pain. Antiinflammatory medication would help ease pain due to costochondritis or musculoskeletal problems.
- If the child has been partaking in new exercises, lifting, or if they carry heavy books to school, consider a possible musculoskeletal cause.
- Ask if there is a family history of sudden death in young adults as there may be a history of hypertrophic obstructive cardiomyopathy or long QT syndrome.
- Check if the child has a history of Kawasaki disease, as this may result in later cardiac problems including a coronary aneurysm.

What to Look for on Examination

- Assess for local tenderness found in costochondritis and musculoskeletal problems.
- Examine the cardiovascular system. Check the peripheral pulses and auscultate for a murmur. If possible check the blood pressure.
- Examine the respiratory and gastrointestinal systems to look for alternative causes of chest pain.

What to Do

- Musculoskeletal causes should be managed with rest and antiinflammatory medication.
- Indications for immediate referral to a paediatric cardiologist include:
  - chest pain on exertion;
  - chest pain with palpitations;
  - chest pain with syncope;
  - a cardiac abnormality found on examination (e.g., a murmur);
  - a family history of sudden death or cardiac problems in a young adult.
- If features suggest a diagnosis of gastrooesophageal reflux, a trial of an acid-blocking drug may be worthwhile.
- Treat respiratory conditions as appropriate.
- Manage anxiety-induced episodes with behavioural techniques.

The Child Who Does Not Walk Aged 15 Months

- Delays in walking may be due to a variety of causes ranging from simple bottom shuffling to cerebral palsy (children have spasticity) and neuromuscular disorders including Duchenne muscular dystrophy and spinal muscular atrophy (children have weakness).

What to Ask About the Child

- Ask about the birth history, including maternal health during pregnancy and prematurity. Check the records for the Apgar scores. Cerebral palsy has many causes but the insult is usually prenatal.
- Ask if the child appears unwell or in pain and whether there is a local cause for the delayed walking (e.g., a swollen or painful joint).
- Assess whether the child has met other gross developmental milestones:
  - Was reaching/grasping delayed (>5 months)?
  - Was sitting delayed (>7 months)?
  - Did the child dislike lying prone (more likely in bottom shufflers)?
  - Did the child crawl (bottom shufflers tend not to crawl)?
- Ask if the child bottom shuffles and if there is a family history of delayed walking or bottom shuffling.

What to Look for on Examination

- Look for dysmorphic features and assess the general development of the child, including vision, hearing, social, and fine motor skills.
- Check the child's truncal tone: Pick up the child under the arms. If the child slides through your hands (like a rag doll), then he or she has truncal hypotonia.
- Check for asymmetry in tone or power in the legs or arms (this may point to an underlying neuromuscular problem).
- Check for tenderness on palpation of the legs or joints.

What to Do

- For children who are bottom shufflers, reassure the parents that the child will walk eventually.
- If you have other concerns regarding the child's neurologic examination or development then refer for further assessment. A physiotherapy assessment is often useful if you are not sure whether there is an underlying problem.

The Child With a Small Head

- *Microcephaly* is defined as an occipital-frontal circumference (OFC) more than 2 standard deviations below the mean. This indicates a small brain, or microcephaly.

- Microcephaly can be caused by a variety of genetic and environmental causes. It is important to distinguish between *primary* microcephaly where an abnormal OFC has been present since birth (corrected appropriately for gestational age and weight and length) and *secondary* or *acquired* microcephaly due to deceleration in the growth of the brain after birth.

What to Ask About the Child

- Ask about the pregnancy and whether the mother was well, whether she had any infections (e.g., cytomegalovirus, rubella, toxoplasmosis), and whether she took any drugs during pregnancy. Consider whether there could have been a prenatal insult.
- Ask about the delivery, including the type of delivery and the Apgar scores, and consider whether there could have been an insult during delivery.
- Enquire whether the parents are consanguineous and consider whether there could be a metabolic or genetic cause (microcephaly may be autosomal recessive).
- Ask whether the infant was unwell during the first 6 weeks of life (e.g., with a serious bacterial infection such as meningitis) and consider whether there has been a postnatal insult.
- Ask about appropriate development milestones: Does the child smile (at 6 weeks), reach/grasp (by 5 months), sit (by 7 months)?

What to Look for on Examination

- Take careful measurements of the weight, length, and OFC and plot on appropriate charts.
- Measure the OFC of the parents and any siblings and plot on appropriate charts.
- Look for any dysmorphic features associated with microcephaly, including primordial dwarfism and Dubowitz syndrome.
- Check if the child is hypertonic or hypotonic.

What to Do

- All children with microcephaly should be referred to secondary care for further assessment.

The Child With a Large Head

- *Macrocephaly* is defined as an occipital-frontal circumference (OFC) more than 2 standard deviations above the mean.
- Macrocephaly does not always indicate a large brain (*megalencephaly*) (e.g., children with hydrocephalus will have a large head but their brain in not enlarged).
- It is important to distinguish between an infant who has always had a large head, whose OFC is tracking appropriately without deviating upward away from previous measurements, and an infant whose OFC was on a lower

centile and is now accelerating and crossing centiles in an upward direction.

- A large head may be familial. Other causes include congenital problems, infections, subdural bleeds, metabolic storage and degenerative diseases, and cranioskeletal dysplasias.

What to Ask About the Child

- Ask about the child's development and whether normal milestones have been reached.
- Check if there are any signs of raised intracranial pressure including poor feeding or irritability.
- Explore whether other members of the family have large heads.
- Enquire whether the child has had any serious illnesses (e.g., meningitis).
- Ask if the parents have any concerns about the child.

What to Look for on Examination

- Take careful measurements of the child's weight, length, and OFC and plot on appropriate charts.
- If possible measure the parents' OFC and plot on an appropriate chart (plot at age 18 years on female and male charts as appropriate).
- Assess the child's development and whether this is age appropriate. In familial macrocephaly the child's development will be normal.
- Palpate the anterior and posterior fontanelles. The anterior fontanelle usually closes by 12–18 months and the posterior fontanelle by 2 months. If they are open beyond this, consider whether the child has raised intracranial pressure.
- Check whether the child's anterior fontanelle is tense and bulging, suggesting raised intracranial pressure.
- Check whether the child has any depigmented or pigmented patches, as neurofibromatosis and tuberous sclerosis are both causes of macrocephaly.

What to Do

- A normally developed child whose OFC is tracking parallel to the 99th centile without deviating in an upward direction, and with a family history of macrocephaly, does not need further investigations. Reassure the parents.
- A child with signs suggesting raised intracranial pressure, or an OFC crossing centiles in an upward direction, should be referred immediately.

The Child With a Febrile Seizure

- Febrile seizures occur when there is a rapid increase in the temperature of a young child, usually between the ages of 1 and 3 years.
- Children who have a seizure below 6 months of age, even if this is associated with fever, should be referred to secondary care for further management and investigation of the source of the fever.
- First febrile seizures do not usually occur in those above 6 years of age.
- The incidence of first febrile seizures is around 1 in 20 children; approximately one third of children who have a febrile seizure will go on to have another febrile seizure.
- Most commonly the duration of febrile seizures ranges from a few seconds to 15 minutes.

What to Ask About the Child

- Ask for a description of the seizure. Febrile seizures may involve a variety of abnormal movements or posturing. Children with focal seizures should be referred to hospital.
- Ask about the length of the seizure and the recovery time. Any child who has not regained consciousness, or whose conscious level is not clearly improving after 30 minutes should be assumed to have increased intracranial pressure and referred for further management.
- Ask about a family history of epilepsy or febrile seizures. If one or both parents have a history of febrile seizures the risk of recurrent febrile seizures for the child increases.
- Try to find a source of the fever by asking about respiratory symptoms, vomiting, diarrhoea, rash, and illness in other family members.

What to Look for on Examination

- Refer any child at high or intermediate risk of a serious illness (see NICE traffic light system for fever in children <5 years earlier in the chapter).
- Take the temperature and give an antipyretic (either orally or per rectum).
- Look for a source of the infection. Specifically examine the throat, ears, chest, abdomen, and skin.

What to Do

- The first priority is to manage the seizure: check airway, breathing, and circulation. If the seizure has lasted for more than 5 minutes give buccal midazolam or rectal diazepam (for doses, see the BNF for Children) and refer the child to hospital.
- You will often be consulted after the seizure and your priority is to determine the cause of, and treat where appropriate, the underlying cause of the fever. See "The Child with a Fever" to guide whether the child should be referred to hospital.
- For children being managed at home reassure the parents that:
  - febrile seizures are common;
  - most children will not have another one;
  - longitudinal studies show that children with febrile seizures have normal school achievement, comparable with their siblings who have not had febrile seizures;

- the majority of children with febrile seizures do not go on to develop epilepsy.
- Refer the child to hospital if there are unusual features associated with the seizure, including a prolonged duration (>15 minutes), asymmetrical movements, a long time (>30 minutes) to return to normal conscious level.

The Child With Seizures

- There are numerous forms of epilepsy, including generalized seizures, focal seizures, absence seizures, infantile spasms, and myoclonic seizures.
- In all children with a seizure, a detailed description of the episode is critical to making a diagnosis. If possible, ask the caregivers to capture the event on video. Providing a detailed description helps to classify the seizure and determine the drugs to use. Approximately 40% of children presenting with a first seizure have nonepileptic events. These include syncope, migraine-related disorders, and self-gratification events (masturbation is normal in infants, although sometimes shocking for the parents).
- Seizures may also be the first indication of raised intracranial pressure and may occur in children with meningitis or with a metabolic derangement, including low blood sugar. These children will be unwell.
- Infants sometimes present with a history of myoclonic jerks. These usually occur either when the child is asleep or when going into or out of sleep. The parents describe rhythmic movements of the limbs. This is not a seizure, does not require investigation or treatment, and the parents should be reassured.

What to Ask About the Child

- Document events preceding the episode(s) including at what time of day/night the events occur, if there are any obvious triggers, and what the child was doing before the seizure.
- Ask for a description of the seizure, from the events preceding the episode to the child recovering completely.
- Ask caregivers to describe any movements or sounds. Explore whether the movements were symmetrical, and if there were any lateralizing signs including eye deviation and tonic/clonic movements of one side of the body only.
- Ask about the length of the episode and whether the child had bladder or bowel incontinence during or after the episode.
- Ask the child, if old enough about the events and what he or she recalls.
- Ask how the child appeared and behaved after the episode.

What to Look for on Examination

- Usually the patient will present to you after the seizure so you are unlikely to witness it.

- If the child has a fever or looks unwell, then assess for signs of meningitis or another cause of febrile illness that may have precipitated the seizure.
- Examine the tone and power and check for symmetry.
- Examine for signs of raised intracranial pressure.

What to Do

- If the child is having a seizure, your first priority is to manage the event. Check airway, breathing, and circulation. If the seizure has lasted for more than 5 minutes, give buccal midazolam or rectal diazepam (for doses, see the BNF for Children) and refer the child to hospital.
- You will often be consulted after the seizure, and your priority is to determine whether the child needs to be urgently referred to hospital (e.g., child not regained consciousness, signs of a serious bacterial infection, seizure was associated with a fever with no obvious cause, or signs of raised intracranial pressure) or whether the child can be referred non-urgently for a clinic appointment.
- It is advisable not to start a discussion about epilepsy, including the prognosis and consequences for lifestyle, until the child has had further investigations (e.g., an EEG) and a diagnosis has been made. Some children may not be started on medication immediately.
- Most neonatal seizures require urgent referral for investigation, as they are often caused by an acute event, including hypoglycaemia, an electrolyte imbalance, or infection.
- Myoclonic jerks are not seizures and do not require investigations or treatment.

The Child With Headaches

Headaches are common in schoolchildren and are usually benign. The challenge is to identify the very small group of children who have serious underlying pathology, including brain tumours.

What to Ask About the Child

- Ask when the headaches first began. A long history of intermittent headaches, and a child who is well in between, suggests a benign aetiology.
- Ask about the frequency of headaches and whether the child is well in between episodes of headache. A headache caused by meningeal stretching (i.e., raised intracranial pressure) is more likely to be constant rather than intermittent.
- Ask about the nature of the headaches:
  - Throbbing headaches are typical of migraines.
  - Feeling as though there is a band around the scalp is typical of tension headaches.
  - Tenderness over the face may suggest inflammation of the sinuses.

- Check whether there are any symptoms suggesting raised intracranial pressure:
  - Have there been recent changes in behaviour?
  - Is the headache made worse on coughing, sneezing, bending over (e.g., to touch the toes), or squatting down?
  - Is the headache worse in the mornings, and is it associated with vomiting?
  - Does the headache wake the child from sleep?
- Enquire whether there have been problems with unsteadiness of the gait, and ask whether the child has had seizures. If the child wears glasses, enquire about recent eye tests or the need for one.
- Explore the social history for any issues that may be causing the child anxiety, including recent separation of parents, change in school, or bullying.

What to Look for on Examination

- Assess whether the child looks well or unwell. A short history of headaches in an unwell child with fever may indicate an infective cause.
- Consider checking the blood pressure.
- Conduct a neurological examination. In particular examine for unsteadiness of the gait and examine the cranial nerves. Specifically assess whether the child can maintain an upward gaze and whether there is *sun setting* of the eyes.
- Examine whether the child's eyes move laterally in both directions and whether there is diplopia.
- Examine the optic fundi for papilloedema. It is often difficult to get a good view of the fundi in young children.
- Palpate the area over the sinuses to check for tenderness.

What to Do

- If the child is acutely unwell refer immediately, including children with fever.
- If the child has abnormalities of the cranial nerves, gait, or neurological examination then refer immediately as these signs are suggestive of raised intracranial pressure.
- If the history and examination are not suggestive of serious underlying pathology, then management will depend on the type of headache:
  - Migraine: reassure, suggest simple analgesia, and if vomiting is a feature, then an antiemetic may be useful. For children with frequent and debilitating migraine, a trial of a migraine prophylaxis (pizotifen or propranolol) may be helpful. Mild hypoglycaemia is a common trigger so encourage the child to eat regularly and healthily. Children often do not drink enough, so encourage an adequate intake of water daily.
  - Tension headaches: reassure, offer advice about avoidance of triggers, and suggest simple analgesia and an adequate fluid intake.
  - Sinusitis: offer a trial of decongestants.
- If headaches are debilitating, then refer to secondary care.

The Child With a Tic

The appearance of facial tics in children, although common, is a source of concern to parents.

What to Ask About the Child

- Ask if there were any triggers for the facial tics, including events that occurred prior to the start of the ticking.
- Enquire whether the tics can be suppressed. Often children can suppress a tic if they are outside the home environment, including at school.
- Ask if the tic is associated with motor or vocal tics suggestive of Tourette's syndrome which requires referral to secondary care.

What to Look for on Examination

- If possible observe the tics or ask the parents to capture them on video.
- Observe for motor and vocal tics.
- Conduct a neurological examination, particularly ensuring the cranial nerves are normal.

What to Do

- Reassurance is the most important management strategy for children with facial tics.
- If the tics are causing excessive distress, psychological interventions may be helpful.
- Suggest that the parents (and teachers) do not reprimand the child, or try to stop the child from ticking, as this is likely to make the tics worse.
- Explain to the parents that the ticking often resolves, although it is difficult to predict if and when the ticking may get better.

The Child With Dysuria and Abdominal Pain

Guideline

National Institute for Health and Care Excellence. Urinary tract infection in under 16s: diagnosis and management. NICE clinical guideline 54. Available at https://www.nice.org.uk/guidance/cg54.

What to Ask About the Child

- In older children ask about fever, dysuria, abdominal and loin pain, symptoms suggestive of UTI.
- Infants with UTI present with nonspecific symptoms, including poor feeding, failure to thrive, irritability, and unexplained fever.
- In all children with a fever and no obvious source of infection, a clean catch urine sample should be obtained for urinalysis, and culture if urinalysis is positive.

- Ask about a history of previous confirmed or unconfirmed UTIs.
- Explore the antenatal history and ask about any antenatal ultrasound scan results.
- Ask about a history of constipation as children who are constipated are prone to UTIs.
- Ask about any family history of renal disease, including vesicoureteric reflux.
- Ask about the child's development and if there are any concerns that the child has a neurological problem.
- Ask if the child has a history of dysfunctional voiding including poor urine flow or diurnal or nocturnal enuresis.
- Assess the child's fluid intake and check for age-appropriate consumption.
- Ask about hygiene including how the child wipes his or her bottom (encourage children to wipe their bottoms from front to back).

What to Look for on Examination

- In most cases examination will be normal.
- Take the child's temperature.
- Plot the child's weight and height on a chart and compare to previous measurements to assess growth.
- Examine the abdomen for tenderness or an enlarged bladder.
- Examine the spine and assess tone and power in the lower limbs and observe the child's gait. Rarely the child may have an underlying neurological condition.
- If appropriate size cuffs are available take the child's blood pressure.

What to Do

- Refer febrile children to secondary care if appropriate according to the NICE guidelines (see above). Children, particularly infants, may need to be referred urgently before you are able to obtain a urine sample if they have a fever and are unwell looking.
- Obtain a clean catch urine sample:
  - Perform urinalysis looking for leukocyte esterase and nitrites. The presence of nitrites with or without leukocyte esterase is indicative of a UTI.
  - Send the urine for culture if urinalysis is positive.
- Try to distinguish between:
  - an upper UTI (acute pyelonephritis): bacteriuria, fever ≥38°C with or without loin pain;
  - a lower UTI: bacteriuria, with no systemic features.
- If the child can be managed at home, treat with antibiotics if the urinalysis is positive for nitrites.
- If the urinalysis is negative for nitrites but positive for leukocyte esterase, only start the antibiotics if there are clinical symptoms of UTI.
- If urinalysis is negative for both nitrites and leukocyte esterase, then do not assume that this is a UTI but search for alternative causes to explain the symptoms.

- Management of a confirmed UTI:
  - Refer all infants, less than 3 months of age, with either upper or lower UTI, for parenteral antibiotics.
  - Refer all infants over 3 months of age for parenteral antibiotics if they are in the high/intermediate risk group (see NICE guideline on page 50) or they are unable to tolerate oral fluids/medication.
  - Refer all children with recurrent UTIs (two upper UTIs or three lower UTIs).
  - For infants over 3 months of age with an upper UTI who are not unwell, manage at home with 10 days of oral antibiotics. Have a low threshold for referral for parenteral antibiotics.
  - For infants over 3 months of age with a lower UTI who are not unwell, manage at home with oral antibiotics as per local guidelines (trimethoprim or a cephalosporin).
  - Infants who are managed at home need an early review to ensure they are responding to treatment. Review the choice of antibiotics once the urine culture and sensitivity results are available.
  - It is not necessary to repeat urine culture at the end of a course of antibiotics if the child responded well.
- Further investigations for children under 3 years of age with a proven UTI:
  - Children under 3 years of age are most at risk of renal damage following UTI. They are also more likely to have underlying pathology leading to the UTI (e.g., vesicoureteric reflux).
  - These will depend on your local guidelines and referral hospital.
  - Children under 6 months of age usually have a renal ultrasound within 6 weeks. Further imaging depends on local guidelines, whether the child responded to treatment within the first 48 hours, and whether the UTI was upper or lower guides further imaging.
- For older children give advice about:
  - cleaning themselves after toileting;
  - encouraging complete bladder emptying and a good fluid intake;
  - managing constipation where appropriate.
- Prophylactic antibiotics are required only in special circumstances (e.g., infants who are waiting for further imaging).
- Most children who require prophylactic antibiotics will have been referred to secondary care, and the antibiotics will have been started there.
- Counsel parents on recognition of the symptoms associated with UTI, particularly in infants who may have nonspecific symptoms.

The Child With Bedwetting (Nocturnal Enuresis)

- Nocturnal enuresis is a distressing condition with significant impact on the lives of the child and the family.
- The prevalence improves with age: approximately 21% at 4 years decreasing to 1.5% at 9 years.

- It is important to establish whether the enuresis is primary (the child has never been dry at night) or secondary (there has been a recent loss of acquired night-time control).

What to Ask About the Child

- Establish whether the child has primary or secondary enuresis.
- If the child has secondary enuresis, consider systemic illness (including UTIs and diabetes mellitus [DM]) and emotional issues.
- Ask about the pattern of the wetting, including how many nights and how many times per night. The latter might be difficult to ascertain if the child does not wake up. Multiple episodes of wetting per night are suggestive of an overactive bladder.
- Enquire the time of night when wetting happens. Wetting often happens after 1 to 2 hours of sleep if the diagnosis is enuresis.
- Ask if the child wakes on wetting.
- Ask about associated daytime symptoms:
  - Ask about daytime wetting, frequency of micturition (>7 times per day), or urgency of micturition, suggestive of an irritable bladder.
  - Enquire whether the child has dysuria or other symptoms of a UTI.
  - Explore symptoms that would suggest DM including thirst, polydipsia, polyuria, weight loss, abnormal breathing.
- If DM is considered in a child, do an immediate capillary blood glucose, and do not wait for a fasting blood glucose or a urine sample.
- Check if the child is having an appropriate, or excessive, fluid intake. Recommended intakes are:
  - age 4 to 8 years: 1000 to 1400 mL/day;
  - age 9 to 13 years: 1200 to 2100 mL/day;
  - age 14 to 18 years: up to 3200 mL/day.
- Explore whether the child has learning difficulties, developmental delay, behavioural or emotional problems, or a family history of DM.

What to Look for on Examination

- In the majority of cases examination will be normal.
- Examine the abdomen for tenderness (possible UTI) and masses, and the spine for abnormalities.
- Observe the child's gait as rarely enuresis may be secondary to a neurological cause.
- Plot the weight and compare against previous measurements. A child with secondary enuresis and weight loss loss must have DM excluded.

What to Do

- Investigations are not normally required unless the child has symptoms of UTI (check urinalysis) or DM (check capillary blood glucose immediately).

- Manage a UTI appropriately.
- General management for nocturnal enuresis includes the following:
  - The child should never be penalized for wetting. A supportive approach should be encouraged.
  - Optimize fluid intake and avoid caffeine.
  - Manage constipation if present.
  - Waking or lifting the child to go to the toilet is a helpful practical measure in the short term but does not influence long-term resolution.
  - Star charts may be helpful for all aspects of management, including adequate fluid intake, regular toileting, and engaging in practical steps (e.g., changing bed sheets).
  - If the child is under 5 years of age, a trial of 2 consecutive nights without wearing a nappy is worthwhile to assess the success of any intervention.
- Alarm systems are often used in children with nocturnal enuresis. Alarms have a high long-term success rate and may be useful if there has been no response to toileting and reward systems. They are less useful if the wetting is infrequent (one or two times per week). Assess the response after 1 month and, if successful, continue until the child has had 2 weeks of uninterrupted dry beds.
- A trial of medication may be used in children from age 5 years. Desmopressin may be used (1) for short-term use (e.g., occasional sleepovers), (2) in conjunction with an alarm system, and (3) if an alarm system is undesirable. Treat for 3 months and then withdraw for 1 week to check if dryness has been achieved. If used longer term, withdraw to assess success every 3 months.

The Child With Protein in the Urine

- Proteinuria may be an incidental finding in a well child but may also be a clue to underlying renal disease.
- A trace of protein is not usually significant; however, 1+ of protein is the equivalent of 30 mg/dL and the urine should be retested to check that the proteinuria has resolved.
- Persistent proteinuria is suggestive of a glomerular lesion and, if associated with haematuria, the likelihood of underlying renal disease increases.

What to Ask About the Child

- In a child with an incidental finding of proteinuria ask if the child has had a recent illness and whether the child has undertaken strenuous exercise. Both are triggers for benign proteinuria.
- For a child with oedema and proteinuria ask if there has been a previous history of oedema, suggesting that the child has had previous episodes of proteinuria.
- Ask if there is a history of a recent upper respiratory infection, as glomerulonephritis may follow a recent infection.

- Check if the child is taking any medications, as some drugs (e.g., penicillamine, gold, and ethosuximide) may be associated with nephrotic syndrome.
- Ask about a family history of renal disease.

What to Look for on Examination

- Check the child's temperature, blood pressure (if an appropriate sized cuff is available), heart rate, and capillary return; assess if the child is haemodynamically stable or acutely unwell.
- Assess for oedema in dependent sites, including the feet, lower back, and face when the child has been recumbent.
- Examine the abdomen for pain.
- If possible, test for orthostatic proteinuria (i.e., check a urinalysis in the recumbent and standing positions). The standing sample will have two to four times more protein in it compared to the recumbent sample. Orthostatic proteinuria may also be diagnosed if an early morning urine specimen is negative for protein but samples taken later in the day are positive.

What to Do

- If there is an incidental finding of proteinuria (1+ or more), repeat urinalysis three times over a period of 2 to 3 weeks, using an early morning urine sample. If proteinuria is persistent then obtain an early morning urine sample and send to the laboratory for a protein to creatinine ratio. The normal range is below 20 mg/mmol.
- If the child has intermittent proteinuria, reassess in 3 to 6 months. If still present refer to secondary care.
- If the child has orthostatic proteinuria, reassure and repeat urinalysis in 1 year. If the child has nonorthostatic proteinuria then refer for further evaluation.
- If the child has associated haematuria or oedema, or a raised protein to creatinine ratio, refer to secondary care.

The Child With Blood in the Urine

- Microscopic haematuria is not visible to the naked eye, but diagnosed on urinalysis and seeing red blood cells on microscopy.
- Macroscopic haematuria is visible to the naked eye.
- It is important to confirm the presence of red blood cells in the urine, as there are other reasons the urine might appear red or brown in colour, including ingestion of some food substances, urates, and the presence of myoglobin or haemoglobin.

What to Ask About the Child

- Ask about the colour of the urine:
  - Bright red or pink urine is suggestive of bleeding from the urinary tract (e.g., UTI, trauma, or a renal calculus).

- Brown or cola coloured urine is suggestive of a glomerular source of bleeding (e.g., poststreptococcal glomerulonephritis, Henoch-Schönlein purpura [HSP], or HUS).
- Ask if there are symptoms of a UTI (dysuria, frequency or urgency of micturition, fever, abdominal or loin pain).
- Enquire whether the child has had a recent upper respiratory tract infection as glomerulonephritis may follow an infection.
- Ask if the child has had a rash, associated with HSP and HUS.
- Ask about any medications, and whether the child is taking rifampicin, which can cause pink urine.
- Ask about the ingestion of specific foods including beetroot.
- Check if there is a family history of deafness (Alport syndrome), renal disease or haematuria, and whether the child has had previous documented episodes of haematuria. Consider benign familial haematuria.
- Enquire whether the child has a history of easy bruising or bleeding and consider a haematological cause.

What to Look for on Examination

- There will be little to find in children with an incidental finding of haematuria.
- Check for oedema suggesting proteinuria.
- Examine the abdomen for a mass (Wilms tumour presents with a mass in a young child) and tenderness (may be present with UTI).
- Examine for a rash, bruising, petechiae, or purpura, which is associated with HSP and HUS.
- Check the joints as swollen and painful joints may be present in HSP.
- Take the temperature and if possible measure the blood pressure, ensuring the correct size cuff is used.

What to Do

- In an asymptomatic child with isolated, microscopic haematuria, repeat urinalysis with microscopy in 2 weeks. If the haematuria persists, check the blood pressure, send urine for a protein–creatinine ratio, arrange to repeat urinalysis again, and ask family members to bring urine samples for urinalysis (considering a diagnosis of benign familial haematuria).
- If haematuria is present on three occasions, refer to secondary care for further investigations.
- If there are symptoms suggestive of UTI, manage appropriately.
- Children with macroscopic haematuria and no obvious cause would have a renal ultrasound performed to exclude a Wilms tumour.
- Refer any child with persistent haematuria to secondary care for further assessment.
- Refer children with haematuria and proteinuria to secondary care, as this is suggestive of glomerulonephritis.

The Child With an Itchy Perineum

- Inflammation or irritation of the vulva is common in young girls and improves at puberty.
- It results from a lack of oestrogen and a thin vaginal/vulval lining that is easily irritated.
- Girls have often had the symptoms for some time before presenting to medical staff.

What to Ask About the Child

- Ask about the frequency and pattern of symptoms (e.g., itch and discharge, both of which are features of vulvovaginitis).
- Ask about urinary symptoms, including burning or stinging on passing urine. If these are present obtain a clean catch urine specimen for urinalysis and culture. Lichen sclerosis is an uncommon condition in children that can present with itch and dysuria, but it has distinct clinical findings (see the upcoming discussion).
- Ask about the following that might be triggers for vulvovaginitis:
  - Irritants, including soap, bubble bath, or shampoo
  - Toilet hygiene, including whether bottom is wiped from front to back
  - Wearing of tight clothing, including jeans and tights
- Ask whether threadworms have been noted. Threadworms cause itch and scratching, which may be the cause of the symptoms, or may have exacerbated an episode of vulvovaginitis.
- Explore carefully whether there are any concerns around child abuse, including whether the child has demonstrated any change in behaviour, if there have been previous social work concerns, how the child is doing at school, and who regularly looks after the child.

What to Look for on Examination

- Examine the external vulval/vaginal area for erythema, discharge, skin changes, and labial adhesions. Vulvovaginitis presents with an erythematous vulva/vagina. Lichen sclerosis also presents with erythema and white patches in a distinctive figure-8 pattern.
- Observe the external anal margin for threadworms.
- Examine for other skin conditions, including eczema.
- Observe for any features of potential concern, including bruising around the perineal area or bleeding.

What to Do

- Investigations are not necessary or helpful. Vaginal thrush is very unusual in an immune-competent, prepubescent girl.
- If the child has symptoms suggestive of a UTI then obtain a clean catch urine for urinalysis and, if positive, a urine culture.
- Advice to prevent recurrence of vulvovaginitis:

- Do not overwash the area.
- Avoid shampoo, soap, and bubble bath; soap substitutes can be used.
- Suggest showers rather than baths, particularly for washing the hair.
- Avoid tight clothing and change wet clothing quickly.
- Use cotton underwear and change regularly.
- Encourage regular toileting and complete emptying of the bladder.
- Use soft toilet paper and encourage good toilet hygiene (wipe from front to back).
- Treat constipation.
- Avoid prolonged sitting if experiencing symptoms (e.g., horse riding or cycling).
- Suggest strategies to manage an episode of vulvovaginitis:
  - Cool compress may soothe the area.
  - Barrier creams (particularly those used for napkin dermatitis) are usually effective.
  - Some experts suggest urinating with the knees open and rinsing with water afterwards.
  - Avoid tight clothing and suggest wearing nightdresses rather than pyjamas to sleep. The exception would be a child with threadworms where pyjamas can decrease the chance of eggs being spread to bedclothes or fingers during the night.
  - Prescribing antibiotic or antifungal treatment is not necessary.
- Management of lichen sclerosis:
  - This is treated in the same way as vulvovaginitis.
  - A steroid cream at night may be helpful.
  - The condition will usually resolve naturally but may cause scarring.
  - If there is doubt about the diagnosis, refer to secondary care.

The Child With Worms in the Stool

- Threadworms affect both pre-school and school-age children, with often more than one family member affected.
- They are spread by the faecal-oral route and the eggs can survive for up to 2 weeks, so repeat infection is common.
- Other worms may be present in the stools, particularly in children who have travelled to areas where other varieties of worms are prevalent.

What to Ask About the Child

- Ask about itch, particularly intense, nocturnal, perineal itching that is common with threadworms.
- Ask about previous episodes.
- Ask about sleep disturbance and irritability at night.
- For girls ask about symptoms of vulvovaginitis.
- Ask about recurrent abdominal pain that may be present.
- Ask if other family members have been affected.

What to Look for on Examination

- Look for small white worms on the perineum or in the stools.
- Examine for evidence of perineal or vulval erythema or irritation.

What to Do

- Investigation for threadworms is not usually necessary. The worms are readily seen at night or in the early morning on the perineum or visible in the stools.
- If the diagnosis is unclear, the *sellotape test* can be conducted: Tape a piece of sellotape over the perineum and then remove. The worms will be seen on the tape.
- Management includes treating all family members, as worms are readily spread within households. Prescribe mebendazole and be aware that a second course may be required.
- Ask all family members to shower; wash all bedclothes, towels, and soft toys. Vacuum all carpets and floors.
- Ensure that fingernails are cut short, encourage good hand washing (including scrubbing of the nails), and avoid thumb sucking.

The Child With A Painful Penis

- *Balanitis* affects prepubescent boys, mostly those who are pre-school age.
- There is inflammation of the glans of the penis, which is painful and sometimes associated with swelling.
- The non-, or partially, retractile foreskin present in this age results in poor hygiene and infection.
- Most boys will only experience a single episode, but balanitis can be chronic or recurrent.
- Aetiology may be grouped into nonspecific dermatitis, infection, irritant, or allergic dermatological, including eczema, and due to manipulation of the foreskin.

What to Ask About the Child

- Ask about penile pain, itch, odour, and any penile discharge suggestive of an infective aetiology.
- Enquire about penile swelling and difficulties with urination and check for a normal urine stream.
- Ask about previous episodes.
- Explore hygiene practices and exposure to irritants, including bubble bath.
- Ask about associated skin conditions, including eczema, and check for symptoms of UTI (dysuria, abdominal/loin pain).

What to Look for on Examination

- Observe for redness of the glans and foreskin with possible swelling.
- Observe for penile exudate and odour.

- Ask an older child to retract the foreskin for you to assess for phimosis.
- Assess for urinary flow if there is a history of problems, and ask about ballooning of the foreskin upon micturition due to a tight meatus.
- In severe phimosis, there may be obstruction to the urinary flow.

What to Do

- If there are symptoms of a UTI, then obtain a clean catch urine for urinalysis and culture.
- Refer for a urological assessment if the child has recurrent episodes of balanitis or phimosis, as a circumcision may be required.
- A subpreputial swab is only required if symptoms are severe or persistent.
- General management of balanitis includes:
    - avoidance of potential irritants, including soap, bubble bath, and wipes;
    - encouragement of good hygiene, including washing the area twice daily with warm water and patting (not rubbing) dry;
    - thorough hand washing;
    - in younger children, encouraging frequent nappy changes;
    - if the foreskin is free, gently retract during washing, but do not forcefully retract the foreskin of an infant.
- Specific management of balanitis will be related to the underlying aetiology.
- Nonspecific dermatitis is treated with a topical hydrocortisone with imidazole cream twice daily for 1 week only.
- If there is no improvement after 1 week, stop the cream and send a swab from the affected area.
- For allergic or irritant balanitis, treat with topical hydrocortisone.
- If a swab has shown candida infection, treat with imidazole cream, but do not treat blindly with an antifungal cream.
- For bacterial infections, treat with a 1-week course of oral flucloxacillin +/- hydrocortisone cream depending on the level of discomfort.

The Child With a Groin Swelling

- The two most common causes of a groin swelling (apart from inguinal lymphadenopathy) are an inguinal hernia and a hydrocele.
- Inguinal hernias may occur in girls but are rare, and also present as a lump in the groin.

What to Ask About the Child

- Ask when the swelling was first noticed. Inguinal hernias are usually noticed during the second or third month of life.

- Enquire whether the swelling comes and goes. Often hernias appear during coughing or crying and reduce spontaneously between such times.

What to Look for on Examination

- Transillumination will help to identify a hydrocele. However, testicular tumours also transilluminate so may be misdiagnosed for a hydrocele.
- Check for cellulitis of the scrotum and groin area, which may indicate an incarcerated hernia. If so, do not try to reduce the hernia but refer immediately to secondary care.

What to Do

- Refer all children with a groin swelling for a surgical opinion (except for a swelling due to enlarged inguinal lymph nodes).
- Urgently refer children with a suspected incarcerated hernia.

The Child With A Painful Scrotum

- It is important not to miss a torsion of the testis in a child presenting with a painful scrotum.
- Other causes include epididymo-orchitis, idiopathic scrotal oedema, trauma, tumour, and a varicocele.

What to Ask About the Child

- Ask whether the pain is in the scrotum and testis or also in the abdomen. A torsion of the testis presents with a painful, swollen testis, and often with pain in the lower abdomen and groin.

What to Look for on Examination

- A painful, swollen testis indicates a torsion of the testis until proven otherwise.
- Examine the scrotum whilst the child is standing up. Do the veins of the testis feel like a bag of worms? If so, the child may have a varicocele.
- Check whether the scrotum and perineal area is red and swollen, with a non tender testis. This may be due to idiopathic scrotal oedema.

What to Do

- Refer all cases of a painful scrotum for surgical review. Torsion of the testis should be referred urgently to a paediatric surgeon.

The Child With a Non-blanching Rash

- The most common causes of a non-blanching rash (petechiae and purpura) include:

- meningococcal disease;
- idiopathic thrombocytopaenic purpura (ITP);
- HSP;
- haematologic malignancy;
- viral illnesses, streptococcal infections, connective tissues disorders, and HUS.
- Any child with a non-blanching rash needs urgent assessment and investigation.
- HSP affects the skin, joints (most commonly the knees and ankles), abdomen, kidneys, and gastrointestinal tract (children may present with gastrointestinal bleeding). Around 1% of children develop end stage renal disease, but mostly the nephritis is self-limiting.
- ITP is an immune mediated thrombocytopenia that is usually acute. Children are usually well and of pre-school age.
- HUS presents with thrombocytopenia, anemia, and renal failure. The child often has bloody diarrhoea, most commonly caused by *E. coli, Shigella,* or echovirus.

What to Ask About the Child

- Ask how long the rash has been present. A rapidly spreading rash in an unwell child suggests meningococcal disease and requires urgent management.
- Check if the child has a fever, which would suggest an infectious cause, but may also be present in malignancy and connective tissue disorders.
- Enquire whether the child had a preceding upper respiratory tract infection as this is often a prodrome to HSP and ITP.
- Ask if the child has bleeding from mucous membranes (e.g., the nose), as this may be present in malignancy and ITP.
- Enquire whether there is a family history of bruising, suggestive of a familial form of thrombocytopenia.
- A history of joint pain, weight loss, or fever may indicate a malignancy or connective tissue disease.
- Abdominal pain and/or arthritis is a common presentation of HSP.
- Check if the child has had bloody diarrhoea as abdominal pain and bloody diarrhoea are often the prodrome to HUS.

What to Look for on Examination

- Assess if the child is acutely unwell. Measure the temperature as a high fever is suggestive of a bacterial infection (e.g., meningococcal or streptococcal disease).
- Check the pattern of petechiae, purpura, and/or bruising:
  - Meningococcal: no specific distribution. There is a widespread, rapidly progressing rash in an ill child.
  - HSP: typical distribution on the lateral malleoli, ventral aspects of feet, buttocks, and extensor aspects of legs. The rash is a palpable, purpuric, rash sometimes with preceding urticaria. The child often has

associated joint swelling/inflammation and a tender abdomen on palpation.

- ITP: widespread petechiae and purpura in a child who is not acutely unwell (note: a child with meningococcal disease is acutely unwell).
- Check if the child has a petechial rash that is only present in the distribution of the superior vena cava (i.e., above the clavicles). In a child with vomiting or a cough, petechiae may be present in this distribution.
- Non-accidental injury may result in non-blanching lesions suggestive of the mechanism of injury (e.g., finger marks or bite marks).
- Check for lymphadenopathy, hepatomegaly, and splenomegaly which may indicate a malignancy.
- In an infant check for signs of a non-accidental injury, including unusual patterns of bruising and petechiae which may be present in the upper body as a result of shaking, a bulging fontanelle indicating raised intracranial pressure, or inflammation of limbs suggestive of a fracture.

What to Do

- Most children with a non-blanching rash should be referred for further investigation and management. Exceptions are when the child has a known respiratory illness, is not acutely unwell, and has petechiae in the distribution of the superior vena cava.
- If the child is acutely unwell, give IM antibiotics prior to transfer.
- In a child with suspected HSP, check the urine for blood and protein and, if possible, check the blood pressure. If HSP is confirmed, it is important to monitor the blood pressure and urine protein at intervals, initially weekly then monthly for 6 months, to detect any renal damage.

The Child With Cervical Lymphadenopathy

- Cervical lymphadenopathy is extremely common in children, a cause of great concern to parents, and a common reason for referral to secondary care.
- The main causes are benign lymphadenopathy secondary to infections and, rarely, granulomatous disease (i.e., TB) and malignancy.
- The most common malignancies causing lymphadenopathy include Hodgkin disease, non-Hodgkin lymphoma, and leukaemia.

What to Ask About the Child

- Ask if the child has had any recent infections, particularly of the throat, ear, nose, and scalp. Benign lymphadenopathy is typically secondary to a recent infection.
- Ask if any of the nodes have recently increased in size. Rapid enlargement of nodes may need further investigation.

- Enquire whether there has been any contact with TB or recent travel to a TB-endemic area, and if the child has night sweats. Night sweats are present with TB or malignancy.
- Ask whether the child has been more lethargic than usual, which may suggest TB or malignancy.
- Ask if the child has a chronic cough that may suggest TB.
- Ask about eczema, as this is a common cause of localized lymphadenopathy.

What to Look for on Examination

- Assess the pattern of the enlarged lymph nodes. Are they only in the cervical region or also in the axillary and inguinal regions?
- Check the appearance of the nodes. Are they red, tender, or fluctuant, suggesting infection and possibly an abscess?
- Check for supraclavicular nodes. A supraclavicular node is not usually associated with a recent infection and is more suggestive of malignancy.
- Nodes that are hard, matted together, or non mobile (i.e., fixed to underlying structures) are more suggestive of non benign lymphadenopathy.
- Examine for hepatosplenomegaly, which may be present in malignancies and also in some viral infections, including Epstein-Barr virus (glandular fever).
- Measure the weight and compare against previous weights. Benign lymphadenopathy does not present with weight loss, and further investigation to rule out TB and malignancy should be undertaken in a child with acute weight loss.
- Examine the mouth for dental caries.

What to Do

- If the child is well, with mobile, small lymph nodes and a recent infection, reassure the parents and arrange to review the patient again.
- If you are suspicious of TB or malignant disease, then refer the patient for further investigations.

The Child With Pica

- Pica (eating substances with no nutritive value) is a common reason for referral to secondary care.
- The main cause of pica is iron deficiency or, rarely, lead poisoning.
- Iron deficiency anemia is common in children, and is usually due to a poor diet or a diet consisting largely of cow's milk.

What to Ask About the Child

- Take a good detailed history, specifically asking about the amount of milk in the child's diet and whether the child eats meat. Iron deficiency anemia is common in children whose diet consists mostly of cow's milk or who

are vegetarian. Red meat and cereals are good sources of dietary iron.
- Ask about the child's gestational age. Preterm infants require supplemental iron, as iron is transferred transplacentally during the last trimester of pregnancy and there is little iron in milk. The iron in breastmilk is more available than that in formula milk.
- Ask if there has been any history of blood loss (e.g., melena, blood in vomit, or menorrhagia in pubertal girls). This is to exclude other causes of iron deficiency, particularly in a child with an apparently good diet.
- Enquire whether the family home is old and consider whether the child has developed lead poisoning from old paint work.
- Check if there is a family history of β-thalassaemia, which also causes a low haemoglobin and low mean corpuscular volume.

What to Look for on Examination

- Examine for pale conjunctivae and pale palmar creases.
- Always examine for lymphadenopathy and hepatosplenomegaly to ensure that the child does not have an underlying pathology accounting for the iron deficiency.
- Examine for a systolic flow murmur often present in iron deficiency.
- Examine the mouth for glossitis or angular cheilitis, both suggesting iron deficiency.

What to Do

- It is often difficult to take blood tests in primary care, so children are often referred to secondary care. If blood testing is possible, take a full blood count and film, ferritin level, and lead level.
  - In iron deficiency anemia there will be a low mean corpuscular volume (MCV) and low haemoglobin.
  - In lead poisoning the blood will be normochromic or slightly hypochromic with characteristic basophilic stippling on the film.
- If relevant for ethnicity, also send blood for a haemoglobinopathy screen.
  - Usually iron deficiency is treated with oral iron supplements after the diagnosis is confirmed.
  - Children with lead poisoning require referral to secondary care and chelation therapy.
  - Premature infants should take oral iron supplements until at least 6 months of age.

The Child Who Is Short

- *Short stature* is defined as a height below the 0.4th centile on a growth chart or less than 2 standard deviations below the mean for gender and age.
- Short stature may be a source of emotional and social distress to both children and parents who often ask for referral to secondary care.

- The vast majority of those referred to secondary care have common variations of normal physiological growth. These include familial short stature and constitutional short stature (also known as constitutional delay).
- Pathological causes are unusual and include endocrine problems, Turner and Noonan syndromes, chronic disease, and malnutrition.

What to Ask About the Child

- Ask for the parents' and siblings' heights and ages of pubertal onset:
  - Children with familial short stature have short parents, a normal growth velocity and pubertal onset, and no signs of physical disease. These children look short but normal.
  - Children with constitutional short stature have parents with normal stature; however, one parent may have had a delay in growth and late puberty. These children look short and normal, have a delayed puberty with late growth spurt, but achieve a final height within the parental target range.
- Ask about nutrition and assess whether the dietary intake is adequate for growth.
- Ask about symptoms of chronic diseases, including diarrhoea, abdominal pain (inflammatory bowel disease, coeliac disease), and uncontrolled asthma.
- Enquire about inhaled steroid therapy, and the length and dose of steroid treatment which may affect growth.
- Explore the social history and whether there are concerns about psychosocial deprivation.
- If relevant ask about signs of puberty.

What to Look for on Examination

- Plot all weight and height measurements on an appropriate chart.
- If the child is less than 2 years of age, also plot the OFC.
- It is useful to measure the height at four monthly intervals to assess the height velocity.
- Conduct a systemic examination for signs of chronic disease.
- Assess if there are any dysmorphic signs (e.g., skeletal disproportion).
- Plot the parents' heights on a growth chart at "age 18 years." This is useful information to provide if you are referring to secondary care, as both parents may not attend the hospital appointment.
- The mean expected adult height is approximately calculated as follows:
  - Boy: The mean of the parents' heights plus 7 cm
  - Girl: The mean of the parents' heights minus 7 cm
- Most growth charts explain how to calculate the midparental height centile and the target range around this mean value.

What to Do

- If you or the parents have concerns about the child then refer to secondary care. However, in most cases monitoring the height velocity and reassurance will be the mainstays of management.
- If referring to secondary care it is useful to provide a detailed history, including measurements of the child, their siblings, and parents.

The Child Who Is Tall

- *Tall stature*, defined as a height greater than 2 standard deviations above the mean for gender and age, is more accepted by society than in previous generations.
- Concern is often expressed by parents about girls who are tall, although most cases will not require investigation. However, repeated measurements to assess growth over a period of 6 to 12 months are important.
- Rarely, tall stature is caused by endocrine problems including hyperthyroidism or precocious puberty.

What to Ask About the Child

- Ask about parental heights and heights of any siblings. Most growth charts explain how to calculate the midparental height centile and the target range around this mean value. Assess whether the child's height is within the expected parental target range. The mean expected adult height is calculated as follows:
  - Boy: The mean of the parents' heights plus 7 cm
  - Girl: The mean of the parents' heights minus 7 cm
- Ask when the parents noticed that the child was tall and try to assess whether the child has been growing constantly or if the growth has accelerated recently.
- Ask about signs of puberty in the child and whether the parents had early puberty:
  - In normal genetic tall stature: one or both parents are tall, and the child looks normal and tall.
  - In constitutional tall stature, the child will have early puberty and grow to his or her final height earlier than peers.
- Ask about symptoms suggestive of hyperthyroidism and whether the child has headaches or visual problems suggestive of a cranial lesion (such as a pituitary tumour in acromegaly).

What to Look for on Examination

- Measure and weigh the child, plot on an appropriate chart, and compare to previous measurements.
- If the child is less than 2 years, measure and plot the OFC.
- Assess if there are features of hyperthyroidism:
  - Weight loss
  - Goiter
  - Tachycardia
  - Exophthalmos

- Plot parental heights on a chart and calculate the expected adult height.
- Check for features of early puberty.

What to Do

- If the cause is thought to be normal genetic tall stature or constitutional tall stature, monitor the growth over 6 to 12 months and reassure the parents and child.
- If the history and examination are not consistent with a normal variant tall stature, refer to secondary care.
- If obesity is an associated issue, provide guidance on weight management.

The Child With Precocious Puberty

- The age of onset of puberty is subject to much variation. Definitions of precocious puberty vary in the literature, but features of sexual development in a girl younger than 8 years and a boy younger than 9 years require assessment.
- The impact of early sexual development can be detrimental to a child both physically and emotionally.
- Precocious puberty can be *true* (i.e., early puberty but under normal hypothalamic control) or *pseudo* (i.e., independent of hypothalamic control).
- True precocious puberty is common in girls, but rare in boys. Therefore it is important to investigate and identify a cause for precocious puberty in all boys.

What to Ask About the Child

- Ask about growth and pubertal onset in the parents and any siblings.
- Ask specifically about different aspects of puberty:
  - Breast enlargement
  - Penile enlargement
  - Development of pubic hair
  - Vaginal bleeding
  - Body odour
  - Mood swings
- Ask about a history of headaches, vomiting, visual disturbance, or polydipsia. These suggest a brain tumour in the presence of precocious puberty.

What to Look for on Examination

- Measure the child and plot weight and height on an appropriate chart and compare to previous measurements.
- If you are confident, perform Tanner staging on the child.
- Examine the optic fundi and the cranial nerves, and observe the gait (very rarely precocious puberty is caused by a brain tumour).
- Neurofibromatosis and McCune-Albright syndrome are both associated with precocious puberty, so check the skin for cafe au lait spots (neurofibromatosis and McCune-Albright syndrome) and axillary freckling (neurofibromatosis).

What to Do

- Refer all girls under 8 years and boys under 9 years with signs of sexual development to secondary care.

The Child With Excess Body Hair

- Excessive or premature hair development can cause significant anxiety and distress for children, particularly girls.
- It is important to establish whether there are associated concerns regarding precocious puberty.
- *Adrenarche*, the adrenal stage of puberty, results in body odour, greasy skin and hair, weight gain, and pubic and axillary hair development without breast development. It is usually seen from 8 years and is considered premature if it occurs before 6 years of age. An exaggerated form can be seen between 6 and 8 years.
- Hirsutism (androgen dependent areas) and hypertrichosis (generalized) are forms of excessive or inappropriate hair growth. They predominate in certain ethnic groups but can also be indicative of polycystic ovary syndrome.

What to Ask About the Child

- Ask about growth and pubertal onset in parents and any siblings.
- Ask about features of adrenal excess including greasy skin and hair, and body odour.
- Enquire about mood swings or behavioural disturbance.
- Explore whether the child has had a recent growth spurt or gain in weight.
- Ask about other pubertal features, including breast and penile enlargement; and in girls, features suggestive of polycystic ovary syndrome, including menstrual disturbance and weight gain.

What to Look for on Examination

- Measure and plot the height and weight and compare to previous measurements. Check the height velocity. Is the child deviating away from his or her previous centile line?
- Look for tall stature.
- Assess the amount and distribution of hair growth.
- If you are confident, perform Tanner staging.
- Observe for greasy hair and skin. Is there body odour?
- Examine the abdomen for masses.
- Check the optic fundi and perform a general neurologic examination.

What to Do

- If pubic or axillary hair is present before 6 years of age, refer for investigation.

- If hair is present at 6 to 8 years and is sparse, refer for assessment. The hair growth will be reviewed every 3 to 4 months over a period of 1 year to ensure that it is appropriate and there is no pubertal development.
- If hair growth is excessive and causing emotional distress, refer for assessment and advice about hair removal, including chemical and laser therapy.
- If features are suggestive of polycystic ovary syndrome, refer for assessment.

The Child With A Painful Limp

- The most common cause of limp due to hip pain is transient synovitis, most common between the ages of 4 and 10 years.
- About 90% of cases resolve in 7 days but, as it cannot be reliably distinguished from more serious causes of hip pain, all children should be referred to secondary care.
- The child who presents with a painful limp and complains of pain in the knee should be assumed to have a problem in the hip until proved otherwise.
- An unwell child who is non–weight bearing is likely to have a more serious underlying pathology, including septic arthritis, osteomyelitis, or leukaemia.

What to Ask About the Child

- Check the child's age as many aetiologies occur in specific age ranges (e.g., synovitis tends to affect pre-school children).
- Ask whether the onset was acute or chronic and whether there was a prodromal illness. Transient synovitis typically presents after a viral illness.
- Ask about a history of trauma and consider a Toddler fracture in a young child.
- Enquire if there has been a history of systemic upset including fever, lethargy, pallor, weight loss, or easy bruising or bleeding, and think about diagnoses including leukaemia, septic arthritis, and osteomyelitis.
- If there is pain at rest or at night consider osteomyelitis, septic arthritis, or malignancy.
- If the child is unable to bear weight, has pain at rest, and is also febrile, then consider septic arthritis or osteomyelitis.
- Take a careful history of the presentation of any injury. If the history is not consistent with the injury, consider a possible non-accidental injury.

What to Look for on Examination

- Assess whether the child looks well or unwell.
- Take the temperature and observe the level of comfort of the child. Children with septic arthritis are in pain at rest.
- Examine for restricted movement, bony tenderness, joint swelling, tenderness, erythema, or deformity and assess the child's gait and spine.

- Remember to examine the feet. Check if there is a local cause for the limp (e.g., a foreign body).
- Examine for a rash, as HSP may present with joint swelling and pain.
- Check for pallor, lymphadenopathy, bruising, or hepatosplenomegaly which may suggest a malignancy.

What to Do

- Refer all children with a painful limp to secondary care to exclude serious pathology.

The Infant Who Vomits or Screams When Feeding

- The complaint of distress or vomiting with feeds is very common in general practice.
- Causes range from relatively benign to potentially life threatening, but the cause can often be elicited through a careful history.

What to Ask About the Child

- For breastfeeding infants, ask about:
  - duration and frequency of feeds (in the first few weeks of life infants will feed at least eight times per 24 hours, and usually more frequently than this);
  - whether the infant appears satisfied after feeding from one breast. If infants are taken off one breast after a few minutes and then offered the second breast, they will only receive foremilk (containing water and lactose) and no hindmilk (containing more fat). These infants may feel hungry again soon after feeding.
- For formula feeding infants ask about:
  - the number and volume of feeds per day;
  - calculating the volume of feeds the infant is receiving. If the total volume of feeds is above 150 mL/kg/24 hours and the infant is thriving, suggest reducing the volume per feed, particularly if the infant is vomiting.
- Ask about vomiting, including the frequency and timing of vomits in relation to feeds, and whether the vomit contains blood or bile. In gastrooesophageal reflux the infant will vomit effortlessly during, after, and sometimes between feeds. Feeding relaxes the lower gastrooesophageal sphincter. The vomit in GOR will not contain bile, and rarely contains blood.
- Ask if the vomiting is projectile and only occurs immediately after a feed. Consider pyloric stenosis and ask about a family history of pyloric stenosis. Infants with pyloric stenosis may have dehydration and failure to thrive, but if diagnosed early enough the only sign may be projectile vomiting.
- Ask about the behaviour of the infant. Infants with GOR will often display certain posturing, including arching of the back, straightening out of the legs, and becoming very distressed when put in a supine or prone position.

What to Look for on Examination

- Assess whether the infant is thriving. Plot the infant's current weight on a chart and compare to previous weights. Infants with GOR are usually thriving. If the infant is not thriving, then consider other diagnoses.
- Examine for pallor, cyanosis, and dehydration. Infants with GOR are usually well looking, normally developed, and thriving. They are miserable and often cry when being fed, but are not acutely unwell looking.
- Always try to observe a feed.
- Conduct a full systematic examination of the infant, including auscultation of the heart and palpation of the abdomen.

What to Do

- If the infant has fever and is unwell, refer to secondary care (see page 39).
- If you suspect that the infant has pyloric stenosis, refer to secondary care.
- If you think the infant has GOR (thriving, well looking, vomiting or screaming with feeds), try the following:
  - Reduced volume but more frequent feeds
  - Thickened feeds in formula-fed babies (e.g., Instant Carobel)
  - Gaviscon. This is easy to give to formula feeding infants where it is added to bottles. For breastfeeding infants, it is not as easy, as it needs to be given before the feed, ideally mixed with breastmilk.
  - A trial of an acid-blocking medication may be useful (ranitidine or omeprazole). Doses are given in the British National Formulary for Children.
  - Children between 1 and 2 years can be considered for a 4-week trial of either omeprazole or ranitidine.
- Arrange for someone to review the infant in a few days' time. GOR can be extremely upsetting for parents, even though they can see that their infant is thriving, and they usually need a lot of support. It is easy for a breastfeeding mother to become discouraged and to stop breastfeeding.
- If the vomiting and screaming does not settle, refer to secondary care. It is not sensible to switch formula milks without a clear reason to do so:
  - Cow's milk protein intolerance presents as excessive crying, vomiting, and sometimes diarrhoea and blood in the stool. Occasionally the infant may have constipation. There is no diagnostic test, but other causes of crying should also be sought. A short trial of a hydrolysed formula will result in a dramatic improvement and reintroduction of cow's milk in resumption of symptoms. Local guidelines are usually available about the brand of milk to prescribe and at what age to rechallenge with cow's milk.

True allergy to cow's milk presents with an urticarial rash or anaphylaxis. There is often a personal or family history of atopy. It is appropriate to refer these children to secondary care for advice. These children need a hydrolysed formula and a milk-free diet for at least the first year of life.

The Infant Who Has Weight Faltering in the First Few Weeks of Life

What to Ask About the Child

- Ask if the mother thinks the baby is unwell. A baby who is failing to thrive may have sepsis.
- Take a thorough feeding history:
  - For breastfed infants, ask about:
    1. frequency of breastfeeds—a young infant who is exclusively breastfed should be taking a minimum of eight feeds per 24 hours;
    2. duration of breastfeeds (Is the baby offered one breast until satisfied and comes off the breast independently? Is the infant offered the second breast?);
    3. whether the baby feeds overnight or sleeps through the night;
    4. whether the baby is given additional fluids or feeds (e.g., Is the infant given drinks of water [with empty calories] between feeds?);
    5. if breastfeeding feels comfortable for the mother.
  - For formula fed infants, ask about:
    1. the frequency of feeds and volume of each feed taken;
    2. the type of milk and how the milk is prepared. If milk is prepared incorrectly and made too dilute, this could be a reason for failure to gain weight.
- In all children ask about vomiting, diarrhoea, and lethargy. Young infants who were initially jaundiced and sleepy are sometimes slower to establish feeding routines.
- Ask about the mother's health in pregnancy, the birth, and delivery.
- Check the mother's antenatal record and make sure that she was screened for infections including HIV. Ask about any infections in the family, including TB.

What to Look for on Examination

- Check the infant thoroughly for symptoms and signs suggestive of a serious infection. If you have any concerns about the infant's general health refer to secondary care.
- Plot weights on an appropriate chart (if the infant was preterm adjust for gestational age). Use growth charts based on the World Health Organization growth charts (including the charts currently used in the United Kingdom) that show the growth of children who have been optimally fed from birth.
- Check the infant's mouth for thrush and the napkin area for rashes.
- Check the infant's tone. Infants who are floppy with poor tone should be referred to secondary care.
- Auscultate the heart and check for a heart murmur.
- Check for signs of a respiratory problem including indrawing, tachypnoea, and nasal flaring

What to Do

- A well infant whom you think has a feeding problem can be dealt with in primary care with support from an experienced health visitor and, if relevant, breastfeeding expert.
- If possible check for a UTI, which may present with failure to thrive in an infant who has few other symptoms.
- If there are concerns about the infant's general health or no obvious cause can be found for the failure to thrive then refer to secondary care.
- Regular review of infants is needed and their families need support and encouragement.

The Infant Who Has Weight Faltering After the First Weeks of Life

- Most cases of failure to thrive or weight faltering are due to poor oral intake and not to underlying pathology. However, sometimes the child has poor intake because of an underlying condition (e.g., children with a UTI may not feed well).
- It is always important to take a detailed dietary history.

What to Ask About the Child

- Take a detailed feeding history, starting from how the child was fed in the first months of life (see The Infant Who Has Weight Faltering in the First Weeks of Life).
- Assess whether there were any problems with feeding in the first few weeks of life.
- Ask about the frequency of complementary feeds and snacks in children over 6 months of age. By 10 months of age, children should be taking three meals and two snacks per day.
- Ask about the consistency of the complementary feeds. Some children are offered very dilute complementary feeds as their parents are concerned about them choking.
- Ask about the quantity of feeds taken and whether they are only taking a mouthful or managing to finish a small bowl of food.
- Find out what milk the child is taking. Ideally breastfeeding should continue after the introduction of complementary feeds.
- Ask about other symptoms the child may have, including fever and dysuria, suggestive of a UTI.
- Ask if the child has abdominal pain suggesting a possible gastrointestinal problem (e.g., coeliac disease).
- Ask about stool patterns and whether the child has constipation (children with constipation often have poor appetites) or diarrhoea.
- Explore whether the child has been drinking more than usual or passing large quantities of urine, as diabetes mellitus (DM) may be the cause of weight loss.
- Ask whether the child has a chronic cough (suggestive of a chronic respiratory condition) or if the child snores

at night with interruptions in breathing (suggestive of obstructive sleep apnoea).

- Check that the mother was tested for HIV in pregnancy.
- Explore whether there are concerns about the child's psychosocial well-being and if there have been previous social work concerns.

What to Look for on Examination

- Weigh and measure the child, including the OFC, plot on an appropriate chart, and compare to previous measurements. Check if the child is tracking appropriately along his or her centile line. If the child's weight and height have always been on the 0.4th centile since birth, and the child is well, then there is no failure to thrive and the child has always been small.
- When assessing a child's weight, a rough rule of thumb is:
  - a child doubles birth weight by 4 to 5 months;
  - a child triples birth weight by 12 to 13 months.
- Examine for pale conjunctivae and palmar creases (suggestive of iron deficiency).
- Examine for loose skin folds (suggestive of recent weight loss).
- Assess whether the child looks neglected, if the child is dirty and ill-kempt, and if there is severe napkin dermatitis.
- Examine the abdomen for masses, including faecal masses, and hepatosplenomegaly.
- Examine the respiratory system to assess if the child has chest signs suggestive of a chronic respiratory problem.
- Examine the tonsils and assess whether the child is a mouth breather. Children with obstructive sleep apnoea are often poor eaters with weight faltering.
- Examine whether the child has any signs suggestive of non-accidental injury, including bruises, and assess how the parent/caregiver interacts with the child. Observe how the child behaves during the consultation (i.e., acting withdrawn or active) and how the caregiver controls the child.

What to Do

- If the problem is a dietary one then address this.
- If possible a home visit by a health visitor may be helpful.
- Give clear counselling around the quantities and frequency of foods to be offered.
- Explain that the child should not be forced to feed but should be fed responsively.
- All children over 1 year of age in the United Kingdom should take a multivitamin supplement (e.g., Healthy Start Vitamins).
- Always encourage a mother who is breastfeeding to continue. It is easy for her to lose confidence in the value of her breastmilk if her child has weight faltering.
- Further management depends on the history and examination:
  - It is useful to obtain a clean catch urine for urinalysis +/− culture to exclude a UTI or glycosuria (DM).

- If DM is suspected, check a capillary blood glucose and refer/discuss immediately if above 8 mmol/l and/or symptomatic of DM.
- Treat constipation.
- If you suspect the child has obstructive sleep apnoea, then refer to an ENT (ears, nose, throat) surgeon.
- If you have concerns about neglect or non-accidental injury, refer to secondary care and contact the social work department.
- Refer children whom you think may have underlying pathology for further investigations.

The Child Who Is Suspected of Having a Non-accidental Injury

- Children can sustain a multitude of injuries during normal, active play. The challenge is to identify those who are at risk of non-accidental injury, and children whose clinical presentation or history is suggestive of non-accidental injury.
- A thorough history and examination is essential.
- Information from other professionals, including health visitors, social workers, and school personnel, who know the family is useful in identifying vulnerable children.

What to Ask About the Child

- Obtain a detailed history of the injury:
  - Was it a witnessed fall or trauma?
  - Is the history describing how the injury occurred consistent with the clinical findings?
  - When did the injury occur and has there been a delay in presentation to medical services?
  - Explore the past medical history, including the perinatal history. Have there been previous injuries, illnesses, visits to the hospital emergency department?
  - Does the child have a history of bleeding or easy bruising and is there a family history of bleeding disorders?
  - Take a detailed social history including who lives in the house, who has contact with the child/children, and whether previous concerns have been raised about the family from the social work department.
  - Ask about the other siblings and how they are growing and developing.
  - Explore whether there are any recent events in the family that could have caused stress, including financial difficulties or separation of the parents.

What to Look for on Examination

- Assess whether the child is thriving. Measure the child and plot his or her weight and height on appropriate charts.
- Observe whether the child is clean and appropriately dressed or unkempt, dirty, and inappropriately clad.

- Examine for features of potential neglect, including untreated skin conditions, severe nappy rash, and lice.
- Assess any injuries and document these carefully and consider whether the injuries are in keeping with the history of how they occurred.
- Injuries of concern:
  - Bruises in the shape of fingers, grip marks, or possibly caused by an implement
  - Any injury in a non-mobile child, unless it was an accident (e.g., a parent falling whilst holding the child)
  - Burns or scalds which appear to have been caused by direct contact being applied to the skin, including immersion in hot water or a cigarette burn
  - A torn frenulum in the mouth of a young infant
  - Injuries on non bony prominences of the head, neck, back, or buttocks
  - Multiple, unexplained lacerations, abrasions, or scars
- In young infants, feel the anterior fontanelle. An infant who has been shaken may have a tense, bulging fontanelle and signs of raised intracranial pressure (irritability, crying, vomiting, poor feeding).
- Assess the child's emotional state and interaction with the parents or caregivers. Is the child wary (frozen watchfulness) or is parental hostility or detachment noted?

What to Do

- Any child who presents with an unexplained injury, unexplained delay in presentation, or whose history is inconsistent with the presentation should be referred for assessment. Local guidelines will dictate further management, but usually this includes:
  - an assessment by a senior paediatrician (including examination and history from the referrer and accompanying adult);
  - consent for taking clinical photographs of any injuries;
  - investigations (blood tests, cranial imaging, x-rays);
  - liaising with other professionals (social workers, police) as required on an individual case basis.
- If you have concerns about any child whom you feel is being neglected, discuss the case with a social worker and senior paediatrician.

References

Books

Beattie, J., & Carachi, R. (Eds.), (2005). *Practical paediatric problems. A textbook for MRCPCH.* London: Hodder Arnold.

Behrman, R., & Kliegman, R. (2002). *Pediatric decision making strategies.* Philadelphia: WB Saunders Company.

Bronzetti, G., & Corzani, A. (2010). The seven "S" murmurs: an alliteration about innocent murmurs in cardiac auscultation. *Clinical Pediatrics, 49*(7), 713.

Cramer, K., & Scherl, S. (2004). *Orthopaedic surgery essential, pediatrics.* Philadelphia: Lippincott Williams and Wilkins.

Raine, J., Donaldson, M., Gregory, J. W., & Van Vliet, G. (2011). *Practical endocrinology and diabetes in children.* Oxford: Wiley-Blackwell.

Guidelines

British Guideline on the Management of Asthma. (2011). *Quick reference guide.* Retrieved from http://www.sign.ac.uk/pdf/qrg101.pdf; http://www.brit-thoracic.org.uk.

British Guidelines on the Management of Community Acquired Pneumonia in Children. (2011). Retrieved from https://www.brit-thoracic.org.uk/standards-of-care/guidelines/bts-guidelines-for-the-management-of-community-acquired-pneumonia-in-children-update-2011/.

National Institute for Health and Care Excellence. (2013). *Clinical knowledge summary. Balanitis in children.* Retrieved from http://cks.org.uk/balanitis.

National Institute for Health and Care Excellence. (2013). *Diarrhoea and vomiting in children under 5. NICE clinical guideline 84.* Retrieved from www.nice.org.uk.

National Institute for Health and Care Excellence. (2013). *Feverish illness in children. NICE clinical guideline 160.* Retrieved from www.nice.org.uk/guidance/cg160/resources/support-for-education-and-learning-educational-resource-traffic-light-table-pdf-189985789.

National Institute for Health and Care Excellence. (2013). *Nocturnal enuresis—the management of bedwetting in children and young people. NICE clinical guideline 111.* Retrieved from www.nice.org.uk.

National Institute for Health and Care Excellence. (2013). *Urinary tract infection in under 16s: Diagnosis and management. NICE clinical guideline 54.* Retrieved from https://www.nice.org.uk/guidance/cgG54.

National Institute for Health and Care Excellence. (2013). *When to suspect child maltreatment. NICE clinical guideline 89.* Retrieved from www.nice.org.uk.

Royal Children's Hospital. (2013). *The management of vulvovaginitis.* Melbourne: Royal Children's Hospital. http://222.rch.org.au.

Resources

The Enuresis Resource and Information Centre (ERIC). www.eric.org.uk.

World Health Organization. (2009). *Infant and young child feeding: Model chapter for textbooks for medical students and allied health professionals.* Retrieved from www.who.int/maternal_child_adolescent/documents/9789241597494/en/.

7

Cardiovascular Problems

DAVID NICHOLAS BLANE

CHAPTER CONTENTS

Hypertension

GUIDELINE

National Institute for Health and Care Excellence. (2011a). *Hypertension: Clinical management of primary hypertension in adults (update). NICE clinical guideline 127.* Available at http://guidance.nice.org.uk/CG127.

- Hypertension is one of the most common conditions treated in primary care in the United Kingdom and one of the most important preventable causes of death worldwide (Krause et al., 2011). It is the main risk factor for development of stroke and ischaemic heart disease and is strongly associated with the development of chronic kidney disease and cognitive impairment.
- *Hypertension*, defined as the presence of persistently raised blood pressure at or greater than 140/90 mm Hg (Box 7.1), affects more than a quarter of all UK adults and over half of those aged 65 years or more (Health and Social Care Information Centre, 2011). The adult prevalence of high blood pressure is even higher in other parts of the world, with over 40% of adults affected in Africa, for example (World Health Organisation [WHO], n.d.).
- Most people with hypertension have no symptoms or clinical findings on examination and their hypertension is identified incidentally or as a result of complications such as angina, myocardial infarction (MI), stroke, and arrhythmias.
- The rule of halves was described in the United States by Wilber and Barrow in 1972. They stated that half of hypertensives are not known to have a raised blood pressure (BP); of those with known hypertension, half are not on treatment and half of those on treatment are poorly controlled. The figures for detection and treatment of hypertension have improved in recent years, but this remains a useful reminder of the challenge posed by hypertension.

● BOX 7.1 | **Definition of Hypertension**

Stage 1 Hypertension

- Clinic BP ≥140/90 mm Hg and subsequent ABPM or HBPM ≥135/85 mm Hg

Stage 2 Hypertension

- Clinic BP ≥160/100 mm Hg and subsequent ABPM or HBPM ≥150/95 mm Hg

Severe Hypertension

- Clinic BP ≥180/110 mm Hg

Note: Where a threshold or target level of blood pressure is given (e.g., 160/100 mm Hg), it means that action should be taken if the systolic is 160 or over OR the diastolic is 100 or over.
ABPM, Ambulatory blood pressure monitoring; *HBPM,* home blood pressure monitoring.
Source: National Institute for Health and Care Excellence. (2011). *Hypertension: Clinical management of primary hypertension in adults (update). NICE clinical guideline 127.* Available at http://guidance.nice.org.uk/CG127.

Detection

- All adults should have their blood pressure measured at least every 5 years up to the age of 80 and at least annually thereafter (Hodgkinson et al., 2011).
- The 2011 NICE guidelines recommended a major shift in how blood pressure measurements are taken and hypertension diagnosed, centering on the use of ambulatory (ABPM) and home (HBPM) blood pressure monitoring to complement clinic measurements (Box 7.2). This is in part a response to the overtreatment of people with so-called *white coat* hypertension.
- The guidelines recommend the following steps to diagnose hypertension:
  1. If a clinic BP is over 140/90 mm Hg, take a second reading in the consultation.
  2. If the second reading is very different from the first, take a third reading.

• BOX 7.2 Definitions of Ambulatory Blood Pressure Monitoring and Home Blood Pressure Monitoring

ABPM is a noninvasive method of measuring blood pressure in a patient's own environment. At least two measurements per hour should be taken during the patient's usual waking hours (e.g., between 8 am and 10 pm). The readings are taken automatically to minimize interference with everyday activities and sleep patterns. By taking regular readings throughout the day, a more accurate estimate of blood pressure can be obtained.

The average value of at least 14 measurements is needed to confirm a diagnosis of hypertension. Patients are most commonly referred to appropriately equipped hospital clinics, though it is possible for general practitioners to establish their own system of ambulatory blood pressure monitoring.

Home blood pressure monitoring requires the patient to measure his or her own blood pressure using an automatic blood pressure monitor, either supplied by the local health service or purchased privately. To confirm a diagnosis of hypertension it is advised that:

1. two consecutive measurements are taken at least 1 min apart, twice daily (ideally in the morning and evening), with the patient seated, for 4–7 days;
2. measurements taken on the first day should be discarded and the average value of all remaining measurements should be used.

---

3. Record the lowest reading; if it is over 140/90 mm Hg, offer 24-hour ABPM to confirm the diagnosis (Hodgkinson et al., 2011).
4. HBPM should be used as an alternative if ABPM is declined or not tolerated, or for practices that lack ABPM equipment (Ritchie, Campbell, & Murchie, 2011).

- There is a growing evidence base for the use of self-monitoring (and, indeed, self-management) of BP by patients (Uhlig, Patel, Ip, Kitsios, Balk, 2013). Guidelines may change to reflect this in the future.
- Other recent research has suggested that blood pressure should be measured in both arms and that subsequent BP monitoring should be done in the arm with the highest reading (Clark, Taylor, Shore, & Campbell, 2012; Clark, Taylor, Shore, Ukoumunne, & Campbell, 2012). If a BP difference of over 10 mm Hg is found, peripheral artery disease is likely and further evaluation (e.g., ankle-brachial pressure measurement) is warranted.

Blood Pressure Targets

- The target of hypertension treatment is to reduce clinic blood pressure levels to below 140/90 mm Hg in people aged under 80, and below 150/90 mm Hg in people aged 80 and over.
- Previous guidance focused on treating those aged under 80, but more recent evidence has shown that treatment is well tolerated and reduces total mortality and cardiovascular events (Beckett et al., 2008, 2011).

- Note that in patients with type 2 diabetes, a stricter target of less than 140/80 mm Hg is the aim (<135/75 mm Hg in those with microalbuminuria).
- Three points should be made about these targets:
  1. *Any* reduction in blood pressure carries benefit, even if the target is not reached (Czernichow et al., 2011).
  2. The lower the blood pressure the greater the benefit (Ettehad et al., 2016).
  3. These BP targets may change in light of more recent research recommending more intensive BP lowering for high risk patients (The SPRINT Research Group, 2015)

Practicalities of Blood Pressure Measurement

1. The patient should be seated, but in older patients and in patients with diabetes check the blood pressure both standing and sitting.
2. On the first occasion measure the BP in both arms. A significant difference is found in 20% of hypertensives. If there is a difference of more than 5 mm Hg, then use the arm with the higher reading for future measurements.
3. Measure the systolic and diastolic pressures to the nearest 2 mm Hg. If over 140/90 mm Hg, repeat the measurement toward the end of the consultation. If markedly different from each other, take at least one more. Take the average. Repeated readings by a nurse give the most reliable clinic results, occasional readings by a doctor the least (Little et al., 2002).
4. *Timing.* In mild uncomplicated hypertension, do not start treatment until three readings have been taken over a 3-month period. About 25% of blood pressures will settle in that time. Those that settle to below treatment levels need lifelong annual follow-up. If the initial diastolic is over 200/110 mm Hg or there is evidence of end organ damage, cardiovascular disease, or diabetes, three readings over 2 weeks would be more appropriate. Consider immediate treatment if the pressure is over 220/120 mm Hg.
5. Follow-up 6 monthly, once the patient is established on treatment. It is as good as monthly.

Workup

1. Check for a history of family and personal risk factors for stroke or coronary heart disease. Check whether relevant drugs (e.g., nonsteroidal antiinflammatory drugs [NSAIDs]) or excess alcohol are taken.
2. Examination, including:
   - fundi (essential only in severe hypertension) (van den Born, Hulsman, Hoekstra, Schlingemann, & van Montfrans, 2005);
   - femoral pulses;
   - palpation of kidneys and auscultation for presence of bruit;
   - signs of left ventricular hypertrophy.
3. Urinalysis for protein and blood

4. Blood:
   - Creatinine and electrolytes
   - Fasting blood sugar
   - Serum lipids
5. Look for left ventricular hypertrophy using electrocardiogram (ECG) and chest x-ray (CXR).
6. Calculate the patient's 10-year cardiovascular disease (CVD) risk using a recognized calculator (e.g., the QRISK®2 cardiovascular disease risk calculator, available at http://www.qrisk.org/). A 20% 10-year CVD risk means that the lower threshold for treatment applies and that primary prevention of CVD is indicated (see section below on Primary Prevention).

Nondrug Treatment

Nondrug treatment can lower the systolic pressure by 4 to 10 mm Hg (Stevens, Obarzanek, & Cook, 2001; Writing Group of the PREMIER Collaborative Research Group, 2003). It lowers the risk of CVD and should be offered to all with hypertension, whether or not drugs are being prescribed.

Consider the following:
1. *Smoking:* Ask about smoking. If appropriate offer advice and refer to the smoking cessation services. Stopping will not reduce the BP but it will lower the cardiovascular risk.
2. *Exercise.* Physical activity lowers the risk of developing hypertension and is an effective treatment for those with established hypertension. Brisk walking for 30 minutes every day is as beneficial as more vigorous exercise three times a week. After only 2 weeks of aerobic exercise, the mean fall in blood pressure is 5/4 mm Hg (Whelton, Chin, Xin, He, 2002).
3. *Weight:* Encourage weight loss if overweight (body mass index [BMI] >25 kg/m^2). Overweight is a significant and independent predictor of the level of BP (Cox et al., 1996). A 10-kg weight loss promotes a reduction of 5 to 20 mm Hg (Chobanian, 2003).
4. *Alcohol:* There is a direct dose–response relationship between alcohol intake and risk of hypertension, particularly when alcohol intake exceeds two drinks per day (Xin et al., 2001). Support patients to reduce excessive consumption.
5. *Salt:* Reduce intake of salt to less than 5.8 g/day or less than 2.4 g sodium. A 2011 Cochrane review was unable to confirm whether reducing dietary salt had significant effects on mortality or cardiovascular morbidity (Taylor, Ashton, Moxham, Hooper, & Ebrahim, 2011) but a subsequent meta-analysis found a significant reduction in cardiovascular events (He & MacGregor, 2011), supporting long-standing public health recommendations to reduce salt consumption in the population. Common sources of salt are nuts, crisps, canned foods, table sauces, and bread. Many processed foods are high in salt, so avoid those with over 1.5 g per 100 g food. Also note that many labels use sodium rather than salt content: 1 g sodium = 2.5 g salt, so more than 0.6 g sodium per 100 g food is high.

6. *Dietary Approaches to Stop Hypertension (DASH) diet:* This is a diet rich in fruit, vegetables, and oily fish and low in sodium and total and saturated fats. It has been shown in a number of trials to reduce BP by up to 11/5 mm Hg (Appel et al., 1997). It is similar to a Mediterranean-style diet (Sacks & Campos, 2010).
7. *Coffee:* Coffee is known to acutely raise BP, but a 2012 systematic review and meta-analysis found no significant effect on BP or the risk of hypertension (Steffen, Kuhle, Hensrud, Erwin, & Murad, 2012). However, standard advice remains to discourage *excessive* coffee drinking.
8. *Contraceptive pill:* Consider stopping but not until other adequate contraceptive measures are in place.
9. *Stress:* The relationship between stress and blood pressure is not well understood, yet anecdotally patients often blame a stressful life for their hypertension. This is an area of ongoing research, with some promising results for stress reduction interventions (Hughes et al., 2013).

Drug Management
Primary Prevention

- *Aspirin:* The use of low-dose aspirin (75 mg daily) in primary prevention is controversial, with ongoing debates about benefits (reducing cardiovascular events) versus risks (bleeding events) (Barnett, Burrill, & Iheanacho, 2010). At the time of writing, aspirin is not licensed for primary prevention in the United Kingdom and should not be routinely started, even in those with risk factors such as hypertension and diabetes (Scottish Intercollegiate Guidelines Network, 2010).
- *Statins:* Give statins if the patient has CVD or diabetes or has a risk of CVD that is sufficiently high. SIGN (2017) recommends a risk threshold of CVD of at or greater than 20% in the next 10 years as an indication for the introduction of statin therapy; however, the NICE guidance from 2014 suggests consideration of primary prevention strategies in those with over a 10% risk in the next 10 years, if lifestyle measures have not proved effective.

Antihypertensives

- About half of patients fail to take their antihypertensives as prescribed. Patients have many reservations about drug treatment (Benson & Britten, 2002). Getting them to voice those reservations gives clinicians a chance to alter any erroneous ideas they may have. A study of black Caribbean patients in London found these common misconceptions (Connell, McKevitt, & Wolfe, 2005):
  - Once the BP was controlled, they were cured and didn't need the medication.
  - They could sense when their BP was raised and so could judge when they needed to take the medication.
- Commonly used drugs produce a similar average fall of 9.1/5.5 mm Hg at standard doses (Law, Wald, Morris, & Jordan, 2003). Most patients with hypertension therefore need more than one antihypertensive drug.

- Combining two drugs from different classes reduces the blood pressure five times more than doubling the dose of one drug (Wald et al., 2009).
- The timing of medication may also be important. There is a morning rise in blood pressure, in keeping with circadian rhythms. A Cochrane review found that advising patients to take their antihypertensives in the evening resulted in small gains in 24-hour BP reduction (mean of 1.7/1.4 mm Hg) (Zhao, Xu, Wan, & Wang, 2011). It is unclear, however, if this translates to a reduction in CV events.
- The choice of drugs should be influenced by age, comorbidity, adverse effects, possible synergistic effects between classes of drugs, and the individual's response to each drug. Ethnic origin also influences the choice of medication; younger white patients tend to have high levels of renin and angiotensin II; older patients and those of African origin tend to have low renin levels and so respond less well to drugs that block the renin–angiotensin system, although the differences are thought to be small.
- Follow the scheme in Table 7.1, but do not persevere with a drug that has produced no benefit (i.e., a drop in BP of <5 mm Hg). Instead, switch to a drug with a different mode of action (e.g., from A to C or D). Persevere with a drug that shows some but inadequate benefit; it may be synergistic with a drug from a different group.
- Divide drugs into those that suppress the renin system (A [ACE inhibitors and angiotensin receptor blockers]) and those that work independently of it (C [calcium channel blockers] and D [diuretics]) (Brown et al., 2003). The following steps are recommended, but tailor them to the needs of the individual patient.
  - Offer step 1 treatment to people aged under 80 with stage 1 hypertension and one or more of the following:
    - Target organ damage
    - Established cardiovascular disease
    - Renal disease
    - Diabetes
    - 10-year cardiovascular risk equivalent to 20% or more

TABLE 7.1	Drug Management in Hypertension	
	Age <55 and Non-Black	Age ≥55 or Black
Step 1	A	C or D
Step 2	A and C or D	
Step 3	A and C and D	
Step 4	Add spironolactone, or, if not tolerated, an alpha-blocker, or a beta-blocker, or another diuretic, or refer	

A 2012 Cochrane review of Randomised Controlled Trials (RCTs) of treatment of mild hypertension in those without preexisting cardiovascular disease found that treatment did not reduce morbidity or mortality (Diao, Wright, Cundiff, & Gueyffier, 2012).

- Offer step 1 treatment to people of any age with stage 2 hypertension.
- Offer people aged under 55 years an ACE inhibitor or a low-cost angiotensin receptor blocker (ARB). If an ACE inhibitor is prescribed and not tolerated (e.g., due to cough), offer a low-cost ARB.
- Offer people aged over 55 years and black people of African or Caribbean family origin of any age a calcium channel blocker (CCB). If a CCB is not suitable (e.g., due to oedema or intolerance), or there is evidence/risk of heart failure, offer a thiazide-like diuretic.

Drug Treatment of Patients With Other Medical Problems

Most individuals (approximately four of five individuals in one study [Barnett et al., 2012]) with hypertension will have additional chronic diseases.

1. *Angina:* Use a beta-blocker or a calcium channel blocker.
2. *Heart failure:* Use a diuretic, an ACE inhibitor, a beta-blocker, then an alpha-blocker.
3. *Diabetes:* Use an ACE inhibitor, a low-dose thiazide, an alpha-blocker, or calcium channel blocker.
4. *Smokers:* Do not use a beta-blocker.
5. *Migraine:* Use a beta-blocker and/or calcium channel blocker, then all other alternatives.
6. *Those active in sports:* Avoid beta-blockers.
7. *Raynaud syndrome:* Use a calcium channel blocker.
8. *Renal failure:* Get specialist advice. ACE inhibitors may improve renal function but will need to be given in lower dosage.
9. *Gout:* Avoid thiazides.
10. *Asthma:* Avoid beta-blockers.

Other Points About the Drugs
Thiazides

- Indapamide (2.5 mg daily) or chlorthalidone (12.5–25 mg daily) has been suggested by NICE to be preferential to bendroflumethiazide.
- Recheck creatinine and electrolytes 1 month after starting a thiazide then repeat annually. Repeat more frequently if the patient is unwell or is taking digoxin or another drug that might affect renal function. A rise of creatinine of up to 30% is acceptable provided it remains less than 200 μmol/L (Martin & Coleman, 2006).
- Diabetes is not a contraindication. In the Systolic Hypertension in the Elderly Program (SHEP) study, a thiazide was associated with the development of diabetes in an extra 4.3% of patients over 4 years, but it protected those who developed diabetes against an increase in cardiovascular mortality (Kostis et al., 2005).

- Ask specifically about erectile difficulties in men. The incidence in patients on thiazides is double that in those on placebo (17% versus 8%), but patients rarely volunteer this information.

Calcium Channel Blockers

- Use a long-acting preparation (e.g., diltiazem 120–180 mg slow release twice a day or verapamil 120–240 mg twice a day or 240–480 mg slow release daily). Their hypotensive effect is the same as nifedipine, with fewer side effects. Use brand names. Different generic products have different bioavailabilities.
- Use a dihydropyridine calcium channel blocker (e.g., nifedipine slow release or amlodipine), if:
  1. beta-blockers are also being given;
  2. there is peripheral vascular disease with skin ischaemia; it will not, however, help intermittent claudication;
  3. there is a risk of heart failure, which might be worsened by a non-dihydropyridine.

ACE Inhibitors and Related Drugs

- Starting them:
  1. The first dose should be taken at night. Even then, first-dose hypotension due to once-daily agents may not occur until 6 to 8 hours after the first dose, and may last for 24 hours.
  2. Recheck serum creatinine and electrolytes 1 week after starting the drug, and after any dose increase, then annually.
- A rise of serum creatinine of less than 30% is acceptable provided it remains under 200 µmol/L (Martin & Coleman, 2006). A greater rise suggests renal artery stenosis or chronic kidney disease. Above that, reduce or stop the drug and recheck weekly till the creatinine has returned to its previous level. Look for underlying renal disease.
- A rise of serum K^+ to 5.5 to 5.9 mmol/L is acceptable but recheck more frequently. Stop the drug if the level reaches 6 mmol/L and refer (WHO, n.d.).
- Use them in patients with insulin-dependent diabetes; they improve insulin resistance (whereas thiazides and beta-blockers may worsen it).
- Avoid them in patients with peripheral vascular disease.
- Use an angiotensin II receptor antagonist in patients who need an ACE inhibitor but cannot tolerate it because of cough.

Beta-Blockers

- Perform a peak flow before and after starting treatment if the history suggests the possibility of chronic obstructive pulmonary disease (COPD). If there is a significant fall, stop the drug. However, cardioselective beta-blockers may be tolerated in mild to moderate reversible airway obstructions (Salpeter, Ormiston, & Salpeter, 2005).

- Warn the patient not to stop a beta-blocker suddenly. Even those without known coronary heart disease (CHD) have a fourfold increased risk of myocardial infarction or angina in the subsequent 4 weeks.

Alpha-Blockers

- Total cholesterol falls by an average of 4%, with a beneficial rise in high-density lipoprotein (HDL) cholesterol.
- Start with a low dose (e.g., terazosin 1 mg or doxazosin 1 mg), taken at night in case of first-dose hypotension.
- Use with caution in the elderly, who may experience continued postural hypotension.

Poor Control

- Gently ask about adherence. A question such as, "How difficult do you find it to take all of your tablets?" is more likely to elicit a truthful answer than "Do you ever forget to take them?"
- Consider the white-coat effect. If the BP seems to fluctuate or the patient seems tense, arrange for home readings (see Box 7.2).
- If neither of these applies, consider this to be resistant hypertension.

Resistant Hypertension

- Resistant hypertension is common, being found in approximately 10% of all treated patients.
- It is defined as *hypertension not controlled by three drugs, at best tolerated doses, where the patient is taking them and the BP is raised at home as well as at the clinic.*
- It is important, as patients with resistant hypertension are very high risk: They are 50% more likely to experience an adverse cardiovascular event compared to other hypertensive patients (Myat, Redwood, Qureshi, Spertus, & Williams, 2012).
- Before a diagnosis of resistant hypertension can be made, check that this is true resistance, not poor adherence or white-coat hypertension
- New evidence suggests adding spironolactone as the 4th line medication (after A + C + D) in patients with an eGFR >45 ml/min (Williams et al., 2015)
- Resistant hypertension is likely to be multifactorial. Consider the following:
  1. Lifestyle factors: obesity, excees alcohol intake, excess dietary sodium, cocaine and amphetamines misuse; of these, obesity is the most common feature of patients with resistant hypertension. One study of over 45,000 primary care patients in Germany found that obese individuals (BMI >40 kg/m²) were more than five times more likely to need three antihypertensive drugs and three times more likely to require four antihypertensive drugs to achieve BP control compared with individuals with a normal BMI (≤25 kg/m²) (Sharma et al., 2004).

2. Medication-related causes: NSAIDs, selective COX-2 inhibitors, steroids, sympathomimetics (e.g., decongestants), oral contraceptives, and liquorice ingestion in sweets or chewed tobacco.
3. An underlying medical cause: Up to 10% of these patients have a previously undiagnosed secondary cause:
   - Renal disorders: the commonest overall cause and least amenable to treatment. Includes diabetic kidney disease, glomerulonephritis, chronic pyelonephritis, obstructive uropathy, and polycystic kidney disease.
   - Primary hyperaldosteronism: the commonest single cause of secondary hypertension, accounting for 5% to 13% of all cases of hypertension (Grasko, Nguyen, & Glendenning, 2010). Suspect if there is low potassium (K) and high sodium (Na), although in many patients these will be normal. The ratio of plasma aldosterone to renin will be raised and warrants referral to confirm the diagnosis and the underlying cause (Conn adenoma or idiopathic). Note that spironolactone, eplerenone, amiloride, and dihydropyridine calcium channel blockers (e.g., amlodipine) should be stopped before doing these tests (Grasko et al., 2010).
   - Obstructive sleep apnoea (OSA): ask about snoring, episodes of apnoea at night, and daytime sleepiness.
   - Vascular disorders: coarctation of the aorta (suspect if significant interarm difference in blood pressure). Check for radio-radial or radio-femoral delay; and renal artery stenosis (common in older hypertensives). Suspect if evidence of peripheral vascular disease. Check for abdominal bruit.
   - Thyroid diseases: hyperthyroidism usually increases systolic blood pressure, whereas hypothyroidism usually increases diastolic blood pressure.
   - Cushing disease: look for the typical clinical features (e.g., centripetal obesity, moon facies, abdominal striae).
   - Phaeochromocytoma: suggested by a history of episodic headaches, sweating, palpitations associated with an often dramatic rise of blood pressure. Check 24-hour urinary catecholamines.
- If a cause for resistance is found that can be managed in primary care, continue management, even if it means proceeding to step 4. Otherwise, refer. Hypertension clinics are capable of controlling half of those referred with resistant hypertension.

Referral

- Refer patients in whom there is reason to suspect secondary hypertension: onset age under 40, fluctuating BP levels, evidence of renal disease, resistant hypertension.
- Refer urgently anyone with accelerated hypertension (grade IV retinopathy).

Chest Pain of Recent Onset

GUIDELINE

National Institute for Health and Care Excellence. (2010a). *Chest pain of recent onset. NICE clinical guideline 95.* Available at www.nice.org.uk.

- Chest pain is very common, accounting for about 1% of all patient encounters in general practice, 5% of visits to the emergency department, and 25% of all emergency hospital admissions (Goodacre, 2005). These encounters represent just a fraction of the number of episodes of chest pain experienced in the community, for which medical attention is not always sought (Elliott, McAteer, & Hannaford, 2011).
- The challenge for GPs is to identify serious cardiac disease while also protecting patients from unnecessary investigations and hospital admissions.
- The 2010 NICE guidelines focus on the assessment and diagnosis of recent onset chest pain or discomfort of suspected cardiac origin. They present two separate diagnostic pathways: one for people with acute chest pain in whom an acute coronary syndrome is suspected; the other for those with intermittent stable chest pain in whom stable angina is suspected (Cooper et al., 2010). Medical history-taking and physical examination will determine which of these pathways to follow, as will be described in the following sections.

Unstable Angina (Acute Coronary Syndrome)

GUIDELINES

Scottish Intercollegiate Guidelines Network. (2016). *Acute coronary syndrome. SIGN publication 148.* Edinburgh: SIGN. Available from http://www.sign.ac.uk.
  National Institute for Health and Care Excellence. (2010). *Unstable angina and NSTEMI: The early management of unstable angina and non-ST-segment-elevation myocardial infarction. NICE clinical guideline 94.* Available from http://www.nice.org.uk/guidance/CG94.

- The definition of acute coronary syndrome (ACS), which includes unstable angina and myocardial infarction, depends on the specific characterstics of each element of the triad (SIGN, 2016):
  - Clinical presentation (including a history of coronary artery disease)
  - ECG changes
  - Biochemical cardiac markers
- Symptoms and signs that may indicate an acute coronary syndrome include the following:
  - Chest pain lasting more than 15 minutes (may be in arms, back, or jaw)

• BOX 7.3 Immediate Management of Suspected Acute Coronary Syndrome

- Admit by emergency ambulance any patient with cardiac pain lasting >15 minutes despite GTN, with an abnormal or unavailable ECG. Start management immediately but **do not delay transfer to hospital.**
- While awaiting admission, give:
  - pain relief:
    1. GTN (e.g., three sprays over 15 minutes) if pain continues.
    2. Consider IV opioid if available: diamorphine 1 mg/min (maximum 5 mg) or morphine 2 mg/min (maximum 10 mg). Administer with IV antiemetic such as metoclopramide 10 mg or cyclizine 50 mg.
  - aspirin 300 mg (unless allergic), written record of administration to go with patient;
  - 12-lead ECG (fax ahead if possible), but do not do if it will delay hospital transfer;
  - ACS if the ECG is normal;
  - pulse oximetry (offer oxygen only if O$_2$ saturation is <94%; aim for 94%–98%);
  - patient monitoring until diagnosis.

- Chest pain with associated nausea and vomiting, sweating, breathlessness
- Chest pain associated with haemodynamic instability
- New onset chest pain, or abrupt deterioration in previously stable angina, with recurrent pain occurring at rest or at significantly lower levels of activity, or that the frequency, duration, or severity of the attacks has substantially worsened
- Subsequent management depends on timing of presentation:
  - If the patient is presenting with current chest pain, proceed with immediate management as outlined in Box 7.3.
  - If the chest pain was in the last 12 hours, but the patient is currently pain free, do an ECG. Arrange emergency admission if the ECG is abnormal or if ECG is unavailable; if ECG is normal, arrange urgent same-day assessment.
  - If the chest pain was 12 to 72 hours ago, arrange urgent same-day assessment.

Myocardial Infarction (MI)

- *Defibrillation:* defibrillate a patient who develops ventricular fibrillation while awaiting transfer to hospital. If no defibrillator is available, perform cardiopulmonary resuscitation while waiting for one to arrive. Out-of-hospital defibrillation has been shown to save lives.
- Primary PCI: patients with an ST-segment-elevation acute coronary syndrome should be treated immediately with primary percutaneous coronary intervention (PCI) (SIGN, 2016).
- When primary PCI cannot be provided within 120 minutes of ECG diagnosis, patients with an ST-segment-elevation acute coronary syndrome should receive immediate (prehospital or admission) thrombolytic therapy (SIGN, 2016).

- *Thrombolysis:* make an initial judgment about the patient's suitability (see the upcoming contraindications). All patients with a typical history of MI and ST segment elevation or left bundle branch block (LBBB) should be considered for thrombolysis, regardless of age, if their quality of life warrants it, and if local policy does not prefer acute percutaneous coronary intervention (PCI).
- Thrombolysis is of benefit in the 24 hours after the onset of symptoms, with more benefit the sooner it is given. Thrombolysis involves hospital admission, whether or not it is given at home first.
- GPs need special training. It should be given outside hospital only if:
  1. there is strong clinical suspicion of acute myocardial infarction;
  2. chest pain, unrelieved by GTN spray, has been present for at least 20 minutes and for no more than 12 hours;
  3. the ECG shows ST elevation or LBBB;
  4. a defibrillator is available, because of the small but significant increase in risk of ventricular fibrillation (VF) after thrombolysis;
  5. no contraindications exist.

Contraindications to Thrombolysis
(Lip, Chin, & Prasad, 2002)

Absolute
1. Aortic dissection
2. Previous cerebral haemorrhage
3. Known cerebral aneurysm or AV malformation
4. Intracranial neoplasm
5. Any cerebrovascular accident in the last 6 months
6. Active internal bleeding (other than menstruation)
7. Streptokinase should not be given to a patient who has received it more than 4 days previously. The development of antibodies may reduce its effectiveness.

Relative
1. Uncontrolled hypertension (BP >180/110 mm Hg) or chronic severe hypertension
2. On anticoagulants or known bleeding diathesis
3. Trauma within past 2 to 4 weeks, including head injury and prolonged (>10 minutes) CPR
4. Aortic aneurysm
5. Recent (within 3 weeks) major surgery, organ biopsy, or puncture of a noncompressible vessel
6. Recent (within 6 months) GI, or GU, or other internal bleeding
7. Pregnancy
8. Active peptic ulcer

Cardiac Rehabilitation

- Most patients following MI will now routinely be enrolled in a cardiac rehabilitation programme. This should be a comprehensive package of support, including exercise, education, and psychologic support.

- *Exercise.* Encourage the continuation of exercise, which will continue to improve cardiac performance and survival and reduce the risk of another infarction by 20%. Exercise can be tennis, jogging, cycling, swimming, or circuit training. NICE (2013) recommends 20 to 30 minutes each day, increasing slowly so that it is sufficiently vigorous to make the patient slightly breathless.
- *Smoking.* Encourage a smoker to stop, with the news that stopping even at this late stage probably reduces mortality by 50%.
- *Weight.* Advise the obese to lose weight.
- *Diet.* Whether the patient needs to lose weight or not, recommend a Mediterranean diet. The elements of the diet that seem to be associated with a lower mortality are moderate alcohol, low meat intake, and high intake of vegetables, fruit, nuts, olive oil, and legumes.
- *Alcohol.* Check that safe limits are not being exceeded.
- *Lipids.* Arrange a test for serum lipids at 3 months postinfarction, unless the lipids were assessed within 24 hours of the onset of the infarct. Once blood has been taken, start a statin regardless of baseline value and continue it long term.
- *Diabetes.* Unless known to be diabetic, or to have had an assessment of glucose metabolism in hospital, check the fasting plasma glucose.
- *Depression.* Look again for depression. Even at 1 year, 25% are depressed.
- *Other drugs.*
  - Check that the patient continues to take an ACE inhibitor (or an angiotensin-11 receptor blocker if not tolerated).
  - A beta-blocker should be taken for at least 12 months post MI in people without left ventricular dysfunction or heart failure, unless contraindicated. A beta-blocker should be carried on indefinitely in those with left ventricular dysfunction.
  - Dual antiplatelet therapy is usually advised for up to 12 months after an MI. This is usually aspirin plus a second antiplatelet drug such as clopidogrel, prasugrel, or ticagrelor. Aspirin is usually carried on lifelong, clopidogrel can be used for those intolerant of aspirin.
- Recommend an annual influenza immunization.
- Check that the patient has a cardiology follow-up appointment for an assessment of the coronary arteries and suitability for invasive treatment (PCI), as well as for an assessment of left ventricular function. The initial screening to assess coronary blood flow is likely to be an exercise (stress) ECG. Patients with a negative stress test are unlikely to require coronary artery surgery, and so an unnecessary angiogram can be avoided.

Other Factual Advice

- Sedentary workers may return to work at 4 to 6 weeks, light manual workers at 6 to 8 weeks, and heavy manual workers at 3 months following MI.
- Do not fly for 2 weeks, and then only if able to climb one flight of stairs without difficulty. A more cautious policy is to advise against flying for 6 weeks.
- Drivers should not drive for 1 month, but no longer required to notify the Driver and Vehicle Licensing Agency (DVLA). They should inform their insurance company. Heavy Goods Vehicle (HGV) and Public Service Vehicle (PSV) licence holders must notify the DVLA, and may only continue vocational driving after individual assessment.

Stable Angina

> **GUIDELINES**
>
> National Institute for Health and Care Excellence. (2011b). *Management of stable angina. NICE clinical guideline 126.* Available at www.nice.org.uk.
>   Scottish Intercollegiate Guidelines Network. (2018). *Management of stable angina. National clinical guideline 151.* Available at www.sign.ac.uk.

- Angina is the main symptom of myocardial ischaemia and is usually caused by atherosclerotic coronary artery disease restricting blood flow (and therefore oxygen delivery) to the heart muscle.
- Stable angina is common, affecting about 8% of men and 3% of women aged 55 to 64 years and about 14% of men and 8% of women aged 65 to 74 years in England (O'Flynn et al., 2011). The diagnosis is clinical, based on the history.
- The history is of pain or constricting discomfort that typically occurs in the front of the chest, but can radiate to the neck, shoulders, jaw, or arms (NICE, 2011). It is usually brought on by physical exertion or emotional stress, but some people can have atypical symptoms such as gastrointestinal discomfort, breathlessness, or nausea.
- Stable angina is unlikely if the pain is:
  - continuous or very prolonged;
  - unrelated to activity;
  - brought on by breathing in;
  - associated with dizziness, palpitations, tingling, or difficulty swallowing.

  In such cases, consider other causes of chest pain such as gastrointestinal or musculoskeletal pain.
- The NICE guidelines present a table to help estimate the likelihood of coronary artery disease in someone presenting with symptoms of angina, but such tables are not yet routinely used in general practice. Put simply, the likelihood of angina increases with age and with the presence of additional cardiovascular risk factors:
  - Smoking
  - Hypertension
  - Diabetes
  - Family history of CHD (first-degree relative: male <55 years/female <65 years)
  - Raised cholesterol (>6.5 mmol/L) and other lipids

- As well as these risk factors, also assess for:
  1. BMI;
  2. hypo/hyperthyroidism;
  3. anaemia/polycythaemia;
  4. arrhythmias;
  5. valvular disease (any aortic systolic murmur needs assessment for aortic stenosis);
  6. depression and social isolation;
  7. physical activity levels.

WORKUP—INVESTIGATIONS

1. Haemoglobin
2. Thyroid function tests (TFTs)
3. Fasting blood sugar
4. Fasting lipid profile
5. Resting ECG. A normal ECG does not exclude the diagnosis but an abnormal ECG makes it more likely. ECG features consistent with coronary artery disease include:
   - pathological Q waves;
   - LBBB;
   - ST segment and T wave abnormalities (e.g., flattening or inversion).

Referral

- Patients with suspected angina should be referred to cardiology (e.g., fast track chest pain clinic) for definitive diagnosis.
- Further investigations will depend on local arrangements but may include exercise ECG or other forms of noninvasive functional testing.

Management

- *Information and support:*
  - Explain stable angina and its long-term course and management, including factors that can provoke an attack (e.g., cold, exertion, stress, heavy meals).
  - Explore fears and misconceptions about angina (e.g., around physical exertion, including sexual activity).
  - Encourage self-management skills (e.g., pacing activities and goal setting).
- *Preventing and treating episodes of angina:*
  - Advise patients to use a short-acting nitrate (e.g., glyceryl trinitrate [GTN]) spray or buccal tablets during episodes of angina and immediately before any planned exertion, including intercourse (except if the patient has just taken Viagra or similar).
  - Explain that side effects such as flushing, headache, and lightheadedness may occur. Patients should sit down or hold onto something if they feel lightheaded or dizzy.
  - Advise patients to repeat the dose after 5 minutes if the pain has not gone, and to call 999 if the pain persists for another 5 minutes.
  - Patients with stable angina should seek professional help if they have a sudden worsening in the frequency or severity of their angina.

Drug Treatment of Stable Angina
(Bass & Mayou, 2002)

- Patients require optimal drug treatment with one or two antiangina drugs as necessary to treat symptoms plus drugs for secondary prevention of cardiovascular disease.
- Explain the purpose of the drug treatment, why it is important to take the drugs regularly, and how side effects of drug treatment might affect the person's daily activities.
- Titrate the drug dosage against the person's symptoms up to the maximum tolerable dosage.
- Review the person's response to treatment, including any side effects, 2 to 4 weeks after starting or changing drug treatment.

Cardiovascular Risk Reduction

- Encourage lifestyle change (i.e., diet, exercise, smoking, alcohol).
- Consider aspirin 75 mg daily. Clopidogrel is preferred if patient has peripheral arterial disease or if aspirin not tolerated. Dual therapy is only recommended in stable angina after PCI for up to one year.
- Offer statin treatment (Atorvastatin 80 mg) and treat high blood pressure in line with NICE guidelines.
- Consider ACE inhibitors or low-cost ARB for people with stable angina and diabetes, previous MI, CKD or LV systolic dysfunction.

Selecting Drugs

1. Offer either a beta-blocker (e.g., atenolol 100 mg, metoprolol 50–100 mg twice daily, or bisoprolol 5–20 mg) or calcium channel blocker (use rate limiting CCB [e.g., diltiazem], unless heart failure or heart block, in which case use amlodipine) as first line treatment.
   - If either is not tolerated, switch to the other.
   - If either is ineffective, switch to the other or combine both (NB: avoid verapamil in combination with beta-blocker).
2. If the person cannot tolerate β-blockers or calcium channel blockers or if both are contraindicated, consider monotherapy with one of the following:
   - A long-acting nitrate
   - Ivabradine
   - Nicorandil
   - Ranolazine
3. If not satisfactorily controlled on two drugs, refer for consideration of revascularization

Revascularization

- Coronary intervention such as percutaneous coronary intervention (PCI) or coronary artery bypass graft (CABG) surgery should only be considered if symptoms are not optimally controlled with medical treatment.

- Refer to cardiology for further assessment, which may include noninvasive investigations and/or coronary angiography.
- Coronary angiography is the traditional investigation for establishing the nature, anatomy, and severity of CHD. It is an invasive investigation and carries a mortality risk of around 0.1% for elective procedures (SIGN, 2018).
- The main purpose of revascularization is to improve the symptoms of stable angina:
  - CABG surgery and PCI are effective in relieving symptoms, but repeat revascularization may be necessary after either procedure, and the rate is lower after CABG surgery.
  - Stroke is an uncommon complication of each of these two procedures (the incidence is similar).
  - There is a potential survival advantage with CABG surgery for some people with multivessel disease.
  - In those for whom both percutaneous and surgical revascularization is feasible, percutaneous revascularization is a more cost-effective approach.

Noncardiac Chest Pain

- Less than half of patients referred to cardiac clinics and accident and emergency (A&E) departments with chest pain are found to have coronary artery disease (Bass & Mayou, 2002). Many of these patients continue to suffer pain and long-term functional impairment. Their management is often inadequate once the diagnosis of cardiac disease is excluded.
- A clinical prediction rule called the Marburg Heart Score (MHS) assists GPs in ruling out chest pain caused by CHD (Haasenritter et al., 2012). Based on five findings from history and examination, the score has a high negative predictive value, but further research is needed to assess its use in routine practice.
- Be clear from the history, investigations, and specialist assessment that the pain is noncardiac. Then resist requests for further cardiac referral.
- Try to make a positive diagnosis of the cause of the pain: musculoskeletal disorders, panic attacks, reflux, depression.
- If a clear diagnosis is possible, treat accordingly (e.g., with NSAIDs for musculoskeletal pain, a PPI for reflux, antidepressants for depression).
- If no clear diagnosis is possible, attempt an explanation along the following lines: that the symptoms are real; that they do not arise from the heart or from any other specific illness; that the brain normally disregards sensations that it receives from all over the body, but that for some reason, in this patient, it is sensitized to sensations from the chest. This explanation might lead on to discussion of how such sensitization may have occurred. The patient may volunteer the memory of some event that seemed to trigger the chest pain.
- Ask who else in the family is worried about the pain and try to see them as well.

- Refer to a psychologist or counsellor patients who accept the above explanation but who still find themselves bothered by the pain.
- Consider a trial of a tricyclic antidepressant or SSRI in a patient sufficiently troubled by pain, even in the absence of depression.

Heart Failure

GUIDELINE

National Institute for Health and Care Excellence. (2010b). *Chronic heart failure: Management of chronic heart failure in adults in primary and secondary care. NICE clinical guideline 108.* Available at www.nice.org.

Scottish Intercollegiate Guidelines Network. (2016a). *Management of chronic heart failure. SIGN guideline 147.* Available at www.sign.ac.uk.

- Heart failure is a complex syndrome of symptoms and signs, caused by structural or functional abnormalities of the heart (NICE, 2010b). It is often divided into heart failure due to left ventricular systolic dysfunction (LVSD, associated with a reduced left ventricular ejection fraction) or heart failure with a preserved ejection fraction (HF-PEF). Most of the evidence on treatment is for heart failure due to LVSD. The most common causes of heart failure in the United Kingdom are coronary artery disease and hypertension, and many patients have had a myocardial infarction in the past.
- Both the incidence and prevalence of heart failure increase steeply with age, and the prevalence is expected to rise in the future as the result of an ageing population, improved survival of people with ischaemic heart disease, and more effective treatments for heart failure (Owan et al., 2006).
- The prognosis remains poor, despite improvements in outcomes in the past decade. In one community-based study, 10-year survival rates ranged from 12% in those with multiple-cause heart failure to around 31% in those with LVSD (Taylor, Roalfe, Iles, & Hobbs, 2012).

Diagnosis

- Making the diagnosis of heart failure can be challenging. Patients may present with a range of symptoms, including fatigue, breathlessness, and ankle swelling; and they may also have other conditions such as CHD, diabetes, hypertension, and COPD, which can confuse the picture (SIGN, 2016a).
- Careful history-taking and examination will help to guide further assessment. The following clinical signs will add to the suspicion of heart failure, though none are diagnostic in isolation:
  - Raised jugular venous pressure (JVP)
  - Presence of a third heart sound (S3)
  - Basal crepitations

- Tachycardia
- Peripheral oedema
- Initial investigations should help to rule out other causes of symptoms and should include full blood count, fasting glucose, thyroid function tests, serum urea and creatinine, urinalysis, ECG, and chest x-ray. NICE and SIGN guidelines also now recommend the widespread use of serum natriuretic peptides as an aid to diagnosis of heart failure.

Serum Natriuretic Peptides

- B-type natriuretic peptide (BNP) and N-terminal-pro-BNP (NT-pro-BNP) are peptide hormones produced in the heart. They are raised with increasing left ventricular volume and pressure and concentrations tend to rise with NYHA class (Table 7.2). Very high levels indicate a worse prognosis and should prompt urgent referral.
- If the test is negative, heart failure is very unlikely (i.e., it has high sensitivity). False negatives may be caused by obesity and by drugs used to treat heart failure (i.e., diuretics, ACE inhibitors, ARBs, and beta-blockers).
- If the test is positive, it does not diagnose heart failure but prompts referral for echo (i.e., it has relatively low specificity). False positives occur with cardiac ischaemia from any causes (e.g., LVH, tachycardia, hypoxia) and in some other chronic conditions (e.g., diabetes, CKD, COPD, cirrhosis) (Al-Mohammad et al., 2010).

How to Use B-Type Natriuretic Peptide

- The first question to ask of someone presenting with possible heart failure is, "Have you previously had an MI?" If so, refer urgently (within 2 weeks) for echo and specialist assessment. There is no need to check BNP in this situation.
- If, however, there is no history of MI, the NICE guidelines suggest checking BNP and referring to cardiology if the level is raised:
  - If very high (BNP >400 pg/mL [116 pmol/L] *OR* NT-pro-BNP >2000 pg/mL [236 pmol/L]): refer urgently (to be seen within 2 weeks)

TABLE 7.2	New York Heart Association Classification of Heart Failure Symptoms
Class I—asymptomatic	No limitations of ordinary activity
Class II—mild	Slight limitation of physical activity but comfortable at rest
Class III—moderate	Marked limitation of physical activity. Comfortable at rest but symptomatic on less than ordinary physical activity
Class IV—severe	Inability to carry on any physical activity without discomfort. Symptoms present at rest

- If raised (BNP 100–400 pg/mL [29–116 pmol/L] *OR* NT-pro-BNP 400–2000 pg/mL [47–236 pmol/L]): refer within 6 weeks
- If levels are normal (BNP <100 pg/mL [29 pmol/L] *OR* NT-pro-BNP <400 pg/mL [47 pmol/L]), a diagnosis of heart failure is unlikely in an untreated patient, and alternative diagnoses should be sought.

Management of Confirmed Chronic Heart Failure

Pharmacologic management of heart failure depends on whether the person has LVSD or preserved ejection fraction (most research has been done on the former), and each will be considered in turn in this section. First, there are a number of general measures that apply to both forms of heart failure.

General Measures

- *Information:* Explain what is going on and what to do if things get worse.
- *Weight:* Encourage to reduce weight, if obese. Recommend daily weighing at roughly the same time and in similar clothes. Patients should report if they gain more than 2 kg over 2 days. Use diuretics flexibly, guided by weight (Arroll, Doughty, & Andersen, 2010).
- *Diet:* Advise a diet with no added salt.
- *Fluid:* Restrict fluid intake to 2 L/day, unless losing fluids from sweat, diarrhoea, or vomiting.
- *Alcohol:* Keep alcohol intake low. In alcoholic heart disease recommend complete cessation.
- *Smoking:* Stop smoking; it causes vasoconstriction. Refer to the smoking cessation services.
- *Exercise:* Rest in the acute phase, but exercise once stable. Regular low intensity physical activity improves mortality and morbidity. Refer to the heart failure rehabilitation service if this facility exists.
- *Sexual activity:* Be prepared to broach sensitive issues with patients, such as sexual activity, as these may not be raised by patients.
- *Vaccination:* Recommend influenza vaccination annually and pneumococcal vaccination once.
- *Air travel:* Air travel will be possible for the majority of patients with heart failure, depending on their clinical condition at the time of travel.
- *Driving regulations:* Advise patients to check with the DVLA, particularly drivers of large goods vehicles (https://www.gov.uk/government/organisations/driver-and-vehicle-licensing-agency).
- *Depression:* Check for depression. It is present in one third and should be treated as thoroughly as if it was not associated with heart failure. Warn patients not to buy St. John wort over the counter (OTC) because of its interaction with prescribed medication, specifically digoxin and warfarin.
- *NSAIDs:* Stop NSAIDs (including COX-2 inhibitors) if taken, unless they are essential. Warn the patient not to buy them OTC.

- *Carers:* Identify the carer or carers and involve them in the management.

Chronic Heart Failure (CHF) With Left Ventricular Dysfunction

Left ventricular systolic dysfunction, assessed by measuring the left ventricular ejection fraction by echocardiography, refers to impaired left ventricular pump (contractile) function. Most evidence to guide management of heart failure is in this group of patients, which make up around half of all heart failure cases (Arroll, Doughty, & Andersen, 2010).

- All patients should be offered *both* ACE inhibitors and beta-blockers, unless there are contraindications.

ACE Inhibitors/Angiotensin-II Receptor Blockers

- ACE inhibitors increase the ability to exercise, improve well-being, and prolong life in all degrees of heart failure (Dargie & McMurray, 1994).
- ARBs (e.g., candesartan and valsartan) may be used in patients intolerant of ACE inhibitors (e.g., with ACEI-related cough).
- If there is a high probability of chronic heart failure (CHF), start treatment before waiting for echo, unless valve disease is suspected, in which case wait.
- Exclude the absolute contraindications of allergy to ACE inhibitors and pregnancy.
- Start at a low dose and titrate upward at short intervals (e.g., every 2 weeks) until the optimal tolerated or target dose is achieved.
- Measure serum urea, creatinine, electrolytes, and eGFR when starting an ACE inhibitor and after each dose increment. Also check blood pressure.
  - ACE inhibitors (and ARBs) should not normally be started if the pretreatment serum potassium concentration is significantly above the normal reference range (typically >5.0 mmol/L). Stop ACEI/ARB therapy if the serum potassium concentration rises to above 6.0 mmol/L and other drugs known to promote hyperkalaemia have been discontinued.
  - If there is a drop in eGFR at or over 25% or an increase in plasma creatinine at or over 30%, investigate other causes of a deterioration in renal function such as volume depletion or concurrent medication (e.g., NSAIDs). If no other cause is found, stop the ACEI/ARB or reduce dose to previously tolerated level.
- Advise the patient to take the first dose before going to bed to reduce the effect of first-dose hypotension.
- Once the dose is stable, repeat creatinine and electrolytes at 3 months then 6 monthly or sooner if further dose titration is necessary or there is intercurrent infection.
- Warn the patient to avoid dehydration, for instance in gastroenteritis or in hot weather, as this can cause a sudden deterioration in renal function. If the weight drops by more than 1 kg because of dehydration, the patient should stop the diuretic and drink more fluid.

Beta-Blockers

- All patients with LVSD should be started on a licensed beta-blocker (e.g., bisoprolol, carvedilol, nebivolol) once heart failure is controlled, provided there are no absolute contraindications (e.g., heart block or asthma).
- In patients already taking another beta-blocker (e.g., atenolol for angina) who develop heart failure, advise switching to one of the above. A study in British general practice found that switching to bisoprolol or carvedilol, mainly from atenolol, was the single most valuable manoeuvre in patients with left ventricular dysfunction (Mant et al., 2008).
- NICE guidelines suggest you should not be put off prescribing beta-blockers in individuals with what were previously considered to be relative contraindications, such as older adults and those with peripheral vascular disease, erectile dysfunction, diabetes mellitus, interstitial pulmonary disease, and COPD without reversibility.
- Take a "start low, go slow" approach. Start at a low dose (e.g., bisoprolol 1.25 mg daily or carvedilol 3.125 mg twice daily), and double the dose every 2 to 4 weeks until the target dose is reached (bisoprolol 10 mg daily, carvedilol 25 mg twice daily).
- Monitor heart rate, BP, and clinical status at each dose titration. If the pulse is less than 50 and symptoms have worsened, halve the dose. Stop and seek specialist advice if symptoms have become severe.
- If at any stage it is necessary to stop the beta-blocker, tail it off gradually to avoid rebound ischaemia and arrhythmias.

Diuretics (Other Than Spironolactone)

- Diuretics should be routinely used for the relief of congestive symptoms and fluid retention in patients with heart failure, and titrated (up and down) according to need following the initiation of first line heart failure therapies. Their only function is symptom relief.
- Avoid overtreatment, which can lead to dehydration and renal dysfunction, particularly with loop diuretics. Hypovolaemia is a common cause of dizziness and lightheadedness.
- Monitor blood pressure and renal function after 4 weeks and then 6 monthly.
- Use a loop diuretic (e.g., furosemide or bumetanide) in moderate to severe heart failure. They will cause less hypokalaemia and impotence than a high-dose thiazide (e.g., bendroflumethiazide). Increase the dose gradually until diuresis occurs.
- Once stable, reduce the dose to as low as possible without oedema or breathlessness occurring. Alternatively, consider stopping or reducing to a thiazide diuretic.
- The addition of a thiazide diuretic or a potassium sparing diuretic such as spironolactone (or both) to loop diuretics can be useful if pulmonary or ankle oedema persists,

because the different classes of diuretic are thought to have an additive effect. However, even in short-term combined use, the diuresis can be excessive and can cause hypokalaemia. Check creatinine and electrolytes after 3 days.

Second Line Pharmacologic Management

- If a patient remains symptomatic despite optimal treatment with ACE inhibitor and beta-blocker, refer for specialist advice on second line treatment which might include:
  - A mineralocorticoid receptor antagonist (MRA), such as spironolactone or eplerenone;
  - an ARB;
  - sacubitril/valsartan (angiotensin receptor neprilysin inhibitor) - stop ACE inhibitor and ARB, continue beta-blocker and MRA;
  - hydralazine plus nitrate (especially for a patient of African or Caribbean descent with moderate to severe heart failure);
  - ivabradine;
  - digoxin.

Mineralocorticoid Receptor Antagonists

- Hyperkalaemia is a potentially fatal adverse effect and is most likely in those with impaired renal function. Only give spironolactone if the creatinine is less than 220 µmol/L.
- Warn the patient to avoid salt substitutes with a high potassium content. Warn males about gynaecomastia.
- If K^+ reaches 5.5 to 5.9 mmol/L or creatinine rises to 200 µmol/L, reduce the dose and monitor closely. If those levels are exceeded, stop and seek specialist advice.

Ivabradine

- Ivabradine was approved by NICE in November 2012 and is an option for patients:
  - with symptomatic stable heart failure (NYHA class II to IV) with LVSD and an ejection fraction of 35% or less;
  - who are in sinus rhythm with a resting heart rate above 75 bpm;
  - who are also receiving standard therapy including beta-blockers, ACE inhibitors, and aldosterone antagonists.
- Ivabradine should be initiated by a heart failure specialist (e.g., specialist nurse) with access to a multidisciplinary heart failure team.

Digoxin

- Consider for patients in sinus rhythm if still symptomatic despite all the above. See the upcoming section on atrial fibrillation for the use of digoxin in patients with AF.

Heart Failure With Preserved Ejection Fraction (HF-PEF)

- As noted, it is thought that up to 50% of patients with heart failure have a preserved ventricular ejection fraction. It has the same symptoms and signs as heart failure with LVSD, and carries a similar mortality risk but has a less clear evidence base for treatment (Jong, McKelvie, & Yusuf, 2010).
- Patients with HF-PEF are more likely than those with LVSD to be older, female, have hypertension, and atrial fibrillation but are less likely to have coronary artery disease.
- NICE recommends the use of diuretics for symptomatic relief.
- ACE inhibitors and beta-blockers should be considered, particularly when there are other compelling indications for their uses (such as coronary artery disease, hypertension, and diabetes mellitus).
- If atrial fibrillation is present, digoxin may be added for rate control, and anticoagulation should be considered.

Grounds for Admission

1. Severe symptoms (e.g., severe dyspnoea or hypotension)
2. Acute myocardial infarction
3. Severe complicating medical illness (e.g., pneumonia)
4. Inadequate social support
5. Failure to respond to treatment
6. Uncontrolled arrhythmia

Referral for Specialist Review

- Refer patients to the specialist multidisciplinary heart failure team for:
  - the initial diagnosis of heart failure;
  - the management of:
    1. severe heart failure (NYHA class IV);
    2. heart failure that does not respond to treatment;
    3. heart failure that can no longer be managed effectively in the home setting.
- Consider specialist review:
  - when renal function continues to deteriorate or deteriorates rapidly;
  - when there are concerns about low blood zpressure;
  - when the patient is pregnant or considering pregnancy.

End-Stage Heart Failure

- Issues of sudden death and living with uncertainty are pertinent to all patients with heart failure. The opportunity to discuss these issues should be available at all stages of care.
- Deciding on prognosis in heart failure is difficult and cardiologic advice may be needed. The palliative needs of patients and carers should be identified, assessed, and managed at the earliest opportunity. There should be access to professionals with palliative care skills within the heart failure team.
- Nonessential treatment should be stopped.
- The focus should be on symptom control (see the upcoming discussion).

Breathlessness

- Morphine is the most effective palliation. Give a low oral dose (2.5–5 mg 4-hourly), as peak plasma levels are higher in heart failure.
- If breathless at rest then consider oxygen therapy at home (40%–80% if there is no COPD).
- Refer for relaxation, breathing exercises, and anxiety management if these are available.

Weakness and Fatigue

- This is usually secondary to a low cardiac output.
- *Drug reduction.* Consider reducing ACE inhibitors and beta-blockers, and diuretics if there is dehydration.
- *Depression.* Avoid tricyclics; SSRIs may be of value.
- *Social factors.* Increase social care if possible and ensure support for the carer(s).

Anorexia/Nausea

- *Digoxin.* Check serum level and renal function.
- Consider increasing diuretics if there is hepatic congestion.
- *Diet.* Advise the patient to have small, appetizing meals more frequently. Allow small amounts of alcohol before meals.
- *Antiemetics.* Use levomepromazine. Avoid cyclizine.

Oedema

- *Mobilization* is advisable in theory but rarely practicable at this stage.
- *Diuretics.* Avoid increasing diuretics at this stage unless doing so gives symptomatic relief. They are unlikely to have much effect on the oedema.
- Be cautious about advising the patient to raise the feet. This may increase the venous return to the heart and worsen the dyspnoea.
- *Compression stockings/bandages.* These may increase tissue damage and are uncomfortable.

Acute Pulmonary Oedema

- When called urgently to the patient *in extremis*, get someone else to dial for an ambulance while you:
  1. sit the patient up with the legs down;
  2. give oxygen if available;
  3. give a GTN tablet or spray sublingually (for its immediate vasodilator effect);
  4. give intravenous (IV) diamorphine 1 mg/min up to 5 mg, or IV morphine 2 mg/min up to 10 mg, mixed with metoclopramide 10 mg IV; do not use cyclizine as it raises systemic arterial pressure;
  5. give a loop diuretic (IV furosemide 50 mg or IV bumetanide 1 mg).
- Look for causes of the heart failure that may need treatment in their own right, especially myocardial infarction.
- Admit once the patient is sufficiently stable, for fuller assessment and for continuing treatment.

- *Note:* Digoxin and aminophylline should not be used in acute failure outside hospital.

Right Heart Failure
Acute Right Heart Failure

- The clinical picture of low output state, no pulmonary oedema, and a raised JVP may be due to massive pulmonary embolism or to acute right heart failure as in a right ventricle myocardial infarction, or acute cor pulmonale.
- Admit urgently. Position the patient however they are the most comfortable. Do not give morphine; respiratory depression and hypotension are very likely to follow. Do not give diuretics as they may precipitate shock.

Chronic Cor Pulmonale

- Treat the lung disease by considering:
  1. antibiotics for exacerbations of infection;
  2. inhaled bronchodilators and steroids via a spacing device;
  3. physiotherapy;
  4. long-term oxygen therapy;
  5. nasal intermittent positive pressure ventilation for those with thoracic deformities and obstructive sleep apnoea.
- Admit readily anyone with an acute exacerbation. Oxygen will dilate the pulmonary vessels and so reduce the pulmonary artery pressure. The danger of hypercapnoea makes this hazardous in the acute situation at home.
- Use diuretics carefully as they may reduce renal blood flow further. They are only required if oedema becomes troublesome.
- Use digoxin only if the patient is in atrial fibrillation.
- Do not start ACE inhibitors outside hospital.

Palpitations and Arrhythmias

- Palpitations are a common presentation in general practice and a frequent reason for cardiology referrals. They often cause considerable distress and anxiety for the patient; however, more often than not they are benign, with less than half of patients with palpitations suffering from an arrhythmia and not every identified arrhythmia being of clinical or prognostic significance (Mayou, Sprigings, Birkhead, & Price, 2003).
- Furthermore, not all arrhythmias present with palpitations. Some may cause no symptoms, while in other cases symptoms include tachycardia, bradycardia, chest pain, breathlessness, lightheadedness, and fainting (syncope) or near fainting.
- As well as arrhythmias, palpitations can be caused by structural heart diseases, psychosomatic disorders, systemic diseases, and effects of medical and recreational drugs (Raviele et al., 2011).

- Careful history-taking and physical examination are important, but further investigation is invariably required (Hoefman et al., 2007).

History

- Ask what the patient means by *palpitations*. It may be more like a pulsatile tinnitus or a chest discomfort.
- Ask about the rate, frequency, and duration of palpitations, as well as exacerbating and relieving factors. The patient may be able to tap out the rate on the consulting desk.
- Are there any associated symptoms, such as sweating, breathlessness, or chest pain? If any of these are present and the patient has palpitations at that time, refer to hospital immediately by 999 ambulance.
- Ask about smoking, alcohol, caffeine consumption, and use of illicit substances such as cocaine, ecstasy, and amphetamines.
- Ask about general well-being. In particular, assess for any life stressors and ask about personal or family history of anxiety or heart problems.

Examination

- Assess for tremor, which may indicate thyrotoxicosis or anxiety. Ask the patient to hold the arms outstretched in front with the palms down and to spread the fingers.
- Assess pulse rate and rhythm and check blood pressure. Is the pulse rate regularly irregular, suggesting ectopic beats, or irregularly irregular, suggesting AF or atrial flutter?
- Examine the heart, assessing for evidence of structural heart disease (e.g., murmurs, abnormal heart sounds, or signs of heart failure).

Investigations

- Blood tests should include full blood count (to exclude anaemia), urea and electrolytes, and thyroid function tests.
- Arrange a 12-lead ECG. Abnormalities to look for include:
  - atrial fibrillation;
  - second- and third-degree AV block;
  - signs of previous myocardial infarction;
  - left ventricular hypertrophy and left ventricular strain patterns;
  - left bundle branch block;
  - abnormal T wave inversion and ST segment changes;
  - signs of preexcitation (short PR interval and delta waves);
  - abnormal QTc interval and T wave morphology.

Next Steps

- There is no validated risk stratification tool that is widely used in practice, although some authors have proposed a traffic light system to guide further management (Wolff & Cowan, 2009).

- Patients with the following features should be referred *urgently* to cardiology:
  - Palpitations with syncope/near syncope
  - Palpitations during exercise
  - Family history of inheritable heart disease/sudden arrhythmic death syndrome (SADS)
  - High-risk structural heart disease
  - High-degree atrioventricular block
- Patients with the following features should be referred routinely to cardiology or to local palpitations assessment service:
  - Palpitations with associated symptoms
  - Abnormal ECG
  - History suggestive of recurrent tachyarrhythmia
  - Structural heart disease
- Patients with the following features may not require referral:
  - History in keeping with extrasystoles/ectopic beats
  - Normal ECG
  - No family history
  - No evidence of IHD or structural heart disease

Ectopic Beats in a Normal Heart

- Explain their benign nature to the patient.
- Advise against caffeine, fatigue, smoking, and alcohol.
- *Beta-blockers* should be used only if the patient is unable to tolerate the ectopics.
- *Frequent ventricular ectopics (>100/hour)* may be grounds for referral. Patients may have a prolapsing mitral valve, or the older patient may have unsuspected ischaemic heart disease.
- For those still troubled by their symptoms, consider referral for cognitive behavioural therapy (CBT) or similar (Mayou, Sprigings, Birkhead, & Price, 2002).

Atrial Fibrillation

GUIDELINE

National Institute for Health and Care Excellence. (2014). *Atrial fibrillation: Management. NICE clinical guideline 180.* Available at www.nice.org.uk.

- Atrial fibrillation (AF) is the most common disorder of heart rhythm with a prevalence that increases with age from about 6% in people aged 65 to 74, to 12% in people aged 75 to 84, and 16% in people aged 85 and over (Fitzmaurice et al., 2007).
- It is associated with increased risk of stroke and heart failure, with higher mortality as a result.
- AF also increases the risk of sudden cardiac death (Chen, Sotoodehnia, & Bůžková, 2013).
- Oral anticoagulation can reduce the risk of stroke by two-thirds (Aguilar & Hart, 2005). However, current

evidence suggests that only about half of patients with AF identified as being at high risk are receiving anticoagulants (Holt et al., 2012).

- The older you are, the more dangerous AF becomes, with strokes being more common and more disabling. Yet underuse of anticoagulation is highest in older people, who have most to gain from treatment (Hobbs et al., 2011).
- Primary care has considerable potential to further reduce the risk of stroke in AF, by identifying high-risk patients and lowering the threshold for offering anticoagulation, as recommended in guidelines.

Identification of Atrial Fibrillation

- The SAFE study in 2005 showed that opportunistic screening (by pulse palpation followed by ECG if pulse irregular) of patients aged over 65 is cost effective for detecting AF (Hobbs et al., 2005). Opportunistic screening is endorsed by the European Society of Cardiology Guidelines.
- Some have gone further, suggesting that a national screening programme should be introduced, using this approach, for all patients over 65 (James & Campbell, 2012).
- Screening of such patients while attending annual influenza vaccination clinics has been piloted, but with mixed results (Gordon, Hickman, & Pentney, 2012; Rhys, Azhar, & Foster, 2013).

WORKUP OF ATRIAL FIBRILLATION

1. History of alcohol intake (either chronic or bingeing)
2. Blood pressure (half of all cases of AF are hypertensive)
3. TFTs, creatinine, and electrolytes
4. Examine for heart failure, valvular heart disease, congenital heart disease, or acute pericarditis or myocarditis
5. ECG (looking for ischaemic heart disease [IHD], left ventricular (LV) strain, and delta waves)
6. NICE recommend performing an echocardiogram in patients for whom:
   - a baseline echocardiogram is important for long-term management;
   - a rhythm control strategy that includes cardioversion is being considered;
   - there is a high risk or a suspicion of underlying structural/functional heart disease (such as heart failure or heart murmur) that influences subsequent management (e.g., choice of antiarrhythmic drug);
   - refinement of clinical risk stratification for antithrombotic therapy is needed.

- Admit if rapid AF is associated with:
  1. chest pain;
  2. hypotension;
  3. more than mild heart failure.
- Refer urgently if seen within 48 hours of the onset of AF and the patient is a candidate for cardioversion (see the upcoming discussion).

Cardioversion Versus Rate Control

- *Rate control* is recommended as the treatment of choice in most patients. It has advantages over rhythm control: fewer hospital admissions, fewer adverse drug reactions, possibly a lower mortality (Atrial Fibrillation Follow-up Investigation of Rhythm Management [AFFIRM], 2002), and it is more cost effective (Hagens, Vermeulen, & TenVergert, 2004).
- *Referral for cardioversion is more appropriate for certain patients*, either because it is more likely to succeed than in others (the first three categories) or because sinus rhythm offers greater chance of clinical benefit than rate control (the last two categories):
  - Younger patients
  - Those presenting for the first time with lone AF
  - Those with AF secondary to a cause that has now been treated
  - Those who are symptomatic
  - Those with congestive heart failure (restoration of sinus rhythm may improve LV function)
- The decision as to whether to use chemical or electrical cardioversion will be made in discussion between the patient and cardiologist. Vernakalant is a new intravenous antiarrhythmic agent approved for cardioversion of AF of 7 days duration or less. Other agents include ibutilide, flecainide, propafenone, and amiodarone.
- Rate control is more appropriate in those in whom cardioversion is less likely to succeed:
  - Those over 65 years old
  - Those with structural heart disease or CHD
  - Those whose AF is longstanding (e.g., >12 months)
  - Those in whom previous attempts at cardioversion have failed or been followed by relapse
  - Those in whom an underlying cause (e.g., thyrotoxicosis) has not yet been corrected
  - Those with a contraindication to antiarrhythmic drugs
- Aim for lenient (HR <110 bpm) rather than strict (HR <80 bpm) rate control, unless patient is symptomatic.
- Use:
  1. a beta-blocker first line (e.g., atenolol, bisoprolol, metoprolol);
  2. a rate-limiting calcium channel blocker second line (e.g., diltiazem or verapamil); avoid both in heart failure, and avoid the combination of verapamil and a beta-blocker;
  3. digoxin if still symptomatic. If digoxin is contraindicated, add diltiazem to the beta-blocker. The usual concern about causing bradycardia or AV block is less of a problem in AF since that is the aim of the treatment.

Risk Stratification for Anticoagulation

- A risk factor-based approach to stroke risk stratification has been promoted for many years (e.g., CHADS2

[Congested heart failure, Hypertension, Age ≥75, Diabetes, Stroke (doubled)]) (Gage et al., 2001), but recent evidence has prompted a shift in focus toward identification of "truly low-risk" patients who *do not* need antithrombotic therapy.

- The CHADS2 score has been replaced by the CHA2DS2-VASc, which has been found to be more accurate (Table 7.3) (Olesen, 2011).
- Using CHA2DS2-VASc, all patients over 75 and all women over 65 are automatically considered at high risk and thus do not need further formal risk assessment, other than consideration of bleeding risk.

Assessment of Bleeding Risk

- Before starting anticoagulation, an assessment of bleeding risk should be undertaken. Major bleeding, especially intracranial haemorrhage (ICH), is the most feared complication of anticoagulation therapy and confers a high risk of death and disability (Connolly et al., 2011).
- Several different guidelines recommend the use of the HAS-BLED score, which has been validated in many cohort studies and correlates well with ICH risk (Table 7.4) (Cairns, Connolly, McMurtry, Stephenson, & Talajic, 2001; Camm et al., 2010; Lip et al., 2011).
- A HAS-BLED score of 3 or more indicates a bleeding risk (ICH or requiring admission) on anticoagulation over the next year sufficient to justify caution with anticoagulation.
- A score of 3 or above does not exclude patients from receiving anticoagulation, but would require extra caution to control bleeding risks (e.g., closer monitoring of renal function and INR, better management of hypertension).

Anticoagulation

- For more than half a century, warfarin has been the primary medication used to reduce the risk of thromboembolic events in patients with atrial fibrillation (Mega, 2011).
- Research has confirmed that warfarin is superior to antiplatelet therapy (e.g., aspirin) in the management of AF in the community, even in older people (Mant et al., 2007). Aspirin should no longer be used for stroke prevention in AF; such patients should be reviewed.
- Despite its clinical efficacy, warfarin has several limitations, including drug interactions and the need for regular blood monitoring (INR should be controlled to between 2 and 3) and dose adjustments. See the accompanying table for contraindications to warfarin.
- As a result, alternative anticoagulants that are at least as efficacious but easier to administer have been developed and widely promoted.
- Four novel oral anticoagulant agents (NOACs) have been approved by NICE as alternatives to warfarin in nonvalvular AF. These are dabigatran, rivaroxaban, apixaban, and edoxaban.
- Dabigatran is a direct thrombin inhibitor and the other three are factor Xa inhibitors.
- The main advantages of these agents are that they are fixed dose, less susceptible to interactions, and do not require monitoring.

TABLE 7.4	The HAS-BLED Bleeding Risk Score (Pisters et al., 2010)	
Letter	**Clinical Characteristic**	**Points**
H	Hypertension	1
A	Abnormal renal and liver function (1 point each)	1 or 2
S	Stroke	1
B	Bleeding	1
L	Labile INRs	1
E	Elderly (over 65)	1
D	Drugs or alcohol (1 point each)	1 or 2

TOTAL

Hypertension is defined as systolic blood pressure >160 mm Hg.
Abnormal kidney function is defined as the presence of chronic dialysis or renal transplantation or serum creatinine ≥200 mmol/L.
Abnormal liver function is defined as chronic hepatic disease (e.g., cirrhosis) or biochemical evidence of significant hepatic derangement (e.g., bilirubin >2 × upper limit of normal, in association with aspartate aminotransferase/alanine aminotransferase/alkaline phosphatase >3 × upper limit normal, etc.).
Bleeding refers to previous bleeding history and/or predisposition to bleeding (e.g., bleeding diathesis, anemia).
Labile INRs refers to unstable/high INRs or poor time in therapeutic range (e.g., <60%).
Drugs/alcohol use refers to concomitant use of drugs, such as antiplatelet agents, nonsteroidal antiinflammatory drugs, or alcohol abuse.
INR, International normalized ratio.

TABLE 7.3	CHA2DS2-VASc		
	Risk Factor	**Score**
C	Congestive heart failure	1
H	Hypertension	1
A_2	Age ≥75	2
D	Diabetes	1
S_2	CVA or TIA	2
V	Vascular disease	1
A	Age ≥65	1
Sc	Sex category (i.e., female)	1

TOTAL SCORE

0 = low risk (0.8% annual stroke rate)
1 = moderate risk (1.75% annual stroke rate)
≥2 = high risk (>2.7% annual stroke rate)
3 = 3.2%; 5 = 6.7%; 7 = 9.6%

- Antidotes have recently been developed for both dabigatran and the factor Xa inhibitors.
- A number of studies have concluded that the NOACs compare favourably to warfarin, in terms of both efficacy (reducing overall mortality and strokes) and safety profile (less intracranial bleeding) (Dentali, Riva, & Crowther, 2012; Rasmussen, Larsen, Graungaard, Skjøth, & Lip, 2012).
- All of the NOACs share these contraindications: significant risk of major bleeding, pregnancy and breast feeding, additional anticoagulant therapy, and concomitant use of itraconazole, ketoconazole and HIV protease inhibitors.
- For patients switching from warfarin to a NOAC, warfarin should be stopped and the NOAC started as soon as the INR is below 2.

Dabigatran

- Dabigatran is recommended by NICE (2012a) as an option for the prevention of stroke in nonvalvular AF in people with one or more of the following risk factors:
  - Heart failure: LVEF less than 40% or symptomatic with NYHA Class 2 or above
  - Previous CVA, TIA, or embolism
  - Age 75 and older
  - Age 65 and older, with diabetes, coronary heart disease, or high blood pressure
- The recommended daily dose is 300 mg taken as one 150-mg capsule twice daily. Therapy is continued long term.
- Patients aged 80 years or older, and those with renal impairment (eGFR 30–49) should be treated with a daily dose of 220 mg taken as one 110-mg capsule twice daily because of the increased risk of bleeding in this population.
- It is contraindicated in people with severe renal impairment (eGFR <30), and those at increased risk of bleeding, including previous GI ulceration, recent surgery, hepatic impairment, or liver disease.
- Check renal function before starting. Do not start in any patient with severe renal impairment (eGFR <30).

Rivaroxaban and Apixaban

- NICE have approved rivaroxaban and apixaban as alternatives to warfarin in people with nonvalvular AF and one or more of the following risk factors (NICE, 2012d, 2013):
  - Heart failure
  - Previous CVA or TIA
  - Hypertension
  - Age over 75 years
  - Diabetes
- The recommended daily dose of rivaroxaban is 20 mg daily, reduced to 15 mg daily in people with renal impairment (eGFR 30–49). It should be taken after food.
- The dose of apixaban is 5 mg twice daily, reduced to 2.5 mg twice daily in renal impairment.

CONTRAINDICATIONS TO WARFARIN IN ATRIAL FIBRILLATION (Man-Son-Hing & Laupacis, 2003)

Absolute Contraindications

- Pregnancy
- Active peptic ulcer or other active source of GI bleeding
- Current major trauma or surgery
- Uncontrolled hypertension
- A bleeding diathesis
- Bacterial endocarditis
- Alcoholism
- Inability to control the INR

Factors Which Increase the Risk of Bleeding Slightly but Only Enough to Alter the Decision in Cases Where the Benefit Is Already Borderline

- Current NSAID use (add gastroprotection or change to a COX-2 inhibitor)
- Activities that involve a high risk of injury

Factors Often Erroneously Thought to Contraindicate Warfarin

- Old age. The INR is no harder to control in the elderly than in younger patients. There is a slight increase in bleeding risk in older patients but with increasing age the benefit from warfarin rises more than the risk
- Past history of peptic ulcer or GI bleeding, now resolved
- Hypertension controlled (<160/90 mm Hg)
- Patients at risk of falling
- Previous stroke
- Alcohol intake of one to two drinks a day

Left Atrial Appendage Closure

- The left atrial appendage (LAA) is considered the main (though not the only) site of thrombus formation leading to ischaemic stroke in people with AF.
- Minimally invasive techniques have been developed to occlude the LAA orifice and thereby reduce stroke risk, with results equivalent to warfarin (Holmes et al., 2009).
- At present, this procedure is only considered for patients in whom oral anticoagulation is contraindicated.

Paroxysmal Atrial Fibrillation

- *Paroxysmal atrial fibrillation* (PAF) is defined as recurrent (two or more) episodes of AF that terminate spontaneously in less than 7 days, and usually less than 24 hours.
- Tailor the treatment to the severity.
- *The patient with infrequent attacks and no serious symptoms, or attacks that can be averted by avoiding a precipitating cause (e.g., alcohol or caffeine),* either give:
  - no drug treatment, or
  - a pill-in-the-pocket, to be taken at the onset of an attack, if the patient is suitable (see the accompanying box).
- *The patient with more frequent attacks or more severe symptoms:*
  - receives a standard beta-blocker.

- If that is ineffective or not tolerated, refer for specialist assessment. Other medications such as sotalol, flecainide, propafenone, or amiodarone may be considered. Dronedarone, which is structurally related to amiodarone, has been approved for the treatment of paroxysmal or persistent AF, but only under specialist initiation and supervision. It should not be given to patients with moderate or severe heart failure, and should be avoided in patients with less severe heart failure, if appropriate alternatives exist.
- NICE warns of the danger of initiating drugs other than standard beta-blockers for paroxysmal AF in general practice without specialist advice because of the risk that the drug will itself cause ventricular arrhythmias. This is most likely in those with underlying heart disease. In practice the patient will often have been assessed already by a cardiologist and had previous experience of an antiarrhythmic drug without adverse effects, obviating the need for re-referral.

NICE RECOMMENDATIONS FOR THE SUITABILITY OF A PATIENT FOR A "PILL-IN-THE-POCKET"

1. Infrequent episodes (e.g., between once per month and once per year)
2. Sufficiently reliable to use the treatment correctly
3. No structural heart disease, coronary heart disease, or left ventricular dysfunction
4. Satisfactory baseline state: systolic blood pressure >100 mm Hg, resting heart rate >70 bpm

- If a paroxysm becomes persistent (arbitrarily defined as lasting at least 7 days), refer for consideration of cardioversion. Refer immediately if the patient develops heart failure or hypotension.

Catheter Ablation

- The European Society of Cardiology (ESC) guidelines recommend that catheter ablation (by pulmonary vein isolation) be considered as a first line therapy for AF rhythm control in selected patients (i.e., those with PAF with a preference for interventional treatment and a low-risk profile for procedural complications) (Kirchhof et al., 2016).
- Studies have shown promising results (Nielsen et al., 2012), but the procedure carries the risk of invasive complications. In one study, complication rates were 0.6% for stroke, 1.3% for tamponade, 1.3% for peripheral vascular complications, and around 2% for pericarditis (Arbelo et al., 2012).

Anticoagulation

A patient with paroxysmal AF should be considered for antithrombotic treatment according to the presence of risk factors (e.g., as assessed by CHA2DS2-VASc). The risk of stroke, although less well defined in paroxysmal AF, is considered to be the same as in persistent or permanent AF,

regardless of the number and severity of paroxysms (Friberg, Hammar, & Rosenqvist, 2010).

Atrial Flutter

- Atrial flutter should be approached in a similar way to atrial fibrillation, with a focus on:
  1. rate control;
  2. rhythm control;
  3. prevention of thromboembolic complications.
- It is much less common than AF and usually less well tolerated, often presenting with palpitations.
- Episodes of atrial flutter and AF can occur in the same person.
- Refer all suspected cases for specialist assessment.
- Radio-frequency catheter ablation is first line treatment (Sawhney & Feld, 2008).

Paroxysmal Supraventricular Tachycardia

- If the patient is seen during the attack, get the patient to perform a Valsalva manoeuvre. This can be described to the patient as trying to breathe out forcefully while keeping the mouth closed and nose pinched, or simulating straining on the toilet (Whinnett, Afzal Sohaib, & Wyn Davies, 2012).
- Apply carotid sinus massage except where the patient:
  1. is elderly;
  2. has ischaemic heart disease;
  3. is likely to be digoxin toxic;
  4. has a carotid bruit;
  5. has a history of transient ischaemic attacks.
  Note: The British National Formulary recommends ECG monitoring during carotid sinus massage.
- Admit if the attack continues and there is no clear history of previous attacks which have terminated themselves. Even if there is such a history, keep the patient at the surgery until the attack indeed terminates.
- Record an ECG and give the patient a copy.
- If SVT is diagnosed from the patient's history or if the attack has terminated before admission was needed:
  - Refer for specialist confirmation and initiation of treatment. Referral should be urgent if attacks are associated with chest pain, dizziness, or breathlessness.
  - Catheter ablation is the first line definitive management option for SVT.
  - Drug treatment is reserved for minimizing symptoms while awaiting catheter ablation or for those who decline catheter ablation or in whom the procedure carries an unacceptably high risk.
  - Discuss with a cardiologist before starting an antiarrhythmic drug (e.g., sotalol, flecainide, verapamil), while awaiting the cardiology appointment.
  - A baseline ECG, with a further ECG before each dose increase, is recommended to look for prolongation of the QT interval, an indicator that there is a risk of drug-induced *torsade de pointes.* A final decision on

the most appropriate drug will depend on the electropathology in the individual patient.

- Instruct the patient in the use of the Valsalva manoeuvre, and check that he or she is not smoking or misusing alcohol or caffeine.

Ventricular Tachycardia

- VT associated with loss of consciousness or hypotension is a medical emergency requiring immediate cardioversion.
- Call 999 emergency ambulance.
- Remember ABCs (airway, breathing, circulation), oxygen, ECG monitoring.
- If the patient is conscious but *in extremis*, consider IV lidocaine 100 mg while waiting for the ambulance.
- After discharge, prophylaxis will be needed. If amiodarone is chosen, 6-monthly TFTs and LFTs are necessary.

Sick Sinus Syndrome

This requires admission for pacing. Drugs are likely to make symptoms worse because of the variability of the rhythms.

Bradycardia

- Refer all patients with a bradycardia, other than sinus bradycardia, even if asymptomatic. A pacemaker is likely to be needed and may be life saving. Untreated second degree and complete atrioventricular (AV) block have a mortality of 25% to 50% in the first year after diagnosis. For this reason, even asymptomatic patients with a rate of 40 or below should be paced.
- Admit a patient in acute AV block with hypotension due to the bradycardia. Give IV atropine if available while waiting for the ambulance.

PATIENT SUPPORT GROUPS

Arrhythmia Alliance: www.heartrhythmcharity.org.uk/
Atrial Fibrillation Association: www.atrialfibrillation.org.uk/
Sudden Adult Death Trust: www.sadsuk.org/
Cardiac Risk in the Young: www.c-r-y.org.uk/

Prophylaxis of Infective Endocarditis

GUIDELINE

National Institute for Health and Care Excellence. (2008). *Prophylaxis against infective endocarditis. NICE clinical guideline 64.* Available at www.nice.org.uk.

- Antibiotic prophylaxis aims to reduce the incidence of infective endocarditis.
- The NICE guidance represented a major shift in advice on antibiotic prophylaxis.

- Do not offer antibiotics to prevent ineffective endocarditis (IE) for any of the following procedures:
  - Any dental procedure
  - An obstetric or gynaecologic procedure, or childbirth
  - A procedure on the bladder or urinary tract
  - A procedure on the oesophagus, stomach, or intestines
  - A procedure on the airways (including ear, nose, and throat and bronchoscopy)
- People with the following cardiac conditions should be regarded as being at risk of developing IE:
  - Acquired valvular heart disease with stenosis or regurgitation
  - Valve replacement
  - Structural congenital heart disease, including surgically corrected or palliated structural conditions, but excluding isolated atrial septal defect, fully repaired ventricular septal defect or fully repaired patent ductus arteriosus, and closure devices that are judged to be endothelialized
  - Hypertrophic cardiomyopathy
  - Previous infective endocarditis
- People at risk of IE should be offered clear and consistent information about prevention, including:
  - the benefits and risks of antibiotic prophylaxis, and an explanation of why antibiotic prophylaxis is no longer routinely recommended;
  - the importance of maintaining good oral health;
  - symptoms that may indicate IE and when to seek expert advice;
  - the risks of undergoing invasive procedures, including nonmedical procedures such as body piercing or tattooing.
- In people at risk of IE, it is important to investigate and treat promptly any episodes of infection to reduce the risk of endocarditis developing.
- If a person at risk of IE is receiving antimicrobial therapy because of undergoing a gastrointestinal or genitourinary procedure at a site where there is a suspected infection, offer an antibiotic that covers organisms that cause infective endocarditis.

PATIENT INFORMATION

There are a range of resources available through the British Heart Foundation website at www.bhf.org.uk. Their helpline (0300 330 3311) is open Monday through Friday, 9 am to 5 pm.

The Prevention of Cardiovascular Disease

GUIDELINE

National Institute for Health and Care Excellence. (2014a). *Cardiovascular disease: Risk assessment and reduction, including lipid modification. NICE clinical guideline 181.* Available at www.nice.org.uk.

- Cardiovascular disease (CVD) describes disease of the heart and blood vessels caused by the process of atherosclerosis and predominantly affects people older than 50 years (NICE, 2014a). There are significant gender differences in cardiovascular risk, including biologic differences associated with pregnancy and menopause (Parikh, 2011), as well as differences in behavioural risk factors (Huxley & Woodward, 2011).
- Worldwide, the two most important modifiable cardiovascular risk factors are smoking and abnormal lipids (SIGN, 2017).
- The next most important are hypertension, diabetes, psychosocial factors (including deprivation), and abdominal obesity, but their relative effects vary in different regions of the world.
- Risk factors tend to cluster and their effects are multiplicative, not additive. The presence of one or more of the following increases the chance that other risk factors will also be present: hypertension, raised cholesterol, inactivity, obesity, smoking, and glucose intolerance (Perry, Wannamethee, & Walker, 1995).
- Strategies for the prevention of cardiovascular disease can be divided into primary and secondary prevention. Primary prevention is concerned with preventing the occurrence of cardiovascular disease in those currently unaffected. Secondary prevention relates to delaying or reversing the progression of disease in those already affected. While targeting those at highest risk is known to be most cost effective, most countries recognize the importance of a multifaceted approach, adopting both population-based and more targeted interventions (Rose, 1981).

Primary Prevention

- For the primary prevention of CVD in primary care, a systematic strategy should be used to identify people who are likely to be at high risk, now considered to be a 10%, 10-year risk after lifestyle modification. The NICE (2014) guidelines remain controversial, reflecting uncertainty in the data that underpins them (Otto, 2016).
- The role of GPs and practice nurses is, first and foremost, to support patients to make and sustain lifestyle changes where appropriate and to help them make an informed decision regarding statins if they are at increased CVD risk. This should be based on an indvidualised assessment of the likely benefits and harms of statins.
- The following groups of people should be assumed to be at high risk based on clinical history alone and do not require risk assessment with a scoring system:
  - People who have had a previous cardiovascular event (angina, MI, stroke, transient ischaemic attack, or peripheral arterial disease)
  - People with diabetes (type 1 or 2) over the age of 40 years
  - People with familial hypercholesterolaemia
- CVD risk should be estimated using information already contained in the patient's records, and using a chart or computer programme based on epidemiologic data such

as the US Framingham heart study data (Anderson, Odell, Wilson, & Kannel, 1991), according to:
  - age;
  - sex;
  - lifetime smoking habit;
  - blood pressure (if treated use pretreatment level);
  - serum lipids if known. If treated use pretreatment level.
- There are a number of different validated resources available to calculate 10-year risk of cardiovascular disease, but NICE now recommends the use of QRISK2 assessment tool.
- Asymptomatic individuals should be considered at high risk if they are assessed as having a 10% or greater risk of a first cardiovascular event over 10 years. Such individuals warrant intervention with lifestyle changes and consideration for drug therapy, to reduce their absolute risk.
- NICE now recommends that the QRISK2 tool is used up to and including age 84 years. Consider people aged 85 and older to be at increased risk of CVD because of their age alone.
- A further consideration when assessing someone's CVD risk is the presence of xanthelasmata. A 2011 study found that xanthelasmata predict an increased risk of CV events, particularly in women, even if serum lipid levels are normal (Christoffersen et al., 2011). The authors suggest xanthelasmata may be a sign of an increased propensity to deposit lipid in soft tissues and is therefore a cutaneous marker of atheroma. There is no such increased risk with arcus corneae.

Lifestyle Changes

- *Stop smoking.* Someone who smokes 20 cigarettes a day or less and stops has a risk of CHD 10 years later almost the same as in one who has never smoked. Recovery is, however, less the longer the person has smoked (Doll, Peto, Boreham, & Sutherland, 2004). Nicotine replacement therapy increases the rate of quitting by 50% to 70%, regardless of the setting and independent of whether support, other than brief advice, is offered (Stead, Perera, Bullen, Mant, & Lancaster, 2008).
- *Alcohol.* Keep alcohol intake within safe limits. Current UK recommendations are 14 units of alcohol or less per week for both men and women.
- *Take exercise..* Encourage the patient to incorporate exercise into his or her daily life, rather than rely on visiting a gym or playing football at the weekend. Simple advice from the GP is unlikely to change behaviour. A more supportive programme is needed.
- *Manage social isolation.* Depression and lack of social support are associated with an increased risk of cardiovascular disease (Bunker et al., 2003), as is the combination of high workload and low autonomy at work (Aboa-Eboule et al., 2007).
- *Control weight.* Central obesity, rather than a raised BMI, carries the greater cardiovascular risk and can be assessed by measuring the waist circumference, with a single cutoff point for each sex. Men with a waist circumference

over 94 cm and women over 80 cm are likely to have other risk factors for cardiovascular disease, and men with a waist circumference over 102 cm (women over 88 cm) are 2.5 to 4.5 times as likely to have other major cardiovascular risk factors (Han et al., 1995). Small losses of weight are possible in primary care if advice on diet and exercise is accompanied by a behavioural programme.

- *Diet.* Encourage patients to:
  - reduce their meat and fat intake;
  - eat oily fish at least twice a week;
  - eat bread, pasta, and potatoes as sources of carbohydrate;
  - eat at least five portions a day of fruit or vegetables;
  - use olive oil and rape seed margarine instead of butter.

Intensive Management When a 10-Year Cardiovascular Disease Risk of At Least 10% Is Detected

Lipid Lowering

- NICE now recommends offering atorvastatin 20 mg for the primary prevention of CVD to people who have a 10% or greater 10-year risk of developing CVD
- Check TFTs, creatinine, LFTs, and fasting sugar. Note that elevated liver enzymes are not a contraindication to the use of a statin. They are not associated with subsequent statin-induced toxicity (Chalasani et al., 2004).
- Check baseline lipids. NICE no longer recommends a fasting test.
- NICE recommends annual medication reviews for patients and consideration of an annual, nonfasting, non-HDL cholesterol blood test to inform the discussion. Aim for a reduction of greater than 40% in non-HDL cholesterol in both primary and secondary prevention.
- Stongly encourage physical activity in all those taking statins. In combination, mortality risk is greatly reduced in those with dyslipidaemia (Kokkinos, Faselis, Myers, Panagiotakos, & Doumas, 2013).
- Warn the patient to report muscle pain or weakness; if present, check creatine kinase (CK) and TSH (Lasker & Chowdhury, 2012).
  - If CK is 10 times or above upper limit of normal then STOP immediately. This is a risk of rhabdomyolysis.
  - If CK is 5 times or below normal, this is rarely clinically significant and is often related to exercise.
  - If CK is not significantly raised, suggest rechallenging with a statin at a lower dose or switching statin (e.g., 10 mg atorvastatin is equivalent to 40 mg simvastatin). If myalgia recurs, try a nonstatin treatment (i.e., ezetimibe 10 mg).
- Continue indefinitely unless adverse effects occur.
- Be aware of interactions:
  - When macrolides (e.g., erythromycin and clarithromycin) have to be prescribed, stop the statin and restart 1 week after the macrolide is finished.
  - Avoid itraconazole and ketoconazole (contraindicated with simvastatin).
  - Reduce statin dose (max 20 mg simvastatin) with amlodipine, diltiazem, verapamil, and amiodarone.
- On subsequent visits, check that the patient is taking the statin. A study from Liverpool found that a quarter of patients took their statin less than 80% of the time and had a higher mortality (Howell, Trotter, Mottram, & Rowe, 2004).

Blood Pressure Control

- Check blood pressure annually.
- Treat if levels are sustained at 140/90 mm Hg or above.
- Aim for a level of below 140/90 mm Hg, or in those with type 2 diabetes below 140/80 mm Hg (and 130/80 mm Hg if microalbuminuria or proteinuria is present).

Talking to the Patient About Absolute Risks When Taking a Statin

NICE have produced guidance on the components of good patient experience in adult NHS services, including recommendations on the communication of risk (NICE, 2014b). Shared decision making is particularly important in the context of CVD prevention, as the benefits to individual patients (of taking a statin, for instance) may be small and are not without the risk of harm. NICE have developed a patient decision aid which provides absolute benefits and harms of taking a statin (NICE, 2014c). Adequate time should be set aside for shared decision making using aids such as this. Discussions should be documented and can be re-visited in the future if patients change their minds.

Secondary Prevention

Consider the following measures in those with cardiovascular disease, diabetes, chronic kidney disease, or primary hyperlipidaemia.
- Recommend *lifestyle changes* as for primary prevention.
- *Lipid-lowering measures:*
  - Order the tests recommended under primary prevention and give the same warnings.
  - Offer a statin regardless of baseline cholesterol level.
  - Start atorvastatin 80 mg in people with CVD. Use a lower dose if there are potential drug interactions, high risk of adverse effects or patient preference.
  - Recheck the serum lipids after 3 months. If TC ≥ 4 mmol/L or LDL ≥2 mmol/L consider intensifying treatment. If targets are still not reached, add ezetimibe. Other options are a fibrate (but with a warning about the increased risk of rhabdomyolysis), nicotinic acid or an omega-3 fatty acid.
  - If adverse effects occur consider reducing the statin dose, or changing to another statin, or using ezetimibe, a fibrate, or nicotinic acid.

- *Blood pressure.* Treat if levels are sustained at 140/90 mm Hg or above. Aim for a level of below 140/90 mm Hg, or in those with diabetes below 130/80 mm Hg.
- *Antiplatelet therapy.* Recommendations for antiplatelet therapy vary in different scenarios. These are now largely specialist-led decisions.
- *ACE inhibition.* Prescribe an ACE inhibitor to all patients with coronary heart disease. Titrate to maximum tolerated doses and continue long term.
- Prescribe a beta-blocker to all those who have had an MI. Start them in patients whose MI was in the last 5 years and who therefore missed the opportunity to have them started in the acute stage. Patients at the highest risk benefit most from beta-blockade (e.g., those aged >50 with angina, hypertension, or heart failure).
- *Eplerenone.* This aldosterone antagonist is now preferred to spironolactone in patients who have LV dysfunction following MI.

Annual Workup at a Coronary Heart Disease Prevention Clinic

- *Check:*
  1. fasting sugar;
  2. total cholesterol;
  3. urine protein;
  4. BP;
  5. weight, height, and BMI.
- Action to be taken when a new abnormal result is found:
  - *Fasting sugar:*
    1. If fasting sugar is 7 mmol/L or higher and the patient has symptoms (thirst, polyuria, lethargy), this is diabetes.
    2. If fasting sugar is 7 mmol/L or higher and the patient has no symptoms, repeat after 1 week. If still 7 mmol/L or higher, diabetes is confirmed.
    3. If fasting sugar is between 6.1 and 6.9 mmol/L inclusive, check blood sugar 2 hours after a 75-g glucose drink (=394 mL of the new Lucozade formulation which contains 73 kcal/100 mL):
       a. If greater than 11 mmol/L, diabetes is confirmed.
       b. If less than 7.8 mmol/L, this is impaired fasting glycaemia (IFG). Warn as for IGT (see the upcoming discussion).
       c. If between 7.8 and 11 mmol/L inclusive, this is impaired glucose tolerance (IGT). Warn that it carries an increased risk of diabetes, which can be reduced by exercise and diet. Recheck fasting sugar annually.
- *Proteinuria.* If + or more, repeat after 1 week on the first morning specimen. If still + or more, send mid-stream urine for culture and sensitivities, serum creatinine and electrolytes, and an albumin to creatinine ratio (ACR) on a single urine sample. If the urine ACR is above 30 or there is haematuria, or the creatinine is raised, this is significant proteinuria (different thresholds apply in diabetes).

Familial Hypercholesterolaemia

GUIDELINE

National Institute for Health and Care Excellence. (2008). *Familial hypercholesterolaemia. NICE clinical guideline 71.* Available at www.nice.org.uk.

- Familial hypercholesterolaemia (FH) is important because it carries a very high risk of premature CV morbidity and mortality. It is generally asymptomatic so is easily missed in general practice (Gill, Harnden, & Karpe, 2012).
- It is present in about 1 in 500 of the population in the United Kingdom and for men carries a 50% risk of a major coronary event by the age of 50. In women the risk is 30% by the age of 60. This risk is far higher than would be predicted from the cholesterol level alone and requires intensive therapy (high-dose statins and ezetimibe).
- Suspect FH as a possible diagnosis in adults with:
  - a total cholesterol level greater than 7.5 mmol/l and/or
  - a personal or family history of premature CHD (an event before 60 years in an index individual or first-degree relative).
- NICE recommends systematically searching primary care records for people:
  - younger than 30 years, with a total cholesterol concentration greater than 7.5 mmol/l and
  - 30 years of older, with a total cholesterol concentration greater than 9.0 mmol/l
- If suspicion of FH is raised:
  - Recheck the serum lipids with a fasting specimen.
  - Check for other causes of raised cholesterol (e.g., hypothyroidism, excess alcohol consumption).
  - Ask about the family history across three generations. Accept that the patient may need to return with these details after consultation with the family.
  - Ask about symptoms of CVD.
  - Examine for evidence of CVD or skin or tendon manifestations of hyperlipidaemia.
- Make a clinical diagnosis of FH according to the Simon Broome criteria:
  - *FH exists* if the total cholesterol is above 7.5 mmol/L or the LDL cholesterol is above 4.9 mmol/L AND tendon xanthoma are present (in the patient or a first or second degree relative).
  - *FH is possible* if:
    1. the total cholesterol is above 7.5 mmol/L or the LDL cholesterol is above 4.9 mmol/L AND there is a first degree relative with a myocardial infarction before the age of 60 or a second degree relative with a myocardial infarction before the age of 50; or
    2. the total cholesterol is above 7.5 mmol/L or the LDL cholesterol is above 4.9 mmol/L in the patient AND also in a first or second degree relative (or

>6.7 mmol/L or >4.0 mmol/L, respectively, in a brother or sister under 16 years old).

- Referral is needed:
  1. *to a specialist with expertise in familial hypercholesterolaemia* for all with a definite or possible clinical diagnosis. Further investigation will include DNA testing for relevant mutations and family screening;
  2. *to a cardiologist* if there are symptoms of CHD. Consider referral if the patient has no symptoms but there is a family history of CHD in early adult life or the patient has two or more other risk factors for CHD.
- *Cholesterol lowering in a patient with a confirmed diagnosis of FH:*
  - Give a high-intensity statin (e.g., atorvastatin 40 mg daily).
  - Aim for a LDL cholesterol over 50% below the pretreated level.
  - If the target is not met, increase the statin to the maximum licensed dose, provided it is tolerated, and/or add ezetimibe.
  - Re-refer if the target is not met.
  - Review annually once stable. Stress that lifestyle changes are even more important in someone with FH than in the general population.

References

Aboa-Eboule, C., Brisson, C., Maunsell, E., et al. (2007). Job strain and risk of acute recurrent coronary heart disease events. *JAMA: The Journal of the American Medical Association, 298,* 1652–1660.

Aguilar, M. I., & Hart, R. (2005). Oral anticoagulants for preventing stroke in patients with non-valvular atrial fibrillation and no previous history of stroke or transient ischemic attacks. *The Cochrane Database of Systematic Reviews, (3),* CD001927.

Al-Mohammad, A., Mant, J., Laramee, P., & Swain, S., on behalf of the Chronic Heart Failure Guideline Development Group. (2010). Diagnosis and management of adults with chronic heart failure: Summary of updated NICE guidance. *British Medical Journal (Clinical Research Ed.), 341,* c4130.

Anderson, K. M., Odell, P. M., Wilson, P. W., & Kannel, W. B. (1991). Cardiovascular disease risk profiles. *American Heart Journal, 121,* 293–298.

Appel, L. J., Moore, T. J., Obarzanek, E., et al. (1997). The effect of dietary patterns on blood pressure: Results from the Dietary Approaches to Stop Hypertension trial. *The New England Journal of Medicine, 336,* 1117–1124.

Arbelo, E., Brugada, J., Hindricks, G., et al. on behalf of the Atrial Fibrillation Ablation Pilot Study Investigators. (2012). ESC-EURObservational research programme: The atrial fibrillation ablation pilot study, conducted by the European Heart Rhythm Association. *Europace: European Pacing, Arrhythmias, and Cardiac Electrophysiology: Journal of the Working Groups on Cardiac Pacing, Arrhythmias, and Cardiac Cellular Electrophysiology of the European Society of Cardiology, 14,* 1094–1103.

Arroll, B., Doughty, R., & Andersen, V. (2010). Investigation and management of congestive heart failure. *British Medical Journal (Clinical Research Ed.), 341,* c3657.

Atrial Fibrillation Follow-Up Investigation of Rhythm Management (AFFIRM) Investigators. (2002). A comparison of rate control and rhythm control in patients with atrial fibrillation. *The New England Journal of Medicine, 347,* 1825–1833.

Barnett, H., Burrill, P., & Iheanacho, I. (2010). Don't use aspirin for primary prevention of cardiovascular disease. *British Medical Journal (Clinical Research Ed.), 340,* c1805.

Barnett, K., Mercer, S. W., Norbury, M., et al. (2012). Epidemiology of multimorbidity and implications for health care, research, and medical education: A cross-sectional study. *Lancet, 380,* 37–43.

Bass, C., & Mayou, R. (2002). Chest pain. *British Medical Journal (Clinical Research Ed.), 325,* 588–591.

Beckett, N., Peters, R., Tuomilehto, J., et al. for the HYVET Study Group. (2011). Immediate and late benefits of treating very elderly people with hypertension: Results from active treatment extension to hypertension in the very elderly randomised controlled trial. *British Medical Journal (Clinical Research Ed.), 344,* d7541.

Beckett, N. S., Peters, R., Fletcher, A. E., et al. for the HYVET Study Group. (2008). Treatment of hypertension in patients 80 years of age or older. *The New England Journal of Medicine, 358,* 1887–1898.

Benson, J., & Britten, N. (2002). Patients' decisions about whether or not to take antihypertensive drugs: Qualitative study. *British Medical Journal (Clinical Research Ed.), 325,* 873–876.

Brown, M., Cruickshank, J., Dominiczak, A., et al. (2003). Better blood pressure control: How to combine drugs. *Journal of Human Hypertension, 17,* 81–86.

Bunker, S., Colquhoun, D., Esler, M., et al. (2003). Stress' and coronary heart disease: Psychosocial risk factors. *The Medical Journal of Australia, 178,* 272–276.

Cairns, J. A., Connolly, S., McMurtry, S., Stephenson, M., & Talajic, M. (2011). Canadian Cardiovascular Society atrial fibrillation guidelines 2010: Prevention of stroke and systemic thromboembolism in atrial fibrillation and flutter. *The Canadian Journal of Cardiology, 27,* 74–90.

Camm, A. J., Kirchhof, P., Lip, G. Y., et al. (2010). Guidelines for the management of atrial fibrillation: The Task Force for the Management of Atrial Fibrillation of the European Society of Cardiology (ESC). *Europace: European Pacing, Arrhythmias, and Cardiac Electrophysiology: Journal of the Working Groups on Cardiac Pacing, Arrhythmias, and Cardiac Cellular Electrophysiology of the European Society of Cardiology, 12,* 1360–1420.

Chalasani, N., Aljadhey, H., Kesterson, J., et al. (2004). Patients with elevated liver enzymes are not at higher risk for statin hepatotoxicity. *Gastroenterology, 126,* 1287–1292.

Chen, L. Y., Sotoodehnia, N., & Bůžková, P. (2013). Atrial fibrillation and the risk of sudden cardiac death. *JAMA Internal Medicine, 173,* 29–35.

Chobanian, A. V., Bakris, G. L., Black, H. R., et al. (2003). The seventh report of the Joint National Committee on Prevention, Detection, Evaluation, and Treatment of High Blood Pressure: The JNC 7 report. *JAMA: The Journal of the American Medical Association, 289,* 2560–2571.

Christoffersen, M., Frikke-Schmidt, R., Schnohr, P., et al. (2011). Xanthelasmata, arcus corneae, and ischaemic vascular disease and death in general population: Prospective cohort study. *British Medical Journal (Clinical Research Ed.), 343,* d5497.

Clark, C. E., Taylor, R. S., Shore, A. C., & Campbell, J. L. (2012). The difference in blood pressure readings between arms and survival: Primary care cohort study. *British Medical Journal (Clinical Research Ed.), 344,* e1327.

Clark, C. E., Taylor, R. S., Shore, A. C., Ukoumunne, O. C., & Campbell, J. L. (2012). Association of a difference in systolic blood pressure between arms with vascular disease and mortality: A systematic review and meta-analysis. *Lancet, 379,* 905–914.

Connell, P., McKevitt, C., & Wolfe, C. (2005). Strategies to manage hypertension: A qualitative study with black Caribbean patients. *The British Journal of General Practice: the Journal of the Royal College of General Practitioners, 55*, 357–361.

Connolly, S. J., Eikelboom, J. W., Ng, J., et al. (2011). ACTIVE (Atrial Fibrillation Clopidogrel Trial with Irbesartan for Prevention of Vascular Events) Steering Committee and Investigators. Net clinical benefit of adding clopidogrel to aspirin therapy in patients with atrial fibrillation for whom vitamin K antagonists are unsuitable. *Annals of Internal Medicine, 155*, 579–586.

Cooper, A., Timmis, A., & Skinner, J., on behalf of the Guideline Development Group. (2010). Assessment of recent onset chest pain or discomfort of suspected cardiac origin: Summary of NICE guidance. *British Medical Journal (Clinical Research Ed.), 340*, c1118.

Cox, K. L., Puddey, I. B., Morton, A. R., et al. (1996). Exercise and weight control in sedentary overweight men; effects on clinic and ambulatory blood pressure. *Journal of Hypertension, 14*, 779–790.

Czernichow, S., Zanchetti, A., Turnbull, F., et al. (2011). Blood Pressure Lowering Treatment Trialists' Collaboration. The effects of BP reduction and of different blood pressure-lowering regimens on major cardiovascular events according to baseline blood pressure: Meta-analysis of randomized trials. *Journal of Hypertension, 29*, 4–16.

Dargie, H., & McMurray, J. (1994). Diagnosis and management of heart failure. *British Medical Journal (Clinical Research Ed.), 308*, 321–328.

Dentali, F., Riva, N., & Crowther, M. (2012). Efficacy and safety of the novel oral anticoagulants in atrial fibrillation: a systematic review and meta-analysis of the literature. *Circulation, 126*, 2381–2391.

Diao, D., Wright, J. M., Cundiff, D. K., & Gueyffier, F. (2012). Pharmacotherapy for mild hypertension. *The Cochrane Database of Systematic Reviews*, (8), CD006742.

Doll, R., Peto, R., Boreham, J., & Sutherland, I. (2004). Mortality in relation to smoking: 50 years' observations on male British doctors. *British Medical Journal (Clinical Research Ed.), 328*, 1519–1528.

Elliott, A. M., McAteer, A., & Hannaford, P. C. (2011). Revisiting the symptom iceberg in today's primary care: Results from a UK population survey. *BMC Family Practice, 12*, 16.

Ettehad, D., Emdin, C. A., Kiran, A., et al. (2016). Blood pressure lowering for prevention of cardiovascular disease and death: a systematic review and meta-analysis. *Lancet, 387*(10022), 957–967.

Fitzmaurice, D. A., Hobbs, F. D. R., Jowett, S., et al. (2007). Screening versus routine practice for detection of atrial fibrillation in people aged 65 or over: Cluster randomised controlled trial. *British Medical Journal (Clinical Research Ed.), 335*, 383–386.

Friberg, L., Hammar, N., & Rosenqvist, M. (2010). Stroke in paroxysmal atrial fibrillation: Report from the Stockholm Cohort of Atrial Fibrillation. *European Heart Journal, 31*, 967–975.

Gage, B., Waterman, A., Shannon, W., et al. (2001). Validation of clinical classification schemes for predicting stroke. *JAMA: The Journal of the American Medical Association, 285*, 2864–2870.

Gill, P. J., Harnden, A., & Karpe, F. (2012). Familial hypercholesterolaemia. *British Medical Journal (Clinical Research Ed.), 344*, e3228.

Goodacre, S., Cross, E., Arnold, J., et al. (2005). The health care burden of acute chest pain. *Heart (British Cardiac Society), 91*, 229–230.

Gordon, S., Hickman, M., & Pentney, V. (2012). Screening for asymptomatic atrial fibrillation at seasonal influenza vaccination. *Primary Care Cardiovascular Journal, 5*, 161–164.

Grasko, J. M., Nguyen, H. H., & Glendenning, P. (2010). Delayed diagnosis of primary hyperaldosteronism. *British Medical Journal (Clinical Research Ed.), 340*, c2461.

Haasenritter, J., Bösner, S., Vaucher, P., Herzig, L., et al. (2012). Ruling out coronary heart disease in primary care: External validation of a clinical prediction rule. *The British Journal of General Practice: the Journal of the Royal College of General Practitioners, 62*, e415–e421.

Hagens, V., Vermeulen, K., & TenVergert, E. (2004). Rate control is more cost-effective than rhythm control for patients with persistent atrial fibrillation - results from the RAte Control versus Electrical cardioversion (RACE) study. *European Heart Journal, 25*, 1542–1549.

Han, T., van Leer, E., Seidell, J., et al. (1995). Waist circumference action levels in the identification of cardiovascular risk factors: Prevalence study in a random sample. *British Medical Journal (Clinical Research Ed.), 311*, 1401–1405.

He, F. J., & MacGregor, G. A. (2011). Comment: Salt reduction lowers cardiovascular risk: Meta-analysis of outcome trials. *Lancet, 378*, 380–382.

Health and Social Care Information Centre. (2011). *Health survey for England – 2011. Hypertension (chap. 3)*. Retrieved from www.hscic.gov.uk/.

Hobbs, F. D., Fitzmaurice, D. A., Mant, J., et al. (2005). A randomised controlled trial and cost-effectiveness study of systematic screening (targeted and total population screening) versus routine practice for the detection of atrial fibrillation in people aged 65 and over. The SAFE study. *Health Technology Assessment, 9*, iii–iv, ix–x, 1–74.

Hobbs, F. D. R., Roalfe, A. K., Lip, G. Y. H., et al. on behalf of the Birmingham Atrial Fibrillation in the Aged (BAFTA) Investigators and Midland Research Practices Consortium (MidReC) Network. (2011). Performance of stroke risk scores in older people with atrial fibrillation not taking warfarin: Comparative cohort study from BAFTA trial. *British Medical Journal (Clinical Research Ed.), 342*, d3653.

Hodgkinson, J., Mant, J., Martin, U., et al. (2011). Relative effectiveness of clinic and home blood pressure monitoring compared with ambulatory blood pressure monitoring in diagnosis of hypertension: systematic review. *British Medical Journal (Clinical Research Ed.), 342*, d3621.

Hoefman, E., Boer, K. R., van Weert, H. C., et al. (2007). Predictive value of history taking and physical examination in diagnosing arrhythmias in general practice. *Family Practice, 24*, 636–641.

Holmes, D. R., Reddy, V. Y., Turi, Z. G., et al. on behalf of PROTECT AF Investigators. (2009). Percutaneous closure of the left atrial appendage versus warfarin therapy for prevention of stroke in patients with atrial fibrillation: A randomised non-inferiority trial. *Lancet, 374*, 534–542.

Holt, T. A., Hunter, T. D., Gunnarsson, C., et al. (2012). Risk of stroke and oral anticoagulant use in atrial fibrillation: A cross-sectional survey. *The British Journal of General Practice: the Journal of the Royal College of General Practitioners, 62*, e710–e717.

Howell, N., Trotter, R., Mottram, D., & Rowe, P. (2004). Compliance with statins in primary care. *The Pharmaceutical Journal, 272*, 23–26.

Hughes, J. W., Fresco, D. M., Myerscough, R., et al. (2013). Randomized controlled trial of mindfulness-based stress reduction for prehypertension. *Psychosomatic Medicine, 75*, 721.

Huxley, R. R., & Woodward, M. (2011). Cigarette smoking as a risk factor for coronary heart disease in women compared with men: A systematic review and meta-analysis of prospective cohort studies. *Lancet, 378*, 1297–1305.

James, M. A., & Campbell, J. L. (2012). Better prevention of stroke through screening for atrial fibrillation. *The British Journal of General Practice: the Journal of the Royal College of General Practitioners, 62*, 234–235.

Jong, P., McKelvie, R., & Yusuf, S. (2010). Should treatment for heart failure with preserved ejection fraction differ from that for heart failure with reduced ejection fraction? *British Medical Journal (Clinical Research Ed.), 341*, c4202.

Kokkinos, P. F., Faselis, C., Myers, J., Panagiotakos, D., & Doumas, M. (2013). Interactive effects of fitness and statin treatment on mortality risk in veterans with dyslipidaemia: A cohort study. *Lancet, 381*, 394–399.

Kostis, J., Wilson, A., Freudenberger, R., et al. (2005). Long-term effect of diuretic-based therapy on fatal outcomes in subjects with isolated systolic hypertension with and without diabetes. *American Journal of Cardiology, 95*, 29–35.

Kirchhof, P., Benussi, S., Kotecha, D., et al. (2016). 2016 ESC guidelines for the management of atrial fibrillation developed in collaboration with EACTS. *European Heart Journal, 37*(38), 2893–2962.

Krause, T., Lovibond, K., Caulfield, M., McCormack, T., & Williams, B., on behalf of the Guideline Development Group. (2011). Management of hypertension: Summary of NICE guidance. *British Medical Journal (Clinical Research Ed.), 343*, d4891.

Lasker, S. S., & Chowdhury, T. A. (2012). Myalgia while taking statins. *British Medical Journal (Clinical Research Ed.), 345*, e5348.

Law, M., Wald, N., Morris, J., & Jordan, R. (2003). Value of low dose combination treatment with blood pressure lowering drugs: Analysis of 354 randomised trials. *British Medical Journal (Clinical Research Ed.), 326*, 1427–1434.

Lip, G. Y., Andreotti, F., Fauchier, L., et al. (2011). Bleeding risk assessment, management in atrial fibrillation patients. Executive summary of a position document from the European Heart Rhythm Association [EHRA], endorsed by the European Society of Cardiology [ESC] Working Group on Thrombosis. *Europace: European Pacing, Arrhythmias, and Cardiac Electrophysiology: Journal of the Working Groups on Cardiac Pacing, Arrhythmias, and Cardiac Cellular Electrophysiology of the European Society of Cardiology, 13*, 723–746.

Little, P., Barnett, J., Barnsley, L., et al. (2002). Comparison of agreement between different measures of blood pressure in primary care and daytime ambulatory blood pressure. *British Medical Journal (Clinical Research Ed.), 325*, 254–257.

Man-Son-Hing, M., & Laupacis, A. (2003). Anticoagulant-related bleeding in older persons with atrial fibrillation. *Archives of Internal Medicine, 163*, 1580–1586.

Mant, D., Hobbs, F., Glasziou, P., et al. (2008). Identification and guided treatment of ventricular dysfunction in general practice using B-type natriuretic peptide. *The British Journal of General Practice: the Journal of the Royal College of General Practitioners, 58*, 393–399.

Mant, J., Hobbs, F. D., Fletcher, K., et al. (2007). Warfarin versus aspirin for stroke prevention in an elderly community population with atrial fibrillation (the Birmingham Atrial Fibrillation Treatment of the Aged Study, BAFTA): A randomised controlled trial. *Lancet, 370*, 493–503.

Martin, U., & Coleman, J. J. (2006). Monitoring renal function in hypertension. *British Medical Journal (Clinical Research Ed.), 333*, 896–899.

Mayou, R., Sprigings, D., Birkhead, J., & Price, J. (2002). A randomized controlled trial of a brief educational and psychological intervention for patients presenting to a cardiac clinic with palpitation. *Psychological Medicine, 32*, 699–706.

Mayou, R., Sprigings, D., Birkhead, J., & Price, J. (2003). Characteristics of patients presenting to a cardiac clinic with palpitations. *The Quarterly Journal of Medicine, 96*, 115–123.

Mega, J. L. (2011). A new era for anticoagulation in atrial fibrillation. *The New England Journal of Medicine, 365*, 1052–1054.

Myat, A., Redwood, S. R., Qureshi, A. C., Spertus, J. A., & Williams, B. (2012). Resistant hypertension. *British Medical Journal (Clinical Research Ed.), 345*, e7473.

National Institute for Health and Care Excellence. (2008). *Prophylaxis against infective endocarditis. NICE clinical guideline 64.* Retrieved from www.nice.org.uk.

National Institute for Health and Care Excellence. (2010a). *Chest pain of recent onset. NICE clinical guideline 95.* Retrieved from www.nice.org.uk.

National Institute for Health and Care Excellence. (2010b). *Chronic heart failure: Management of chronic heart failure in adults in primary and secondary care. NICE clinical guideline 108.* Retrieved from www.nice.org.

National Institute for Health and Care Excellence. (2011a). *Hypertension: Clinical management of primary hypertension in adults (update). NICE clinical guideline 127.* Retrieved from http://guidance.nice.org.uk/CG127.

National Institute for Health and Care Excellence. (2011b). *Stable angina: management. NICE clinical guideline 126.* Retrieved from www.nice.org.uk.

National Institute for Health and Care Excellence. (2012a). *Dabigatran etexilate for the prevention of stroke and systemic embolism in atrial fibrillation. NICE TA249.* Retrieved from www.nice.org.uk.

National Institute for Health and Care Excellence. (2012d). *Rivaroxaban for the prevention of stroke and systemic embolism in people with atrial fibrillation. NICE TA256.* Retrieved from www.nice.org.uk.

National Institute for Health and Care Excellence. (2013). *Apixaban for preventing stroke and systemic embolism in people with nonvalvular atrial fibrillation. NICE TA275.* Retrieved from www.nice.org.uk.

National Institute for Health and Care Excellence. (2014a). *Cardiovascular disease: risk assessment and reduction, including lipid modification. NICE clinical guideline 181.* Retrieved from www.nice.org.uk.

National Institute for Health and Care Excellence. (2014b). *Patient experience in adult NHS services: improving the experience of care for people using adult NHS services. NICE clinical guideline 138.* Retrieved from www.nice.org.uk.

National Institute for Health and Care Excellence. (2014c). *Statins to reduce the risk of CHD and stroke: patient decision aid.* Retrieved from www.nice.org.uk/guidance/cg181/resources/patient-decision-aid-pdf-243780159.

Nielsen, J. C., Johannessen, A., Raatikainen, P., et al. (2012). Radiofrequency ablation as initial therapy in paroxysmal atrial fibrillation. *The New England Journal of Medicine, 367*, 1587–1595.

O'Flynn, N., Timmis, A., Henderson, R., Rajesh, S., & Fenu, E., on behalf of the Guideline Development Group. (2011). Management of stable angina: Summary of NICE guidance. *British Medical Journal (Clinical Research Ed.), 343*, d4147.

Olesen, J. B., Lip, G. Y., Hansen, M. L., et al. (2011). Validation of risk stratification schemes for predicting stroke and thromboembolism in patients with atrial fibrillation: Nationwide cohort study. *British Medical Journal (Clinical Research Ed.), 342*, d124.

Otto, C. M. (2016). Statins for primary prevention of cardiovascular disease. *British Medical Journal (Clinical Research Ed.), 355*.

Owan, T. E., Hodge, D. O., Herges, R. M., et al. (2006). Trends in prevalence and outcome of heart failure with preserved ejection fraction. *The New England Journal of Medicine, 355*, 251–259.

Parikh, N. I. (2011). Sex differences in the risk of cardiovascular disease. *British Medical Journal (Clinical Research Ed.), 343*, d5526.

Perry, I., Wannamethee, S., & Walker, M. (1995). Prospective study of risk factors for development of non-insulin dependent diabetes in middle-aged British men. *British Medical Journal (Clinical Research Ed.), 310,* 560–564.

Pisters, R., Lane, D. A., Nieuwlaat, R., et al. (2010). A novel user-friendly score (HAS-BLED) to assess 1-year risk of major bleeding in patients with atrial fibrillation: The Euro Heart Survey. *Chest, 138,* 1093–2000.

Rasmussen, L. H., Larsen, T. B., Graungaard, T., Skjøth, F., & Lip, G. Y. H. (2012). Primary and secondary prevention with new oral anticoagulant drugs for stroke prevention in atrial fibrillation: Indirect comparison analysis. *British Medical Journal (Clinical Research Ed.), 345,* e7097.

Raviele, A., Giada, F., Bergfeldt, L., et al. (2011). Management of patients with palpitation: A position paper from the European Heart Rhythm Association. *EP Eurospace, 13,* 920–934.

Rhys, G. C., Azhar, M. F., & Foster, A. (2013). Screening for atrial fibrillation in patients aged 65 years or over attending annual flu vaccination clinics at a single general practice. *Quality in Primary Care, 21,* 131–140.

Ritchie, L. D., Campbell, N. C., & Murchie, P. (2011). New NICE guidelines for hypertension. *British Medical Journal (Clinical Research Ed.), 343,* d5644.

Rose, G. (1981). Strategy of prevention: Lessons from cardiovascular disease. *British Medical Journal (Clinical Research Ed.), 282,* 1847–1851.

Sacks, F. M., & Campos, H. (2010). Dietary therapy in hypertension. *The New England Journal of Medicine, 362,* 2102–2112.

Salpeter, S., Ormiston, T., & Salpeter, E. (2005). Cardioselective beta-blockers for chronic obstructive pulmonary disease. *Cochrane Database of Systematic Reviews,* (4), CD003566, doi:10.1002/14651858.CD003566.pub2.

Sawhney, N. S., & Feld, G. K. (2008). Diagnosis and management of typical atrial flutter. *The Medical Clinics of North America, 92,* 65–85.

Scottish Intercollegiate Guidelines Network. (2017). *Risk estimation and the prevention of cardiovascular disease: A national clinical guideline.* Retrieved from www.sign.ac.uk.

Scottish Intercollegiate Guidelines Network. (2010). *Management of diabetes: A national clinical guideline.* Retrieved from www.sign.ac s.uk/pdf/sign116.pdf.

Scottish Intercollegiate Guidelines Network. (2016a). *Management of chronic heart failure. SIGN publication 147.* Retrieved from www.sign.ac.uk.

Scottish Intercollegiate Guidelines Network. (2016b). *Acute coronary syndromes. SIGN publication 148.* Retrieved from www.sign.ac.uk.

Scottish Intercollegiate Guidelines Network (2018). *Management of stable angina. SIGN publication 151.* Retrieved from www.sign.ac.uk.

Sharma, A., Wittchen, H., Kirch, W., et al. (2004). High prevalence and poor control of hypertension in primary care: Cross-sectional study. *Journal of Hypertension, 22,* 479–486.

Stead, L. F., Perera, R., Bullen, C., Mant, D., & Lancaster, T. (2008). Nicotine replacement therapy for smoking cessation. *Cochrane Database of Systematic Reviews,* (1), CD000146.

Steffen, M., Kuhle, C., Hensrud, D., Erwin, P. J., & Murad, M. H. (2012). The effect of coffee consumption on blood pressure and the development of hypertension: A systematic review and meta-analysis. *Journal of Hypertension, 30,* 2245–2254.

Stevens, V., Obarzanek, E., & Cook, N. (2001). Long-term weight loss and changes in blood pressure: Results of the Trials of Hypertension Prevention, phase 2. *Annals of Internal Medicine, 134,* 1–11.

Taylor, C. J., Roalfe, A. K., Iles, R., & Hobbs, F. D. R. (2012). Ten-year prognosis of heart failure in the community: Follow-up data from the Echocardiographic Heart of England Screening (ECHOES) study. *European Journal of Heart Failure, 14,* 176–184.

Taylor, R. S., Ashton, K. E., Moxham, T., Hooper, L., & Ebrahim, S. (2011). Reduced dietary salt for the prevention of cardiovascular disease. *The Cochrane Database of Systematic Reviews,* (7), CD009217.

The SPRINT Research Group. (2015). A randomized trial of intensive versus standard Blood-pressure control. *The New England Journal of Medicine, 373*(22), 2103–2116.

Uhlig, K., Patel, K., Ip, S., Kitsios, G. D., & Balk, E. M. (2013). Self-measured blood pressure monitoring in the management of hypertension: a systematic review and meta-analysis. *Annals of Internal Medicine, 159*(3), 185–194.

van den Born, B. J. H., Hulsman, C. A. A., Hoekstra, J. B. L., Schlingemann, R. O., & van Montfrans, G. A. (2005). Value of routine funduscopy in patients with hypertension: Systematic review. *British Medical Journal (Clinical Research Ed.), 331,* 73–76.

Wald, D., Law, M., Morris, J., et al. (2009). Combination therapy versus monotherapy in reducing blood pressure: Meta-analysis on 11,000 participants from 42 trials. *The American Journal of Medicine, 122,* 290–300.

Whelton, S., Chin, A. V., Xin, X., & He, J. (2002). Effect of aerobic exercise on blood pressure: A meta-analysis for randomised controlled trials. *Annals of Internal Medicine, 136,* 493–503.

Whinnett, Z. I., Afzal Sohaib, S. M. A., & Wyn Davies, D. (2012). Diagnosis and management of supraventricular tachycardia. *British Medical Journal (Clinical Research Ed.), 345,* e7769.

Wilber, J., & Barrow, J. (1972). Hypertension: Community problem. *The American Journal of Medicine, 52,* 653–663.

Williams, B., MacDonald, T. M., Morant, S., et al. (2015). Spironolactone versus placebo, bisoprolol, and doxazosin to determine the optimal treatment for drug-resistant hypertension (PATHWAY-2): a randomised, double-blind, crossover trial. *Lancet, 386*(10008), 2059–2068.

Wolff, A., & Cowan, C. (2009). 10 steps before your refer for palpitations. *The British Journal of Cardiology, 16,* 182–186.

World Health Organisation. (n.d.). *Global Health Observatory. Raised blood pressure.* Retrieved from www.who.int/gho/ncd/risk_factors/blood_pressure_prevalence_text/en/.

Writing Group of the PREMIER Collaborative Research Group. (2003). Effects of comprehensive lifestyle modification on blood pressure control. *JAMA: The Journal of the American Medical Association, 289,* 2083–2093.

Xin, X., He, J., Frontini, M. G., Ogden, L. G., Motsami, O. I., & Whelton, P. K. (2001). Effects of alcohol reduction on blood pressure: A metaanalysis of randomized controlled trial. *Hypertension, 38,* 1112–1117.

Zhao, P., Xu, P., Wan, C., & Wang, Z. (2011). Evening versus morning dosing regimen drug therapy for hypertension. *The Cochrane Database of Systematic Reviews,* (10), CD004184.

8

Respiratory Problems

HILARY PINNOCK

CHAPTER CONTENTS

Asthma

Diagnosis (see Appendices)

- The probability of asthma is assessed from a structured clinical assessment, supported by lung function tests and the diagnosis confirmed by response to treatment (BTS/SIGN, 2016). The process should be clearly documented so that the evidence for the diagnosis is clear to future users of the clinical record.
- Structured clinical assessment:
  1. Variable symptoms of coughing, wheezing, chest tightness, and shortness of breath.
  2. Symptoms are episodic, often worse at night and are commonly triggered by viral infections, exercise, and allergy.
  3. An historical record of significantly lower peak flows during symptomatic episodes provides objective evidence of variability.
  4. A personal or family history of atopy supports the diagnosis.
  5. Absence of symptoms, signs or clinical history to suggest alternative diagnoses.
- *Lung function tests:*
  1. *Evidence of airflow obstruction.* The presence and severity of airflow obstruction can be assessed by spirometry,

93

GUIDELINES

BTS/SIGN, 2016

British Thoracic Society/Scottish Intercollegiate Guideline Network. (2016). *British guideline on the management of asthma. SIGN guideline 153.* Available at www.brit-thoracic. org.uk; See https://www.sign.ac.uk/assets/sign153_figure1_ diagnostic_algorithm.pdf. See also Appendices 11A–D.

GINA, 2018

The Global Initiative on Asthma. (2018). *Asthma prevention and management: A practical guide for public health officials and health care professionals.* Available at www.ginasthma.com.

NICE, 2017

National Institute for Health and Clinical Excellence. (2017). *Asthma: diagnosis, monitoring and chronic asthma management.* Available from nice.org.uk/guidance/ng80.

ARIA, 2010

Brożek, J. L., Bousquet, J., Baena-Cagnani, C. E., et al. (2010). Allergic Rhinitis and its Impact on Asthma (ARIA) guidelines: 2010 revision. *Journal of Allergy and Clinical Immunology, 126,* 466–476. Available at http://www.euforea .eu/assets/pdfs/aria/2010-ARIA-Report.pdf.

BSACI, 2017

Scadding, G. K., Kariyawasam, H. H., Scadding, G., et al. (2017). BSACI guideline for the diagnosis and management of allergic and non-allergic rhinitis (Revised Edition 2017; 2007). *Clinical & Experimental Allergy, 47,* 856–889. Available from http://www.bsaci.org/Guidelines/rhinitis-2nd-edition-guideline.

BTS Emergency Oxygen Guidelines, 2017

O'Driscoll, B. R., Howard, L. S., Earis, J., et al. (2017). BTS guideline for oxygen use in adults in healthcare and emergency settings. *Thorax, 72*(Suppl 1), ii1–ii90.

but because asthma is a variable condition, asymptomatic patients will commonly have normal lung function. This does not exclude asthma.

2. *Objective evidence of variability.* Diurnal variation greater than 20% may conveniently be demonstrated by recording morning and evening peak flows over 2 weeks and demonstrating the typical sawtooth pattern. A fall in peak flow exceeding 20% when the patient next meets his or her trigger, or an increase over 20% in response to treatment, may be noted as part of home charting. Note that a normal peak flow at a consultation does not exclude the diagnosis of asthma. Asthma is a variable condition, and readings need to be taken over time to check for variability.

3. *A formal reversibility test.* If the presenting lung function is obstructive or the patient is symptomatic, it may be possible to demonstrate a significant response to a single dose of a β-2 agonist or a 6-week course of inhaled steroids. An increase in forced expiratory volume in 1 second (FEV_1) greater than 400 mL or an increase in peak flow over 20% suggests asthma.

4 *Fractional exhaled nitric oxide* (FeNO) can be measured if facilities are available. Levels of exhaled nitric oxide are raised in conditions that cause eosinophilic inflammation, and therefore raised levels support, but do not prove, a diagnosis of asthma.

- The probability of asthma is based on a structured clinical assessment supported by investigations:

  1. *High probability of asthma.* Commence a carefully monitored initiation of treatment with a moderate dose of inhaled steroids, and monitor the response, both symptomatically and with repeated measures of lung function. A good response confirms a diagnosis of asthma. A poor response, if inhaler technique and compliance are good, should lead to reconsideration of the diagnostic possibilities.

  2. *Low probability of asthma.* Investigate and treat for the more probable diagnosis, reconsidering asthma in those who do not respond.

  3. *Intermediate probability of asthma.* If the diagnosis is not clear, or the response to asthma treatment is poor, arrange further investigations. Spirometry is the pivotal test as the differential diagnosis and approach to management depends on whether the patient has airflow obstruction. Consider referral for further tests, potentially including FeNO, if the diagnosis remains unclear.

Diagnosis of Asthma in Children

The diagnosis of asthma in children follows a similar process of establishing probabilities and observing the response to a trial of treatment (BTS/SIGN, 2016). There are, however, some specific caveats:

- Clarify what parents mean when they use the word *wheeze* (Cane, Ranganathan, & McKenzie, 2000).
- Assess on the basis of symptoms supplemented by lung function tests. Children under 7 cannot reliably use a peak flow meter, though school-age children can usually perform spirometry if encouraged by a skilled technician.
- A period of watchful waiting may be appropriate for children who cannot perform spirometry and who are minimally symptomatic.

Diagnosis of Asthma in Infants

Wheezy infants present particular diagnostic difficulties, and there is little evidence-based data to guide decisions.

- *Exclude serious pathology* (e.g., cystic fibrosis, congenital heart defects, inhaled foreign body, oesophageal problems). Referral to a paediatrician is appropriate if the diagnosis is in doubt.
- *Distinguish between asthma and viral-associated wheeze* (Table 8.1). This can be a difficult distinction to make, and the diagnosis may only be clear in retrospect, as children with viral-associated wheeze will usually lose that tendency by the time they reach school age.

  1. Consider risk factors and the clinical history.
  2. Record the presence of wheeze heard by a health professional.
  3. A carefully supervised trial of treatment (e.g., inhaled steroids for 8 weeks) may be helpful (Bush, 2000;

TABLE 8.1	Distinguishing Between Asthma and Viral-Associated Wheeze	
Suggestive of Asthma	**Suggestive of Viral-Associated Wheeze**
Family or personal history of atopy	Prematurity, small for dates
	Maternal smoking
Cough and wheeze not associated with viral illness	Cough and wheeze only with viral infections
Good response to treatment and relapse on cessation of treatment	Poor response to treatment

Cochran, 1998). Doses up to beclomethasone 200 μg daily, budesonide 200 μg daily, or fluticasone 100 μg daily via a spacer ± mask may be needed to overcome practical problems with delivering inhaled therapy to very young children.

4. A poor response to therapy makes asthma unlikely, and treatment should be stopped.

5. A good response to therapy should be confirmed by a stepped withdrawal of treatment to exclude coincidental improvement.

Management

General Measures

- Advise on the avoidance of triggers:
  1. Asthma UK and Allergy UK produce useful information for patients about allergen avoidance.
  2. Common allergens include pets, especially cats, house dust mite, and pollen.
  3. Current chemical and physical measures for reducing house dust mite allergen have not been shown to be effective (Gøtzsche & Johansen, 2008).
  4. Rhinitis is a common comorbidity and may be effectively treated with intranasal steroids (Scadding, 2017; Taramarcaz & Gibson, 2003).
  5. Adults in whom an occupational cause for their symptoms is suspected should be referred.
- Encourage smoking cessation. Both active and passive smoking status should be documented and support offered to those wishing to quit.
- Consider drug effects:
  1. Beta-blockers (systemic or topical eye drops) are contraindicated.
  2. Asthmatics sensitive to aspirin should not use nonsteroidal antiinflammatory drugs (NSAIDs).

Therapeutic Management (see Appendices 11A and 11B)

- Patients should start treatment at the step most appropriate to the severity at presentation (see Appendices 11A–C) (BTS/SIGN, 2016; GINA, 2018).

- *Inhaled steroids* are are recommended as the first treatment step for almost all people with symptomatic asthma (BTS/SIGN, 2016). Regular treatment improves lung function, reduces symptoms, reduces use of rescue bronchodilation, and reduces the risk of exacerbations (Adams, Bestall, & Jones, 1999; Adams, Bestall, Lasserson, Jones, & Cates, 2008; Adams et al., 2005).

- The correct dose of inhaled steroids is the lowest dose compatible with asthma control. Many adults will be controlled on a low dose: beclomethasone or budesonide 400 μg daily or fluticasone 250 μg daily. BTS/SIGN, 2016 has a useful table of comparative doses.

- Discuss attitudes to regular treatment. Compliance with inhaled steroid treatment is poor (van Staa, 2003) and may be improved by strategies such as simplifying regimes, regular supportive review, and reminders (Nieuwlaat, 2014).

- Explain ways of avoiding local side effects. Candidiasis may be reduced by rinsing the mouth after administration or using a spacer device; dysphonia may be improved by reducing the dose.

- Reassure patients that important systemic side effects are unlikely at moderate doses (beclomethasone or budesonide <800 μg daily, fluticasone <500 μg daily). In children, despite an initial reduction in growth velocity, final height is not significantly affected (Agertoft & Pedersen, 2000; Childhood Asthma Management Program Research Group, 2000). High-dose inhaled steroids (beclomethasone or budesonide >1500 μg daily, fluticasone >750 μg daily) have an increased risk of adrenal suppression, cataracts, reduced bone density, and bruising (Adams et al., 2008), and risks should be balanced against benefits (e.g., in people using frequent/regular oral steroids to treat exacerbations).

- *β-2 agonists* provide symptomatic relief and should be prescribed on an *as required* basis (BTS/SIGN, 2016; Walters, Walters, Gibson, & Jones, 2003).

- Patients requiring relief medication more than three times a week, waking with asthma on more than one night a week, or who have had an exacerbation in the last 2 years should be offered regular prevention with inhaled steroids.

- Exercise-induced asthma that persists despite good asthma control with inhaled steroids may be prevented by using a β-2 agonist prior to exercise.

- *Long-acting β-2 agonists* are given regularly twice a day as add-on therapy to people whose asthma is not controlled on inhaled steroids (BTS/SIGN, 2016). The addition of long-acting β-2 agonists improves lung function and symptom control compared with increasing the dose of inhaled steroids (Pauwels et al., 1997; Walters, Gibson, Lasserson, & Walters, 2007).

- In response to concerns about a very small increased risk in patients on long-acting β-2 agonists of asthma deaths (Nelson et al., 2006), and serious adverse events (Cates & Cates, 2008; Cates, Cates, & Lasserson, 2012; Cates, Oleszczuk, Stovold, & Wieland, 2012), guidelines emphasize the importance of maintaining an adequate dose of inhaled steroids. Patients should be counselled appropriately.

- Combination inhalers have the advantage of ensuring that patients cannot take long-acting β-2 agonists without taking inhaled steroids and simplify treatment regimes, but with the disadvantage of that it is more difficult to adjust the dose of individual components.
- Flexible use of a budesonide/formoterol combination as a rescue medication in addition to regular use as a pre-venter therapy is an effective treatment option for selected adult patients who are poorly controlled with inhaled corticosteroids (ICS) and β-2 agonists. Careful self-management education about this strategy is required.

Leukotriene Antagonists

- Leukotriene antagonists are mediator antagonists that are an option as an add-on therapy (BTS/SIGN, 2016; Chauhan, 2017; NICE 2017). A review concluded that although they were less effective than long-acting β-2 agonists in relieving symptoms over 12 weeks, the reduc-tion in exacerbations over 2 years was similar, with some studies showing an improved safety profile (Joos et al., 2008).
- A trial in primary care demonstrated that, in real-life practice, when factors such as patient preference for inhal-ers or tablets, ability to use inhalers, attitudes to steroids, and adherence may all influence effectiveness, there may be little difference between long-acting β-2 agonist or leukotriene antagonist treatment options (Price et al., 2011).
- Leukotriene antagonists are recommended as the first line add-on therapy for children under 5 years.

Other Therapeutic Options

- Sodium cromoglicate may have a small overall treatment effect but should not be first line treatment for the pre-vention of asthma (van der Wouden et al., 2008).
- A short rescue course of oral steroids may be needed at any time and at any step, but frequent use should prompt referral to a respiratory physician.

Management of Adults and Children 5 Years and Over Not Controlled on a Moderate Dose of Inhaled Steroids and Initial Add-on Therapy

- There is little evidence to guide treatment in patients poorly controlled on moderate doses of inhaled steroid/long-acting β-2 agonists. Options include a trial of a second add-on treatment (e.g. a long acting muscarinic receptor antagonist [NICE 2017; BTS/SIGN 2016) or high dose inhaled steroid.
- Consider referring patients requiring additional add-on therapy for specialist advice, especially if control remains poor.

Devices

The effectiveness of inhaled therapy depends on inhaler technique and the particle size produced by the device. Inhaler devices should be selected for individual patients, taking the following into consideration (Table 8.2):

1. *The patient's ability to use a device.* This should always be checked before an inhaler is prescribed and rechecked regularly. Only a minority of patients using a metered dose inhaler have adequate inhaler technique, with slightly better performance for other devices (Brocklebank et al., 2001). Technique should be observed for:
   - the patient's inspirational flow rate compared to flow rate recommended by the manufacturer for efficient actuation and inhalation;
   - hand/breath coordination;
   - ability to follow the instructions for correct use.
2. *The drug and dosage required.* High doses of inhaled steroid should be given by a spacer device.
3. *National Institute for Health and Care Excellence (NICE) guidelines* recommend the use of spacers (with masks for infants) for children under the age of 5 (NICE, 2000). Older children will need careful assessment of ability to use inhalers, and more portable options will be appro-priate especially for bronchodilators (NICE, 2002).
4. *Patient preference* and lifestyle issues may be relevant.
5. *Cost of the device.*

TABLE 8.2 Choice of Inhaler Device for Different Age Groups

Age	Devices to Consider	Comments
Preschool	MDI + spacer (with a mask for infants)	NICE (2000) recommendation
School-age	MDI + spacer	Recommended for inhaled steroids because it reduces oral deposition (NICE, 2002)
	Dry powder devices	Once a child has adequate inspiration and can be relied on not to blow by mistake
	Breath-actuated devices	Once inspiration is adequate
Adults	MDI	If technique is adequate. Should be used with a spacer to deliver high doses of inhaled steroid
	Breath-actuated devices Dry powder devices	

MDI, Metered dose inhaler.

Regular Review

Patients receiving treatment for asthma should be reviewed regularly by a general practitioner (GP) or trained asthma nurse. Reviews in primary care, conducted face to face or, if a patient is well controlled, by telephone (Pinnock et al., 2003, 2007), should encompass the following three steps (Pinnock et al., 2010):

1. Assessing current symptom control and risk of future exacerbations
   - *Specific morbidity questions.* Patients underreport symptoms (Haughney, Barnes, Partridge, & Cleland, 2004), and control should be assessed by asking standard morbidity questions at every asthma review consultation. The Royal College of Physicians' "three questions" (RCP3Qs) is an example of a suitable morbidity score (Table 8.3) (Pearson & Bucknall, 1999). A negative response to all three questions suggests good control; two or more positive answers indicate poor control (Pinnock et al., 2012). Interpret responses in the light of other indicators of control (such as exacerbations and use of reliever inhalers).
   - *Patient reported outcomes: control questionnaires.* Short questionnaires for measuring asthma control include the Asthma Control Questionnaire (Juniper, Bousquet, Abetz, & Bateman, 2006) and the Asthma Control Test (Nathan et al., 2004). They are validated for patient self-completion: completion with the assistance of the clinician may influence the result (Honkoop et al., 2013).
   - *Use of relief medication.* Good asthma control is associated with little or no need for short-acting β-2 agonists. At the other extreme, use of 12 or more canisters a year is a marker for at-risk asthma (RCP, 2104).
   - Assessing risk of future attacks. A history of acute attacks, poor current symptom control, over-reliance of short-acting beta agonists are key predictors of future risk (Buelo 2018).

2. Responding to the assessment by identifying reasons for poor control and adjusting the management strategy accordingly (Ryan, 2013):
   - Systematically consider reasons for poor control (Haughney, 2008):
     - *Review the diagnosis.* Failure to respond to treatment may indicate an incorrect diagnosis or the development of a comorbid cause for symptoms.
   - *Check and correct inhaler technique.*
   - *Assess and address adherence.* Patients and their healthcare professionals both overestimate compliance with regular medication. Nonjudgmental questioning and achieving concordance about treatment goals may improve compliance (Nieuwlaat, 2014).
   - *Ask about and treat rhinitis.* Three quarters of people with asthma have symptoms of rhinitis, which should be treated with nasal steroids (Brożek, 2010; Scadding, 2017; Thomas & Price, 2008).
   - *Assess smoking status, and offer cessation advice.* Smoking adversely affects asthma control. This may be because of a comorbid diagnosis of chronic obstructive pulmonary disease (COPD) or because smoking reduces the effectiveness of inhaled steroids. Persistent smokers need relatively high doses of inhaled steroids.
   - *Adjust therapy according to evidence-based guidelines.*

3. Exploring patients' ideas, concerns, and expectations and supporting self-management to facilitate ongoing control:
   - *Supported self-management.* Every asthma consultation is an opportunity to review, reinforce, and extend asthma knowledge and skills (BTS/SIGN, 2016). Education should aim to empower patients to be in control of their asthma and should include the provision of written personalised asthma action plans (Pinnock, 2015).

Personal Asthma Action Plans

Education involving self-monitoring and written action plans reduces hospitalizations, emergency consultations, days off work or school, and nocturnal asthma (Pinnock, 2017; Pinnock, 2015).

- Offer all people with asthma a written asthma action plan, which should (Gibson & Powell, 2004):
  1. be tailored to the individual patient, taking into account his or her clinical condition and preference for autonomy;
  2. involve self-monitoring, based on symptoms and/or peak flows;
  3. provide information about features that would indicate the patient's asthma is worsening;
  4. advise what action the patient should take, including information about increasing inhaled steroids and starting oral steroids. A recent trial in adults shows that a four fold increase in ICS at the onset of an attack reduces the risk of need a course of oral steroids by 20% (McKeever, 2018).

TABLE 8.3	Royal College of Physicians Three Questions (Pearson & Bucknall, 1999)	
In the past week (or month):		
1	Have you had difficulty sleeping because of your asthma symptoms (including cough)?	Yes/No
2	Have you had your usual asthma symptoms during the day (cough, wheeze, tight chest, or breathlessness)?	Yes/No
3	Has your asthma interfered with your usual activities (housework, work or school, etc.)?	Yes/No

An example of a PAAP can be found on the Asthma UK website: www.asthma.org.uk.

Indications for Outpatient Referral

Referral to a respiratory physician or paediatrician should be considered if:

1. the diagnosis is not clear;
2. the patient is not controlled with moderate doses of inhaled steroids ± add-on therapy and inhaler technique is satisfactory;
3. there is a possibility of occupational asthma;
4. there is a history of life-threatening attacks or brittle asthma.

Acute Asthma

Acute Asthma in Adults and Schoolchildren (See Appendices 11C and D)

Delay is the most common factor identified as contributing to asthma deaths, often related to a failure on the part of the patient or the healthcare professional to appreciate the severity of the attack (British Thoracic Association, 1982; RCP, 2014). The presence of psychosocial problems is an important risk factor for fatal asthma (Mohan et al., 1996).

- Assess severity and record the following:
  1. *General condition.* Inability to speak, exhaustion, cyanosis, and a silent chest indicate life-threatening asthma.
  2. *Peak flow.* Peak flow (PF) at presentation should be compared with the patient's best (or predicted, if best is not known):
     - PF <75% of best = moderate asthma exacerbation;
     - PF <50% of best = acute severe asthma;
     - PF <33% of best = life-threatening asthma.
  3. *Respiratory rate (RR).* More than 25/min in adults, more than 30/min in children over 5 years indicates severe asthma.
  4. *Heart rate (HR).* More than 110/min in adults, more than 125/min in children over 5 years indicates severe asthma.
  5. *Oximetry.* Oxygen saturation below 92% should alert the clinician to the severity of the attack.
- Act promptly to provide relief:
  1. *Bronchodilation.* Administer multiple (10) doses of a β-2 agonist through a large-volume spacer, or 5 mg salbutamol/by oxygen-driven nebulizer (Cates, Welsh, & Rowe, 2013). Nebulizers require flow rates of 6 to 8 L/min. Consider adding ipratropium in severe or life-threatening asthma.
  2. *Oxygen.* Give at high flow rates for severe or life-threatening asthma aiming to maintain oxygen saturation between 94% and 98% (O'Driscoll, 2017).
  3. *Systemic steroids.* Steroids reduce mortality, relapses, subsequent hospital admission, and the requirement for β-2 agonist therapy (Rowe, Spooner, Ducharme, Bretzlaff, & Bota, 2001; Smith, Iqbal, Rowe, &

N'Diaye, 2003). Early administration improves outcomes; prednisolone 40 to 50 mg for adults, 30 mg for children should therefore be given at the consultation. The number needed to treat (NNT) to prevent one admission in patients with severe asthma is five (95% confidence interval [CI] 4 to 7).
  4. *Assess response.*

Note: Infective triggers for acute asthma are usually viral. Routine prescribing of antibiotics is not appropriate.

- Arrange further care.
  - Admit:
    1. patients with life-threatening asthma;
    2. patients with severe asthma who do not respond to emergency bronchodilation.

    Other factors (e.g., time of day, social situation, previous history of severe attacks) will influence the decision to admit.
  - Instructions:
    1. Bronchodilation may be repeated 3 to 4 hourly. Ideally, progress should be monitored by peak flow.
    2. Prednisolone 40 to 50 mg daily for at least 5 days or until recovery (adults); 30 mg daily for 3 days (children).
    3. Increase (or recommence) inhaled steroids until full control is regained.
    4. Ensure the patient knows when and how to call further medical help.
- Provide early follow-up. Arrange to assess progress within 24 hours (severe asthma) or 48 hours (uncontrolled asthma).
- Review. Arrange for a review of overall asthma control and revision of wriiten Personal Asthma Action Plan.

Acute Asthma in Preschool Children (See Appendix 11D)

- *Assess severity and record:* exhaustion, agitation, drowsiness, too breathless to feed, use of accessory muscles, RR over 40/min or HR over 140/min are signs of severe asthma.
- *Act promptly to provide relief*
  1. *Bronchodilation:* multiple (10) doses of a β-2 agonist through a large volume spacer ± mask or 2.5 mg salbutamol or 5 mg terbutaline by nebulizer.
  2. *Oxygen* should be given at high flow rates.
  3. *Systemic steroids:* Consider soluble prednisolone 20 mg.
  4. *Assess response:* RR, HR, and general condition.
- Arrange further care. Admit:
  1. children with any features of severe or life-threatening asthma;
  2. children who do not respond to bronchodilation or who relapse within 3 hours.
- Poor social circumstances or a previous history of a severe attack should lower the threshold for admission.
- Children not admitted should be given prednisolone 20 mg for 3 days and clear instructions for review.

Lower Respiratory Tract Infection

GUIDELINES

NICE (RTI), 2008

National Institute for Health and Clinical Excellence. (2008). *Prescribing of antibiotics for self-limiting respiratory tract infections in adults and children in primary care. NICE clinical guideline 69.* Available at www.nice.org.uk/cg69.

BTS (CAP), 2009

Lim, W. S., Baudouin, S. V., George, R. C., et al. (2009). BTS guidelines for the management of community acquired pneumonia in adults: Update 2009. *Thorax, 64,* Siii1–55. [A primary care summary is available at https://www.nature.com/articles/pcrj201014.]

- The majority of previously well patients who present to their GP with acute respiratory symptoms have a self-limiting illness (Macfarlane et al., 2001).
- Fewer than half have evidence of a bacterial infection (Macfarlane et al., 1993, 2001).
- Without a chest x-ray (CXR), identification of the 6% of patients with lower respiratory tract infection who have community-acquired pneumonia is imprecise, with no individual sign or symptom being reliably predictive (Macfarlane et al., 2001; Metlay, Kapoor, & Fine, 1997).

Clinical Assessment

The aim of the initial history and examination is to identify patients with, or at risk of developing, severe or complicated illness.

- *Identify high-risk groups.* The risk of pneumonia increases with age and in institutionalized patients. Clinical features are less reliable in the elderly.
- *Ask about comorbidity.* Premorbid conditions that increase the risk of pneumonia include COPD (with increased risk in patients using inhaled steroids), congestive heart failure, neurologic disease, diabetes, alcoholism, and chronic renal or hepatic failure (Farr et al., 2000).
- *Examine the chest.* The presence of localized chest signs is positively correlated with radiographic evidence of pneumonia, but their absence does not exclude the diagnosis (Macfarlane et al., 2001; Metlay et al., 1997).
- *Assess severity.* Fever above 40°C, RR over 30/min, BP below 90/60, pleuritic chest pain, or confusion indicate severe infection (Ewig, Schafer, & Torres, 2000; Fine et al., 1996) and should prompt referral.
- *Assess oximetry.* An oxygen saturation below 92% indicates significant hypoxia and should prompt referral.

Investigations

Investigations are rarely needed in primary care, but consider:
1. CXR may be indicated if there are focal chest signs and in high-risk patients or those with signs of severe disease even in the absence of focal chest signs. Persistence of systemic illness, the development of unexpected symptoms (e.g., haemoptysis or pleuritic pain), or failure of respiratory symptoms to resolve should prompt investigation;
2. a raised C-reactive protein (CRP) (>50 mg/L) is positively correlated with radiographic evidence of pneumonia, but is of no value in assessing severity;
3. a raised blood urea (>11 mmol/L) and a leukocytosis (>20,000 white blood cells [WBC]/mL) or leukopenia (<4000 WBC/mL) indicate severe infection and should prompt urgent referral (Ewig et al., 2000; Fine et al., 1996).

Management of *Well* Patients With Lower Respiratory Tract Symptoms Without Focal Chest Signs

- Once patients with, or at risk of developing, severe or complicated illness have been excluded, well patients with lower respiratory tract infections can be managed with explanation, self-management of symptoms, and safety netting.

- *Discuss the natural history of lower respiratory tract illness.* The provision of leaflets explaining the nature of a cough and the expected duration (up to 3 weeks) can reduce reconsultation rates (Macfarlane, Holmes, & Macfarlane, 1997). Advise that failure to improve as expected, deterioration, or development of new symptoms should prompt reconsultation.
- *Provide advice on symptomatic treatment:*
  - Paracetamol, extra fluids, hot lemon, and bed rest are commonly recommended in the acute phase, although there are no studies to validate these common remedies.
  - Zinc used within 24 hours of the onset of symptoms may improve the resolution rate of upper respiratory tract symptoms (Hemilä, 2011).
  - The use of vitamin C supplements to prevent or treat respiratory infection is unproven (Hemilä, 2013).
  - Cough medicines are often bought over the counter, but there is no evidence to support effectiveness (Chang, Cheng, & Chang, 2014).
- *Avoid prescribing antibiotics in well patients with no additional risk factors.* Benefits from antibiotics are modest and, for most patients, will not outweigh the risk of adverse effects, the costs, or the negative consequences of antibiotic resistance (Smith, Fahey, Smucny, & Becker, 2017).
  - Antibiotics increase the resolution of symptoms by about half a day.
  - Patients who also have the typical symptoms of upper respiratory tract infection (URTI) and have been ill for less than 1 week may be least likely to benefit from antibiotics.
  - Declining the request for antibiotics and educating patients on the limitations and disadvantages of treatment is effective in reducing antibiotic use, does not increase reattendance rates for the same episode, and reduces the likelihood that the patient will consult with a subsequent self-limiting respiary infection.
  - Use the opportunity to provide smoking cessation advice.

Management of Patients With Lower Respiratory Tract Symptoms With Focal Chest Signs or Where the Patient Is at High Risk of Pneumonia or Is Systemically Ill

- Community-acquired pneumonia is a potentially serious condition with a mortality in the community of less than 1%, In people admitted with pneumonia, mortality rises to between 5% and 14%.
- *Consider the need for a CXR* if the diagnosis is in doubt, there is concern about underlying pathology, or there is a poor response to treatment (Levy et al., 2010).
- *Assess oxygen saturation* and consider referral if previously healthy patients have an oxygen saturation below 94% (Levy et al., 2010).

- *Prescribe antibiotics.* Antibiotic treatment should not be delayed if a diagnosis of pneumonia is suspected:
  - Use amoxicillin 500 mg to 1 g three times a day for 5 to 7 days (doxycycline 200-mg loading dose then 100 mg daily or clarithromycin 500 mg twice a day are alternatives).
  - Doxycycline or clarithromycin are first choice for mycoplasma pneumonia.
  - Local microbiologists can provide information about local resistance patterns.
- *Consider the need for admission.* Admission is recommended in the presence of (Levy et al., 2010):
  1. signs of severe disease (fever >40°C, RR >30/min, BP <90/60, pleuritic chest pain, confusion). These parameters may be combined in the CRB-65 score to inform the decision to admit (see upcoming discussion);
  2. high-risk conditions (e.g., pneumonia associated with influenza, chickenpox);
  3. suspected complications (e.g., pleural effusion, malignancy);
  4. diagnostic uncertainty.
- *Factors that may contribute to the decision to admit are:*
  1. comorbidity (COPD, CCF, diabetes, alcoholism, chronic renal or hepatic failure);
  2. unsatisfactory social circumstances;
  3. failure to respond to first line antibiotics.
- *Arrange follow-up.* Consider investigating or admitting patients who fail to respond. Fever should settle within 2 days, but some symptoms such as cough may persist for a few weeks after the antibiotic course has finished. If symptoms persist and the initial CXR was abnormal, it should be repeated 6 weeks later to exclude underlying malignancy, especially in patients who smoke.

CRB-65 Score

CRB-65 is a validated score for assessing severity of pneumonia (Bauer et al., 2006). Score 1 point for each of the following parameters: confusion, respiratory rate over 30/min, BP below 90/60, 65 years or older.
- CRB-65 0: Low risk. Referral to hospital not indicated for clinical reasons.
- CRB-65 1 or 2: Increased risk. Consider the need for hospital assessment.
- CRB-65 3 or 4: High risk of death. Arrange urgent hospital admission.

Vaccination

- Influenza vaccine is recommended for the following groups of patients:
  - all children aged two to nine
  - those aged six months to under 65 years in clinical risk groups
  - pregnant women
  - those aged 65 years and over
  - those in long-stay residential care homes

- carers
- frontline health and social care workers

Three forms of vaccine are available:

- a quadrivalent live attenuated influenza vaccine (LAIV), administered as a nasal spray for children (excluding those with immunodeficiency or severe asthma)
- A trivalent inactivated flu vaccine for adults 65 years and over
- A quadrivalent influenza vaccines for adults under 65years.

For further details see Public Health England: Flu plan 2017/18.

- Pneumococcal vaccination is recommended for people over 65 and those with comorbidities.

Tuberculosis

GUIDELINES

National Institute for Health and Care Excellence. (2016). *Tuberculosis. NICE clinical guideline 33.* Available at https://www.nice.org.uk/guidance/ng33.

Patients with tuberculosis (TB) should be managed by physicians or paediatricians with specialist expertise in the management of TB and supported by TB nurse specialists or health visitors. The role of primary care is to:

- *Be alert to the possibility of TB.* The incidence of TB is particularly high among people born in countries with a high TB burden, with almost two-thirds of TB cases in migrants occurring within 6 years of entering the country (Public Health England, 2017). New patient medicals may be an opportunity to check the bacillus Calmette-Guérin (BCG) status of immigrants (Griffiths et al., 2007). Other high-risk groups include patients with impaired immunity (including human immunodeficiency virus [HIV]), patients on steroids, the homeless, and those dependent on alcohol or drugs.
- *Consider the diagnosis.* Symptoms of fever and night sweats, cough, weight loss, and haemoptysis should prompt investigation, though primary care clinicians should be alert to the wide range of nonspecific symtoms that occur in people with TB (Metcalf, Davies, Wood, & Butler, 2007). A CXR should be arranged and three sputum samples may be sent for microscopy, culture, and sensitivity and should be marked as "suspected TB."
- *Ensure prompt referral.* Most patients can be treated as outpatients. Inpatient care may be considered because of clinical severity or to ensure compliance with treatment regimes.
- *Encourage compliance.* Treatment regimes will involve a combination of drugs and will continue for at least 6 months. Supervision will be arranged by the hospital clinic in accordance with local policy. Directly observed therapy may be needed to ensure compliance.
- *Support the patient and family.* Information for clinicians and answers to frequently asked questions in a range of languages are available on the British Lung Foundation website (https://shop.blf.org.uk/collections/lung-health-information/products/tuberculosis) and from TB Alert (https://www.thetruthabouttb.org/professionals/patient-support/).
- *Be prepared for concerned enquiries from contacts.* Contact tracing is undertaken according to defined procedures usually by a respiratory nurse specialist. Close contacts are defined as people from the same household, close friends, or frequent visitors to the household. Most other contacts are usually casual contacts and are at considerably lower risk of infection. In the event of a local outbreak, the local Consultant in Communicable Disease can provide advice.

Chronic Obstructive Pulmonary Disease

GUIDELINES

NICE (COPD), 2010

National Institute for Health and Care Excellence. (2010). *Management of chronic obstructive pulmonary disease in adults in primary and secondary care. NICE clinical guideline 101.* Available at www.nice.org.uk/cg101.

GOLD, 2013

Global Initiative for Chronic Obstructive Lung Disease. (2018). *Global strategy for the diagnosis, management and prevention of chronic obstructive pulmonary disease.* Available at www.goldcopd.com.

Diagnosis

- The aim is to make an objective diagnosis of COPD as early as possible in the course of the disease to encourage smoking cessation and prevent progression.
- *Ask about smoking.* Smoking history may be recorded as *pack years* (i.e., 1 pack year = 20 cigarettes a day for 1 year). Note any occupational exposure (e.g., coal mining).
- *Ask about symptoms of cough, sputum production, wheeze, and breathlessness* and their impact on lifestyle. These symptoms have an insidious onset, usually after the age of 35 years, and progress slowly with little variability. Suspect bronchial carcinoma if there is haemoptysis.
- *Examine the chest.* The chest will usually be clear in mild COPD; rhonchi may develop during exacerbations and as the disease progresses. Localized signs may indicate an underlying carcinoma.
- *Record body mass index (BMI).* Low BMI is associated with a poor prognosis.
- *Check for signs of chronic hypoxia.* Cyanosis and confusion can occur with the onset of respiratory failure; ankle oedema suggests cor pulmonale.
- *Arrange spirometry.* The diagnosis should be confirmed by spirometry, which should be undertaken when the patient is stable (i.e., at least 6 weeks should have elapsed since an exacerbation). Spirometry in COPD demonstrates an obstructive pattern (forced expiratory volume in 1 second/forced vital capacity [FEV_1/FVC] <70%).

- *Consider the need to exclude asthma.* In most cases the diagnosis of COPD will be suggested by the combination of clinical history, signs, and spirometry that does not return to normal with drug therapy. In some cases, to exclude asthma, it will be important to confirm the lack of reversibility. This may be demonstrated by:
  1. a poor response (<400 mL increase in FEV_1) to bronchodilators, inhaled, or oral steroids;
  2. serial peak flow measurements showing less than 20% variability. This may be undertaken as a therapeutic trial or as a formal reversibility test.
- *Consider the need for other investigations:*
  1. A CXR should be considered at initial presentation to exclude other pathology.
  2. An oxygen saturation of less than 92%, the presence of polycythaemia or peripheral oedema suggests chronic hypoxia and should prompt referral for blood gas estimations.

Assessment of Severity

- *Postbronchodilator FEV₁* expressed as a percentage of predicted may be used to classify the severity of airflow obstruction:
  - Mild COPD is defined as FEV_1 >80% of predicted in a symptomatic patient
  - Moderate COPD is defined as FEV_1 <80% of predicted
  - Severe COPD is defined as FEV_1 <50% of predicted
  - Very severe COPD is defined as FEV_1 <30% of predicted
- *Use the MRC dyspnoea scale* to grade the degree of breathlessness (Table 8.4) (Fletcher et al., 1959).
- *Patient-reported outcomes.* Short validated questionnaires for assessing the symptomatic burden of COPD and the impact on quality of life include the COPD Assessment Test (CAT; www.catestonline.org) (Jones et al., 2009) and the Clinical COPD Questionnaire (CCQ; www/ccq/nl/) (van der Molen et al., 2003).

TABLE 8.4	MRC Dyspnoea Scale (Fletcher et al., 1959)
Grade	**Degree of Breathlessness Related to Activities**
1	Not troubled by breathlessness except on strenuous exercise
2	Short of breath when hurrying or walking up a slight hill
3	Walks slower than contemporaries on level ground because of breathlessness or has to stop for breath when walking at own pace
4	Stops for breath after walking about 100 m or after a few minutes on ground level
5	Too breathless to leave the house, or breathless when dressing or undressing

- *Composite indices.* There is increasing interest in multi-component assessments. For example, the DOSE index (D = dyspnoea, O = airflow obstruction, S = smoking status, E = exacerbation frequency) is designed for use in primary care and predicts use of healthcare resources (Jones et al., 2009). An alternative, more suited to use in secondary care, is the BODE index (B = body mass index, O = airflow obstruction, D = dyspnoea, E = exercise capacity measured by the 6-minute walk test) predicts mortality (Celli et al., 2004).

Management

- Treatment is aimed at providing the best possible relief of symptoms, preventing exacerbations, and improving quality of life. As the disease progresses, treatment levels and professional support should be stepped up to provide adequate palliation.
- *Use every opportunity to encourage the patient to stop smoking.* This is the only intervention that can prevent the accelerated decline in lung function that occurs in patients with COPD (Anthonisen, 1994; Fletcher & Peto, 1977; Kohansal et al., 2009). It is essential that patients understand the implications of continuing to smoke and the benefit of quitting—even with severe disease. Combine pharmacotherapy with appropriate support to aid quit attempts (NICE, 2006; van Schayck, Pinnock, Ostrem, Litt, & IPCRG, 2008).
- *Encourage exercise.* Exercise is a key component of all pulmonary rehabilitation programmes which have been shown to improve exercise capacity and the quality of life. Explain that breathlessness is uncomfortable but not dangerous.
- *Stress the importance of good nutrition in all patients.* Refer patients with an abnormal BMI for dietetic advice. Nutritional supplements may be recommended for underweight patients (Ferreira, Brooks, White, & Goldstein, 2012).
- *Advise vaccination.* Influenza vaccination reduces the number of patients who experience an exacerbation (Poole, Chacko, Wood-Baker, & Cates, 2006). Reactions to the vaccine are mild and transient. COPD patients are at increased risk of pneumonia and pneumococcal vaccination is recommended.
- *Provide information.* The British Lung Foundation publishes patient information about COPD (www.blf.org.uk). They also run Breathe Easy clubs in many areas.

Drug Management

Bronchodilators

- These are the cornerstone of treatment to reduce symptoms. They reduce breathlessness, improve quality of life, and reduce need for oral steroids, but have a only small effect on lung function.
- *Start with a short-acting β-2 agonist or antimuscarinic.* Both are effective in treating COPD, and there may be

a small additive effect (Appleton, Jones, et al., 2006). They should be prescribed on an *as required* basis.

- *Introduce a new drug as a therapeutic trial*, accepting improved lung function or subjective improvement, such as reduced breathlessness, improved exercise capacity, or activities of daily living as end points.
- *Add a long-acting bronchodilator* if still symptomatic. Long-acting β-2 agonists or long-acting antimuscarinics can produce a small increase in lung function and result in a reduction in breathlessness and symptom scores, and improved quality of life (Appleton, Poole, et al., 2006; Barr, Bourbeau, & Camargo, 2005; Chong, Karner, & Poole, 2012). Consider using a long-acting bronchodilator in patients who have two or more exacerbations a year. Both long-acting β-2 agonists and long-acting antimuscarinics have been shown to reduce exacerbation rates (NNT for 1 year to prevent an exacerbation: with a long-acting β-2 agonist = 24; with tiotropium = 14) (Appleton, Poole, et al., 2006; Barr et al., 2005; Chong et al., 2012).
- *Check inhaler technique* before prescribing an inhaler, choosing a device the patient is able to use (Brocklebank et al., 2001).
- *Consider using a theophylline* if control is still poor or in patients unable to use inhaled therapy. They have a modest effect on lung function and a variable effect on symptoms and exercise capacity. Side effects are frequent, limiting their value (Ram et al., 2002).

Inhaled Steroids

- Consider whether inhaled steroids are indicated:
  - Inhaled steroids do not consistently reduce the underlying rate of decline in lung function (Yang, Clarke, Sim, & Fong, 2012).
  - Inhaled steroids have been shown to reduce the exacerbation rate by 25% in patients with severe or very severe COPD (FEV$_1$ <50% predicted) and are therefore of most benefit in patients who have two or more exacerbations a year (Yang et al., 2012).
  - Prescribe inhaled steroids in patients who have both asthma and COPD (GINA & GOLD, 2017).
  - Bruising occurs more frequently in patients on inhaled steroids. There is a potential risk of osteoporosis in patients using high-dose inhaled steroids.
  - Inhaled steroids increase the risk of pneumonia with a 3-year number needed to harm (NNH) of 17 (Nannini, Lasserson, & Poole P, 2012).

Combination Therapy

- Prescribe inhaled steroids in combination with long-acting bronchodilators for patients in whom both drugs are indicated as these simplify the treatment regime and are generally cost effective.

Mucolytic Therapy

- Consider mucolytic therapy in patients with a chronic productive cough. Mucolytic therapy can improve symptoms and reduce exacerbations (Poole, Chong, & Cates, 2015).

Severe and Very Severe Chronic Obstructive Pulmonary Disease

- Patients with COPD become progressively more disabled. Regular monitoring of symptoms (e.g., with the MRC dyspnoea score) and lung function should prompt increasingly aggressive therapy.
- Offer referral to pulmonary rehabilitation. All patients with functional disability (e.g., MRC dyspnoea score 3 or more) should be encouraged to attend pulmonary rehabilitation. Rehabilitation, which may be hospital or community based, provides a multidisciplinary, holistic approach to the care of patients with COPD and has been shown to increase exercise tolerance, relieve breathlessness, and improve quality of life (McCarthy, Casey, Devane, Murphy, Murphy, & Lacasse, 2015).
- Consider the need for a high-dose bronchodilator for symptomatic relief. If this is not possible by multiple doses through a spacer device, consider referral for assessment for a home nebulizer.
- Consider referral for assessment for long-term oxygen therapy. Patients with oxygen saturation at rest below 92%, and/or with polycythaemia or peripheral oedema, should be referred for assessment for oxygen therapy. The criteria depend on lung function, blood gas estimations, and the presence of complications. In patients who are chronically hypoxic, oxygen therapy for at least 15 hours a day has been shown to improve 5-year survival (Cranston, Crockett, Moss, & Alpers, 2005). The evidence to support the use of short bursts of oxygen to relieve exercise-induced breathlessness is less clear (Nonoyama, Brooks, Lacasse, Guyatt, & Goldstein, 2007). Advice on air travel with oxygen is available from the European Lung Foundation (http://www.europeanlung.org/en/).
- Look for depression. Depression is common in COPD. Psychological treatments (e.g. cognitive behavioural therapy) and/or lifestyle interventions that include an exercise component significantly improve symptoms (Coventry et al., 2013). Some patients may require treatment with antidepressants.
- Advise disabled patients that they may qualify for benefits. Advice may be obtained from the Department of Work and Pensions.
- Offer referral for practical help as disability increases. People with severe COPD are often silent about their disease and do not ask for help (Habraken, 2008; Giacomini, DeJean, Simeonov, & Smith, 2012; Pinnock et al., 2011). Provision of appliances such as walking aids, stair lifts, and bath aids may be appropriate. Support with domestic care may be needed. A wheelchair and a disabled parking permit may prevent the COPD patient becoming housebound, and daycare may provide a break for both the patient and the carer.
- Even though accurate prognosis is difficult, consider the need for holistic assessment and supportive care. Repeated hospital admissions, comorbidity, chronic hypoxia, low BMI, and being housebound are all indicators of poor prognosis, though the slow deterioration (over years)

may make it very difficult to identify the moment for inclusion on a palliative care register (Giacomini et al., 2012; Pinnock et al., 2011). COPD patients, however, need the same attention to symptom control (especially relief of breathlessness) and support as patients dying of cancer.

- Consider therapeutic options for palliating symptoms:
  - Morphine (initial dose: morphine 5 mg 4 hourly) relieves intractable breathlessness without increasing hypoxia (Jennings, Davies, Higgins, & Broadley, 2001).
  - Cool air (e.g., from a fan) sometimes reduces the sensation of breathlessness.
  - Benzodiazepines may relieve anxiety (though first remember that high doses of β-2 agonists can aggravate anxiety).
  - Oxygen may reduce confusion due to hypoxia.
  - Chlorpromazine or haloperidol may ease confusion and restlessness.
- Offer the opportunity to discuss their prognosis and consider their preferences in the event of future exacerbations.

Indications for Referral for Specialist Advice

- For an objective diagnosis if the diagnosis is not clear, or if spirometry is not available in primary care
- Aged under 40 or rapid deterioration in symptoms of lung function
- Frequent infective exacerbations
- Onset of cor pulmonale
- Assessment for long-term oxygen therapy or regular nebulizer use
- Assessment for pulmonary rehabilitation
- The possibility of industrial disease (e.g., pneumoconiosis) or an occupational cause for the COPD

Acute Exacerbations of COPD

Although commonly due to infection, worsening of previously stable COPD may be due to the development of other pathology, including pneumonia, lung cancer, left ventricular failure, pulmonary embolism, and pneumothorax.

Assessment

- In the history ask about:
  1. onset and duration of current exacerbation;
  2. increased volume and purulence of sputum;
  3. increased wheeze and shortness of breath;
  4. increasing confusion or decreasing conscious level;
  5. condition when stable, especially the need for long-term oxygen;
  6. severity of previous exacerbations and previous admissions.
- When examining the patient look for signs of a severe exacerbation:
  1. Cyanosis, confusion, exhaustion, decreased level of activity
  2. Severity of breathlessness, use of accessory muscles, respiratory rate

3. Peripheral oedema, right heart failure
4. Low (<92%) oxygen saturation, or a reduction from the patient's normal levels
- Consider:
  1. the patient's social circumstances;
  2. the possibility of other respiratory pathology (e.g., carcinoma or TB);
  3. the possibility of nonrespiratory comorbidity. In one study, 40% of patients with an exacerbation of COPD were found to have other conditions (e.g., hypertension, CHD, diabetes); 14% had more than one condition (O'Brien et al., 2000).

Initial Treatment

- Bronchodilators to relieve breathlessness:
  1. Increase or add a β-2 agonist and/or anticholinergic drugs (McCrory & Brown, 2003).
  2. Check inhaler technique (MDI + spacer may be easiest for the breathless patient).
  3. Consider nebulized therapy for the severely breathless.
- Antibiotics are only indicated if there is increased purulence of sputum (Anthonisen et al., 1987; Ram et al., 2006). Recommended antibiotic is amoxicillin, tetracycline, or erythromycin, but prescribers should take into account any guidance issued by local microbiologists.
- *Oral steroids* increase the rate of lung function improvement over the first 72 hours of an exacerbation (Niewoehner et al., 1999; Walters, Tan, White, Gibson, Wood-Baker, & Walters, 2014). In general practice, patients with moderate or severe COPD (i.e., baseline FEV_1 <50% predicted) who have a significant increase in breathlessness should be given prednisolone in a dose of 30 mg daily for 7 to 14 days for severe exacerbations unless contraindicated.
- Diuretics may be given for peripheral oedema due to cor pulmonale.

Arrange Further Care

- Consider admission if there is:
  1. confusion, or deteriorating general condition; or
  2. cyanosis, SaO_2 below 90%, or the patient is already on long-term oxygen therapy; or
  3. severe breathlessness and poor response to treatment; or
  4. worsening peripheral oedema; or
  5. social circumstances are poor or there is an inability to cope at home.
- Arrange follow-up bearing in mind the following points:
  1. Failure to make a recovery should prompt a CXR.
  2. Smoking cessation should be encouraged and lifestyle advice given.
  3. Regular treatment should be optimized.
- Hospital at home. About one in four patients presenting to hospital emergency departments with acute exacerbations of COPD can be safely and successfully treated at home with support from respiratory nurses (Jeppesen et al., 2012). Both patients and carers preferred this *hospital at home* scheme to inpatient care.

References

Adams, N. P., Bestall, J. C., & Jones, P. (1999). Budesonide versus placebo for chronic asthma in children and adults. *Cochrane Database of Systematic Reviews*, (4), CD003274, doi:10.1002/14651858.CD003274.

Adams, N. P., Bestall, J. C., Jones, P., et al. (2008). Fluticasone at different doses for chronic asthma in adults and children. *Cochrane Database of Systematic Reviews*, (4), CD003534, doi:10.1002/14651858.CD003534.pub3.

Adams, N. P., Bestall, J. C., Lasserson, T. J., Jones, P., & Cates, C. J. (2008). Fluticasone versus placebo for chronic asthma in adults and children. *Cochrane Database of Systematic Reviews*, (4), CD003135, doi:10.1002/14651858.CD003135.pub4.

Adams, N. P., Bestall, J. C., Malouf, R., et al. (2005). Beclomethasone versus placebo for chronic asthma. *Cochrane Database of Systematic Reviews*, (1), CD002738, doi:10.1002/14651858.CD002738.pub2.

Agertoft, L., & Pedersen, S. (2000). Effect of long-term treatment with inhaled budesonide on adult height in children with asthma. *New England Journal of Medicine*, 343, 1064–1069.

Anthonisen, N. R. (1994). The Lung Health Study. Effects of smoking intervention and the use of an inhaled anticholinergic bronchodilator on the rate of decline of FEV1. *JAMA: The Journal of the American Medical Association*, 272, 1497–1505.

Anthonisen, N. R., Manfreda, J., Warren, C. P. W., et al. (1987). Antibiotic therapy in exacerbations of chronic obstructive pulmonary disease. *Annals of Internal Medicine*, 106, 196–204.

Appleton, S., Jones, T., Poole, P., Pilotto, L., Adams, R., Lasserson, T. J., et al. (2006). Ipratropium bromide versus short acting beta-2 agonists for stable chronic obstructive pulmonary disease. *Cochrane Database of Systematic Reviews*, (2), CD001387, doi:10.1002/14651858.CD001387.pub.

Appleton, S., Poole, P., Smith, B., et al. (2006). Long-acting beta2-agonists for poorly reversible chronic obstructive pulmonary disease. *Cochrane Database of Systematic Reviews*, (3), CD001104, doi:10.1002/14651858.CD001104.pub2.

Barr, R. G., Bourbeau, J., & Camargo, C. A. (2005). Tiotropium for stable chronic obstructive pulmonary disease. *Cochrane Database of Systematic Reviews*, (2), CD002876, doi:10.1002/14651858.CD002876.pub2.

Bauer, T. T., Ewig, S., Marre, R., Suttorp, N., Welte, T., & the CAPNETZ Study Group. (2006). CRB-65 predicts death from community-acquired pneumonia. *Journal of Internal Medicine*, 260, 93–101.

British Thoracic Association. (1982). Death from asthma in two regions of England. *British Medical Journal (Clinical Research Ed.)*, 285, 1251–1255.

British Thoracic Society/Scottish Intercollegiate Guideline Network. (2016). *British guideline on the management of asthma. SIGN guideline 153.* Available at www.brit-thoracic.org.uk; www.sign.ac.uk.

Brocklebank, D., Ram, F., Wright, J., et al. (2001). Comparison of the effectiveness of inhaler devices in asthma and chronic obstructive airways disease: A systematic review of the literature. *Health Technology Assessment*, 5, 1–149.

Brożek, J. L., Bousquet, J., Baena-Cagnani, C. E., et al. (2010). Allergic Rhinitis and its Impact on Asthma (ARIA) guidelines: 2010 revision. *Journal of Allergy and Clinical Immunology*, 126, 466–476. Available at http://www.euforea.eu/assets/pdfs/aria/2010-ARIA-Report.pdf.

Buelo, A., McLean, J., Julious, S., Flores-Kim, J., Bush, A., Henderson, J., et al. (2018). Pinnock H on behalf of the ARC group. Identifying the child (5–12 years) with asthma at increased risk of attacks: the At-Risk Child with asthma (ARC) systematic review of risk factors. *Thorax*, 73, 813–824.

Bush, A. (2000). Diagnosis of asthma in children under five. *British Journal of General Practice*, 8, 4–6.

Cane, R. S., Ranganathan, S. C., & McKenzie, S. A. (2000). What do parents of wheezy children understand by "wheeze"? *Archives of Disease in Childhood*, 82, 327–332.

Cates, C. J., & Cates, M. J. (2008). Regular treatment with salmeterol for chronic asthma: Serious adverse events. *Cochrane Database of Systematic Reviews*, (3), CD006363, doi:10.1002/14651858.CD006363.pub2.

Cates, C. J., & Cates, M. J. (2012). Regular treatment with formoterol for chronic asthma: serious adverse events. *Cochrane Database of Systematic Reviews*, (4), CD006923, doi:10.1002/14651858.CD006923.pub3.

Cates, C. J., Oleszczuk, M., Stovold, E., & Wieland, L. S. (2012). Safety of regular formoterol or salmeterol in children with asthma: An overview of Cochrane reviews. *Cochrane Database of Systematic Reviews*, (10), CD010005, doi:10.1002/14651858.CD010005.pub2.

Cates, C. J., Welsh, E. J., & Rowe, B. H. (2013). Holding chambers (spacers) versus nebulisers for beta-agonist treatment of acute asthma. *Cochrane Database of Systematic Reviews*, (9), CD000052, doi:10.1002/14651858.CD000052.pub3.

Celli, B. R., Cote, C. G., Marin, J. M., et al. (2004). The body-mass index, airflow obstruction, dyspnea, and exercise capacity index in chronic obstructive pulmonary disease. *New England Journal of Medicine*, 350, 1005–1012.

Chang, C. C., Cheng, A. C., & Chang, A. B. (2014). Over-the-counter (OTC) medications to reduce cough as an adjunct to antibiotics for acute pneumonia in children and adults. *Cochrane Database of Systematic Reviews*, (3), CD006088, doi:10.1002/14651858.CD006088.pub4.

Chauhan, B. F., Jeyaraman, M. M., Singh Mann, A., Lys, J., Abou-Setta, A. M., Zarychanski, R., et al. (2017). Addition of anti-leukotriene agents to inhaled corticosteroids for adults and adolescents with persistent asthma. *Cochrane Database of Systematic Reviews*, (3), CD010347, doi:10.1002/14651858.CD010347.pub2.

Childhood Asthma Management Program Research Group. (2000). Long term effects of budesonide or nedocromil in children with asthma. The CAMP study. *New England Journal of Medicine*, 34315, 1054–1063.

Chong, J., Karner, C., & Poole, P. (2012). Tiotropium versus long-acting beta-agonists for stable chronic obstructive pulmonary disease. *Cochrane Database of Systematic Reviews*, (9), CD009157, doi:10.1002/14651858.CD009157.pub2.

Cochran, D. (1998). Diagnosing and treating chesty infants. *British Medical Journal (Clinical Research Ed.)*, 316, 1546–1547.

Coventry, P. A., Bower, P., Keyworth, C., et al. (2013). The effect of complex interventions on depression and anxiety in chronic obstructive pulmonary disease: Systematic review and meta-analysis. *PLoS ONE*, 8, e60532.

Cranston, J. M., Crockett, A., Moss, J., & Alpers, J. H. (2005). Domiciliary oxygen for chronic obstructive pulmonary disease. *Cochrane Database of Systematic Reviews*, (4), CD001744, doi:10.1002/14651858.CD001744.pub.

Ewig, S., Schafer, H., & Torres, A. (2000). Severity assessment in community acquired pneumonia. *European Respiratory Journal*, 16, 1193–1201.

Farr, B. M., Woodhead, M. A., MacFarlane, J. T., et al. (2000). Risk factors for community-acquired pneumonia diagnosed by general practitioners in the community. *Respiratory Medicine*, 94, 422–427.

Ferreira, I. M., Brooks, D., White, J., & Goldstein, R. (2012). Nutritional supplementation for stable chronic obstructive pulmonary disease. *Cochrane Database of Systematic Reviews*, (12), CD000998, doi:10.1002/14651858.CD000998.pub3.

Fine, M. J., Smith, M. A., Carson, C. A., et al. (1996). Prognosis and outcome measures of patients with community acquired pneumonia: A meta analysis. *JAMA: The Journal of the American Medical Association*, *275*, 134–141.

Fletcher, C., & Peto, R. (1977). The natural history of chronic airflow obstruction. *British Medical Journal (Clinical Research Ed.)*, *1*, 1645–1648.

Fletcher, C. M., Elmes, P. C., Fairbairn, M. B., et al. (1959). The significance of respiratory symptoms and the diagnosis of chronic bronchitis in a working population. *British Medical Journal (Clinical Research Ed.)*, *2*, 257–266.

Giacomini, M., DeJean, D., Simeonov, D., & Smith, A. (2012). Experiences of living and dying with COPD: A systematic review and synthesis of the qualitative empirical literature. *Ontario Health Technology Assessment Series*, *12*, 1–47. www.hqontario.

Gibson, P. G., & Powell, H. (2004). Written action plans for asthma: An evidence-based review of the key components. *Thorax*, *59*, 94–99.

GINA & GOLD. (2017). *Asthma, COPD and Asthma-COPD Overlap*. Available from https://ginasthma.org/. (Accessed October 2018).

Global Initiative for Chronic Obstructive Lung Disease. (2013). *Global strategy for the diagnosis, management and prevention of chronic obstructive pulmonary disease*. Available at www.goldcopd.com.

Gøtzsche, P. C., & Johansen, H. K. (2008). House dust mite control measures for asthma. *Cochrane Database of Systematic Reviews*, (2), CD001187, doi:10.1002/14651858.CD001187.pub3.

Griffiths, C., Sturdy, P., Brewin, P., et al. (2007). Educational outreach to promote screening for tuberculosis in primary care: A cluster randomised controlled trial. *Lancet*, *369*, 1528–1534.

Habraken, J. M., Pols, J., Bindels, P. J. E., & Willems, D. L. (2008). The silence of patients with end-stage COPD: A qualitative study. *British Journal of General Practice*, *58*, 844–849.

Haughney, J., Barnes, G., Partridge, M., & Cleland, J. (2004). The living & breathing study: A study of patients' views of asthma and its treatment. *Primary Care Respiratory Journal*, *13*, 28–35.

Haughney, J., Price, D., Kaplan, A., et al. (2008). Achieving asthma control in practice: Understanding the reasons for poor control. *Respiratory Medicine*, *102*, 1681–1693.

Hemilä, H. (2011). Zinc Lozenges may shorten the duration of colds: a systematic review. *Open Respiratory Medicine Journal*, *5*, 51–58.

Hemilä, H., & Chalker, E. (2013). Vitamin C for preventing and treating the common cold. *Cochrane Database of Systematic Reviews*, (1), CD000980, doi:10.1002/14651858.CD000980.pub4.

Honkoop, P. J., Loijmans, R. J. B., Termeer, E. H., et al. for the ACCURATE Study Group. (2013). Comparison between an online self-administered and an interviewer-administered version of the Asthma Control Questionnaire: A cross-sectional validation study. *Primary Care Respiratory Journal*, *22*, 284–289.

Jennings, A. L., Davies, A. N., Higgins, J. P. T., & Broadley, K. E. (2001). Opioids for the palliation of breathlessness in terminal illness. *Cochrane Database of Systematic Reviews*, (3), CD002066, doi:10.1002/14651858.CD002066.

Jeppesen, E., Brurberg, K. G., Vist, G. E., Wedzicha, J. A., Wright, J. J., Greenstone, M., et al. (2012). Hospital at home for acute exacerbations of chronic obstructive pulmonary disease. *Cochrane Database of Systematic Reviews*, (5), CD003573, doi:10.1002/14651858.CD003573.pub2.

Jones, P. W., Harding, G., Berry, P., et al. (2009). Development and first validation of the COPD Assessment Test. *European Respiratory Journal*, *34*, 648–654.

Jones, R. C., Donaldson, G. C., Chavannes, N. H., et al. (2009). Derivation and validation of a composite index of severity in chronic obstructive pulmonary disease. *American Journal of Respiratory Critical Care Medicine*, *180*, 1189–1195.

Joos, S., Miksch, A., Szecsenyi, J., et al. (2008). Montelukast as add-on therapy to inhaled corticosteroids in the treatment of mild to moderate asthma: a systematic review. *Thorax*, *63*, 453–462.

Juniper, E. F., Bousquet, J., Abetz, L., & Bateman, E. D. (2006). Identifying 'well-controlled' and 'not well-controlled' asthma using the Asthma Control Questionnaire. *Respiratory Medicine*, *100*, 616–621.

Kohansal, R., Martinez-Ca, P., Agustı, A., et al. (2009). The natural history of chronic airflow obstruction revisited. An analysis of the Framingham Offspring Cohort. *American Journal of Respiratory Critical Care Medicine*, *180*, 3–10.

Levy, M. L., Le Jeune, I., Woodhead, M. A., Macfarlaned, J. T., & Lim, W. S., on behalf of the British Thoracic Society Community Acquired Pneumonia in Adults Guideline Group. (2010). Primary care summary of the British Thoracic Society Guidelines for the management of community acquired pneumonia in adults: 2009 update. *Primary Care Respiratory Journal*, *19*, 21–27.

Lim, W. S., Baudouin, S. V., George, R. C., et al. (2009). BTS guidelines for the management of community acquired pneumonia in adults: update 2009. *Thorax*, *64*, Siii1–Siii55.

Macfarlane, J., Holmes, W., Gard, P., et al. (2001). Prospective study of the incidence, aetiology and outcome of adult lower respiratory tract illness in the community. *Thorax*, *56*, 109–114.

Macfarlane, J. T., Colville, A., Guion, A., et al. (1993). Prospective study of aetiology and outcome of adult lower-respiratory-tract infections in the community. *Lancet*, *341*, 511–514.

Macfarlane, J. T., Holmes, W. F., & Macfarlane, R. M. (1997). Reducing reconsultations for acute lower respiratory illness with an information leaflet: A randomised controlled study of patients in primary care. *British Journal of General Practice*, *47*, 719–722.

McCarthy, B., Casey, D., Devane, D., Murphy, K., Murphy, E., & Lacasse, Y. (2015). Pulmonary rehabilitation for chronic obstructive pulmonary disease. *Cochrane Database of Systematic Reviews*, (2), CD003793, doi:10.1002/14651858.CD003793.pub3.

McCrory, D. C., & Brown, C. D. (2003). Anticholinergic bronchodilators versus beta2-sympathomimetic agents for acute exacerbations of chronic obstructive pulmonary disease. *Cochrane Database of Systematic Reviews*, (1), CD003900, doi:10.1002/14651858.CD003900.

McKeever, T., Mortimer, K., Wilson, A., et al. (2018). Quadrupling inhaled glucocorticoid dose to abort asthma exacerbations. *The New England Journal of Medicine*, *378*, 902–910.

Metcalf, E. P., Davies, J. C., Wood, F., & Butler, C. C. (2007). Unwrapping the diagnosis of tuberculosis in primary care: A qualitative study. *British Journal of General Practice*, *57*, 116–122.

Metlay, J. P., Kapoor, W. N., & Fine, M. J. (1997). Does this patient have community acquired pneumonia? Diagnosing pneumonia by history and physical examination. *JAMA: The Journal of the American Medical Association*, *278*, 1440–1445.

Mohan, G., Harrison, B. D., Badminton, R. M., et al. (1996). A confidential enquiry into deaths caused by asthma in an English health region: Implications for general practice. *British Journal of General Practice*, *46*, 529–532.

Nannini, L. J., Lasserson, T. J., & Poole, P. (2012). Combined corticosteroid and long-acting beta2-agonist in one inhaler versus long-acting beta2-agonists for chronic obstructive pulmonary disease. *Cochrane Database of Systematic Reviews*, (9), CD006829, doi:10.1002/14651858.CD006829.pub2.

Nathan, R. A., Sorkness, C. A., Kosinski, M., et al. (2004). Development of the asthma control test: A survey for assessing asthma control. *Journal of Allergy and Clinical Immunology, 113,* 59–65.

National Institute for Health and Care Excellence. (2000). *Guidance on the use of inhaler systems (devices) in children under the age of 5 years with chronic asthma.* Technology Appraisal Guidance No. 10. http://www.nice.org.uk.

National Institute for Health and Care Excellence. (2002). *Inhaler devices for routine treatment of chronic asthma in older children (aged 5–15 years).* Technology Appraisal Guidance No. 38. http://www.nice.org.uk.

National Institute for Health and Care Excellence. (2006). *Brief interventions and referral for smoking cessation. NICE public health guidance 1.* Retrieved from http://www.nice.org.uk.

National Institute for Health and Care Excellence. (2008). *Prescribing of antibiotics for self-limiting respiratory tract infections in adults and children in primary care.* Retrieved from www.nice.org.uk.

National Institute for Health and Care Excellence. (2010). *National clinical guideline management of chronic obstructive pulmonary disease in adults primary and secondary care.* Retrieved from www.nice.org.uk/cg101.

National Institute for Health and Care Excellence. (2016). *Tuberculosis. NICE clinical guideline 33.* Available at www.nice.org.uk; https://www.nice.org.uk/guidance/ng33.

National Institute for Health and Care Excellence. (2017). *Asthma: diagnosis, monitoring and chronic asthma management.* Available from nice.org.uk/guidance/ng80.

Nelson, H. S., Weiss, S. T., Bleecker, E. R., et al; & the SMART Study Group. (2006). The salmeterol multicenter asthma research trial: A comparison of usual pharmacotherapy for asthma or usual pharmacotherapy plus salmeterol. *Chest, 129,* 15–26.

Nicholson, P. J., Cullinan, P., Burge, P. S., & Boyle, C. (2010). *Occupational asthma: Prevention, identification & management: Systematic review & recommendations.* London: British Occupational Health Research Foundation.

Nieuwlaat, R., Wilczynski, N., Navarro, T., Hobson, N., Jeffery, R., Keepanasseril, A., et al. (2014). Interventions for enhancing medication adherence. *Cochrane Database of Systematic Reviews*, (11), CD000011, doi:10.1002/14651858.CD000011.pub4.

Niewoehner, D. E., Erbland, M. L., Deupree, R. H., et al. (1999). Effect of systemic glucocorticoids on exacerbations of chronic obstructive pulmonary disease. *New England Journal of Medicine, 340,* 1941–1947.

Nonoyama, M., Brooks, D., Lacasse, Y., Guyatt, G. H., & Goldstein, R. (2007). Oxygen therapy during exercise training in chronic obstructive pulmonary disease. *Cochrane Database of Systematic Reviews*, (2), CD005372, doi:10.1002/14651858.CD005372.pub2.

O'Brien, C., Guest, P. J., Hill, S. L., et al. (2000). Physiological and radiological characterisation of patients diagnosed with chronic obstructive pulmonary disease in primary care. *Thorax, 55,* 635–642.

O'Driscoll, B. R., Howard, L. S., Earis, J., et al. (2017). BTS guideline for oxygen use in adults in healthcare and emergency settings. *Thorax, 72*(Suppl. 1), ii1–ii90.

Pauwels, R. A., Lofdahl, C. G., Postma, D. S., et al. (1997). Effect of inhaled formoterol and budesonide on exacerbations of asthma. *New England Journal of Medicine, 337,* 1405–1411.

Pearson, M., & Bucknall, C. (1999). *Measuring clinical outcome in asthma: A patient focussed approach.* London: Royal College of Physicians.

Pinnock, H., Adlem, L., Gaskin, S., et al. (2007). Accessibility, clinical effectiveness and practice costs of providing a telephone option for routine asthma reviews: Controlled implementation study. *British Journal of General Practice, 57,* 714–722.

Pinnock, H., Bawden, R., Proctor, S., et al. (2003). Accessibility, acceptability, and effectiveness in primary care of routine telephone review of asthma: Pragmatic, randomised controlled trial. *British Medical Journal (Clinical Research Ed.), 326,* 477–479.

Pinnock, H., Burton, C., Campbell, S., et al. (2012). Clinical implications of the Royal College of Physicians three questions in routine asthma care: A real-life validation study. *Primary Care Respiratory Journal, 21,* 288–294.

Pinnock, H., Fletcher, M., Holmes, S., et al. (2010). Setting the standard for routine asthma consultations: a discussion of the aims, process and outcomes of reviewing people with asthma in primary care. *Primary Care Respiratory Journal, 19,* 75–83.

Pinnock, H., Kendall, M., Murray, S., et al. (2011). Living and dying with severe chronic obstructive pulmonary disease: Multi-perspective longitudinal qualitative study. *British Medical Journal (Clinical Research Ed.), 342,* d142.

Pinnock, H. (2015). Supported self-management for asthma. *Breathe, 11,* 98–109.

Pinnock, H., Epiphaniou, E., Pearce, G., Parke, H. L., Greenhalgh, T., Sheikh, A., et al. (2015). Implementing supported self-management for asthma: a systematic review of implementation studies. *BMC Medicine, 13,* 127.

Pinnock, H., Parke, H. L., Panagioti, M., Daines, L., Pearce, G., Epiphaniou, E., et al.; for the PRISMS group. (2017). Systematic meta-review of supported self-management for asthma: a healthcare service perspective. *BMC Medicine, 15,* 64.

Poole, P., Chong, J., & Cates, C. J. (2015). Mucolytic agents versus placebo for chronic bronchitis or chronic obstructive pulmonary disease. *Cochrane Database of Systematic Reviews*, (7), CD001287, doi:10.1002/14651858.CD001287.pub5.

Poole, P., Chacko, E. E., Wood-Baker, R., & Cates, C. J. (2006). Influenza vaccine for patients with chronic obstructive pulmonary disease. *Cochrane Database of Systematic Reviews*, (1), CD002733, doi:10.1002/14651858.CD002733.pub2.

Price, D., Musgrave, S. D., Shepstone, L., et al. (2011). Leukotriene antagonists as first-line or add-on asthma-controller therapy. *New England Journal of Medicine, 364,* 1695–1707.

Public Health England. *Tuberculosis in England. 2017 report (presenting data to end of 2016).* https://assets.publishing.service.gov.uk/government/uploads/system/uploads/attachment_data/file/686185/TB_Annual_Report_2017_v1.1.pdf.

Ram, F. S. F., Jones, P., Jardim, J., Castro, A. A., Atallah, Á. N., Lacasse, Y., et al. (2002). Oral theophylline for chronic obstructive pulmonary disease. *Cochrane Database of Systematic Reviews*, (3), CD003902, doi:10.1002/14651858.CD003902.

Ram, F. S. F., Rodriguez-Roisin, R., Granados-Navarrete, A., Garcia-Aymerich, J., & Barnes, N. C. (2006). Antibiotics for exacerbations of chronic obstructive pulmonary disease. *Cochrane Database of Systematic Reviews*, (2), CD004403, doi:10.1002/14651858.CD004403.pub2.

Rowe, B. H., Spooner, C., Ducharme, F., Bretzlaff, J., & Bota, G. (2001). Early emergency department treatment of acute asthma with systemic corticosteroids. *Cochrane Database of Systematic Reviews*, (1), CD002178, doi:10.1002/14651858.CD002178.

Rowe, B. H., Spooner, C., Ducharme, F., Bretzlaff, J., & Bota, G. (2007). Corticosteroids for preventing relapse following acute exacerbations of asthma. *Cochrane Database of Systematic Reviews*, (3), CD000195, doi:10.1002/14651858.CD000195.pub2.

Ryan, D., Murphy, A., Stallberg, B., Baxter, N., & Heaney, L. G. (2013). SIMPLES': A structured primary care approach to adults with difficult asthma. *Primary Care Respiratory Journal, 22,* 365–373.

Scadding, G. K., Kariyawasam, H. H., Scadding, G., et al. (2017). BSACI guideline for the diagnosis and management of allergic and non-allergic rhinitis (Revised Edition 2017; 2007). *Clinical & Experimental Allergy, 47,* 856–889. Available from http://www.bsaci.org/Guidelines/rhinitis-2nd-edition-guideline.

Smith, M., Iqbal, S. M. S. I., Rowe, B. H., & N'Diaye, T. (2003). Corticosteroids for hospitalised children with acute asthma. *Cochrane Database of Systematic Reviews,* (1), CD002886, doi:10.1002/14651858.CD0028.

Smith, S. M., Fahey, T., Smucny, J., & Becker, L. A. (2017). Antibiotics for acute bronchitis. *Cochrane Database of Systematic Reviews,* (6), CD000245, doi:10.1002/14651858.CD000245.pub4.

Taramarcaz, P., & Gibson, P. G. (2003). Intranasal corticosteroids for asthma control in people with coexisting asthma and rhinitis. *Cochrane Database of Systematic Reviews,* (3), CD003570, doi:10.1002/14651858.CD003570.

The Global Initiative on Asthma. (2018). *Asthma prevention and management: A practical guide for public health officials and health care professionals.* Available at www.ginasthma.com.

The Royal College of Physicians. (2014). *Why asthma still kills The National Review of Asthma Deaths (NRAD) Confidential Enquiry report.* RCP London. Available at https://www.rcplondon.ac.uk/projects/outputs/why-asthma-still-kills.

Thomas, M., & Price, D. (2008). Impact of co-morbidities on asthma. *Expert Review of Clinical Immunology, 4,* 731–774.

van der Molen, T., Willemse, B. W., Schokker, S., et al. (2003). Development, validity and responsiveness of the Clinical COPD Questionnaire. *Health Quality Life Outcomes, 1,* 13.

van der Wouden, J. C., Uijen, J. H. J. M., Bernsen, R. M. D., et al. (2008). Inhaled sodium cromoglycate for asthma in children. *Cochrane Database of Systematic Reviews,* (4), CD002173, doi:10.1002/14651858.CD002173.pub2.

van Schayck, O. C. P., Pinnock, H., Ostrem, A., & Litt, J., for the IPCRG. (2008). IPCRG consensus statement: Tackling the smoking epidemic -practical guidance for primary care. *Primary Care Respiratory Journal, 17,* 185–193.

van Staa, T. P., Cooper, C., Leufkens, H. G. M., et al. (2003). The use of inhaled corticosteroids in the United Kingdom and the Netherlands. *Respiratory Medicine, 97,* 578–585.

Walters, E. H., Gibson, P. G., Lasserson, T. J., & Walters, J. A. E. (2007). Long-acting beta2-agonists for chronic asthma in adults and children where background therapy contains varied or no inhaled corticosteroid. *Cochrane Database of Systematic Reviews,* (1), CD001385.

Walters, E. H., Walters, J. A. E., Gibson, P. G., & Jones, P. (2003). Inhaled short acting beta2-agonist use in chronic asthma: Regular versus as needed treatment. *Cochrane Database of Systematic Reviews,* (1), CD001285, doi:10.1002/14651858.CD001285.

Walters, J. A. E., Tan, D. J., White, C. J., Gibson, P. G., Wood-Baker, R., & Walters, E. H. (2014). Systemic corticosteroids for acute exacerbations of chronic obstructive pulmonary disease. *Cochrane Database of Systematic Reviews,* (9), CD001288, doi:10.1002/14651858.CD001288.pub4.

World Health Organisation. (2010). *Allergic rhinitis and its impact on asthma (ARIA) pocket guide.* Retrieved from www.whiar.org.

Yang, I. A., Clarke, M. S., Sim, E. H. A., & Fong, K. M. (2012). Inhaled corticosteroids for stable chronic obstructive pulmonary disease. *Cochrane Database of Systematic Reviews,* (7), CD002991, doi:10.1002/14651858.CD002991.pub3.

9

Gastroenterologic Problems

JOHN PAUL SEENAN, HEATHER LAFFERTY

CHAPTER CONTENTS

Dyspepsia, *Helicobacter Pylori*, and Gastrooesophageal Reflux Disease

> ### GUIDELINE
> National Institute for Health and Care Excellence. (2014). *Gastro-oesophageal reflux disease and dyspepsia in adults: Investigation and management. NICE clinical guideline 184.* Retrieved from www.nice.org.uk/guidance/cg184.
>   NICE Clinical Guideline. (2015). *Suspected cancer: recognition and referral.* Retrieved from www.nice.org.uk/guidance/ng12.

- Dyspepsia is not a diagnosis but rather describes a range of symptoms which should prompt doctors to consider underlying disease of the upper gastrointestinal (GI) tract. These symptoms may include upper abdominal/epigastric pain, nausea, vomiting, belching, bloating, and borborygmi (NICE, 2014b).
- Upper gastrointestinal symptoms are extremely common in the general population and the vast majority of patients have benign disease (Maconi, Manes, & Porro, 2008).
- In Western coutries, one-third of the population has symptoms of dyspepsia but of these only 25% seek medical attention; 10% will be investigated by endoscopy with only 2% of patients undergoing endoscopy being diagnosed with gastric cancer (NICE, 2004).
- In 90% of patients (including 75% of patients with *Helicobacter pylori* infection) the final diagnosis is functional dyspepsia and most disease is managed symptomatically (Briggs et al., 1996).

Alarm Symptoms

- Although benign disease predominates, the possibility of cancer is often a significant concern for patients, families, and treating clinicians.
- Alarm features have been shown to be sensitive, but not specific, in screening for upper GI carcinoma. In a UK study of 1852 patients referred to a rapid access upper GI cancer service, only dysphagia, weight loss, and age over 55 were independent significant predictors of cancer. Furthermore, age over 55 was only a significant predictor if at least one other alarm feature was present (anemia, anorexia, vomiting, dysphagia, weight loss, or high-risk features). Simple dyspepsia, even if new or continuous,

was *inversely* correlated with the finding of cancer in these older patients (Kapoor, Bassi, Sturgess, & Bodgeret, 2005).

Initial Management in Primary Care

- If a previous diagnosis has been made at endoscopy with no new alarm symptoms, then manage as previously advised.
- Encourage lifestyle modification with avoidance of food triggers, alcohol reduction, smoking cessation, and weight loss.
- Check that the patient is not taking a drug that can cause dyspepsia (e.g., aspirin or nonsteroidal antiinflammatory drug [NSAID], calcium antagonist, nitrate, theophylline, bisphosphonate, or steroid).
- Offer to test and treat *H. pylori* infection.
- Consider a 4-week empirical trial of a proton pump inhibitor (PPI) such as omeprazole 20 mg once daily in *Helicobacter*-negative patients. If symptoms recur after initial treatment, step down PPI to the lowest dose required to control symptoms. Encourage self-management and discuss using treatment on an *as required* basis.
- Offer histamine-2 (H_2) antagonists (e.g., ranitidine 150 mg twice daily) in patients with inadequate response to a PPI.

Investigation and Referral

- Patients presenting with dyspepsia and significant acute gastrointestinal bleeding require immediate (same day) specialist referral for endoscopy.
- Consider referral to exclude upper GI cancer in the following circumstances:
  - Consider a suspected cancer pathway referral (for an appointment within 2 weeks) for people with an upper abdominal mass consistent with gastric cancer.
  - Offer urgent direct access upper GI endoscopy (to be performed within 2 weeks) to assess for oesophago-gastric cancer in people with dysphagia or aged 55 and older with weight loss and upper abdominal pain, reflux, or dyspepsia.
  - Consider nonurgent direct access upper GI endoscopy to assess for oesophagogastric cancer in people with haematemesis.
  - Consider nonurgent direct access upper GI endoscopy to assess for oesophagogastric cancer in people with:
    - treatment-resistant dyspepsia, or
    - upper abdominal pain with low haemoglobin levels, or

- raised platelet count with nausea, vomiting, weight loss, reflux, dyspepsia, or upper abdominal pain, or
- nausea/vomiting with weight loss, reflux, dyspepsia, or upper abdominal pain.

H. pylori

- Gram-negative bacterium identified in 1982 by Australian scientists Barry Marshall and Robin Warren (Marshall & Warren, 1984) and recognized to affect at least 50% of the population worldwide.
- Infection usually occurs in the first few years of life and tends to persist indefinitely unless treated.
- *H. pylori* infection is recognized as a risk factor for peptic ulcer disease (reported to develop in 1% to 10% of infected patients) and gastric cancer (occurring in 0.1% to 3%) (McColl, 2010).

Testing for H. pylori

- *H. pylori* serology testing is cheap, convenient, and widely available. However, a meta-analysis of commercially available antibody assays demonstrates a sensitivity and specificity of only 85% and 79%, respectively (Loy, Irwig, Katelaris, & Talley, 1996). A further limitation is that this test has little value in confirming eradication of the infection because the antibodies persist for many months, if not longer, after eradication.
- The urea breath test (UBT) involves drinking ^{13}C- or ^{14}C-labeled urea, which is converted to labelled carbon dioxide by the urease in *H. pylori*. The infection can also be detected by identifying *H. pylori*–specific antigens in a stool sample. These tests have much better sensitivity (95%) and specificity (95%) than serologic testing (Gisbert & Pajares, 2004; Vaira & Vakil, 2001).

For both the breath test and the faecal antigen test, the patient should stop taking PPIs 2 weeks before testing, should stop taking H_2-receptor antagonists for 24 hours before testing, and should avoid taking antimicrobial agents for 4 weeks before testing, since these medications may suppress the infection and reduce the sensitivity of testing.

Test and Treat

- The rationale for *test and treat* is that *Helicobacter* eradication can effectively treat undiagnosed peptic ulcer disease in uninvestigated dyspepsia without alarm symptoms. A large randomized control study found this to be cost effective due to the reduction in unnecessary endoscopy despite having a number needed to treat (NNT) of seven patients (Ford et al., 2005).
- *H. pylori* eradication is likely to be helpful in patients with duodenal ulcer (DU), gastric ulcer (GU), gastritis, duodenitis, and (marginally) in functional dyspepsia (NNT = 15) (McColl, 2010).

Eradicating H. pylori

- NICE recommends a 1-week triple therapy regimen as first line eradication therapy. The optimum regimen consists of a full dose PPI, with amoxicillin 1 g and either clarithromycin 500 mg, or (in the case of penicillin hypersensitivity) metronidazole 400 mg and clarithromycin 250 mg, all given twice daily.
- Eradication is effective in 80% to 85% of patients on triple therapy using either antibiotic combination.
- Prescribing amoxicillin and tetracycline rarely results in *H. pylori* resistance, whereas resistance occurs after limited exposure to clarithromycin and quinolones. Exposure to metronidazole also results in *H. pylori* resistance, but this has less of an impact on the effectiveness of treatment regimens.
- *First-line therapy.* Choose the treatment regimen with the lowest acquisition cost and consider previous exposure to clarithromycin or metronidazole (it is not necessary to consider previous metronidazole exposure in patients with penicillin allergy).
- *Second-line therapy.* Should use different antibiotics to first-line therapy.
- Seek advice from a gastroenterologist if eradication of *H. pylori* is not successful with second line therapy.
- Before prescribing further therapy with quadruple or sequential therapy, it will be important to confirm that the infection is still present and to consider whether additional antimicrobial treatment is appropriate (e.g., patients with confirmed peptic ulcer disease). This is likely to require endoscopy with rapid-urease testing or gastric histology used to confirm persistent infection. It may also allow tissue to be sent for culture and sensitivity to guide antibiotic prescribing where appropriate (McColl, 2010).
- However, patients with no endoscopic evidence of significant *Helicobacter*-related pathology are likely to have functional dyspepsia and given the marginal benefit of *Helicobacter* eradication in this group (NNT =15) symptomatic management with long-term acid suppression may be more appropriate (McColl, 2010).

Confirmation of Successful Eradication

- Not routinely required but should be performed in the following circumstances:
  1. Ongoing or recurrent symptoms following eradication therapy
  2. Partial resection for gastric cancer
  3. Mucosa-associated lymphoid tissue (MALT) lymphoma
  4. Complicated peptic ulcer disease (e.g., following perforation or ulcer bleed)
- Wait 4 weeks after eradication before repeating UBT or faecal antigen.

Other Considerations and Controversies

- *H. pylori and reflux.* Chronic *Helicobacter* infection may result in atrophic gastritis and reduced acid secretion, which is protective against significant reflux disease. Most epidemiologic studies have demonstrated a negative association between *H. pylori* infection and gastroesophageal reflux disease (GORD) or its complications with the prevalence of *H. pylori* infection being lower in reflux patients than in controls. Numerous studies have now reported a strong negative association between *H. pylori* infection and the risk of adenocarcinoma of the oesophagus or gastrooesophageal junction.

- *Population screening.* Despite being identified as a carcinogen, there is no consensus that population screening and eradication of asymptomatic individuals is beneficial. Given the negative association of *Helicobacter* with oesophageal adenocarcinoma, it has been postulated that eradication might increase the risk of oesophageal adenocarcinoma due to increased acid secretion and reflux, thus potentially trading one cancer risk for another (Islami & Kamangar, 2008).
- *Other people to test and treat.* European guidelines recommend eradicating *H. pylori* infection in first-degree relatives of patients with gastric cancer and in patients with atrophic gastritis, unexplained iron deficiency anemia, or chronic idiopathic thrombocytopenic purpura (Malfertheiner et al., 2007).
- *Reinfection.* This rarely occurs and many reported cases may simply represent recrudescence (i.e., failure of initial eradication) (van der, van der Hulst, Dankert, & Tytgat, 1997).

Functional Dyspepsis

- Functional dyspepsia (FD) is defined as the presence of symptoms thought to originate in the gastroduodenal region, in the absence of any organic, systemic, or metabolic disease that is likely to explain the symptoms (Tack et al., 2006).
- Significant overlap may occur with the symptoms of irritable bowel syndrome. FD should be diagnosed based on the ROME III diagnostic criteria* and must include:
  1. One or more of the following:
     a. Bothersome postprandial fullness
     b. Early satiation
     c. Epigastric pain
     d. Epigastric burning
     AND
  2. No evidence of structural disease (including at upper endoscopy) that is likely to explain the symptoms
- Treatment of FD begins with reassurance and explanation regarding the diagnosis. The evidence base in FD is limited by high placebo response rates (20%–60%) and many small, heterogenous studies, but acid suppression remains the first line management. Meta-analyses have shown PPIs and H_2 antagonists to be effective with a NNT of 7 and 8, respectively (Moayyedi et al. 2003b). However, some of the benefit with these drugs may be from treating undiagnosed reflux. Helicobacter eradication provides only marginal benefit (NNT = 17) (Moayyedi et al., 2003a). Prokinetics (e.g., domperidone and metoclopramide) appear efficacious but are limited by risk of

---

*Criteria fulfilled for the last 3 months with symptom onset at least 6 months before diagnosis.

cardiac arrhythmia and extrapyramidal side effects such that they are largely restricted to use for short-term symptomatic relief (Moayyedi et al., 2003b).

Peptic Ulcer Disease

- The vast majority of peptic ulcer disease is caused by *H. pylori* infection or use of NSAIDs.
  - *H. pylori*–positive patients should receive eradication therapy.
  - Offer *H. pylori*–negative patients who are not taking NSAIDs a full dose PPI (e.g., omeprazole 20 mg daily) or H_2-receptor agonist for 4 to 8 weeks.
- Patients taking NSAIDs should stop where possible and be offered full dose PPI (e.g., omeprazole 20 mg daily) or H_2-receptor agonist for 8 weeks.
- Patients continuing NSAIDs should be coprescribed a PPI, counselled regarding the risk with the need for treatment reviewed regularly, and a switch to COX-2 selective NSAID considered.
- Patients with gastric ulcer should undergo repeat endoscopy after 6 to 8 weeks +/− biopsy to ensure healing and exclude malignancy.
- Consider repeat testing to confirm successful eradication in *H. pylori*–positive patients with complicated PUD (e.g., perforation or bleeding) and depending on size/extent of ulceration.

Gastrooesophageal Reflux Disease

- Is the most common chronic disease in Western countries with 25% experiencing monthly symptoms and 5% having reflux daily (Moayyedi & Talley, 2006).
- Typically presents with heartburn and regurgitation.
- Patients should be advised regarding lifestyle modification with the avoidance of food triggers (e.g., chocolate, red wine, caffeine), smoking cessation, and weight loss while acid suppression is the mainstay of pharmacologic treatment.
- In general, the differences between available PPIs are small. However, patients with an insufficient therapeutic response to the standard dose of one PPI may benefit from one of the other PPIs, an increased dose of the same PPI, or a twice-a-day PPI regimen (Boeckxstaens, El Serag, Smout, & Kahrilas, 2014).
- Consider referral for laparoscopic fundoplication in patients who have confirmed reflux unresponsive to acid suppression or in whom long-term acid suppression is not tolerated or desired.
- Complications of reflux include oeosphagitis, peptic stricture formation, columnar metaplasia (Barrett oesophagus), and oesophageal adenocarcinoma.
- Screening for Barrett oesophagus with endoscopy is not feasible or justified for an unselected population with reflux symptoms but can be considered in patients with chronic GORD symptoms and multiple risk factors (at least three of age ≥50 years, white race, male sex, obesity).

The threshold should be lowered if there is a family history of Barrett or oesophageal adenocarcinoma in one or more first-degree relatives (Fitzgerald et al., 2014).

- Due to the increased risk of oesophageal adenocarcinoma in patients with Barrett oesophagus, surveillance endoscopy is recommended (Fitzgerald et al., 2014). High-grade and persistent low-grade dysplasia may now be treated endoscopically with radio-frequency ablation (RFA), often avoiding the need for oesophagectomy (NICE, 2014a).

Dysphagia

- As discussed, urgent direct-access endoscopy should be considered in all patients presenting with dysphagia. However, many will subsequently have a normal examination or be found to have benign disease, so an approach to further investigation is required (Abdel Jalil, Katzka, & Castell, 2015).
- Patients with peptic oesophageal strictures may require balloon dilatation (perforation risk of approximately 1%) and should be maintained on long-term PPI to prevent recurrence.
- Eosinophilic oesophagitis typically presents as food bolus obstruction in young men with a history of atopy. Characteristic endoscopic appearances have been described but it should be considered in patients presenting with dysphagia even with a normal endoscopy. Proximal and distal oesophageal biopsies (showing >20 eosinophils per high-powered field) may help to confirm or refute the diagnosis. Many patients respond to acid suppression, but in others elimination diets and/or topical steroids may be required.
- Chest x-ray (CXR), should be considered in smokers to exclude extrinsic compression from a bronchial neoplasm +/− mediastinal mass.
- Barium swallow may identify the presence of a pharyngeal pouch or oesophageal dysmotility in patients with persistent dysphagia.
- Oesophageal manometry (+/− pH monitoring to exclude significant reflux) helps to diagnose motor disorders of the oesophagus (e.g., diffuse oesophageal spasm or achalasia).
- Oesophageal spasm often presents with chest pain, while achalasia is characterized by weight loss and frequent regurgitation. Heller myotomy, pneumohydralic balloon dilatation, and Botox injection to the lower oesophageal sphincter are therapeutic options that may be considered in confirmed achalasia.
- NB: Patients with *high* dysphagia (i.e., above the level of the suprasternal notch) should be considered for otorhinolaryngology referral and nasendoscopy particularly if current or ex-smokers.

Biliary/Pancreatic Disease

- Consider an urgent direct access computerized tomography (CT) scan (to be performed within 2 weeks), or an urgent ultrasound scan if CT is not available, to assess for pancreatic cancer in people aged 60 and over with weight loss and diarrhoea, back pain, abdominal pain, nausea, vomiting, constipation, or new-onset diabetes.
- If endoscopy is negative and symptoms do not respond to *H. pylori* eradication or acid suppression, consider alternative investigations such as abdominal ultrasound, amylase, and liver function tests (LFTs) which may point to biliary or pancreatic disease.
- Cholecystitis typically presents with persistent pain (lasting >6 hours) and fever. In contrast, the pain from biliary colic is intermittent and lasts from a few minutes to 1 hour before subsiding after up to 6 hours. In both cases pain classically occurs postprandially.
- Ultrasound is effective in detecting cholecystitis and/or gallstones (sensitivity >95%) (Shea et al., 1994) but inferior to magnetic resonance cholangiopancreatography (MRCP) for identifying biliary obstruction (e.g., common bile duct stones) (Singh, Mann, Thukral, & Singh, 2014).
- If biliary colic/cholecystitis is suspected or confirmed, then surgical referral should be considered. Endoscopic retrograde cholangiopancreatography (ERCP) +/− sphincterotomy is required for bile duct stones. Cholecystectomy should subsequently be performed and is also indicated for chronic cholecystitis.
- Functional disorders can also affect the gallbladder (e.g., biliary dyskinesia) and biliary tree (sphincter of Oddi dysfunction). Pharmacologic therapy seems to be ineffective, and ERCP with sphincterotomy may be required (Sgouros & Pereira, 2006).

Irritable Bowel Syndrome

GUIDELINES

National Institute for Health and Care Excellence. (2008). *Irritable bowel syndrome in adults: Diagnosis and management. NICE clinical guideline 61 (updated 2017).* Retrieved from www.nice.org.uk/guidance/cg61.
    Spiller, R., Aziz, Q., Creed, F., Emmanuel, A., Houghton, L., Hungin, P., et al. (2007). Guidelines on the irritable bowel syndrome: Mechanisms and practical management. *Gut, 56,* 1770–1798

- Irritable bowel syndrome (IBS) is a common, chronic gastrointestinal condition of unknown cause (Spiller et al., 2007).
- Of the UK population, 10% to 20% are estimated to be affected with the condition; it is twice as common in women, and the peak incidence is between ages 20 and 30 years (NICE, 2008).
- It is characterized by abdominal pain or discomfort associated with defaecation, abdominal bloating, and bowel dysfunction (constipation, diarrhoea, or both).
- IBS can also affect sleep and cause stress, anxiety, and lethargy. It is associated with reduced work productivity and quality of life.

Diagnosis and Referral

- Consider IBS in patients presenting with 6 months or more of *a*bdominal pain/discomfort, *b*loating, or *c*hange in bowel habit (think *ABC*).
- It is defined by the ROME III diagnostic criteria as recurrent abdominal pain or discomfort at least 3 days/month in the last 3 months associated with two or more of the following:
  1. Improvement with defecation
  2. Onset associated with a change in frequency of stool
  3. Onset associated with a change in form (appearance) of stool
- Symptom onset should be at least 6 months prior to diagnosis. Refer to secondary care patients with any of the following red flags:
  1. Unintentional and unexplained weight loss
  2. Rectal bleeding
  3. Family history of bowel or ovarian cancer
  4. Change in bowel habit to looser and/or more frequent stools for 6 or more weeks in patients over 60 years
  5. anaemia
  6. Abdominal/rectal masses
  7. Raised inflammatory markers

Investigation

- Full blood count (FBC), erythrocyte sedimentation rate (ESR), C-reactive protein (CRP), and antibody testing for coeliac disease (tissue transglutaminase or endomysial antibodies) should be performed in all patients with suspected IBS (NICE, 2008).
- Faecal calprotectin (FC) has been shown to be a useful screening test to differentiate between inflammatory bowel disease (IBD) and IBS. It is a calcium and zinc-binding protein within the cytosol of neutrophils and a sensitive but nonspecific marker of inflammation within the GI tract.
- NICE (2013a) recommends using FC to support the diagnosis of IBS where cancer is not suspected.
- Some studies suggest the manufacturer's FC cutoff values are too low for utilization in clinical practice with levels less than 200 μg/g rarely associated with any organic disease (Seenan, Thomson, Rankin, Smith, & Gaya, 2014).

IBS Subtypes

- Irritable bowel syndrome can be classified based on the predominant symptoms into:
  - constipation-predominant IBS (IBS-C);
  - diarrhoea-predominant IBS (IBS-D);
  - mixed-type IBS (IBS-M).
- This allows treatment to be tailored to the most troublesome symptom (Longstreth et al., 2006).

Treatment

- A positive diagnosis of IBS should be made with emphasis on reassurance and explanation.

- Patient self-management should be encouraged. This should include information on general lifestyle, physical activity, and diet (including limiting intake of insoluble fibre) (NICE, 2008).
- More detailed dietary advice is provided in the British Dietetic Association's Food Facts for IBS Factsheet, available at www.bda.uk.com/foodfacts/IBSfoodfacts.pdf. Referral to a specialist dietitian for more detailed advice and/or supervision of a low FODMAP diet may also be helpful.
- The evidence for probiotics is weak, but they may help bloating and flatulence in some patients (Didari, Mozaffari, Nikfar, & Abdollahi, 2015; DuPont, 2014; Zhang et al., 2016).
- Consider prescribing antispasmodic agents (e.g., peppermint oil) for patients with IBS (Ruepert et al., 2011).
- Laxatives should be considered for constipated patients but lactulose avoided as it may exacerbate bloating and discomfort (NICE, 2008).
- Loperamide should be the first choice antimotility agent in IBS-D.
- Consider tricyclic antidepressants (TCAs) as second line treatment for patients with IBS if laxatives, loperamide, or antispasmodics have not helped. Start at a low dose (e.g., amitriptyline 10 mg nocte) to minimize sedation. Increase dose if necessary and tolerated (but not usually >30 mg). TCAs are effective (NNT = 3) and primarily reduce pain but also have an antimotility effect with a suggestion that patients with IBS-D obtain the greatest benefit (Ruepert et al., 2011).
- Consider selective serotonin reuptake inhibitors (e.g., fluoxetine 20 mg daily) only if TCAs are ineffective (Ruepert et al., 2011).
- Linaclotide (290 μg once daily) is a guanylate cylcase C agonist (GCCA) which elevates cyclic guanosine monophosphate (cGMP), accelerating transit in the GI tract through increased fluid transit and reducing visceral hypersensitivity. It improves pain, bloating, and constipation in IBS-C and should be considered if optimal or maximum tolerated doses of laxatives from different classes have not helped in patients with constipation for 12 or more months (Chey et al., 2012; Quigley et al., 2013).
- Prucalopride (1–2 mg daily) is a highly selective serotonin 5-HT4 agonist that stimulates gut motility. It has been shown to be effective in patients (85% women) suffering from chronic constipation with an expected onset of effect within 4 weeks (Camilleri, Kerstens, Rykx, & Vandeplassche, 2008; Camilleri et al., 2010, 2016).

Inflammatory Bowel Disease

Ulcerative Colitis

- Ulcerative colitis (UC) is the most common form of inflammatory bowel disease with an incidence of 10 per 100,000 and prevalence of 240 per 100,000. This means there are an estimated 146,000 patients with UC across the United Kingdom.

GUIDELINES

National Institute for Health and Care Excellence. (2012). *Crohn's disease: Management. NICE clinical guideline 152* (updated 2016). Retrieved from www.nice.org.uk/guidance/cg152.

National Institute for Health and Care Excellence. (2013). *Ulcerative colitis: Management. NICE clinical guideline 166.* Retrieved from www.nice.org.uk/guidance/cg166.

- Presentation peaks between the ages of 15 and 25 years, with a smaller peak later in life from 55 to 65 years of age.
- UC typically affects the colon continuously from the rectum to a variable distance proximally.
- It usually presents with bloody diarrhoea, urgency, and abdominal pain. Weight loss and extraintestinal symptoms can also occur (NICE, 2013c).

Crohn's Disease

- Crohn's disease affects an estimated 115,000 people in the United Kingdom.
- One-third of cases present before the age of 21 years.
- Unlike UC, it causes transmural inflammation and can affect anywhere in the GI tract from mouth to anus.
- Historically 50% to 80% of patients require surgery due to complications such as perforation, obstruction due to stricture formation, or fistulization.
- Smoking and genetic predisposition are potential aetiological factors (NICE, 2012).

Inflammatory Bowel Disease Pharmacologic Treatment

Topical Therapy

- *Indication.* Induction and maintenance of remission in patients with UC and Crohn's colitis.
- Particularly effective in distal disease. Consider using suppositories in proctitis and enemas in patients with distal or left-sided colitis. Various enema preparations are available including liquid, foam, and retention enemas. Choice of preparation depends on patient preference.
- Topical therapy can also provide additional benefit to oral therapy in patients with extensive colitis (inflammation that extends beyond splenic flexure).
- Studies suggest aminosalicylate preparations are more effective than steroid suppositories or enemas (Marshall & Irvine, 1997; Munkholm, Michetti, Probert, Elkjaer, & Marteau, 2010).
- Topical therapy may be used to treat acute exacerbations, as *as required therapy* in patients with limited disease (proctitis) or as regular maintenance therapy.
- *Typical doses.* Mesalazine suppositories 0.75 to 1.5 g daily, mesalazine enemas 1 to 2 g daily, prednisolone rectal foam 20 to 40 mg daily (for up to 4 weeks).
- *Monitoring.* Nil required.

Oral Aminosalicylates

- *Indications:* Induction and maintenance of remission in patients with mild to moderate or moderate to severe (high dose) UC.
- Sulphasalazine and oral aminosalicylates are effective therapy for both inducing and maintaining remission in UC.
- Oral aminosalicylates are preferred due to an improved side effect profile. Diarrhoea (3%), headache (2%), nausea (2%), and rash (1%) are reported, but a systematic review has shown adverse events are similar to placebo for mesalazine.
- All aminosalicylates have been associated with nephrotoxicity (including interstitial nephritis and nephrotic syndrome). Patients receiving oral aminosalicylates should have renal function monitored at commencement and then annually (Mowat et al., 2011).
- Studies suggest that doses over 2 g are more effective at inducing remission in patients with moderate to severe disease (Ford et al., 2011). Higher doses (4.8 g versus 2.4 g daily) are associated with increased rates of response and earlier mucosal healing (Hanauer et al., 2005, 2007; Lichtenstein, Ramsey, & Rubin, 2011).
- Oral therapy can be combined with topical aminosalicylates if required.
- Except in patients with proctitis, treatment is continued indefinitely to reduce the risk of relapse (Feagan & MacDonald, 2012) and mitigate colorectal cancer risk (van Staa, Card, Logan, & Leufkens, 2005). The threshold dose to reduce colorectal cancer risk appears to be 1.2 g/day (Rubin, LoSavio, Yadron, Huo, & Hanauer, 2006). Modified release preparations should be used to reduce the pill burden, minimize dosing, and improve patient compliance.
- There is limited evidence to support the use of aminosalicylates in active Crohn's disease. However, they may have a role in reducing the risk of colorectal neoplasia in Crohn's colitis (van Staa et al., 2005) and the prevention of postoperative recurrence (Gordon, Naidoo, Thomas, & Akobeng, 2011).
- *Typical doses.* Mesalazine 2.4 to 4.8 g daily (active disease) and 1.2 to 2.4 g (maintenance).
- *Recommended monitoring.* Renal function annually.

Oral Steroids

- *Indication.* Induction of remission in patients with both UC and Crohn's disease.
- Effective in inducing remission but maintenance therapy avoided due to side effects of long-term use (e.g., hypertension, diabetes, osteoporosis, cataracts, and glaucoma).
- Patients receiving systemic steroids should be coprescribed calcium and vitamin D as bone protection.
- Budesonide can be used in both UC (Cortiment, Ferring, Budesonide MMX, colonic release) and mild to moderate ileocaecal Crohn's disease (Entocort, Tillotts or Budenofalk, Dr Falk terminal ileal release). It may be preferred due to high first-pass metabolism, low systemic absorption, and better side effect profile.

- Consider prescribing steroids in patient unresponsive or intolerant to aminosalicylates.
- *Typical doses:*
  a. Prednisolone 40 mg daily, reducing by 5 mg per week over 8 weeks to stop
  b. Budesonide MMX (Cortiment) 9 mg for 8 weeks then stop
  c. Budesonide (Entocort, Budenofalk) 9 mg for 8 weeks then 6 mg for 2 weeks and 3 mg for further 2 weeks
- *Monitoring.* Consider risk of diabetes in symptomatic patients and screening for osteoporosis, hypertension, cataracts, and glaucoma with high cumulative doses.

Thiopurines

- *Indication:* Maintenance of remission in moderate to severe UC and Crohn's disease.
- Thiopurines have demonstrated efficacy in maintaining remission for both UC (Gisbert, Linares, McNicholl, Mate, & Gomollon, 2009) and Crohn's disease (Chande, Tsoulis, & MacDonald, 2013). They may also have a role in preventing postoperative recurrence in Crohn's disease (Gordon, Taylor, Akobeng, & Thomas, 2014).
- Check thiopurine methyltransferase (TPMT) activity prior to starting. One in 300 will have absent TPMT activity, putting them at risk of life-threatening myelosuppression (Mowat et al., 2011).
- Other side effects (e.g., pancreatitis, hepatitis, myalgia, nausea, vomiting) appear to be independent of TPMT activity. Patients should also be advised regarding the increased relative risk (approximately two- to threefold) of nonmelanoma skin cancer (NMSC) and lymphoma. Advice to reduce the risk of NMSC by avoiding excessive sun exposure should be offered (see www.bad.org.uk).
- Mercaptopurine may be used in patients with normal TPMT activity who are intolerant of azathioprine without pancreatitis (Hindorf, Johansson, Eriksson, Kvifors, & Almer, 2009; Lees, Maan, Hansoti, Satsangi, & Arnott, 2008).
- Thiopurine metabolite monitoring can identify noncompliance and patients in whom coprescription of allopurinol to low-dose azathioprine may be beneficial to improve efficacy and prevent drug-induced hepatitis (Smith et al., 2012).
- Given the potential side effects of long-term use, cessation should be considered after 4 years of remission with the benefits and risks of continuing azathioprine discussed with individual patients.
- Typical doses:
  1. Azathioprine 2 to 2.5 mg/kg
  2. Mercaptopurine 1 to 1.5 mg/kg
- *Monitoring.* Please refer to local *shared-care protocol* but typically requires Full Blood Count FBC Urea and Electrolytes, U&Es, and Liver Function Tests LFTs weekly for 8 weeks then monthly for 3 months and 3 monthly thereafter.

Methotrexate

- *Indication.* Induction and maintenance therapy in patients with Crohn's disease.

- Methotrexate (MTX) has been shown to be effective as both induction (Alfadhli, McDonald, & Feagan, 2003; McDonald, Wang, Tsoulis, MacDonald, & Feagan, 2014) and maintenance therapy for Crohn's disease (Feagan et al., 2000).
- It is often used in patients who are intolerant to thiopurines.
- Coprescription of folic acid 5 mg (once a week, taken 3 days after MTX) limits GI side effects of nausea, vomiting, diarrhea, and stomatitis. Long-term concerns are hepatotoxicity, pneumonitis, and opportunistic infections.
- MTX is teratogenic and should not be used in women or men considering conception. It may persist in tissues for long periods; therefore conception should be avoided for 3 to 6 months after withdrawal of therapy (Mowat et al., 2011).
- *Monitoring.* Please refer to local shared-care protocol. Measurement of full blood count and liver function tests are generally advisable before and within 4 weeks of starting therapy, then monthly.

Biologics

- *Indication.* Induction and maintenance therapy in patients with moderate to severe UC and Crohn's disease who are unresponsive to, or intolerant of, or unsuitable for conventional therapy.
- Infliximab, adalimumab (anti–tumor necrosis factor-alpha [anti-TNFα]), and vedolizumab (antiadhesion) are now approved for use in both UC and Crohn's disease. Golimumab (anti-TNFα) is only approved for use in UC.
- Prior to initiation patients are screened for tuberculosis (TB) based on history, CXR, and blood testing (interferon gamma release assays [IGRAs]—e.g., T-SPOT or QuantiFERON-TB Gold). Human immunodeficiency virus (HIV) and hepatitis B and C serology should also be performed.
- Anti-TNFs are avoided in patients with a history of confirmed or suspected demyelination.
- *Monitoring:* Please refer to local shared-care protocol.

Surgery

Ulcerative Colitis

- *Indications:*
  1. Severe colitis refractory to medical therapy—may be emergency or semielective procedure
  2. Dysplasia/cancer
- Acutely patients will usually undergo subtotal colectomy. In some cases, an ileal pouch anal anastomosis (IPAA) will be considered at a later stage (e.g., 6 months after initial surgery).
- In UC surgery can generally be considered *curative* and removes both the risk of colorectal cancer and need for colonoscopic surveillance. Laparascopic surgery with enhanced recovery and early discharge is increasingly available.
- However, there is a morbidity and mortality attached to surgery. Furthermore, IPAA will not always be possible, and some patients may require a permanent stoma. Pouch function may be variable and increased stool frequency/ volume is expected.

- After proctocolectomy with IPAA, the median stool frequency is four to eight motions per day with a volume of around 700 mL (compared to 200 mL in healthy subjects).
- Pouchitis (nonspecific inflammation of the pouch) occurs in up to 50% of patients after 10 years. Once confirmed (endoscopically and histologically) antibiotics (metronidazole and/or ciprofloxacin) will often induce remission. This can be maintained with the probiotic VSL#3 (Singh, Stroud, Holubar, Sandborn, & Pardi, 2015). Other treatments for refractory pouchitis include Infliximab (IFX), steroids (e.g., budesonide), and removal of the pouch (van Assche et al., 2013).

Crohn's Disease

- *Indications:*
  1. Severe colitis refractory to medical therapy—subtotal colectomy or panproctocolectomy without IPAA
  2. Stricturing disease causing obstruction
  3. Crohn's mass/abscess
  4. Fistulizing disease (including perianal disease with associated sepsis)
  5. Colonic dysplasia/cancer
- Patients with perianal sepsis associated with Crohn's disease should undergo an examination under anaesthesia (EUA), ideally by a colorectal surgeon experienced in managing IBD. This will often involve drainage of any abscess/collection, laying open of fistula tracts +/− insertion of a noncutting Seton suture to allow drainage and prevent recurrent sepsis.
- Perianal disease may also be treated with antibiotics (e.g., metronidazole or ciprofloxacin). However, long-term use of these drugs is limited by concerns regarding antibiotic resistance, antibiotic-associated diarrhoea, and other side effects (e.g., neuropathy with metronidazole and seizures with ciprofloxacin).

Indications for Admission

- Patients with acute severe colitis require hospital admission for intravenous steroids +/− rescue medical therapy with infliximab (or, in cases where this is contraindicated, cyclosporin). The rate of colectomy (nonelective) for inpatients with UC remains relatively high at 10% to 15% (Royal College of Physicians, 2014). Acute severe colitis is defined according to Truelove and Witts (1955) criteria as follows:

Bowel movements (no. per day)	≥6 plus at least one of the features of systemic upset (marked with an*)
Blood in stools	Visible blood
Pyrexia (temperature >37.8°C)*	Yes
Pulse rate >90 bpm*	Yes
Anemia*	Yes
Erythrocyte sedimentation rate (mm/h)*	>30

- Other indications for admission include:
  - acute obstruction;
  - suspected intrabdominal or perianal sepsis;
  - significant GI bleeding.

Cancer Surveillance

- Patients with UC and Crohn's disease are considered to have an equivalent increased risk of colorectal cancer (CRC) provided there is a similar extent and duration of colonic inflammation.
- Risk factors for CRC in patients with IBD include:
  - duration and extent of disease;
  - family history of CRC (patients with an affected first-degree relative have a twofold increased risk);
  - primary sclerosing cholangitis;
  - young age at diagnosis;
  - evidence suggesting persistent inflammation, which increases the risk of colorectal cancer; this is now considered when determining surveillance intervals. This emphasizes the importance of compliance to treatment and good disease control.
- All patients should undergo a repeat colonoscopy at 10 years from initial diagnosis. This should ideally be performed as a dye-spray chromoendoscopy with the patient in clinical remission and will guide the need for further surveillance, which may be at 1, 3, or 5 years dependant on the estimated risk.

Fertility and Pregnancy

- Patients with inactive IBD can be expected to have normal fertility levels, but this is reduced by active disease.
- Both male and female patients undergoing surgery are at risk of resultant infertility (via impotence/ejaculatory problems and impaired tubular function, respectively). This is of particular concern when pouch formation and/or rectal excision is performed. Sulphasalazine (but not other aminosalicylates or thiopurines) cause a reversible and dose-dependent decrease in sperm motility and count.
- Methotrexate is teratogenic and therefore should not be used in females wishing to conceive (van Assche et al., 2010).
- Patients should be in clinical remission before conception as this will be associated with better pregnancy outcomes.
- Folate supplementation (about 2 mg/day) is important to prevent neural tube defects. This is particularly important when sulphasalazine is used since this may interfere with folate absorption.
- IBD is a risk for preterm birth and low birth weight but not stillbirth or congenital malformations.
- If conception occurs when disease is quiescent, then the risk of relapse during pregnancy is the same as in nonpregnant women. However, in patients who conceive when the disease is active, the majority will continue to have active disease during pregnancy (e.g., in Crohn's disease two-thirds of those with active disease at conception continue to have active disease with the majority [two-thirds] deteriorating clinically during their pregnancy).

- Medical treatment (except MTX) should generally be continued throughout pregnancy as the benefits of good disease control outweigh the risks of therapy.
- Specific guidance:
  - Metronidazole should be used with caution and only if there is no alternative due to the risk of prematurity. Ciprofloxacin or co-amoxiclav is preferable but to minimize risk, the shortest possible course should always be used.
  - Suppositories and enemas are safe until the third trimester.
  - Despite having an FDA rating D, which is extrapolated from animal studies, human studies suggest azathioprine and mercaptopurine are safe and well tolerated (Alstead, Ritchie, Lennard-Jones, Farthing, & Clark, 1990; Francella et al., 2003; Norgard, Pedersen, Fonager, Rasmussen, & Sorensen, 2003; Zlatanic et al., 2003).
  - Anti-TNF drugs are recognized to cross the placenta in the late second and third trimesters. To minimize foetal exposure and subsequent immunosuppression, consideration may be given to discontinuing these drugs at 24 weeks of gestation if patients are in remission. If continued throughout pregnancy, a neonatologist should be consulted and live vaccines avoided in the foetus until at least 6 months old.
- Flares should be treated aggressively and similar to nonpregnant patients.
- Patients with uncomplicated IBD can deliver vaginally. Caesarean section should be preferred in perianal Crohn's disease, active rectal disease, or when an ileoanal pouch anastomosis is present. Colectomy or ileostomy patients can deliver vaginally.
- Close collaboration between gastroenterologists and obstetricians is encouraged and in complex cases, consideration should be given to early referral via pregnancy planning or medical obstetric clinics (van Assche et al., 2010).

Breastfeeding

- Sulphasalazine, other aminosalicylates, thiopurines, and anti-TNF therapy are all considered safe in breastfeeding.
- Metronidazole and ciprofloxacin should be avoided as they are excreted into breast milk.
- Steroids appear in low concentrations in breast milk. To minimize exposure, a 4-hour delay after oral dosing may be considered (van Assche et al., 2010).

Vaccinations

- A vaccine and infection history, including TB exposure, chickenpox history, and risk of hepatitis B, should be obtained at diagnosis in patients with IBD.
- Varicella zoster serology should be checked if there is no history of infection and immunization considered before initiation of steroids/immunosuppressants.
- Hepatitis B serology should be checked in high-risk patients (please refer to *Immunisation Against Infectious Diseases: The Green Book*, Department of Health, United Kingdom) and vaccination considered before initiation of steroids, immunosuppressants, or anti-TNF monoclonal antibody therapy in the nonimmune.
- Influenza, pneumococcal, and human papillomavirus (HPV) (females) vaccination is recommended for immunosuppressed adults and is best considered for all patients with IBD, given the frequent need for steroid and immunosuppressive therapy. Booster vaccinations are appropriate for influenza (annually) and pneumococcus (after 3 years).
- Live vaccines should be avoided in patients on immunosuppression or steroids (measles, mumps, rubella [MMR], oral polio, yellow fever, live typhoid, varicella, bacillus Calmette-Guérin [BCG]).
- Immunoglobulin postexposure prophylaxis of nonimmune individuals on high-dose steroid or immunosuppression should be considered after exposure to varicella or measles. Acyclovir prophylaxis may also be used for varicella (van Assche et al., 2010).

Chronic Diarrhoea

> **GUIDELINE**
>
> Thomas, P.D., Forbes, A., Green, J., Howdle, P., Long, R., Playford, R., et al. (2003). Guidelines for the investigation of chronic diarrhea (2nd ed.). *Gut, 52*, S1–15.

- Chronic diarrhoea may be defined as the abnormal passage of three or more loose or liquid stools per day for more than 4 weeks and/or a daily stool weight greater than 200 g/day.

Further Investigation

- NB: Refer to secondary care for further investigation patients over 60 years of age with a change in bowel habit to looser and/or more frequent stools.
- Stool culture (including analysis for ova, cysts, and parasites) should always be considered.
- Coeliac disease occurs in approximately 1 in 100 patients in the United Kingdom. Therefore serologic testing for coeliac disease should be performed in all patients presenting with diarrhoea:
  - Immunoglobulin A (IgA) tissue transglutaminase (tTG) antibody testing is most common. In patients with IgA deficiency (2%–3% of coeliac patients) an IgG antiendomysial antibody can be tested (both have >95% sensitivity and specificity).
  - Serology testing and histologic confirmation with duodenal biopsy must be performed on a gluten-rich diet to avoid false negative results.
- Microscopic colitis (lymphocytic or collagenous colitis) is increasingly recognised as a cause of chronic watery diarrhoea. The aetiology is unclear and it may occur as a postinfectious phenomenon but is often drug induced.

Commonly implicated drugs include lansoprazole, NSAIDs, and selective serotonin reuptake inhibitors (SSRIs), which should be withdrawn if possible. Budesonide (9 mg daily for 6 weeks) is effective at controlling diarrhoea in approximately 80%, but symptoms often recur on discontinuation. Other therapeutic options include antidiarrhoeals, bismuth, prednisolone, and aminosalicylates +/− bile acid sequestrants. However, microscopic colitis is distinct from conventional IBD and, importantly, is not associated with any long-term complication, so it should be managed symptomatically (Nguyen, Smalley, Vege, & Carrasco-Labra, 2016).

- Malabsorption is often accompanied by steatorrhoea and the passage of bulky, malodorous, pale stools. It may be associated with biochemical or haematologic abnormalities suggesting nutritional deficinecy (e.g., electrolyte deficiencies, hypocalcaemia, low vitamin D, elevated prothrombin time suggesting vitamin K deficiency, macrocytosis, or haematinic deficiencies).
- In patients with a history or investigations suggestive of malabsorption, consider the following:
  - Faecal elastase (normal >500, low if pancreatic exocrine failure) +/− CT pancreas.
  - Hydrogen breath test or empiric trial of antibiotics for small bowel bacterial overgrowth (SBBO)—particularly in patients with increased risk of this, such as those with gut dysmotility or altered anatomy (e.g., blind loop) due to previous surgery.
  - Small bowel imaging (e.g., CT enterography or MRI small bowel) to exclude small bowel Crohn disease (Headstrom & Surawicz, 2005; Schiller, 2004).
- Bile salt malabsorption may occur following terminal ileal resection but has also been described following cholecystectomy and in postinfectious or idiopathic diarrhoea. A ^{75}Se homocholic acid-taurine (75Se-HCAT) scan demonstrating poor retention (<5% at 7 days) or an elevated serum 7-alpha cholestenone suggests the diagnosis. However, a therapeutic trial of bile acid sequestrant (e.g., cholestyramine 4 g twice a day or colesevelam 3.75 g daily) is often preferred.
- Other rare causes of diarrhoea include:
  - carcinoid syndrome—may be associated with flushing and diagnosed by demonstrating elevated urinary 5-hydroxyindoleacetic acid (5-HIAA);
  - gastrointestinal neuroendocrine tumours (GI NETs)—consider gut hormone analysis;
  - facticious diarrhoea (e.g., laxative abuse) (Thomas et al., 2003).

Coeliac Disease

- Coeliac disease is an autoimmune condition causing inflammation of the proximal small bowel induced by the ingestion of gluten.
- It affects around 1% of the world's population but incidence varies geographically.
- The prevalence of coeliac disease has increased in the last 50 years but most patients are undiagnosed.

GUIDELINES

National Institute for Health and Care Excellence. (2015). *Coeliac disease: Recognition, assessment and management. NICE clinical guideline.* Retrieved from www.nice.org.uk/guidance/ng20.

Ludvigsson, J.F., Bai, J. C., Biagi, F., Card, T. R., Ciacci, C., Ciclitira, P. J., et al. (2014). The diagnosis and management of adults with coeliac disease: Guidance from the British Society of Gastroenterology. *Gut, 63,* 1210–1228.

- Human leukocyte antigen (HLA) types DQ2 (95%) or DQ8 are present in over 99% of individuals affected by coeliac disease.
- Histologic features on duodenal biopsy are subtotal villous atrophy associated with crypt hyperplasia and increase in intraepithelial lymphocytes.
- Coeliac disease is associated with increased risk of non-Hodgkin lymphoma and small bowel adenocarcinoma but not an overall increase in malignant conditions (Mooney, Hadjivassiliou, & Sanders, 2014).
- The interest in gluten as a factor in other conditions has increased and many individuals without coeliac disease may identify themselves as gluten sensitive. The mechanism for gluten sensitivity is unclear (Aziz et al., 2014; Lebwohl, Ludvigsson, & Green, 2015).

Initial Testing and Referral

- Many individuals with coeliac disease are asymptomatic but presenting symptoms which should prompt testing for coeliac disease include:
  - *In children:*
    a. recurrent abdominal pain;
    b. failure to thrive or short stature;
    c. diarrhoea (only in 10%).
  - *In adults:*
    a. diarrhoea (<50% of patients);
    b. nonspecific abdominal symptoms often mimicking IBS;
    c. anemia (around 50% of patients at diagnosis may be iron deficient but B_{12} and folate may also be low);
    d. elevated liver enzymes;
    e. osteoporosis;
    f. dermatitis herpetiformis (itchy, blistering rash on trunk). May precede clinical evidence of intestinal involvement, but duodenal biopsies are abnormal;
    g. aphthous stomatitis;
    h. unexplained neurologic symptoms (may relate to micronutrient deficiency);
    i. subfertility and low birthweight offspring.
- In addition to the above patients with a clinical picture suggesting possible coeliac disease, testing is recommended in the following groups:
  - First-degree relatives of patients with coeliac disease (risk is 10%)

- Patients with type 1 diabetes (risk is 4%–7%)
- Patients with other autoimmune disease with unexplained symptoms
- Individuals with Down or Turner syndrome
- IgA tTG antibody has 98% specificity and 95% sensitivity and is the initial investigation of choice.
- Where IgA deficiency is present, IgG antiendomysial antibody should be tested.
- Adult patients with positive antibody screening should be referred for oesophagogastroduodenoscopy (OGD) and duodenal biopsy.
- Patients referred for biopsy should be told to continue to take gluten in at least one meal per day in the interim.
- In symptomatic children an IgA tTG titre more than 10 times the upper limit of normal may be sufficient for diagnosis without biopsy (Murch et al., 2013).
- HLA typing should only be carried out in specialist settings to exclude coeliac disease:
  - in patients who exclude gluten prior to biopsy and are not willing to reintroduce it;
  - to minimise future testing in high-risk individuals such as first-degree relatives (NICE, 2015a).

Further Management

- Where coeliac disease is confirmed by duodenal biopsy, patients should be advised on lifelong exclusion of gluten from their diet.
- Patients diagnosed with coeliac disease should be referred to a dietitian.
- Patients should be advised to avoid all wheat, rye, and barley.
- Guidance on prescription of gluten-free products can be found in the document "Gluten Free Foods: A Revised Prescribing Guide" online at www.coeliac.org.uk. Prescribing of gluten-free products may be restricted according to local policy.
- Oats should be avoided initially but certified gluten-free oats may be introduced after 6 to 12 months with follow-up assessment and serologic testing to assess tolerance (NICE, 2015a).
- Patients should have a repeat biopsy if tTG titre has not fallen to normal range after 12 months on gluten-free diet (Ludvigsson et al., 2014).
- Patients should be encouraged to join a national coeliac support group (e.g., Coeliac UK).
- Patients with coeliac disease should be vaccinated against:
  - pneumococcus;
  - meningitis C;
  - Haemophilus influenza B;
  - influenza annually.

Ongoing Management

- Patients should be seen on an annual basis to:
  - measure weight and height;
  - assess symptoms;

- assess diet and adherence to gluten-free diet and consider the need for specialist dietetic advice.
- Suggested investigations:
  - Measure tTG titre.
  - Measure FBC, ferritin, folate, B$_{12}$.
  - Check calcium levels, alkaline phosphatase, and vitamin D levels (Ludvigsson et al., 2014).
- Bone densitometry scan should be offered to patients with two or more of these: BMI less then 20, weight loss over 10%, age older than 70 years, persistent symptoms, poor adherence to gluten-free diet (British Society of Gastroenterology [BSG], 2007).
  - If osteopenia, repeat after 3 years on gluten-free diet.
  - Repeat at age 55 years for men or at menopause for women if normal at baseline.
  - Patients with osteoporosis should be treated according to current guidelines.
  - All patients should be encouraged to ensure adequate calcium intake, taking supplements if necessary, to achieve this.
- Other autoimmune conditions are common in individuals with coeliac disease and these should be tested for where there are symptoms.

Refractory or Recurrent Symptoms

- Patients with refractory symptoms or recurrence of symptoms should be referred to gastroenterology for assessment.
- Causes of ongoing diarrhoea include:
  - noncompliance with gluten-free diet or inadvertent gluten ingestion;
  - lymphocytic colitis;
  - small bowel bacterial overgrowth;
  - lactose intolerance;
  - hyperthyroidism;
  - pancreatic insufficiency;
  - refractory coeliac disease;
  - small bowel lymphoma or adenocarcinoma (Mooney et al., 2014).

Refractory Coeliac Disease

- Refractory coeliac disease (RCD) is diagnosed when clinical and histologic features of coeliac disease persist despite strict gluten exclusion for at least 6 to 12 months.
- The incidence is uncertain but rare.
- *Type 1 RCD* small bowel lymphocytes are polyclonal and express typical CD3/CD8 positivity. Response to treatment with steroids and immunosuppression is good and 5-year survival is over 90%.
- *Type 2 RCD* have aberrant or clonal T-cell lines with loss of CD3/CD8 positivity.
  - Response to treatment is poor and progression to lymphoma is common; 5-year survival is 40% to 60% (Al Toma et al., 2007; Rubio-Tapia & Murray, 2010).
  - There are no guidelines for treatment of this condition, so patients should be referred to a tertiary centre.

Lymphoma and Cancer Risk

- Individuals with coeliac disease should be reassured that life expectancy is not reduced.
- Patients with coeliac disease have around a two- to fourfold increased risk of non-Hodgkin lymphoma equating to about 1 in 2000 per year (Mooney et al., 2014).
- Enteropathy associated T-cell lymphoma (type 1)
  - This is a rare form of lymphoma associated with coeliac disease particulary type 2 RCD.
  - Prognosis is poor with 2-year survival less than 20% (Al Toma et al., 2007).
  - Highest rate of diagnosis is in first year after diagnosis, and risk reduces with compliance to a gluten-free diet.
- Risk of small bowel adenocarcinoma is more than 30 times higher in patients with coeliac disease, although it is still rare (Howdle, Jalal, Holmes, & Houlston, 2003; Mooney et al., 2014).
- Gluten-free diet is thought to reduce the risk of lymphoma and small bowel cancer.

Noncoeliac Gluten Sensitivity

- Many people without coeliac disease perceive that there are health benefits to excluding gluten from diet (Lebwohl et al., 2015).
- In a population study of 1002 people in the United Kingdom, 13% reported gluten sensitivity and 3.7% avoid eating gluten (Aziz et al., 2014).
- Some patients with IBS improve when gluten is restricted.
- Some of these patients will have IBS and be sensitive to FODMAPs.
- The biologic basis for noncoeliac gluten sensitivity is not established, therefore a frank discussion with patients regarding risks and benefits of dietary restriction is recommended.

Iron Deficiency Anemia

> **GUIDELINE**
>
> Goddard, A.F., James, M.W., McIntyre, A.S., & Scott, B.B. (2011). Guidelines for the management of iron deficiency anaemia. *Gut, 60,* 1309–1316.

- Iron deficiency is common affecting up to 2% to 5% of men and postmenopausal women in developed countries (Goddard, James, McIntyre, & Scott, 2011).
- Causes of iron deficiency include dietary deficiency, lack of absorption from the diet, and chronic loss of blood.
- Endoscopic investigation of iron deficiency in the absence of anemia rarely yields a diagnosis of malignancy. Risks and benefits of investigation should be discussed with the individual patient and should only be considered in patients aged over 50 or with GI symptoms (Goddard et al., 2011).

Causes of Iron Deficiency Anemia

- Coeliac disease is the most common cause of iron deficiency from malabsorption (prevalance 4%–6%). Other causes including postgastrectomy, *Helicobacter* colonization, gut resection, and small bowel bacterial overgrowth are less common.
- Benign sources of gastrointestinal blood loss include aspirin and NSAID use, which account for 10% to 20% of patients.
- Prevalence of GI tract cancers are in the region of:
  - colonic 5% to 10%;
  - gastric 5%;
  - oesophageal 2%;
  - small bowel tumours 1% to 2%;
  - ampullary carcinoma <1% (Goddard et al., 2011)
- Non-GI sources of blood loss include menstruation (20%–30%), blood donation (5%), and haematuria (1%); if persistent warrants urology referral (Goddard et al., 2011).

History

- Should include dietary review, careful history for any source of blood loss, and/or associated symptoms (e.g., dyspepsia, altered bowel habit, and weight loss).
- Ask about previous history of anemia and investigation.
- Ask about family or personal history of haemoglobinopathies, telangiectasia, or other bleeding disorders.
- Enquire about family history of GI tract cancer, IBD, or coeliac disease.
- Check drug history (e.g., anticoagulants, antiplatelets, NSAIDs).
- Ask about previous surgical history (e.g., gastrectomy).

Examination

- Clinical signs of iron deficiency are unusual, but patients should be examined to exclude an abdominal mass and those with rectal bleeding or tenesmus should have a digital rectal examination (Goddard et al., 2011).

Initial Investigation

- Full blood count with mean cell volume, blood film, ferritin level.
  - Low serum ferritin is recognised as the best indicator of iron deficiency.
  - Ferritin is elevated in inflammatory states, so iron deficiency can exist in the presence of normal ferritin.
  - Iron studies may help to clarify iron deficiency but can be difficult to interpret. The accompanying table may help interpretation.
- IgA tTG antibody for coeliac disease.
- Urinalysis in all patients (Goddard et al., 2011).
- The 2015 NICE guidelines for recognition of lower GI cancers suggest considering faecal occult blood (FOB) testing in those with iron deficiency anemia without rectal bleeding who are under the age of 60 years.

Test	Iron Deficiency Anemia	Anemia of Chronic Disease
MCV/MCH	Low	Low/normal
Ferritin	Low	Normal/high
Iron	Low	Low
TF	High	Low
TF saturation	Low	Normal

MCV/MCH, Mean corpuscular volume/mean corpuscular haemoglobin; *TF*, transferrin

Further Investigation

- Menstruating women with no GI symptoms should be screened for coeliac disease with IgA tTG antibody.
- More invasive gastrointestinal investigation is only warranted where there are GI symptoms or other high-risk factors (i.e., age >50 years or strong family history of GI tract malignancy) (Goddard et al., 2011).
- Women who are not menstruating and not pregnant, and men of any age should have both upper and lower GI investigation (Goddard et al., 2011).
- Endoscopy is the best test for investigation of the upper GI tract.
- Distal duodenal biopsies should be taken to exclude coeliac disease unless tTG is negative.
- Colonoscopy is the optimal lower GI investigation because of high sensitivity and ability to biopsy or remove polyps.
- CT virtual colonoscopy is (up to 90%) sensitive for lesions larger than 1 cm but does not allow for biopsy and histologic diagnosis. This investigation usually still involves full bowel preparation but can be performed with minimal preparation and/or without contrast on request (Spada et al., 2014).
- Following CT colonoscopy, flexible sigmoidoscopy may be required for completion as views of the rectum can be suboptimal.
- Small bowel investigation is not indicated in every patient with iron deficiency anemia but should be considered in those who become anemic again after iron replacement, particularly if the patient is young or transfusion dependent despite iron supplementation (Goddard et al., 2011; Sidhu, Sanders, Morris, & McAlindon, 2008).
- In such cases:
  - Capsule endoscopy has a high diagnostic yield but is not a therapeutic modality, so it may need to be followed up by push or balloon enteroscopy.
  - MR or CT enterography is sensitive for diagnosing inflammation and mucosal thickening but may not show small vascular abnormalities or flat lesions.

Treatment

- Elemental iron 120 mg/day (e.g., ferrous fumarate 210 mg 3 doses/day) is required until haemoglogin is normal, then for 3 months to replenish iron stores (Goddard et al., 2011; Short & Domagalski, 2013).
- A haemoglobin rise of 1 g in 4 weeks indicates adequate response to treatment.
- Lack of response should prompt assessment of compliance and/or consideration of ongoing blood loss or problems with absorption.
- Parenteral iron can be used where oral preparations are not tolerated or not absorbed adequately (Goddard et al., 2011).

Weight Loss

GUIDELINES

National Institute for Health and Care Excellence. (2015). Suspected cancer: Recognition and referral. NICE clinical guideline 12. Retrieved from www.nice.org.uk/guidance/ng12.
National Institute for Health and Care Excellence. (2006). Nutrition support for adults: Oral nutrition support, enteral tube feeding and parenteral nutrition. NICE clinical guideline 32 (updated 2017). Retrieved from www.nice.org.uk/guidance/cg32.

- Unintentional weight loss is common, particularly in elderly patients with 15% to 20% of those aged over 65 years, but as many as 50% to 60% of those residing in nursing homes are affected (McMinn, Steel, & Bowman, 2011; NICE, 2006).
- Weight loss of 5% of body weight over 6 to 12 months is generally accepted as significant, but smaller losses in frailer patients may also be important.
- Weight loss may be due to reduced calorie intake and conditions causing malabsorption, but in other conditions such as weight loss in malignancy the mechanism is less well understood.
- Weight loss is not exclusively a symptom of gastrointestinal disease, which is the cause in around one-third of cases, so a holistic approach to the patient is important.
- Exclusion of malignancy is often the primary concern for both patient and doctor. Referral via urgent suspicion of cancer pathway for assessment or investigation should be offered (NICE, 2015b).
- No cause may be found in up to 25% of older adults. Malignancy may be the cause in a similar proportion. Data for younger adults are lacking (Gaddey & Holder, 2014; McMinn et al., 2011).
- The incidence of eating disorders is increasing. Both genders can be affected and a wide range of age from childhood upwards (Micali, Hagberg, Petersen, & Treasure, 2013).
- Patients with eating disorders have significantly increased mortality rates (Arcelus, Mitchell, Wales, & Nielsen, 2011), therefore it is important to have a high index of suspicion.

History and Examination

- Many conditions and medications can lead to reduced appetite. Careful history of what the Patient eats as well as factors associated with their ability to access, prepare, and consume food is important (Gaddey & Holder, 2014).

- Medication side effects including nausea and altered sense of taste may be important (Alibhai, Greenwood, & Payette, 2005).
- Thorough systematic review is key to elicit other symptoms which can guide referral pathway.
- It is *essential* to document the patient's weight, as self-reporting of weight is often not reliable.
- Full examination of all systems and examination for lymphadenopathy is indicated.

Investigation

- There are no guidelines specifically for the investigation of weight loss in all patients but there are many recommendations for investigation of suspected cancer. Patients' symptoms should guide initial investigation.
- Laboratory investigation:
  - tTG antibody
  - FBC
  - Thyroid function tests (TFTs)
  - CRP
  - Glucose
  - There is some evidence that in older patients elevated serum LDH is predictive of organic cause (McMinn et al., 2011).
  - Tumour markers are generally unhelpful but CA125 should be tested in women with weight loss, loss of appetite, or early satiety (NICE, 2015b).
  - HIV test should be performed (British HIV Association, 2008).
  - Faecal elastase if diarrhoea or risk factors for pancreatic disease
  - Faecal calprotectin if diarrhoea

Endoscopy

- Oesophagogastroscopy (OGD) in any patients with unintentional weight loss. Patients aged over 55 years with abdominal pain, dyspepsia, reflux, or nausea and vomiting with weight loss should be referred for urgent direct access OGD.
- Patients with weight loss associated with altered bowel habits, rectal bleeding, or iron deficiency anemia should be referred for urgent assessment or direct access colonoscopy (NICE, 2015b).

Imaging

- Ultrasound scan pelvis in women over 40 years especially if bloating.
- CXR all ever smokers or any respiratory symptom.
- CT abdomen as urgent direct access in patients aged 60 or over with diarrhoea, constipation, nausea, and vomiting or abdominal or back pain or new onset diabetes (NICE, 2015b).

Further Management

- In elderly patients who have been investigated along the lines above with negative results, malignant diagnosis is uncommon.

- The yield from further blind investigation is low and an approach of watchful waiting over 3 to 6 months may be appropriate at this stage particularly in elderly patients (Alibhai et al., 2005; McMinn et al., 2011).
- In younger patients and where malignancy is still strongly suspected, CT thorax abdomen and pelvis may be the next investigation of choice.

Treatment

- Nutrition support is advised in patients with body mass index below 18.5 kg/m^2, loss of 10% body weight in 3 to 6 months, or BMI less than 20 and loss of over 5% body weight in 3 to 6 months.
- Dietetic input is essential to ensure micronutrient needs are met as well as energy and protein needs (NICE, 2006).
- Social support, aids, and equipment may be just as important for some patients, so a full multidisciplinary approach is required.
- No pharmacologic treatments have a proven benefit in improving weight gain.
- In patients with depression mirtazapine may be appropriate. Megestrol is sometimes used in patients with poor appetite, but the evidence base for this is poor and side effects may limit use (Alibhai et al., 2005; McMinn et al., 2011).

Jaundice and Abnormal Liver Function Tests

GUIDELINES AND REVIEWS

Williams, R., et al. (2014). Addressing liver disease in the UK: A blueprint for attaining excellence in health care and reducing premature mortality from lifestyle issues of excess consumption of alcohol, obesity, and viral hepatitis. *Lancet, 384,* 1953–1997.

Lilford, R., et al. What is the best strategy for investigating abnormal LFTs in primary care? *BMJ Open, 3,* e003099.

Dyson, J.K., et al. (2014). Non-alcoholic fatty liver disease: A practical approach to treatment. *Frontline Gastroenterology, 5,* 277–286.

National Institute for Health and Care Excellence. (2016). Assessment and management of cirrhosis. NICE clinical guideline 50. Retrieved from www.nice.org.uk/guidance/ng50.

- Liver disease is increasing in prevalence and general practitioners will see many patients with abnormal liver function tests.
- In England and Wales, 600,000 people have some form of liver disease, with around 60,000 with cirrhosis (Williams et al., 2014).
- Death from liver disease is increasing and is the third most common cause of premature death in the United Kingdom.
- General practitioners are best placed to identify patients at risk of liver disease and intervene to modify risk factors.

- Less than 5% of people with abnormal liver tests will have a specific liver disease and less will require treatment (Lilford et al., 2013a; Lilford, Bentham, Armstrong, Neuberger, & Girlinget, 2013b).
- Conversely many individuals will be developing liver fibrosis with normal liver function tests (Williams et al., 2014).

Special Situations

- Patients with jaundice and fever with right upper quadrant pain may have ascending cholangitis and require urgent admission for antibiotics and definitive management with ERCP.
- All patients aged over 40 with jaundice should be referred as urgent to be seen within 2 weeks by a specialist (NICE, 2015b).
- Patients with evidence of impending liver failure such as altered mental status or in whom paracetamol overdose is suspected should be admitted as emergency (Bernal, Auzinger, Dhawan, & Wendon, 2010).
- Jaundice or abnormal LFT in the pregnant patient, particularly in the third trimester, may indicate acute fatty liver of pregnancy, preeclampsia, or HELLP syndrome and requires urgent admission to an obstetric unit (Hay, 2008).
- Decompensation of chronic liver disease with jaundice, encephalopathy, tense ascites, or evidence of bleeding is likely to require emergency admission.
- Patients with isolated elevation of bilirubin are likely to have Gilbert syndrome and should have levels of conjugated and unconjugated bilirubin measured and be screened for evidence of haemolysis.

History

History of the Presenting Complaint

- May give the diagnosis (e.g., where right upper quadrant pain is associated with dark urine and pale stools in choledocholithiasis).
- Hepatitis may present with general malaise and nonspecific symptoms.
- Many patients with abnormal LFTs are entirely asymptomatic and are picked up incidentally.

Drug History

- Incidence of drug-induced liver injury (DILI) is in the region of 20 per 100,000 per year (Bjornsson, Bergmann, Bjornsson, Kvaran, & Olafsson, 2013).
- Careful drug history should go back at least 6 months prior to the abnormality.
- Ask about nonprescribed drugs, Chinese, herbal, and other complementary therapies and dietary supplements.
- Common causes of DILI:
  a. Antibiotics; co-amoxiclav, nitrofurantoin
  b. NSAID; diclofenac
  c. Immunomodulators; azathioprine, infliximab
  d. Diet and weight loss supplements increasingly (Bjornsson et al., 2013)

(For more information on DILI, go to www.livertox.nih.gov.)

Social History

- Alcohol history (units per day or week):
  a. The UK Department of Health (2016) recommends that to reduce the risk of harm from alcohol all adults drink no more than 14 units of alcohol per week spread evenly over 3 days of the week.
  b. Daily alcohol of less than 20 g for a woman or less than 30 g for a man are unlikely to be the cause of liver disease.
  c. Patients with harmful drinking should be offered interventions to reduce this (NICE, 2016a).
- Risk factors for bloodborne and sexually transmitted infections
- Travel history
- Family history (e.g., haemochromatosis, Gilbert syndrome)

Past Medical History

- Comorbidities: diabetes and metabolic syndrome, autoimmune diseases

Examination

- This may reveal evidence of underlying chronic liver disease, tender hepatomegaly in acute hepatitis, right upper quadrant tenderness, and Murphy sign in cholecystitis.
- It is useful to document the patient's weight and BMI.

Initial Investigations

- *Blood tests:*
  - Initial LFT panel. Alanine transaminase (ALT) and alkaline phosphatase are most useful to guide whether this is a hepatitis or cholestatic picture (Lilford et al., 2013b).
  - Coagulation. Prolongation of prothombin time may indicate liver failure or vitamin K deficiency in cholestasis).
  - Full blood count. Thrombocytopaenia may indicate chronic liver disease and portal hypertension.
- *Initial liver screen:*
  - A prospective cohort study has shown that repeating abnormal LFTs after a period of time is an inefficient use of resources and suggests that individuals are instead tested for significant liver diagnoses directly (Lilford et al., 2013b).
  - The following panel is suggested:
    a. Hepatitis B and C serology (Hep A, E, Epstein-Barr virus [EBV], and cytomegalovirus [CMV] in an acute hepatitis)
    b. Immunoglobulin levels
    c. Antinuclear antibody (ANA), antimitochondrial antibody (AMA), antismooth muscle antibody (SMA), antinucleolar cytoplasmic antibody (ANCA), liver kidney microsomal antibody (LKM), and soluble liver antigen

d. Ferritin and (if elevated) transferrin saturation and HFE gene

e. caeruloplasmin

f. Alpha-1 antitrypsin level

g. Tissue transglutaminase antibody

h. HIV test (particularly where risk factors are identified)

- *Imaging:*
  - Ultrasound scan of the liver and biliary system is often a useful first line investigation, especially where biliary obstruction is suspected. MRCP is indicated for abnormal biliary dilatation or persistent cholestatic LFTs.
  - ERCP is reserved for patients in whom intervention is planned and is no longer regarded as a diagnostic procedure.
  - Ultrasound may also be useful as a screening tool to identify steatosis.
- *Transient elastography (fibroscan):*
  - Gives a measurement of liver stiffness, which correlates with severity of liver fibrosis, and can be a useful tool in staging liver disease and prognosticating. It is particularly well validated for viral hepatitis. It may be less accurate in patients with high BMI (Castera, 2010; Castera et al., 2010; Czul & Bhamidimarri, 2016).
  - NICE recommends the use of transient elastography (TE) to screen for cirrhosis in high-risk groups including individuals with hepatitis B, hepatitis C, and those who drink in excess of 50 units of alcohol per week.
- *Serum biomarkers of fibrosis:*
  - These include direct markers such as hyaluronic acid or procollagen III propeptide (PIIINP), proprietary panels of tests such as enhanced liver fibrosis (ELF) or FibroTest, or scoring systems based on a range of laboratory results (e.g., aspartate aminotransferase to platelet ratio index [APRI] score or fibrosis-4 [FIB-4]). Again these are validated against biopsy scores and can help to stage liver disease without the need for biopsy (Castera, Vilgrain, & Angulo, 2013; Czul & Bhamidimarri, 2016).
  - NICE has recommended ELF for identifying advanced fibrosis in patients with nonalcoholic fatty liver disease (NICE, 2016b).
- *Liver biopsy:*
  - Mainly required when there is diagnostic uncertainty rather than for staging of liver disease; however, it may be carried out when surrogate markers for fibrosis are borderline. Liver biopsy carries significant risks of haemorrhage (0.05%–0.1%) and death (0.1%–0.01%). In patients with coagulopathy or ascites, transjugular approach may be undertaken which reduces risk but gives smaller samples.

Specific Liver Diseases
Viral Hepatitis

- Chronic viral hepatitis B and C are important long-term conditions with significant morbidity and mortality and highly effective available treatments. Patients at risk should be encouraged to have testing (NICE, 2013b; NICE 2016a; Williams et al., 2014).

Hepatitis B

- Hepatitis B has a prevalence of 0.1% to 0.5% in the United Kingdom. But this varies between individual communities. Worldwide an estimated 350 million people are infected. Transmission is predominantly vertical in developing countries. The majority of patients diagnosed in the United Kingdom have migrated from endemic areas.
- All pregnant women in the United Kingdom should be screened antenatally. Any patient with positive HBV serology should be referred to a specialist for further management.
- Not all patients require treatment at diagnosis but should have monitoring by a specialist to determine if and when treatment should be started.
- Treatment when required is with a finite course of 48 weeks of pegylated interferon monotherapy or with (usually indefinite) treatment with antivirals, now usually tenofovir or entecavir (NICE, 2013b).
- Patients should be given advice on prevention of transmission of the virus and testing, and vaccination should be offered to sexual partners and the patients' children.
- Hepatitis B is associated with increased risk of hepatocellular carcinoma (HCC) in certain groups even in the absence of cirrhosis and surveillance will be offered (European Association for the Study of the Liver [EASL], 2012).

Hepatitis C

- The number of people in the United Kingdom with chronic HCV is in the region of 215,000.
- Injecting drug use is the main risk factor but migration from endemic areas and receipt of blood products prior to 1991 are also important risk factors.
- HCV rarely causes an acute hepatitis and 75% to 85% of patients develop chronic active hepatitis.
- Treatment of HCV has advanced rapidly in recent years with the advent of a range of direct acting antivirals. These used in combination, 'are well tolerated and offer high cure rates with short treatment durations of between 8 and 16 weeks. Treatment regimens including pegylated interferon are no longer recommended' (EASL, 2018)
- All patients with chronic hepatitis C infection should be considered for treatment of the virus and should be referred to specialist care. Hepatitis C is now seen as an inf.

Hepatitis A

- This faecal-oral transmitted virus is a cause of acute hepatitis often in the returning traveller.
- Vaccination with 2 doses 6 months apart is effective for prevention in high-risk groups including travellers to endemic areas, individuals who work in high-risk occupations, and men who have sex with men with high-risk sexual behaviours. Intravenous drug users and their close contacts should also be considered high risk.

- The illness is usually self-limiting with mild symptoms occasionally lasting up to 6 months. In a minority (<1%) of cases fulminant hepatitis may occur (Rezende et al., 2003).

Hepatitis E

- Also transmitted through the faecal-oral route, HEV usually causes a mild self-limiting acute hepatitis or subclinical infection.
- It can present with fulminant hepatic failure in pregnant women.
- HEV is linked to outbreaks in places with contaminated water supply in the developing world. In the United Kingdom more recently, incidence is rising and may be linked to a reservoir of infection among animal populations, including pigs.
- Chronic infection with rapid progression to cirrhosis has been documented in immunosuppressed groups (e.g., post liver transplant), and in these groups treatment using ribavirin may be indicated.
- The virus has been detected in donated blood from asymptomatic donors; however, the risk of transmission to immunocompetent individuals is unclear and the role for screening of blood products has not been established.
- Patients may present with extrahepatic features including up to 5% with neurologic syndromes such as Guillain-Barré syndrome (Dalton, Hunter, & Bendall, 2013).

Autoimmune Hepatitis (AIH)

- Presentation of this condition can range from a minor elevation of transaminases with or without symptoms of general malaise through acute hepatitis to subacute liver failure, athough the latter is rare. A relapsing remitting course may mean LFTs fluctuate with repeat testing.
- One-third of patients will have cirrhosis at diagnosis.
- There is a female preponderance (2:1) and there may be a history of other associated autoimmune conditions including rheumatoid arthritis, Graves disease, and coeliac disease.
- Diagnosis is usually based on typical biochemistry along with positive autoantibodies and elevated IgG.
- Liver biopsy is regarded as a prerequisite to confirm the diagnosis and for staging and prognosis. The validity of noninvasive fibrosis markers is not well stablished (EASL, 2015).
- Treatment is with steroids initially which may be in the form of prednisolone or budesonide before introducing a steroid sparing agent, usually a thiopurine.
- Occasionally second line immunosupressive agents are required, including mycophenolate mofetil or tacrolimus.
- Withdrawl of treatment should be undertaken with caution as up to 50% to 90% of patients relapse. Treatment should be for at least 3 years and at least 24 months from normalization of LFTs. Biopsy should be repeated prior to treatment withdrawal to exclude disease activity (EASL, 2015).

Primary Sclerosing Cholangitis (PSC)

- Male predominance and strong association with inflammatory bowel disease (in 80% of cases).
- Diagnosis usually made by MRCP characteristic stricturing and dilatation—typical beading appearance.
- No specific treatment shown to prevent progression. Some studies report improvement in biochemistry with certain doses of ursodeoxycholic acid; however, evidence is insufficient to recommend universally, and American guidelines state this treatment should not be used due to an excess mortality in a study of higher doses (Chapman et al., 2010; EASL, 2009).
- PSC carries a significant increased risk of cholangiocarcinoma which can be difficult to diagnose, colon cancer, and gallbladder cancer.
- Surveillance is recommended with:
  - annual colonoscopy (chromoendoscopy where possible) with biopsies;
  - annual abdominal ultrasound for gallbladder (cholecystectomy if any abnormality). Some clinicians may perform interval MRCP; however, the evidence base for this is lacking.
  - If dominant stricture is identified, then ERCP with brushings +/− intervention may be required.

Primary Biliary Cholangitis (PBC)

- Female preponderance (3:1) and association with other autoimmune conditions.
- Symptoms of itch and fatigue are typical.
- Cholestatic LFTs IgM elevated and positive antimitochondial antibody.
- Typical phenotype associated with positive serology is sufficient for the diagnosis, and biopsy is not always necessary (EASL, 2009; Lindor et al., 2009).
- Treatment with ursodeoxycholic acid at a dose of 13 to 15 mg/kg/day has been shown to improve long-term prognosis in patients who respond biochemically.
- Treatment of itch initially is with antihistamines. Bile sequestrants can be used (patients must be advised not to take ursodeoxycholic acid within 2–4 hours of taking these) and in some cases rifaxim or naltrexone (Lindor et al., 2009).
- Hyperlipidaemia occurs but may not reflect increased cardiovascular risk.
- Osteoporosis is increased and should be screened for by dual-energy x-ray absorptiometry (DEXA) (Lindor et al., 2009).

Overlap Syndromes

- Patients may have features of two or more of the above-mentioned conditions. Treatment often follows the predominant condition or patients may receive a combination of immunosupression and ursodeoxycholic acid.

Nonalcoholic Fatty Liver Disease

- This is the most common liver disease in the Western world and with increasing prevalence, possibly the biggest challenge in liver disease in the developed world in the next decades; 17% to 40% of adults have some degree of nonalcoholic fatty liver disease.

- Spectrum from steatosis to steatohepatitis to fibrosis and cirrhosis.
- Death in these patients is mostly from cardiovascular disease and cancer, but there is significant risk of progression to liver cirrhosis (Angulo et al., 2015).
- Fibrosis on biopsy is still the best predictor of prognosis but in practice noninvasive tests are usually preferred (Angulo et al., 2015; EASL, 2016).
- No specific treatments are available, but patients should be counselled on lifestyle and risk factors.
- Weight loss of 7% to 10% of body weight has been shown to improve fibrosis but the optimum method has not been proven.
- There is some evidence of benefit from pioglitazone, vitamin E, or obeticholic acid; however, these should only be used within specialist settings (NICE, 2016b; Rinella, 2015).
- Statins are generally safe in this patient group and may be beneficial, therefore should not usually be discontinued.

Alcoholic Hepatitis

- Alcohol is a common cause of cirrhosis. Alcoholic hepatitis presents with jaundice and carries a very high mortality when severe. Diagnosis is usually based on the history of excessive alcohol consumption within 4 weeks prior to presentation and typical biochemistry with bilirubin greater than 80 and aspartate aminotransferase/alanine transaminase (AST/ALT) typically less than 500.
- Treatment with corticosteroids may be considered under specialist supervision (Thursz et al., 2015).

Hereditary Haemochromatosis

- Autosomal recessive inherited condition with homozygosity of C282Y mutation most common.
- H63D /C282Y *compound* heterozygote is associated with some risk of iron overload.
- Associated with iron overload from the third or fourth decade. Later in women due to menstrual blood loss.
- Patients may present with joint pain or fatigue (van Bokhoven, van Deursen, & Swinkels, 2011).
- Genetic testing is not recommended as a screening test due to low penetrance of the condition (EASL, 2010).
- Ferritin level below 1000 with normal LFTs has a good negative predictive value for cirrhosis.
- Treatment with venesection until iron stores (ferritin) depleted to less than 50 and, as required, venesection thereafter (target ferritin 50–100).
- In patients in whom cirrhosis is suspected biopsy should be performed.

Wilson Disease

- Rare genetic condition with associated neuropsychiatric features.
- Can present as fulminant hepatic failure typically associated with haemolytic anemia.
- Ceruloplasmin measurement is a useful screening test (levels will be low) but diagnosis requires liver biopsy and urinary copper.
- Treatment with chelating agents (i.e., penicillamine or trientene) (Ferenci, 2004).

Chronic Liver Disease

> **GUIDELINE**
>
> National Institute for Health and Care Excellence. (2016). *Cirrhosis in over 16s: Assessment and management. NICE clinical guideline 50.* Retrieved from www.nice.org.uk/guidance/ng50.

- Cirrhosis results from injury (due to a variety of mechanisms or disease processes) leading to necroinflammation and fibrinogenesis within the liver. Histologic features of liver cirrhosis include diffuse nodular regeneration, fibrous septa, collapse of the normal liver architecture, and distortion of vascular structures.
- Clinical examination findings in advanced liver disease may include:
  - palmar erythema, spider naevi (>5 considered abnormal);
  - caput medusae;
  - loss of body hair in men;
  - gynaecomastia;
  - testicular atrophy;
  - all or none of these signs.
- Patients at risk of cirrhosis include individuals with a BMI over 30, those who misuse alcohol, patients with type 2 diabetes, and patients with hepatitis B or C infection, as well as patients with other forms of liver disease as previously discussed.
- NICE recommends testing for cirrhosis with transient elastography in all men drinking more than 50 units of alcohol per week (women >35 units) or anyone diagnosed with alcohol-related liver disease. (NICE, 2016a)

Staging of Advanced Liver Disease

- Liver cirrhosis or advanced liver disease can be thought of as a spectrum of clinical states from early disease with compensated disease and absence of oesophageal varices, through the development of portal hypertension, to decompensated liver disease with complications of varices and ascites.
- Prognosis varies between these stages with 1-year mortality of 1% per year for early stage to more than 50% for decompensated disease (Tsochatzis, Bosch, & Burroughs, 2014).
- Child-Pugh classification (see accompanying table) can be used to describe the stage or severity of liver cirrhosis.

The Model for End-stage Liver Disease (MELD) and UK Model for End-stage Liver Disease (UKELD) scores are used in the transplant assessment process to risk-stratify patients and select those in whom risk of transplant is outweighed by risk of death without transplant.

Child-Pugh Classification of Chronic Liver Disease

Measure	1 Point	2 Points	3 Points
Total bilirubin (μmol/L)	<34	34–50	>50
Prothrombin time prolongation(s)	<4.0	4.0–6.0	>6.0
Ascites	None	Mild	Moderate to severe
Hepatic encephalopathy	None	Grade I–II (or suppressed with medication)	Grade III–IV (or refractory)
Serum albumin (g/L)	<28	28–35	>35

Management of Patients With Cirrhosis

- Patients with stable compensated cirrhosis will usually be seen at a liver clinc every 6 to 12 months for monitoring and to arrange surveillance for HCC:
  - Currently recommended 6 monthly ultrasound of liver as HCC surveillance (Bruix & Sherman, 2011).
  - Patients should receive appropriate treatment depending on the underlying aetiology of liver disease (e.g., antiviral therapy or venesection in haemochromatosis).
  - Patients should be advised on lifestyle (weight reduction in obesity, management of type 2 diabetes, smoking cessation, and abstinence from alcohol).

Ascites

- Half of patients with compensated cirrhosis will develop ascites within a 10-year period.
- The development of ascites marks progression of liver disease and associated 2-year mortality of up to 50%. The development of ascites should prompt consideration of assessment for transplantation.
- Treatment is with low sodium diet (<2000 mg/day), aldosterone antagonist (e.g., spironolactone 100 mg increasing in increments of 100 mg to maximum 300 mg) with the addition of loop diuretics (e.g., furosemide 40–120 mg) in some cases.
- Fluid restriction is not indicated unless hyponatraemia.
- Hyponatraemia is common and may limit diuretic use. Diuretics should be reduced or stopped if serum sodium is below 125 mmol/L (Moore & Aithal, 2006).
- NSAIDs should be avoided in patients with ascites due to cirrhosis.
- Angiotensin converting enzyme inhibitors (ACEi) and angiotensin receptor blockers (ARBs) may be harmful in patients with ascites and should be stopped.

- Rapid accumulation of ascites may be due to development of portal vein thrombosis or HCC and should prompt referral and consideration of imaging.
- Spontaneous bacterial peritonitis (SBP) may present with decompensation without specific symptoms and should prompt urgent admission. Signs of peritonism are usually absent. In hospital, mortality from SBP is around 20%.
- After one episode of SBP, patients should receive long-term antibiotic prophylaxis. Antibiotic choice is usually a quinolone or cotrimoxazole but will be guided by local protocols and sensitivities.

Hepatic Encephalopathy

- Hepatic encephalopathy (HE) will affect 30% to 40% of patients with cirrhosis at some time in their clinical course.
- HE can be classified according to the West Haven Criteria. Minimal hepatic encephalopathy (MHE) may be apparent only on psychometric testing; however, it may still lead to a reduction in quality of life for patients.
- Overt hepatic encephalopathy (OHE) classically presents with deficit in attention, reduced visiospatial awareness, disorientation, alteration of sleep-wake cycle, change in personality, and in later stages reduced concious level. OHE usually has a precipitant such as variceal bleeding or infection.
- It is important in acute confusion to consider other causes and to be aware that patients with advanced liver disease are at risk of intracranial bleeding. There should be a low threshold for referral for urgent assessment and imaging in new confusion (EASL & American Association for the Study of Liver Diseases [AASLD], 2014).
- Lactulose is usually given to treat and prevent encephalopathy and rifaxamin is added in as a second line treatment. Both treatments are usually continued indefinitely.

Varices

- All patients at risk of varices should have a screening endoscopy. Until recently this included all patients with cirrhosis; however, evidence now suggests that those with lower fibrosis scores (i.e., TE with stiffness <20 with platelet count >150) may not require screening (Bosch & Sauerbruch, 2016; Tripathi et al., 2015).
- Grade 1 varices without red spots do not require primary prophylaxis but should have further endoscopy after 1 year.
- Patients with Grade 2 or 3 varices receive nonselective beta blocker (NSBB) as primary prophylaxis (e.g., carvedilol 6.25 mg daily increasing to 12.5 mg daily after 1 week if tolerated or propanolol 40 mg twice daily increased to maximum tolerated dose). Patients on NSBB for primary prophylaxis do not require routine endoscopy.
- Where NSBB is contraindicated, patients should have primary prophylaxis by endoscopic band ligation (EBL).
- Patients who have had a variceal bleed should undergo a program of EBL every 2 to 4 weeks until varices are

obliterated. They should also receive NSBB unless there is a contraindication.

- Transjugular intrahepatic portosystemic shunt (TIPSS) may be required as a recue therapy in acute variceal bleeding.
- Bleeding from gastric varices can be more difficult to manage endoscopically and more commonly requires TIPSS.
- There is controversy regarding the treatment with NSBB in advanced decompensated liver disease, with some studies indicating loss of benefit or harm from NSBB in more advanced disease but others showing benefit. More research is needed in this area and the decision to stop or restart NSBB should be made by the specialist (Krag & Madsen, 2015).

TIPSS

- Indicated as a rescue therapy in acute variceal haemorrhage or for high-risk gastric varices.
- May be indicated for refractory ascites in appropriate patients.
- Main adverse effect is encephalopathy which occurs in up to 10% to 50% of patients, therefore careful patient selection is very important (EASL & AASLD, 2014).

Hepatocellular Carcinoma

- Diagnosed by characteristic contrast-enhanced imaging on one or two modalities. Biopsy not usually required.
- Treatment options depend on the stage of liver disease as well as the number, size, and site of tumours by the Barcelona Clinic Liver Cancer (BCLC) staging.
- Resection is reserved for those with Child-Pugh A with one small (<2 cm) lesion.
- Transplant is considered for those with three or fewer lesions all less than 3 cm in size who are otherwise candidates for transplantation.
- Transarterial chemoembolization (TACE) and radiofrequency ablation are effective palliative treatment but not suitable for patients' Child-Pugh A or B cirrhosis and good performance status.
- Sorafenib is an oral kinase inhibitor used as a palliative treatment in selected patients.

Liver Transplant

- Liver transplant should be considered in all patients with advanced liver disease.
- Many patients will not be suitable due to comorbidity or risk of recidivism.
- After transplant the vast majority of patients will remain on lifelong immunosuppression.
- They will be seen at least 6 monthly by a specialist who will review immunosuppression and aim to minimise toxicity. Changes to immunosuppression should not be made by nonspecialists (AASLD & AST, 2012).
- In the first year, complications of surgery, rejection, and infections are the greatest cause of morbidity and mortality.

- In patients who survive after 1 year from transplant, renal disease and cardiovascular disease are the main causes of morbidity and malignancy; and cardiovascular disease accounts for most deaths. Many patients undergoing transplant have multiple risk factors including obesity, metabolic syndrome, and type 2 diabetes (AASLD & AST, 2012).
- Patients should be given the following lifestyle advice:
  - Diet: Avoid unpasteurized dairy products and raw or undercooked meat or eggs.
  - Avoid smoking.
  - Use high factor sun protection and stay out of strong sunlight. Patients should also be counselled to self-examine their skin for suspicious lesions (AASLD & AST, 2012).
- Cardiovascular risk factors should be addressed, including weight management, hypertension, and diabetes.
- Bone density should be considered and appropriately managed according to protocols.

References

American Association for the Study of Liver Disease & American Society of Transplantation. (2012). *Long-term management of the successful adult liver transplant: 2012 practice guideline by AASLD and the American Society of Transplantation.*

Abdel Jalil, A. A., Katzka, D. A., & Castell, D. O. (2015). Approach to the patient with dysphagia. *American Journal of Medicine, 128,* 1138.e17–1138.e23.

Al Toma, A., Verbeek, W. H., Hadithi, M., von Blomberg, B. M., & Mulder, C. J. (2007). Survival in refractory coeliac disease and enteropathy-associated T-cell lymphoma: Retrospective evaluation of single-centre experience. *Gut, 56,* 1373–1378.

Alfadhli, A. A., McDonald, J. W., & Feagan, B. G. (2003). Methotrexate for induction of remission in refractory Crohn's disease. *Cochrane Database of Systematic Reviews,* (1), CD003459.

Alibhai, S. M., Greenwood, C., & Payette, H. (2005). An approach to the management of unintentional weight loss in elderly people. *CMAJ, 172,* 773–780.

Alstead, E. M., Ritchie, J. K., Lennard-Jones, J. E., Farthing, M. J., & Clark, M. L. (1990). Safety of azathioprine in pregnancy in inflammatory bowel disease. *Gastroenterology, 99,* 443–446.

Angulo, P., Kleiner, D. E., Dam-Larsen, S., Adams, L. A., Bjornsson, E. S., Charatcharoenwitthaya, P., et al. (2015). Liver fibrosis, but no other histologic features, is associated with long-term outcomes of patients with nonalcoholic fatty liver disease. *Gastroenterology, 149,* 389–397.

Arcelus, J., Mitchell, A. J., Wales, J., & Nielsen, S. (2011). Mortality rates in patients with anorexia nervosa and other eating disorders. A meta-analysis of 36 studies. *Archives of General Psychiatry, 68,* 724–731.

Aziz, I., Lewis, N. R., Hadjivassiliou, M., Winfield, S. N., Rugg, N., Kelsall, A., et al. (2014). A UK study assessing the population prevalence of self-reported gluten sensitivity and referral characteristics to secondary care. *European Journal of Gastroenterology and Hepatology, 26,* 33–39.

Bernal, W., Auzinger, G., Dhawan, A., & Wendon, J. (2010). Acute liver failure. *Lancet, 376,* 190–201.

Bjornsson, E. S., Bergmann, O. M., Bjornsson, H. K., Kvaran, R. B., & Olafsson, S. (2013). Incidence, presentation, and outcomes in patients with drug-induced liver injury in the general population of Iceland. *Gastroenterology, 144,* 1419–1425.

Boeckxstaens, G., El Serag, H. B., Smout, A. J., & Kahrilas, P. J. (2014). Symptomatic reflux disease: The present, the past and the future. *Gut, 63*, 1185–1193.

Bosch, J., & Sauerbruch, T. (2016). Esophageal varices: Stage-dependent treatment algorithm. *Journal of Hepatology, 64*, 746–748.

Briggs, A. H., Sculpher, M. J., Logan, R. P., Aldous, J., Ramsay, M. E., & Baron, J. H. (1996). Cost effectiveness of screening for and eradication of *Helicobacter pylori* in management of dyspeptic patients under 45 years of age. *British Medical Journal (Clinical Research Ed.), 312*, 1321–1325.

British HIV Association. (2008). *UK national guidelines for HIV testing.*

British Society of Gastroenterology. (2007). *Guidelines for osteoporosis in inflammatory bowel disease and coeliac disease.*

Bruix, J., & Sherman, M. (2011). Management of hepatocellular carcinoma: An update. *Hepatology (Baltimore, Md.), 53*, 1020–1022.

Camilleri, M., Kerstens, R., Rykx, A., & Vandeplassche, L. (2008). A placebo-controlled trial of prucalopride for severe chronic constipation. *New England Journal of Medicine, 358*, 2344–2354.

Camilleri, M., Piessevaux, H., Yiannakou, Y., Tack, J., Kerstens, R., Quigley, E. M., et al. (2016). Efficacy and safety of prucalopride in chronic constipation: An integrated analysis of six randomized, controlled clinical trials. *Digestive Diseases and Sciences.*

Camilleri, M., Van Outryve, M. J., Beyens, G., Kerstens, R., Robinson, P., & Vandeplassche, L. (2010). Clinical trial: The efficacy of open-label prucalopride treatment in patients with chronic constipation—follow-up of patients from the pivotal studies. *Alimentary Pharmacology and Therapeutics, 32*, 1113–1123.

Castera, L. (2010). Diagnosing cirrhosis non-invasively: Sense the stiffness but don't forget the nodules! *Journal of Hepatology, 52*, 786–787.

Castera, L., Sebastiani, G., Le Bail, B., de Ledinghen, V., Couzigou, P., & Alberti, A. (2010). Prospective comparison of two algorithms combining non-invasive methods for staging liver fibrosis in chronic hepatitis C. *Journal of Hepatology, 52*, 191–198.

Castera, L., Vilgrain, V., & Angulo, P. (2013). Noninvasive evaluation of NAFLD. *Nature Reviews. Gastroenterology and Hepatology, 10*, 666–675.

Chande, N., Tsoulis, D. J., & MacDonald, J. K. (2013). Azathioprine or 6-mercaptopurine for induction of remission in Crohn's disease. *Cochrane Database of Systematic Reviews, (4)*, CD000545.

Chapman, R., Fevery, J., Kalloo, A., Nagorney, D. M., Boberg, K. M., Shneider, B., et al. (2010). Diagnosis and management of primary sclerosing cholangitis. *Hepatology (Baltimore, Md.), 51*, 660–678.

Chey, W. D., Lembo, A. J., Lavins, B. J., Shiff, S. J., Kurtz, C. B., Currie, M. G., et al. (2012). Linaclotide for irritable bowel syndrome with constipation: A 26-week, randomized, double-blind, placebo-controlled trial to evaluate efficacy and safety. *American Journal of Gastroenterology, 107*, 1702–1712.

Czul, F., & Bhamidimarri, K. R. (2016). Noninvasive markers to assess liver fibrosis. *Journal of Clinical Gastroenterology, 50*, 445–457.

Dalton, H. R., Hunter, J. G., & Bendall, R. P. (2013). Hepatitis E. *Current Opinions on Infectious Disease, 26*, 471–478.

Didari, T., Mozaffari, S., Nikfar, S., & Abdollahi, M. (2015). Effectiveness of probiotics in irritable bowel syndrome: Updated systematic review with meta-analysis. *World Journal of Gastroenterology, 21*, 3072–3084.

DuPont, H. L. (2014). Review article: Evidence for the role of gut microbiota in irritable bowel syndrome and its potential influence on therapeutic targets. *Alimentary Pharmacology and Therapeutics, 39*, 1033–1042.

European Association for the Study of the Liver. (2009). EASL clinical practice guidelines: Management of cholestatic liver diseases. *Journal of Hepatology, 51*, 237–267.

European Association for the Study of the Liver. (2010). EASL clinical practice guidelines for HFE hemochromatosis. *Journal of Hepatology, 53*, 3–22.

European Association for the Study of the Liver. (2012). EASL-EORTC clinical practice guidelines: Management of hepatocellular carcinoma. *Journal of Hepatology, 56*, 908–943.

European Association for the Study of the Liver. (2015). EASL clinical practice guidelines: Autoimmune hepatitis. *Journal of Hepatology, 63*, 971–1004.

European Association for the Study of the Liver. (2016). EASL-EASD-EASO clinical practice guidelines for the management of non-alcoholic fatty liver disease. *Journal of Hepatology, 64*, 1388–1402.

European Association for the Study of the Liver and the American Association for the Study of Liver Diseases. (2014). *Hepatic encephalopathy in chronic liver disease: 2014 practice guideline by the EASL and the AASLD.*

European Association for the study of the Liver. (2018). EASL recommendations on treatment of hepatitis C 2018. *Journal of Hepatology, 2018.*

Feagan, B. G., Fedorak, R. N., Irvine, E. J., Wild, G., Sutherland, L., Steinhart, A. H., et al. (2000). A comparison of methotrexate with placebo for the maintenance of remission in Crohn's disease. North American Crohn's Study Group Investigators. *New England Journal of Medicine, 342*, 1627–1632.

Feagan, B. G., & MacDonald, J. K. (2012). Oral 5-aminosalicylic acid for maintenance of remission in ulcerative colitis. *Cochrane Database of Systematic Reviews, (10)*, CD000544.

Ferenci, P. (2004). Review article: Diagnosis and current therapy of Wilson's disease. *Alimentary Pharmacology and Therapeutics, 19*, 157–165.

Fitzgerald, R. C., di Pietro, M., Ragunath, K., Ang, Y., Kang, J. Y., Watson, P., et al. (2014). British Society of Gastroenterology guidelines on the diagnosis and management of Barrett's oesophagus. *Gut, 63*, 7–42.

Ford, A. C., Achkar, J. P., Khan, K. J., Kane, S. V., Talley, N. J., Marshall, J. K., et al. (2011). Efficacy of 5-aminosalicylates in ulcerative colitis: Systematic review and meta-analysis. *American Journal of Gastroenterology, 106*, 601–616.

Ford, A. C., Qume, M., Moayyedi, P., Arents, N. L., Lassen, A. T., Logan, R. F., et al. (2005). *Helicobacter pylori* "test and treat" or endoscopy for managing dyspepsia: An individual patient data meta-analysis. *Gastroenterology, 128*, 1838–1844.

Francella, A., Dyan, A., Bodian, C., Rubin, P., Chapman, M., & Present, D. H. (2003). The safety of 6-mercaptopurine for child-bearing patients with inflammatory bowel disease: A retrospective cohort study. *Gastroenterology, 124*, 9–17.

Gaddey, H. L., & Holder, K. (2014). Unintentional weight loss in older adults. *American Family Physician, 89*, 718–722.

Gisbert, J. P., Linares, P. M., McNicholl, A. G., Mate, J., & Gomollon, F. (2009). Meta-analysis: The efficacy of azathioprine and mercaptopurine in ulcerative colitis. *Alimentary Pharmacology and Therapeutics, 30*, 126–137.

Gisbert, J. P., & Pajares, J. M. (2004). Stool antigen test for the diagnosis of *Helicobacter pylori* infection: A systematic review. *Helicobacter, 9*, 347–368.

Goddard, A. F., James, M. W., McIntyre, A. S., & Scott, B. B. (2011). Guidelines for the management of iron deficiency anaemia. *Gut, 60*, 1309–1316.

Gordon, M., Naidoo, K., Thomas, A. G., & Akobeng, A. K. (2011). Oral 5-aminosalicylic acid for maintenance of surgically-induced remission in Crohn's disease. *Cochrane Database of Systematic Review, (1)*, CD008414.

Gordon, M., Taylor, K., Akobeng, A. K., & Thomas, A. G. (2014). Azathioprine and 6-mercaptopurine for maintenance of surgically-induced remission in Crohn's disease. *Cochrane Database of Systematic Reviews*, (8), CD010233.

Hanauer, S. B., Sandborn, W. J., Dallaire, C., Archambault, A., Yacyshyn, B., Yeh, C., et al. (2007). Delayed-release oral mesalamine 4.8 g/day (800 mg tablets) compared to 2.4 g/day (400 mg tablets) for the treatment of mildly to moderately active ulcerative colitis: The ASCEND I trial. *Canadian Journal of Gastroenterology*, 21, 827–834.

Hanauer, S. B., Sandborn, W. J., Kornbluth, A., Katz, S., Safdi, M., Woogen, S., et al. (2005). Delayed-release oral mesalamine at 4.8 g/day (800 mg tablet) for the treatment of moderately active ulcerative colitis: The ASCEND II trial. *American Journal of Gastroenterology*, 100, 2478–2485.

Hay, J. E. (2008). Liver disease in pregnancy. *Hepatology (Baltimore, Md.)*, 47, 1067–1076.

Headstrom, P. D., & Surawicz, C. M. (2005). Chronic diarrhea. *Clinical Gastroenterology and Hepatology*, 3, 734–737.

Hindorf, U., Johansson, M., Eriksson, A., Kvifors, E., & Almer, S. H. (2009). Mercaptopurine treatment should be considered in azathioprine intolerant patients with inflammatory bowel disease. *Alimentary Pharmacology and Therapeutics*, 29, 654–661.

Howdle, P. D., Jalal, P. K., Holmes, G. K., & Houlston, R. S. (2003). Primary small-bowel malignancy in the UK and its association with coeliac disease. *QJM: Monthly Journal of the Association of Physicians*, 96, 345–353.

Islami, F., & Kamangar, F. (2008). *Helicobacter pylori* and esophageal cancer risk: A meta-analysis. *Cancer Prevention Research (Philadelphia)*, 1, 329–338.

Kapoor, N., Bassi, A., Sturgess, R., & Bodger, K. (2005). Predictive value of alarm features in a rapid access upper gastrointestinal cancer service. *Gut*, 54, 40–45.

Krag, A., & Madsen, B. S. (2015). To block, or not to block in advanced cirrhosis and ascites: That is the question. *Gut*, 64, 1015–1017.

Lebwohl, B., Ludvigsson, J. F., & Green, P. H. (2015). Celiac disease and non-celiac gluten sensitivity. *British Medical Journal (Clinical Research Ed.)*, 351, h4347.

Lees, C. W., Maan, A. K., Hansoti, B., Satsangi, J., & Arnott, I. D. (2008). Tolerability and safety of mercaptopurine in azathioprine-intolerant patients with inflammatory bowel disease. *Alimentary Pharmacology and Therapeutics*, 27, 220–227.

Lichtenstein, G. R., Ramsey, D., & Rubin, D. T. (2011). Randomised clinical trial: Delayed-release oral mesalazine 4.8 g/day vs. 2.4 g/day in endoscopic mucosal healing—ASCEND I and II combined analysis. *Alimentary Pharmacology and Therapeutics*, 33, 672–678.

Lilford, R. J., Bentham, L., Girling, A., Litchfield, I., Lancashire, R., Armstrong, D., et al. (2013a). Birmingham and Lambeth Liver Evaluation Testing Strategies (BALLETS): A prospective cohort study. *Health Technology Assessment*, 17, i307.

Lilford, R. J., Bentham, L. M., Armstrong, M. J., Neuberger, J., & Girling, A. J. (2013b). What is the best strategy for investigating abnormal liver function tests in primary care? Implications from a prospective study. *British Medical Journal Open*, 3.

Lindor, K. D., Gershwin, M. E., Poupon, R., Kaplan, M., Bergasa, N. V., & Heathcote, E. J. (2009). Primary biliary cirrhosis. *Hepatology (Baltimore, Md.)*, 50, 291–308.

Longstreth, G. F., Thompson, W. G., Chey, W. D., Houghton, L. A., Mearin, F., & Spiller, R. C. (2006). Functional bowel disorders. *Gastroenterology*, 130, 1480–1491.

Loy, C. T., Irwig, L. M., Katelaris, P. H., & Talley, N. J. (1996). Do commercial serological kits for *Helicobacter pylori* infection differ in accuracy? A meta-analysis. *American Journal of Gastroenterology*, 91, 1138–1144.

Ludvigsson, J. F., Bai, J. C., Biagi, F., Card, T. R., Ciacci, C., Ciclitira, P. J., et al. (2014). Diagnosis and management of adult coeliac disease: Guidelines from the British Society of Gastroenterology. *Gut*, 63, 1210–1228.

Maconi, G., Manes, G., & Porro, G. B. (2008). Role of symptoms in diagnosis and outcome of gastric cancer. *World Journal of Gastroenterology*, 14, 1149–1155.

Malfertheiner, P., Megraud, F., O'Morain, C., Bazzoli, F., El Omar, E., Graham, D., et al. (2007). Current concepts in the management of *Helicobacter pylori* infection: The Maastricht III Consensus Report. *Gut*, 56, 772–781.

Marshall, B. J., & Warren, J. R. (1984). Unidentified curved bacilli in the stomach of patients with gastritis and peptic ulceration. *Lancet*, 1, 1311–1315.

Marshall, J. K., & Irvine, E. J. (1997). Rectal corticosteroids versus alternative treatments in ulcerative colitis: A meta-analysis. *Gut*, 40, 775–781.

McColl, K. E. (2010). Clinical practice. *Helicobacter pylori* infection. *New England Journal of Medicine*, 362, 1597–1604.

McDonald, J. W., Wang, Y., Tsoulis, D. J., MacDonald, J. K., & Feagan, B. G. (2014). Methotrexate for induction of remission in refractory Crohn's disease. *Cochrane Database of Systematic Reviews*, (8), CD003459.

McMinn, J., Steel, C., & Bowman, A. (2011). Investigation and management of unintentional weight loss in older adults. *British Medical Journal (Clinical Research Ed.)*, 342, d1732.

Micali, N., Hagberg, K. W., Petersen, I., & Treasure, J. L. (2013). The incidence of eating disorders in the UK in 2000-2009: Findings from the General Practice Research Database. *British Medical Journal Open*, 3.

Moayyedi, P., Soo, S., Deeks, J., Delaney, B., Harris, A., Innes, M., et al. (2003a). Eradication of *Helicobacter pylori* for non-ulcer dyspepsia. *Cochrane Database of Systematic Reviews*, (1), CD002096.

Moayyedi, P., Soo, S., Deeks, J., Delaney, B., Innes, M., & Forman, D. (2003b). Pharmacological interventions for non-ulcer dyspepsia. *Cochrane Database of Systematic Reviews*, (1), CD001960.

Moayyedi, P., & Talley, N. J. (2006). Gastro-oesophageal reflux disease. *Lancet*, 367, 2086–2100.

Mooney, P. D., Hadjivassiliou, M., & Sanders, D. S. (2014). Coeliac disease. *British Medical Journal (Clinical Research Ed.)*, 348, g1561.

Moore, K. P., & Aithal, G. P. (2006). Guidelines on the management of ascites in cirrhosis. *Gut*, 55, vi1–vi12.

Mowat, C., Cole, A., Windsor, A., Ahmad, T., Arnott, I., Driscoll, R., et al. (2011). Guidelines for the management of inflammatory bowel disease in adults. *Gut*, 60, 571–607.

Munkholm, P., Michetti, P., Probert, C. S., Elkjaer, M., & Marteau, P. (2010). Best practice in the management of mild-to-moderately active ulcerative colitis and achieving maintenance of remission using mesalazine. *European Journal of Gastroenterology and Hepatology*, 22, 912–916.

Murch, S., Jenkins, H., Auth, M., Bremner, R., Butt, A., France, S., et al. (2013). Joint BSPGHAN and Coeliac UK guidelines for the diagnosis and management of coeliac disease in children. *Archive of Disease in Childhood*, 98, 806–811.

Nguyen, G. C., Smalley, W. E., Vege, S. S., & Carrasco-Labra, A. (2016). American Gastroenterological Association Institute guideline on the medical management of microscopic colitis. *Gastroenterology*, 150, 242–246.

National Institute for Health and Care Excellence. (2004). *Dyspepsia: Managing dyspepsia in adults in primary care. NICE clinical guideline 17.*

National Institute for Health and Care Excellence. (2006). *Nutrition support for adults: Oral nutrition support, enteral tube feeding and parenteral nutrition. NICE clinical guideline 32.*

National Institute for Health and Care Excellence. (2008). *Irritable bowel syndrome in adults: Diagnosis and management. NICE clinical guideline 61.*

National Institute for Health and Care Excellence. (2012). *Crohn's disease: Management. NICE clinical guideline 152.*

National Institute for Health and Care Excellence. (2013a). *Faecal calprotectin diagnostic tests for inflammatory diseases of the bowel. NICE diagnostic guidance 11.*

National Institute for Health and Care Excellence. (2013b). *Hepatitis B (chronic): Diagnosis and management. NICE clinical guideline 165.*

National Institute for Health and Care Excellence. (2013c). *Ulcerative colitis: Management. NICE clinical guideline 166.*

National Institute for Health and Care Excellence. (2014a). *Endoscopic radiofrequency ablation for Barrett's oesophagus with low-grade dysplasia or no dysplasia. NICE interventional procedures guidance 496.*

National Institute for Health and Care Excellence. (2014b). *Gastro-oesophageal reflux disease and dyspepsia in adults: Investigation and management. NICE clinical guideline 184.*

National Institute for Health and Care Excellence. (2015a). *Coeliac disease: Recognition, assessment and management. NICE clinical guideline 29.*

National Institute for Health and Care Excellence. (2015b). *Suspected cancer: Recognition and referral. NICE Guideline 12.*

National Institute for Health and Care Excellence. (2016a). *Assessment and management of cirrhosis. NICE Guideline 49.*

National Institute for Health and Care Excellence. (2016b). *Non-alcoholic fatty liver disease (NAFLD): Assessment and management. NICE Guideline 49.*

Norgard, B., Pedersen, L., Fonager, K., Rasmussen, S. N., & Sorensen, H. T. (2003). Azathioprine, mercaptopurine and birth outcome: A population-based cohort study. *Alimentary Pharmacology and Therapeutics, 17*, 827–834.

Quigley, E. M., Tack, J., Chey, W. D., Rao, S. S., Fortea, J., Falques, M., et al. (2013). Randomised clinical trials: Linaclotide phase 3 studies in IBS-C—a prespecified further analysis based on European Medicines Agency-specified endpoints. *Alimentary Pharmacology and Therapeutics, 37*, 49–61.

Rezende, G., Roque-Afonso, A. M., Samuel, D., Gigou, M., Nicand, E., Ferre, V., et al. (2003). Viral and clinical factors associated with the fulminant course of hepatitis A infection. *Hepatology (Baltimore, Md.), 38*, 613–618.

Rinella, M. E. (2015). Nonalcoholic fatty liver disease: A systematic review. *JAMA: The Journal of the American Medical Association, 313*, 2263–2273.

Royal College of Physicians. (2014). *UK inflammatory bowel disease audit.*

Rubin, D. T., LoSavio, A., Yadron, N., Huo, D., & Hanauer, S. B. (2006). Aminosalicylate therapy in the prevention of dysplasia and colorectal cancer in ulcerative colitis. *Clinical Gastroenterology and Hepatology, 4*, 1346–1350.

Rubio-Tapia, A., & Murray, J. A. (2010). Classification and management of refractory coeliac disease. *Gut, 59*, 547–557.

Ruepert, L., Quartero, A. O., de Wit, N. J., van der Heijden, G. J., Rubin, G., & Muris, J. W. (2011). Bulking agents, antispasmodics and antidepressants for the treatment of irritable bowel syndrome. *Cochrane Database of Systematic Reviews*, (8), CD003460.

Schiller, L. R. (2004). Chronic diarrhea. *Gastroenterology, 127*, 287–293.

Seenan, J. P., Thomson, F., Rankin, K., Smith, K., & Gaya, D. R. (2014). Are we exposing patients with a mildly elevated faecal calprotectin to unnecessary investigations? *Frontline Gastroenterology.*

Sgouros, S. N., & Pereira, S. P. (2006). Systematic review: Ssphincter of Oddi dysfunction—non-invasive diagnostic methods and long-term outcome after endoscopic sphincterotomy. *Alimentary Pharmacology and Therapeutics, 24*, 237–246.

Shea, J. A., Berlin, J. A., Escarce, J. J., Clarke, J. R., Kinosian, B. P., Cabana, M. D., et al. (1994). Revised estimates of diagnostic test sensitivity and specificity in suspected biliary tract disease. *Archives of Internal Medicine, 154*, 2573–2581.

Short, M. W., & Domagalski, J. E. (2013). Iron deficiency anemia: Evaluation and management. *American Family Physician, 87*, 98–104.

Sidhu, R., Sanders, D. S., Morris, A. J., & McAlindon, M. E. (2008). Guidelines on small bowel enteroscopy and capsule endoscopy in adults. *Gut, 57*, 125–136.

Singh, A., Mann, H. S., Thukral, C. L., & Singh, N. R. (2014). Diagnostic accuracy of MRCP as compared to ultrasound/CT in patients with obstructive jaundice. *Journal of Clinical & Diagnostic Research, 8*, 103–107.

Singh, S., Stroud, A. M., Holubar, S. D., Sandborn, W. J., & Pardi, D. S. (2015). Treatment and prevention of pouchitis after ileal pouch-anal anastomosis for chronic ulcerative colitis. *Cochrane Database of Systematic Reviews*, (11), CD001176.

Smith, M. A., Blaker, P., Marinaki, A. M., Anderson, S. H., Irving, P. M., & Sanderson, J. D. (2012). Optimising outcome on thiopurines in inflammatory bowel disease by co-prescription of allopurinol. *Journal of Crohns and Colitis, 6*, 905–912.

Spada, C., Stoker, J., Alarcon, O., Barbaro, F., Bellini, D., Bretthauer, M., et al. (2014). Clinical indications for computed tomographic colonography: European Society of Gastrointestinal Endoscopy (ESGE) and European Society of Gastrointestinal and Abdominal Radiology (ESGAR) guideline. *Endoscopy, 46*, 897–915.

Spiller, R., Aziz, Q., Creed, F., Emmanuel, A., Houghton, L., Hungin, P., et al. (2007). Guidelines on the irritable bowel syndrome: Mechanisms and practical management. *Gut, 56*, 1770–1798.

Tack, J., Talley, N. J., Camilleri, M., Holtmann, G., Hu, P., Malagelada, J. R., et al. (2006). Functional gastroduodenal disorders. *Gastroenterology, 130*, 1466–1479.

Thomas, P. D., Forbes, A., Green, J., Howdle, P., Long, R., Playford, R., et al. (2003). Guidelines for the investigation of chronic diarrhoea, 2nd edition. *Gut, 52*, S1–S15.

Thursz, M. R., Richardson, P., Allison, M., Austin, A., Bowers, M., Day, C. P., et al. (2015). Prednisolone or pentoxifylline for alcoholic hepatitis. *New England Journal of Medicine, 372*, 1619–1628.

Tripathi, D., Stanley, A. J., Hayes, P. C., Patch, D., Millson, C., Mehrzad, H., et al. (2015). UK guidelines on the management of variceal haemorrhage in cirrhotic patients. *Gut, 64*, 1680–1704.

Truelove, S. C., & Witts, L. J. (1955). Cortisone in ulcerative colitis; final report on a therapeutic trial. *British Medical Journal (Clinical Research Ed.), 2*, 1041–1048.

Tsochatzis, E. A., Bosch, J., & Burroughs, A. K. (2014). Liver cirrhosis. *Lancet, 383*, 1749–1761.

Vaira, D., & Vakil, N. (2001). Blood, urine, stool, breath, money, and *Helicobacter pylori*. *Gut, 48*, 287–289.

van Assche, G., Dignass, A., Reinisch, W., van der Woude, C. J., Sturm, A., De Vos, M., et al. (2010). The second European evidence-based Consensus on the diagnosis and management of Crohn's disease: Special situations. *Journal of Crohns and Colitis, 4*, Sfir–101.

van Assche, G., Dignass, A., Bokemeyer, B., Danese, S., Gionchetti, P., Moser, G., et al. (2013). Second European evidence-based consensus on the diagnosis and management of ulcerative colitis part 3: Special situations. *Jouranl of Crohns and Colitis, 7,* 1–33.

van Bokhoven, M. A., van Deursen, C. T., & Swinkels, D. W. (2011). Diagnosis and management of hereditary haemochromatosis. *British Medical Journal (Clinical Research Ed.), 342,* c7251.

van der Ende, A., van der Hulst, R. W., Dankert, J., & Tytgat, G. N. (1997). Reinfection versus recrudescence in *Helicobacter pylori* infection. *Alimentary Pharmacology and Therapeutics, 11,* 55–61.

van Staa, T. P., Card, T., Logan, R. F., & Leufkens, H. G. (2005). 5-Aminosalicylate use and colorectal cancer risk in inflammatory bowel disease: A large epidemiological study. *Gut, 54,* 1573–1578.

Williams, R., Aspinall, R., Bellis, M., Camps-Walsh, G., Cramp, M., Dhawan, A., et al. (2014). Addressing liver disease in the UK: A blueprint for attaining excellence in health care and reducing premature mortality from lifestyle issues of excess consumption of alcohol, obesity, and viral hepatitis. *Lancet, 384,* 1953–1997.

Zhang, Y., Li, L., Guo, C., Mu, D., Feng, B., Zuo, X., et al. (2016). Effects of probiotic type, dose and treatment duration on irritable bowel syndrome diagnosed by Rome III criteria: A meta-analysis. *BMC Gastroenterology, 16,* 62.

Zlatanic, J., Korelitz, B. I., Rajapakse, R., Kim, P. S., Rubin, S. D., Baiocco, P. J., et al. (2003). Complications of pregnancy and child development after cessation of treatment with 6-mercaptopurine for inflammatory bowel disease. *Journal of Clinical Gastroenterology, 36,* 303–309.

10
Surgical Problems

IAIN WILSON

CHAPTER CONTENTS

Gallstone Disease

GUIDELINES

European Association for the Study of the Liver (EASL) Clinical Practice Guidelines. (2016). The prevention, diagnosis and treatment of gallstones. https://easl.eu/publication/prevention-diagnosis-and-treatment-of-gallstones/.
    National Institute for Health and Care Excellence. (2014). Gallstone disease. Diagnosis and management of cholelithiasis, cholecystitis and choledocholithiasis. NICE clinical guideline 188. https://www.nice.org.uk/guidance/cg188/evidence/cg188-gallstone-disease-full-guideline3

- Gallstone disease is the most common gastrointestinal disorder causing hospital admission in European countries (Farthing et al., 2014).

- 80% of gallstones are asymptomatic; 2% to 4% of people with asymptomatic gallstones will develop symptoms or complications each year (Gurusamy & Davidson, 2014).
- Complications of gallstones include biliary colic, cholecystitis, pancreatitis, choledocholithiasis, cholangitis, obstructive jaundice, and gallbladder cancer.

Investigation

- Take bloods, including full blood count (FBC) and liver function tests (LFTs) (National Institute for Health and Care Excellence [NICE], 2014). Serum amylase is only required if there is suspicion of pancreatitis.
- Arrange an abdominal ultrasound.
- Consider referring for magnetic resonance cholangiopancreatography (MRCP) if there are dilated bile ducts and/or abnormal liver function tests.

- Consider referring for MRCP or endoscopic ultrasound (EUS) if there is a strong suspicion of gallstones with a negative abdominal ultrasound (AUS).

Management

- Laparoscopic cholecystectomy is not recommended for patients with asymptomatic gallbladder stones in a normal gall bladder.
- Refer all patients with symptomatic gallstones for consideration of laparoscopic cholecystectomy.
- Advise patients to avoid food and drink that triggers their symptoms until they have had their gallbladder removed (NICE, 2014).

Biliary Colic

- Patients with biliary colic require analgesia with paracetamol and, if appropriate, nonsteroidal antiinflammatory drugs (NSAIDs).
- Patients with severe symptoms may benefit from opioid analgesia and spasmolytics.
- Cholecystectomy should be performed as early as possible for patients with uncomplicated biliary colic (European Association for the Study of the Liver [EASL], 2016).

Cholecystitis

- Antibiotics should be commenced if there is evidence of sepsis, cholangitis, abscess, or perforation (EASL, 2016). These patients should usually have been admitted emergently. *Note:* Patients with cholecystitis are usually prescribed antibiotics. There is however some evidence to suggest that not all patients benefit from antibiotics. A small randomized controlled trial could not demonstrate that intravenous antibiotic treatment improved outcomes of patients with mild acute cholecystitis (Mazeh et al., 2012).
- Patients with acute cholecystitis should be offered early laparoscopic cholecystectomy by the admitting surgical team (to be carried out within 1 week of diagnosis) (NICE, 2016). A Cochrane review has shown that early laparoscopic cholecystectomy for acute cholecystitis shortens the total length of hospital stay (Gurusamy, Davidson, Gluud, & Davidson, 2013).

Choledocholithiasis

- Common bile duct (CBD) stones should be suspected in patients with acute cholangitis, acute pancreatitis, deranged liver function tests (LFTs), or a dilated biliary tree.
- Bile duct clearance and laparoscopic cholecystectomy should be offered to people with symptomatic or asymptomatic common bile duct stones (NICE, 2014).

Gallbladder Polyps

- Polypoid lesions of the gallbladder are found in 4% to 7% of patients who undergo abdominal ultrasound (Chou, Chen, Shyr, & Wang, 2019).

GUIDELINE

EASL Clinical Practice Guidelines. (2016). The prevention, diagnosis and treatment of gallstones. https://easl.eu/publication/prevention-diagnosis-and-treatment-of-gallstones/.

- Most polypoid lesions are benign, but a small number are malignant or premalignant. The likelihood of a polypoid lesion being malignant or premalignant increases with polyp size.
- Cholecystectomy should be performed in patients with gallbladder polyps 1 cm or larger.
- Cholecystectomy should also be considered in patients with asymptomatic gallbladder stones and gallbladder polyps 6 to 10 mm and in case of growing polyps.
- Cholecystectomy is not indicated in patients with asymptomatic gallbladder stones and gallbladder polyps 5 mm or smaller.

Diverticular Disease

GUIDELINES

Association of Coloproctology of Great Britain and Ireland (ACPGBI) Commissioning Guide. (2014). Colonic diverticular disease. https://www.acpgbi.org.uk//content/uploads/2017/02/Commissioning-guide-colonic-diverticular-disease-RCS-2014.pdf.
    National Institute for Health and Care Excellence. (2017). Suspected cancer: Recognition and referral. NICE clinical guideline 12. https://www.nice.org.uk/guidance/ng12.
    National Institute for Health and Care Excellence (NICE) Clinical Knowledge Summary. (2017). Diverticular disease. https://cks.nice.org.uk/diverticular-disease#!rightTopic.
    World Society of Emergency Surgery (WSES) Guidelines. (2016). WSES guidelines for the management of acute left sided colonic diverticulitis in the emergency setting. https://www.ncbi.nlm.nih.gov/pmc/articles/PMC4966807/.

Definitions

- Diverticulosis: presence of diverticula that are asymptomatic. The presence of diverticula is rare in individuals under the age of 40; 50% of the population aged over 50 years is affected, 70% aged over 80 years of age is affected (Association of Coloproctology of Great Britain and Ireland [ACPGBI], 2014).
- Diverticular disease: diverticula that are symptomatic.
- Diverticulitis: diverticula that become inflamed and/or infected. Classic symptoms include left iliac fossa pain, fever, and a change in bowel habit.
- Uncomplicated diverticulitis refers to localised diverticular inflammation.

Complications

- Complications of diverticulitis include rectal bleeding, local and generalised peritonitis, perforation, abscess, fistula, and stricture formation.

- About 4% of people with diverticulosis will develop acute diverticulitis (Shahedi, Fuller, & Bolus, 2013).
- Approximately 15% of people will have rectal bleeding from their diverticula (ACPGBI, 2014).

Diverticulosis

- Advise patients to maintain a healthy, balanced, high-fibre diet with adequate fluid intake (NICE, 2017).

Diverticular Disease

- Advise patients to maintain a healthy, balanced, high-fibre diet with adequate fluid intake.
- Consider prescribing bulk-forming laxatives.
- Patients should be referred to secondary care in the following circumstances:
  - To confirm a suspected diagnosis of diverticular disease
  - If symptoms affect quality of life
  - If pain is not controlled by paracetamol
  - If there are symptoms that are suspicious for a colorectal cancer (see upcoming guidelines).
- Patients with the following symptoms should be referred for an appointment within 2 weeks under the NICE suspected cancer: recognition and referral pathway:
  - Aged 40 and over with unexplained weight loss and abdominal pain
  - Aged under 50 with rectal bleeding and unexplained abdominal pain, change in bowel habit, weight loss, and/or iron-deficiency anaemia
  - Aged 50 and over with unexplained rectal bleeding
  - Aged 60 and over with iron-deficiency anaemia, changes in bowel habit, or tests show occult blood in faeces
  - Finding of a rectal or abdominal mass

Acute Mild Uncomplicated Diverticulitis

Investigation

- Consider checking blood for raised white cell count and C-reactive protein (CRP). CRP is a useful tool in the prediction of the clinical severity of acute diverticulitis. Patients with a CRP value higher than 150 mg/L have a significant risk of complicated diverticulitis (Mäkelä, Klintrup, Takala, & Rautio, 2015).

Management

- Referral to hospital is not mandatory for all patients with acute uncomplicated diverticulitis (ACPGBI, 2014).
- In selected patients without significant comorbidities, management includes:
  - a diet of clear liquids only. Reintroduce solid food as symptoms improve over 2 to 3 days;
  - regular paracetamol for pain. Avoid NSAIDs and opioid analgesics;
  - considering prescribing broad-spectrum oral antibiotics that cover anaerobes and Gram-negative bacilli (e.g., co-amoxiclav or ciprofloxacin and metronidazole). Treatment should last for at least 7 days (NICE, 2017).

- There is evidence to suggest that selected patients with acute uncomplicated diverticulitis do not require antibiotics. A multicentre randomised trial comparing antibiotic treatment versus no antibiotic treatment of computed tomography (CT) proven acute uncomplicated diverticulitis showed that antibiotics did not expedite recovery or prevent complications (Chabok et al., 2012).
- Reassess the patient within 48 hours, or sooner if symptoms deteriorate, and thereafter depending on response to treatment.
- An emergency surgical admission should be arranged in the following circumstances:
  - There is suspicion of perforation or abscess.
  - Symptoms cannot be managed in primary care.
  - The patient is unable to take or tolerate oral fluids at home.
  - The patient is unable to tolerate oral antibiotics at home.
  - The patient is frail and/or has significant comorbidities and/or is immunocompromised (NICE, 2017).

Further Management

- All patients require investigation of the colonic lumen by endoscopy, barium enema, or CT colonography after the acute episode of diverticulitis has resolved (ACPGBI, 2014).
- Indications for referral to secondary care include:
  - frequent or severe recurrent episodes of acute diverticulitis;
  - symptoms that affect quality of life;
  - pain that is not controlled by paracetamol; and
  - the presence of red flag symptoms (i.e., change in bowel habit, weight loss, symptoms suggestive of anaemia) (ACPGBI, 2014).
- Patient-related factors and not the number of episodes of diverticulitis should dictate if elective sigmoid resection in indicated (World Society of Emergency Surgery [WSES], 2016).
- Patients were previously offered elective bowel resection following two episodes of diverticulitis. The risk or recurrent diverticulitis is lower than previously thought. A systematic review has shown that complicated diverticulitis following an attack of uncomplicated diverticulitis is rare (<5%) (Regenbogen, Hardiman, Hendren, & Morris, 2014).
- Clear indications for elective sigmoid resections are symptomatic stenosis, fistulas, and recurrent diverticular bleeding.

Rectal Bleeding

> **GUIDELINE**
>
> ACPGBI Commissioning Guide. 2017. Rectal bleeding.
> https://www.acpgbi.org.uk//content/uploads/2014/03/
> Commissioning-Guide-for-Rectal-Bleeding-Dec-2017.pdf.

- Rectal bleeding is a common problem. In the United Kingdom the 1-year prevalence in adults is about 10% (ACPGBI, 2017).

- Most rectal bleeding is due to benign conditions such as haemorrhoids, anal fissure, and diverticular disease.
- Rectal bleeding can be a manifestation of more sinister problems such as inflammatory bowel disease and colorectal cancer. Clinicians should take care not to miss proximal colorectal disease in the presence of benign anorectal pathology (ACPGBI, 2017). Rectal bleeding has a positive predictive value (PPV) for colorectal malignancy of 8% in patients aged over 50 (Astin et al., 2011).

Assessment

- Ask about perianal symptoms (pain, lump, prolapse, itch, leakage, incomplete evacuation, and discharge).
- Enquire about bleeding, including colour of the blood (bright red, dark red) and where blood was observed (on the paper, coating stool, or in the pan).
- Enquire about any family history of colorectal cancer and inflammatory bowel disease.
- Ask about red flag symptoms, including weight loss, symptoms suggestive of anaemia, and change in bowel habit.
- Perform an abdominal examination to exclude an abdominal mass.
- Examine the external anus. Spread the buttocks and look for fissures, prolapsed mucosa, or haemorrhoids.
- Perform a digital rectal examination (DRE). DRE will provide useful information about the presence of perianal disease, the prostate, sphincter tone, and the presence of any pelvic masses. The cervix can commonly be palpated anteriorly in women. Haemorrhoids are vascular structures and cannot usually be palpated on DRE. Patients with a fissure may not tolerate a DRE.
- If experience and logistics permit, undertake proctoscopy.

Investigation

- Blood tests are not routinely indicated in patients with rectal bleeding.
- Consider FBC if there are signs and symptoms of anaemia.
- Other bloods tests may be indicated if bleeding is associated with problems such as weight loss or change in bowel habit.
- If inflammatory bowel disease is suspected in a young, low-risk patient consider a test for faecal calprotectin. A positive faecal calprotectin result has a high positive predictive value for finding inflammatory bowel disease at colonoscopy.
- Tumour markers and faecal occult blood testing are not indicated in patients with rectal bleeding (ACPGBI, 2017).

Management

- The management of specific conditions will be discussed later in this chapter.
- Most bleeding resolves spontaneously. It is reasonable to manage low-risk patients with rectal bleeding with a "watch and wait" policy (ACPGBI, 2017).
- Emergency surgical referral should be arranged in the presence of haemodynamic instability, significant blood loss, and the potential requirement for blood transfusion (ACPGBI, 2017).

- Clinicians should consider an emergency referral in patients who are elderly, on oral anticoagulation, and unable to monitor bleeding.
- Direct access flexible sigmoidoscopy provides the best reassurance for patients with rectal bleeding who are primarily concerned about malignancy (ACPGBI, 2017).

Indications for Referral

- Patients with the following symptoms should be referred for an appointment within 2 weeks under the NICE suspected cancer: recognition and referral pathway:
  - Aged under 50 with rectal bleeding and any unexplained abdominal pain, change in bowel habit, weight loss, iron-deficiency anaemia
  - Aged 50 and over with unexplained rectal bleeding
- Patients with rectal bleeding who do not fulfil the above-mentioned criteria should be considered for urgent referral if there is:
  - a strong family history of colorectal malignancy;
  - anxiety about colorectal malignancy;
  - persistent rectal bleeding despite treatment for haemorrhoids;
  - rectal bleeding in patients with a past history of pelvic radiotherapy; and
  - suspected inflammatory bowel disease (ACPGBI, 2017).

Haemorrhoids

GUIDELINES

American Society of Colon and Rectal Surgeons (ASCRS) Clinical Practice Guidelines. (2018). Management of haemorrhoids. https://www.fascrs.org/sites/default/files/downloads/publication/cpg_management_of_hemorrhoids.pdf. NICE Clinical Knowledge Summary. (2016). Haemorrhoids. https://cks.nice.org.uk/haemorrhoids.

- Haemorrhoids arise when the circular venous plexuses in the anus become persistently dilated.
- Haemorrhoids that originate above the dentate line are internal haemorrhoids. Haemorrhoids that originate below the dentate line are external haemorrhoids.
- Factors that contribute to the development of haemorrhoids include constipation, straining, ageing, heavy lifting, chronic cough, pregnancy, and childbirth (NICE, 2016).

Assessment

- It is important for the clinician to establish that haemorrhoids are the cause of a patient's symptoms and exclude the presence of more proximal and sinister colorectal disease.
- See "Assessment" under "Rectal Bleeding."
- Bleeding classically presents as bright red blood on the toilet paper. Blood can also be seen in the toilet bowl or coating the faeces.
- Other possible symptoms include itching or irritation, a feeling of rectal fullness, discomfort, incomplete evacuation, and soiling.

- Ask about prolapse. Internal haemorrhoids can be classified according to their degree of prolapse:
  - Grade I: project into the anal canal only
  - Grade II: prolapse on straining but reduce spontaneously
  - Grade III: prolapse on straining but require manual reduction
  - Grade IV: persistently prolapsed and cannot be reduced

Investigation

- See "Investigation" under "Rectal Bleeding."

Management

- Diet and lifestyle modification are the first line for all patients with symptomatic haemorrhoids (American Society of Colon and Rectal Surgeons [ASCRS], 2018).
- Recommend a diet with enough fluid and fibre intake so stools are soft and easy to pass.
- Advise that patients minimise time spent sitting on the toilet and straining.
- The anal region should be kept clean and dry.
- Consider prescribing a bulk-forming laxative if there is constipation.
- Consider prescribing a topical haemorrhoidal preparation (NICE, 2016).

Topical Haemorrhoidal Preparations

- A variety of topical treatments are available to manage the symptoms of haemorrhoids. These may contain one or a combination of mild astringents, lubricants, local anaesthetic, or corticosteroids.
- There is no evidence to suggest that one topical preparation is more effective than another, although lidocaine is the preferred topical anaesthetic agent.
- Generally, haemorrhoidal preparations should be used in the morning and night, and after a bowel movement.
- Prolonged use of any agent is not recommended; anaesthetic-containing preparations may cause sensitization of the anal skin. Corticosteroid-containing preparations should be used for no longer than 7 days because prolonged use may lead to skin atrophy, contact dermatitis, and skin sensitisation (NICE, 2016).

Indications for Referral

- Consider an emergency admission with acutely thrombosed external haemorrhoids (see upcoming discussion) and incarcerated and thrombosed internal haemorrhoids.
- Refer all patients for an urgent 2-week appointment if anal or colorectal cancer is suspected.
- Indications for routine referral to secondary care include:
  - patients who do not respond to conservative treatment;
  - third-degree or fourth-degree haemorrhoids that are too large for nonoperative measures (haemorrhoidectomy may be needed);
  - combined internal and external haemorrhoids with severe symptoms (surgery may be required);
  - the presence of chronic irritation or leakage; and

- large skin tags (surgical excision may be required) (NICE, 2016).
- Most patients with grade I, II, and selected patients with grade III internal hemorrhoidal disease who fail medical treatment can be effectively treated with office-based procedures. Hemorrhoidal banding is typically the most effective option (ASCRS, 2018).

Thrombosed External Haemorrhoid

- Patients are usually advised to manage symptoms with oral analgesia, topical analgesia, and laxatives. Most patients treated nonoperatively will experience eventual resolution of their symptoms.
- Selected patients with thrombosed external haemorrhoids may benefit from early surgical excision (ASCRS, 2018).
- One paper has shown that patients who underwent surgical management of their thrombosed haemorrhoid achieved resolution of symptoms faster than those managed conservatively (3.9 days vs. 24 days) (Greenspon, Williams, Young, & Orkin, 2004).

Anal Fissure

GUIDELINES

ASCRS Clinical Practice Guidelines. (2017). Clinical practice guideline for the management of anal fissures. https://www.fascrs.org/sites/default/files/downloads/publication/cpg_for_the_management_of_anal_fissures_jan_2017_dcr_issue.pdf.
　NICE Clinical Knowledge Summary. (2017). Anal fissure. https://cks.nice.org.uk/anal-fissure.

- An anal fissure is a longitudinal tear in the skin of the anal canal.
- Primary anal fissures are thought to arise due to spasm of the internal anal sphincter causing localised ischaemia.

Assessment

- Spread the buttocks and inspect the anus.
- Of anal fissures, 90% occur in the posterior midline.
- Features of chronic fissures include a hypertrophied anal papilla at the proximal aspect of the fissure, a sentinel skin tag at the distal aspect of the fissure, and exposed internal anal sphincter muscle within the base of the fissure (NICE, 2017).
- DRE may not be possible in patients with a fissure owing to pain.

Management

- Advise patients increase the amount of fibre and fluid in their diet.
- Consider prescribing a bulking agent.
- Advise taking paracetamol and ibuprofen for analgesia.
- Avoid opiate analgesia.
- Consider prescribing a topical anaesthetic for a few days. Avoid prolonged use as it can desensitise the anal skin.

- Advise that sitting in a shallow, warm bath several times a day (if possible, particularly after a bowel movement) may help relieve pain.
- Recommend the anal region is kept clean and dry.
- Almost half of patients who have an acute anal fissure will resolve their symptoms with non-operative measures (Stewart et al., 2017).

Topical Medications
- Anal fissures may be treated with topical nitrates.
- Consider prescribing topical glyceryl trinitrate (GTN) 0.4% ointment. Advise the patient to use twice a day for 6 to 8 weeks. Consider prescribing a second course if the fissure remains unhealed but there has been an improvement in symptoms (NICE, 2017).
- The main side effect of topical GTN is headaches, which often leads to patients stopping treatment. Headaches with GTN have been observed in up to 70% of patients in one paper (Berry, Barish, & Bhandari, 2013).
- Topical GTN is associated with healing in approximately 50% of chronic anal fissures (Berry et al., 2013).
- Topical 2% diltiazem is an alternative treatment for anal fissure but is unlicensed.
- GTN and diltiazem have been shown to be equally effective in treating fissures (Sanei, Mahmoodieh, & Masoudpour, 2009), although diltiazem is associated with fewer side effects.

Indications for Referral
- Refer all patients for an urgent 2-week appointment if anal or colorectal cancer is suspected.
- Consider referral for examination under anaesthesia if the diagnosis is unclear or if spasm and pain make diagnosis impossible.
- Refer patients who remain symptomatic and/or have an unhealed fissure despite adherence to conservative measures and topical agents.
- Consider referring patients whom you are considering starting topical diltiazem.
- Refer with the presence of a fissure in an elderly patient.
- Further options for the management of anal fissure in secondary care include injection of botulinum toxin and lateral internal sphincterotomy.

Inguinal Hernia

> **GUIDELINES**
>
> British Hernia Society (BHS) Commissioning Guide. (2016). Groin hernia. https://www.rcseng.ac.uk/standards-and-research/commissioning/commissioning-guides/topics/.
> HerniaSurge Group. (2018). International guidelines for groin hernia management. https://www.ncbi.nlm.nih.gov/pubmed/29330835.

- Groin hernia repair is one of the most commonly performed operations in the world.

- Inguinal hernias are almost always symptomatic.
- Asymptomatic hernias tend to become symptomatic. One study has shown that 70% of patients managed with a "watch and wait" strategy will eventually require surgery within 5 years (Fitzgibbons et al., 2013).

Investigation
- The gold standard for hernia diagnosis is clinical examination.
- The British Hernia Society (BHS) advises that diagnostic imaging should not be arranged at primary care level.
- Dynamic ultrasound scan is recommended as the first line investigation for patients with groin pain or swelling of an unclear origin (BHS, 2016).

Management
- The only cure for groin hernia is surgery.

Indications for Referral
- All patients with an overt or suspected primary or recurrent inguinal or femoral hernia should be offered routine referral to secondary care.
- Patients with strangulated or obstructed groin hernia should be emergency referrals.
- Irreducible and partially reducible inguinal hernias, and all groin hernias in women, should be urgent referrals.
- Patients with bilateral groin hernias should be referred to a surgeon who performs both open and laparoscopic repair.
- Patients with recurrent inguinal or femoral hernias meeting referral criteria should be referred to a surgeon who performs both open and laparoscopic repair and where possible to the named surgeon who performed the first repair (providing the patient does not request otherwise).
- Patients with multiple recurrent (more than one recurrence) groin hernias should be referred to a named surgeon who has subspecialty interest in hernia repair and performs both open and laparoscopic repair.
- Patients with minimally symptomatic inguinal hernias who have significant comorbidity *and* do not want to have surgical repair (after appropriate information has been provided) do not need to be referred (BHS, 2016).

Vascular Problems

Varicose Veins

> **GUIDELINE**
>
> National Institute of Health and Care Excellence. (2013). Varicose veins: Diagnosis and management. NICE clinical guideline 168. www.nice.org.uk.

- Varicose veins occur when the valves within the veins become incompetent allowing blood to reflux, which results in tortuous, dilated veins.

- For some patients varicose veins are primarily a cosmetic concern, but they can be complicated by discomfort, thrombophlebitis, deep vein thrombosis, bleeding, and skin changes (including lipodermatosclerosis, venous eczema, and ulceration).
- For management of skin changes or ulcers in the context of varicose veins, see Chapter 22.

Management

- If bleeding, then apply first aid and admit urgently. Bleeding from varicose veins can sometimes be life threatening.
- If not bleeding offer reassurance that complications are rare but warn about signs and symptoms of thrombosis, bleeding, and ulceration.
- Give lifestyle advice, including:
  - weight loss;
  - light or moderate exercise; and
  - avoiding prolonged periods of sitting and standing.
- If referral is not indicated (see upcoming discussion) or if the patient declines referral, consider compression stockings, although note that NICE advises that compression hosiery should only be offered if interventional treatment is thought to be inappropriate.
- If considering compression hosiery:
  - assess whether the patient is able to use the hosiery correctly;
  - explain that class 2 stockings may be more effective than class 1 but are less well tolerated (see Chapter 22 for more detail); and
  - exclude underlying arterial disease, which is a contraindication to compression, with ankle brachial pressure index (ABPI).

Referral

- Many areas have specific referral criteria for varicose veins but NICE recommends that referral be considered for:
  - symptomatic veins;
  - thrombophlebitis; and
  - skin changes, including active or healed ulceration.
- Treatment options in secondary care include endothermal ablation, endovenous laser treatment, ultrasound-guided foam sclerotherapy, or surgery.

Peripheral Arterial Disease (PAD)

GUIDELINES

National Institute of Health and Care Excellence. (2012, updated 2018). Peripheral arterial disease: Diagnosis and management. NICE clinical guideline 147. www.nice.org.uk.
   NICE Clinical Knowledge Summaries. (2015). Peripheral arterial disease. cks.nice.org.uk.

- Peripheral arterial disease results from the narrowing or occlusion of peripheral arteries due to atherosclerotic disease.

- PAD is associated with the same risk factors as other cardiovascular disease, including increasing age, smoking, obesity, diabetes mellitus, and hypercholesterolaemia.
- Limb ischaemia may be acute or chronic.

Diagnosis

- Suspect acute ischaemia in a limb that has become painful over a period of minutes, hours, or days that is pallid with a loss of distal pulses. The limb may also be cold, cyanotic, with a loss or alteration of sensation and muscle power. This is a threat to limb viability and is thus an emergency. Admit immediately.
- Suspect chronic limb ischaemia if the patient reports the cramp-like pain on exercise typical of intermittent claudication. Pain is usually in the calf if there is narrowing of the femoral or popliteal arteries. It is less commonly in the hip, thigh, or buttock if the common iliac artery is affected. Chronic limb ischaemia may also be indicated by non healing wounds on the leg (including arterial ulcers) or distal pulses are difficult to palpate.
- Measure the ankle brachial pressure index if PAD is suspected:
  - ABPI <0.9 suggests PAD.
  - ABPI <0.5 suggests the patient is at risk of critical limb ischaemia. Refer urgently.
  - A value between 0.9 and 1.3 makes PAD less likely.
  - A value >1.3 suggests arterial stiffening particularly in patients with diabetes mellitus or renal failure.
  - *Note: NICE advises not to exclude PAD in patients with diabetes mellitus based on a normal or raised ABPI alone.*

Management

- Offer treatment for secondary prevention of cardiovascular disease, including:
  - smoking cessation;
  - advice on diet and exercise;
  - lipid modification with a statin;
  - management of hypertension;
  - management of diabetes; and
  - antiplatelet therapy (NICE recommends clopidogrel 75 mg once daily as first line).
- If available, offer a supervised exercise programme for patients with intermittent claudication. This involves 2 hours of supervised exercise per week for 3 months. Patients should be encouraged to exercise to the point of maximum pain.
- Unsupervised exercise may be recommended in suitable patients with advice to patients to exercise for 30 minutes, three to five times each week, exercising until the onset of symptoms and then resting until recovered.
- See Chapter 22 for management of arterial ulcers.
- Consider referral to a vascular surgeon if the above mentioned measures are ineffective.
- Refer urgently if ABPI is below 0.5 due to the risk of critical limb ischaemia.
- Consider naftidrofuryl oxalate if the patient declines referral or is not appropriate for angioplasty or bypass surgery. Treat for 3 to 6 months and discontinue if there is no benefit.

References

Association of Coloproctology of Great Britain and Ireland (ACPGBI). (2014). *Commissioning guide: Rectal bleeding.* https://www.acpgbi.org.uk//content/uploads/2017/02/Commissioning-guide-colonic-diverticular-disease-RCS-2014.pdf.

Association of Coloproctology of Great Britain and Ireland (ACPGBI). (2017). *Commissioning guide: Colonic diverticular disease.* https://www.acpgbi.org.uk//content/uploads/2014/03/Commissioning-Guide-for-Rectal-Bleeding-Dec-2017.pdf.

Astin, M., Griffin, T., Neal, R., et al. (2011). The diagnostic value of symptoms for colorectal cancer in primary care: A systematic review. *British Journal of General Practice, 61,* e231–e243.

Berry, S., Barish, C., & Bhandari, R. (2013). Nitroglycerin 0.4% ointment vs placebo in the treatment of pain resulting from chronic anal fissure: A randomized, double-blind, placebo-controlled study. *BMC Gastroenterology, 13,* 106.

British Hernia Society. (2016). *Commissioning guide: Groin hernia.* https://www.rcseng.ac.uk/standards-and-research/commissioning/commissioning-guides/topics/.

Davis, B., Lee-Kong, S., Migaly, J., et al. (2018). *The American Society of Colon and Rectal Surgeons clinical practice guidelines for the management of hemorrhoids.* https://www.fascrs.org/sites/default/files/downloads/publication/cpg_management_of_hemorrhoids.pdf.

Chabok, A., Påhlman, L., Hjern, F., et al. (2012). Randomized clinical trial of antibiotics in acute uncomplicated diverticulitis. *British Journal of Surgery, 99,* 532–539.

Chou, S., Chen, S., Shyr, Y., & Wang, S. (2019). Polypoid lesions of the gallbladder: Analysis of 1204 patients with long-term follow-up. *Surgical Endoscopy, 31,* 2776–2782.

European Association for the Study of the Liver (EASL). (2016). EASL clinical practice guidelines on the prevention, diagnosis and treatment of gallstones. *Journal of Hepatology, 65,* 146–181. https://easl.eu/publication/prevention-diagnosis-and-treatment-of-gallstones/.

Farthing, M., Roberts, S., Samuel, D., et al. (2014). Survey of digestive health across Europe: Final report. Part 1: The burden of gastrointestinal diseases and the organisation and delivery of gastroenterology services across Europe. *United European Gastroenterology Journal, 2,* 539–543.

Fitzgibbons, R., Ramanan, B., Arya, S., et al. (2013). Long-term results of a randomized controlled trial of a nonoperative strategy (watchful waiting) for men with minimally symptomatic inguinal hernias. *Annals of Surgery, 258,* 505–508.

Greenspon, J., Williams, S., Young, H., & Orkin, B. (2004). Thrombosed external haemorrhoids: Outcome after conservative or surgical management. *Diseases of the Colon & Rectum, 47,* 1493–1498.

Gurusamy, K., & Davidson, B. (2014). Gallstones. *British Medical Journal, 348,* g2669.

Gurusamy, K., Davidson, C., Gluud, C., & Davidson, B. (2013). Early versus delayed laparoscopic cholecystectomy for people with acute cholecystitis. *The Cochrane Database of Systematic Reviews, (6),* CD005440.

HerniaSurge Group. (2018). International guidelines for groin hernia management. *Hernia: The Journal of Hernias and Abdominal Wall Surgery, 22,* 1–65.

Mäkelä, J., Klintrup, K., Takala, H., & Rautio, T. (2015). The role of C-reactive protein in prediction of the severity of acute diverticulitis in an emergency unit. *Scandinavian Journal of Gastroenterology, 50,* 536–541.

Mazeh, H., Mizrahi, I., Dior, U., et al. (2012). Role of antibiotic therapy in mild acute calculus cholecystitis: A prospective randomized controlled trial. *World Journal of Surgery, 36,* 1750–1759.

National Institute for Health and Care Excellence (NICE). (2014). *Gallstone disease: Diagnosis and management of cholelithiasis, cholecystitis and choledocholithiasis. NICE clinical guideline 188.* https://www.nice.org.uk/guidance/cg188/evidence/cg188-gallstone-disease-full-guideline3.

National Institute for Health and Care Excellence Clinical Knowledge Summaries. (2016). *Haemorrhoids.* https://cks.nice.org.uk/haemorrhoids.

National Institute for Health and Care Excellence Clinical Knowledge Summaries. (2017). *Diverticular disease.* https://cks.nice.org.uk/diverticular-disease#!rightTopic.

National Institute for Health and Care Excellence Clinical Knowledge Summaries. (2017). *Diverticular disease: Anal fissure.* https://cks.nice.org.uk/anal-fissure.

Regenbogen, S., Hardiman, K., Hendren, S., & Morris, A. (2014). Surgery for diverticulitis in the 21st century: A systematic review. *JAMA Surgery, 149,* 292–303.

Sanei, B., Mahmoodieh, M., & Masoudpour, H. (2009). Comparison of topical glyceryl trinitrate with diltiazem ointment for the treatment of chronic anal fissure: A randomized clinical trial. *Acta Chirurgica Belgica, 109,* 727–730.

Sartelli, M., Catena, F., Ansaloni, L., et al. (2016). WSES guidelines for the management of acute left sided colonic diverticulitis in the emergency setting. *World Journal of Emergency Surgery, 11,* https://www.ncbi.nlm.nih.gov/pmc/articles/PMC4966807/.

Shahedi, K., Fuller, G., & Bolus, R. (2013). Long-term risk of acute diverticulitis among patients with incidental diverticulosis found during colonoscopy. *Clinical Gastroenterology and Hepatology, 11,* 1609–1613.

Stewart, D., Gaertner, W., Glasgow, S., et al. (2017). *Clinical practice guidelines for the management of anal fissures.* https://www.fascrs.org/sites/default/files/downloads/publication/cpg_for_the_management_of_anal_fissures_jan_2017_dcr_issue.pdf.

11

Musculoskeletal Problems

JOHN MACLEAN

CHAPTER CONTENTS

Osteoarthritis

> **GUIDELINE**
>
> National Institute for Health and Care Excellence. (2014).
> *Osteoarthritis: Care and management. NICE clinical guideline
> 177.* Available at www.nice.org.uk/Guidance/CG177.

- The aims of management are to:
  - empower the patient in self-management;
  - control symptoms (mainly pain and stiffness);
  - prevent progression of joint damage;
  - reduce disability and improve function.

Management Strategy

- Make a holistic assessment of the impact of osteoarthritis on the patient in terms of:
  - function, occupation, leisure activities;
  - quality of life;
  - mood and sleep;
  - relationships;
  - comorbidities.

TABLE 11.1	Management of Osteoarthritis		
Core treatment	These should be considered for all patients	Education Exercise Weight loss for the overweight
Relatively safe pharmaceutic options	These should be considered before adjunctive treatments	Paracetamol Topical nonsteroidal antiinflammatory drugs
Adjunctive treatments	This refers to treatments which have less proof of efficacy or involve more risk to the patient	Pharmaceutical • Nonsteroidal antiinflammatory drugs • Opioids • Intraarticular steroids • Capsaicin Self-management • Local heat and cold • Assistive devices Other nonpharmacologic • Supports and braces • Shock-absorbing shoes and insoles • Transcutaneous electrical nerve stimulation • Manual therapy • Surgery

- Elicit the patient's understanding of the illness and concerns.
- Discuss the risks and benefits of treatment options.
- Formulate a management plan with the patient based on the above and taking account of the patient's values and preferences.
- Screen for depression which is more common in patients with long-term disability.

Management can be divided into three domains (Table 11.1).

Education and Self-Management

- Address concerns and counter any misconceptions (e.g., that the disease inevitably progresses to joint replacement). Patient-centred consultations result in better outcomes and better use of resources (such as fewer unhelpful investigations).
- Explain the disease in appropriate language and back this up with an offer of written information.

PATIENT INFORMATION

Arthritis Research UK. *Osteoarthritis: An information booklet.* Available from www.arthritisresearchuk.org.

Arthritis Care. *Living with osteoarthritis (information booklet).* Available from www.arthritiscare.org.uk/do-i-have-arthritis/publications/223-living-with-osteoarthritis.

- Encourage exercise:
  - Local muscle strengthening
  - General aerobic exercise
- Refer to physiotherapy for exercise according to local policies.

- Encourage weight loss in the overweight. This improves function, though whether it reduces pain is not certain.

Relatively Safe Pharmaceutical Options

- Recommend paracetamol. Regular doses, namely 1 g four times daily, might be better than taking a dose *as required*.
- For some joints, such as the knee, recommend topical nonsteroidal anti-inflammatory drugs (NSAIDs) before progressing to adjunctive drugs with their associated risks.

Adjunctive Nonpharmacologic, Nonsurgical Management

- Consider the following for pain relief:
  - Local application of heat or cold
  - Referral for manipulation or stretching
  - Transcutaneous electrical nerve stimulation (TENS)
- Refer to the most appropriate agency according to local policies (e.g., physiotherapy or occupational therapy) for:
  - assessment for bracing, joint supports, or insoles in those with biomechanical joint pain or instability;
  - assistive devices such as walking sticks.
- Advise on footwear. Shock-absorbing shoes (trainers) and insoles (which can be purchased from pharmacies) may help weightbearing joints.
- Advise the patient to keep active and to pace oneself, take planned rest periods, and avoid bursts of overactivity.
- Look out for depression. If present, treating it not only improves mood but results in less pain and improved function at 12 months (Lin et al., 2003).
- Recommend tricyclic antidepressants if sleep or mood disturbance is present.
- Do not recommend electroacupuncture. Consider the use of acupuncture when there are few options left.

Adjunctive Pharmacologic Management

- Prescribe either a weak opioid or an oral NSAID (see NSAID section) depending on patient preferences and comorbidities.
- Educate the patient in the self-management of analgesics so that he or she can step up or down the scale of treatment:
  - Recommend that NSAIDs be used for the shortest period possible.
  - Explain that paracetamol or co-codamol can be used with ibuprofen, but that co-codamol should *never* be taken with paracetamol because it contains the same drug.
  - Ensure the patient is not on more than one NSAID, including over-the-counter (OTC) preparations (e.g., aspirin).
- Consider intraarticular steroid injections.
- Consider topical capsaicin.
- Do not prescribe glucosamine or chondroitin (Towheed et al., 2005).

Local Injections

- Intraarticular corticosteroid injections provide short-term pain relief and may give patients the opportunity to begin other interventions such as exercise.
- Intraarticular hyaluronic acid injections have been shown to have only a weak effect.
- Consider a steroid injection for moderate to severe pain and for flareups.
- Do not refer for intraarticular hyaluronic acid injections for knees.

Disability

- Consider the patient's need for aids (e.g., bath aids) and refer as appropriate.
- Consider eligibility for benefits (e.g., Attendance Allowance, a disabled driver's badge) and refer to the appropriate agency for advice.
- Consider the need for support and rehabilitation. Refer, according to local circumstances, to social services, a rehabilitation team, or hospital-based multidisciplinary team.

X-Rays

- Plain x-rays are not routinely indicated. They cannot confirm the diagnosis because degenerative changes in several joints (e.g., spine and knees) start in middle age and x-ray appearances correlate poorly with the symptoms (Royal College of Radiologists, 2003). Diagnosis is mainly clinical in many syndromes and plain x-rays do not differentiate between disease and nondisease (e.g., shoulder impingement syndrome).
- Refer for x-ray when:
  - soft tissue calcification is suspected (e.g., shoulder) and when the result might inform the choice to use an NSAID or steroid injection;

- referral for joint replacement is being considered;
- there is knee pain with locking: x-ray may show radiopaque loose bodies;
- there is diagnostic doubt.

Referrals to a Specialist

- Consider referral for joint replacement surgery when a patient experiences joint symptoms, whether pain, stiffness, or reduced function, that impact substantially on his or her quality of life and have not responded to core and adjunctive treatments. Referral is best made before prolonged functional limitation and severe pain become established.
- Follow local referral thresholds, which vary, but age, gender, smoking, obesity, and comorbidities should not be barriers to referral.

Postoperative Care

Patients will occasionally ask their general practitioner (GP) about their return to normal activities:

- Advise the patient who has had a hip replacement not to cross the legs or drive for 6 weeks. The danger of dislocation is greatest in the first 6 weeks and occurs when the hip is flexed, especially if internally rotated and adducted.
- Advise patients that they may resume activities, including walking, swimming, bicycling, and tennis, *after 6 weeks*, provided they take care not to fall. Contact sports and use of ladders are not advised.

Recurrence of Pain

- Arrange for an x-ray, erythrocyte sedimentation rate (ESR), and white blood cell (WBC) count in any patient with a hip prosthesis who develops pain. This may show loosening, infection, stress fracture, or dislocation. Refer any of these to the surgeon urgently. Refer anyway if the pain does not settle with rest. Any of the above may be present despite a normal x-ray.

Antibiotic Prophylaxis

Patients with prosthetic joint implants including total hip replacements do not need antibiotic prophylaxis for dental treatment (Uçkay, 2008).

Low Back Pain

> **GUIDELINE**
>
> National Institute for Health and Care Excellence. (2016). *Low back pain and sciatica in over 16s: Assessment and management.* NICE clinical guideline 59. Available from www.nice.org.uk/guidance/NG59.

- Low back pain (LBP) can be defined as:
  - acute LBP: duration of 6 weeks or less
  - subacute LBP: duration of 6 to 12 weeks
  - chronic LBP: duration of 3 months or more

- LBP is extremely common. At any one time, 15% of adults have it and 60% will have it some time in their lives (Mason, 1994). Back pain is the most common cause of long-term sickness: 52 million working days are lost each year from back pain.
- Mechanical LBP is self-limiting: 80% to 90% of patients recover spontaneously within 3 months.
- At presentation triage patients into one of the three following groups based on history and examination:
  - Mechanical back pain
  - Nerve root compression
  - Possible serious spinal pathology—look for *red flags* (see upcoming discussion) and act accordingly
- Note any psychological or social influences that might retard recovery: so-called *yellow flags*.

Aims of Management

- Reduce pain and the length of sickness in mechanical back pain.
- Identify early the small minority with serious pathology needing immediate or urgent attention.
- Prevent acute back pain becoming chronic.

Managing Acute Mechanical Low Back Pain

- Features of mechanical back pain include:
  - presentation at age 20 to 55;
  - pain felt over lumbosacral area, buttocks, or thighs;
  - pain alters with posture and activity;
  - the patient is well.
- Take time to listen and examine, explain, and reassure. These have beneficial effect on pain and anxiety.
- Encourage continued activity, including work if appropriate. Bedrest worsens outcome and should only be taken if pain is severe, and then for no longer than necessary (Waddell, Feder, & Lewis, 1997).
- Prescribe analgesics or NSAIDs.
- Avoid prescribing muscle relaxants (e.g., diazepam). They control pain, but the abuse potential and the availability of other analgesic options means that it should not be common practice.
- Ensure the patient has a medium-firm mattress (5 on the European Committee for Standardisation scale). This has been shown to be more effective than a firm one (Kovacs et al., 2003).
- Demonstrate stretching exercises or give written instructions (e.g., "Back Pain" booklet from the Association for Real Change [ARC] is available from www.arc.org.uk). Many exercises are available and some have fanatical supporters, but there is no evidence that any specific type of exercise is best (Tulder et al., 2000).
- Offer a follow-up consultation after 2 to 6 weeks:
  - If activity and function are improving, encourage return to normal activities even if pain is still present. Stress that activity will not damage the back.

- If not improving, advise graded return to normal activity and set a return date to work.
- If not improving, also consider referral to another health professional with expertise in LBP, usually a physiotherapist, or possibly a manipulative therapist.
- Reassess for *red flags* (to come).
- Reassess for *yellow flags* (to come). If present, be positive, schedule regular reviews, encourage a programme of activity, and consider early referral.
- If there has been a failure to progress at 6 weeks then continue and intensify current management and consider referral to specialist services.

Psychosocial Blocks to Recovery (Yellow Flags)

- Yellow flags include:
  - a belief that back pain is harmful or potentially disabling;
  - fear-avoidance behaviour (avoiding a movement or activity due to misplaced anticipation of pain) and reduced activity levels;
  - a tendency to low mood and withdrawal from social interaction; an expectation that passive treatments rather than active participation will help;
  - awaiting compensation;
  - a history of absence from work for back pain or other problems;
  - poor job satisfaction, long hours, heavy work;
  - an overprotective family or a lack of support at home.
- Note that these yellow flags should not be used pejoratively. They are a guide to those patients in whom early intervention and early return to work are especially important.

Management of Chronic Low Back Pain

- The prevalence of LBP is not increasing but the level of disability and claims for long-term sickness benefits are. The management of chronic LBP therefore encompasses several approaches:
  - Appropriate referral for physical treatments (see upcoming discussion)
  - Principles of chronic pain management
  - Attention to psychosocial issues
- Recommend regular physical exercise. This should start as soon as possible in the course of the illness. A light mobilization programme for patients who have had back pain for 8 to 12 weeks has been shown to improve outcomes initially and at 3 years (Hagen, Eriksen, & Ursin, 2000).
- Treat underlying anxiety or depression if present.
- Consider prescribing a tricyclic antidepressant at low doses, even if depression is not present (Staiger et al., 2003).
- Explore work-related issues. If return to former employment is unlikely, advise the patient to see the disability employment adviser at the job centre.
- Consider referral to a multidisciplinary team; this can be effective in resistant cases (Guzmán et al., 2001).

Nerve Root Compression

- Mechanical back pain can be referred down the leg so not all sciatica arises from a prolapsed disc; nerve root compression is more likely if pain extends down to the foot. Conversely, not all prolapsed discs cause sciatica since they can be demonstrated in 50% of asymptomatic adults.
- Sciatica arising from a prolapsed disc that causes significant disability has a lifetime prevalence of 5%.
- Recognizing nerve root compression is important because surgery leads to quicker recovery than natural resolution, although there may be no difference in long-term outcomes (Peul et al., 2007).
- Chymopapain (discolysis) is also effective but not widely used in the United Kingdom.
- At presentation, test for limitation of straight leg raising. If straight leg raising is not impaired and pain does not radiate below the knee then nerve root compression is very unlikely (Vroomen, de Krom, & Knotterus, 1999).
- Look for neurological deficit from L5/S1 compression: loss of sensation over the lateral border of the lower leg and foot, weakness of dorsiflexion and plantarflexion of foot, and impairment of the ankle reflex. In L3/4 compression the knee reflex may be impaired.
- Manage sciatica as you would acute LBP.
- Refer patients whose pain is not settling (the timescale will depend on local circumstances) or where there is increasing neurological deficit.

Referrals

Whom to refer to will depend on local availability and agreed care pathways: physiotherapist, pain clinic, multidisciplinary team, orthopaedic physicians, or orthopaedic surgeons.

Failure to Progress in Acute Low Back Pain

- All guidelines are consistent in recommending early referral (≤2 weeks) for physiotherapy or manipulation to prevent acute LBP becoming chronic. However, there is conflicting evidence about whether this makes a difference to long-term outcome, although a large UK trial shows evidence of modest benefit at 3 and 12 months from manipulation (UK BEAM Trial Team, 2004). This held whether the manipulation was in National Health Service (NHS) or private facilities. Conversely, it is now clear that, even in sciatica, epidural corticosteroid injection offers no long-term benefit, although there may be transient benefit at 3 weeks (Arden et al., 2005).
- Be prepared (Hazard et al., 1997) to discuss manipulation; many patients take themselves to osteopaths or chiropractors and many physiotherapists practice a related treatment, mobilization. The evidence for manipulation is of low quality but it may lead to quicker recovery in the first few weeks without making any difference to long-term outcomes (Koes et al., 1996).

- There is insufficient evidence for physical agents and passive modalities (e.g., ice, heat, short-wave diathermy, massage, ultrasound, TENS, acupuncture), but they remain popular.

Failure to Progress With Neurological Symptoms or Signs, and Other Serious Situations

- Evidence of benefit from discectomy, which may be long term, is accumulating for patients with disc herniation, spinal stenosis, and spondylolisthesis (Gibson, 2007).
- *Sciatica.* The ideal timing of referral to an orthopaedic surgeon of patients with sciatica which is not improving is not clear. A *British Medical Journal (BMJ)* leading article suggests 8 weeks (Fairbank, 2008); patients with severe pain will be referred earlier.
- *Cauda equina syndrome* (see upcoming discussion). Refer immediately to an orthopaedic surgeon.
- *Other red flags.* Refer urgently where appropriate and, if a malignancy is suspected, refer urgently according to the recommendations of the Department of Health (DOH, 2000).

X-Rays

- Explain to patients with mechanical LBP why x-rays are unhelpful: Degenerative changes are common; most disorders are of soft tissue, which cannot be shown on x-ray; and the dose of radiation is high (60 times that of a chest x-ray) (Royal College of Radiologists, 2003).
- Consider x-rays in the presence of red flags, alongside urgent referral.

Possible Serious Spinal Pathology

- Red flags include:
  - cauda equina syndrome (features include urinary retention, bilateral neurological symptoms and signs, saddle anaesthesia—urgent referral is indicated);
  - significant trauma (risk of fracture);
  - weight loss (suggestive of cancer);
  - history of cancer (suggestive of metastases);
  - fever (suggestive of infection);
  - intravenous drug use (suggestive of infection);
  - steroid use (risk of osteoporotic collapse);
  - patient aged over 50 years (cancer unlikely below this age);
  - severe, unremitting nighttime pain (suggestive of cancer);
  - pain that gets worse when patient is lying down (suggestive of cancer).

The Elderly With Acute Back Pain

These patients are a special case because osteoporotic collapse and malignancy are more likely and they need an early x-ray. Half will have definite abnormality, and 10% will have a malignancy (Frank, 1993).

Advice/Exercises for Low Back Pain

The following is taken from the BackCare leaflet "Exercise for a Better Back" and from the ARC leaflet "Back Pain" (see upcoming discussion).

- Pay attention to sitting, lifting, and bending to avoid aggravating pain and to prevent recurrence.
  - *Sitting:* Avoid prolonged sitting. A rolled towel in the small of the back may ease pain.
  - *Lifting:* Always lift with a straight back and bent knees.
  - *Bending:* Avoid spending too long at a task that requires bending (e.g., ironing).
- Exercise regularly.
  - Stretching exercises to maintain flexibility—daily. You may start these early on in an attack and should keep them up long term.
  - Muscle strengthening exercises—daily. You should start these as your pain improves and keep them up long term.
  - Take up aerobic exercise for general fitness (e.g., swimming).
- Suitable exercises (there are many others):
  - Starting position: on all fours with hands shoulder width apart, arms and thighs vertical:
    1. Arch the back and look down. Then lower the stomach toward the floor, hollowing the back.
    2. Slowly walk the hands around to one side, back to the starting position, then around to the other side.
    3. Raise one hand off the floor, reach underneath your body as far as you can. On the return, swing the arm out to the side as far as you can then return to the starting position. Follow the moving hand with the eyes. Repeat with the other arm.
    4. Draw alternate knees to the opposite elbow.
    5. Stretch one arm forward in front, at the same time stretching the opposite leg out behind. Repeat on the other side.
    6. Swing the seat from side to side.

All exercises should be repeated 10 times. Exercises that hurt should be set aside and returned to with fewer repetitions on another occasion.

Neck Pain

- The principles of management of low back pain apply to neck pain (Nachemson & Jonsson, 2000).
- Triage neck pain into mechanical, nerve root compression (often termed *radiculopathy*), and potential serious pathology (*red flags*).
- In mechanical neck pain, keeping active is more effective than immobilization.
- Similar medication may be prescribed.
- Psychosocial factors are important (see previous discussion).
- Imaging is not routinely indicated.
- Manipulation or mobilization may be effective in the short term (Gross et al., 2004).
- Acupuncture is not effective (Trinh et al., 2006).

Mechanical Pain

- Recognize by:
  - aged 18 to 55;
  - absence of signs of radiculopathy or red flags;
  - made worse by posture/activity.
- Advise the patient to stay active (Aker et al., 1996). Collars should only be worn for a limited period.
- Give regular analgesia.
- Advise or refer for exercises (Kay et al., 2005).
- Treat hyperextension injuries (including whiplash injuries) in the same way but avoid a collar as this prolongs symptoms.

Daily Stretching and Strengthening Exercises

Advise the patient to hold the neck for 10 seconds in each of the six positions (right and left lateral flexion and rotation, flexion and extension) within the pain-free range. Repeat 10 times. (Based on the ARC information leaflet "Pain in the Neck.")

Radiculopathy

- Distinguish radiculopathy from neck pain that is referred to the shoulder and arm.
- Look for the following signs, though their sensitivity and specificity have not been adequately assessed:
  - Diminished reflexes (triceps, biceps, supinator)
  - Diminished power
  - Diminished sensation along dermatomes
  - Axial compression test: Extend the neck and rotate the head to the side of the pain, then apply pressure to the head. Reproducing pain or paraesthesiae in the arm signifies likely radiculopathy.
- Treat as for mechanical neck pain but refer if there is no improvement after 4 weeks. Refer earlier if there is loss of power and refer immediately if deterioration is rapid. However, warn the patient that surgery is no better than conservative treatment except in severe cases (Kadanka et al., 2002).

Red Flags

- Red flags for malignancy, infection, and inflammation are as for LBP.
- A red flag specific for neck pain is evidence of cervical myelopathy (the equivalent of the cauda equina syndrome). Neck pain may be absent but the syndrome should be suspected when any of the following features are present:
  - Sensory disturbances in upper and lower limbs
  - Weakness in upper and lower limbs
  - Clumsiness and gait disturbance
  - Spasticity of lower limbs (upper limbs may be normal, spastic, or flaccid)
  - Increased tendon reflexes
  - Lhermitte sign: paraesthesiae in limbs on neck flexion indicates neck instability and warrants *immediate* admission.
- Refer patients with one or more red flags urgently for a specialist opinion.

PATIENT INFORMATION

Arthritis Research UK. *Pain in the neck: An information booklet.* Available at www.arthritisresearchuk.org.

Problems With the Upper Limbs

Acute Shoulder Pain

REVIEW

Mitchell, C., Adebajo, A., Hay, E., & Carr, A. (2005). Shoulder pain: Diagnosis and management in primary care. *British Medical Journal, 331*, 1124–1128.

Acute Onset With Injury

- Clinical fracture or dislocation: send to the emergency department.
- If there is no clinical fracture or dislocation then x-ray and send to the emergency department if a fracture or dislocation is shown.
- If the x-ray is normal: control pain for 3 weeks with analgesia and a sling.
- If pain or loss of movement continues beyond 3 weeks consider performing the local anaesthetic (LA) test if you feel confident to do so (see below).
  - If pain and movement are both improved refer for physiotherapy.
  - If pain is improved but not movement refer urgently to an upper limb specialist (fracture clinic) as suspected rotator cuff tear. Repair, if needed, should be performed within 6 to 8 weeks of the injury.
- The LA test helps to distinguish pain from a tear as the cause of an inability to raise the arm. Instill 2 mL of local anaesthetic (e.g., 1% lidocaine) anterolaterally into the subacromial bursa. Pain should be relieved within 5 minutes. If indicated, steroid (e.g., 40 to 80 mg Depo-Medrone) can be given through the same needle.

Acute Onset Without Injury

- If there is a sudden onset of desperate pain then refer to accident and emergency (A&E) department. This may indicate acute decalcification of an area of calcification in the rotator cuff which would need urgent decompression.
- If the situation is less desperate then x-ray:
  - If normal, give local anaesthetic and steroid injection and advice on cuff strengthening exercises (or refer to physiotherapy for this advice). If that fails, refer to outpatient department (OPD). If it helps substantially but is followed by relapse give further injections with a maximum of three per year.
  - If abnormal, refer according to diagnosis (see upcoming discussion).

Arthritis of Acromioclavicular Joint or Glenohumeral Joint

- If symptoms are mild then give analgesia, an NSAID, heat, shoulder exercises, or refer to physiotherapy.
- If symptoms are more severe then support as above and refer to OPD.

Calcification in the Rotator Cuff

- Refer to OPD. They are more likely to need surgery at some stage. They may benefit from a subacromial injection of local anaesthetic and steroid meanwhile.

Red Flags for Systemic Disease

- Investigate further if the patient is systemically unwell (e.g., with fever or weight loss), has a history of cancer, has arthritis elsewhere, has a mass or neurological symptoms or signs in that arm.

Chronic Shoulder Pain

Is It Acromioclavicular Joint Pain?

- Characteristics:
  - Pain is localized to the acromioclavicular joint (ACJ).
  - The joint may be swollen and tender with crepitus.
  - Abduction is painful in the final 20 degrees.
- Inject local anaesthetic and steroid and give analgesia. If not better in 2 weeks, refer to physiotherapy. If still no better, check the diagnosis and refer.

Is It a Rotator Cuff Lesion?

- Characteristics:
  - Pain is usually felt at the deltoid insertion.
  - Any or all movements are painful.
  - Active movements are more painful than passive movements.
  - Pain is felt on resisted active elevation (this is the impingement sign).
- If pain is mild then give analgesia and advice on cuff strengthening exercises. If no improvement after 3 weeks refer to physiotherapy (Green, Buchbinder, & Hetrick, 2003). If physiotherapy is unhelpful give a subacromial injection of LA. Subacromial injection of steroid has

been shown to be no better than the same injection into the buttock (Koes, 2009).

- If pain is moderate or severe consider performing the LA test.
  - If the pain is improved and power is full, refer to physiotherapy. If still unresolved, refer.
  - If pain is improved but there is weakness, refer urgently as a suspected rotator cuff tear.
  - If pain is not improved, refer.
  - If pain and power improve substantially but return, give further injections up to a maximum of three per year.

Is It Chronic Capsulitis (Frozen Shoulder)?

- Characteristics:
  - There is tenderness anteriorly between the coracoid process and the head of the humerus.
  - All movements are painful and restricted, whether active or passive, but there is less pain on resisted active movement (when the joint does not move).
  - Characteristically, the loss of external rotation is the most marked, there is no crepitus, and no arthritis elsewhere.
- Explain the nature of the condition and the fact that spontaneous resolution can be expected, with a mean duration of 30 months. However, explain that some long-term restriction of movement is usual (Dias, Cutts, & Massoud, 2005).
- Order mobilization physiotherapy, designed to keep the shoulder mobile within the limits of pain (Green et al., 2003).
- At the same time, give a single steroid injection into the glenohumeral joint (GHJ). The earlier the injection is given, the more effective it is (Dias et al., 2005).
- Refer refractory cases that have not resolved after 30 months for consideration of manipulation under anaesthesia or arthroscopic release.

Is It Glenohumeral Joint Arthrosis?

- The characteristics are the same as in chronic capsulitis, but crepitus may be felt and there may be arthritis elsewhere.
- Confirm with an x-ray. Management depends on both the degree of pain and functional loss:
  - If mild, give analgesia and advice on exercises.
  - If moderate or severe, refer with a view to replacement surgery.

Is the Glenohumeral Joint Unstable?

- Characteristics:
  - There may be a history of subluxation or dislocation.
  - There are two tests for this:
    1. Fix the shoulder girdle with one hand and, with the other, try to rock the head of the humerus backward and forward in the glenoid fossa.
    2. Hold the arm abducted to 90 degrees with the upper arm pointing forward. Does external rotation cause apprehension and pain?
- Refer for consideration of specialist physiotherapy or surgery.

- *Note:* Nerve root compression in the neck frequently presents as shoulder pain, coexists with it, and can cause it!
- *Note:* Young sports people with shoulder pain frequently have occult instability; refer them readily.

Simplified Guide to Cover Most Cases of Shoulder Pain

- If the patient is unwell or has other disorders that could cause shoulder pain, investigate further.
- If the pain is acute and the patient cannot raise the arm actively but you can raise it passively, refer urgently as a suspected rotator cuff tear.
- If there is a history of partial or complete dislocation, refer for assessment of instability.
- Otherwise, decide between:
  - acromioclavicular joint pain (tender over the ACJ with restriction of moving the arm across the front of the chest);
  - GHJ pain (active and passive movements of the shoulder painful and restricted).
- In both those conditions recommend:
  - analgesia and rest until the acute pain eases;
  - exercises within the limits of pain to keep the joint mobile;
  - the ARC booklet (see upcoming discussion) and explain the likely outcome; and possibly steroid/local anaesthetic injection into the appropriate joint.

Exercises for the Shoulder

Flexibility

- Demonstrate pendular exercises:
  1. Stand up and lean forward with arm of affected side hanging perpendicularly.
  2. Sweep the arm around in a circle within the pain-free range. Do this 20 to 30 times.
  3. As time goes on, increase the range of the movement and length of time.

Strengthening the Rotator Cuff

1. Hold your arm outstretched at shoulder height and out to the side.
2. Bring your arm forward then up, push to the back then down to the starting position.
3. Repeat 10 times. As time goes on, build up to doing three sets of 10 repetitions.

PATIENT INFORMATION

Arthritis Research UK. *Shoulder pain*. Available from www.arthritisresearchuk.org.

Tennis Elbow (Lateral Epicondylitis)

- A randomized trial has now clarified the benefits of therapy (Bisset et al., 2006).

- Recommend that the patient avoid or reduce the provoking action. They should not be attempted to resume the activity until the pain has gone.
- Recommend an analgesic or NSAID either topically or orally. There is evidence for short-term but not long-term benefit.
- *Explain that waiting for recovery* is as effective as any other approach, with 89% of patients recovered within 1 year. Refer for a brace if the pain is troublesome enough to warrant it.
- *Consider referral to physiotherapy* for manipulation and exercises: in the short term it is superior to a wait-and-see approach although at 1 year it shows no benefit.
- *Do not offer corticosteroid injection.* Despite some benefit at 6 weeks the relapse rate is high (72%) and the results at 1 year are worse than physiotherapy and worse even than a wait-and-see approach.
- *Consider referral for surgery* if the patient's life is sufficiently disturbed 1 year after onset. There is some evidence for benefit (Verhaar et al., 1993).

Carpal Tunnel Syndrome

> **PATIENT EDUCATION**
>
> Ashworth, N. (2014). *Carpal tunnel syndrome.* Retrieved from www.clinicalevidence.com (search "carpal tunnel").

- Advise the patient to rest the joint if possible and avoid provoking activities.
- Advise the patient to try a night splint (Futuro, Ace) to reduce the flexion of the joint.
- Do not give diuretics. Although commonly prescribed, there is no evidence that they are of value.
- Refer for steroid injection or surgical treatment, if:
  - there is thenar wasting or constant sensory impairment; or
  - symptoms are severe; or
  - there has been no improvement after 3 months. Surgical decompression is more effective than splinting (Verdugo et al., 2003).
- Consider oral steroids while waiting for the appointment. There is evidence of benefit after 2 weeks.

De Quervain Tenosynovitis

- Consider injection of steroid into the tendon sheath, although accurate placing of the needle is difficult.

Ganglion

- Explain to the patient that the lesion is harmless, that 40% resolve spontaneously, and that surgery has its problems:
  - Excision does not always relieve pain.
  - Recurrence after surgery is common.
  - The scar may be unsightly.

- Consider aspiration with a wide bore needle under local anaesthesia.
- Refer the following if they are painful:
  - Dorsal wrist ganglia (over the scapholunate ligament). Recurrence after surgery is 5% to 10%.
  - Palmar digital ganglia (from the flexor tendon sheath at the base of the finger). Recurrence after surgery is rare.
- Try to avoid referring palmar wrist ganglia. Recurrence after surgery is 45%.

Problems With the Lower Limbs

Acute Knee Injury

- The Ottawa Knee Rules reduce the need for an x-ray after acute knee injury by 26%. They are as reliable in children as in adults (Bulloch et al., 2003). Patients with major trauma are not suitable candidates for the use of the decision rule.
- The economic impact of adopting this approach could be a cost saving to the NHS of nearly £2 million (Nichols et al., 1999).
- The rules state that a knee x-ray series is only required for knee injury patients with any of these findings:
  - Age 55 or older
  - Isolated tenderness of the patella (i.e., no bone tenderness of the knee other than the patella)
  - Tenderness at the head of the fibula
  - Inability to flex to 90 degrees
  - Inability to bear weight both immediately and when examined (they should be able to take four steps [i.e., take their weight on each leg twice even if they limp])

If There Is No Fracture
- Mobilize as soon as pain permits.
- Encourage quadriceps exercises (see upcoming discussion).
- Provide suitable analgesia.

Anterior Knee Pain
Where There Is a Past History of Injury
- Refer to the next fracture clinic if pain and effusion have persisted for more than 2 weeks.
- If no grounds for immediate referral, arrange an x-ray. Request anteroposterior (AP), lateral, and skyline views.
- If the x-ray is abnormal, refer to the next fracture clinic. This applies whether the fracture is of the patella or a flake of bone from an osteochondral fracture.
- If the x-ray is normal, refer to orthopaedic outpatients if there is a good history of patella dislocation or the patella is unstable on examination.
- If neither of these applies, give advice (see upcoming discussion) and review after 8 weeks. Most young patients with anterior knee pain will have improved spontaneously in that time (Heintjes et al., 2003a).

Where There Is No History of Injury

- Examine for gross abnormalities that might warrant immediate attention.
- Reassure the patient if it is Osgood-Schlatter disease (see upcoming discussion). Otherwise advise as below.

Patients Still in Pain After 8 Weeks (With or Without History of Injury)

- Arrange an x-ray, if not already done.
  - *If abnormal,* refer to OPD for assessment.
  - *If normal,* refer for physiotherapy. If still no progress, refer to OPD for assessment. Advise the patient that it may mean specialist physiotherapy or a brace rather than surgery.

General Advice for Patellofemoral Pain

1. Avoid provoking activities (e.g., stairs, walking up and down hill, the breaststroke kick, skiing, cycling, exercise bikes, and high impact aerobics).
2. Recommend quads exercises (see upcoming discussion) and hamstring stretching exercises. There is some evidence that exercise may reduce anterior knee pain (Heintjes et al., 2003b).
3. Recommend simple analgesics. NSAIDs may reduce pain in the short term but not after 3 months.
4. Recommend a support bandage.

Knee Exercises

- Stretching the hamstrings:
  1. Stand up with the affected leg slightly in front.
  2. Place both palms over the knee cap and push toward the ground. Keep this position for 30 seconds.
  3. Repeat four times. As time goes on, try to increase the stretch by pointing your toes upward.
- Strengthening the quadriceps:
  1. Lying down on your back, lift the leg with the knee straight to a position about 45 degrees off the horizontal.
  2. Hold this position for a count of 10 seconds.
  3. Lower the leg, then rest.
  4. Repeat 10 times. As time goes on, build up to doing three sets of 10 repetitions.

Steroid Injections at the Knee

- Consider injections for:
  - anserine bursitis;
  - the knee joint;
  - the medial ligament of the knee.

Acute Ankle Injury

- The Ottawa Ankle Rule reduces the need for x-rays following ankle injury by 30% to 40% (Table 11.2) (Bachmann et al., 2003). Note that the rule is very good at identifying patients who do not need an x-ray (high sensitivity). It is poor at identifying those who have a fracture (low specificity).

TABLE 11.2 | Reliability of the Ottawa Ankle Rules for Identifying Ankle and Foot Fractures or Avulsion Fractures

Patient Groups	Sensitivity (95% CI)	Specificity (Interquartile Range)	LR
All patients	96% (94%–99%)	26% (19%–34%)	0.10
Ankle injuries	98% (96%–99%)	40% (30%–48%)	0.08
Midfoot injuries	99% (97%–100%)	38% (25%–70%)	0.08

LR, the likelihood ratio for a negative result.

- An *ankle x-ray* is required if there is any pain in the malleolar zone and:
  - there is bone tenderness at the posterior edge or tip of the lateral malleolus; or
  - there is bone tenderness at the posterior edge of the medial malleolus; or
  - the patient is unable to weight bear both at injury and when seen.
- A *foot x-ray* is required if there is pain in the midfoot zone and:
  - there is bone tenderness at the navicular; or
  - there is bone tenderness at the base of the fifth metatarsal; or
  - the patient is unable to weight bear both at injury and when seen.
- The immediate treatment of an ankle sprain (as for any injured joint or limb) is rest, ice, compression, elevation (RICE). Of these, compression appears to be the most important and, with elevation, must be maintained for at least 48 hours (Smith, 2003). Ice should be applied no more than 20 minutes at a time, three times a day; and the skin should be separated from the ice by a wet towel (Institute for Clinical Systems Improvement [ICSI], 2003). It is an approach based on experience rather than evidence.
- Analgesia, support with mobilization, immobilization, and surgical repair are all used in inversion injuries of the ankle. There is no robust evidence to guide the clinician in their use although the use of support and early mobilization seems to result in faster recovery and better long-term outcomes (Kerkhoffs et al., 2002).

Rehabilitation After Ankle Injuries

- Recommend active mobilization to restore proprioception. This can be achieved by regular exercises:
  - Imagine writing the alphabet with the foot, first capitals then small letters.

- Balance on the injured leg while moving the free leg forward and backward and side to side; initially with eyes open then with eyes shut.
- Use a wobble board.

Heel Pain

Plantar Fasciitis

- Characteristics include:
  - isolated plantar heel pain on initiation of weight bearing either in the morning on rising or after a period of sitting;
  - pain tends to decrease after a while but increases as time on the feet increases.
- Examine to confirm heel tenderness and to check the range of movements. There may be associated tightness of the Achilles tendon.
- Do not x-ray. The presence of a calcaneal spur does not alter treatment.
- Advise the patient about weight reduction, if appropriate, and the use of cushioned shoes.
- Give analgesics. There is no evidence that NSAIDs are more effective than simple analgesics.
- Advise the patient about stretching exercises (plantar fascia and Achilles tendon) although there is no evidence of effectiveness (Digiovanni et al., 2003).
- Refer to a podiatrist if there is no improvement after 6 weeks.
- The benefit of steroid injection is likely to be temporary, if any, and not worth the possible harms (Crawford, 2004). There is evidence of benefit from shock-wave application if it is available (Rompe et al., 2003).

Plantar Stretching for Plantar Fasciitis

1. Sit with the affected foot crossed over the other knee.
2. Grasp the toes and pull toward the shin until the plantar fascia is stretched.
3. Hold each stretch for a count of 10 and repeat 10 times, three times a day, for 8 weeks.

Achilles Tendonopathy

- Characteristics of Achilles tendonpathy include:
  - an insidious onset leading to chronic posterior heel pain and swelling;
  - worsened pain with activity and pressure from shoes;
  - swelling medially and laterally to the insertion of the Achilles tendon.
- There is insufficient evidence to determine which treatment is most appropriate. However, the following are commonly tried:
  - Open backed footwear
  - Stretching exercises to lengthen the Achilles tendon
  - Simple analgesia. The condition is not one of inflammation and there is no reason to prefer an NSAID (Khan et al., 2002).

Achilles Tendon Rupture

- There may be a history of a sharp snap felt in the tendon on exertion or on injury (e.g., slipping off a ladder). Up to 20% of ruptures are missed (Maffulli, 1999).
- Consider the possibility of rupture in those with an acute history (as above) and all those who have a longer standing Achilles swelling or ankle injury that is slow to resolve.
- Diagnose rupture by lying the patient face down with the feet over the end of the couch. Squeeze the calf firmly. If the tendon is intact this will cause plantar flexion of the foot. If the tendon is ruptured there will be, at most, a small flicker of the foot (Thompson test).
- Refer any patient with a suspected rupture to be seen within 24 hours.

Problems With the Feet

Bunions

- Although a percentage of bunions are inherited by an autosomal dominant gene this is of variable penetrance and hence not a reason for early referral or assessment.
- Examine to exclude heel valgus deformity and flatfoot and refer to a podiatrist if either is found. Orthoses may help reduce pain (Ferrari, 2003). While awaiting the appointment teach the patient calf and foot exercises.
- Refer only those whose lives are severely affected by the bunion. They should be aware that:
  - after the operation they will not be able to wear a shoe for 8 weeks; and
  - recovery of function will take at least 6 months.

Hallux Rigidus

- Advise the patient to wear a shoe with a rigid sole or to insert a rigid insole into the shoe.
- Refer if pain is interfering with work or sleep. Advise the patient that surgery is similar to bunion surgery, as is the recovery time.

Metatarsalgia

- Examine for a high arch and the presence of corns or calluses beneath the metatarsal heads.
- Refer to a podiatrist.
- Advise the patient to wear a metatarsal pad on the foot (just behind the site of the pain) or an adhesive pad inserted into the shoe to relieve the pressure on the metatarsal heads.
- Refer those not responding and patients with severe lancinating pain radiating down the cleft between two toes (Morton neuroma).

Steroid Injections in Soft Tissue Lesions

- The poor quality of many studies means that evidence of long-term benefit of steroid injections is lacking.

However, it is used because clinical experience demonstrates at least short-term relief for which there is evidence (Speed, 2001).

- The following potential harms are found in injections of the shoulder (Speed & Hazelman, 2001) and similar figures will apply to injections in other sites:
  - Infection in 1 in 14,000 to 50,000 injections
  - Tendon rupture in less than 1%
  - Local scarring in less than 1%
- Discuss with the patient the benefits and harms.
- Familiarize yourself with the common techniques (Silver, 1999).

Indications

- Intensive use of other approaches for at least 2 months has failed.
- Rehabilitation is inhibited by symptoms.

Good Practice

- Obtain the patient's consent.
- Check that you can define the local anatomy.
- Select the finest needle that will reach the lesion.
- Clean your hands and the patient's skin.
- Use a no-touch technique.
- Use short-acting or medium-acting corticosteroid preparations in most cases, with local anaesthetic.
- Injection should be peritendinous; avoid injection into tendon substance.
- Minimum interval between injections should be 6 weeks.
- Use a maximum of three injections at one site.
- Soluble preparations may be useful in those patients who have had hypersensitivity/local reaction to a previous injection.
- Record details of the injection.
- Do not repeat if two injections do not provide at least 4 weeks of relief.

Postinjection Advice

- Warn the patient of early postinjection local anaesthesia and to avoid initial overuse.
- Advise resting for at least 2 weeks after injection and avoid heavy loading for 6 weeks.
- The patient should inform the doctor if there is any suggestion of infection or other serious adverse event.

Contraindications to Corticosteroid Injection in Soft Tissue Lesions

- If pain relief and anti-inflammatory effects can be achieved by other methods
- Local or systemic infection
- Coagulopathy
- Tendon tear
- Young patients

Oral Nonsteroidal Antiinflammatory Drugs

- NSAIDs have good analgesic action but many patients with acute or chronic pain can be managed with paracetamol or weak opioids such as codeine.
- NSAIDs taken *regularly at full dosage* have an antiinflammatory action which is beneficial in controlling swelling and stiffness, as well as pain, in inflammatory diseases such as rheumatoid arthritis (RA), spondyloarthropathies (SpA), and in some cases advanced osteoarthritis.
- Unlike opioids, they do not cause constipation, drowsiness, or dependence. Against this must be set serious cardiovascular and gastrointestinal risks, particularly in the elderly.

Which Oral Nonsteroidal Antiinflammatory Drug?

- The clinical effects of NSAIDs vary from patient to patient. There are important differences between NSAIDs in their relative cardiovascular and gastrointestinal toxicity.
- Selective cyclooxygenase-2 (coxibs) have a lower risk of serious gastrointestinal effects than traditional NSAIDs. However, this advantage may be lost if prophylactic low-dose aspirin is also prescribed.
- Of the traditional NSAIDs, low-dose ibuprofen (1.2 g daily) has the lowest gastrointestinal toxicity.
- Coxibs increase the risk of thrombotic events and are therefore contraindicated in established cardiovascular disease. Diclofenac has the same thrombotic risk as coxibs.
- Low-dose ibuprofen and naproxen 1000 mg daily have the lowest risk of thrombotic events.
- The choice of NSAID, therefore, should take account of the individual's risk profile.

Adverse Drug Reactions

- Upper gastrointestinal (GI) disease: peptic ulceration, bleeding, nonulcer dyspepsia
- Fluid retention, leading to aggravation of heart failure
- Renal failure, precipitated in preexisting renal impairment
- Hypersensitivity
- Worsening of hypertension control

Contraindications and Cautions

- Absolute contraindications to all NSAIDs:
  - Active peptic ulceration
  - Hypersensitivity (rhinoconjunctivitis, bronchospasm, urticaria, angioedema, and laryngeal oedema) to aspirin or another NSAID; avoidance is essential to prevent life-threatening reactions
  - Pregnancy—third trimester
  - Severe heart failure

- Absolute contraindications to coxibs:
  - Ischaemic heart disease
  - Cerebrovascular disease
  - Peripheral arterial disease
  - Moderate heart failure
- Cautions for all NSAIDs:
  - Breastfeeding—largely due to manufacturer warnings. The British National Formulary (BNF) states the amounts in breast milk for most NSAIDs are insignificant. See individual NSAIDs in Appendix 3 of the BNF.
  - Renal, cardiac, or liver failure—renal failure may worsen; monitor urea and electrolytes (U&Es).
  - Asthma—worsening of asthma may be due to prescribed or OTC NSAIDs.
  - Coagulation defects—includes anticoagulation therapy.
  - The elderly.
  - Previous peptic ulceration.
  - Concomitant use of medications that increase GI risk (e.g., steroid therapy or anticoagulants)
- Cautions for the use of coxibs:
  - Left ventricular dysfunction
  - Hypertension
  - Oedema for any other reason
  - Patients with risk factors for heart disease

Prescribing Practice

- Before prescribing an oral NSAID, consider using a topical NSAID.
- Weigh the risks and benefits (Table 11.3) for the individual and involve the patient in the decision.
- Prescribe the lowest effective dose for the shortest period to control symptoms.
- If the patient has not responded after 3 weeks, consider changing to an NSAID from another class.
- Advise patients to take their tablets with meals and to report dyspepsia immediately.
- For patients at high risk of developing GI complications, whether prescribing a traditional NSAID or a coxib,

coprescribe a gastroprotective drug. Use a proton pump inhibitor (PPI) though side effects (colic and diarrhoea) may limit its use. Misoprostol is an alternative. Old age is one such high-risk factor. Indeed, NICE (2014) guidance on osteoarthritis recommends the routine prescription of a PPI for all patients on oral NSAIDs or coxibs.
- Review the patient's continued need for NSAIDs regularly.

Managing Nonsteroidal Antiinflammatory Drug-Induced Gastrointestinal Complications
(New Zealand Guideline Group, 2004)
Uninvestigated Dyspepsia

- Review risk factors for NSAID-induced ulcer. These are:
  - past history of proven peptic ulcer disease or serious GI complications;
  - on medications likely to increase GI complications such as steroids or anticoagulants or bisphosphonates;
  - patients with significant comorbidity, such as heart failure;
  - *Helicobater pylori* infection;
  - previous NSAID gastropathy;
  - high dose of NSAID or taking an NSAID plus aspirin.
- Consider as being at increased risk patients who are:
  - aged over 65 years plus one risk factor;
  - aged under 65 years plus two risk factors.
- *If at increased risk then:*
  - refer patients for endoscopy if risk factor for ulcer present; stop the NSAID pending the outcome (NICE, 2004);
  - test and treat for *H. pylori* if positive.
- *If not at increased risk then:*
  - stop the NSAID if possible, or reduce the dose, or change to a less toxic NSAID or to a coxib;
  - if there is a need to continue an NSAID, prescribe a PPI—misoprostol is an alternative;
  - proceed to endoscopy and testing for *H. pylori* as above only if there is no improvement.

TABLE 11.3	**Comparative Risks of Traditional Nonsteroidal Antiinflammatory Drugs and Coxibs** (National Prescribing Centre, 2007)	
	Traditional NSAID	**Coxibs**
Thrombotic risk	RRs compared to placebo are diclofenac 1.63* (equivalent to a coxib), low-dose ibuprofen 1.51 (not statistically significant), naproxen 0.92 (not statistically significant)	RR 1.42 NNH compared to placebo = 300 per annum The risk remains constant for the period of use
GI risk	RRs compared to placebo (from RCTs) are diclofenac 1.7, ibuprofen 1.2, naproxen 1.8. Risk is highest during first week	RR compared to traditional NSAIDs: 0.39; however, coxibs still carry some GI risk, probably equivalent to low-dose ibuprofen

*Meaning that diclofenac increases the risk of a thrombotic event by 63%. The absolute increase in risk depends on the baseline risk.
GI, Gastrointestinal; *NNH*, number needed to harm (the number who need to take the drug for one of them to have an excess adverse effect); *NSAID*, nonsteroidal antiinflammatory drug; *RR*, relative risk.

Proven Peptic Ulcer
- If NSAID treatment needs to be continued after ulcer healing:
  - coprescribe a PPI or misoprostol; and
  - consider switching to a coxib.

Classes of Nonsteroidal Antiinflammatory Drugs

- Salicylates: aspirin, diflunisal, benorylate
- Acetic acids: diclofenac, etodolac, indomethacin, sulindac, tolmetin
- Propionic acids: fenbufen, fenoprofen, flurbiprofen, ketoprofen, ibuprofen, naproxen, tiaprofenic acid
- Fenamic acids: flufenamic, mefenamic
- Enolic acids: piroxicam, tenoxicam
- Nonacidic acids: nabumetone
- Selective COX-2 inhibitors: celecoxib, etoricoxib

Monitoring Patients Taking Disease Modifying Antirheumatic Drugs

See following discussion and Appendix 13.

Biologic Therapy Monitoring

- Patients receiving biologicals will be monitored in secondary care. Disease modifying antirheumatic drugs (DMARDs) may be coprescribed; if so, monitoring should be in line with the recommendation for the DMARDs.
- Patients receiving biologicals are at increased risk of serious infections. They also have an increased risk of malignancies and possibly autoimmune diseases, including demyelinating and lupuslike syndromes.
- Therefore for GPs it is more important to be alert for the appearance of symptoms suggestive of these complications than to rely on routine monitoring.
- Warn patients of the risk of infection and advise them to report symptoms other than minor illnesses.
- Pay particular attention to the risk of tuberculosis. If the patient develops a productive cough or haemoptysis, weight loss, and fever, stop treatment and send a sputum sample to be tested for acid-fast bacilli.
- Warn patients who are not immune to varicella of the need to avoid contact with chickenpox and shingles, and of the need to report any inadvertent contact.
- Ensure that the patient has had a single immunization against pneumococcus and annual influenza vaccine.
- If the patient develops a lupuslike rash, take blood for antinuclear antibodies (ANA) and double stranded DNA (dsDNA) binding and inform the rheumatologist.

Gout

GUIDELINE

Hui, M., Carr, A., Cameron, S., et al. (2017). The British Society for Rheumatology guideline for the management of gout. *Rheumatology, 56*(7), e1–20. https://academic.oup.com/rheumatology/article-lookup/doi/10.1093/rheumatology/kex156.
National Institute for Health and Care Excellence. (2015). *Clincial knowledge summaries: Gout.* Available from https://cks.nice.org.uk/gout.

Aims of Management

- To terminate an attack
- To prevent recurrent attacks
- To prevent complications

Treatment of the Acute Attack

- Consider the possibility of septic arthritis and refer urgently if this is suspected.

Nonpharmacological
- Advise resting of the affected joint(s).
- Advise the application of a cold pack.

Pharmacolocgical
- Prescribe a fast-acting NSAID at maximum dose providing there are no contraindications.
- Advise that the NSAID should be continued until symptoms subside and for 1 to 2 weeks thereafter.
- Prescribe additional analgesia in the form of opiates, if needed for severe pain.

Patients With Comorbidity
- For patients at increased risk of GI complications, follow advice under NSAID section or consider an alternative.
- For patients on a diuretic for hypertension, consider changing to another hypertensive.
- For patients with heart failure, do not stop the diuretic.
- For patients with heart failure or renal failure, limit the use of NSAID or consider an alternative.

Alternatives to an Nonsteroidal Antiinflammatory Drugs
- Prescribe colchicine at a dose of 500 μg two to four times per day. Do not use higher doses because of the risk of adverse effects (vomiting, diarrhea, and abdominal cramps). The drug should be stopped when the attack abates or if side effects outweigh the benefit. Caution is urged in breastfeeding, the elderly, in hepatic and renal impairment, and in GI and cardiac disease.
- Prescribe prednisolone 35 mg daily until the attack is settling, then reduce to zero so that the total course is 7 to 10 days (Janssens et al., 2008).

Patients Not Responding to the Above

- Consider an intraarticular injection of methylprednisolone (40 or 10 mg for a small joint) as a single dose.

Management After an Attack

- Review the patient at 4 to 6 weeks.
- Educate the patient regarding self-management. Advise the patient to start treatment *as soon as possible* after the onset of any future attacks and to have a standby supply of NSAID or alternative.
- Assess all patients for conditions associated with hyperuricaemia:
  - Obesity
  - Alcohol consumption
  - Blood pressure
  - Hyperlipidaemia
  - Diabetes
  - Renal failure

Investigations

- Uric acid—check this after the attack has settled because it may be lowered during an attack. A raised level does not prove the diagnosis nor does a low level exclude it. The main value is in determining and monitoring prevention.
- Blood tests—check renal function, serum glucose, and cholesterol.
- Consider joint aspiration when the diagnosis is in doubt (e.g., knee monoarthritis when the differential diagnosis may be gout or pseudogout [urate crystals and calcium pyrophosphate dihydrate crystals seen respectively on microscopy]). Send the aspirate immediately in a plain glass bottle for polarizing microscopy (by prior arrangement).
- X-rays are rarely helpful but can sometimes confirm pseudogout (chondrocalcinosis seen on plain films) or demonstrate joint damage from chronic gout, which is more likely to happen as an insidious process in the elderly.

Prevention of Recurrence and Complications

- Advise patients to:
  - lose weight if obese but to avoid rapid weight loss, which can precipitate an attack;
  - restrict alcohol to recommended limits, have three alcohol-free days each week, and avoid beer and fortified wines;
  - avoid excessive amounts of purine-rich foods (e.g., offal, red meat, yeast extract, oily fish, and shellfish);
  - take skimmed milk, lowfat dairy products (e.g., yoghourt, vegetable sources of protein such as beans and cherries);
  - maintain a fluid intake over 2 litres/day;
  - consider stopping drugs that reduce uric acid excretion or reduce them to the lowest effective dose. They are aspirin (though not low-dose aspirin used in cardiovascular protection), thiazides, and loop diuretics.

Consider drug prophylaxis according to the following indications:
1. If a second or further attacks occur within a year
2. Polyarticular gout
3. The presence of tophi
4. Clinical or radiologic signs of chronic gouty arthritis
5. Prophylaxis when cytotoxic therapy is given for haematologic malignancy
6. Recurrent uric acid renal stones

- Asymptomatic hyperuricaemia is not considered an indication for drug prophylaxis.
- Wait until the acute attack has subsided for at least 2 weeks before starting prophylaxis, otherwise the attack may be prolonged.

Prophylactic Drugs

Allopurinol

- Prescribe allopurinol as the first choice because it is effective and does not increase the risk of uric acid stone formation (unlike uricosurics, see upcoming discussion).
- Prescribe allopurinol starting at 50 to 100 mg daily, increasing by 50 to 100 mg every few weeks until the serum uric acid is below 300 μmol/L. The maximum dose is 900 mg/day. Doses above 300 mg daily should be divided.
- Check uric acid and creatinine yearly.
- If minor side effects occur (e.g., rash) stop allopurinol and then reintroduce it at as low a dose as the patient can cut from a 100-mg tablet (e.g., 10 mg). If this is tolerated, increase the dose slowly.
- Do not restart if the rash was exfoliative dermatitis or if it was associated with fever or involvement of another organ.
- Give colchicine or an NSAID for the first 3 to 6 months; attacks may be precipitated in the early stages of allopurinol treatment. Use colchicine 500 μg twice a day for the first 3 to 6 months or a standard dose of an NSAID for up to 6 weeks.
- If an attack occurs during prophylaxis, continue to use allopurinol at the same dose and treat the attack in its own right.

Febuxostat

- Febuxostat is an alternative xanthine-oxidase inhibitor that can be used in patients who cannot tolerate allopurinol or whose renal function is prohibitive to its use.
- Start with a dose of 80 mg daily and increase to 120 mg daily after 4 weeks if necessary.
- When starting febuxostat use colchicine 500 μg twice a day for at least 6 months or a standard dose of an NSAID for up to 6 weeks (and consider gastroprotection). A low dose of oral prednisolone can be considered for 4 to 12 weeks if both colchicine and NSAIDs are contraindicated.

If the Above Fails

- Check compliance and review lifestyle (e.g., alcohol consumption).
- Consider referral for uricosuric drugs.

Indications for Referral (National Library for Health, 2008)

- Septic arthritis is suspected: referral is urgent.
- The diagnosis is uncertain.
- There is a suspicion of an underlying systemic illness (e.g., rheumatoid arthritis or connective tissue disorder).
- Gout occurs during pregnancy or in a young person (<25 years of age).
- Allopurinol is contraindicated or not tolerated, or is being started but NSAIDs and colchicine are contraindicated or not tolerated.
- Allopurinol at maximum dose has been ineffective.
- A person has persistent symptoms during an acute attack despite maximum doses of antiinflammatory medication (alone or in combination).
- An intraarticular steroid injection is indicated but the facilities or expertise are not available.
- Complications are present, including urate kidney stones or urate nephropathy.

PATIENT EDUCATION

Arthritis Research UK. *Gout: An information booklet.* Available from www.arthritisresearchuk.org.

Rheumatoid Arthritis

GUIDELINES

Luqmani, R., Hennell, S., Estrach, C., et al. (2006). British Society for Rheumatology and British Health Professionals in Rheumatology guideline for the management of rheumatoid arthritis (the first 2 years). *Rheumatology, 45,* 1167–1169.
    National Institute for Health and Care Excellence. (2009). *Rheumatoid arthritis: The management of rheumatoid arthritis in adults. NICE clinical guideline 79, updated 2015.* Available from www.nice.org.uk.

Aims of Management

- To suppress or minimize disease progression
- To control symptoms (pain and stiffness)
- To preserve function
- To minimize drug side effects
- To promote independence and quality of life

General

- The impact of early intensive treatment with DMARDs has raised hopes that they may suppress rheumatoid disease. However, complete disease suppression is limited by side effects.
- Treatment needs to be started as soon as possible before joint damage occurs. This window of opportunity is within 3 months of the onset of symptoms. Yet early diagnosis is difficult even for specialists.

- Therefore, the GP has a vital role in referring patients as soon as the suspicion of RA arises, when they have *undifferentiated inflammatory arthritis* and before the diagnosis is confirmed; 12% to 15% of such patients will eventually turn out to have RA.
- The GP has a continuing role in managing the patient in the long term, within protocols shared with secondary care. The GP also has a role in managing the illnesses that accompany RA.
- Patients with RA have an increased risk of cardiovascular disease and mortality.
- Patients with RA have an increased risk of osteoporosis.

Model of Care

- Early referral from primary care for suspected RA for early diagnosis
- Early intervention with DMARDs in the window of opportunity before joint erosion occurs
- Intense initial secondary care management and patient education
- Patient access and primary care management when the disease is stabilized
- Regular review by a specialist nurse in secondary care

Patient Assessment

- Assess the impact on the patient's mental health, sleep, fatigue, acts of daily living, and social function.
- Screen for and treat cardiovascular risk factors.
- Check for extraarticular manifestations including constitutional upset.

Referral

- Refer when any of the following are present for over 6 weeks (Scottish Intercollegiate Guidelines Network [SIGN], 2000):
  - Three or more joints are swollen.
  - The metacarpophalangeal or metatarsophalangeal joints are involved.
  - Early morning stiffness lasts longer than 30 minutes.
  The secondary care service should provide:
- formal assessment of the severity of disease as baseline for monitoring;
- a range of responses from a multidisciplinary team of nurses, physiotherapists, occupational therapist, social workers, dieticians, orthopaedic surgeons, and podiatrists;
- a specialist nurse to review patients and to provide a telephone helpline. Secondary care may provide an educational programme.

Prereferral Investigations

- Follow local protocols and investigate in accordance with the availability of tests at the local laboratory.

- Consider ordering the following with results to accompany the referral:
  - ESR and C-reactive protein (CRP), as an indication of disease activity.
  - Rheumatoid factor—do this because a positive result early in the disease has prognostic significance. However, the sensitivity and specificity are not sufficiently high to make a diagnosis.
  - The anticyclic citrullinated peptide (anti-CCP) (Maddison & Huey, 2006). It is highly specific (>95%) for rheumatoid at all stages of the disease. This means that a positive finding makes the diagnosis almost certain. However, the sensitivity is not sufficiently high in early disease (45%–60%) to rule out disease so, if it is negative, referral should still be made on clinical grounds.
  - Full blood count (FBC), because the anaemia of chronic disease is common and to get a baseline because some DMARDs and biologicals affect the blood count.
  - Liver function tests (LFTs), because some DMARDs and biologicals affect the liver.
  - U&Es and dip testing of urine because some DMARDs and biologicals affect renal function.
  - Viral serology if recent illness suggests a viral arthritis.
  - Consider x-ray of affected joints and of the hands and feet because rheumatologists usually request them as a baseline for future progression. However, x-rays are unlikely to be helpful in diagnosis because erosive changes are not usually apparent early in the disease (Royal College of Radiologists, 2003).

Patients With Poor Prognosis

The following carry a poor prognosis if present early in the disease:
- Persistent synovitis
- High ESR or CRP
- Positive rheumatoid factor
- Male sex

Shared Care: Pharmacologic Treatment

Pain Control

- Recommend paracetamol as a first line analgesic. It is effective and safe.
- Weigh and discuss the risks and benefits of additional strategies for controlling pain: NSAIDs (which are superior to paracetamol in controlling stiffness and swelling) and opiates.
- Choose an NSAID or coxib according to the patient's risk and comorbidities. It is customary to try a patient on one NSAID or coxib for a period of several weeks and then to switch to an alternative if it is ineffective.
- If NSAIDs or coxibs are needed for the long term, prescribe the lowest effective dose.
- Start with a weak opiate such as codeine.

- If necessary, prescribe stronger opiates.
- Bear in mind the effects of pain and of side effects on the individual's lifestyle.

Steroids

- Consider using systemic steroids in the following situations:
  - Bridging disease control between different DMARD therapies
  - To achieve rapid control of symptoms but only once the diagnosis has been established
- Recommend local steroid injections for localized flareups.
- Caution is required in long-term steroid use. (See Steroids in sections on polymyalgia and temporal arteritis and section on osteoporosis.)

Disease Modifying Antirheumatic Drugs

- They include antimetabolites, antimalarials, and biologic agents (Table 11.4).
- The choice of DMARD will be made by the patient and consultant.
- Methotrexate has emerged as the most commonly prescribed DMARD closely followed by sulfasalazine.
- Cytokine modulators (anti–tumor necrosis factor [anti-TNF] drugs) are indicated in patients who have failed to respond to at least two DMARDs, including methotrexate (unless contraindicated).

The General Practitioner's Role

- Support patients during the initiation of therapy. There may be no benefit for 2 to 6 months.
- Counsel patient to report potential adverse effects promptly (see Table 11.4).
- Ensure patients know about the dangers to conception:
  - Several DMARDs are contraindicated in pregnancy.
  - Both male and female patients may need to delay conception until a period has elapsed after stopping cytotoxics. The period depends on the DMARD (e.g., 3 months for methotrexate, 2 years for women on leflunomide).
- Follow local protocols for monitoring the adverse effect of these drugs, as protocols vary between institutions. See Appendix 13 for a proposed protocol.

Methotrexate

- The National Patient Safety Agency reports errors in prescribing and dispensing.
- State clearly on prescriptions for methotrexate that the dose is to be taken *weekly*.
- Prescribe *only one strength* (usually 2.5 mg).
- Prescribe folic acid 5 mg to be taken on a separate day of the week to reduce nausea.

Antidepressants

- Ask about sleep disturbance and fatigue.
- Prescribe an antidepressant to aid sleep and reduce pain as well as to treat depression, if present.

TABLE 11.4	Disease Modifying Antirheumatic Drugs, Usual Dose, and Selected Toxicity (See British National Formulary for Full List of Adverse Effects)	
Drug	**Usual Maintenance Dose**	**Toxicity**
Methotrexate	7.5–15 mg/week	GI symptoms, stomatitis, rash, alopecia, infrequent myelosuppression, hepatotoxicity, rare but serious (even life-threatening) pulmonary toxicity
Sulfasalazine	1000 mg twice or three times daily	Rash, myelosuppression (infrequent), GI intolerance
Leflunomide	Maintenance, 10–20 mg once daily	Hepatotoxicity, myelosuppression, GI symptoms, rashes including Stevens-Johnson syndrome, toxic epidermal necrolysis
Cytokine modulators, anti-TNF drugs (etanercerpt, adalimumab, infliximab)	Etanercerpt, weekly or fortnightly subcutaneous injection Infliximab intravenous infusion every 8 weeks Adalimumab fortnightly s.c. injection	Infections, sometimes severe, including tuberculosis, septicaemia, and hepatitis B reactivation. Hypersensitivity reactions, including lupus erythematosus–like syndrome, pruritus, injection-site reactions, and blood disorders, myelosuppression. Worsening heart failure
Hydroxychloroquine	200 mg twice daily	Rash (infrequent), diarrhoea, retinal toxicity (rare)
Injectable gold salts	25–50 mg intramuscular every 2–4 weeks	Rash, stomatitis, myelosuppression, thrombocytopenia, proteinuria
Oral gold	3 mg daily or twice daily	Same as injectable gold but less frequent, plus frequent diarrhoea
Azathioprine	50–150 mg daily	Myelosuppression, hepatotoxicity (infrequent), early flulike illness with fever, GI symptoms, elevated liver function tests
Penicillamine	250–750 mg daily	Rash, stomatitis, loss of taste, proteinuria, myelosuppression, infrequent but serious autoimmune disease

GI, Gastrointestinal; *TNF*, tumor necrosis factor.

Nondrug Management

- Education, physiotherapy, and related interventions remain at the centre of care.
- Constantly review patients not under the care of the multidisciplinary hospital team for the need for referral to any of the following:
  - Physiotherapists—for education, exercise programmes, and splints
  - Occupational therapists—for mobility and daily living aids
  - Nurse specialists
  - Orthotic and prosthetic departments
  - Chiropodists
  - Orthopaedic surgeon

Education

- Education improves knowledge, symptom control, adherence, and self-management.
- Consider every consultation an opportunity to educate the patient.
- Provide information leaflets (see box).

Exercise

- Advise patients to keep active and exercise. This improves mood and encourages self-sufficiency.

- Advise the patient to pace activities to a realistic level.
- Explain the benefits of the different forms of exercise:
  - Range-of-movement or stretching exercises relieve stiffness and maintain flexibility.
  - Strengthening exercises maintain muscle strength, needed for function and joint support.
  - Aerobic exercise improves cardiovascular risk and aids weight control and overall function.

Transcutaneous Electrical Nerve Stimulation, Heat, and Cold Applications

- There is no evidence that they do harm, though cold rather than heat application is usually recommended for actively inflamed joints.
- There is evidence they may provide short-term relief.

Surgery

Surgery can be highly effective in selected cases (Scott et al., 1998) and covers tendon transfers, arthroplasties (including upper limb and small joints), and arthrodeses.

Alternative Therapies/Diet

- Of RA patients, 60% have tried alternative therapies and diets. Be prepared to discuss alternative and complementary strategies.
- Complementary therapies that may help but require further research:
  - Gamma-linolenic acid (GLA) containing plant oils, such as evening primrose, borage, and blackcurrant. GLA may relieve pain and morning stiffness. Side effects include flatulence, nausea, and diarrhoea. Some plant oils can cause liver damage or interact with medications.
  - Fish oils containing eicosapentaenoic acid (EPA) or docosahexaenoic acid (DHA). EPA and DHA may reduce pain and stiffness. Side effects include flatulence and nausea. Fish oil can interact with medication (Mayo Clinic, 2008).
  - *Acupuncture.* Electroacupuncture may relieve pain but acupuncture has no effect on symptoms, function, or quality of life (Casimiro et al., 2005).

Disability

- Historically, over 80% of patients would have been at least moderately disabled after 20 years. This may change with the use of DMARDs.
- Manage the disability according to the guidance in the section on disability.

Spondyloarthropathies

- The spondyloarthropathies (SpA) are a group of conditions characterized by inflammatory spinal pain and enthesitis. They are associated with the HLA-B27 tissue type. The category includes:
  - ankylosing spondylitis (AS);
  - reactive arthritis (following an infection, usually bowel or genitourinary, the latter often termed *Reiter syndrome*);
  - psoriatic arthritis;
  - inflammatory bowel disease–associated arthritis;
  - undifferentiated spondyloarthropathy.

Aims of Management

- Control symptoms (pain, stiffness, and disability)
- Prevent deformity and disability
- Manage nonskeletal complications: fatigue, anterior uveitis, pulmonary and thoracic restriction (AS), aortic incompetence (AS), and inflammatory bowel disease

Diagnosis of Ankylosing Spondylitis

- Early diagnosis is important to establish an exercise programme and to start effective pharmacotherapy to prevent deformity. The average delay in diagnosis is 5 to 7 years.
- A history suggestive of inflammatory back pain (see upcoming discussion) has both a sensitivity and specificity of about 75% for AS.
- Features of inflammatory back pain (Sieper & Rudwallet, 2005):
  - Morning stiffness of longer than 30 minutes duration
  - Improvement in back pain with exercise
  - Pain at night or on early wakening
  - Good response to NSAIDs

Diagnosis of Other Spondyloarthropathies

- Search for clues in the personal and family histories and on examination for diseases of bowel and skin and sexually transmitted disease.
- Investigations:
  - CRP and ESR are frequently raised but may be normal.
  - HLA-B27 does not confirm the diagnosis since the background incidence is 6% to 8% in the general population. However, a negative result makes the diagnosis unlikely because 95% of AS sufferers are positive.
  - X-rays of the sacroiliac joints (SIJs) give a high dose of radiation with little benefit because diagnostic changes take years to develop. MRIs are more accurate than x-rays.
- Ask for CRP and ESR to assess inflammation.
- Check FBC for the anaemia of chronic disease.
- Check U&Es and LFTs if referring as DMARD or anti-TNF therapy may be considered.
- Explain why a plain x-ray is unlikely to help early in the disease. Consider x-ray of the sacroiliac joints if symptoms have been present for several years.
- Consider referral for diagnosis.

Management

- Prescribe an NSAID at full dose. Choose one with a long half-life to ease morning stiffness (e.g., naproxen). Prescribe an alternative NSAID if response after 4 to 6 weeks is insufficient.
- Prescribe or advise OTC analgesics for use as needed.
- Explain the need for regular, daily exercise: It helps to control pain, prevents increasing stiffness, and prevents deformity (Elyan & Khan 2008). Swimming is a good all-round exercise, but specific daily exercises have been developed for maintenance of posture.
- Refer to physiotherapy for exercises or to the local National Ankylosing Spondylitis Society (NASS) group (see accompanying box), or both.
- During flareups, advise patients to continue exercises within the limits of pain.

- Advise patient to lie on the floor prone or supine for 20 minutes each day.
- Prescribe low-dose antidepressants for nocturnal pain and fatigue (Koh et al., 1997).
- Advise the patient to stop smoking. Limitation of chest expansion occurs over time.
- Prescribe or advise hypromellose eye drops for conjunctival disease (dry gritty eyes).
- Watch out for and warn the patient of the symptoms of acute iritis.
- Consider local steroid injections for peripheral joint disease or enthesitis for short-term relief during flareups.

Referrals

To a Rheumatologist

- Refer suspected new cases:
  - Age under 45 years at onset; and
  - Pain present for over 3 months; and
  - Inflammatory back pain features or sacroiliitis shown on x-ray or MRI (Sieper & Rudwaleit, 2005).
- Refer if flareups fail to settle.
- Refer established patients if NSAIDs alone are insufficient. Options which can be initiated in secondary care include DMARDs (methotrexate and sulfasalazine) and biologicals (adalimumab and etanercept).

To Other Specialities

- Refer immediately for an ophthalmologic opinion if you suspect acute iritis.
- Refer to a gastroenterologist in presence of symptoms of inflammatory bowel disease (NICE, 2008b).

PATIENT INFORMATION

National Ankylosing Spondylitis Society. *About AS.* Available at www.nass.co.uk.

Connective Tissue Diseases

- The connective tissue diseases are:
  - systemic lupus erythematosus (SLE);
  - systemic sclerosis;
  - polymyositis;
  - dermatomyositis;
  - Sjögren syndrome;
  - Raynaud disease;
  - mixed connective tissue disorder.
- The term *connective tissue diseases (CTDs)* covers a group of inflammatory diseases affecting multiple systems that have a variable presentation and course and whose features overlap. They are strongly associated with several autoantibodies.
- Complications can be serious and fatal (e.g., lung fibrosis, renal failure, gangrene).
- Many features, especially early in the disease, are nonspecific.

- A group practice with 8000 patients may have 50 to 80 patients with Sjögren syndrome, 4 patients with SLE, and 4 to 8 with other CTDs. They are uncommon but the GP has a special role in both diagnosis and treatment because of their multisystem and chronic nature.
- Evidence-based guidelines are not available for CTDs in general; however, many of the management issues overlap with those of other inflammatory rheumatic conditions already mentioned.

Diagnosis

- Most present with either arthralgia or Raynaud phenomenon.
- Suspect a CTD when:
  - there is arthralgia but no evidence of clinical synovitis;
  - a rash is present (malar rash of SLE spares the nasolabial fold, the rash of dermatomyositis affects face and hands);
  - muscle weakness, rather than the stiffness of polymyalgia rheumatica (PMR), is present;
  - symptoms suggest multiple system involvement. The more suggestive features there are, the greater is the likelihood of disease being present, especially if combined with nonspecific features.
- Review the medical history for salient features which may have been overlooked in the past (e.g., miscarriages).
- Order the following tests:
  - FBC: leucopenia, lymphopenia, thrombocytopenia, or haemolysis suggest a CTD;
  - Urine dipstick and U&Es to screen for renal disease;
  - Creatine kinase;
  - ESR/CRP: they are usually raised in a CTD (but note that the CRP is often normal in SLE in the absence of infection);
  - Serum ANA: it is positive in over 90% of many CTDs; however, it should *not* be relied on as a diagnostic test in the absence of clinical features as it is positive in 5% of the general population and over 30% of people with rheumatoid arthritis.

Management

- Refer suspected cases early to a rheumatologist for diagnosis and a management plan.
- Share care for monitoring progress and therapy with the hospital specialist (as for RA).
- Screen for and manage other cardiovascular risk factors (e.g., hypertension) especially when renal disease is present or high-dose steroid therapy is used.
- *Women's health:* consider the increased risk of thromboses and drug therapy (e.g., cytotoxics) for CTD in preconception counselling, contraception, pregnancy, and hormone replacement therapy (HRT).
- Treat infections promptly in SLE as they may lead to flareups. Consider the possibility of atypical organisms in the immunocompromised.

- Maintain a high index of suspicion for malignancy which may underlie the disease, complicate the disease, or complicate immunosuppressive treatment.

Osteoporosis

GUIDELINES

National Osteoporosis Guideline Group. (2017). *Clinical guideline for the prevention and treatment of osteoporosis.* Available at www.shef.ac.uk/NOGG/downloads.html.
  The NOGG guidelines have been used in this section because:
- they cover both men and women;
- they include corticosteroid-induced osteoporosis;
- they give explicit guidance on risk calculation.

- Osteoporosis is a disorder of diminished bone density and degenerate microarchitecture leading to fragility and increasing the risk of fracture.
- Osteoporosis causes over 200,000 fractures each year in the United Kingdom.
- Most fractures occur in the larger group with lesser degrees of demineralization (osteopenia) through interaction with other risk factors (see upcoming discussion).
- A fragility fracture occurs on minimal trauma (e.g., falling when standing on the ground) after the age of 40, in a typical site, including the vertebral bodies, distal radius, proximal femur, and the proximal humerus.

Definitions of Osteopenia and Osteoporosis

- These conditions are defined by the result of dual-energy x-ray absorptiometry (DXA) measurements of bone mineral density (BMD):
  - T score below −2.5 = *osteoporosis.* The BMD is greater than 2.5 standard deviations below the young adult mean.
  - T score between −1 and −2.5 = *osteopenia.* The BMD is between 1 and 2.5 standard deviations below the young adult mean.
  - T score above −1 = *normal.*
- Where more than one site is scanned, the lowest score is used.

General Principles

- Diagnosis is based on case finding—namely, identifying those likely to be at risk because of either:
  - a previous fragility fracture; or

- the presence of significant clinical risk factors in postmenopausal women or men over the age of 50.
- The risk of future fracture is used as a *guide* to further management. Clinical judgment still has a place. Calculators do not take account of a tendency to falls, the greater prognostic risk attached to vertebral relative to other fractures, or the greater risk after more than one fragility fracture.
- There is geographic variation in how services are organized and which speciality leads them. The GP's role, referral routes, and prereferral workup will vary accordingly and local protocols need to be observed.
- Assessment in general practice includes the search for a possible cause of secondary osteoporosis and a differential diagnosis, according to the individual's age, sex, and clinical features.
- Take a history, perform an examination, and order investigations appropriate to the individual's clinical picture (see box).
- Refer younger men with osteoporosis for further investigation since there is a greater chance of secondary osteoporosis in this group.

Procedures Proposed in the Investigation of Osteoporosis

- Perform the following investigations:
  - Blood cell count, ESR or CRP, serum calcium, albumin, creatinine, phosphate, alkaline phosphatase, and liver transaminases
  - Thyroid function tests
  - Bone densitometry (DXA)
- Consider the following investigations if indicated by history and examination:
  - Lateral radiographs of lumbar and thoracic spine/DXA-based vertebral imaging
  - Protein immunoelectrophoresis and urinary Bence Jones proteins
  - Serum testosterone, sex hormone–binding globulin (SHBG), follicle stimulating hormone (FSH), luteinizing hormone (LH) (in men)
  - Serum prolactin
  - Screening tests for coeliac

Approach to Prognosis and Intervention

- Be alert to patients at risk with a previous fragility fracture or significant clinical risk factors (see upcoming discussion).
- Consider pharmacological intervention in postmenopausal women with a fragility fracture without performing a DXA scan (NICE recommendations differ, suggesting this strategy for women over 75).
- For all other cases, use the FRAX tool to assess the patient's 10-year probability of a major osteoporotic fracture (www.sheffield.ac.uk/FRAX/index.htm). The tool will place the patient in one of three bands: *low, intermediate,* or *high risk.*

- If the risk is intermediate, arrange for a DXA scan because the results may alter management. Recalculate the risk using the FRAX tool and the result of the DXA. The tool will now place the patient in one of two bands: *low* or *high risk.*
- *Low risk:* Give general advice (see upcoming discussion).
- *High risk:* Offer pharmacological intervention (see upcoming discussion).

Clinical Risk Factors for Osteoporosis

- Age
- Sex
- Low body mass index ($\leq$19 kg/m^2)
- Previous fragility fracture, particularly of the hip, wrist, and spine including morphometric vertebral fracture
- Parental history of hip fracture
- Current glucocorticoid treatment (any dose, by mouth for 3 months or more)
- Current smoking
- Alcohol—dose dependent, risks start at daily intake of three or more units
- Causes of secondary osteoporosis, including:
  - rheumatoid arthritis;
  - untreated hypogonadism in men and women;
  - prolonged immobility;
  - organ transplantation;
  - type I diabetes;
  - hyperthyroidism;
  - gastrointestinal disease;
  - chronic liver disease;
  - chronic obstructive pulmonary disease.
- Falls (not used in the FRAX calculation)

General Management

- Assess the risk of falls and refer to local falls prevention services as appropriate.
- Encourage exercise: resistance exercises (lifting weights) and weight-bearing impact exercise (skipping, dancing) (SIGN, 2003).
- Advise a diet that provides a daily intake of 1000 mg calcium and 800 IU of vitamin D$_3$. The recommended calcium intake can be achieved with 1 pint of semiskimmed milk plus one of: 3 oz hard cheese, three slices white bread (or six of wholemeal bread), one small pot of yoghourt, or 3 oz canned sardines. The National Osteoporosis Society has a list of calcium and vitamin D contents which can be useful for vegans and religious observances.
- Give the same dietary advice to those receiving pharmacological intervention.
- Prescribe calcium and ergocalciferol 1 tablet twice daily to the housebound elderly.

Pharmacological Intervention

- Prevention and treatment relate to the prevention of osteoporosis and treatment of established osteoporosis, not the prevention and treatment of fractures.

- Prescribe alendronate as a first line agent because of a good evidence base for the prevention of fractures at several sites and its cost effectiveness. Risedronate is an alternative. It is suitable in both men and women for the:
  - treatment of postmenopausal osteoporosis, 10 mg daily or 70 mg once weekly;
  - treatment of osteoporosis in men, 10 mg daily;
  - prevention of postmenopausal osteoporosis, 5 mg daily;
  - prevention and treatment of corticosteroid-induced osteoporosis, 5 mg daily but for postmenopausal women not receiving hormone replacement therapy, 10 mg daily.

The Practicalities of Prescribing Bisphosphonates

- Advise the patient to swallow the tablets whole with plenty of water, half an hour before breakfast and to remain upright for half an hour afterward.
- Correct disturbances of calcium and mineral metabolism (e.g., vitamin D deficiency, hypocalcaemia) before starting. Monitor serum calcium concentration during treatment.
- Advise the patient on good dental hygiene during and after treatment to avoid the rare complication of osteonecrosis of the jaw. If remedial dental treatment is needed, advise the patient to consider having it done before starting alendronate.
- If alendronate is not tolerated or contraindicated, consider an alternative bisphosphonate such as risedronate. If this is not tolerated consider intravenous bisphosphonate or denosumab. Raloxifene is an alternative for postmenopausal osteoporosis (advise the patient it does not reduce menopausal vasomotor symptoms).
- The bisphosphonates have similar contraindications and side effects. If GI side effects are prominent, a weekly formulation (alendronate 70 mg or risedronate 35 mg) may be tried.
- Contradindications to bisphosphonates are:
  - abnormalities of the oesophagus that delay emptying (alendronate, risedronate);
  - inability to stand or sit upright for at least 30 minutes;
  - hypocalcaemia;
  - pregnancy;
  - breastfeeding.
- Bisphosphonates should be used with caution if there is:
  - other upper GI problems;
  - significant renal failure (creatinine clearance <30 mL/min). Treatment should be reviewed after 3 years with intravenous (IV) zoledronate and after 5 years of oral bisphosphonate. Continuing treatment beyond this period is generally recommended for those with a history of hip or vertebral fracture, those who have had a fracture on treatment, those taking corticosteroids, and people over age 75.

Corticosteroid-Induced Osteoporosis

- Keep doses of oral corticosteroids as low as possible and courses as short as possible.

- Consider the risk of osteoporosis in patients with cumulative doses from intermittent courses. Long-term use of high-dose inhaled corticosteroids may also carry a risk.

Polymyalgia Rheumatica

Management Objectives

- To control symptoms of stiffness and pain (plus associated constitutional symptoms such as fatigue and weight loss)
- To reduce the risk of the complication of temporal arteritis (TA)
- To minimize the risks of steroid therapy

Diagnosis

- The patient is being committed to at least 2 years of steroid therapy. As no single test reliably confirms the diagnosis, the history is important.
- The typical history in PMR is of pain, stiffness, or both, affecting the upper arms and upper legs with diurnal variation, that is to say, worse in the mornings. This history is present in 95% of cases (Bahlas, Ramos-Remos, & Davis, 1998).
- Confidently diagnose PMR if three or more of the diagnostic criteria (see box) are present or if one criterion is associated with a clinical or pathologic abnormality of the temporal artery. The sensitivity for this criterion-based test is 92% (i.e., it will correctly identify 92% of all cases) and the specificity is 80% (i.e., it will correctly exclude 80% of normals) (Bird et al., 1979).

Features of Polymyalgia Rheumatica

- Bilateral shoulder pain or stiffness
- Onset of illness <2 weeks duration
- Initial ESR above 40 mm/h.
- Age 65 years or older
- Depression and/or weight loss
- Bilateral tenderness in the upper arms

Investigations

- Check ESR or CRP. Note that the ESR may be normal in 20% of cases.
- Consider tests to rule out alternative diagnoses as appropriate:

- TFTs for hypothyroidism
- Creatinine kinase for polymyositis and statin-induced myositis
- CXR, as malignancy, especially lung cancer, can cause polymyalgia
- Protein electrophoresis to exclude multiple myeloma

Initial Management

- Check FBC; a normocytic normochromic anaemia is common.
- Measure weight, blood pressure (BP), and check serum glucose before starting steroids.
- Prescribe prednisolone 15 mg daily. Higher starting doses are rarely needed and are more likely to cause adverse effects (Kyle & Hazleman, 1989a).
- Review within a fortnight. Expect a dramatic response within days.
- If there is no response to steroids, review alternative diagnoses as above plus:
  - cervical spondylosis (the most common differential diagnosis);
  - rheumatoid arthritis.
- Raise the dose of prednisolone to 30 mg daily if you have confidently excluded other diagnoses.

Maintenance Steroid Therapy

- The risk of relapse is highest early on in treatment and at doses below prednisolone 10 mg. Temporal arteritis is more likely to develop at doses below 10 mg daily.
- Treatment needs to be maintained for at least 2 years. Even then, only a quarter of patients can stop steroids after this time (Kyle & Hazleman, 1993).
- Over half of patients with PMR (and giant cell arteritis [GCA]) will develop complications of steroids, the most common being weight gain (Kyle & Hazleman, 1989b).
- The principle: reduce the prednisolone dose to the lowest possible to maintain control.
- *A suggested routine is as follows* (Clinical Knowledge Summaries, 2009):
  - Prescribe 15 mg daily for the first month. Check inflammatory markers after 2 to 6 weeks.
  - Reduce by 2.5 mg each fortnight until 10 mg daily is reached, providing there is no relapse of symptoms or rise in inflammatory markers.
  - Review the patient 1 week after each dose reduction.
  - Reduce the daily dose by 1 mg every 6 weeks until 5 to 7 mg daily is reached.
  - Maintenance dose: 5 to 7 mg for 12 months providing there is no relapse of symptoms or inflammatory markers.
  - Final reduction: reduce the daily dose by 1 mg every 6 to 8 weeks, until 3 mg daily is reached, then by 1 mg every 12 weeks, providing symptoms and (less importantly) inflammatory markers remain controlled.

- If symptoms suggest continuing disease in the presence of normal inflammatory markers, give more weight to the former.
- Warn patients that symptoms may return and advise early consultation. A return of symptoms is a more reliable early indication of relapse than inflammatory markers.

Referral

- Refer patients when:
  - symptom control requires a high maintenance dose of steroids or the patient develops significant adverse steroid effects on lower doses (steroid sparing drugs may be considered);
  - there is doubt about the diagnosis, particularly when there is synovitis and anaemia suggestive of rheumatoid arthritis.

Patient Education

- Advise patients to seek urgent attention if they develop symptoms suggestive of GCA:
  - Unilateral headache
  - Tenderness in the scalp
  - Jaw claudication (facial pain on chewing)
- Advise patients about the risks of steroids (see upcoming discussion) and precautions to take.
- Offer the ARC booklet, available at www.arc.org.uk (search for "polymyalgia rheumatica").

Temporal Arteritis

- TA is the most common form of giant cell arteritis, but other arteries may be involved. After headache or pain in the temple, the next most common syndrome is jaw claudication.
- It is almost exclusively a disease of white people.
- A normal ESR, CRP, or negative temporal artery biopsy does not rule out the disease. The chance of obtaining a positive biopsy after 1 week of steroid therapy falls to 10% (Pountain & Hazleman, 1995).
- Steroid therapy should not be delayed pending the results of investigations because untreated GCA carries a risk of visual loss in 40% of patients.

Diagnostic Criteria: American College of Rheumatology

- The presence of three of the following has a sensitivity and specificity greater than 90%:
  - Age at onset over 50 years
  - New type of headache
  - Clinically abnormal temporal artery; thickened, tender, or nodular with decreased pulsation
  - ESR greater than 50 mm/h
  - Positive arterial biopsy

Initial Management (Pountain & Hazleman, 1995)

- *Likely clinical diagnosis according to ACR criteria with visual loss:* If vision is impaired, give prednisolone up to 80 mg immediately and make an urgent referral to an ophthalmologist. If there is likely to be a delay, continue that dose daily.
- *Likely clinical diagnosis according to American College of Rheumatology criteria without visual loss:*
  - Take blood for an ESR, CRP, and FBC.
  - Start prednisolone 40 mg daily.
  - See the patient after 48 hours.
- If there is no response, review the diagnosis.
- *Suspected diagnosis:* Check ESR or CRP, start steroids 40 mg daily, and arrange for the patient to be seen within 48 hours by a rheumatologist/ophthalmologist.
- Opinion varies on the use of routine temporal artery biopsy. Follow local guidance with regard to referral.

Maintenance Treatment

- Reduce the dose by 5 mg every 4 weeks down to 10 mg daily, then as for polymyalgia rheumatica.
- If long-term maintenance is needed, keep the dose as low as possible (e.g., about 3 mg daily).

Steroids

Adverse effects will develop in up to 50% of patients. The risk is positively associated with the dose.
- Educate the patient about the risks:
  - Weight gain
  - Hypertension
  - Osteoporosis
  - Development of diabetes/worsening of diabetic control
  - Infection risk
  - Risk of GI perforation in combination with NSAIDs
  - Adrenal suppression
- Ensure the patient has an up-to-date steroid card.
- Follow guidance on steroid-induced osteoporosis.
- Advise the patient not to stop steroids suddenly.
- Advise the patient that it may be necessary to increase the dose of steroids during intercurrent illness and to seek medical advice.
- Warn the patient to avoid contagious contacts with chickenpox and shingles (there is a risk of fatal disseminated chickenpox if not immune). Advise them to seek urgent medical advice if they are exposed. Obtain specialist advice if such exposure occurs.
- Consider testing immune status for chickenpox when commencing steroid therapy.
- Check weight, BP, and urine (or blood) for glucose every 3 months.
- Patients are likely to be on 7.5 mg or more prednisolone daily for 6 months so should be started on prophylaxis against osteoporosis (see Osteoporosis earlier in chapter).
- Recommend pneumococcal and flu vaccination.

Fibromyalgia

GUIDELINE

Macfarlane, G. J., Kronisch, C., Dean, L. E., et al. (2017). European League Against Rheumatism (EULAR) revised recommendations for the management of fibromyalgia. *Annals of the Rheumatic Diseases, 76,* 318–328. www.eular.org (choose "Recommendations").

- This is a distinct syndrome of widespread, chronic pain. The mechanism for the pain is thought to be driven primarily by central sensitization. Criteria for diagnosis (Wolfe et al., 1990):
  1. A history of widespread pain: pain must be present in all four quadrants of the body and in the spine.
  2. Pain should be elicited in at least 11 of 18 specified tender point sites on digital palpation. These are:
     - *occiput:* suboccipital muscle insertions;
     - *low cervical:* anterior aspects of the intertransverse spaces at C5 to C7;
     - *trapezius:* midpoint of the upper border;
     - *supraspinatus:* origins, above the scapula spine near the medial border;
     - *second rib:* at the second costochondral junctions, just lateral to the junctions on upper surfaces;
     - *lateral epicondyle:* 2 cm distal to the epicondyles;
     - *gluteal:* in upper outer quadrants of buttocks in anterior fold of muscle;
     - *greater trochanter:* posterior to the trochanteric prominence;
     - *knee:* the medial fat pad proximal to the joint line.
  3. Symptoms have been present for over 3 months.

Management

- Find out the patient's concerns and worries and answer appropriately. A patient-centred approach has been found to be associated with less pain and less distress 1 year later (Alamo, Moral, & de Torres, 2002).
- Explain that there is no serious pathology and that pain arises from abnormal processing of pain signals.
- Prescribe simple analgesics and weak opiates. Do not prescribe steroids or strong opiates.
- Refer for heated pool treatment with or without exercise if available.
- Advise gradually increasing aerobic exercise of the sort recommended for cardiovascular fitness (Busch et al., 2007).
- Explain the value of antidepressants in raising the pain threshold and improving sleep and function.
- Prescribe low-dose amitriptyline 25 mg at night and increase according to the response (O'Malley et al., 2000). There is no evidence that any one antidepressant is better than any other.
- In severe unremitting cases, consider referral to a multidisciplinary team. The EULAR guideline recommendations include a multidisciplinary approach on the basis of expert opinion; there is no evidence that it is better in the majority of cases (Karjalainen et al., 2000).
- Consider referral for cognitive behavioural therapy.
- Complementary and alternative remedies are often tried. The one systematic review was not of sufficient quality to draw conclusions (Holdcraft et al., 2003).

PATIENT INFORMATION

Arthritis Research UK. *Fibromyalgia.* Available at https://www.arthritisresearchuk.org/arthritis-information/conditions/fibromyalgia.aspx.

Patient Support

Fibromyalgia Association UK, PO Box 206, Stourbridge, DY9 8YL, helpline 0845 345 2322; benefits helpline 0845 345 2343, http://www.fmauk.org.

References

Aker, P., Gross, A., Goldsmith, C., et al. (1996). Conservative management of mechanical neck pain: Systematic overview and meta-analysis. *British Medical Journal (Clinical Research Ed.), 313,* 1291–1296.

Alamo, M., Moral, R., & de Torres, L. (2002). Evaluation of a patient-centred approach in generalised musculoskeletal chronic pain/fibromyalgia patients in primary care. *Patient Education and Counseling, 48,* 23–31.

Arden, N., Price, C., Reading, I., et al. (2005). A multicentre randomized controlled trial of epidural corticosteroid injections for sciatica: The WEST study. *Rheumatology, 44,* 1399–1406.

Bachmann, L., Kolb, E., Koller, M., et al. (2003). Accuracy of Ottawa ankle rules to exclude fractures of the ankle and mid-foot: Systematic review. *British Medical Journal (Clinical Research Ed.), 326,* 417–419.

Bahlas, A., Ramos-Remos, C., & Davis, P. (1998). Clinical outcome of 149 patients with polymyalgia rheumatica and giant cell arteritis. *Journal of Rheumatology, 25,* 99–104.

Bird, H., Esselinckx, W., Dixon, A., et al. (1979). An evaluation of criteria for polymyalgia rheumatica. *Annals of Rheumatic Diseases, 38,* 434–439.

Bisset, L., Beller, E., Jull, G., et al. (2006). Mobilisation with movement and exercise, corticosteroid injection, or wait and see for tennis elbow: Randomised trial. *British Medical Journal (Clinical Research Ed.), 333,* 939–941.

Bulloch, B., Neto, G., Plint, A., et al. (2003). Validation of the Ottawa knee rule in children: A multicenter study. *Annals of Emergency Medicine, 42,* 48–52.

Busch, A., Schachter, C., Peloso, P., et al. (2007). Exercise for treating fibromyalgia syndrome. *Cochrane Database of Systematic Reviews,* (4), CD003786.

Casimiro, L., Barnsley, L., Brosseau, L., et al. (2005). Acupuncture and electroacupuncture for the treatment of rheumatoid arthritis. *Cochrane Database of Systatic Reviews,* (4), CD003788, doi:10.1002/14651858.CD003788.pub2

Clinical Knowledge Summaries. (2009). *How do I treat someone with polymyalgia rheumatica? National Library for Health.* Retrieved from www.cks.library.uk/polymyalgia.

Crawford, F. (2004). *Plantar heel pain (including plantar fasciitis). Clinical evidence.* Tavistock Square: BMJ Publishing Group. www.clinicalevidence.com.

Dias, R., Cutts, S., & Massoud, S. (2005). Frozen shoulder. *British Medical Journal (Clinical Research Ed.), 331*, 1453–1456.

Digiovanni, B., Nawoczenski, D., Lintal, M., et al. (2003). Tissue-specific plantar fascia-stretching exercise enhances outcomes in patients with chronic heel pain. *The Journal of Bone and Joint Surgery, 85*, 1270–1277.

Department of Health. (2000). *Guidelines for the urgent referral of patients with suspected cancer*. Retrieved from www.dh.gov.uk/cancer/referral.htm.

Elyan, M., & Khan, M. (2008). Does physical therapy still have a place in the treatment of ankylosing spondylitis? *Current Opinion in Rheumatology, 20*, 282–286.

Fairbank, J. (2008). Prolapsed intervertebral disc. *British Medical Journal (Clinical Research Ed.), 336*, 1317–1318.

Ferrari, J. (2003). Bunions. *Clinical Evidence*, Retrieved from www.clinicalevidence.com.

Frank, A. (1993). Low back pain. *British Medical Journal (Clinical Research Ed.), 306*, 90.

Gibson, J. (2007). Surgery for disc disease. *British Medical Journal (Clinical Research Ed.), 335*, 949.

Green, S., Buchbinder, R., & Hetrick, S. (2003). Physiotherapy interventions for shoulder pain. *Cochrane Database of Systematic Reviews*, (2), CD004258, www.thecochranelibrary.com.

Gross, A., Hoving, J., Haines, T., et al. (2004). Manipulation and mobilisation for mechanical neck disorders. *Cochrane Database of Systematic Reviews*, (1), CD004249.

Guzmán, J., Esmail, R., Karjalainen, K., et al. (2001). Multidisciplinary rehabilitation for chronic low back pain: Systematic review. *British Medical Journal (Clinical Research Ed.), 322*, 1511–1516.

Hagen, E., Eriksen, H., & Ursin, H. (2000). Does early intervention with a light mobilization program reduce long-term sick leave for low back pain? *Spine (Phila Pa 1976), 28*, 2309–2316.

Hazard, R., Haugh, L., Reid, S., et al. (1997). Early physician notification of patient disability risk and clinical guidelines after low back injury: A randomized, controlled trial. *Spine (Phila Pa 1976), 22*, 2951–2958.

Heintjes, E., Berger, M., Bierma-Zeinstra, S., et al. (2003a). Pharmacotherapy for patellofemoral pain syndrome. *Cochrane Database of Systematic Reviews*, (3), CD003470, www.thecochranelibrary.com.

Heintjes, E., Berger, M., Bierma-Zeinstra, S., et al. (2003b). Exercise therapy for patellofemoral pain syndrome. *Cochrane Database of Systematic Reviews*, (4), CD003472, www.thecochranelibrary.com.

Holdcraft, L., Assefi, N., Buchwald, D., et al. (2003). Complementary and alternative medicine in fibromyalgia and related syndromes. *Best Practices & Research: Clinical Rheumatology, 7*, 667–683.

Institute for Clinical Systems Improvement. (2003). *Ankle sprain: Bloomington (MN)*. www.ngc.gov/anklesprain.

Janssens, H., Janssen, M., van de Lisdonk, E., et al. (2008). Use of oral prednisolone or naproxen for the treatment of gout arthritis: A double-blind, randomised equivalence trial. *Lancet, 371*, 1854–1860.

Kadanka, Z., Mares, M., Bednarik, J., et al. (2002). Approaches to spondylotic cervical myelopathy. *Spine (Phila Pa 1976), 27*, 2205–2211.

Karjalainen, K., Malmivaara, A., Van Tulder, M., et al. (2000). Multidisciplinary rehabilitation for fibromyalgia and musculoskeletal pain in working age adults. *Cochrane Database of Systematic Reviews*, (2), CD001984.

Kay, T., Gross, A., Goldsmith, C., et al. (2005). Exercises for mechanical neck disorders. *Cochrane Database of Systematic Reviews*, (3), CD004250.

Kerkhoffs, G., Rowe, B., Assendelft, W., et al. (2002). Immobilisation and functional treatment for acute lateral ankle ligament injuries in adults. *Cochrane Database of Systematic Reviews*, (3), CD003762.

Khan, K. M., Cook, J. L., Kannus, P., et al. (2002). Time to abandon the "tendinitis" myth. *British Medical Journal (Clinical Research Ed.), 324*, 626–627.

Koes, B. (2009). Corticosteroid injection for rotator cuff disease. *British Medical Journal (Clinical Research Ed.), 338*, 245–246.

Koes, B., Assendelft, W., van der Heijden, G., et al. (1996). Spinal manipulation for low back pain: An updated systematic review of randomized clinical trials. *Spine (Phila Pa 1976), 21*, 2860–2871.

Koh, W., Pande, I., Samuels, A., et al. (1997). Low dose amitriptyline in ankylosing spondylitis: A short term, double blind, placebo controlled study. *Journal of Rheumatology, 24*, 2158–2161.

Kovacs, F., Abraira, V., Pena, A., et al. (2003). Effect of firmness of mattress on chronic non-specific low-back pain: Randomised, double-blind, controlled, multicentre trial. *Lancet, 362*, 1599–1604.

Kyle, V., & Hazleman, B. (1989a). Treatment of polymyalgia rheumatica and giant cell arteritis. I. Steroid regimens in the first two months. *Annals of the Rheumatic Diseases, 48*, 658–661.

Kyle, V., & Hazleman, B. (1989b). Treatment of polymyalgia rheumatica and giant cell arteritis. II. Relation between steroid dose and steroid-associated side effects. *Annals of the Rheumatic Diseases, 48*, 662–666.

Kyle, V., & Hazleman, B. (1993). Clinical and laboratory course of polymyalgia rheumatica/giant cell arteritis after the first two months of treatment. *Annals of the Rheumatic Diseases, 52*, 847–850.

Lin, E., Katon, W., Von Korff, M., et al. (2003). Effect of improving depression care on pain and functional outcomes among older adults with arthritis: A randomized controlled trial. *JAMA: The Journal of the American Medical Association, 290*, 2428–2429.

Maddison, P., & Huey, P. (2006). *Rheumatic diseases: Serological aids to early diagnosis: Arthritis Research Campaign: Reports on the rheumatic diseases series 5: Topical reviews*. www.arc.org.uk.

Maffulli, N. (1999). Rupture of the Achilles tendon. *The Journal of Bone and Joint Surgery, 7*, 1019–1036.

Mason, V. (1994). *The prevalence of back pain in Great Britain*. London: OPCS HMSO.

Mayo Clinic. (2008). *Rheumatoid arthritis*. Retrieved from www.mayoclinic.com/health/rheumatoid-arthritis/DS00020/DSECTION=11.

Nachemson, A., & Jonsson, E. (Eds.), (2000). *Neck and back pain*. Philadelphia, PA: Lippincott Williams & Wilkins.

National Iinstitute for Health and Care Excellence. (2004). *Dyspepsia: Managing dyspepsia in adults in primary care*. www.nice.org.uk/guidelines.

National Institute for Health and Care Excellence (2008b). *Adalimumab, etanercept and infliximab for ankylosing spondylitis (no. 143)*. London: Technology Appraisal Guidance.

National Library for Health. (2008). *Clinical knowledge summaries: Gout management*. Retrieved from http://cks.library.nhs.uk/gout/management/detailed_answers/when_to_refer.

National Prescribing Centre. (2007). *Cardiovascular and gastrointestinal safety of NSAIDs. MeReC extra issue No 30*. Retrieved from www.npc.co.uk/MeReC_Extra/2008/no30_2007.html.

New Zealand Guideline Group. (2004). *Management of dyspepsia and heartburn*. www.nzgg.org.nz.

Nichols, G., Stiell, I., Wells, G., et al. (1999). An economic analysis of the Ottawa knee rule. *Annals of Emergency Medicine, 34*, 438–447.

O'Malley, P., Balden, E., Tomkins, G., et al. (2000). Treatment of fibromyalgia with antidepressants: A meta-analysis. *Journal of General Internal Medicine, 15*, 659–666.

Peul, W., van Houwelingen, H., van den Hout, W., et al. (2007). Surgery versus prolonged conservative treatment for sciatica. *The New England Journal of Medicine, 356*, 2245–2256.

Pountain, G., & Hazleman, B. (1995). Polymyalgia rheumatica and giant cell arteritis. *British Medical Journal (Clinical Research Ed.), 310*, 1057–1059.

Rompe, J., Decking, J., Schoellner, C., et al. (2003). Shock wave application for chronic plantar fasciitis in running athletes. *American Journal of Sports Medicine, 31*, 268–275.

Royal College of Radiologists (2003). *Making the best use of a department of clinical radiology* (5th ed.). London: RCR.

Scott, D., Shipley, M., Dawson, A., et al. (1998). The clinical management of rheumatoid arthritis and osteoarthritis: Strategies for improving clinical effectiveness. *British Journal of Rheumatology, 37*, 546–554.

Scottish Intercollegiate Guidelines Network. (2000). *Management of early rheumatoid arthritis. Guideline 48.* Retrieved from www.sign.ac.uk.

Sieper, J., & Rudwaleit, M. (2005). Early referral recommendations for ankylosing spondylitis (including pre-radiographic and radiographic forms) in primary care. *Annals of the Rheumatic Diseases, 64*, 659–663.

Silver, T. (1999). *Joint and soft tissue injection, injecting with confidence* (2nd ed.). London: Radcliffe Medical Press.

Smith, G. (2003). Sprains and soft tissues injuries: Do you know the latest priorities? *The New Generalist, 1*(4), 21–22.

Speed, C. (2001). Corticosteroid injections in tendon lesions. *British Medical Journal (Clinical Research Ed.), 323*, 382–386.

Speed, C., & Hazleman, B. (2001). *Shoulder pain. Clinical evidence.* London: BMJ Publishing Group.

Staiger, T., Gaster, B., Sullivan, M., et al. (2003). Systematic review of antidepressants in the treatment of chronic low back pain. *Spine (Phila Pa 1976), 28*, 2540–2545.

Towheed, T., Maxwell, L., Anastassiades, T., et al. (2005). Glucosamine therapy for treating osteoarthritis. *Cochrane Database of Systematic Reviews*, (2), CD002946, doi:10.1002/14651858. CD002946.pub2

Trinh, K., Graham, N., Gross, A., et al. (2006). Acupuncture for neck disorders. *Cochrane Database of Systematic Reviews*, (3), CD004870.

Tulder, M., Malmivaara, A., Esmail, R., et al. (2000). Exercise therapy for low back pain (Cochrane Review). In *The Cochrane Library.* Oxford: Update Software. Issue 2.

Uçkay, I. (2008). Antibiotic prophylaxis before invasive dental procedures in patients with arthroplasties of the hip and knee. *Journal of Bone and Joint Surgery, 90*, 833–838.

UK BEAM Trial Team. (2004). United Kingdom back pain exercise and manipulation (UK BEAM) randomised trial: Effectiveness of physical treatments for back pain in primary care. *British Medical Journal (Clinical Research Ed.), 329*, 1377–1381.

Verdugo, R., Salinas, R., Castillo, J., et al. (2003). Surgical versus nonsurgical treatment for carpal tunnel syndrome. *The Cochrane Database of Systematic Reviews*, (3), CD001552, www.thecochranelibrary.com.

Verhaar, J., Walenkamp, G., Kester, A., et al. (1993). Lateral extensor release for tennis elbow. *Journal of Bone and Joint Surgery, 75A*, 1034–1043.

Vroomen, P., de Krom, M., & Knotterus, J. (1999). Diagnostic value of history and physical examination in patients suspected of sciatica due to disc herniation: A systematic review. *Journal of Neurology, 246*, 899–906.

Waddell, G., Feder, G., & Lewis, M. (1997). Systematic reviews of bed rest and advice to stay active for acute low back pain. *British Journal of General Practitioners, 47*, 647–652.

Wolfe, F., Smythe, H., Yunus, M., et al. (1990). The American College of Rheumatology 1990 criteria for the classification of fibromyalgia: Report of the multicenter criteria committee. *Arthritis & Rheumatology, 33*, 160–172.

12

Neurological Problems

DECLAN NUGENT

CHAPTER CONTENTS

Headache

Headache accounts for 4.4% of consultations in primary care and 30% of neurology outpatient appointments. They are a cause of pain and disability, a substantial societal burden, and an important cause of absence from work and school.

For details of assessment of headaches refer to guidelines below or National Institute of Health and Care Excellence (NICE) Pathways.

GUIDELINES

British Association for the Study of Headache (2010). *Guidelines for all healthcare professionals in the diagnosis and management of migraine, tension-type, cluster and medication-overuse headache.* www.bash.org.uk.

National Institute for Health and Care Excellence (2012). *Headaches in over 12s: Diagnosis and management. Clinical guideline, 150,* updated 2015. www.nice.org.uk.

Scottish Intercollegiate Guidelines Network (2008). *The diagnosis and management of headache in adults. Guideline, 107.* www.sign.ac.uk.

- Where a positive diagnosis of primary headache has been made, a patient-centred approach to treatment should be adopted to include:
  - explanation of diagnosis and reassurance that other pathology has been excluded;
  - options for management;
  - recognition that headache is a valid medical disorder that can have a significant impact on the person, his or her family, or carers;
  - written and oral information about headache disorders, including information about support organizations;
  - explanation of the risk of medication overuse for people using acute treatments for their headache disorder.
- Do not refer people diagnosed with tension-type, migraine, or cluster headaches for neuroimaging solely for reassurance.
- Consider use of a headache diary to record the frequency, duration, and severity of headache; to monitor the effectiveness of headache interventions; and as a basis of discussion with the person about the headache disorder and its impact.

Migraine (With or Without Aura)

- Migraine occurs in 15% of the UK adult population and more than 100,000 people are absent from work or school as a result of migraine every working day. The current management of migraine in primary care is far from satisfactory.
- Correct treatment can relieve the symptoms of migraine and improve quality of life. Increasingly it is being demonstrated that undertreatment is not cost effective. Previously people with migraine would have been treated with a stepped-care approach; however, evidence now suggests that combination therapy is the most effective first line treatment for migraine.

Once the Diagnosis Is Made

- Explain that the large majority of patients can be successfully treated but finding the best treatment can take time.
- Discuss lifestyle changes that might make a difference (see upcoming discussion).
- Discuss the possibility of nondrug therapies (see upcoming discussion).
- Make a follow-up appointment at a time calculated to give the patient a chance to have had three or four further attacks.

Acute Treatment

- Of the various symptoms of migraine only the headache and nausea respond to drug treatment. Acute use of drugs has therefore nothing to offer the patient who is most troubled by the aura.
  NICE guidelines suggest:
- Offer combination therapy with an oral triptan and a nonsteroidal anti-inflammatory drug (NSAID), or an oral triptan and paracetamol, as first line treatment taking into account person's preference, comorbidities, and risk of adverse events.
- For people aged 12 to 17 years consider a nasal triptan in preference to an oral triptan.
- For people who prefer to take only one drug, consider monotherapy with:
  a. an oral triptan (see upcoming discussion);
  b. NSAID: British Association for the Study of Headache (BASH) recommends ibuprofen 400 to 600 mg, up to four doses in 24 hours. Alternatives include tolfenamic acid rapid release, naproxen, and diclofenac. Where nausea and vomiting exist the use of diclofenac suppositories 100 mg can be considered;
  c. aspirin (900 mg): Should not be offered to patients under 16 years due to the association with Reye syndrome;
  d. paracetamol (1 g): There is little evidence for the use of paracetamol on its own.
- Consider an antiemetic in addition to other acute treatment for migraine even in the absence of nausea and vomiting. There is evidence that antiemetics also enhance the efficacy of simultaneously administered oral analgesics (Drug and Therapeutics Bulletin [DTB], 1998). Scottish Intercollegiate Guidelines Network (SIGN) and BASH suggest use of:
  - prochlorperazine 3 to 6 mg buccal tablets or domperidone 10 mg orally or 30 mg rectally for nausea and vomiting;
  - metoclopramide 10 mg and domperidone 20 mg are also useful as a prokinetic to promote gastric emptying.

- Do not offer ergots or opioids for the acute treatment of migraine. Ergots have been found to be less effective than other treatments with a more concerning side effect profile. Opioids offer little benefit to headache pain and it is at the expense of increased side effects such as nausea, plus the risk of medication overuse headache.
- For people in whom oral preparations (or nasal preparations in those ages 12–17 years) for the acute treatment of migraine are ineffective or not tolerated:
  a. Offer a nonoral preparation of metoclopromide or prochlorperazine.
  b. Consider adding a non-oral NSAID or triptan if these have not been tried.

Use of Triptans

- Triptans vary in individual response and tolerability. NICE recommends to start with the triptan with lowest cost, and if consistently ineffective try one or more alternative triptans. BASH adds that ideally each triptan should be tried in three attacks before being rejected. Different dosage and route of administration should be considered.
- Should be taken at the start of the headache phase. There is evidence of greater efficacy if taken while pain is still mild, but triptans appear to be ineffective if administered during aura.
- Contraindicated in ischemic heart disease (IHD), previous myocardial infarction, uncontrolled/severe hypertension, coronary vasospasm, peripheral vascular disease (PVD), and in those with previous cerebral vascular accident (CVA) or transient ischemic attack (TIA).
- Not indicated for hemiplegic, basilar, or ophthalmoplegic migraine.
- Warn patients regarding side effects (tingling, heat, heaviness, pressure or tightness in any part of body including chest and throat); discontinue if intense, flushing, dizziness, vomiting.

Patients Who Respond and Then Relapse

- Repeat the medication that worked earlier provided that doing so does not exceed dosage limits. All triptans are associated with a return of symptoms within 48 hours in 20% to 50% of those who initially responded.
- In those who can be predicted to relapse, give naproxen 500 mg or tolfenamic acid 200 mg, along with sumatriptan 100 mg.

Prevention

- Encourage the patient to discover the triggers of an attack and see how they can be altered (e.g., stress, excitement, certain foods, alcohol, hunger, fatigue, exertion, oversleeping, menstruation). However, food may be unfairly blamed as a migraine trigger. Only accept the suggestion if attacks occur within 6 hours of ingestion, the association is repeated, and avoiding that food reduces the frequency of attacks.
- Encourage physical fitness, provided exercise does not trigger attacks. Fitness can reduce the frequency of attacks.

- Stop combined oral contraceptives (COCs) in a woman whose migraine starts or worsens when taking them, especially if focal symptoms develop. Their use is associated with an increased risk of cerebral thrombosis.
- Discuss non-drug therapies, even though most are not available on the NHS. Limited evidence exists for benefit from psychological therapies, stress management, and manual therapy such as chiropractic treatment. NICE highlights a low risk of cervical artery dissection/stroke with neck manipulation, although evidence for this is poor at present.
- Evidence exists for benefit from acupuncture in chronic migraine and NICE suggests considering this if first line drug prophylaxis is unsuitable or ineffective.
- Advise people that riboflavin 400 mg/day may be effective in reducing migraine frequency and intensity for some people.
- Reconsider the diagnosis in a patient who uses rescue medication more than once a week.
- Consider drug prophylaxis in anyone whose life is sufficiently disturbed by attacks.

Drug Prophylaxis

Two or more attacks per month is the usual criterion for prophylaxis, but a patient with severe attacks may choose prophylaxis with fewer than that.

- Discuss the benefits and risks of prophylactic treatment, taking into account the person's preferences, comorbidities, risk of adverse events, and impact of the headache on quality of life.
- NICE recommends use of topiramate or propranolol as first line prophylactic agents.
  1. Topiramate: Initially 25 mg at night for 1 week, then increase in steps of 25 mg at weekly intervals. The usual dosage is 50 to 100 mg daily in two divided doses and the maximum dosage is 200 mg daily. Not licensed for those under 18 years of age.
     - Advise women and girls with childbearing potential that topiramate is associated with fetal malformations and can impair the effectiveness of hormonal contraception. Ensure women are on appropriate contraception.
     - The drug should not be stopped rapidly. If the patient suffers from any visual problems reduce and stop the drug as rapidly as possible while seeking urgent advice from an ophthalmologist; acute myopia and secondary angle-closure glaucoma can occur.
  2. Propranolol: Initially 80 mg daily (either 40 mg twice a day or 80 mg MR once daily). The dose may be increased to 160 mg daily and subsequently to 240 mg daily if necessary (either in divided doses or once daily if MR). BASH however recommend the use of atenolol 25 to 100 mg twice a day or metoprolol 50 to 100 mg twice a day over propranolol.
- Titrate each drug up to an effective dose or to the maximum recommended dose.
- Try each for 6 to 8 weeks at full dose before abandoning it. Ask the patient to monitor attacks with a diary.

- Continue a drug that is effective for 6 months then review as the migraine may be in remission. Withdrawal is best achieved by tapering the dose over 2 to 3 weeks.
- If both topiramate and propranolol are unsuitable or ineffective, NICE suggests considering a course of up to 10 sessions of acupuncture over 5 to 8 weeks.
- For people who are already having treatment with another form of prophylaxis, such as amitriptyline, and whose headache is well controlled, continue the current treatment as required.
- Use only one prophylactic drug at a time, except as an extreme measure, although the combination of a beta blocker and amitriptyline may be useful in a patient who also has tension-type headaches.
- Alternative options:
  1. *Tricyclic antidepressants.* The drug most studied is amitriptyline 10 to 150 mg at night and is recommended by NICE. They are likely to be especially helpful in patients with a combination of migraine and tension headaches. Venlafaxine 75 to 150 mg/day is an alternative. To avoid misunderstanding, explain that you are not giving them for their antidepressant effect.
  2. *Sodium valproate* is helpful both in migraine and tension-type headache. Initially 200 mg twice a day, increased if necessary to 1.5 g in divided doses.
  3. *Pizotifen* has been used for many years, particularly in children and young people but clinical trials show little evidence of efficacy.
  4. *Methysergide* still has a role where all other prophylaxes have failed, but it should be given under specialist supervision for 4 months at a time with 1 month between courses to reduce the risk of retroperitoneal fibrosis.
  5. *Calcium channel blockers.* Nifedipine, verapamil, and diltiazem are thought to be effective in conventional doses, but there is a lack of evidence.

Botulinum Toxin Type A in Chronic Migraine

In separate guidance NICE (2012) has recommended the use of botox as an option for prophylaxis of headache in adults with chronic migraine (defined as headaches on at least 15 days/month of which at least 8 days are with migraine):

- that has not responded to at least three prior pharmacologic prophylaxis therapies; and
- whose condition is appropriately managed for medication overuse.

SELF-HELP GROUP

Migraine Action Association, 27 East Street, Leicester LE1 6NB, Tel. 0116 275 8317; www.migraine.org.uk.

Migraine in Women of Reproductive Age
Menstrual Migraine

- Suspect if migraine occurs predominantly between 2 days before and 3 days after the start of menstruation in at least two of three menstrual cycles. Use a headache diary to diagnose.
- If standard acute treatment fails to give an adequate response, consider intermittent prophylaxis.
- *Frovatriptan* (2.5 mg twice a day) or zolmitriptan (2.5 mg twice or three times a day) on the days migraine is expected is recommended by NICE. Warn the patient that she may experience rebound headache after stopping the triptan.
- *An NSAID*, traditionally mefenamic acid 500 mg three times a day or naproxen starting 2 days before the migraine is expected and ending after the risk has passed, usually 2 to 3 days after the onset of menses. Though widely used there is limited evidence for this.
- *Oestrogen supplementation.* Some evidence exists for the use of transdermal oestrogen in the form of patches or gel in the perimenstrual period. This is limited and not recommended within NICE/SIGN guidelines.
- *Women already on the COC.* Consider the tricycle regimen to reduce the frequency of menstruation to once every 10 weeks (i.e., take the pill continuously for 9 weeks rather than 3, followed by the usual 7-day pill-free interval). If migraine with aura occurs while on the COC, it must be stopped.

Migraine and Oral Oestrogens

- *Migraine with aura.* NICE advise not to use combined hormonal contraceptives for contraception in women with migraine with aura. This supports the UK Medical Eligibility Criteria (UKMEC) advice that this would present an unacceptable risk to the individual due to increased risk of ischaemic stroke.
- *Migraine without aura.* Use the COC up to the age of 35, provided there are no other risk factors for vascular disease, and the patient is not using ergotamine.
- *The menopause.* Use hormone replacement therapy (HRT) if indicated. There is no evidence that its use increases stroke risk, although the migraine itself may be exacerbated. If so, consider changing HRT, and SIGN suggests if taking oral HRT to consider transdermal as an alternative.

Migraine in Pregnancy and Lactation

- Most women find that their migraine improves in pregnancy. In those still troubled by attacks, the treatment options are limited.
- Offer paracetamol for acute treatment. Consider use of a triptan or NSAID, after discussing the need for treatment and risks associated with medication use. Aspirin or an NSAID are felt to be safe except in the third trimester. For nausea, metoclopramide or domperidone are unlikely to cause harm throughout pregnancy and lactation.
- Triptans: limited evidence for use during pregnancy and as such cannot be recommended as routine. British National Formulary (BNF) states avoid unless potential benefit outweighs the risk.
- Be wary of making a new diagnosis of migraine in a pregnant woman. Cerebral venous thrombosis may mimic migraine.

- In lactating women use paracetamol, ibuprofen, diclofenac, and/or domperidone. Sumatriptan is probably safe.
- Seek specialist advice if prophylactic treatment is needed during pregnancy. This is not commonly required.

Cluster Headaches (Migrainous Neuralgia)

Acute Treatment

- Discuss the need for neuroimaging for people with a first bout of cluster headache with a specialist.
- Offer oxygen and/or subcutaneous or nasal triptan as acute treatment.
- *A triptan, given parenterally* (e.g., sumatriptan 6 mg subcutaneously), relieves pain in 73% to 96% of people within 15 minutes. Intranasal zolmitriptan 5 to 10 mg has a delayed bioavailability but evidence of efficacy with relief at 30 minutes in 50% to 63% of people (2008).
- *100% oxygen* at a flow rate of at least 12 L/min through a non-rebreathing mask and reservoir bag for 10 to 20 minutes aborts an attack in some people. If found to be useful in the accident and emergency department (A&E), arrange provision of home and ambulatory oxygen.
- Do not offer paracetamol, NSAIDs, opioids, ergots, or oral triptans.

Prevention

- Attacks are so devastating that prevention is needed in most cases. BASH recommends specialist referral, but the GP is likely to be involved in initiating or changing treatment before or between specialist appointments.
- Prophylaxis should be continued for 2 weeks after the last attack then tailed off.
- Trial evidence for the treatments below is scanty; it is probably best for verapamil.
- Consider *verapamil 80 mg* three times a day increasing as high as 320 mg three times a day for prophylaxis during a bout of cluster headache. Seek specialist advice regarding dosage regimes and need for electrocardiogram (ECG) monitoring (risk of atrioventricular [AV] block). Beta blockers should not be given concomitantly. It will stop two-thirds of episodes once attacks begin.
- Seek specialist advice for cluster headache that does not respond to verapamil. There is a lack of controlled evidence for other prophylactic agents but prednisolone, lithium carbonate, and methysergide have been used previously.

PATIENT ORGANISATION

Organisation for the Understanding of Cluster Headache (OUCH), OUCH (UK), Pyramid House, 956 High Road, London, N12 9RX. Tel. 01646 651979; www.ouchuk.org.

Non-migrainous Headache

- A history and simple examination (blood pressure [BP], fundi, and a search for focal neurologic signs) permit a clinical diagnosis in most patients. An erythrocyte sedimentation rate (ESR) may be needed in patients over 50 to exclude giant cell arteritis. Cervical spondylosis, sinusitis, intracranial haemorrhage, and other conditions of which headache is a symptom will need treatment in their own right.
- *Analgesic headache* may complicate management and is most likely to occur in patients taking analgesics combined with benzodiazepines or opioids.

Tension-Type Headache

- Exclude conditions associated with tension-type headache (e.g., cervical spondylosis, poor neck posture, temporomandibular [TM] joint dysfunction, sinus pain, eye muscle disorders).
- Explain that the condition is real and benign, and that treatment aims at reducing the frequency and severity of symptoms rather than cure. Reassurance is very important.
- Explore the tensions in the patient's life.
- Advise exercise (tension-type headache is more commonly seen in sedentary people) and relaxation methods.
- Assess whether depression is present.
- Check whether medication overuse is contributing to the headache.
- Consider aspirin, paracetamol, or an NSAID as acute treatment, taking into account the person's preference, comorbidities, and risk of adverse events. Episodic tension headaches occurring more than 2 days/week should prompt consideration of prophylaxis rather than acute treatments.
- Do not offer opioids in the acute treatment of tension-type headaches.
- Consider prophylaxis in those whose attacks are sufficiently severe and frequent:
  - NICE recommends considering a course of acupuncture, up to 10 sessions over a period of 5 to 8 weeks.
  - NICE felt there was not sufficient evidence to recommend pharmacologic prophylaxis but SIGN has previously recommended the use of tricyclic antidepressants (TCAs). This was supported by a systematic review which found some evidence for their use in tension-type headaches with a number needed to treat (NNT) of approximately 10 (Jackson et al., 2010).
  - Amitriptyline 25 to 150 mg at night. Low doses are effective. Explain that it is not being given for its antidepressant effect. A significant effect can be expected in 25% to 50% of patients.
- Aim to tail off prophylactic treatment after 4 to 6 months if remission has occurred.
- *Naproxen 250 to 500 mg* twice a day for 3 weeks to break a pattern of particularly troublesome and frequent attacks may be helpful. Should not be repeated in case of treatment failure.

Medication-Overuse Headache

- Establish the diagnosis. Headache may be daily or at least 15 days/month in people overusing acute relief medication for an underlying headache disorder. This does not occur in people using analgesia for other painful conditions such as arthritis. Consider it in a patient who has taken simple analgesics on 15 or more days/month for at least 3 months, or who has taken a triptan, ergotamine, opioids, or combination analgesics for 10 or more days/month for at least 3 months.

- Explain the diagnosis to the patient. Patients are often hard to convince, especially the minority whose headache takes up to 2 months without analgesics to resolve.
- Explain that it is treated by withdrawing overused medications. Advise people to stop taking all overused acute headache medications for at least 1 month and to stop abruptly rather than gradually.
- Advise that headache symptoms are likely to get worse in the short term before they improve and that there may be associated withdrawal symptoms. Offer close follow-up and support.
- Consider specialist referral/advice if using strong opioids, or have relevant comorbidities, or in whom repeated attempts at withdrawal have been unsuccessful. Relapse is common with 40% estimated to relapse within 1 year (DTB, 2010).
- Consider prophylactic treatment for the underlying primary headache disorder in addition to stopping overused medication.
- Review the diagnosis of medication overuse headache and further management at 4 to 8 weeks after the start of withdrawal of overused medications.
- Withdrawal headaches can be managed with naproxen 250 mg three times a day or 500 mg twice a day. Some specialists recommend a prolonged period of this treatment for 3 to 4 weeks, and not repeated, but there are no studies to support this. Where nausea and vomiting are present, antiemetics can be used.

Chronic Daily Headache

This is said to exist when headache lasts for at least 4 hours and occurs at least 15 days a month. Most patients are suffering from one or more of the following: migraine, tension-type headache, and analgesic-overuse headache. Management is of the underlying cause. If analgesic-overuse headache is present, tackle that first.

Chronic Paroxysmal Hemicrania

- These are repeated attacks of unilateral headache lasting less than 45 minutes.
- Indomethacin 25 to 75 mg three times a day reducing to 25 mg daily should prevent attacks. Indeed, if it does not, reconsider the diagnosis.

Exertional and Coital Headache

- Give an NSAID or propranolol before attacks once a pattern is established. This should be a diagnosis of exclusion, having ruled out subarachnoid bleeding for example.

Severe Headache of Sudden Onset

- Refer urgently if the first attack is sufficiently severe to present acutely. It may be a subarachnoid haemorrhage, presaging a more severe bleed.

Raised Intracranial Pressure

- This is rarely the cause of headache in a patient without vomiting, papilloedema, or neurological signs. However, exceptions occur.
- Refer patients with a short history of headache (<4 months), especially if it is localized, worse on waking, worse on coughing or straining, and especially in the older patient.

Epilepsy

GUIDELINES

National Institute for Health and Care Excellence (2012). Epilepsies: Diagnosis and management. *NICE clinical guideline, 137*, updated 2016. www.nice.org.uk.
  Scottish Intercollegiate Guidelines Network. (2015) Diagnosis and management of epilepsy in adults. *SIGN guideline, 143*. www.sign.ac.uk.

Management of a Major Fit

1. Protect them from injury.
2. Prevent onlookers from restraining the fitting patient or putting anything in his or her mouth.
3. Do not give drugs initially. The fit is likely to have stopped before the person can act. Give drugs if the fit is continuing without signs of abating after 5 minutes or if three seizures occur within 1 hour.
4. When seizure stops, check the airway and put in the recovery position.
5. Check the patient's cardiovascular and neurologic status.
6. Admit any patient with a fit if:
   - there is suspicion that the fit is secondary to an other illness;
   - this is his or her first seizure;
   - the patient fails to recover completely after the fit (other than feeling sleepy);
   - there is status epilepticus.

Emergency Management of Prolonged or Repeated Seizures, Including Status Epilepticus in the Community

- Initiate treatment if a seizure lasts longer than 5 minutes or there are more than three in one hour:
  1. Check airway, breathing, circulation (ABC).
  2. Provide high flow oxygen if available.
  3. Check the blood glucose with a test strip.

4. NICE recommends administering buccal midazolam as first line treatment for children, young people, and adults in the community. Use rectal diazepam if preferred or if buccal midazolam is not available.
   - *Adults*:
     a. Administer buccal midazolam 10 mg first line.
     b. Provide rectal diazepam as an alternative: 10 to 20 mg rectally, repeating 15 minutes later if necessary.
   - *Children.* Give buccal midazolam: 0.5 mg/kg, to a maximum of 10 mg. The BNF for Children suggests:
     a. 0 to 3 months: 0.3 mg (300 µg)/kg up to a maximum of 2.5 mg
     b. 3 months to 1 year: 2.5 mg
     c. 1 to 5 years: 5 mg
     d. 5 to 10 years: 7.5 mg
     e. 10 to 18 years: 10 mg
   - All doses can be repeated once after 10 minutes if necessary.
   - At the time of writing, midazolam oromucosal solution is not licenced for use in children under 3 months of age.
5. Call an ambulance (this will depend on response to treatment, the individual's situation, and any personalized care plan) particularly if:
   - seizure is continuing 5 minutes after the emergency medication has been given;
   - history of frequent episodes of serial seizures or status epilepticus;
   - this is first seizure;
   - there are difficulties monitoring person's ABC.

- *Convulsive status epilepticus* exists where a convulsive seizure continues for a prolonged period (>5 minutes) or when convulsive seizures occur one after the other with no recovery in between. This is a medical emergency.

Subsequent Management

- A single fit is not necessarily epilepsy. Risk of a second seizure occurring within 2 years is about 50%. After a second seizure the risk of a third is about 70% (Rugg-Gunn & Sander, 2012). Initial screening will generally take place in A&E with onward referral for specialist assessment. Some patients may present to the general practitioner (GP) after the event.
- Urgently refer for neurological assessment to be seen, if possible, within 2 weeks, because of the need to exclude an underlying cause and because of the implications for work and driving. Refer more urgently if there are multiple seizures or focal neurologic signs. The only patient who need not be referred is a child aged 18 months to 5 years who has recovered promptly from a febrile convulsion.
- The NICE guideline recommends that referral without drug treatment should be the norm. Initiation of antiepileptic treatment should only be considered in exceptional circumstances following discussion with specialist services.

- Once the diagnosis of epilepsy has been made and a decision taken about drug treatment, the role of the GP depends on who else is on the team. An epilepsy nurse specialist may be best suited to act as key worker but the GP is best placed to see the epilepsy in the context of the patient's other medical needs, and will be the only professional in the community available out of hours.
- Whoever undertakes it, follow-up must be structured, with a review at least annually, and defaulters sought out.
- Repeat prescriptions of drugs and a policy of waiting until a patient complains of problems are inadequate. The NICE guideline recommends that the care plan be in writing; that it should be agreed by professionals, patient, and carers; and that it should include details of how to access care, about drug treatment including benefits and possible adverse effects, and lifestyle issues such as employment, driving, and swimming.
- Re-referral is needed where:
  - control is poor or the drugs are causing side effects;
  - seizures have continued for 5 years;
  - there are pointers to a previously unsuspected cause for the fits;
  - concurrent illness complicates management;
  - the patient needs preconceptual advice for withdrawal of antiepileptic drugs (AEDs).

Initial Management

- Find out how much the patient and family/carers understand about epilepsy and answer their questions. Issues to include in discussions are:
  - *support:* offer verbal and written information about epilepsy and signpost to support groups (see box);
  - *risk management:* first aid and safety at home/school/work;
  - *prognosis:* in 80% of patients with epilepsy, fits can be controlled by drug treatment (Rugg-Gunn & Sander, 2012).
- Acknowledge the distress and anger the patient and family feel at the disruption this diagnosis has brought to their lives.
- *Driving.* Advise the patient of the need to notify the Driver and Vehicle Licensing Agency (DVLA) and the insurance company of any seizure, however minor. Document this advice. A licence is likely to be withdrawn until:
  - free from fits for 1 year; or
  - if the patient's fits in the last year have been while asleep *and* the patient has had fits while asleep for more than 3 years with no fits while awake in that time. Fits at the time of waking or falling asleep count as "daytime" fits.
- *Employment.* Advise the patient not to work at heights or near dangerous machinery. A heavy goods vehicle (HGV) or public service vehicle (PSV) license will be lost until fit-free for 10 years.

- *Lifestyle.* Stress the positive side of how few changes there need to be. Swimming is possible provided someone else is present who could life save if necessary, provided the patient is not in one of the higher risk categories (see upcoming discussion). Avoid bathing a baby alone. Cycling in traffic is probably unwise. Counsel the patient about disclosing the diagnosis to friends and employers.

SELF-HELP GROUPS

Epilepsy Action, New Anstey House, Gate Way Drive, Yeadon, Leeds LS19 7XY, helpline 0808 800 5050, www.epilepsy.org.uk.

Epilepsy Society, Chesham Lane, Chalfont St Peter, Bucks SL9 ORJ, helpline 01494 601400 for details of local groups and also as an excellent source of information. www.epilepsysociety.org.uk

The Joint Epilepsy Council website has links to all the UK and Irish patient organisations: http://www.jointepilepsycouncil.org.uk.

The Danger of Swimming

- The danger of swimming for a patient with epilepsy varies according to clinical situation, as follows, compared to the general population:
  - All types of epilepsy: ×15
  - Prevalent epilepsy: ×18
  - Epilepsy and learning disability: ×26
  - Temporal lobe excision performed: ×41
  - Epilepsy and institutional care: ×97

Drug Treatment

- Epilepsy is not a single condition but an umbrella term for a number of conditions. First line treatment and adjuvant therapy are outlined by NICE based on the type of epilepsy diagnosed. This will be a specialist decision following discussion with the patient and family/carers to include risks and side effects.
- Treatment with AEDs is generally started after the second epileptic seizure and diagnosis is confirmed with a specialist. Exceptions to this do occur.
- Consistent use of the same manufacturer's preparations is recommended.
- NICE recommends monotherapy wherever possible. If this fails, monotherapy with a different drug is advised. Only where control is not achieved with any first line drug should an add-on drug be given as well.
- Antiepileptic treatment is associated with a small increased risk of suicidal thoughts and behaviour. Patients and caregivers should be alert to signs of this throughout treatment (Medicines and Healthcare Products Regulatory Agency [MRHA], 2008).
- Be alert to the use of sodium valproate in women of childbearing age because of the risk of congenital malformation and neurodevelopmental effects.

National Institute of Health and Care Excellence Recommendations for Treatment in Epilepsy

- *Tonic-clonic or generalized seizures:*
  - First line treatment: sodium valproate; initially 300 mg twice a day, increased gradually (in steps of 150–300 mg) every 3 days. Usual maintenance 1 to 2 g, max 2.5 g with specialist advice.
  - Lamotrigine: if sodium valproate not suitable, initially 25 mg once a day, as monotherapy, increased fortnightly to 100 to 200 mg daily.
  - Adjunctive treatment options include clobazam, lamotrigine, levetiracetam, sodium valproate, or topiramate.
- *Focal seizures:*
  - First line is carbamazepine or lamotrigine.
  - Carbamazepine: initially 100 to 200 mg once or twice daily, increased slowly (100–200 mg every 2 weeks). Usual dose 0.8 to 1.2 g daily in divided doses.
  - Levetiracetam, oxcarbazepine, or sodium valproate can be used if first line choices are unsuitable or not tolerated.
  - Adjunctive treatment options include carbamazepine, clobazam, gabapentin, lamotrigine, levetiracetam, oxcarbazepine, sodium valproate, and topiramate.
- *Petit mal or absence seizures:*
  - May require treatment with ethosuximide, lamotrigine, or sodium valproate.
- *Myoclonic seizures:*
  - Sodium valproate

Practical Points

- *Adverse effects.* Before starting a new drug note the adverse effects listed, for instance, in the BNF and discuss them with the patient.
- *Compliance.* Explain the importance of not missing doses and, especially, of not stopping treatment abruptly. Poor compliance may be a sign that the patient does not fully accept the diagnosis.
- *Alcohol.* Explain that moderate drinking of 1 to 3.5 units/day twice a week has no effect on seizure control. One to 2 units a day is probably safe. Heavier drinking may induce a fit as well as interact with antiepileptic drugs.
- *Drugs bought over the counter*
  - *Aspirin.* Warn patients taking sodium valproate against taking intermittent aspirin. It displaces valproate from protein-binding sites and so potentiates it. If regular aspirin is needed, the dose of valproate may need to be reduced to allow for this.
  - *St John's wort.* It reduces plasma concentrations of carbamazepine and phenytoin.

Special Considerations for Women and Girls' Epilepsy

- Careful counselling, with their partners if appropriate, about contraception, conception, pregnancy, and breastfeeding are required.
- Be aware of interactions with contraception.

- AEDs and risk to developing foetus—most notably sodium valproate.
- *Planning pregnancy and pregnancy:*
  - Early specialist referral is indicated, ideally preconception, for advice regarding the risks and benefits of medication adjustment. Risk associated with inadequate seizure control is considered more detrimental to the foetus than use of AEDs. For unplanned pregnancies patients should be advised not to stop any AEDs and be referred urgently.
  - Offer all women on AEDs 5 mg folic acid daily. This should be continued throughout the first trimester.
  - Risk of seizure during labour is low, but sufficient to recommend delivery in an obstetric led unit.
  - Vitamin K is indicated for the baby on delivery (1 mg intramuscular (IM)) due to risk of neonatal haemorrhage associated with antiepileptics.
  - Most women on monotherapy should be encouraged to breastfeed. If on combination therapy or other risk factors, such as premature birth, seek specialist advice.
- *Contraception and AED therapy:*
  - Enzyme-inducing AEDs may reduce the effect of combined oral contraceptive pill (COCP), progestin-only pill (POP), and progesterone implants.
  - Enzyme-inducers have no effect on intrauterine devices (IUDs), whether copper coil or Mirena, or depot medroxyprogesterone injection. Possible impact to effectiveness of norethisterone enanthate (Noristerat) injection.
  - If using COC, increased doses of oestrogen are required.
  - Emergency contraception: IUD is the preferred option. Otherwise use of levonorgestrel at double dose (3 g as a single dose) as soon as possible within the first 72 hours.
  - Refer to Faculty of Sexual and Reproductive Healthcare (FSRH, 2017): Drug Interactions with Hormonal Contraception for further details.

Follow-Up

- NICE recommends a structured routine review in general practice should take place once a year with specialist review depending on individual circumstances. This should include:
  a. *seizure control* and adverse effects of treatment. Encourage the use of a seizure diary to record seizure frequency and severity. Seizure type for those who have more than one type of seizure and any changes in pattern since last review;
  b. *social or psychological issues* related to epilepsy. This may include driving, work, family planning, attitude to diagnosis, and depression;
  c. *review drug compliance* by checking the frequency of repeat prescriptions. Ensure person understands risks of poor control of seizures and sudden unexpected death in epilepsy (SUDEP), to be discussed;

d. *person's information needs.* May involve signposting to websites (as discussed) or information sources such as www.patient.co.uk where a range of information leaflets are available;
  e. *carer skills.* Review knowledge of first aid for people having a seizure and any agreed treatment protocols for the treatment of prolonged or recurrent seizures;
  f. *other considerations.* SIGN does not recommend routine blood tests as part of review.

Adverse Effects of Anticonvulsant Drugs

Acute: Rash (usually seen shortly after starting the drug). Tail off the drug. If combined with fever and lymphadenopathy the rash may represent a severe hypersensitivity syndrome. Usually starts between 1 and 8 weeks of exposure. Multiple organ failure can occur. If the patient is systemically ill, admit.

Chronic: Weight gain and sedation are the adverse effects of most common complaints. Check that the patient is taking the lowest effective dose of as few drugs as possible. There is some evidence that the quality of life is better on the newer drugs but the NICE review did not consider the evidence to be strong. What is clear is that each drug has a different side effect profile and individuals respond to a drug in different ways. A small increased risk of suicidal thoughts and behaviour has been reported.

Some AEDs are known to reduce bone mineral density and increase fracture risk with long-term use. SIGN recommends dietary and lifestyle advice be given at review to minimize the risk of osteoporosis. Consider supplementation for those at increased risk.

Avoiding SUDEP

- The deaths of 500 people a year in the United Kingdom are attributed to (Sudden unexpected death in epilepsy) SUDEP.
- In adults 33% are thought to be avoidable and the result of inadequate treatment.
- Failure to collect prescriptions for antiepileptic drugs has been identified as a warning sign (Neligan, Bell, & Sander, 2011).
- To reduce this risk, observe the following rules:
  - Titrate a drug up to the maximum tolerated dose, or until seizures are controlled.
  - When discontinuing a drug, titrate a new drug up to an effective dose first and then tail the old drug off slowly. The only exception to this is the patient having a life-threatening reaction to a drug, in which case abrupt cessation (with immediate introduction of a new drug) is justified.

Stopping Treatment

- Specialist advice is wise before withdrawing drugs in a patient who has been free from fits for a number of years. Ultimately it is the patient who must make the decision, weighing the problems of drug-taking against the upset of a further fit with its implications for driving, employment, and family distress.

- SIGN recommends this be discussed with patients who have been seizure free for at least 2 years. A risk table is found within the SIGN guideline to aid discussions.
- In adults with epilepsy who have been seizure free for 2 years, about 60% will have no further seizures when medication is withdrawn (DTB, 2003).
- There is an increased likelihood of recurrence if there has been:
  - epilepsy since childhood;
  - the need for more than one medication to control epilepsy;
  - seizures while on medication;
  - myoclonic or tonic-clonic seizures;
  - an abnormal EEG in the last year (DTB, 2003).
- Reduction should be gradual and SIGN recommends for those on carbamazepine, lamotrigine, phenytoin, sodium valproate, or vigabatrin, the dose should be reduced by 10% every 2 to 4 weeks.
- *Driving when stopping medication.* The DVLA recommends that patients should be advised not to drive during withdrawal and for 6 months after cessation of treatment. Patients must be counselled regarding the need to satisfy driving regulations before resuming driving if seizure does occur.

Parkinson Disease

> **GUIDELINES**
>
> Scottish Intercollegiate Guidelines Network (2010). *Diagnosis and pharmacological management of Parkinson's disease. SIGN guideline, 113.* www.sign.ac.uk.
> National Institute for Health and Care Excellence (2017). *Parkinson's disease in adults. NICE clinical guideline, 71.* www.nice.org.uk.
> Clinical Knowledge Summaries (2016). *Parkinson's disease.* Available at www.cks.nice.org.uk/parkinsons-disease.

- Parkinson's disease (PD) is a progressive neurodegenerative condition resulting from the loss of dopamine-containing cells in the substantia nigra. The disease should be confirmed by a specialist in all cases and patients referred untreated.
- Parkinsonism is a clinical syndrome involving bradykinesia plus one or more of tremor (4–6 Hz when at rest), rigidity, and postural instability. Parkinson's disease is the most common form of parkinsonism. Diagnosis of PD also involves the absence of atypical features, a slow clinical progression, and response to drug treatment.
- Other causes of parkinsonism include drug-induced cerebrovascular disease, other forms of dementia, multisystem atrophy, and supranuclear palsy.
- Clinical diagnosis has poor specificity in the early stages of PD. Regular specialist review is needed to review diagnosis and response to treatment.

- Routine use of functional imaging is not recommended by SIGN, but may be considered by specialists in certain situations. Single-photon emission computed tomography (SPECT) can be considered as an aid to clinical diagnosis in patients where there is uncertainty between PD and nondegenerative parkinsonism/tremor.
- Acute dopamine challenge testing is not recommended in diagnosis of PD.

Management

- The diagnosis of Parkinson's disease has huge medical, psychological, and social implications for the patient and family. The medical aspects of care will be shared between specialist and GP. The role of primary care in management of confirmed PD has been outlined by NICE Clinical Knowledge Studies (CKS).
- GPs should enable appropriate access to:
  - a Parkinson's disease specialist physician, generally a neurologist or a geriatrician;
  - a Parkinson's disease specialist nurse if available;
  - speech and language therapy, physiotherapy, occupational therapy, social services, community nursing, continence and urology specialists, palliative care specialists, and psychology and mental health services;
  - the Parkinson's Disease Society local branch and regional support (see upcoming discussion).
- Liaise with specialist services, particularly in relation to changes in medication. Only start or alter antiparkinsonian medication on the advice of specialist, ensure that changes to repeat medications are made promptly, and titrate therapy between specialist reviews according to the recommendations of secondary care.
- Do not suddenly stop any antiparkinsonian medication as this can precipitate acute akinesia or neuroleptic malignant syndrome.
- Identify worsening motor symptoms and motor complications (which may be caused by the disease itself or by antiparkinsonian medication), and manage these appropriately. This will usually require specialist advice or an interim referral.
- Identify and appropriately manage nonmotor symptoms and complications, which may be caused by the disease itself or by antiparkinsonian medication.
- Manage comorbidities. Avoid or use with caution any drugs that could exacerbate parkinsonism or interact with antiparkinsonian medications. For example, avoid use of metoclopramide, prochlorperazine, and antipsychotics.
- Advise care staff in nursing or residential homes of the need for correct timing of antiparkinsonian medication.
- Offer a regular medication review, including adherence and adverse effects.
- Other considerations:
  - *Financial benefits.* Many patients are eligible for benefits for the disabled.
  - *Carers.* Assess, and reassess, the ability of the carer to cope.

- *Driving.* Advise drivers to notify the DVLA and their insurance company at the point of diagnosis.

SELF-HELP GROUP

The Parkinson's Disease Society, 215 Vauxhall Bridge Road, London SW1V 1EJ, tel. 020 7931 8080, has information for patients and carers and organizes local groups. Helpline: 0808 800 0303; www.parkinsons.org.uk.

Drug Treatment

- Choice of medication is a specialist decision and should be made taking into account patient preferences.
- Drug therapy does not prevent disease progression but improves most patients' quality of life.
- When initiating treatment, patients should be advised about its limitations and possible side effects. About 5% to 10% of patients with PD respond poorly to treatment.
- Claims that certain drugs are neuroprotective and should be started before the development of disabling symptoms are not supported by clinical evidence.
- The old practice of *drug holidays* is contraindicated because sudden cessation may give rise to acute akinesia or to neuroleptic malignant syndrome.
- It is not possible to identify a universal first-choice therapy for early PD or as adjuvant therapy for later PD according to guidelines.
- Early disease can be considered the point at which a diagnosis of idiopathic PD has been made and a clinical decision has been made to start treatment (based on a functional disability requiring symptomatic treatment). Possible first choice therapies include levodopa, nonergot-derived dopamine agonists, or monoamine oxidase B (MAO-B) inhibitors. Most people will eventually require levodopa.
- Later disease refers to people with PD and on levodopa who have developed motor complications. Possible first choice therapies are dopamine agonists, MAO-B inhibitors, and catechol-*O*-methyltransferase (COMT) inhibitors.

Treatment Options for Early Parkinson Disease

- *Levodopa:*
  - Given with a dopa decarboxylase inhibitor to reduce peripheral availability of levodopa and reduce side effects such as nausea, vomiting, and cardiovascular effects (e.g., co-beneldopa and co-careldopa). Slow release preparations may also reduce side effects.
  - Use the lowest effective dose to maintain good function to reduce the development of motor complications. This may include individual realistic goal setting with specialist team (e.g., being able to walk to the shop).
  - Warn patients about the immediate side effects (e.g., nausea, postural hypotension, and sleepiness). Give the tablets after food to avoid nausea. Be aware however that a protein meal can compete with levodopa for absorption. If an antiemetic is needed, use domperidone. Check the standing blood pressure before and after starting the drug.
  - Over time, the response to treatment may decrease and motor complications may occur in approximately 40% after 4 to 6 years, including motor fluctuations such as unpredictable switching between *on* and *off* states, wearing off between doses, and dose failures; or dyskinesia may occur such as athetosis (slow, writhing motions of fingers and hands) and dystonia (involuntary spasms of muscle contraction that cause abnormal movements and postures).
  - There is some debate about use of levodopa as first line and some specialists employ alternative first line treatments to delay starting levodopa and thereby reduce the onset of disabling dyskinesia.
- *Dopamine agonists:*
  - Used as monotherapy as either oral or transdermal preparations. These are found to be slightly less effective than levodopa in terms of treating motor impairment and disability but may delay motor complications.
  - Two groups exist:
    1. Nonergot-derived dopamine receptor agonists (e.g., pramipexole, ropinirole, and rotigotine); can be used as first line treatment
    2. Ergot-derived dopamine receptor agonists (e.g., bromocriptine, cabergoline, and pergolide). Both NICE and SIGN advise these are not used as first line treatment due to the risk of fibrotic reactions (pulmonary, retroperitoneal, and pericardial). Specific baseline investigations and follow-up are recommended if used, as outlined in the BNF and SIGN guidance. Be alert for symptoms such as persistent cough, chest pain, cardiac failure, and abdominal pain.
  - Patients should be warned that treatment with dopamine agonists and levodopa is associated with:
    1. impulse control disorders (including pathological gambling, binge eating, and hypersexuality); and
    2. excessive daytime somnolence; be informed of the implications for driving/operating machinery.
  - Other side effects include hallucinations, especially in older people, and postural hypotension, often worse at the start of treatment.
  - Dopamine agonists are very likely to cause initial nausea or vomiting and domperidone may be needed.
- *MAO-B inhibitors:*
  - Such as rasagiline and selegiline
  - NICE and SIGN state may be considered as a first-choice therapy. When used as a monotherapy has been found to:
    1. improve motor symptoms, improve activities of daily living, and delay the need for levodopa. It is less clear whether they delay the onset of motor complications;

2. cause or worsen dopaminergic side effects such as dyskinesia, hallucinations, or vivid dreaming;
3. demonstrate a levodopa sparing effect (i.e., a lower dose is required).

- Other drugs available:
  - *Anticholinergics.* Occasionally used when tremor predominates. It is not recommended as first choice treatment due to limited efficacy and the propensity to neuropsychiatric side effects.
  - *Amantadine.* SIGN found there to be insufficient evidence to support its use in early PD. Relatively weak efficacy and mechanism of action has not been established.

Treatment Options in Later Parkinson Disease

- Most people with PD will develop, with time, motor complications and will eventually require levodopa. Adjuvant drugs to take alongside levodopa have been developed with aim of reducing motor complications and improving quality of life.
- There are three main strategies when managing motor complications:
  - Manipulation of oral/topical drug therapy
  - More invasive drug treatments (such as apomorphine infusions or intraduodenal levodopa)
  - Neurosugery, most commonly deep brain stimulation
- Patients with complex and disabling motor complications should be reviewed regularly by their specialist team. In the later stages of disease, as nonmotor complications begin to dominate quality of life, the withdrawal of some drugs is often appropriate. These decisions should be made by specialist in consultation with carers and patients.
- SIGN recommend the following options may be considered in people with advanced PD:
  - MAO-B inhibitors (selegiline or rasagiline)
  - Dopamine agonists (oral or transdermal); nonergot agonists (ropinirole, pramipexole, and rotigotine) are preferable
  - COMT inhibitors (entacapone or tolcapone); may aid reduction of *off* time in patients who have motor fluctuations.
  - Intermittent subcutaneous apomorphine; may aid reduction of *off* time.
  - Subcutaneous apomorphine infusions; for severe motor complications in specialist units.

Nonmotor Complications of Parkinson Disease

- It is important to be alert to nonmotor symptoms at patient reviews and manage them appropriately. An extensive list of these is available in NICE CKS, which will include postural hypotension, falls, and pain.
- *Depression* is of particular importance:
  - May be part of the disease rather than a reaction to the disease. Mood disorders including depression are thought to affect up to 50% of patients. There is significant overlap in symptoms of depression, cognitive impairment, and PD which makes diagnosis difficult. Screening using self-rating or clinician rating scales may be of benefit. Information from relatives and carers should also supplement any assessment.
  - In general terms, treatment of depression is the same as those without PD. There is limited evidence from trials but selective serotonin reuptake inhibitors (SSRIs) are most frequently used.
  - Tricyclic antidepressants may be more effective than SSRIs but use is limited due to adverse effects of the medication.
  - Both classes should be avoided if on MAO-B inhibitors and with cautions if using a COMT inhibitor. Seek specialist advice if necessary.
- *Dementia* is more common in people with PD.
  - Treatable causes should be investigated and treated (e.g., acute infection and depression).
  - Consider safely reducing or discontinuing (on specialist advice if necessary) any drugs which may be causing or worsening symptoms. This includes antimuscarinics such as tricyclic antidepressants, tolterodine or oxybutynin, H2 antagonists such as ranitidine, benzodiazepines, amantadine, and dopamine agonists.
  - Refer for specialist assessment and management.

PATIENT INFORMATION

Parkinson's Dementia Information Sheet. PDS UK 2013. www.parkinsons.org.uk.

- *Psychosis* is a key neuropsychiatric feature of PD and associated with a high degree of disability. This includes hallucinations, delusions, and paranoid beliefs.
  - Management should include treating any reversible causes and reviewing medication.
  - Liaise with specialist services early.
  - Mild symptoms that are well tolerated may not need treatment. More severe symptoms may require gradual withdrawal of precipitating anti-parkinsonian medications or the use of an atypical antipsychotic.
  - Evidence supports the use of clozapine, but this requires weekly blood monitoring which may be difficult in some patients. There is some evidence of benefit from quetiapine, but it is not licensed for treatment of psychosis in PD.
- *Excessive daytime somnolence* is found in up to 54% of PD patients. Aetiology is felt to be multifactorial and increases with age.
  - Management should centre around finding a reversible cause such as depression, poor sleep hygiene, and drugs associated with altered sleep pattern.
  - Other conditions associated with PD that may affect sleep include restless legs syndrome, periodic leg movement of sleep, nocturnal akinesia, and nocturia.

Palliative Care of the Terminal Patient

- A time will come when no further alteration in drugs will be helpful, and the patient and family will need an increased amount of support.
- Check that the patient and family have been given a chance to state how they want this stage of the patient's life to be managed.
- Adequate analgesia and sedation of the patient will be needed, as in any palliative situation.

Main Drugs to Avoid in Parkinson Disease

- *Antipsychotics* (e.g., chlorpromazine, haloperidol, flupentixol). Atypical antipsychotics maybe less likely to cause problems. Use clozapine cautiously.
- *Antiemetics* (e.g., metoclopramide, prochlorperazine). Use domperidone.
- *Baclofen* may cause agitation and confusion. Use with caution.

Stroke

GUIDELINES

National Institute for Health and Care Excellence (2008). *Stroke and transient ischaemic attack in over 16s: Diagnosis and initial management. NICE clinical guideline*, 68, updated 2017. www.nice.org.uk.
    National Institute for Health and Care Excellence (2010). *Clopidogrel and modified-release dipyridamole for the prevention of occlusive vascular events. NICE clinical guideline*, 210. www.nice.org.uk/ta210.
    National Institute for Health and Care Excellence (2017). Stroke and TIA. NICE Clinical Knowledge Summaries. www.cks.nice.org.uk.
    Scottish Intercollegiate Guidelines Network (2008). *Management of patients with stroke or TIA: Assessment, investigation, immediate management and secondary prevention. SIGN guideline*, 108. www.sign.ac.uk/guideline108.

Stroke is a preventable and treatable disease. Stroke is the third biggest cause of death in the United Kingdom and it is estimated that 10% of the world's population dies from a stroke.

Acute Stroke

- NICE recommends all people with suspected stroke be admitted directly to a specialist stroke unit, after initial assessment, either from the community or from A&E. In certain circumstances this may be inappropriate, for instance the patient is already in the terminal stage of another illness.
- Admit by dialling 999, without seeing the patient if necessary. This will trigger the local protocol for the management of acute stroke.
- Assessment of the patient by paramedics using a validated tool such as face arm speech time (FAST) (see upcoming

discussion) to diagnose stroke or TIA is supported by NICE stroke quality standards. Those people with persistent neurological symptoms who screen positive using a validated tool, in whom hypoglycaemia has been excluded and who have a possible diagnosis of stroke, should be transferred to specialist stroke unit within 1 hour.
- Patients with acute stroke should receive brain imaging within 1 hour of arrival in hospital if they meet the indications for immediate imaging. These include:
  - those who are candidates for thrombolysis (i.e., they are within 3 hours of the start of symptoms, although SIGN highlights evidence for up to 4.5 hours) or early anticoagulation;
  - patients on anticoagulants or with a bleeding tendency;
  - those with a depressed level of consciousness (Glasgow Coma Score <13);
  - those with progressive or fluctuating symptoms;
  - those with signs of alternative pathology (neck stiffness, papilloedema, fever);
  - those whose stroke begins with severe headache of sudden onset.

Face Arm Speech Time

This was initially developed to aid paramedics to recognize people with stroke but has become a widely publicized part of the Act FAST campaign, which was launched in the United Kingdom in 2009 to aid public awareness:
- Face: ask patient to smile and note if there is a new droop of the mouth or eye on one side
- Arm: a new inability to hold one arm out for 5 seconds compared to the other arm
- Speech: new slurred speech or new inability to understand or say words
- Time: time to dial 999 immediately if you see any of these signs

Longer-Term Management

- Follow-up arrangements will be based on individual need and response to treatment. It is recommended to have a primary care review within 6 weeks of discharge, again at 6 months, and then annually.
- Management should include:
  - assess need for further specialist review, advice, information, support, and rehabilitation;
  - assess social care needs over time, including carer needs;
  - assess health care needs;
  - check and optimize lifestyle measures and drug treatments for secondary prevention.
- Ensure involvement of the community rehabilitation team, if they are not already involved. This team will manage the rehabilitation process but may need support from the GP.
- Check that a multidisciplinary assessment has been performed, including assessment of conscious level, swallowing, speech, pressure sore risk, nutritional status, cognitive impairment, movement, and handling needs.
- *Depression.* Monitor for depression with a screening questionnaire. Mood disturbance is common post stroke, which

includes depression, anxiety, and emotional lability. Consider a therapeutic trial of an SSRI if depression is present and continue for at least 6 months if a benefit is achieved.

- *Bowel and bladder problems.* Disturbance of control of excretion is common in the acute phase of a stroke and remains a problem for a significant minority of patients. Support and continence aids should have been put in place prior to discharge, including carer training, but this will require ongoing support in the community.
- For further information on specific issues refer to NICE CKS Stroke—Long-Term Care and Support.

Secondary Prevention

- *Lifestyle changes.* Assist smokers to stop and urge weight reduction, dietary change to include lowfat diet with two portions of oily fish a week, increased fruit and vegetable intake, and reduced salt intake if hypertensive. Reduction of alcohol intake to no more than 14 units of alcohol per week spread over at least 3 days. Encourage daily physical activity.
- *Antiplatelet therapy.* Following an ischaemic stroke all patients should be given clopidogrel 75 mg daily for life. This is based on evidence from the Clopidogrel versus Aspirin in Patients at Risk of Ischemic Events (CAPRIE) trial and outlined in updated guidelines from NICE in 2010. If clopidogrel is not tolerated then aspirin and dipyridamole MR should be used in combination. If either aspirin or dipyridamole MR is contraindicated or not tolerated, the other agent should be given alone.
- *Blood pressure.* Once the initial phase of the stroke is over (usually about 2 weeks), control any hypertension to achieve a target blood pressure of less than 130/80. Treatment of hypertension in the immediate poststroke period is thought to potentially cause extension of stroke.
- *Atrial fibrillation.* People with disabling ischaemic strokes should be treated with aspirin 300 mg daily for 2 weeks before considering anticoagulant treatment with warfarin or an alternative anticoagulant.
- *Cholesterol.* Statin therapy is recommended for all people following an ischaemic stroke. This should be initiated 48 hours after stroke symptoms onset. NICE recommends atorvastatin 20 to 80 mg daily as first line statin.
- *Carotid artery surgery.* Check that the patient has been considered for carotid endarterectomy or angioplasty, if the stroke was in the appropriate carotid artery territory, and a good recovery from the stroke is likely. NICE recommends surgery should occur within 2 weeks of acute non-disabling stroke or TIA, as benefit is greatest within this timeframe.

Other Routine Matters

- Explain the prognosis if requested; 65% are likely to achieve independence but the GP can modify this figure according to the individual patient's clinical state. Patients with a better prognosis are those who are continent, who have regained power on the affected side within 1 month, and who are progressing toward walking within 6 weeks. Improvement is likely to continue for some months.
- *Driving.* Explain that the patient should not drive for at least 1 month after a stroke or TIA and that the DVLA and the insurance company should be informed.
- *Influenza.* Arrange for annual immunization, as well as pneumococcal immunization in those aged 65 and over.
- Check that the patient knows about the relevant statutory and voluntary organizations.
- Arrange relief admissions and other support for the carers (e.g., attendance allowance) in consultation with the stroke team.

Transient Ischaemic Attack

- A TIA is a sudden focal neurological disturbance lasting less than 24 hours. Early recurrent stroke is common. It is estimated that 10% to 15% have a second TIA/CVA in the first week, with a high proportion being in the first 48 hours (Markus, 2007).
- The likelihood of a subsequent stroke must be assessed so that urgent investigation can be provided for those most at risk.
- Check that the symptoms are due to a TIA. Differentiate TIA from:
  - transient cerebral symptoms caused by hypoperfusion due to cardiac disease;
  - cerebral tumour. Patients with sensory TIAs, jerking TIAs, loss of consciousness, or speech arrest should be assumed to have a tumour until proved otherwise;
  - epilepsy. A careful history of the attacks from an observer is important;
  - migraine;
  - traumatic brain injury;
  - subdural haematoma;
  - subarachnoid haemorrhage.
- Note that a patient with a TIA who seems to be in the vertebrobasilar distribution, as manifested for instance by vertigo, bilateral visual loss, or diplopia, should be managed in the same way as one with a TIA in the carotid distribution, except that the ABCD (Tsivgoulis et al., 2006) score is likely to be lower.

Assess the Urgency of Referral Using ABCD (Tsivgoulis et al., 2006)

Score the patient's risk of stroke after a TIA as follows:
1. Age 60 and older: 1 point
2. Blood pressure 140/90 or above: 1 point if either systolic or diastolic reaches those levels
3. Clinical features: 2 points if unilateral weakness; if not, 1 point if speech affected
4. Duration: 2 points if event lasted 60 minutes or more; 1 point if 10 to 59 minutes; 0 points if less than 10 minutes
5. Diabetes: 1 point

Significance of the Score

A study of patients admitted to the Oxford Neurology Department found, using the 6-point ABCD score (omitting diabetes), an overall stroke risk at 30 days of 9.7%. None of the strokes occurred in those with a score of 2 or less. Above this the stroke risks were as follows:

- a score of 3: stroke risk 3.5%
- a score of 4: stroke risk 7.6%
- a score of 5: stroke risk 21.3%
- a score of 6: stroke risk 31.3% (Tsivgoulis et al., 2006)

Referral

- **Score of 4 or more:** these patients are at high risk of subsequent stroke. Refer to the rapid access TIA clinic (or equivalent local facility) to be seen within 24 hours of the onset of symptoms. This may involve admission in some areas.
- **Score of less than 4 but other worrying features:** for example, crescendo TIAs with two or more TIAs occurring in 1 week. Refer to the rapid access TIA clinic (or equivalent local facility) to be seen within 24 hours of the onset of symptoms.
- **Score of less than 4:** or the TIA occurred over a week before presentation. Refer to the rapid access TIA clinic (or equivalent local facility) to be seen within 7 days.
- **Admission also required where uncontrolled atrial fibrillation (AF) is present or if a TIA has occurred in a patient on warfarin, as urgent computed tomography (CT) is required to rule out a bleed.**

Other Measures

- *Aspirin.* Give 300 mg daily to be started immediately unless contraindicated. Continue while awaiting specialist assessment. Consider use of a proton pump inhibitor if there is a history of dyspepsia associated with aspirin. If there is a history of intolerance to aspirin, then an alternative antiplatelet should be given, generally clopidogrel 75 mg daily should be used, although this is an unlicensed use.
- *Long-term antiplatelet therapy.* Initiated in secondary care following diagnosis. Generally, clopidogrel 75 mg (unlicensed use). NICE recommends use of a combination of aspirin 75 mg daily and dipyridamole MR 200 mg BD if clopidogrel is not tolerated. Aspirin 75 mg alone can be used if clopidogrel and dipyridamole are both not tolerated or contraindicated.
- *Secondary prevention.* Manage as for stroke.
- *Driving.* Advise as for stroke.

Recurrent Transient Ischemic Attacks

- If the TIA occurred in a patient already taking aspirin 75 mg daily, options would include change to clopidogrel.
- Check that a treatable cardiac or carotid cause has been excluded.
- Tighten control of other risk factors for stroke (BP, cholesterol, glucose, etc.).
- Admit if the TIAs assume a crescendo pattern.
- Refer if recurrent attacks continue despite the above measures.

Motor Neurone Disease

- Refer every patient for confirmation of the diagnosis.
- Explain what little is known about the disease. Offer referral to the Motor Neurone Disease (MND) Association regional care development adviser.
- Support the patient and family as you would in any terminal illness. The median survival is only 3 to 4 years, with older patients having the worst prognosis. Always make a further appointment rather than waiting for the patient or family to contact you with a problem.
- *Ventilation.* Discuss at an early stage with the patient and family the fact that ventilation may become necessary. Noninvasive ventilation (i.e., via facemask), at night only, in those with good bulbar function prolongs life by a median of 7 months with improvement in the quality of life (McDermott & Shaw, 2008). If bulbar function fails, tracheostomy or ventilation may become necessary. Discuss this well before it becomes necessary; there is often no time to discuss it with them during a crisis.
- *Nutrition.* In the early stages of dysphagia, refer to a speech therapist and a dietician. Offer referral for consideration of insertion of a gastrostomy tube or a nasogastric tube *before* the patient becomes weak through malnutrition. Standard criteria for tube feeding are when over 10% of premorbid weight has been lost or when the patient finds eating an ordeal because of choking or because it takes too long (McDermott & Shaw, 2008).
- Refer for physiotherapy, occupational therapy, speech therapy for help with speech as well as eating, district nursing, and social work assistance as appropriate. In each case do this pro-actively, not when a serious problem has developed.
- *Hospice care.* Introduce this idea well before it is needed. Short-term admission as respite care will establish a link with the hospice and help the patient to make a decision about what he or she wants to happen in the terminal stages.
- *Drug treatment.* Riluzole is recommended by NICE (2001) for the amyotrophic lateral sclerosis (ALS) form of motor neurone disease. Treatment should be initiated by a

specialist, but it can then be supervised under a shared-care arrangement with GPs. Riluzole prolongs life in ALS by an average of 3 to 4 months (McDermott & Shaw, 2008).

End-of-Life Care in Motor Neurone Disease

- *Musculoskeletal pain.* Consider physiotherapy to relieve the stiffness associated with prolonged immobility. Treat with NSAIDs and opioids. Use opioids early rather than late in patients with pain, as well as to ease the distress of terminal respiratory failure. Treat muscle spasms with baclofen, tizanidine, or diazepam, although evidence for their use in MND is lacking.
- *Dribbling.* Treat dribbling with anticholinergics (e.g., sublingual hyoscine 0.3 mg three times a day or hyoscine hydrobromide transdermal patches).
- *Dry mouth.* Try pineapple chunks or apple or lemon juice to stimulate saliva.
- Consider referral for tracheostomy for sputum retention or stridor, or for recurrent aspiration of food or drink.
- *Choking spasms.* Give sublingual lorazepam (0.5–2.5 mg) and leave a supply with the patient for future occasions. They relieve the laryngeal spasm associated with inhalation of food, drink, or saliva.
- *Respiratory failure.* Consider referral for ventilatory support if the quality of life is otherwise sufficiently good. Be prepared to ease the distress of more prolonged dyspnoea with oral morphine (start with 2.5 mg four to six times a day and titrate up) while the patient is able to swallow and subcutaneous morphine in the terminal stage. More than 90% of patients die in their sleep as a result of increasing hypercapnia. Choking to death is not seen in clinical practice (McDermott & Shaw, 2008).

PATIENT ORGANIZATION

Motor Neurone Disease Association, PO Box 246, Northampton NN1 2PR; 08457 626262; www.mndassociation.org.

Multiple Sclerosis

GUIDELINE

National Institute for Health and Clinical Excellence (2014). *Multiple sclerosis in adults: Management.* NICE clinical guideline, 186. www.nice.org.uk.

- The NICE guidance sets out the following principles regarding multiple sclerosis (MS):
  - Diagnosis should be made rapidly by a specialist neurologist; and every patient, once diagnosed, should have access to neurologist and specialist neurological rehabilitation services as the need arises.
  - The patient should be actively involved in all decisions. To do this the patient needs clear verbal and written information.
  - The patient and any family or other carers need emotional as well as practical support from the medical services.
  - Whenever the patient is assessed, attention should be paid to any *hidden* factors (e.g., emotional state, fatigue, bladder and bowel problems) as well as to the presenting symptom. The NICE guidance includes a useful checklist of issues to consider.
  - The GP should be proactive in the prevention of avoidable morbidity (e.g., contractures, inhalation, pressure sores, renal infections).
- The MS Society booklet for GPs stresses the role of the GP as patient's advocate. The GP may not know how to manage every problem raised by this complex illness but he or she should know someone who does and should make the referral.
- Even if the patient is already authorized to self-refer directly, the GP may be needed to expedite the appointment if the first offer of an appointment is not sufficiently prompt.

Prognosis

- MS follows an unpredictable course, but a better prognosis is associated with:
  - young age at onset;
  - female gender;
  - a relapsing and remitting course;
  - initial symptoms (sensory or optic neuritis);
  - first manifestations affecting only one CNS region;
  - high degree of recovery from initial bout;
  - longer interval between first relapses;
  - low number of relapses in the first 2 years;
  - less disability at 5 years after onset.
- Explain what is known about the disease and how good the prognosis is; the average life expectancy is 25 years after onset of the disease; 5 years after diagnosis approximately 70% of people are still employed and 50% need some help with walking. Approximately 25% of patients have a non-disabling form of MS but up to 15% of patients are severely disabled within a short period (Confavreux, Vukusic, Moreau, & Adeleine, 2000). Point out the positive prognostic features (see box) if they apply.

Management of Acute Relapses

- Diagnose a relapse if new symptoms develop or existing symptoms worsen and these last for longer than 24 hours and occur after a stable period of longer than 1 month.
- Prior to treatment, possible precipitants, particularly infections, should be sought. Urine dipstick should be done on all patients.
- Liaise with the specialist team; frequency of relapse may influence decisions regarding disease modifying treatment.

- At the start of an acute disabling relapse give methylprednisolone 500 mg orally daily for 5 days, after discussion with the patient of the risks and benefits. Intravenous treatment may be necessary if the relapse is severe enough to warrant admission or the patient cannot tolerate oral steroids.
- Give gastric protection with ranitidine 150 mg twice a day or omeprazole 20 mg once daily.
- Also consider what help the patient needs, in the way of care and equipment, because of the relapse and whether referral to the specialist neurological rehabilitation service is needed.
- Giving the same dose intravenously is not feasible in primary care because the high-dose intravenous preparation should be given over 30 minutes.
- Steroids can hasten recovery, but there is no evidence that the long-term course is altered.
- No more than three courses should be given in 1 year.
- Do not give patients a prescription for steroids to keep on standby.

Disease Modifying Treatment

First Line Treatments
- There are currently five first line drugs: the beta interferons (Avonex, Betaferon, Extavia, and Rebif) and glatiramer acetate (Copaxone). These should be started and supervised by a consultant neurologist, preferably one with a specialist interest in MS.
- All drugs must be given by injection.
- Prescribing decisions in the United Kingdom are determined by the criteria for NHS funding. NICE did not recommend the use of these drugs but in the United Kingdom, under the *risk-sharing* scheme set out in Health Service Circular 2002/004 (Department of Health [DOH], 2002) they were available for funding for patients who met the specified criteria. The Association of British Neurologists (2009) updated their guidelines and supported their use, taking into account some revisions in the diagnostic criteria for MS.
- Flulike symptoms are common with both beta-interferon and glatiramer acetate after treatment. These lessen over time. Injection site reactions are also common.
- Any woman receiving disease modifying therapy (e.g., interferon) must stop treatment for at least 12 months before trying to conceive.

Second Line Therapies
- NICE (2007) has recommended natalizumab as an option only for the treatment of rapidly evolving severe relapsing-remitting MS. Fingolimod is the first oral therapy for MS and has also been approved by NICE as an option in the treatment of highly active relapsing-remitting MS (NICE, 2012). In expert centres other treatments may be considered.
- *Other treatment.* Sativex oromucosal spray, a cannabis extract, is licenced for use in the United Kingdom on a named patient basis, via specialists, for moderate to severe spasticity. Percutaneous venoplasty is being used in some centres but the evidence for this is currently lacking. NICE (2012) recommends that this procedure should only be used in the context of research.

Regular Review

- Check that there is a key worker to whom the patient has immediate access and who is coordinating all members of the multidisciplinary team. If there is no such person then, by default, the role falls to the GP.
- *Fatigue*, which is common and not the same as sleepiness. The fatigue may be physical or mental, so that the patient can concentrate for only a short period of time. Check for an underlying cause (e.g., depression, chronic pain, disturbed sleep). The most useful manoeuvre is to explain that the fatigue is real and that it is a part of the syndrome.
- *Spasticity.* Treat any precipitating cause, such as infection or pain. Otherwise management should be supervised by the specialist rehabilitation service. The components of a treatment programme are:
  - stretching exercises by physiotherapist, patient, or family;
  - a skeletal muscle relaxant: baclofen or gabapentin is often used first line; or if these fail, tizanidine, diazepam, and dantrolene are options. Start low and increase the dose slowly. Up to 100 mg/day of baclofen may be required. If stopping, reduce the dose over several weeks. Abrupt withdrawal of baclofen may result in hallucinations or seizures;
  - consider an evening dose of diazepam if spasms or clonus interfere with sleep;
  - refer if spasticity is still uncontrolled for consideration of other treatments. This may include use of Sativex (cannabis extract) spray or botulinum toxin as an intramuscular injection.
- *Weakness.* Refer to the specialist rehabilitation service for training in exercises and techniques to maximize strength.
- *Contractures.* These may develop around any joint whose muscles are weak or spastic. Contractures lead to further reductions in mobility and difficulties in handling. Prevent them by instructing the patient or carer in passive stretching of the joint. Refer to the specialist team if a contracture develops.
- *Pressure sores.* Check that all wheelchair users have been assessed for pressure sore risk and appropriate preventive measures are in place.
- *Depression and anxiety.* A major depressive episode occurs in over 50% at some stage. Search for it and treat it as actively as in a patient without MS.
- *Emotionalism.* Consider a trial of an antidepressant (a TCA or SSRI).
- *Dysphagia.* If the patient has bulbar signs (dysarthria, ataxia, or abnormal eye movements), or if there has been a chest infection, assess swallowing formally.
- *Dysarthria.* If communication is affected refer to a speech and language therapist.

- *Pain* may be neuropathic or musculoskeletal. The former needs a trial of carbamazepine, gabapentin, or amitriptyline; the latter needs physiotherapy and analgesics.
- *Visual problems* that are not corrected with glasses need assessment by an ophthalmologist. Optic neuritis is the most common cause of visual loss.
- *Cognitive impairment*, if suspected, should be formally assessed and the results used to inform the management of every aspect of the patient's care.
- *Bladder problems* (see upcoming discussion).
- *Constipation.* Can usually be managed with adequate fluid, bulk laxatives, and stool softeners. More severe constipation may require osmotic agents, bowel stimulants, anal stimulation, suppositories, or enemas.
- *Sexual problems.* The precise nature of the sexual dysfunction will determine the treatment. Physical difficulty from spasticity may be alleviated by premedication with baclofen, and a fast-acting anticholinergic such as oxybutynin may calm urinary urgency. Sexual dysfunction should not be automatically attributed to MS. It may be necessary to investigate hormonal levels and to obtain urological or gynaecological consultation. Manual lubrication with gel is a ready solution to vaginal dryness. Erectile dysfunction may be treated by sildenafil at NHS expense in the United Kingdom. If it fails, older treatments may succeed (vacuum devices, intracavernous injections, or a penile implant).
- *The health and state of mind of any carers* should also be explored.

The Bladder

- *Urgency.* See whether access to the toilet can be made easier and give an anticholinergic (e.g., oxybutynin or tolterodine).
- *Minor incontinence.* Consider desmopressin for nighttime incontinence. It works by reducing the volume of urine produced. The same dose once in any 24-hour period may be useful to tide a patient over a time when there is no toilet within reach (e.g., on a journey). Padding may help a patient of either sex.
- *More severe incontinence*, occurring more than once a week: refer to a continence service. The patient needs ultrasound assessment for a residual urine and consideration of intermittent or even long-term catheterization. Meanwhile, supply pads for a woman and a penile drainage device for a man.
- *Urinary infection.* Once treated, order an ultrasound scan for residual urine, if not already performed. Residuals in excess of 15 mL are abnormal. If the residual is above 50 mL, or if there have been more than three confirmed infections in a year, refer to a continence service. If catheterization is needed, intermittent self-catheterization is better than an indwelling catheter if the patient can manage it.

Other Issues

- *Pregnancy* does not appear to influence the course of the disease overall. There may be fewer relapses during the pregnancy with a slight increase in the risk of relapse after delivery.
- *Immunisations.* A patient should have all routine immunizations as well as an annual influenza vaccination. There is no evidence that they precipitate relapse.
- *Employment.* Check that the patient knows about the assistance that is available from disability employment advisors and the Access to Work scheme.

End-of-Life Care

While MS is not often fatal in itself, life is shortened by an average of 6 to 11 years and it may complicate a death from another condition. See Motor Neurone Disease for a discussion of end-of-life care.

PATIENTS' ORGANIZATION

The Multiple Sclerosis (MS) Society, 372 Edgware Road, London NW2 6ND. National helpline: 0808 800 8000; www.mssociety.org.uk.

Huntington's Disease

- Diagnosis should always be made by a specialist.
- Genetic testing may be requested by people who are at risk because of their family history. The arguments in favour and against are complex and the discussion is best handled by experienced staff at a genetics centre.
- Management should be in the hands of a specialist team; but the GP may be the first person to detect a new problem and needs to understand the principles of management.

Management

- Involuntary movements may be helped by three groups of drugs: neuroleptics, benzodiazepines, and dopamine depleting agents. They have the problems respectively of parkinsonism and tardive dyskinesia; of drowsiness and ataxia; and of depression and sedation. Some patients can be managed by ensuring an environment free from stress, with padding of chair and bed and weights on wrists and ankles to reduce movements.
- The impairment of voluntary movements does not respond to medication, but useful improvement can be achieved by behavioural methods. Dysphagia can improve with a change of food type, usually to a slightly more liquid food, and by developing a habit of eating slowly. A speech therapist can help with speech and with dysphagia. An occupational therapist can make the home safer for a patient at risk of falling.
- The problems posed by cognitive impairment can be reduced by training the family to communicate with the patient in a simple way. Explain that a patient who seems to be unaware of his or her disability may have a neurological basis for the unawareness and is not being difficult.

- The specific psychiatric disorders that are associated with Huntington's disease (HD), namely depression, mania, and obsessive-compulsive disorder, may respond to the same treatment as would be appropriate for a patient without HD.

Coping With the Cognitive Impairment

- Explain to the family, and to the patient if the impairment is not too advanced, the principles of coping with cognitive impairment.
- Explain that HD has certain specific problems and suggest solutions to them:
  - Difficulty with initiating and organizing tasks: use lists and prompt the patient to do things.
  - Perseveration of thoughts or actions: gently ease the patient on to something else.
  - Impulsivity and irritability: reduce stress with a regular schedule, respond with calmness, and try to find out what has prompted it.
  - Difficulty with attention: do one thing at a time.
  - Lack of insight: it is a feature of the disease, not a sign that the patient is being difficult.
- Advise the patient of the need to notify the DVLA and insurance company of the condition once it is diagnosed (though not when a genetic diagnosis has been made in an asymptomatic patient).
- Raise the question of an advance directive. It can be a great help if the patient decides certain key issues, and records the decision, when still competent to do so. Some key issues are preferred place of terminal care when the need arises, whether to be given a gastrostomy tube when no longer able to swallow, whether to be resuscitated when in a terminal state.
- Check what the family has been told about who else is at risk of developing the disease and what decision has been made about genetic testing. Record this in those patients' records.

PATIENT GROUPS

Huntington's Disease Association, Neurosupport Centre, Liverpool L3 8LR. Tel. 0151 298 3298; www.hda.org.uk.

Scottish Huntington's Association, Suite 135, St James Business Centre, Linwood Road, Paisley PA3 3AT, Scotland. Tel. 0141 848 0308; www.hdscotland.org.

Huntington's Disease Association, Northern Ireland, C/O Dept of Medical Genetics, Belfast City Hospital Trust, Lisburn Road, Belfast BT9 7AB, Northern Ireland. www.hdani.org.uk.

Paraplegia

Every patient with paraplegia will be under the care of a consultant. The GP however is likely to be the doctor to whom certain problems present. A proactive approach can make a difference to the patient's quality of life.

Spasticity

- Four types of oral drugs are licenced for the treatment of spasticity in the United Kingdom. These are benzodiazepines, baclofen, dantrolene, and tizanidine. The Drugs and Therapeutic Bulletin (2000) reported that tizanidine was slightly better tolerated than other oral drugs (baclofen and diazepam) and caused less muscle weakness.
- Attempts to control troublesome spasticity should include referral for consideration of intrathecal injection of baclofen, botulinum toxin, or nerve blocks.

Urinary Tract Infection

- Always confirm suspected urinary tract infections with a midstream specimen of urine (MSU).
- Do not give antibiotics if the patient is catheterized unless there are systemic symptoms.

Autonomic Dysreflexia

- This is reflex sympathetic overactivity, giving rise to vasoconstriction resulting in hypertension, severe headache, visual disturbance, anxiety, and pallor. The parasympathetic system slows the heart and causes flushing and sweating above the lesion. It only occurs in patients with lesions above T6. This should be considered a medical emergency.
- If this occurs do the following:
  a. Sit the patient up.
  b. Remove the cause (e.g., distended bladder, UTI, loaded colon, or anal fissure). If catheterizing or disimpacting, allow the lidocaine jelly at least 2 minutes to act. Both activities can exacerbate autonomic dysreflexia. If flushing a catheter through, use fluid at body temperature.
  c. It is essential that prompt action is taken to reduce blood pressure to avoid serious or life-threatening complications. Do not ignore headaches. Give nifedipine 10 mg sublingual. Get the patient to bite the capsule. Alternatively, use glyceryl trinitrate (GTN) one to two sprays sublingually. Note that a spinal injury patient may normally have low blood pressure (e.g., 90/60 mm Hg) and a rise to *normal* level of 120/80 mm Hg may represent a significant elevation.
  d. Monitor the BP at least every 5 minutes. It may fluctuate rapidly. If hypotension occurs, lie the patient down and raise the legs.
  e. Admit urgently to hospital if not settling.
  f. If it does settle, warn the patient that it may recur as the medication wears off, and that he or she should call for help at the first sign of recurrence (The Queen Elizabeth National Spinal Injuries Unit, 1999).

Pressure Ulcers

- Avoid prolonged (>2 hours) immobilization in the same position.
- Identify pressure areas and protect them.

- Ensure that someone inspects at-risk areas daily (ischii, sacrum, trochanters, heels).
- Refer for an exercise programme to retain posture, muscle strength.
- Refer to a dietician to ensure adequate nutrition.
- Treat sores or ulcers intensively and admit early if not resolving (e.g., within 2–4 weeks).

Psychological Aspects

- Be aware of the fact that patients may be suffering:
  - a severe grief response to the loss of function and independence;
  - a feeling of fear and vulnerability;
  - difficulties with their changing relationships with those around them.
- Be prepared to raise the issue of sexuality. Avoid the temptation to think of the individual as asexual. Sexual function and fertility are possible with appropriate support. Recommend publications from the Spinal Injuries Association (see box).

ADVICE FOR PATIENTS AND PROFESSIONALS

Spinal Injuries Association, SIA House, 2 Trueman Place, Oldbrook, Milton Keynes MK6 2HH
Helpline: 0800 980 0501; www.spinal.co.uk.

Essential Tremor

SYSTEMATIC REVIEW

Deuchl, G., Raethjen, J., et al. (2011). Treatment of patients with essential tremor. *Lancet Neurology.*

- Ask what effect the tremor is having. A quarter of those who consult about tremor retire early or change jobs because of it.
- *Mild cases:* Patients may choose not to take any medication. Check that they are not exacerbating the tremor with, for instance, caffeine. They may have noticed the improvement given by alcohol that is seen in 50% to 70% of patients.
- *Cases where the patient is more bothered:* Propranolol and primidone have established efficacy and produce a mean tremor reduction of about 50%.
  - Use propranolol 30 to 60 mg/day, increased to 60 to 240 mg three times a day if necessary.
  - Primidone 50 mg daily initially, increased gradually over 2 to 3 weeks if necessary. Side effects are common and frequently dose limiting (e.g., drowsiness, dizziness, or disequilibrium).
- *Cases not responding to propranolol/primidone or in whom they are contraindicated:* Consider one of atenolol, sotalol, alprazolam, topiramate, or gabapentin although the evidence of efficacy is less convincing.
- *Severe cases uncontrolled by medication:* Consider referral for neurosurgery; deep brain stimulation has shown significant reductions in tremor but further studies are required. Botulinum toxin injection has been used in some studies, but limited evidence exists to support use.

References

Association of British Neurologists. (2009). *Revised guidelines for prescribing in multiple sclerosis.* www.theabn.org.uk.

Confavreux, C., Vukusic, M. D., Moreau, M. D., & Adeleine, P. (2000). Relapses and progression of disability in multiple sclerosis. *NEJM, 343,* 1430–1438.

Department of Health. (2002). Health Service Circular 2002/004: Cost Effective Provision of Disease Modifying Therapies for People with Multiple Sclerosis.

Drug and Therapeutics Bulletin. (1998). Managing migraine. *DTB, 36*(6), 41–44.

Drugs and Therapeutics Bulletin. (2000). The management of spasticity. *DTB, 38,* 44–46.

Drugs and Therapeutics Bulletin. (2003). When and how to stop antiepileptic drugs in adults. *DTB, 41,* 41–43.

Drug and Therapeutics Bulletin. (2010). Management of medication overuse headache. *DTB, 48,* 2–6.

Faculty of Sexual and Reproductive Health. (2017). *Clincial Guidance: Drug Interactions with Hormonal Contraception.* Available www.fsrh.org. Accessed: 2nd October 2018.

Jackson, J. L., Shimeall, W., Sessums, L., et al. (2010). Tricyclic antidepressants and headaches: Systematic review and meta-analysis. *British Medical Journal (Clinical Research Ed.), 341,* c5222.

Markus, H. (2007). Improving the outcomes of stroke. *British Medical Journal (Clinical Research Ed.), 335,* 359–360.

McDermott, C. J., & Shaw, P. J. (2008). Diagnosis and management of motor neurone disease. *British Medical Journal (Clinical Research Ed.), 336,* 658–662.

Medicines and Healthcare Products Regulatory Agency. (2008). *Antiepileptics: Risk of suicidal thoughts and behaviour.* www.mrha.gov.uk.

National Institute for Health and Care Excellence. (2001). *Guidance on the use of riluzole for the treatment of motor neurone disease. NICE technology appraisal guidance, 20.* www.nice.org.uk.

National Institute for Health and Care Excellence. (2007). *Natalizumab for the treatment of adults with highly active relapsing-remitting multiple sclerosis. NICE technology appraisal guidance, 127.* www.nice.org.uk.

National Institute for Health and Care Excellence. (2012a). *Botulinum toxin type a for the prevention of headaches in adults with chronic migraine. NICE technology appraisal guidance, 260.* www.nice.org.uk.

National Institute for Health and Care Excellence. (2012b). *Fingolimod for the treatment of highly active relapsing-remitting multiple sclerosis. NICE technology appraisal guidance, 254.* www.nice.org.uk.

National Institute for Health and Care Excellence. (2012c). *Percutaneous venoplasty for chronic cerebrospinal venous insufficiency for multiple sclerosis. NICE interventional procedure guidance, 420.* www.nice.org.uk.

Neligan, A., Bell, G., & Sander, J. W. (2011). Sudden death in epilepsy. *British Medical Journal (Clinical Research Ed.), 343,* d7303.

Rugg-Gunn, F. J., & Sander, J. W. (2012). Management of chronic epilepsy. *British Medical Journal (Clinical Research Ed.), 345,* e4576.

Scottish Intercollegiate Guidance Network. (2008). *Diagnosis and Management of Headache in Adults*. SIGN Guidance 107. Available www.sign.ac.uk. Accessed 2nd October 2018.

The Queen Elizabeth National Spinal Injuries Unit. (1999). *Management of autonomic dysreflexia*. Retrieved from www.spinalunit.scot.nhs.uk.

Tsivgoulis, G., Spengos, K., Manta, P., et al. (2006). Validation of the ABCD score in identifying individuals of high risk of early stroke after a transient ischaemic attack. A hospital based case series study. *Stroke; a Journal of Cerebral Circulation, 37*, 2892–2897.

13

Women's Health

LINDSEY POPE

CHAPTER CONTENTS

Dysmenorrhoea

GUIDELINE

Royal College of Obstetricians and Gynaecologists. (2012). *The initial management of chronic pelvic pain. 'Green Top' guideline*, 41. www.rcog.org.uk.

Primary Dysmenorrhoea

- Dysmenorrhoea is common. In about 20% of women it is severe enough to interfere with daily activities.
- Dysmenorrhoea is more common in women with an early age of menarche, longer duration of menstruation, and in those who smoke.
- Reassure the patient that this is not a sign of disease. An examination of the abdomen is worthwhile as part of that reassurance as well as to exclude gross pelvic pathology. The need for a vaginal examination will depend on the individual circumstances. It should be performed if the patient has been sexually active.
- Give a nonsteroidal antiinflammatory drug (NSAID) alone or in addition to an analgesic. These work by inhibiting the synthesis of prostaglandins, and if the cycle is regular they should be started the day before the onset of menstruation until pain subsides. NSAIDs are effective in up to 70% of cases. Examples are ibuprofen 1200 mg daily, mefenamic acid 750 to 1500 mg daily, or naproxen, although adverse effects may be more common with the latter (Marjoribanks, Proctor, & Farquhar, 2006).
- Simple analgesics such as paracetamol can be helpful, especially for patients in whom NSAIDs are contraindicated (Zhang & Po, 1998).
- Consider a trial of the combined oral contraceptive (COC). It is commonly used despite the lack of evidence either way about its benefit.
- Complementary and alternative therapy options:
  - Non drug measures that may help include locally applied heat (e.g. a hot water bottle) and transcutaneous electrical nerve stimulation (TENS).
  - Alternative and complementary therapies such as herbal remedies, dietary supplements and acupuncture lack good quality evidence to support their use (Khan et al, 2012).
  - *Toki-shakuyaku-san*, a herbal remedy, which may reduce pain after 6 months.
  - Acupressure, which may be as effective as ibuprofen and high-frequency transcutaneous electrical nerve stimulation (TENS).
- Lifestyle and self-help techniques which could be helpful include smoking cessation, warmth to the abdomen, lying supine, tea, and a warm bath.
- *Women who are still in pain.* Consider referral for all those not responding.

Secondary Dysmenorrhoea

- Perform an abdominal, vaginal and pelvic examination. Take a high vaginal swab (HVS) and swabs for *Chlamydia*. Consider a pelvic ultrasound scan.
- Suspect a serious cause if there is persistent intermenstrual bleeding, post coital bleeding or an abnormal looking cervix.
- Refer for laparoscopy women in whom there is suspicion of pelvic pathology.
- *Chronic pelvic pain.* This affects about one in six women. It is a symptom with a number of contributory factors including gynaecological factors and non-gynaecological factors (e.g., irritable bowel syndrome, nerve entrapment) as well as psychologic and social factors.
  - Allow enough time for the woman to tell her story.
  - Recommend a pain diary and review.
  - Refer women who also have dyspareunia and low-grade pain throughout the cycle; they may have subclinical endometriosis, adenomyosis, or low-grade pelvic inflammatory disease (PID) despite a normal pelvic examination.
- Otherwise, treat symptomatically as for primary dysmenorrhoea, although symptom control is less likely to be successful.
- A levonorgestral releasing intrauterine system (IUS) may be beneficial, especially as up to 50% of women will be amenorrhoeic after 12 months. This option depends on the suitability for the patient (Vercellini, Cortesi, & Crosignani, 1997).
- *Intrauterine contraceptive device (IUD).* Consider removing an IUD, if present.
- Refer all women, if the pain persists, to a gynaecologist.

Endometriosis

GUIDELINES

National Institute of Health and Care Excellence. (2017). *Endometriosis: Diagnosis and Management. NICE Guideline* 73. Available: www.nice.org.uk.
  Royal College of Obstetricians and Gynaecologists. *The investigation and management of endometriosis. "Green Top" clinical guideline*, 24. www.rcog.org.uk/endometriosis.

- In addition to dysmenorrhoea, consider the diagnosis particularly in those with deep dyspareunia, chronic pelvic pain, ovulation pain, subfertility, and those with cyclical symptoms without excessive bleeding.
- Refer for laparoscopy patients in whom you suspect the diagnosis as examination is likely to be normal. The interpretation of the finding of endometriosis can, however, be difficult. It is found in about half of women presenting with dysmenorrhoea. In some of these it may be coincidental, in that it is present in 2% to 22% of women who have no symptoms.

- *Where endometriosis has been diagnosed*, treatment should be guided by a number of factors: wishes of the woman, severity and duration of symptoms, requirements for fertility, previous treatment, and any abnormalities identified on pelvic ultrasound or clinical examination.
- Patients not wishing to become pregnant consider:
  - *a combined oral contraceptive*. First line is usually a monophasic COC containing 30 to 35 μg ethinyloestradiol, and either norethisterone or levonorgestrel. A 3-month trail of this treatment is recommended. A further option may be to use a tricycling regime to control endometrioisis (Moore, Kennedy, & Prentice, 2001);
  - *progestogens* continuously for 6 months (e.g., norethisterone 10–20 mg daily). Dydrogesterone appears to be no better than placebo (Farquhar, 2001; Vercellini et al., 1997);
  - *danazol*, an androgen that is less commonly used now. Most often initiated in secondary care, the patient should be maintained on the lowest effective dose for 6 months. Warn the patient about the possible side effects of acne, weight gain, muscle cramps, oedema, and irreversible voice changes (Drug Therapy Bulletin [DTB], 1999; Pattie et al., 1998). Nonhormonal contraception is essential if the patient is sexually active;
  - *gonadorelin analogues*, but prescribed only under the supervision of a gynaecologist. These are available in a number of different preparations (e.g., goserelin subcutaneous [SC] injection every 28 days, buserelin intranasal every day). Oral contraceptives should be stopped prior to starting treatment and a nonhormonal form of contraception should be recommended as ovulation may occur if the treatment is interrupted at any point. Usual treatment is a single course of up to 6-month duration, though there is some evidence for repeated and shorter duration courses. It is important to warn patients about the possibility of menopausal type symptoms with this treatment and these may necessitate addback treatment in the form of tibolone (licensed) or hormone replacement therapy (HRT; continuous combined, off licence);
  - *levonorgestrel-releasing intrauterine system (LNG-IUS)*. This may reduce pain when maintained for at least 3 years.
- Patients wishing to become pregnant should:
  - consider using NSAIDs, as in primary dysmenorrhea; or
  - refer for consideration of surgical ablation or excision of endometriosis. This is an effective alternative to medical management (Sutton et al., 1994).

PATIENT ADVICE

National Endometriosis Society, 50 Westminster Palace Gardens, Artillery Row, London SW1P 1RL, tel. 020 7222 2781; helpline 0808 808 2227; www.endo.org.uk.
    Royal College of Obstetricians and Gynaecologists. (2016). *Endometriosis: Information for you*. www.rcog.org.uk.

Menorrhagia

GUIDELINES

National Institute for Health and Care Excellence. (2007). *Heavy menstrual bleeding. NICE clinical guideline, 44*, updated 2016. www.nice.org.uk.
    National Institute for Health and Care Excellence. (2017). *CKS menorrhagia*. cks.nice.org.uk/menorrhagia.

- Menorrhagia is regular, excessive menses occurring over consecutive cycles in an otherwise normal menstrual cycle that interferes with the woman's quality of life.
- Two thirds of women who have a blood loss of more than 80 mL per month have to limit normal activities and have anaemia.
- Menorrhagia is suggested by a history of bleeding that cannot be controlled with tampons alone and by having to get up during the night to change.
- The presence of other menstrual symptoms may influence a woman's assessment of the severity of her blood loss; 50% of women referred for menorrhagia have depression or anxiety as their primary problem (DTB, 1994a).
- One in 20 women aged 30 to 55 years consults her general practitioner (GP) each year with menorrhagia (Royal College of Obstetricians and Gynaecologists [RCOG], 1999) with one-third of women quantifying their periods as heavy.
- In 40% to 60% no underlying cause is found.

Clinical Assessment

- Check that there is no intermenstrual or postcoital bleeding.
- Check that there are no other menstrual symptoms, such as pain or pelvic pressure, which might suggest an underlying pathology.
- Check that the patient has had a recent smear as offered by the current recall system.
- Ascertain the impact the bleeding is having on the patient's life.
- Perform a pelvic and abdominal examination particularly if the history suggests an underlying pathology, initial treatment has proved ineffective, or an IUS is being considered.
- Check haemoglobin (Hb); two-thirds of patients will be anaemic.
- Exclude hypothyroidism only if there are signs or symptoms.
- Consider haematologic abnormalities (e.g., von Willebrand disease or thrombocytopenia), especially in women who have a family history of easy bleeding or who have bled heavily since the menarche.
- Refer to a gynaecologist for assessment if:
  - the patient is over 45; or

- there is suspicion of an organic cause (fibroids, pelvic pain, dyspareunia); or
- there is any postcoital, intermenstrual, or irregular bleeding, or any sudden change in blood loss; or
- medical treatment is unsuccessful.

Treatment

- *LNG-IUS (Mirena)*. This appears to be the most effective nonsurgical treatment (National Institute for Health and Care Excellence [NICE], 2007), is licensed for the treatment of menorrhagia, and is now suggested as the preferred first-choice treatment. The ECLIPSE trial found that the LNG-IUS resulted in greater improvements in quality of life than usual medical treatment after 2 years but the difference at 5 years was no longer significant (Gupta et al, 2015).
- If the LNG-IUS is to be used, the patient should be warned that irregular bleeding may occur in the first 6 months and that progestogen-type adverse effects are possible: breast tenderness, acne, and headaches. A pelvic examination is needed before insertion.
- *Tranexamic acid (TXA)*. Start on the first day of each cycle and continue until heavy bleeding has ceased. TXA 1 g four times a day decreases bleeding by up to 70% (NICE, 2007).
- *NSAIDs*. Give mefenamic acid 500 mg three times a day or naproxen 500 mg twice daily. Taken shortly before or at the start of menstruation and continued during heavy loss, they can decrease bleeding by 20% to 50%. They are especially useful if there is dysmenorrhoea.
- *The COC* is commonly used but there is insufficient evidence at present to adequately assess its effectiveness (NICE, 2007). It is especially useful if there is also dysmenorrhoea and if contraception is required.
- *Progestogens*. Give them in tablet form for 21 days of each cycle (days 5–26). Giving them for the second half of each cycle only is no better than placebo (Lethaby, Irvine, & Cameron, 2001). This is not an effective form of contraception. Alternatively, they can be given by injection in the same way as for contraception.
- *IUD*. If an IUD is in situ, either give an NSAID or an antifibrinolytic or change to a progestogen-releasing IUD.
- *Women not responding*. Consider referral for:
  - ultrasound and if inconclusive, hysteroscopy to exclude endometrial polyps and other pathology such as fibroids. Also consider endometrial sampling in patients over 40 years of age;
  - endometrial ablation or hysterectomy. Endometrial ablation has a shorter hospital stay and less time off work, but a proportion of women will have further bleeding and will require further surgery (Gannon et al., 1991). It is not suitable for women who may wish to conceive in the future;

- *gonadotropin-releasing hormone (GnRH) analogues* are effective at treating menorrhagia but have significant side effects. These should not be initiated in primary care and are time limited in their use.

Flooding

- Give norethisterone:
  - 15 mg twice a day for 2 days, then 10 mg twice a day for 2 days, then 15 mg once daily for 2 days, followed by 10 mg once daily for 14 days. The patient should expect a bleed 2 to 3 days after stopping the norethisterone; or
  - 20 mg twice a day for 5 days.

Delaying a Period

- Give norethisterone 5 mg two or three times a day 3 days prior to the expected period. If that fails, double the dose on the next occasion. Continue until it is convenient to have the period. The next period can be expected 2 to 3 days after stopping norethisterone.

Irregular Periods

Teenagers

- *Reassure* the patient that irregular periods are common after the menarche and that a regular cycle will probably establish itself without treatment.
- *If the patient is sufficiently bothered*. Give a progestogen cyclically, from day 10 to 25 or day 1 to 21, for 3 months. There is, however, no reason to think that this will speed up the establishment of normal periods.
- *COC* can be considered especially if contraception is required or the patient has dysmenorrhoea.
- *Very infrequent periods*. These patients need assessment (see upcoming discussion).

Women in Their Reproductive Years

- Exclude pregnancy.
- Check whether irregular periods or amenorrhoea have always been a feature. They may have polycystic ovary syndrome (PCOS; see upcoming discussion).
- Check whether the irregularity is due to the progestogen-only pill (POP).
- Look for weight loss, excessive exercise, recent stress, hirsutism, galactorrhoea, or infertility.
- Take blood for thyroid function tests (TFTs), prolactin, free androgen index, luteinizing hormone (LH), and follicle-stimulating hormone (FSH) on day 2 of the cycle.
- If results are normal and the patient wishes to become pregnant, consider referral for clomiphene.
- If the results are normal and pregnancy is not desired, COC or cyclical progestogens can be considered.

- If the results are abnormal, refer to an endocrinologist or gynaecologist, as appropriate.

Older Women

- Distinguish the irregularity due to ovarian failure from the pathological pattern of intermenstrual bleeding (IMB), which should be referred.
- Consider cyclical progestogens if the patient is sufficiently bothered.
- The COC will regulate bleeding and provide contraception. The known risks of thrombosis and breast carcinoma should be discussed with the patient and documented.
- HRT can be considered if there are other symptoms of the menopause and the bleeding is not pathological.

Postmenopausal Women

GUIDELINES

National Institute of Health and Care Excellence. (2015). *Suspected cancer: Recognition and referral. NICE clinical guideline, 12.* www.nice.org.uk.
Scottish Intercollegiate Guidelines Network. (2002). *Investigation of postmenopausal bleeding. SIGN guideline, 61.* www.sign.ac.uk.

- Postmenopausal bleeding is generally accepted as an episode of bleeding 12 months or more after the last period.
- Refer (to be seen within 2 weeks) if:
  - there has been an episode of postmenopausal bleeding
  - the patient is on tamoxifen, especially for more than 5 years. There is a fourfold increase in incidence in endometrial cancer.
- For the management of bleeding in women taking HRT, see the section on HRT.

Intermenstrual Bleeding

- Examine:
  - for anaemia;
  - the pelvis for abnormalities with a bimanual examination;
  - the cervix for abnormalities, and take swabs;
  - the vulva and vagina.
- Check smear history and past results.
- Take a pregnancy test, if appropriate.
- Refer urgently (to be seen within 2 weeks) any woman with abnormalities on examination suspicious for cancer.
- Consider urgent referral for any patient with persistent IMB despite normal examination findings.
- *Premenstrual spotting* reassure the patient if the loss is light and premenstrual. It is probably due to failure of the corpus luteum, and should settle within a few cycles.

Give cyclical progestogens from day 12 to 26 (i.e., in the luteal phase), to women sufficiently troubled by the symptoms.
- *Women on the COC:* Check compliance. If the examination is normal and bleeding persists, consider changing the pill (see section on COC).
- *Women with an IUD:*
  - Take endocervical swabs and a HVS.
  - If there is no infection, remove the IUD but remember to discuss alternative contraception.
  - Reassess in 3 months.

Amenorrhoea

REVIEW

National Institute of Health and Care Excellence. (2009/2014). *CKS: Amenorrhoea.* https://cks.nice.org.uk.

Primary Amenorrhoea
Girls Aged 14 to 16 Years

- Refer any girl aged 14 who has no secondary sexual characteristics.
- Refer any girl whose breast development began more than 2 years ago and who has not yet menstruated.

Girls Aged 16 and Over

- Examine her for evidence of endocrine disorders, chronic systemic illness, and eating disorders.
- Look at the external genitalia and secondary sexual characteristics, and check for an imperforate hymen (associated with cyclical pain).
- Refer to a gynaecologist or endocrinologist as indicated by likely diagnosis.

Secondary Amenorrhoea

- Secondary amenorrhoea exists when a woman has not menstruated for 6 months, having had a previously established cycle.
- In the history, note particularly:
  - any weight loss (if the patient's weight is <45 kg and she is of average height, she is unlikely to menstruate);
  - contraception. Amenorrhoea may occur with use of the LNG-IUS system, with depot medroxyprogesterone, or following use of the COC;
  - excessive exercise;
  - recent stress;
  - the character of the cycles prior to the amenorrhoea.
- Exclude pregnancy.
- Take blood for LH and FSH, free testosterone, prolactin, oestradiol, and TFTs.

- Refer to a gynaecologist or endocrinologist, as appropriate, if:
  - the FSH and LH are persistently high and the patient is under the age of 40. This indicates premature ovarian failure; or
  - the free testosterone is raised. This suggests PCOS (see upcoming discussion); or
  - the prolactin is over 1000 mIU/L or 500 to 1000 mIU/L on two occasions. This suggests a pituitary adenoma. Check for drugs that can cause hyperprolactinaemia (e.g., selective serotonin reuptake inhibitors [SSRIs]); or
  - the oestradiol is low; or
  - there is a recent history of uterine or cervical surgery. This may indicate Asherman syndrome.
- Osteoporosis risk needs to be considered in patients with persistent amenorrhoea. Measurement of bone density may be required and if symptoms have persisted over 12 months then consideration should be given to treatment with cyclic combined HRT (off-label use). Advice on adequate dietary intake of calcium should be given.

Polycystic Ovary Syndrome

GUIDELINES

National Institute for Health and Care Excellence. (2013). *CKS: Polycystic ovary syndrome.* cks.nice.org.uk/polycystic-ovary-syndrome.
    Royal College of Obstetricians and Gynaecologists. (2014). *Long-term consequences of polycystic ovary syndrome.* "Green Top" clinical guideline, 33. www.rcog.org.uk.

- Polycystic ovaries are a common ultrasound finding affecting up to 33% of women of reproductive age in the United Kingdom, only a third of whom have clinical or biochemical features of PCOS.
- The characteristic features include:
  - truncal obesity;
  - oligomenorrhoea/amenorrhoea/dysfunctional uterine bleeding;
  - hirsutism;
  - acne;
  - raised serum-free testosterone or free androgen index;
  - male-pattern hair loss
- Patients with PCOS are twice as likely to develop diabetes (Wild et al., 2000). By the age of 40, up to 40% will have type 2 diabetes (Lord, Flight, & Norman, 2003). They have a higher prevalence of features associated with metabolic syndrome: hypertension, dyslipidaemia, visceral obesity, insulin resistance, and hyperinsulinaemia.

Diagnosis

Consider the diagnosis if two of the following three criteria are met:

1. Polycystic ovaries on ultrasound scan (USS) (either ≥12 follicles in at least one ovary or increased ovarian volume [>10 mL]). The diagnosis can be made in the absence of polycystic ovaries on USS; and the appearance of polycystic ovaries on USS, without the other criteria, is not enough to make the diagnosis.
2. Oligoovulation or anovulation: as suggested by menstrual cycles longer than 35 days or less than 10 periods a year.
3. Clinical and/or biochemical signs of hyperandrogenism. Clinical signs include acne, hirsutism, and androgenic alopecia. The biochemical confirmation required is a raised total or free testosterone. A raised LH/FSH ratio is no longer considered useful in the diagnosis because of its inconsistency.

- Exclude adrenal hyperplasia, hyperprolactinaemia, androgen secreting tumours, and Cushing syndrome. If the latter is suspected on clinical grounds, refer to an endocrinologist.
- Check TFTs, serum prolactin, and free testosterone. If there is clinical evidence of hyperandrogenism and the total testosterone is greater than 5 nmol/L, check the level of 17-hydroxyprogesterone.
- If one of the previous two criteria is met but not the other, order a pelvic USS for ovarian cysts.

Management

- Explain what little is known about the syndrome: that the pituitary produces excess LH, which stimulates the ovary to produce excess testosterone which in turn causes acne and hirsutism. Associated with this is a tendency to insulin resistance, manifested by overweight and the development of diabetes.
- *Cardiovascular disease (CVD) risk.* Check the serum lipids, blood pressure, waist circumference, and body mass index (BMI) regularly in women over 35. NICE recommends calculating the CVD risk score but it should be noted that cardiovascular risk calculators have not been validated in PCOS. Hypertension should be treated, but lipid-lowering agents should only be introduced by a specialist. Advice should be given on weight loss, diet, and exercise, as appropriate.
- *Diabetes.* Screen all women with PCOS for impaired glucose tolerance and type 2 diabetes mellitus (DM). Initially offer an oral glucose tolerance test to all women. Consider repeating this annually for women at higher risk (impaired glucose tolerance, strong family history of DM, BMI >30 kg/m^2 or 25 kg/m^2 in Asian women, and those with a history of gestational diabetes). Those not offered an annual oral glucose tolerance test (OGT) should be offered their fasting glucose checked annually or should be offered a OGT every second year.
- *Snoring.* Ask about snoring and sleep apnoea. PCOS appears to be a risk factor independently of BMI in sleep apnoea.
- *Weight.* Advise about weight loss through diet (especially with a low gastrointestinal [GI] diet) and exercise. Loss of weight has been reported to result in resumption of

ovulation, improvement in fertility, increased sex hormone binding globulin (SHBG), and reduced risk of diabetes and cardiovascular disease.

Management of Symptoms

- *Acne.* See section on acne, but consider using COC pill or co-cyprindiol (Dianette) (NICE CKS, 2013).
- *Hirsutism.* Physical methods of hair removal (e.g., waxing, intense pulsed light [IPL]) and topical treatment with eflornithine may be helpful but will not treat the underlying cause. Eflornithine has been reported as resulting in marked improvement in 32% of women. Women who are overweight should be advised to lose weight. First line drug treatment is with a combination of cyproterone acetate and ethinylestradiol (as Dianette) although a desogestrel-containing COC may be as effective. Second line treatments include spironolactone, finasteride, GnRH analogues, and metformin. Contraception is required while on spironolactone as there is a theoretical risk of feminizing a male foetus (Farquhar et al., 2000). Warn that benefit is unlikely before about 6 months of any of these treatments.
- *Lack of regular periods.* This may predispose to endometrial hyperplasia and later carcinoma and so all women who have been amenorrhoeic should have their endometrial thickness assessed. RCOG (UK) recommends that a withdrawal bleed be induced every 3 to 4 months with progestogens (for at least 12 days) or the COC. Women who do not have withdrawal bleeds should be referred to a gynaecologist.
- *Lack of ovulation.* Refer to a gynaecologist. Metformin 500 mg three times a day, although unlicensed for this use, can induce ovulation and reduce fasting insulin concentrations, blood pressure, and low density lipoprotein (LDL) cholesterol. However, RCOG (UK) states "long term use of insulin sensitizing agents cannot as yet be recommended." Patients are increasingly aware and ask for metformin treatment but this is ahead of the evidence and outside the product licence (Harborne et al., 2003).
- *Infertility.* Refer. Other treatments recommended by NICE are metformin and clomiphene in combination, ovarian drilling and gonadotrophins (NICE, 2013).

SELF-HELP GROUP

Verity. The polycystic self-help group; www.verity-pcos.org.uk.

Vaginal Discharge

- Ask about the type of discharge, the timing, whether it smells, whether it itches, and whether there is pelvic pain.
- Ask the woman what she thinks it is and, when asking whether it seems related to sexual activity, ask tactfully about the number of sexual partners.
- Examine the vulva and test the vaginal pH using narrow range pH paper. Bimanual examination is needed if the history raises the possibility of pelvic infection; swabs are needed in those at risk of sexually transmitted infections and in those in whom the clinical picture does not suggest bacterial vaginosis or candida.
- In those who are at low risk of sexually transmitted infection and who decline examination, treatment can be given based on clinical history.
- *Interpretation of findings:*
  - Smelly white discharge with pH above 4.5: bacterial vaginosis.
  - White curdy discharge, usually with vulval soreness and itch, erythema, possibly fissuring and satellite lesions; pH below 4.5: candidiasis.
  - Smelly yellow or green frothy discharge with pH above 4.5, perhaps with dysuria: trichomonas.
- When the clinical picture is not typical of bacterial vaginosis or candidiasis, or the patient is under age 25 or has had a new sexual partner in the last year, take swabs:
  - HVS for *Trichomonas*, the clue cells of bacterial vaginosis, and *Candida*.
  - Endocervical swab for chlamydia and gonorrhoea testing with nucleic acid amplification test (NAAT).
- Patients with sexually transmitted infections are best managed in the genitourinary medicine (GUM) clinic.

Management: Candida

GUIDELINE

Clinical Effectiveness Group (Association for Genitourinary Medicine and Medical Society for the Study of Venereal Disease). (2007). *Management of vulvovaginal candidiasis.* www.bashh.org/guidelines.

- Give general advice to avoid local irritants, and avoid tight-fitting synthetic clothing (Bingham, 1999).
- Treat only if symptomatic.
- Prescribe a topical imidazole. Cure rates are 80% to 95%. Give it either as a single dose or as a short course at night, usually for 3 nights. Oral imidazoles are no more effective (Watson et al., 2002) but they have more side effects. In addition, they are contraindicated in pregnancy.
- *Male partners.* There is no evidence to support the treatment of asymptomatic male sexual partners (Bisschop et al., 1986).
- COC. Do not stop the COC. Its use is not associated with candidiasis.
- *Pregnancy.* Asymptomatic colonization is more common in pregnancy (30%–40%). Treat symptomatic patients with topical azoles, but a longer course may be necessary.

Recurrent Candidiasis (Four or More Symptomatic Episodes per Year)

- Check the urine for glucose approximately 2 hours after a meal or glucose load. Note that this would be inadequate as a screening test for diabetes in any other situation.

- Exclude other risk factors: iron deficiency anaemia, thyroid disease, frequent antibiotic use, corticosteroid use, immunodeficiency.
- Screen for other vaginal infections.
- Give either:
  - an imidazole pessary daily for 2 weeks then weekly for 6 months; or use a pessary only when an infection is most likely (e.g., after intercourse or when taking a broad-spectrum antibiotic). These treatment regimens are empirical and are not based on randomized controlled trials; or
  - fluconazole 150 mg orally every 3 days for three doses then weekly for 6 months. Approximately 90% of women remain disease free for 1 year. If there is relapse between doses, consider giving twice weekly fluconazole 150 mg.
- Consider giving cetirizine 10 mg daily for 6 months or zafirlukast 20 mg twice a day for 6 months. Allergy may be an important component especially in women with atopy.
- *Candida of the gut.* There is no evidence to suggest that eradication of candida from the gut is helpful.
- *Probiotics/Lactobacillus.* Evidence does not support the use of oral or topical *Lactobacillus* in prevention of vulvovaginal candidiasis.
- *Alteration of vaginal pH.* Suggest a trial of a pH-lowering agent (e.g., AciGel).

Management: Bacterial Vaginosis

GUIDELINE

British Association for Sexual Health and HIV (2012). *UK National Guideline for the management of bacterial vaginosis.* www.bashh.org.uk/guidelines.

- Bacterial vaginosis is characterized by a reduction in lactobacilli and an overgrowth of predominantly anaerobic organisms (*Gardnerella vaginalis, Mycoplasma hominis, Prevotella* species, *Mobiluncus* species).
- Approximately 50% of women with the condition are asymptomatic.
- It is not regarded as sexually transmitted. It can arise and remit spontaneously in women regardless of sexual activity. However, it is more common in women liable to sexually transmitted infections.
- *Partners.* No evidence has been found supporting the treatment of partners of women affected by bacterial vaginosis (Potter, 1999).
- Treatment is indicated for:
  - symptomatic women;
  - pregnant women with a history of recurrent miscarriage;
  - women undergoing termination of pregnancy. They are at greater risk of PID if the bacterial vaginosis is untreated.
- Give metronidazole 400 to 500 mg twice a day for 5 to 7 days; or intravaginal metronidazole gel (0.75%) once daily for 5 days; or metronidazole 2 g as a single oral

dose: or intravaginal clindamycin cream (2%) once daily for 7 days. The cure rate is 70% to 80%.
- *Pregnancy and lactation.* Symptomatic women in pregnancy should be treated with metronidazole. Lactating women should be treated with intravaginal metronidazole.

Pelvic Inflammatory Disease

GUIDELINE

British Association for Sexual Health and HIV. (2011). *UK National Guideline for the management of pelvic inflammatory disease.* www.bashh.org.

- PID is usually the result of ascending infection from the endocervix. *Neisseria gonorrhoeae* and *Chlamydia trachomatis* have been identified as causative agents, whilst *Mycoplasma genitalium*, anaerobes, and other organisms commonly found in the vagina may also be implicated.
- PID has a high morbidity; about 20% of affected women become infertile, 20% develop chronic pelvic pain, and 10% of those who conceive have an ectopic pregnancy (Metters et al., 1998).
- Repeated episodes of PID are associated with a four- to sixfold increase in the risk of permanent tubal damage (Hills et al., 1997).
- PID may be asymptomatic.
- Of women with PID, 10% to 20% will develop perihepatitis.
- A delay of only a few days in receiving treatment markedly increases the risk of long-term sequelae (Hills et al., 1993). Because of this, and the lack of definitive diagnostic criteria, a low threshold for the empirical treatment of PID is recommended.

Diagnosis

- Symptoms can include fever, lower abdominal pain, deep dyspareunia, abnormal bleeding, abnormal vaginal or cervical discharge. On examination there may be cervical excitation and adnexal tenderness.
- Clinical diagnosis is correct in only 65% to 90% of cases compared to laparoscopy. Even laparoscopy can miss mild cases but it remains the most reliable investigation. In the United Kingdom, it is not recommended in all cases but should be performed when there is diagnostic doubt.
- If not referring, perform the following:
  - Endocervical swabs for gonococcus and chlamydia. Negative microbiological tests do not exclude a diagnosis of PID; in at least 50% of cases no specific organism is identified. Screen for the same diseases in any sexual partners.
  - Urinalysis, pregnancy test, and mistream specimen of urine (MSU) to look for other causes of lower abdominal pain.

- Blood for erythrocyte sedimentation rate (ESR) or C-reactive protein (CRP). A raised level would support the diagnosis (Miettinen et al., 1993).
- Recommend rest and provide adequate analgesia.
- Recommend that unprotected intercourse be avoided until the woman and her partner(s) have completed treatment and follow-up. If it is not possible to screen for gonorrhoea and chlamydia in the sexual partner(s) give empirical treatment for both gonorrhoea and chlamydia (Groom et al., 2001; Haddon et al., 1998).
- If an IUD is in situ, and this is the preferred method of contraception, leave it in place. Remove it only if the condition fails to respond to treatment and other causes of pain have been excluded (Larsson & Wennergren, 1981; Soderberg & Lingren, 1981; Teisala, 1989).
- Drug treatment:
  - Ofloxacin 400 mg twice a day plus metronidazole 400 mg twice a day for 14 days.
  - In women at high risk of gonococcal infection: ceftriaxone 500 mg intramuscularly as a single dose then 14 days of oral doxycycline 100 mg twice a day and metronidazole 400 mg twice a day.
- Review daily in case admission becomes necessary.

Admission

- Admit patients if:
  - the illness is severe;
  - not responding after 3 days of oral therapy;
  - unable to tolerate oral drugs;
  - a pelvic mass is present;
  - the patient is pregnant;
  - there is diagnostic uncertainty;
  - the patient suffers from immunodeficiency;
  - the patient is above the usual age for PID. An alternative diagnosis (e.g., ovarian carcinoma) is more likely.

Follow-Up for All Patients

- Review within 72 hours. Refer if there is little improvement.
- Review again in 4 weeks to:
  - ensure there is adequate clinical response;
  - ensure there was compliance with the antibiotics;
  - trace, investigate, and treat the woman's partner(s) if a sexually transmitted disease (STD) is diagnosed (Robinson & Kell, 1995). A study found that 60% of contacts had relevant infections, and that in most of these it was asymptomatic (Kamwendo et al., 1993). Consider referral to a GUM clinic for contact tracing;
  - stress the significance of the disease and the sequelae.
- Discuss with the patient her need for safer sex.
- Advise the patient to ask for antibiotic cover (e.g., doxycycline 200 mg stat or metronidazole 2 g stat) if she ever needs a termination of pregnancy (TOP) or a dilatation and curettage (D&C).
- Advise the patient to seek advice promptly if the symptoms return.

> **PATIENT INFORMATION**
>
> Download the RCOG leaflet "Acute Pelvic Inflammatory Disease". Available at www.rcog.org.uk.

Premenstrual Syndrome (PMS)

> **GUIDELINE**
>
> National Institute for Health and Care Excellence. (2014). *CKS: Premenstrual syndrome.* cks.nice.org.uk/premenstrual-syndrome.
> Royal College of Obstetricians and Gynaecologists. (2016). *Management of Premenstrual Syndrome.* Green-top Guidline No. 48.

- Ninety-five percent of women have symptoms related to their menstrual cycle; in 5% they are disabling. More than 150 symptoms have been reported.
- Diagnosis depends not on the type of symptom but on the timing of the symptoms and their cyclicity. Symptoms present 1 to 14 days prior to menstruation and disappear at the onset or by the day of the heaviest flow. If behavioural symptoms persist throughout the cycle, then consider a psychological/psychiatric disorder.
- Ask the patient to keep a menstrual and symptom diary for at least 2 months. She can score symptoms according to their severity.
- Listen sympathetically. It is a real entity. This alone can be therapeutic.
- Give simple advice:
  - *Dietary advice.* Explain that some women seem more sensitive to blood sugar changes at this time of the cycle, and this may be the cause of food cravings, panic reactions, irritability, and aggression. Advise patients to reduce their refined sugar intake as well as their caffeine intake. Small frequent carbohydrate snacks seem effective in about 30% of women.
  - *Stress management.* Explain that although it is not the cause of the syndrome, stress is harder to cope with during the premenstrual period. Relaxation methods, yoga, meditation, and exercise can be of benefit.

Therapeutic Options

- *SSRI.* Consider using an SSRI. There is good evidence of their efficacy (Wyatt, Dimmock, & O'Brien, 2002) and they may be effective if used in the luteal phase alone. Side effects may limit their acceptability.
- *Breast tenderness, bloating, and irritability* may be improved by taking spironolactone 100 mg daily from day 12 until the onset of menstruation.
- *NSAIDs* given for 7 days prior to menses and 4 days after the onset have been shown to improve a number of symptoms but not breast tenderness.

- *Aerobic exercise.* Low and moderate exercise (50%–70% of maximum) three times a week for 45 minutes has been shown to reduce symptoms.
- *Oestrogens* may improve or in some cases worsen the situation. The COC can prove helpful, especially in those women requiring contraception. Women who experience symptoms during their pill-free week can take three consecutive packets back to back. A lower dose of oestrogen, as HRT, may help some women but cyclical progestogens must also be used in women with an intact uterus.
- *Danazol* has been shown to be effective. Adverse effects are common (masculinization and weight gain) with continuous use but may not occur with luteal phase use alone. Danazol should normally be initiated by a specialist.
- *Vitamin B$_6$ (pyridoxine)* 50 to 100 mg daily. This recommendation is based on limited information from poor quality trials, but the evidence suggests that B$_6$ may be of benefit.

    Breast tenderness. Consider bromocriptine 1.25 mg twice a day, but adverse effects are common.

    Note: Progestogens have been found unhelpful in the treatment of PMS.

    Note: Evening primrose oil. There is no evidence that it is helpful in PMS.

Patients Not Responding

- Refer to a gynaecologist for the consideration of suppression of ovarian function. Treatment options include high-dose danazol, high-dose oestrogen, and GnRH analogues with addback HRT.

PATIENT SUPPORT

National Association for Premenstrual Syndrome (NAPS), www.pms.org.uk.
   Premenstrual Society, PO Box 429, Addlestone, Surrey KT15 1DZ, helpline 01932 872560 (11 am–6 pm, weekdays only).

Ovarian Cancer Screening

- Many women will request screening for ovarian cancer on the basis of their family history. Some useful figures can be used to reassure many women (Table 13.1).
- There is currently no national screening programme for ovarian cancer. Despite early promising results, the UK Collaborative Trial of Ovarian Cancer Screening (UKTOCS) has so far failed to show clearcut evidence of benefit from a screening programme.
- Women at higher risk may be eligible for screening and genetic testing; and if they fall into one of the following groups, may be referred to the UK Familial Ovarian Cancer Screening Study (UKFOCSS) or for genetic testing by the local genetics service. Women considered at higher risk are those with:

TABLE 13.1   Ovarian Cancer Risk

Number of First-Degree Relatives With Ovarian Cancer	Lifetime Risk of Developing Ovarian Cancer
0	1%
1	5%
2	15%
>2	50%

a. two or more first-degree relatives with ovarian cancer; or

b. one first-degree relative with ovarian cancer and one first-degree relative with breast cancer diagnosed under 50 years of age; or

c. one ovarian cancer and two breast cancers diagnosed under 60 years in first-degree relatives;

- known BRCA-1 or BRCA-2 mutations in the family; or
- three colorectal cancers, at least one diagnosed under 50 years of age, and one ovarian cancer, all first-degree relatives of each other;
- affected relatives with any of the above combinations who are related by second degree through an unaffected male and there is an affected sister (i.e., paternal transmission is occurring).

Note: A first-degree relative is a parent, sibling, or child; a second-degree relative is a grand-parent, aunt or uncle, or cousin.

- *Weak family history.* Women with one close relative with epithelial ovarian cancer diagnosed before the age of 50 may also wish to be referred for advice but may not be offered regular screening.

PATIENT INFORMATION

Cancer Research UK. *Ovarian cancer screening.* www.cancerresearchuk.org.

Gestational Trophoblastic Hydatidiform Mole and Choriocarcinoma

GUIDELINE

Royal College of Obstetricians and Gynaecologists. (2010). *The management of gestational trophoblastic disease.* "Green Top" clinical guideline, 38. www.rcog.org.uk.

- Gestational trophoblastic disease is uncommon in the United Kingdom, with a calculated incidence of 1/714 live births. The incidence is highest in women from Asia (incidence 1/387) compared to non-Asian women (incidence 1/752).

- In the United Kingdom, there is an effective registration and treatment programme with high cure rates.
- Once the diagnosis of hydatidiform mole has been made, follow-up will be needed for between 6 months and 2 years. The aim is to detect the occurrence of choriocarcinoma.
- Once treated, serum estimations of levels of human chorionic gonadotrophin (HCG) should be performed according to protocols from the regional expert units (London, Sheffield, and Dundee).
- The COC pill and hormone replacement are safe to use once HCG levels have reverted to normal.
- Women should be advised not to conceive until the HCG level has been normal for 6 months or follow-up has been completed (whichever is the sooner). The risk of further recurrence is 1 in 55. After any further pregnancy, urine and blood samples should be taken to exclude disease recurrence.
- Women who undergo chemotherapy should not attempt to conceive until a year after completion of treatment.
- Refer all women with persistent bleeding:
  - after the evacuation of retained products of conception;
  - after normal pregnancy;
  - after miscarriage.
- Send for histology any products of conception passed at home.
- If no products of conception are available, check HCG 4 weeks after the loss of the pregnancy.

PATIENT INFORMATION

The Hydatidiform Mole and Choriocarcinoma UK information service, www.hmole-chorio.org.uk.

SCREENING CENTRES

Trophoblastic Tumour Screening and Treatment Centre. Department of Oncology, Charing Cross Hospital, Fulham Palace Road, London W6 8RF, tel. 020 8846 1409, fax 020 8748 5665.

Trophoblastic Tumour Screening and Treatment Centre. Weston Park Hospital, Whitham Road, Sheffield S10 2SJ, tel. 0114 226 5202, fax 0114 226 5511.

Hydatidiform Mole Follow-Up (Scotland) Department of Obstetrics and Gynaecology, Ninewells Hospital, Dundee DD1 9SY, tel. 01382 632748, fax 01382 632096.

The Menopause

Establishing the Diagnosis

- No investigations are routinely indicated. FSH levels fluctuate markedly during the perimenopause and so are of limited value in symptomatic women in whom a clinical history can form the basis of diagnosis. There is little place for LH, oestradiol, and progesterone estimation in clinical practice (Hope, Rees, & Brockie, 1999).

- Consider taking serial FSH measurements in the following circumstances:
  - Women with symptoms under the age of 40 because of the implications of premature ovarian failure
  - Women with symptoms who have had a hysterectomy with ovarian conservation, who thus are at risk of an early menopause
- Take FSH levels:
  - 4 to 8 weeks apart when the woman is not on HRT or hormonal contraception. FSH levels of greater than 30 IU/L are generally considered to be in the postmenopausal range;
- *Abnormal bleeding.* Refer women, without starting HRT, if they give a history of abnormal bleeding (e.g., sudden change in menstrual pattern, intermenstrual bleeding, postcoital bleeding, or a postmenopausal bleed) (Hope et al., 1999; Korhonen et al., 1997).

Initial Management

- Counsel women about the menopause. Ideally all perimenopausal women should be given the opportunity to discuss the menopause, with particular reference to the symptomatology, common misconceptions, and treatment options.
- Take the opportunity to discuss lifestyle issues (smoking cessation, diet, and exercise). HRT is no longer recommended as a general prophylactic measure because of the increased risk of breast cancer, but individual women may judge that, for them, the benefit outweighs the risks (discussed later).
- *Osteoporosis.* Identify those patients at high risk of osteoporosis and investigate and treat, if appropriate. HRT is no longer indicated for the prevention of osteoporosis except in those with an early menopause.
- *Vasomotor symptoms:*
  - *HRT* is extremely effective in controlling these symptoms (MacLennan, Lester, & Moore, 2001). Because of the possible harms, use the lowest effective dose for the shortest time possible (see upcoming discussion).
  - *SSRIs and related drugs.* A meta-analysis has found some evidence of benefit, with paroxetine performing best. However, even paroxetine reduced flushes by only one or two a day compared to placebo (Nelson et al., 2006). Venlafaxine has also been shown to be superior to placebo for treating vasomotor symptoms (Caan et al, 2015).
  - *Gabapentin.* A trial of 12 weeks of 900 mg/day reduced the hot flash composite score by 54% against 31% with placebo (Guttuso et al., 2003). The use of gabapentin for menopause is currently restricted to specialist centres.
  - *Consider clonidine* for those unable to take HRT or an SSRI (Edington & Chagnon, 1980; Nagamani, Kelver, & Smith, 1987).
  - *Black cohosh,* with or without other natural remedies, has been shown to be ineffective (Newton et al., 2006).

- *Vaginal dryness.* Treatment options include:
  - HRT (see upcoming discussion);
  - local oestrogens. These can be given per vaginum daily until symptoms have ceased, then twice weekly for 3 to 6 months. Systemic progestogens do not need to be given alongside local oestrogens as there is no evidence that they cause endometrial proliferation;
  - vaginal lubricants. These include K-Y jelly, Replens (a nonhormonal aqueous moisturizer), and Senselle (a water-based lubricant).
- *Urinary symptoms:*
  - Symptoms related to urogenital atrophy will respond to oestrogen by any route. Maximum benefit will not be seen for at least the first month, and may take up to a year (Cardozo et al., 1998).
  - Stress incontinence is unlikely to respond to oestrogen replacement therapy alone. Refer patients who are sufficiently troubled to a gynaecologist.
- *Psychological symptoms.* Psychological symptoms may relate to a woman's hormonal status but, equally, the menopause may become a scapegoat for patients with underlying emotional problems (Hunter, 1996). Counselling may be helpful but many will improve when their physical symptoms improve (Gath & Iles, 1990). Depression may need treatment in its own right.

Hormone Replacement Therapy

GUIDELINE

National Institute for Health and Care Excellence. (2015). *Menopause: Diagnosis and management. NICE clinical guideline, 23.* www.nice.org.uk.

- HRT may be indicated in the following:
  - Women with an early menopause (<45 years of age) mainly for the prevention of osteoporosis. It may also give some protection in this young age group against CVD. It is usually given until age 50.
  - Women under the age of 65 with severe vasomotor and other symptoms of the menopause who understand the risks and are prepared to take HRT for a limited period. Analysis of the Women's Health Initiative results has shown no increase in breast cancer, myocardial infarction, or stroke in women under 60 years of age who use HRT for 5 years or less (Rossouw et al., 2007).
- Record that the risks of HRT have been explained and an informed decision taken by the patient. Review the decision at least annually.

Benefits and Risks
Benefits

- *Symptom relief.* Improvement in vasomotor symptoms occurs in a few weeks and in vaginal symptoms in 3

TABLE 13.2	Minimum Doses of Oestrogen Needed for Bone Conservation		
Drug	Dosage	Frequency	
Oestradiol	1–2 mg	Daily*	
Oral conjugated equine oestrogens	0.625 mg	Daily	
Transdermal oestradiol patch	50 mg	Daily	
Oestradiol gel	1.5 g (two measures)	Daily	
Oestradiol implants	50 mg	6 monthly	

*Although 1 or 2 mg oral oestradiol can be used for prevention of osteoporosis, the bone protective effect is dose related. Some products are licensed for osteoporosis prevention at 2 mg only, while others are licensed at 1 and 2 mg.

months. Improvement in mental function is less certain. The mental health of women with vasomotor symptoms seems to improve on HRT but those without vasomotor symptoms worsen, with poorer physical functioning and lower energy levels compared to those on placebo (Hlatky et al., 2002). Overall, HRT does not improve the quality of life (Hays et al., 2003).

- *Osteoporosis.* Combined HRT protects against hip fracture in unselected postmenopausal women and reduces the risk of all fractures. This represents five fewer hip fractures per 10,000 person-years, a number needed to treat (NNT) of 2000 for 1 year (Rossouw et al., 2002). In women at high risk of fracture the absolute benefit will be greater. The benefit is dose related (Table 13.2). However, the benefit on fracture risk is lost within 3 years of stopping HRT (Heiss et al., 2008).
- *Prevention of carcinoma of the colon.* HRT appears to reduce the risk of developing colonic carcinoma by 20% (RR 0.80 [95% CI 0.74–0.86]) (Nelson et al., 2002).

Risks

- *CVD.* HRT does not increase risk of CVD when given to women under the age of 60 nor does it affect the risk of dying from CVD. If cardiovascular risk factors are well managed, then they are not a contraindication to using HRT. Oral oestrogen appears to be associated with a small increased risk of stroke but no increase is seen with the transdermal route.
- *Breast cancer.* The use of combined HRT in healthy postmenopausal women is associated with an increase in breast cancer risk (RR 1.24 [95% CI 1.01–1.54]) (Rossouw et al., 2002) but this is not the case with oestrogen-only treatment. The increase in risk is related to the duration of treatment and the risk decreases again after stopping treatment.
- *Endometrial cancer.* Unopposed oestrogen is associated with an extra five cases per 1000 women over 5 years.

The use of combined preparations reduces but does not eliminate this risk, with an estimated risk of two extra cases per 1000 women over 10 years.

- *Ovarian cancer.* Long-term combined or oestrogen-only HRT is associated with a small increased risk of ovarian cancer. This excess risk disappears within a few years of stopping HRT.
- *Venous thromboembolism (VTE).* Oral HRT increases the risk of VTE but transdermal HRT does not increase risk above the baseline population risk. Therefore consider the transdermal route for women with additional risk factors for VTE e.g. women with a BMI over 30. Consider referring women who are at high risk of VTE (e.g., due to family history of hereditary thrombophilia or VTE) to a haematologist for assessment.
- *Dementia.* The affect of HRT on dementia risk is unknown.

Other Issues to Discuss

- Explain that taking HRT means that cyclical bleeding will return if the woman has an intact uterus and a cyclical preparation is used. Irregular bleeding is common with continuous preparations.
- Explain that evidence from randomized trials suggests that HRT does not cause extra weight gain in addition to that normally gained at the time of the menopause (Norman, Flight, & Rees, 2001).

Contraindications

- Oestrogen replacement therapy is absolutely contraindicated in very few patients. Even in women in whom treatment appears contraindicated, oestrogen therapy may be prescribed under supervision of a specialist menopause clinic if the woman's symptoms are particularly severe (Rees & Purdie, 1999).
- Absolute contraindications include:
  - acute-phase myocardial infarction, pulmonary embolism, or deep vein thrombosis (DVT);
  - active endometrial or breast cancer;
  - pregnancy;
  - undiagnosed breast mass;
  - uninvestigated abnormal vaginal bleeding;
  - severe active liver disease.

Note: Many contraindications given in prescribing data sheets are derived from high-dose combined oral contraceptives and are, in the view of most experts, not applicable to HRT (Rees & Purdie, 1999).

HRT Use in Women With Comorbidity (Relative Contraindications)

- *History of thromboembolic disease.* Women with a personal or family history of thromboembolism should be offered screening for thrombophilia before starting. Those with a personal history of VTE should not take HRT unless the woman decides that, for her, the benefits outweigh the risks (RCOG, 2004). She may choose prophylactic anticoagulation, though that has its own risks. A transdermal route may reduce the risk of VTE. A specialist opinion would be wise in those with thrombophilia.
- *Past history of endometrial cancer.* Refer women who want to consider HRT to the appropriate specialist. Although conventional advice is that oestrogens are contraindicated, small studies of endometrial cancer survivors have not shown an adverse effect on survival.
- *Diabetes and gall bladder disease.* Use a transdermal preparation.
- *Liver disease.* Refer to a specialist clinic.
- *Endometriosis.* Refer to a specialist clinic.
- *Fibroids.* HRT may enlarge fibroids, causing heavy or painful withdrawal bleeds. Warn patients to report pain or pressure effects on the bladder or bowel.
- *Migraine* is not a contraindication to HRT. There is no evidence that the risk of stroke is increased by the use of HRT in women with migraine (Bousser et al., 2000).
- *Hypertension.* There is no evidence that HRT raises blood pressure (Rees & Purdie, 1999).

Initial Assessment

- Take a history and assess the woman's menopausal status.
- Check for contraindications to HRT therapy, especially a history of breast cancer or VTE.
- Check blood pressure (BP), BMI, and serum lipids.
- Advise the woman about breast awareness. Check that mammography screening is in place if over 50 years. Mammography is not needed before commencing HRT unless the woman is at high risk of breast cancer (Hope et al., 1999).
- Check that regular cervical screening is taking place.
- Give lifestyle advice, as discussed.

Treatment
Oestrogens

- Start at the lowest possible dose of oestrogen (especially in older women who tend to get more oestrogenic side effects) and increase at 3-monthly intervals, if necessary, to achieve optimum symptom control.
- Give oestrogens continuously, and only give them without progestogens if the woman has had a hysterectomy.

Progestogens

- These must be added for endometrial protection in women with a uterus. Most products contain either C-19 derivatives (norethisterone/levonorgestrel), which are more androgenic, or C-21 derivatives (medroxyprogesterone acetate/dydrogesterone), which are less androgenic.
- Change to a less androgenic preparation if the patient is troubled by progestogenic side effects.

Perimenopausal Women With an Intact Uterus

- Use a cyclical regimen (monthly or 3-monthly). The majority of women will have a bleed toward the end of the progestogen phase.

Postmenopausal Women With an Intact Uterus

- Use:
  - a cyclical regimen; or
  - a continuous combined regimen. Continuous regimens induce an atrophic endometrium and so do not produce a withdrawal bleed, although irregular bleeding can occur in the first 4 to 6 months. Bleeding should be investigated if it persists for longer than 6 months, becomes heavier rather than less, or occurs after amenorrhoea; or
  - tibolone. This combines oestrogenic and progestogenic activities, and weak androgenic activity. It must only be started at least 1 year after the menopause. There is evidence that it improves libido (Kokcu et al., 2000).

Alternative Modes of Delivery

- *Oestrogen implants.* Repeat every 4 to 8 months. Occasionally vasomotor symptoms can return despite supraphysiologic plasma concentrations of oestradiol (tachyphylaxis). Check that plasma oestradiol levels have returned to normal (<1000 pmol/L) before inserting a new implant.
- *Transdermal patches and gels.* These avoid the first-pass metabolism in the liver and deliver a more constant level of hormone. Patches come as either reservoir or matrix patches. Skin reactions are less common with the matrix patches.
- *IUS.* The LNG-IUS is licensed for 4-year usage for the delivery of progestogen to protect the endometrium. A 5-year follow-up concludes that the LNG-IUS effectively protects against endometrial hyperplasia (Varila, Wahlstrom, & Rauramo, 2001). It provides contraception, and it is the only way a nonbleed regimen may be achieved in the perimenopause.

Managing the Side Effects of HRT

Bleeding

Patients on HRT should only be referred urgently (in the United Kingdom under the 2-week rule) if the bleeding continues after the HRT has been stopped for 4 weeks.

Bleeding on Cyclic Combined Therapy

- Check when the bleeding occurs. These regimens should produce regular predictable bleeds starting toward or soon after the end of the progestogenic phase.
- Consider poor compliance, drug interactions, or GI upset.
- Try stopping HRT to see if it is the cause of the bleeding.
- If bleeding problems are due to HRT, alter the progestogen:
  - Heavy or prolonged bleeding: increase the dose or duration of progestogen or change the type of progestogen to a more androgenic type (see previous discussion).
  - Bleeding early in the progestogenic phase: increase the dose or change the type of progestogen.
  - Painful bleeding: change the type of progestogen.
  - Irregular bleeding: change the regimen or increase the dose of progestogen.

- *No bleeding* whilst taking a cyclic regime reflects an atrophic endometrium and occurs in 5% of women, but pregnancy needs to be excluded in perimenopausal women.
- Refer if there is:
  - a change in the pattern of withdrawal bleeds and breakthrough bleeding that persists for more than 3 months;
  - unexpected or prolonged bleeding that persists for more than 4 weeks after stopping HRT: refer urgently.

Bleeding on Continuous Combined Therapy or Tibolone

- Explain to patients that the risk of bleeding is 40% in the first 4 to 6 months.
- Make sure the patient was at least 1 year postmenopausal before she started the regimen.
- Bleeding beyond 6 months requires further investigation.
- Bleeding that occurs after a period of amenorrhoea requires further investigation.

Oestrogen-Related Side Effects

- Oestrogenic side effects include fluid retention, bloating, breast tenderness and enlargement, nausea, headache, leg cramps, and dyspepsia.
- Encourage the patient to persist with therapy for 12 weeks, as most side effects resolve with time.
- For persistent side effects consider:
  - reducing the dose; or
  - changing the oestrogen type (swap between the two main forms of oestrogen: oestradiol and conjugated equine oestrogens); or
  - changing the route of delivery.
- *Nausea and gastric upset.* Change the timing of the oestrogen dose (e.g., try taking it with food or at bedtime).

Progestogen-Related Side Effects

- Progestogen-related side effects tend to occur in a cyclic pattern during the progestogenic phase of cyclical HRT. Continuous combined products contain lower doses of progestogens and side effects are less likely. Side effects include fluid retention, breast tenderness, headaches, mood swings, depression, acne, lower abdominal pain, and backache.
- Encourage the patient to persist with therapy for about 12 weeks as some side effects will resolve.
- Various changes in the progestogens may be helpful, but remember not to reduce the dose or duration below that which protects the endometrium. Options:
  a. Reduce the duration but not below 10 days per cycle.
  b. Reduce the dose of progestogen, or
  c. Change the progestogen type (either C-19 or C-21 derivatives; see earlier discussion), or
  d. Change the route of progestogen (oral, transdermal, vaginal, or intrauterine), or
  e. Reduce the frequency of how often the progestogen is taken by switching to a long-cycling regime in which progestogens are administered for 14 days every 3 months. This is only suitable for women with scant periods or who are postmenopausal, or

f. Change to a continuous combined therapy, which often reduces progestogenic side effects with established use; it is suitable only for postmenopausal women however.

Follow-Up of Women on Hormone Replacement Therapy

- See after 3 months, then every 6 months.
- Check for compliance, bleeding patterns, and side effects.
- Check that the patient is up to date with her cervical smears and mammograms.

Note: There is no need to check the BP except as good practice in any well-person screening.

How Long to Continue?

- *Symptomatic relief.* Guidelines recommend that HRT be given "for the shortest possible time" but there is no way of predicting how long this is. Most authorities recommend that HRT given for symptom relief be stopped within 5 years. In the World Health Organisation (WHO) trial, HRT was stopped after 5.7 years. Half the women with vasomotor symptoms at the start of the trial reported moderate or severe symptoms after stopping (Ockene et al., 2005). If troublesome symptoms recur on withdrawal, HRT can be restarted for 6 to 12 months at a time.
- *Osteoporosis prevention when no more appropriate alternatives exist.* Five-year treatment is the minimum period for which benefit has been shown, yet after this the risks, especially of breast cancer, rise. The fact that the benefit rapidly drops off after stopping HRT must be set against the risks associated with longer term use.

Stopping Treatment

- HRT may be stopped abruptly or gradually. There is no evidence that either approach is better in terms of preventing the return of symptoms.
- For gradual reduction, reduce the strength of oestrogen every 1 to 2 months, then take it on alternate days for 1 to 2 months, then stop. At this stage:
  - if using a calendar pack, take alternate tablets from the pack so that the regimen includes progestogen for the second half of the cycle;
  - if using a patch, cut the patch in half once the lowest dose has been reached. If using the half-patch cyclically, use the progestogen-containing half-patch for the second half of the cycle.
- Review after a few months. If troublesome symptoms have recurred, consider restarting therapy at the lowest possible dose and titrating up as necessary. If only local symptoms persist, use a vaginal preparation.
- *Stopping HRT prior to surgery.* The RCOG (2004) does not consider that this is necessary but recommends prophylactic measures instead: antithromboembolic stockings and low molecular weight heparin.

Hormone Replacement Therapy and Contraception

- Perimenopausal women cannot be assumed to be infertile.
- Routine HRT preparations do not suppress ovulation and are not contraceptive.
- Contraception should be continued for 1 year after the last menstrual period (LMP) for women over 50 years, or for 2 years after the LMP for women under the age of 50 years.
- Perimenopausal women may use:
  a. barrier methods, IUD, or LND-IUS, as well as HRT; or
  b. the low-dose COC instead of HRT; or
  c. the POP, possibly combined with HRT, although there are theoretical concerns that the oestrogen component of HRT may interfere with the action of the POP on the cervical mucus (Pitkin, 2000).

When Has the Menopause Occurred When Masked by Hormone Replacement Therapy or Combined Oral Contraceptive?

- It is important to know this so that a realistic idea of how long the woman needs to remain on contraception can be calculated (see previous discussion); 80% of women are postmenopausal by the age of 54 years (DTB, 1994b).
- Discontinue HRT or COC for 6 to 8 weeks, then check FSH, and repeat after a further 4 to 8 weeks (Gebbie, 1998). If both FSH levels are above 30 IU/L, stop contraception after a further year. If a spontaneous period occurs, or FSH is less than 30 IU/L, continue contraception and repeat the test in 1 year.
- *Women on the POP.* Check the FSH without stopping the POP.

PATIENT ORGANIZATIONS

British Menopause Society. 4-6 Eton Place, Marlow, Bucks SL7 2QA, tel. 01628 890199; www.thebms.org.

Cervical Screening

GUIDELINES

A summary of updated national guidelines within the cervical screening programme is available at www.cancerscreening.nhs.uk/cervical.
National Institute for Health and Care Excellence. (2017). *CKS: Cervical screening*. cks.nice.org.uk/cervical-screening.

- The NHS screening programme requires that all women between the ages of 25 and 64 are offered a smear:
  - Aged 25: first invitation
  - 25–49: 3 yearly
  - 50–64: 5 yearly

- 65+: only screen those who have not been screened since the age of 50 or have had a recent abnormal test.
- The advisory committee on cervical screening reviewed the policy on screening (June 2009) and concluded that there should be no change in policy on age of starting screening and that the harms of screening under this age outweigh the benefits.
- Evidence for the programme:
  - In 2000, there were 2424 new registrations for invasive cervical cancer in England (National Statistics, Cancer registrations in England, 2000).
  - Cervical cancer incidence fell by 42% between 1988 and 1997 (England and Wales). This fall was directly related to the cervical screening programme (National Statistics, 2000).
  - In 1995, there were 10.4/100,000 newly diagnosed cases, by 1999 this had fallen to 9.3/100,000 (National Statistics, 1999).
  - Cervical cancer screening saves approximately 4500 lives in England and prevents 3900 cases per year in the United Kingdom (Peto et al., 2004; Sasieni et al., 1996).
- The major risk groups are:
  - women with many sexual partners or whose partners have had many partners;
  - smoking. It doubles a woman's risk.
- Liquid-based cytology (LBC) has reduced the number of inadequate samples from over 9% to 2.9% in 2008. Results are received faster and there is less pressure on the workforce. The changeover to LBC was completed in October 2008.

Action According to the Smear Result

An Inadequate Smear

- Smears cannot be interpreted (inadequate) if the specimen is obscured by inflammatory cells/blood, does not contain the right type of cells, or is incorrectly labelled.
- Repeat an inadequate smear after between 6 weeks and 3 months. Repeating the smear within 6 weeks does not allow adequate tissue regrowth. Refer if there are two further inadequate smears, repeated at 3-monthly intervals (preferably midcycle).

Borderline or Mild Dyskaryosis ±Human Papillomavirus

- The laboratory will test the sample for human papillomavirus (HPV):
  - If positive, the woman will be offered a colposcopy appointment.
  - If negative, the woman can be returned to routine recall.

Moderate or Severe Dyskaryosis

- The woman will be referred urgently (Table 13.3) (within 2 weeks) to colposcopy. Stress that this is part of the screening process and does not mean that the patient has cancer.

TABLE 13.3	**Terminology Used During Cervical Screening**
Cytological terms	Histological equivalent*
Mild dyskaryosis	CIN 1 (mild dysplasia) outer 1/3 of epithelium
Moderate dyskaryosis	CIN 2 (moderate dysplasia) 1/3 to 2/3 of epithelium
Severe dyskaryosis	CIN 3 (severe dysplasia or carcinoma in situ) full thickness of the epithelium with breakdown of structure between basement membrane and epithelium

CIN, Cervical intraepithelial neoplasia.
*The correlation between status on smear and on histology is not close.

- Advise the woman to continue her contraception, including the COC; pregnancy makes management more difficult.

Follow-Up After Colposcopy and Treatment

- Follow-up at 6 months (by gynaecologist).
- If this is normal, then a smear will be performed yearly for up to 10 years (GP or gynaecologist).
- If normal, then revert to 3-yearly smears.

Follow-Up After Hysterectomy

- Routine smears for 10 years prior to hysterectomy and negative for cervical intraepithelial neoplasia (CIN) at hysterectomy, vault cytology not required.
- Less than 10 years routine smears prior to hysterectomy and negative for CIN at hysterectomy, single vault smear required, then no further follow-up required.
- CIN present at hysterectomy but fully excised, vault smears at 6 and 18 months, then no further follow-up, if negative.
- CIN present at hysterectomy with incomplete or uncertain excision, follow-up as if cervix still in situ.

References

ALTS Group. (2003). A randomized trial on the management of low-grade squamous intraepithelial lesion cytology interpretations. *American Journal of Obstetrics and Gynaecology, 188*, 1393–1400.

Bingham, J. S. (1999). What to do with patients with recurrent vulvovaginal candidiasis. *Sexually Transmitted Infections, 75*, 225–227.

Bisschop, M. P., Merkus, J. M., Scheyground, H., et al. (1986). Cotreatment of the male partner in vaginal candidosis: A double blind randomised controlled study. *British Journal of Obstetrics and Gynaecology, 93*, 79–81.

Bousser, M. G., Conard, J., Kittner, S., et al. (2000). Recommendations on the risk of ischaemic stroke associated with use of combined oral contraceptives and hormone replacement therapy in women with migraine. The international headache society task force on combined oral contraceptives & hormone replacement therapy. *Cephalalgia: An International Journal of Headache, 20*, 155–156.

Caan, B., La Croix, A., Joffe, H., et al. (2015). Effects of Estrogen or Venlafaxine on Menopause Related Quality of Life in Healthy Postmenopausal Women with Hot Flashes: A Placebo-Controlled Randomized Trial. *Menopause*, 2015 Jun;*22*(6), 607–615.

Cardozo, L., Bachmann, G., McClish, D., et al. (1998). Meta-analysis of estrogen therapy in the management of urogenital atrophy in postmenopausal women: Second report of the hormones and urogenital therapy committee. *Obstetrics & Gynecology, 92*, 722–727.

Drug Therapy Bulletin. (1994a). Surgical management of menorrhagia. *DTB, 32*, 70–72.

Drug Therapy Bulletin. (1994b). Hormone replacement therapy. *DTB, 34*, 81–84.

Drug Therapy Bulletin. (1999). Managing endometriosis. *DTB, 37*, 25–29.

Duckitt, K., & Collins, S. (2008). Menorrhagia. *British Medical Journal Clinical Evidence*, 2008 Sep 18;2008. pii: 0805.

Edington, R. F., & Chagnon, J. P. (1980). Clonidine for menopausal flushing. *Canadian Medical Association Journal, 123*, 23–26.

Farquhar, C. (2001). *Endometriosis. Clinical evidence* (Issue 5). London: British Medical Journal Publishing Group. www.clinicalevidence.org.

Farquhar, C., Lee, O., Toomath, R., et al. (2000). Spironolactone versus placebo or in combination with steroids for hirsutism and/or acne (cochrane review). In *The Cochrane Library* (Issue 4). Oxford: Update Software.

Gannon, M. J., Holt, E. M., Fairbank, J., et al. (1991). A randomised trial comparing endometrial resection and abdominal hysterectomy for the treatment of menorrhagia. *British Medical Journal (Clinical Research Ed.), 303*, 1362–1364.

Gath, D., & Iles, S. (1990). Depression and the menopause. *British Medical Journal (Clinical Research Ed.), 300*, 1287–1288.

Gebbie, A. E. (1998). Contraception for women over 40. In J. Studd (Ed.), *The management of the menopause, annual review* (pp. 67–80). London: Parthenon Publishing.

Groom, T. M., Stewart, P., Kruger, H., et al. (2001). The value of a screen and treat policy for *Chlamydia trachomatis* in women attending for termination of pregnancy. *Journal of Family Planning and Reproductive Health Care, 27*, 69–72.

Gupta, J. K., Daniels, J. P., & Middleton, L. J. (2015). A randomised controlled trial of the clinical effectiveness and cost-effectiveness of the levonorgestrel-releasing intrauterine system in primary care against standard treatment for menorrhagia: the ECLIPSE trial. *Health Technol Assess*, 2015 Oct;*19*(88), i–xxv.

Guttuso, T., Kurlan, R., McDermott, M. P., et al. (2003). Gabapentin's effects on hot flashes in postmenopausal women: A randomized controlled trial. *American College of Obstetricians and Gynaecologists, 101*, 337–345.

Haddon, L., Heason, J., Fay, T., et al. (1998). Managing STIs identified after testing outside genitourinary medicine departments: One model of care. *Sexually Transmitted Infections, 74*, 256–257.

Harborne, L., Fleming, R., Lyall, H., et al. (2003). Descriptive review of the evidence for the use of metformin in polycystic ovary syndrome. *Lancet, 361*, 1894–1901.

Hays, J., Ockene, J. K., Brunner, R. L., et al. (2003). Women's health initiative investigators. Effects of estrogen plus progestin on health-related quality of life. *New England Journal of Medicine, 348*, 1839–1854.

Heiss, G., Wallace, R., Anderson, G. L., et al. (2008). Health risks and benefits 3 years after stopping randomized treatment with estrogen and progestin. *JAMA: The Journal of the American Medical Association, 299*, 1036–1045.

Hills, S. D., Joesoef, R., Marchbanks, P. A., et al. (1993). Delayed care of pelvic inflammatory disease as a risk factor for impaired fertility. *American Journal of Obstetrics and Gynecology, 168*, 1503–1509.

Hills, S. D., Owens, L. M., Marchbanks, P. A., et al. (1997). Recurrent chlamydial infections increase the risks of hospitalisation for ectopic pregnancy and pelvic inflammatory disease. *American Journal of Obstetrics and Gynecology, 176*, 103–107.

Hlatky, M. A., Boothroyd, D., Vittinghoff, E., et al. (2002). Quality-of-life and depressive symptoms in postmenopausal women after receiving hormone therapy: Results from the heart and estrogen/progestin replacement study (HERS) trial. *JAMA: The Journal of the American Medical Association, 287*, 591–597.

Hope, S., Rees, M., & Brockie, J. (1999). *Hormone replacement therapy—a guide for primary care*. Oxford: Oxford University Press.

Hunter, M. S. (1996). Depression and the menopause. *British Medical Journal (Clinical Research Ed.), 313*, 350–351.

Kamwendo, F., Johansson, E., Moi, H., et al. (1993). Gonorrhoea, genital chlamydia infection and non-specific urethritis in male partners of hospitalized women treated for acute pelvic inflammatory disease. *Sexually Transmitted Diseases, 20*, 143–146.

Khan, K. S., Champaneria, R., & Latthe, P. M. (2012). How effective are non-drug, non-surgical treatments for primary dysmenorrhoea? *British Medical Journal, 344*, e3011.

Kokcu, A., Cetinkaya, M. B., Yanik, F., et al. (2000). The comparison of effects of tibolone and conjugated estrogen medroxyprogesterone acetate therapy on sexual performance in postmenopausal women. *Maturitas, 36*, 75–80.

Korhonen, M. O., Symons, J. P., Hyde, B. M., et al. (1997). Histological classification and pathological findings for endometrial biopsy specimens obtained from 2964 perimenopausal and postmenopausal women undergoing screening for continuous hormone replacement therapy. *American Journal of Obstetrics and Gynaecology, 176*, 377–380.

Larsson, B., & Wennergren, M. (1981). Investigation of copper-intrauterine device (Cu-IUD) for possible effect on frequency and healing of pelvic inflammatory disease. *Contraception, 24*, 137–149.

Lethaby, A., Irvine, G., & Cameron, I. (2001). Cyclical progestogens for heavy menstrual bleeding (cochrane review). In *The Cochrane Library* (Issue 3). Oxford: Update Software.

Lord, J. M., Flight, I. H. K., & Norman, R. J. (2003). Metformin in polycystic ovary syndrome: Systematic review and meta-analysis. *British Medical Journal (Clinical Research Ed.), 327*, 951–955.

MacLennan, A., Lester, S., & Moore, V. (2001). Oral oestrogen replacement therapy versus placebo for hot flushes (cochrane review). In *The Cochrane Library* (Issue 3). Oxford: Update Software.

Marjoribanks, J., Proctor, M. L., & Farquhar, C. (2006). Nonsteroidal anti-inflammatory drugs for primary dysmenorrhoea. *Cochrane Database of Systematic Reviews*, www.library.nhs.uk/Cochranelibrary.

Metters, J. S., Catchpole, M., Smith, C., et al. (1998). *Chlamydia trachomatis: Summary and conclusions of CMO's expert advisory group*. London: Department of Health.

Miettinen, A. K., Heinonen, P. K., Laippala, P., et al. (1993). Test performance of erythrocyte sedimentation rate & C-reactive protein in assessing the severity of acute pelvic inflammatory disease. *American Journal of Obstetrics and Gynecology, 169*, 1143–1149.

Moore, J., Kennedy, S., & Prentice, A. (2001). Modern combined oral contraceptives for pain associated with endometriosis (cochrane review). In *The Cochrane Library* (Issue 3). Oxford: Update Software.

Nagamani, M., Kelver, M. E., & Smith, E. R. (1987). Treatment of menopausal flashes with transdermal administration of clonidine. *American Journal of Obstetrics and Gynecology, 156*, 561–565.

National Institute for Health and Care Excellence. (2007). *Heavy menstrual bleeding. NICE clinical guideline, 44*, www.nice.org.uk.

National Institute for Health and Care Excellence. (2013). *Acne Vulgaris. NICE CKS*.

National Institute of Care Excellence. (2013, updated 2017). *Fertility problems: Asessment and Treatment. NICE Clinical Guideline, 156.* Available: www.nice.org.uk.

National Statistics (1999). *MB1 No 28 Cancer Statistics Registrations 1995–1997; National Statistics MB1 No 30 Registrations of cancer diagnosed in 1999.*

National Statistics (2000). *Health Quarterly Statistics 07, Autumn.*

Nelson, H. D., Humphrey, L. L., Nygren, P., et al. (2002). Postmenopausal hormone replacement therapy: Scientific review. *JAMA: The Journal of the American Medical Association, 288,* 872–881.

Nelson, H. D., Vesco, K. K., Haney, E., et al. (2006). Nonhormonal therapies for menopausal hot flashes. *JAMA: The Journal of the American Medical Association, 295,* 2057–2071.

Newton, K. M., Reed, S. D., LaCroix, A. Z., et al. (2006). Treatment of vasomotor symptoms of menopause with black cohosh, multibotanicals, soy, hormone therapy or placebo. *Annals of Internal Medicine, 145,* 869–879.

Norman, R. J., Flight, I. H. K., & Rees, M. C. P. (2001). Oestrogen and progestogen hormone replacement therapy for perimenopausal and post-menopausal women: Weight and body fat distribution (cochrane review). In *The Cochrane Library* (Issue 3). Oxford: Update Software.

Ockene, J. K., Barad, D. H., Cochrane, B. B., et al. (2005). Symptom experience after discontinuing use of estrogen plus progestin. *JAMA: The Journal of the American Medical Association, 294,* 183–191.

Pattie, M. A., Murdoch, B. E., Theodoros, D., et al. (1998). Voice changes in women treated for endometriosis and related conditions: the need for comprehensive vocal assessment. *Journal of Voice, 12,* 366–371.

Peto, J., Gilham, C., Fletcher, O., et al. (2004). The cervical cancer epidemic that screening has prevented in the UK. *Lancet, 364,* 249–256.

Pitkin, J. (2000). Contraception and the menopause. *Maturitas, 1,* S29–S36.

Potter, J. (1999). Should sexual partners of women with bacterial vaginosis receive treatment? *British Journal of General Practice, 49,* 913–918.

Royal College of Obstetricians and Gynaecologists (1999). *The initial management of menorrhagia. Evidence-based clinical guidelines* (no. 1). London: RCOG.

Royal College of Obstetricians and Gynaecologists. (2004). *Hormone replacement therapy and venous thromboembolism. RCOG guideline, 19,* www.rcog.org.uk.

Rees, M., & Purdie, D. W. (1999). *Management of the menopause.* London: BMS Publications. The Handbook of the BMS.

Robinson, A. J., & Kell, P. (1995). Male partners of women with pelvic infection should be traced (letter). *British Medical Journal (Clinical Research Ed.), 311,* 630.

Rossouw, J. E., Anderson, G. L., Prentice, R. L., et al. (2002). Writing group for the Women's health initiative investigators. Risks and benefits of estrogen plus progestin in healthy postmenopausal women: principal results from the Women's health initiative randomized controlled trial. *JAMA: The Journal of the American Medical Association, 288,* 321–333.

Rossouw, J. E., Prentice, R. L., Manson, J. E., et al. (2007). Postmenopausal hormone therapy and risk of cardiovascular disease by age and years since menopause. *JAMA: The Journal of the American Medical Association, 297,* 1465–1477.

Sasieni, P. D., Cuzick, J., Lynch-Farmery, E., et al. (1996). Estimating the efficacy of screening by auditing smear histories of women with and without cervical cancer. *British Journal of Cancer, 73,* 1001–1005.

Soderberg, G., & Lingren, S. (1981). Influence of an intrauterine device on the course of acute salpingitis. *Contraception, 24,* 137–143.

Sutton, C. J., Ewen, S. P., Whiltelaw, N., et al. (1994). Prospective, randomized, double-blind, controlled trial of laser laparoscopy in the treatment of pelvic pain associated with minimal, mild, and moderate endometriosis. *Fertility and Sterility, 62,* 696.

Teisala, K. (1989). Removal of an intrauterine device and the treatment of acute pelvic inflammatory disease. *Annals of Medicine, 21,* 63–65.

Varila, E., Wahlstrom, T., & Rauramo, I. (2001). A 5-year study of the use of a levonorgestrol intra-uterine system in women receiving hormone replacement therapy. *Fertility and Sterility, 76,* 969–973.

Vercellini, P., Cortesi, I., & Crosignani, P. G. (1997). Progestogens for symptomatic endometriosis—a critical analysis of the evidence. *Fertility and Sterility, 68*(3), 393–401.

Watson, M. C., Grimshaw, J. M., Bond, C. M., et al. (2002). Oral versus intra-vaginal imidazole and triazole anti-fungal treatment of uncomplicated vulvovaginal candidiasis (thrush) (cochrane review). In *The Cochrane Library* (Issue 1). Oxford: Update Software.

Wild, S., Pierpoint, T., Mckeigue, P., et al. (2000). Cardiovascular disease in women with polycystic ovary syndrome at long term follow up: A retrospective cohort study. *Clinical Endocrinology, 52,* 595–600.

Wyatt, K. M., Dimmock, P. W., & O'Brien, P. M. S. (2002). Selective serotonin reuptake inhibitors for premenstrual syndrome. *Cochrane Database of Systematic Reviews.*

Zhang, W. Y., & Po, A. L. (1998). Efficacy of minor analgesics in primary dysmenorrhoea: A systematic review. *British Journal of Obstetrics and Gynaecology, 105*(7), 780–789.

14

Obstetric Problems

LINDSEY POPE

CHAPTER CONTENTS

Prepregnancy Care

- Whilst prepregnancy counselling offers an opportunity to reinforce good health habits and identify potential problems for pregnancy early, there is no evidence from randomized controlled trials that women who attend such visits have better health or pregnancy outcomes. In one large cohort study, only a small proportion of women planning pregnancy followed recommendations for nutrition and lifestyle (Inskip et al., 2009).
- General practitioners (GPs) may have the opportunity to identify risk factors before conception. This can be done either at a specific consultation or when the opportunity arises (e.g., as part of contraceptive care) or when seeing patients with diabetes or hypertension.
- If a woman presents for a prepregnancy visit this can be used as a time to encourage her to:
  - stop smoking;
  - take 400 μg of folic acid a day for the first 12 weeks of pregnancy (explain that folic acid supplements have been shown to reduce the risk of neural tube defects by 50%–70%) (Rush, 1994);
  - avoid alcohol or at most take 2 units a week;
  - take a healthy diet; particularly avoiding soft cheeses and liver.
- At the same time the doctor can:
  - consider the risk of inherited disorders;
  - assess medical conditions (e.g., hypertension, diabetes, epilepsy, hyperthyroidism);
  - assess whether the woman has an eating disorder or is overweight;
  - check that the patient is immune to rubella and has an up-to-date cervical smear;
  - warn the patient to avoid contact with chickenpox or exposed shingles. In the United States and Australia, varicella vaccination is offered to non-immune women.
- Consider offering flu vaccination.

Genetic Disorders

- All couples should be referred for genetic counselling if they request it or there are risk factors that need further investigation. The list of identifiable conditions is increasing, and studies suggest that clinicians across specialties are poor at appreciating which conditions have identifiable genetic components (Harris et al., 1999).
- If there is any doubt, contact the nearest department of clinical genetics for advice. Children or adults with a major abnormality or disease, even if not at present thought to be genetic in origin, should have blood stored at a regional genetics laboratory for later analysis.
- Those at higher risk include the following:
  1. Couples with a personal or family history of an abnormality that is presumed to be genetic in origin. They should be referred for genetic counselling or have blood taken by the GP on the advice of the geneticist. Important examples are:
     - cystic fibrosis;
     - Huntington chorea;
     - Duchenne and other muscular dystrophies;
     - polycystic kidneys;
     - intellectual disability, which may be due to fragile-X syndrome.
  2. Couples belonging to a high-risk ethnic group (discussion to come).
  3. *Older women.* The risk of having a baby with Down syndrome is 1:400 at age 35, rising to 1:100 at age 40, and 1:30 at age 45. Around the age of 37, the risk of chromosomal abnormality is greater than the risk of miscarriage after amniocentesis. Recommend the leaflet "Screening for ., Edwards' and Patau's Syndromes" from www.nhs.uk/.
  4. *Consanguineous couples.* First-degree cousins have a slight but significant increase in congenital malformations. This is likely to be higher if there is a family history of congenital disease. Caucasian first-degree cousins should be offered screening for cystic fibrosis even when there is no family history.

Diseases in High-Risk Ethnic Groups
Sickle Cell and Thalassaemia

- Women from areas where malaria has been common are at increased risk of carrying the sickle cell or thalassaemia traits: Africa, the Caribbean, the Middle East, the Indian subcontinent, South America, South and Southeast Asia, and the Mediterranean.

- In the United Kingdom, all pregnant women are offered screening for thalassaemia using the mean corpuscular haemoglobin (MCH) measurement as part of the routine blood count.
- Women, or potential fathers, from an ethnic group at risk are also offered a test for sickle cell and related haemoglobin variants.
- At a prenatal consultation, a couple may choose to undergo screening because of the ethnic group to which they belong or because of a positive family history. When assessing ethnic origin try to go back at least two generations. Discuss the appropriate test with the laboratory and send the completed Family Origin Questionnaire with the blood samples. This is available from the sickle cell and thalassaemia screening programme (www.gov.uk, then search for "Family origin questionnaire").
- Refer to the obstetrician all couples who are both heterozygous for sickle cell or thalassaemia, or when the mother is and the father is unknown.

PATIENT INFORMATION

Sickle Cell Society, 54 Station Road, London NW10 4UA, tel. 020 8961 7795, helpline 0800 001 5660, www.sicklecellsociety.org.

UK Thalassaemia Society, 19 The Broadway, Southgate Circus, London N14 6PH, tel. 020 8882 0011, free adviceline 0800 731 109, www.ukts.org.

Jewish Population: Tay-Sachs

- Tay-Sachs disease is an incurable neurodegenerative disorder that begins around 6 months of age. Babies born with it live for only a few years. People of Ashkenazi (Eastern European) Jewish descent are most at risk.
- Consider referral of both prospective parents to the regional genetics centre for testing for *Tay-Sachs* trait. One in 25 of Jewish descent is positive.

Previous Obstetric History

- *Down syndrome.* Make certain that all women who have had a previous pregnancy affected by Down syndrome have received genetic counselling, regardless of the age at which they conceived.
- *Previous miscarriages* (see upcoming discussion). Inform all patients, if asked, that the overall incidence of miscarriage is around 15%. However, women whose last pregnancy was normal have a risk of miscarriage of only 5%, whereas women whose last pregnancy ended in miscarriage have a 20% to 25% chance of a miscarriage (Regan et al., 1989). Women with three consecutive miscarriages have a 40% chance of the next pregnancy ending in miscarriage.

- *Recurrent miscarriages.* Refer to a gynaecologist for assessment all women who have had three consecutive miscarriages. Reassure them, however, that they still have a 60% chance of a normal pregnancy and that it is common for no cause to be identified. Consider earlier referral if:
  - the woman requests it;
  - there is a family history of miscarriage or of congenital disease;
  - there is a relevant medical problem; or
  - there is an urgency to achieve a live birth, as in the older woman.

Investigations to Consider Undertaking Prior To Referral for Recurrent Miscarriage

- Pelvic ultrasound
- Luteinizing hormone (LH) on day 7
- Blood group and antibodies
- Anticardiolipin antibodies (IgM and IgG)
- Lupus anticoagulant
- Protein C, protein S, factor V Leiden
- Karyotyping of both partners (and of foetal products, if available)
- Family history or previous infant with neural tube defects:
  - All women in this category should receive folic acid prior to conception.
  - Give 5 mg daily, starting 1 month prior to stopping contraception, and continue throughout the first trimester.
  - Women should also receive advice about antenatal diagnosis (see upcoming discussion).
- Size, gestation, and maturity of previous infants:
  - *Previous baby less than 2500 g:* Stress the importance of not smoking and drinking alcohol and explain that she is at increased risk of intrauterine growth retardation. Careful symphysis–fundal measurements should be performed at each visit, ideally by the same experienced practitioner. The woman should be referred early in pregnancy for assessment by a specialist obstetrician.
  - *Large previous baby:* Check that a modified glucose tolerance test has been performed.

Medical History
Hypertension (Discussion to Come)

- This should be assessed before a woman gets pregnant, as it may be masked by the fall in blood pressure (BP) in the first half of pregnancy.
- Discuss the most appropriate drug with the relevant specialist before conception.

Diabetes (Discussion to Come)

- Explain that diabetes is associated with an increase in congenital abnormalities (about double), but that this can be decreased significantly by good control of the blood sugar prior to and during pregnancy (Nachum et al., 1999; Steel et al., 1990).

Epilepsy

- Women with epilepsy are more likely to have unplanned pregnancies due to contraceptive failure and twice as likely to have a foetal malformation.
- Not all malformations may be attributable to antiepileptic drugs (Fairgrieve et al., 2000).
  - Sodium valproate increases the risk of neural tube defects 50 times, to about 1.5%.
  - With carbamazepine, the rate is 1%.
  - There are few data on the safety of newer drugs.
  - The evidence of safety of one drug over another is limited (RCOG, 2016).
- Discuss with the neurologist:
  - whether to stop anticonvulsants in any woman who has been free of seizures for 2 years; but counsel the patient about the risks of untreated epilepsy in pregnancy. Seizures may lead to stillbirth; or
  - whether to change anticonvulsants or reduce their dose in those in whom they cannot be stopped.
- Make it clear that even on anticonvulsants there is a 90% chance of a normal outcome that prenatal diagnosis is effective in picking up neural tube defects (see upcoming discussion), and that many defects can be corrected after birth.
- Ensure that all women with epilepsy are offered:
  - *folic acid.* Those continuing antiepileptic medication should take folic acid 5 mg daily from 3 months before conception until the end of week 12. Those stopping their drugs need only take 400 µg daily from 1 month before conception;
  - an anomaly ultrasound examination at 18/19 weeks; and
  - There is insufficient evidence to recommend the maternal use of oral vitamin K to prevent haemorrhagic disease of the newborn, but all babies born to mothers using anti-epileptic medication should be offered 1 mg vitamin K IM (RCOG, 2016).
- Educate a woman's partner about what to do should she have a seizure, as epilepsy may be less predictable.

Asthma

- Asthma is one of the most common chronic medical conditions and around 5% of pregnant women will require asthma medication during pregnancy (Olesen et al., 1999).
- Asthma increases the risk of intrauterine growth restriction (IUGR) by 24% overall, and by 47% in those with severe asthma (Bracken et al., 2003).
- Women with asthma should continue on their asthma medication, including preventers, as the risk of uncontrolled asthma poses a greater risk to the fetus than continuing preventive medication (Martel et al., 2005).

Other Medication

- A decision should be taken about the need to stop other drugs that are associated with foetal abnormalities (e.g., warfarin and lithium).

- The National Institute for Heath and Care Excellence (NICE) guideline "Antenatal and Postnatal Mental Health: Clinical Management and Service Guidance" (available at www.nice.org.uk) discusses the risks associated with psychotropic medication.

Psychiatric History

Mental illness is a common indirect cause of maternal mortality. Seeking a history early in pregnancy and ensuring effective follow-up in late pregnancy and the early postnatal period is essential. See Chapter 18, *Psychiatric Problems*, for management of mental health problems during pregnancy.

Infection

- *Rubella.* All women should have rubella antibodies tested before each pregnancy; immunity can be lost between one pregnancy and the next.
- *Hepatitis B.* All women should be offered screening for hepatitis B early in pregnancy as selective screening has been shown to miss cases of hepatitis B virus (HBV) due to the time pressures of routine clinical practice.
- *Listeria.* Advise women to avoid soft cheeses, chilled ready-to-eat foods (unless thoroughly reheated), and patés prior to and during pregnancy. They should avoid contact with sheep at lambing time, and with silage. Advise women to reheat food to steaming hot and thaw frozen foods in a microwave or refrigerator. Listeriosis is rare but can occur in outbreaks.
- *Toxoplasmosis.* Women contemplating pregnancy should be warned about the risks of handling soil, cat faeces, or raw meat and of eating undercooked meat and unwashed vegetables and fruit; 80% of British women are not immune at the time of pregnancy. Routine screening is not recommended.
- *Human immunodeficiency virus (HIV).* All women should be offered screening for HIV early in pregnancy by midwives or doctors trained in pretest and post test counselling (Brocklehurst, 2000).
- *Genital herpes and warts.* Management is only an issue in the last weeks of pregnancy.

Prenatal and Antenatal Advice

Lifestyle

- *Alcohol.* Counsel the woman to reduce her alcohol consumption to a minimum (at the most 1 or 2 units once or twice a week). Complete abstinence is now recommended by the Department of Health, the British Medical Association (BMA), the Royal College of Obstetricians and Gynaecologists (RCOG), and the World Health Organisation (WHO). However, the evidence relating to the possibility of foetal damage from very low levels of alcohol intake does not provide a clear answer about the risk. A more powerful argument in favour of total abstinence is that women who drink a little in pregnancy may easily overstep the limits without realizing it (O'Brien, 2007).

- *Smoking.* Rather than asking women, "Do you smoke?" a better question is, "What best describes your smoking? Daily, Every once in a while, or I don't currently smoke?" All women who smoke should be offered a smoking cessation intervention. Advise about the risks. Provide information. Assess willingness to quit. Assist to quit using a cognitive behavioural intervention. Arrange for additional support if unsuccessful.
- *Coffee.* Heavy coffee drinking (8 or more cups a day) is associated with a tripling of the risk of stillbirth (OR 3.0 [95% CI 1.5–5.9]) (Wisborg et al., 2003). One study found that caffeine intake as low as 200 mg (2 cups of coffee or 5 cups of tea or 5 cans of caffeinated fizzy drinks) was associated with a doubling of the rate of miscarriage and that lower intakes were not without risk (Weng, Odouli, & Li, 2008). However, a Danish randomized trial failed to show any effect on birth weight or length of gestation from reducing caffeine intake, suggesting that the association of caffeine with poor outcomes may be due to one or more confounding factors (Bech et al., 2007).
- *Other drugs.* All women should be asked about their use of prescription and non-prescription drugs. Women using non-prescription drugs should be referred to the appropriate drug service for assistance in quitting.

Nutrition

- Recommend a balanced diet low in fat with adequate iron, fresh fruits, and vegetables. Avoid soft cheeses (see Listeria earlier).

Anaemia

- Check haemoglobin (Hb) in all women with a previous history or at high risk of anaemia (e.g., vegans, multiple pregnancies, and those with a short interval between pregnancies).
- Check the serum ferritin in those women who have a history of iron deficiency anaemia, even if the Hb is normal.

Vitamin D

- Evidence for the importance of vitamin D in pregnancy is conflicting but low levels may be implicated in preeclampsia, low birth weight, and impaired glucose tolerance (RCOG, 2014).
- All women should be counselled about the importance of adequate vitamin D intake during pregnancy and whilst breastfeeding.
- It is recommended that all pregnant women take 400 units of vitamin D daily and high risk women (such as those with dark skin, little sun exposure, or BMI >30) should take at least 1000 units daily.
- Deficiency should be treated over 4–6 weeks with either cholecalciferol 20,000 international units (iu) per week or ergocalciferol 10,000 iu twice weekly (RCOG, 2014).

Folic Acid

- Recommend that all women take 400 μg of folic acid a day from before conception until the end of week 12. This will prevent 95% of neural tube defects (DTB, 1994b).
- Higher dose folic acid supplementation (5 mg daily) should be offered to women who have one of the following:
  - The woman or her partner is affected by spina bifida.
  - The woman has had a previous pregnancy affected by neural tube defects.
  - Women taking epilepsy medication (see earlier).
  - The woman suffers with diabetes or coeliac disease.
  - BMI above 30.
  - Women who suffer from sickle cell disease or thalassaemia.

Vitamin A

- Advise all women to limit intake of vitamin A to 700 μg/day and not to eat liver or liver products (e.g., sausage or paté) because of their high vitamin A content. High levels of vitamin A may be teratogenic.

Exercise

- Advise women that beginning or continuing a moderate course of exercise during pregnancy is not associated with adverse outcomes.
- Inform women about sports that have a danger: contact sports, high-impact sports, and vigorous racquet sports that may involve the risk of abdominal trauma, falls, or excessive joint stress; and scuba diving, which may result in foetal birth defects and foetal decompression disease.

Sexual Intercourse in Pregnancy

- Advise women that sexual intercourse in pregnancy is not known to be associated with any adverse outcomes.

Car Travel

- Advise about the correct use of seatbelts in pregnancy:
  - Above and below the bump, not over it.
  - Use three-point seatbelts with the lap strap placed as low as possible beneath the bump, lying across the thighs with the diagonal shoulder strap above the bump lying between the breasts.
  - Adjust the fit to be as snug as comfortably possible.

Travel Overseas

- See Chapter 17 for information about overseas travel.
- For advice about immunization in pregnancy, see Appendix 19.
- *Malaria.* Pregnant women are advised to avoid travel to malarious areas. However, advice is available for those whose travel is essential: See the Health Protection Agency

document "Malaria Prevention Guidelines for Travellers from the UK" available at www.gov.uk.

Routine Antenatal Care

GUIDELINE

National Institute for Health and Care Excellence. (2008). *Antenatal care for uncomplicated pregnancies. NICE clinical guideline 62.* Updated 2017. Retrieved from www.nice.org.uk.

- The woman should be the focus of maternity care.
- Midwifery and GP-led models of maternity care are safe for low-risk women.
- Women with the following conditions may require specialist care:
  - Current medical problem (e.g., diabetes, epilepsy, hypertension)
  - Psychiatric disorder (on medication)
  - Drug use such as heroin, cocaine (including crack cocaine), and ecstasy
  - HIV or HBV infected
  - Autoimmune disorder
  - Obesity (BMI ≥35 at first contact) or underweight (BMI <18 at first contact)
  - Women who are particularly vulnerable (e.g., teenagers) or who lack social support
  - Multiple pregnancies
- Women who have experienced any of the following in previous pregnancies also need specialist care:
  - Recurrent miscarriage (three or more consecutive pregnancy losses) or a midtrimester loss
  - Severe preeclampsia, HELLP (hemolysis [H], elevated liver enzymes [EL], and low platelet count [LP]) syndrome, or eclampsia
  - Rhesus isoimmunisation or other significant blood group antibodies
  - Uterine surgery including caesarean section, myomectomy, or cone biopsy
  - Antenatal or postpartum haemorrhage on two occasions
  - Retained placenta on two occasions
  - Puerperal psychosis
  - Grand multiparity (more than six pregnancies)
  - Stillbirth or neonatal death
  - Small-for-gestational-age infant (<5th centile)
  - Large-for-gestational-age infant (>95th centile)
  - Baby weighing less than 2500 g or more than 4500 g
  - Baby with a congenital anomaly (structural or chromosomal)
- Women at risk of gestational diabetes should be offered an oral glucose tolerance test (OGTT) at 16 to 18 weeks and at 28 weeks. Those at high risk are women with a high BMI, previous gestational diabetes, a previous macrosomic baby, a family history of diabetes, and an ethnic origin with a high prevalence of diabetes.

- Risk factors for postnatal depression should be noted at this stage, to facilitate earlier detection should it occur. There is little evidence that it can be prevented by intervention in the antenatal period (NICE, 2014).
- Care providers should:
  - ensure that pregnancy care is woman-centred and that they use effective communication skills to ensure that women make informed choices about their care;
  - be aware that there is a huge amount of information presented to women during pregnancy and they should provide written information and resources in plain language;
  - ensure women are given an opportunity to discuss information at antenatal visits.
- Because of the increase in information to be processed by pregnant women, early antenatal appointments should be scheduled to allow discussion time.

Booking—Prior to 12 Weeks

- Take a full medical and obstetric history if the patient is new to the practice.
- Recommend folic acid 400 μg daily until week 12 if the patient is not already taking it.
- Assess risk and discuss the model of maternity care appropriate for the woman.
- Estimate end due date (EDD). Offer early ultrasound (10–13 weeks) to determine gestation. Offer 18- to 20-week ultrasound for structural anomalies.
- Provide information on diet and lifestyle. Routine iron supplementation is not recommended. Advise about reducing the risk of listeriosis, toxoplasmosis, and salmonellosis.
- Offer a smoking cessation programme, if a smoker.
- Check blood group and rhesus D (RhD) status.
- Offer screening for anaemia, red-cell autoantibodies, HBV, HIV, rubella, asymptomatic bacteriuria, and syphilis. Tests for sickle cell trait and thalassaemia, if at risk.
- Offer screening for Down syndrome.
- Measure BMI and BP and test urine for proteinuria.
- Assess psychosocial well-being. Ask about feelings and fears. Ask about relationships and supports. Consider asking about intimate partner violence. Ask the two screening questions for depression (see upcoming discussion) and, if the answers are positive, ask if this is something the patient would like help with (NICE, 2014).
- Offer Pertussis vaccination to protect the newborn prior to routine immunisation at 8 weeks.
- Offer influenza vaccination if the woman has not been vaccinated in the current influenza season.
- Advise women about the Healthy Start Scheme if they are under 18 years old or over 18 and in receipt of certain benefits.

Follow-Up Appointments

- Reducing the number of visits is not associated with worse outcomes, except that women may be less satisfied (Sikorski et al., 1996; Villar et al., 2001). Ten visits can provide essential care (booking, and weeks 16, 18–20, 25, 28, 31, 34, 36, 38, 40). Visits should be long enough to allow women to have concerns voiced and addressed. Some women will require more visits. Multiparous women may need as few as six visits (booking and 28, 34, 36, 38, 41 weeks).

- Current evidence does NOT support the following *as routine*:
  - Repeated maternal weighing
  - Breast examination
  - Pelvic examination
  - Antenatal screening to predict postnatal depression using Edinburgh Postnatal Depression Scale (EPDS)
  - Iron supplementation
  - Screening for cytomegalovirus (CMV), hepatitis C virus, group B streptococcus, toxoplasmosis, bacterial vaginosis, gestational diabetes mellitus
  - Formal foetal movement counting
  - Antenatal electronic cardiotocography
  - Ultrasound scanning after 24 weeks
  - Umbilical artery Doppler ultrasound scan (USS)
  - Uterine artery Doppler USS to predict preeclampsia

At Each Appointment Check

- Patient's general health and psychosocial well-being
- BP
- Symphysis–fundal height, plotted in centimeters on a chart
- Foetal movements or foetal heart sounds
- Presentation (after 34 weeks)
- Check urine for proteinuria or signs of infection.

Prenatal Diagnosis and Screening

Screening Tests

Pregnant women should be offered screening for structural anomalies and chromosomal abnormalities by appropriately trained staff. If there is a family history of another genetic disorder, the woman should be referred to a specialist service for genetic counselling.

Structural Abnormalities

- *Ultrasonography* should be offered between 18 and 20 weeks. Routine ultrasonography can detect the more obvious forms of congenital abnormality (e.g., cranial and neural tube defects, severe skeletal dysplasia, and abnormalities of the heart, chest, and abdominal organs). Hydrocephalus may be detected later. As technology and training improve, the range of anomalies detectable before birth continues to increase.
- *Fetoscopy.* Visualization of the foetus is necessary for the assessment of some external malformations. It is also used for laser treatment of twin-to-twin transfusion syndrome.

Chromosomal Abnormalities

- Women need:
  - to understand that screening is a risk assessment and not a diagnostic test;
  - to be informed that diagnostic tests are invasive and have a risk of miscarriage;
  - information about the performance of a screening test based on *their* age, as maternal age is a key component of all screening tests: younger women (<25) having screening tests will have a low screen positive rate (1%) and a 30% detection rate whilst older women (>40) will have a high screen positive rate (50%) and a 90% detection rate (Three Centres Consensus Guidelines on Antenatal Care Project, 2001);
  - to be informed that most women having a screen positive result will *not* have a pregnancy affected by Down syndrome.

Types of Screening Tests for Chromosomal Abnormalities

- A number of screening tests exist, yet availability varies between countries and centres. Check with your local maternity unit to confirm availability.
- Tests with detection rates greater than 75% and false positive rates less than 3% are:
  - *combined first trimester screening* (nuchal translucency at 11.5–14 weeks, human chorionic gonadotropin [hCG], and pregnancy-associated plasma protein A [PAPP-A] at 8–12 weeks);
  - *second trimester maternal serum screening—the quadruple test* (hCG, alpha-fetoprotein [AFP], unconjugated estriol [uE3], inhibin A) performed between 14 and 20 weeks;
  - *the integrated test* (nuchal translucency, PAPP-A + hCG, AFP, uE3, inhibin A);
  - *the serum integrated test* (PAPP-A + hCG, AFP, uE3, inhibin A) can be performed between 11 and 20 weeks.
  - Maternal blood cell-free DNA testing at 10 weeks is currently not offered on the NHS in the UK. It has a detection rate of >99% for trisomy 21 and one study has shown it would be feasible for use as a screening tool (Gil et al., 2013).
- The first, third, and fourth methods involve tests at different stages of pregnancy. A result is only reported when all tests have been performed.

Diagnostic Tests for Chromosomal Abnormalities

- *Chorionic villus biopsy (CVB).* This is usually performed after 11 weeks and allows women to consider termination of pregnancy in the first trimester, but has a miscarriage rate of 1.2%. There is also a further 1% to 2% chance of needing an amniocentesis to establish the diagnosis. CVB performed before 10 weeks may rarely cause limb abnormalities (Lilford, 1991).
- *Amniocentesis.* This is usually performed at 15 to 16 weeks, which will allow women to consider termination by 20 weeks. It is associated with a miscarriage rate of 1%. Polymerase chain reaction technology allows results for Down and Edward syndromes in 48 hours, usually backed by culture results for other chromosomal anomalies available 2 weeks later.

Problems in Pregnancy

Nausea and Vomiting

- Around 80% of pregnant women experience nausea during the first trimester and around 50% experience vomiting. These problems can vary from being minor to severe and disabling.
- Reassure the woman that most cases of nausea and vomiting settle by 20 weeks and that it does not harm the foetus.
- Consider over-the-counter or prescribed treatment if the vomiting has severe consequences on the quality of life (on day-to-day activities, including interfering with household activities, restricting interaction with children, greater use of healthcare resources, and time lost off work). Ensure that women remain adequately hydrated, avoid exhaustion, and consider the following (Jewell & Young, 2003):
  - Acupressure at P6 (seabands) and ginger may be of benefit.
  - Antihistamines (such as promethazine or cylcizine) or prochlorperazine reduce nausea and vomiting but can cause drowsiness. There is no evidence that they are teratogenic. NICE CKS advise metoclopramide or ondansetron as second line options but advise that their use should not be continued beyond 5 days.
- If associated with reflux, advise:
  - a biscuit before getting up;
  - small frequent meals;
  - a low-sodium, low-sugar antacid for heartburn;
  - stop iron, if it is making symptoms worse.
- Prescribe an H_2 receptor antagonist (e.g. ranitidine 150 mg twice a day) or a proton pump inhibitor to patients with reflux not controlled by the above measures (RCOG, 2016).
- In late pregnancy exclude urinary tract infection (UTI), preeclampsia, and surgical causes of vomiting.
- *Hyperemesis gravidarum.* Admit if the weight loss is more than 5% with ketosis. Thiamine supplementation, either orally or intravenously should be given (RCOG, 2016).

Heartburn

- Heartburn is common in pregnancy and becomes more common as the pregnancy progresses.
- Suggest lifestyle modifications (see upcoming discussion).
- Alginate antacids (e.g., Gaviscon).
- H_2 receptor antagonists or proton pump inhibitors can be used as discussed above.

Pelvic Pain

- Symphysis pubis dysfunction is a collection of signs and symptoms of discomfort and pain in the pelvic area, including pelvic pain radiating to the upper thighs and perineum. It can be debilitating.
- There is no evidence that any treatment helps, but referral to a physiotherapist and pelvic support may be of value.

Vaginal Bleeding and Miscarriage

GUIDELINE

Stillbirth and Neonatal Death Society. (2016). *Pregnancy loss and the death of a baby: Guidelines for professionals* (4th ed.). SANDS. Retrieved from www.uk-sands.org.

- *Rhesus status.* If a rhesus-negative patient bleeds, anti-D immunization is recommended. The dose depends upon the preparation used. Give it within 72 hours of the start of bleeding, although if a longer period has elapsed it may still give some protection.

Ectopic Pregnancy

- Ectopic pregnancy is usually associated with mild vaginal bleeding as well as pain. A negative pregnancy test (i.e., an hCG level <50 IU/L) virtually excludes it.
- Intrauterine pregnancies should be visible on transvaginal ultrasound when serum hCG exceeds 1000 IU/L.
- Admit any patient in whom the possibility of an ectopic is anything more than remote. It is the most common cause of death in the first trimester.

Suspected Miscarriage Up to 14 Weeks Pregnancy

GUIDANCE

National Institute for Health and Care Excellence. (2012). *Ectopic pregnancy and miscarriage: Diagnosis and initial management. NICE clinical guideline 154.* Retrieved from www.nice.org.uk.

- If provided with appropriate counselling, most women who miscarry in the first trimester will choose expectant management. About 81% of these complete their miscarriage without intervention (Luise et al., 2002).
- Assess haemodynamic stability. Admit women who are not haemodynamically stable.
- Perform a pregnancy test if pregnancy has not previously been confirmed.
- Perform an abdominal exam looking for tenderness; unilateral tenderness is suggestive of an ectopic pregnancy.
- Perform a pelvic exam for cervical motion tenderness or pelvic tenderness (suggestive of an ectopic pregnancy), provided there is no abdominal pain or tenderness. Do not palpate for adnexal masses as this may risk rupturing an ectopic pregnancy.
- If they are over 6 weeks of gestation, arrange admission to an early pregnancy assessment unit (EPAU); the urgency of admission will depend on the clinical situation.
- If they are less than 6 weeks of gestation:
  - Repeat a pregnancy test after 7 to 10 days to confirm miscarriage if bleeding stops before 6 weeks of gestation.
  - Arranged admission to the EPAU if bleeding continues beyond 6 weeks of gestation or if the patient develops signs suggestive of an ectopic pregnancy.

- If miscarriage is confirmed but not completed, then management may be expectant, medical (with vaginal or oral misoprostol), or surgical (by manual vacuum aspiration under local anaesthetic, or surgically under general anaesthetic).
- Women who have been managed medically should take a pregnancy test 3 weeks later. If it is still positive, they need to be reassessed for molar or ectopic pregnancy.
- Rhesus-negative women who have undergone surgical management should be offered anti-D rhesus prophylaxis.

Follow-Up After Miscarriage
- Arrange to meet all patients who have miscarried about 4 weeks afterwards. Be aware that the patient has suffered a bereavement, and may need counselling; 50% are still likely to feel depressed (Friedman, 1989).
- Attend to any physical issues and the possible need for contraception. The traditional advice to have two normal periods before trying to conceive again may be more important to allow time for the grieving process than for any physical reason.
- Be aware that women are distressed by the fact that no reason for the miscarriage can usually be given. Many feel unreasonable guilt and feel brushed off by being reassured that miscarriage is common (Wong et al., 2003). Explain that early miscarriage is due either to an abnormality of foetal development or to a failure of implantation.
- Explain that one miscarriage is followed by a slight or even no increase in risk of subsequent miscarriages (Everett, 1997). Investigations are unlikely to be fruitful unless three or more pregnancies have miscarried. Having three consecutive miscarriages gives a patient a subsequent risk of 40%. Referral for investigation is then traditional, but earlier referral may be justified as discussed earlier.

Suspected Miscarriage After 14 Weeks of Pregnancy

- The more advanced the pregnancy, the more advisable it is to admit the patient to hospital at the onset of bleeding, regardless if pain is present.
- After 14 weeks, painless bleeding is due to placenta praevia until proved otherwise.
- Bleeding with severe pain is likely to be due to abruptio placentae.
- Do not do a vaginal examination in these patients.

Abdominal Pain
- Abdominal pain may be due to a variety of causes, some of which are serious and may present in an atypical way. Any cause that could occur outside pregnancy (e.g., renal calculus) must be considered.
- *In the first 20 weeks*, consider:
  - miscarriage;
  - ectopic pregnancy;
  - urinary infection;
  - appendicitis;
  - impaction of a retroverted uterus;
  - red degeneration of a fibroid (the maximum incidence is 12–18 weeks, but it may occur at any time);
  - torsion of an ovary or tube;
  - haematoma of the round ligament;
  - accident to an ovarian cyst.
- *After 20 weeks*, consider, in addition:
  - labour;
  - abruptio placentae;
  - haematoma of the rectus abdominis;
  - red degeneration of a fibroid;
  - uterine rupture;
  - dehiscence of the pubic symphysis.

Infection or Contact With Infectious Disease
Rubella Contact
- If a pregnant woman is infected with rubella, the risk to the foetus is greatest up to 11 weeks but 30% of foetuses between 11 and 16 weeks are affected.
- Women experiencing infection before 16 weeks should be offered counselling regarding termination of pregnancy.
- If a pregnant woman is affected between 16 and 19 weeks, the risk of foetal damage is less than 2%. Deafness is the most likely problem.
- After 19 weeks, the risk appears very low (Jones, 1990).
- Accidental immunization in pregnancy has not been associated with embryopathy.

Rubella Contact Before 16 Weeks
If the pregnancy is less than 16 weeks, regardless of whether the woman has had rubella or the vaccination or antibodies were previously detected, do the following:
- Take blood for rubella antibodies:
  - If IgG is present and the blood was taken within 12 days of contact, inform the woman that she is immune and that there is little need to worry.
  - If IgG is present but the blood was taken more than 12 days after contact, request IgM levels. If IgM shows

recent infection, discuss the risks of foetal abnormality and the question of termination of pregnancy.

- If IgG is absent, repeat IgM 2 weeks later. If she has seroconverted, discuss the question of termination of pregnancy as mentioned. The value of immunoglobulin in protecting the foetus is doubtful.
- Any IgG-negative woman should be immunized in the puerperium.

Note: If a woman contracts rubella and decides to continue the pregnancy, foetal blood sampling (from the umbilical vein) from 20 weeks onwards can indicate whether the baby has contracted it by assessing foetal IgM.

Note: IgM can persist for up to a year after rubella. Only act on an IgM result, if it is consistent with the clinical picture or with a reliable history of exposure (Best et al., 2002).

Varicella (Chickenpox)

GUIDELINE

Royal College of Obstetricians and Gynaecologists. (2015). *Chickenpox in pregnancy.* RCOG "Green Top" clinical guideline 13. Retrieved from www.rcog.org.uk.

- A congenital varicella syndrome, including limb deformities and scarring, may occur in 1–2% of pregnancies where the mother contracts chickenpox (though not shingles) up to, but not after, 20 weeks of gestation.
- Exposure to chickenpox after 20 weeks and before 36 weeks does not appear to be associated with foetal abnormalities.
- *A woman who is not known to be immune* and who is in contact with chickenpox in the first trimester: Check her varicella antibodies urgently and give varicella zoster immune globulin (VZIG), if not immune.
- *Give acyclovir* to a pregnant woman who develops chickenpox at a gestation of over 20 weeks, starting within 24 hours of the appearance of the rash. Monitor any pregnant woman with chickenpox carefully, as 10% develop pneumonia.
- Offer an ultrasound anomaly scan to women contracting chickenpox before 20 weeks of gestation.
- If a mother contracts chickenpox in the 5 days prior to giving birth or within 2 days of giving birth, the baby should be given VZIG.

Cytomegalovirus

- CMV infection is now the most common congenital infection worldwide. The birth incidence is between 0.2–2.5%, and 10% of these infections will produce an affected neonate.
- Consequences of infection can include deafness and developmental disability; this is more common with primary infection and occurs in up to 20% of cases.
- Two-thirds of congenital infections are thought to result from primary maternal infection and one-third from recurrent infection in the mother.

- Ganciclovir is effective in the neonate but has not been proven to be of benefit, if given to the mother during pregnancy.
- Advice to a woman who seroconverts to CMV during pregnancy is difficult and such cases should be referred for tertiary centre advice.

Toxoplasmosis

- Toxoplasmosis causes fetal infection in about 15% of cases in the first trimester, rising to 70% in the third. The risk of serious fetal damage if the fetus is infected is, however, greater in early pregnancy. Overall, up to 90% of infected babies escape long-term damage. Most maternal cases are asymptomatic. The incidence of children born with definite or probable toxoplasmosis is very low.
- Where there is concern, check serology as soon as possible after conception and monthly thereafter. IgM may stay positive for months; timing infection in relation to pregnancy stage requires IgG avidity testing at the National Reference Laboratory.
- In the case of infection, the woman may be offered USS and amniocentesis to detect foetal abnormality, and foetal blood sampling between 20 and 24 weeks. Even if FBS demonstrates foetal infection, it cannot indicate whether the foetus has been damaged (Robinson, 1991). Treatment with spiramycin in pregnancy is safe but of unproven benefit.

Listeria

- Maternal infection may be asymptomatic or associated with fever. The infection carries a risk of miscarriage, stillbirth, or the birth of an infected baby.
- Symptoms in the mother are so nonspecific that the diagnosis is rarely made during the acute illness, especially since the only useful diagnostic test is blood culture.
- Women with fever for 48 hours who are pregnant and who have no obvious other source of infection should have a blood culture specifying listeria. Treatment is with intravenous ampicillin.

Group B Streptococcal Infection (RCOG, 2017)

- Group B streptococcal (GBS) is the most common severe infection in infants in the first 7 days of life.
- Routine screening for GBS is not recommended.
- If performed (e.g., in women considered at high risk), screening should be performed 3 to 5 weeks prior to the expected delivery.
- Situations in which neonatal GBS infection is more likely are:
  - neonatal GBS infection in a previous baby;
  - vaginal, urinary, or intestinal GBS present in the woman in this pregnancy;
  - preterm (<37 weeks) labour;
  - prolonged (>18 hours) rupture of membranes;
  - fever during labour (>38°C).
- Consider women at risk, as above, for intravenous antibiotics during labour, or the newborn baby for antibiotics until blood cultures show that there is no BGS present.

- Recommend to the woman the excellent leaflet available from Group B Strep Support on www.gbss.org.uk.

Hepatitis A

Reassure the mother that the infant will not be harmed although it may be infected if occurring shortly before term.

Hepatitis B

- Hepatitis B is not influenced by pregnancy, but if the mother is infected there is a risk of acute infection of the foetus or neonate.

Herpes Simplex

Genital Herpes (BASSH & RCOG, 2014)

- Primary infection at delivery gives a 20% to 50% risk of neonatal herpes, which is frequently fatal. Recurrent herpes at delivery gives a risk of 0% to 3%. Lower segment caesarean section (LSCS) is therefore only recommended if the patient is suffering her first attack during labour.
- Viral shedding is less in subsequent attacks and maternal IgG crosses the placenta to provide some foetal protection. There is little value in taking viral swabs in the last month of pregnancy in those with a history of infection but without active lesions.
- Aciclovir (400 mg three times daily) in the last month of pregnancy reduces viral shedding and vertical transmission (Braig et al., 2001).

Labial Herpes

The mother, and indeed any family or friends with labial herpes, should refrain from direct contact with the baby (i.e., kissing) once born.

Genital Warts

Respiratory papillomatosis in the child is strongly related to maternal genital warts during pregnancy. However, the risk is small (6.9 cases per 1000 live births, against a risk of 0.03 per 1000 live births with no such maternal history) and is not reduced by caesarean section (Silverberg et al., 2003).

Human Immunodeficiency Virus

- A mother who is HIV positive has a risk of foetal infection of 15% to 25%, but this can be substantially reduced by caesarean section delivery and/or antiretroviral therapy. Vaginal delivery is recommended for those with a low viral load.
- All HIV positive women should be on anti-retroviral treatment during pregnancy, either continuing their current regime or starting it once they fall pregnant (BHIVA, 2018).
- Screening should be offered to all women. Some babies will be HIV antibody positive at birth due to maternal antibody, but will become negative as maternal antibody is cleared.
- Breastfeeding doubles the chance of vertical transmission and is not recommended. If a woman must breastfeed, then exclusive breastfeeding rather than mixed feeding should be recommended as neonatal seroconversion may be greatest with the bowel inflammation secondary to artificial feeds.
- Pregnancy does not appear to hasten the onset of acquired immunodeficiency syndrome (AIDS) in women who are HIV positive.

Parvovirus B19 Infection (Fifth Disease/ Slapped Cheek Syndrome) (Morgan-Capner & Crowcroft, 2002)

- This is common in schools and nurseries, especially in April and May. If a woman is exposed in the first 20 weeks of pregnancy, there is an increased risk of intra-uterine death (excess risk 9%) and if infection occurs between 9 and 20 weeks, foetal anaemia leads to hydrops foetalis (3% of whom die [included in the excess 9%]). The consequences usually occur within 3 to 5 weeks of maternal infection.
- Maternal asymptomatic infection is as likely to damage the foetus as symptomatic infection.
- Check antibodies in all women exposed as soon as possible, informing the lab of the clinical details.
  - If specific IgG is detected and specific IgM not detected, the woman can be reassured that she has had past infection.
  - If specific IgM is detected but specific IgG is not, a further sample should be tested immediately. Refer all women who are positive to an obstetrician.
  - If specific IgG and IgM are not detected, a further sample should be tested after 1 month.

Zika Virus

- Mosquito borne illness, linked to microcephaly, especially in the first trimester.
- Advise women to avoid traveling to Zika areas until after pregnancy.
- If travel is unavoidable take strict precautions to avoid mosquito bites.
- Get specialist advice if potential infection.
- Zika is transmitted in semen. Use condoms for 28 days after return from Zika area if no symptoms and 6 months if symptomatic or infection confirmed.

Pruritis

- Pruritis, without jaundice, is the most common manifestation of obstetric cholestasis, which in turn is associated with premature birth in 60%, foetal distress in up to 33%, and intrauterine death in up to 2% (Milkiewicz et al., 2002). Although most women with pruritis in pregnancy do not have obstetric cholestasis, it should be considered in every case because of its serious implications.
- Check liver function tests (LFTs). Transaminases are raised in 60% of cases of obstetric cholestasis, though only 25% have a raised bilirubin.
- Refer all affected patients. Most obstetricians will deliver the baby at 37 weeks.

Excessive Weight Gain

- A woman's BMI should be calculated at the first booking appointment.
- The average weight gain in pregnancy is 10 to 12.5 kg (0.65 kg first quarter, 4 kg by midpregnancy, 8.5 kg by the third quarter, 12.5 kg by term). Over a quarter of the total gain is due to fat deposition in the middle two quarters of pregnancy.
- The ideal weight gain depends on the pre-pregnancy BMI. A woman with a BMI that is low or normal has fewest obstetric and neonatal adverse outcomes if her weight gain is less than 10 kg. A woman with a BMI 25 to 30 does best if her weight gain is less than 9 kg and an obese woman does best with a weight gain less than 6 kg (Cedergren, 2007). Excessive weight gain may be associated with an increased incidence of pre-eclampsia. Check BP, urine, and the presence of oedema.
- Despite the above, there is no evidence that the regular weighing of patients is of benefit and it is not recommended.
- *Obesity.* Obesity is associated with an increase in congenital malformations and first trimester abortions, gestational diabetes, hypertension, macrosomia, stillbirth, prolonged labour, and caesarean birth. All women with obesity should be seen by an obstetrician and monitored closely for weight gain, BP, and diabetes (Stotland, 2009).
- *Eating disorders* are common in pregnancy; the disorder may worsen or improve as the pregnancy progresses (Ward, 2008). Women with a recognized eating disorder should be referred to an obstetrician and the eating disorder service, early in pregnancy. Suggested screening questions at each antenatal visit:
  - What is your current eating pattern? Are you restricting your dietary intake? Do you binge? Do you vomit or take laxatives after eating?
  - How do you feel about your shape and weight?
  - What is your weight? Are you gaining weight appropriately?
  - What is your mood like? Do you feel low or anxious?
  - What exercise are you taking? Are you exercising too much?

Fundal Height

- At 22 weeks, the fundus should have reached the umbilicus, and at 32 weeks the lower rib border.
- The symphysis-to-fundus height in centimetres should be within two of the number of weeks gestation between 20 and 36 weeks; after 36 weeks it should be within ±3 cm.
- If the fundus is over 3 cm less than dates, refer for exclusion of foetal IUGR, or oligohydramnios.
- If the fundus is 3 cm more than dates, refer for assessment for possible multiple pregnancy or hydramnios.

Hypertension

- BP falls early in the first trimester as the fall in peripheral resistance exceeds the rise in cardiac output. BP reaches its nadir by 16 weeks, plateaus until 22 weeks, and then increases toward term.
- *Pregnancy-induced hypertension (PIH):* BP which rises to exceed 90 mm Hg diastolic on more than one occasion, in the second half of pregnancy, resolves after delivery and is *not* complicated by proteinuria. The International Society for the Study of Hypertension in Pregnancy has chosen this definition, rather than one based on a relative rise in diastolic pressure, because any rise in pressure varies according to when the baseline was taken and because a relative rise seems to correlate less well with outcomes than the use of an absolute cut off point.
- *Pre-eclampsia:* This is defined in the same way as above, but is associated with proteinuria of more than 300 mg/24 h. It may be further complicated by the HELLP syndrome in which there is haemolysis, elevated liver enzymes and low platelets. The terms *PIH* and *pre-eclampsia* should not be used interchangeably as the former is not associated with poor maternal or foetal outcome, whilst pre-eclampsia is a leading cause of maternal and foetal morbidity.
- *Antihypertensives* do not lessen the risk of developing pregnancy-induced hypertension or alter its progression, but protect against stroke and possibly placental abruption.
- *Aspirin* prophylaxis (75 mg daily) may prevent the development of pre-eclampsia and moderate the condition once it has started (Askie et al., 2007).
- *Measuring the BP.* Use phase 4 diastolic pressure and not phase 5, which may be misleadingly low in pregnancy (MacGillivray & Thomas, 1991).
- *Chronic hypertension* predates pregnancy or appears prior to 20 weeks of gestation. A BP of 140/90 and above before 20 weeks suggests pre-existing hypertension and needs specialist assessment.

Pre-eclampsia

GUIDELINE

National Institute of Health and Care Excellence. (2010). *Hypertension in Pregnancy: the management of hypertensive disorders during pregnancy. NICE clinical guideline 107.*

- *Women with any of the following should be referred for specialist assessment before 20 weeks of gestation:*
  - Previous pre-eclampsia
  - Multiple pregnancy
  - Underlying medical conditions:
    1. Pre-existing hypertension or booking diastolic BP 90 mm Hg or above
    2. Pre-existing renal disease or booking proteinuria (increased on more than one occasion or ≥300 mg/24 h)
    3. Pre-existing diabetes
    4. Presence of antiphospholipid antibodies
- *Women with any two or more of the following should be referred for specialist assessment before 20 weeks of gestation and offered aspirin 75 mg from 12 weeks:*

- First pregnancy
- More than 10 years since last baby
- Age more than 40 years
- BMI 35 and above
- Family history of pre-eclampsia (mother or sister)
- Multiple pregnancy

- Any woman with suspected pre-eclampsia should be managed in conjunction with specialist advice. This will usually be undertaken in a special day assessment centre.
- *Action to be taken if new hypertension is discovered after 20 weeks:*
  - BP 140/90 - 149/99: monitor blood pressure weekly and test for proteinuria at each visit.
  - BP 140/90 - 149/99 plus a symptom associated with preeclampsia: refer for same-day assessment
  - BP 140/90 - 149/99 plus proteinuria: refer for same-day assessment
  - BP 150/100 - 159/109: measure blood pressure at least twice weekly, check for proteinuria at each visit and check renal function, liver function tests (including bilirubin) and full blood count. Treat using oral labetolol as first line.
  - BP 160/110 or higher: admit to hospital.

Note: Symptoms associated with preeclampsia include headache, visual disturbance, nausea, vomiting, and epigastric pain.

Note: Management of hypertension in pregnancy as outlined above should be in conjunction with the obstetric team.

Long-Term Follow-Up *(NICE, 2010)*

- Women who have had pre-eclampsia are at higher long-term risk of cardiovascular disease (CVD) and also higher risk that the disease may occur earlier.
- Inform them that their risk of CVD when young is still low but that they should concentrate on prevention.
- Counsel all women who have had pre-eclampsia about a healthy lifestyle.
- Screen for the emergence of other risk factors for CVD at an earlier stage than usual.

Eclampsia

- This is a medical emergency with a high maternal mortality. The patient must be resuscitated and transferred to hospital as fast as possible. The anticonvulsant of choice to prevent further fits is magnesium sulphate.
- *Recurrence and follow-up:* Many women will have posttraumatic stress disorder when their normal physiological pregnancy has been taken from them. It is important to explain what happened and the relatively low chance of recurrence in future pregnancies (20%). Many units offer uterine artery Doppler as a screening test in subsequent pregnancies, with the possibility that aspirin can reduce this rate further.

Proteinuria

A trace of protein is acceptable. It may be due to contamination with vaginal secretions or to a delay since the urine was passed.

Proteinuria in the Absence of Raised Blood Pressure
(NICE, 2010)

- *One plus (+).* Arrange for a midstream urine for culture and microscopy and check the urinary spot protein to creatinine ratio. Review in 1 week. If culture and microscopy are negative but the protein to creatinine ratio is positive, check the serum creatinine, the 24-hour urinary protein or spot protein:creatinine ratio, and refer. Continue to look for preeclampsia; 10% of patients who develop eclampsia have proteinuria without a raised BP (Douglas & Redman, 1994).
- More than +. Seek specialist advice with a view to obstetric assessment.
- At least + with a symptom associated with preeclampsia. Refer for same-day assessment.

Using the Different Tests for Proteinuria
(Chappell & Shennan, 2008)

- *The protein dipstick* is prone to both false negatives and false positives. Although recommended by NICE for the routine assessment of urinary protein in antenatal care, it is the least useful of the available tests.
- *The urinary spot protein to creatinine ratio* has few false negatives and more false positives. It is therefore a good screening test (if it is negative, the patient almost certainly does not have significant proteinuria) but a more accurate test is required to confirm a positive finding. A positive result is considered to be at or above 30 mg/mmol.
- *A 24 hour-urinary protein* remains the most accurate test available, with a cutoff of 300 mg/24 h. False negatives occur when women forget to collect every sample; and different laboratories use different assays and so get different results.

Bacteriuria

- Of pregnant women, 2% to 10% have asymptomatic bacteriuria. If untreated, 30% will develop a urinary infection. Antibiotics are very effective in preventing pyelonephritis (Smaill, 2001).
- Treat with amoxicillin, cephalosporin, or nitrofurantoin according to sensitivities.
- Repeat the MSU 2 weeks after treatment.

Glycosuria

- This occurs in 70% of pregnant women.
- If there is 2+ of glucose in urine or + on two occasions, then arrange for a modified glucose tolerance test. If the sugar level is raised (fasting sugar ≥5.6 mmol/L or the 2-hour sugar ≥7.8 mmol/L), refer the patient urgently.

Gestational Diabetes

GUIDELINE

National Institute for Health and Care Excellence. (2015). *Diabetes in pregnancy: Management from preconception to the postnatal period. NICE guideline 3.* Retrieved from www.nice.org.uk.

- A patient should be managed intensively if her 2-hour sugar is over 7.6 mmol/L or her fasting glucose is over 5.6 mmol/L. For most patients, however, diet will be sufficient to control blood sugars. Active management with diet, blood glucose monitoring, and, if necessary, metformin or insulin has been shown to reduce the risk of serious perinatal complications (Crowther et al., 2005). Recheck fasting glucose 6 to 13 weeks postpartum to be sure that it has returned to normal.
- Warn the patient of her 20% to 30% chance of developing diabetes in the next 5 years. This risk can be decreased by maintenance of a diabetic diet after pregnancy.

Anaemia

- As the plasma volume increases in pregnancy, the Hb falls. Only a Hb below 11 g/dL (WHO) in the first trimester, or below 10.5 g/dL at 28 weeks, is considered to be anaemia.
- Routine iron supplementation is not recommended.
- A low serum ferritin is not a reliable guide to iron deficiency in pregnancy. It may reflect a shift of iron stores to the increased red cell mass rather than a low total body iron. However, there is no better non-invasive test.

Anaemia Developing in Pregnancy

- Check full blood count, film, and serum ferritin. Check B$_{12}$ and red cell folate if there is macrocytosis.
- Start iron in treatment doses if the Hb is below 10 g/dL or mean corpuscular value (MCV) is below 82 fL (e.g., give ferrous sulphate 200 mg three times a day and folic acid 5 mg daily). The addition of folate can almost double the rise in Hb regardless of the patient's folate status (Juarez-Vazquez, Bonizzoni, & Scotti, 2002).
- Repeat Hb in 2 weeks. It should rise by about 0.8 g/dL per week.
- If there has been no response:
  - exclude occult infection, especially urinary; and either
  - consider arranging for parenteral iron; or
  - if the serum ferritin is normal, check the serum B$_{12}$ and red cell folate (if not already checked) and continue combined iron and folate.
- If Hb remains low, seek expert advice. Consider an Hb electrophoresis regardless of the apparent ethnic origin.

Rhesus-Negative Women

- Check antibodies at booking and in primagravida at 28 and 36 weeks; in multigravida, monthly from 24 weeks. If the maternal anti-D levels are 0.5 to 10.0 IU, antibody levels are needed every 2 weeks. A level above 10 means that foetal blood sampling is needed and referral to a foetal medicine unit is indicated. If gestation allows, delivery, rather than intrauterine transfusion, may be the preferred option. It is important to realize (and explain) that subsequent pregnancies may behave similarly.

- Offer routine anti-D immunization to all Rhesus-negative women at 28 and 34 weeks, if nonsensitized, except where the patient:
  - is certain she will not have another child after the present pregnancy; or
  - is in a stable relationship with the father of the child and the father is known to be RhD negative (NICE, 2002).
- In addition to routine antenatal anti-D immunization, offer it postnatally and if a sensitizing event occurs antenatally, namely:
  - abdominal trauma including external cephalic version;
  - chorionic villus biopsy and amniocentesis;
  - antepartum haemorrhage;
  - ectopic pregnancy;
  - termination of pregnancy or endoscopic retrograde cholangiopancreatography (ERCP);
  - threatened or complete miscarriage after 12 weeks;
  - intrauterine death.
- Use 250 IU up to 20 weeks of pregnancy. Give 500 IU thereafter, followed by a Kleihauer test for foetal Hb. If the foetomaternal haemorrhage exceeds 4 mL red cells, a further dose will be needed.

Abnormal Lie

- Check the lie from 32 to 34 weeks onward. If a transverse lie is found at 32 weeks or later, then either:
  - refer; or
  - arrange a scan and reassess at 36 weeks. Refer if still transverse.

  Note: A breech presentation should be seen at the hospital by 37 to 38 weeks.

High Head

- A *high head* is one that lies completely out of the pelvis. Make sure that the bladder and rectum are empty before accepting that the head is high.
- *Primipara:* refer by 36 weeks.
- *Multipara:* refer if still high at 38 weeks.

Premature Rupture of Membranes

All women suspected of rupturing membranes should be referred for specialist assessment. After 35 weeks of gestation, the specialist is likely to recommend induction of labour. Before 35 weeks, a short inpatient stay with antibiotic cover is more likely.

Postmaturity

- If the expected date of delivery was established by USS in early pregnancy, routine induction of labour at 41 weeks reduces perinatal mortality (Crowley, 2002). Routine induction does not cause a rise in the rate of LSCS nor in lower maternal satisfaction.

- Women who have not given birth by 41 weeks should be offered a pelvic examination and membrane sweep and discussion and information about induction of labour.

Specific Medical Conditions and Pregnancy

Asthma

- Deterioration occurring during pregnancy is usually due to a reduction in therapy because of a fear that it will harm the foetus.
- Explain that poorly controlled asthma has been linked to IUGR.
- Explain that beta-sympathomimetics, inhaled steroids, and ipratropium are safe, while oral steroids and theophylline have been linked to preterm delivery.

Diabetes (Types 1 and 2)

- Optimum control of blood sugars should be achieved by the time of conception to reduce the risk of congenital malformation.
- The GP should emphasize the importance of good control throughout pregnancy, even if the majority of the management will be done by the hospital.
- Because of the higher risk of neural tube defects, women with diabetes should take 5 mg (instead of 400 µg) of folate daily before conception until the end of week 12.
- Patients should be referred to the diabetes clinic and seen 2-weekly before 28 weeks and then weekly.
- Insulin dose may need to be doubled or tripled, and will need to be reduced immediately after delivery to the pre-pregnant dose.
- Patients on oral hypoglycaemic drugs should be changed to insulin.
- Blood sugar profiles should show the majority of readings (pre-meals) below 6 mmol/L.
- Aim to keep the HbA_{1c} at 6% (42 mmol/mol) or below.
- Discontinue angiotensin converting enzyme I (ACE-I) and angiotensin receptor blockers before conception or as soon as pregnancy is confirmed. Substitute with a more suitable drug.
- Discontinue statins before pregnancy or as soon as pregnancy is confirmed.
- Women should have serial USSs to exclude macrosomia and placental insufficiency. They should have examination of the foetal heart at 18 to 20 weeks.

Thyroid Disorders

Pre-existing Thyroid Disease

- *Hypothyroidism.* Women should be advised to delay conception until thyroid function is stable on levothyroxine. Thyroid function should be checked at booking, at least once in each trimester, and after any dose changes. Thyroxine requirements may increase during pregnancy. Liaise with an endocrinologist as soon as the patient falls pregnant with regards to changes in thyroxine doses.
- *Hyperthyroidism.* Refer all pregnant women with hyperthyroidism to an endocrinologist as soon as they present. It is important that they remain euthyroid throughout the pregnancy. Propylthiouracil is the preferred drug during pregnancy, given at the lowest effective dose to reduce the risk of foetal hypothyroidism and goitre (Marx, Amin, & Lazarus, 2008).

Postpartum Thyroiditis

- Up to 10% of women develop transient autoimmune thyroiditis after delivery. This is usually between 1 and 3 months and may present with features of hyperthyroidism, but more commonly with those of hypothyroidism (i.e., fatigue and lethargy), at a time when she is understandably tired anyway. Thyroxine is necessary for 6 months, followed by repeat TFTs. Antithyroid drugs are not usually needed for the hyperthyroid state, but beta-blockers may be given to control symptoms.
- Follow the patient with yearly TFTs. Up to 20% develop hypothyroidism in the subsequent 4 years (DTB, 1995).

Epilepsy

- 20% of patients have an increase of fits during pregnancy due either to poor compliance or to a fall in serum levels because of the physiological changes of pregnancy. Fits are more common when tired.
- Do not stop anticonvulsants or reduce their dose if a woman presents already pregnant. Any teratogenic effect will have already occurred. Liaise with her neurologist to plan the rest of the pregnancy. In general, it is not necessary to monitor serum levels of anticonvulsant in pregnancy, but be guided by the clinical condition, and only increase the dose of a drug if the frequency of fits increases.
- Encourage the patient to take her treatment correctly. Poor compliance is the main reason for fits in pregnancy.
- Ensure that an anomaly ultrasound is performed at 18 to 19 weeks.
- Recommend folic acid 5 mg daily to all epileptic women until the end of week 12. This is particularly important in patients taking sodium valproate or carbamazepine or who have a history of a previous baby with a neural tube defect.
- Reassure women that the majority have a normal delivery and that epilepsy is not an indication for elective caesarean section.

Inflammatory Bowel Disease
(Fergusson, Mahsu-Dornan, & Patterson, 2008)

- Inflammatory bowel disease (IBD) is not worsened by pregnancy and may improve. If the disease is quiescent at the time of conception, it remains so in two-thirds of patients. If the disease is active, two-thirds of patients will have ongoing active disease.
- Women with inactive disease have no increased risk of an adverse outcome. Women with active disease have up

to a 35% miscarriage rate. Crohn's disease has an increased risk of low birth weight, preterm delivery, and adverse perinatal outcome.

- Assessment of IBD in pregnancy is based on clinical factors (e.g., abdominal pain, stool frequency, and bleeding). Pregnancy affects Hb concentration, erythrocyte sedimentation rate (ESR), and serum albumin. C-reactive protein is not altered by pregnancy.
- Reassure the woman that it is most important to achieve the best control of the disease possible and that this seems to give the best outcome. All women should be seen urgently by the gastroenterology and obstetric team.
- For the safety of commonly used drugs for inflammatory bowel disease, see Caprilli et al. (2006).

Depression

> ### GUIDELINE
>
> O'Keane, V., & Marsh, M. S. (2007). Depression during pregnancy. *BMJ (Clinical Research Ed.), 334*, 1003–1005. National Institute for Health and Care Excellence. (2014). *Antenatal and postnatal mental health: Clinical management and service guidance. NICE clinical guideline 45.* Retrieved from www.nice.org.uk.

- Rates of depression are higher during pregnancy than at any other point in a woman's life.
- About half of postnatal depression starts during pregnancy.
- Two-thirds of women with recurrent depression will relapse during pregnancy if they stop their antidepressants after conception.
- Depression during pregnancy is associated with poorer outcomes, especially preterm delivery.
- Women depressed during pregnancy are more likely to drink alcohol and smoke and less likely to attend antenatal appointments.
- For a discussion about drug treatment for depression during pregnancy see Chapter 18, *Psychiatric Problems*.

Drug Misuse

- Liaise with local substance misuse services.
- *Amphetamines and cocaine:* stop the drugs immediately.
- *Benzodiazepines:* withdraw over 4 weeks.
- *Barbiturates:* arrange admission. If there is any delay, maintain the patient on phenobarbital.
- *Opiates:* arrange an urgent outpatient appointment. Maintain the patient on oral methadone meanwhile.

Postnatal Care

Mother

- *Examine* fundal height, perineum, lochia, and breasts.
- *Feeding.* If necessary, reinforce the midwife's advice on breastfeeding (see upcoming discussion).

- *Contraception.* Hormonal methods should not be started before 4 weeks or before bleeding has stopped.
- *Rest.* Stress the need for rest in the first week, but the mother should also be encouraged to mobilize gently as soon as possible to prevent deep vein thrombosis (DVT).
- *Pelvic exercises.* Urge the patient to perform pelvic exercises from the first day.
- Warn the patient that she will inevitably receive conflicting advice from professionals, family, and friends. Parents need to develop their own solutions.
- *Depression.* Ensure there is time to talk about her emotional well-being.

Baby

- Examine the baby, unless this has already been done in hospital.
- Vitamin K. If it has not already been given intramuscularly, give it orally according to local guidelines. If the baby is breastfed, it will need to be repeated at 1 and 4 weeks.
- Registration. Encourage early registration of the baby with the registrar; the start of Child Allowance is dependent on this. Register the baby with the practice.

At 6 Weeks

- Does she have any outstanding questions about what happened during labour or birth?
- Is she getting enough sleep? Who is sharing in the work of caring for the baby? How is she feeling in herself? Is she feeling depressed? How is she getting along with her partner (if she has one)? Is she getting any time away from the baby?
- Ask about pain in her breasts, back, perineum.
- Ask about urinary and faecal incontinence, haemorrhoids, constipation.
- Ask about sex. Around 90% of women will report having sex by 10 weeks postpartum, while 2% report not attempting sex by 1 year (Glazener, 1997). An explanation that libido is often low in the first year may relieve a couple who are finding that this is the case.
- Perform a vaginal examination only if symptoms dictate or if a smear is due.
- Offer contraceptive advice.
- *Prevention of sudden infant death syndrome.* Reinforce the importance of:
  - the sleeping position (on the back);
  - not smoking;
  - not giving the baby a duvet.

Breastfeeding
Advantages of Breastfeeding

- *Advantages for the baby:* less infection, less chance of atopy or diabetes, better bonding.
- *Advantages for the mother:* a lower risk of breast and ovarian cancer, weight loss, and less postpartum bleeding. It is also cheaper.

Problems With Breastfeeding

The majority of problems centre round the infant's attempts to remove milk. The baby needs to be in a comfortable position to allow jaw and tongue to drain the milk ducts under the areola.

- Check that mother and baby are managing the following:
  - Baby's chest against the mother's chest, with baby's chin to the breast
  - Mouth wide open
  - Both lips curled back
  - Lower lip at the junction of the areola and breast
  - Rhythmic movements of jaw muscles

Sore Nipples

> **GUIDANCE**
>
> The Breastfeeding Network. (2009). *Differential diagnosis of nipple pain.* Retrieved from www.breastfeedingnetwork.org.uk.

- These are usually due to the baby's tongue rubbing the nipple rather than the areola.
- Check that the nipple is positioned in an upward direction toward the roof of the baby's mouth.
- Allow breast milk to dry on the nipple when not feeding or, if the skin is broken, use white soft paraffin.

Skin Infection

> **GUIDANCE FOR PATIENTS AND HEALTH PROFESSIONALS**
>
> The Breastfeeding Network. (2009). *Thrush and breastfeeding.* Retrieved from www.breastfeedingnetwork.org.uk.

- This may be due to candida infection and may present as localized soreness, as pain around the areola and nipple, or as pain in the breast after a feed.
- Treat the mother with miconazole cream and the baby with miconazole oral gel, whether the baby has signs of infection or not. It is unnecessary for the mother to remove the cream before feeding.
- Consider using oral fluconazole if local treatment alone is not working. This use is not licensed but WHO recognizes fluconazole as compatible with breastfeeding. Download the leaflet "Thrush and Breastfeeding" for guidance on dosing. The unlicensed use must be discussed with the mother and documented.

Blocked Duct

- This presents as a hard lump anywhere in the breast.
- Get the mother to massage the breast while feeding the baby from that breast.
- The baby's position should be altered so that the lower lip is nearer the blocked duct.

Breast Engorgement

- The pain of engorgement is one of the most common reasons for stopping breastfeeding in the first 2 weeks. Treatment is disappointing with cabbage leaves, ultrasound, and cold packs being no better than placebo (Snowden, Renfrew, & Woolridge, 2001).
- Give simple analgesia and support.
- Attempt to prevent engorgement by removing any obstacles to easy breastfeeding.

Mastitis

- Early mastitis is inflammatory, not infectious, and may respond to effective emptying of the breast plus a nonsteroidal antiinflammatory drug (NSAID).
- Reassess the feeding position of the baby to ensure that milk is removed completely.
- Prescribe an NSAID.
- Treat with flucloxacillin for 10 to 14 days if the patient is unwell, febrile, or there is any suspicion of abscess formation. Use erythromycin if the patient is allergic to penicillin. Warn mothers that the milk will change in taste and feeding may be harder initially, or that the baby may develop diarrhoea and need to feed more frequently.
- Consider admission for any woman who is systemically unwell with mastitis.
- *Breast abscess.* If an abscess forms which is large enough to need draining, admit the patient for incision and drainage.

Suppression of Lactation

This usually takes 4 to 5 days after stopping breastfeeding. It may be very painful and require analgesia and a supportive bra. It is usually not necessary to use drugs. However, after stillbirth, or if there is another good reason to stop lactation, use bromocriptine 2.5 mg at night for 2 nights, then 2.5 mg twice a day for 3 weeks. If used for a shorter period, a number of patients relapse.

Vaginal Bleeding After 24 Hours

- The traditional management of excessive bleeding more than 24 hours after delivery (secondary postpartum haemorrhage [PPH]) is surgical. However, ERCP yields placental tissue in less than 30% of these cases and so the majority of patients do not benefit.
- *Mild bleeding.* Give:
  - ergometrine 0.5 mg intramuscularly, then 0.5 mg three times a day orally for 4 days; and
  - antibiotics (e.g., amoxicillin/erythromycin ± metronidazole for 5 days).
- *Severe bleeding,* or if the os still admits one finger after 7 days: admit. Admit more readily if there is no one at home to look after the patient, if she is already anaemic, febrile, or otherwise unwell.

Fever

- *Endometritis.* Patients with fever, pain, and foul-smelling lochia are likely to need admission, but early cases could be treated at home with amoxicillin/erythromycin and metronidazole.
- Be aware that DVT and UTI can cause fever without localized symptoms.

Depression

- Depression after birth is experienced by one in seven women in the year after childbirth. It is distinct from the transient blues of the first 10 days and from a puerperal psychosis, which is likely to need admission.
- For a discussion of the management of postnatal depression please see Chapter 18, *Psychiatric Problems.*

Management of Postnatal Depression

- Antenatal and postnatal interventions offered routinely to all women in an effort to prevent postnatal depression have been ineffective (Lumley, Austin, & Mitchell, 2004) apart from the IMPACT programme consisting of a redesigned community midwifery model of care (MacArthur et al., 2002).
- Antenatal and postnatal interventions offered only to those women perceived to be at a higher risk of developing depression have been ineffective (Lumley et al., 2004).
- Interventions offered to women identified as experiencing depression have been effective and there is strong evidence that postnatal counselling (from active listening to cognitive behavioural therapy) will reduce depression with a number needed to treat of two to three (Lumley et al., 2004). Simple nondirective counselling by health visitors, weekly for 8 weeks, doubles the recovery rate (Holden, Sagovsky, & Cox, 1989).
- Check for physical health problems. Women experiencing the common postnatal physical problems are more likely to be depressed. Ask about:
  - tiredness. Consider checking Hb and ferritin, and TFTs;
  - backache;
  - sexual problems;
  - perineal pain;
  - mastitis and feeding problems;
  - urinary and faecal incontinence;
  - constipation and haemorrhoids.
- *Offer counselling/psychotherapy.* Cognitive behavioural therapy is as effective as fluoxetine in reducing postnatal depression. The choice of treatment can be made by the woman herself (Appleby, Warner, Whitton, & Faragher, 1997).
- *Offer an antidepressant* to the 3% to 5% of women whose depression is moderate or severe (Oates, 2003) and for whom an effective form of counselling/psychotherapy is not immediately available, or who chooses an antidepressant. An SSRI is recommended. If she is breastfeeding, the choice is between an SSRI which is present in breast milk at low levels (e.g., sertraline but not fluoxetine or citalopram) and a TCA which, with the exception of doxepin, appears safe in lactation (Spigset & Martensson, 1999). Prescribing antidepressants for a lactating woman is a case-specific, risk-benefit decision (Wisner, Perel, & Findling, 1996).
- Consider referral if a multidisciplinary mental health team is able to offer more than the primary healthcare team. Ideally, if the woman requires admission, this should be to a mother and baby facility.
- Refer urgently, to be seen within 24 hours, any woman with ideas of suicide or of harming the baby.

PATIENT INFORMATION AND SUPPORT

Association for Postnatal Illness, 145 Dawes Road, London SW6 EB, helpline 020 7386 0868, www.apni.org.

Exhaustion

- Around 70% of women will experience extreme tiredness and exhaustion in the 6 months after giving birth (Watson et al., 1984).
- Tiredness is common, even among women who are not depressed. It is uncommon to find a specific cause, but anaemia, iron deficiency, and thyroid problems should be considered.
- Lack of sleep is one of the most common causes. Taking note of the baby's sleep patterns, excluding depression, offering time to talk, encouraging time-out from childcare, and encouraging sharing the work of looking after the baby are all simple support strategies.

Common Physical Problems

- Physical problems are common: around 44% of women will experience backache, 26% sexual problems, 21% haemorrhoids, 21% perineal pain, 17% mastitis, 13% bowel problems, 11% urinary incontinence, 6% faecal incontinence (Brown & Lumley, 1998; MacArthur, Bick, & Keighley, 1997).
- Unfortunately, there is little evidence to guide our management of postpartum incontinence or perineal pain. Three quarters of women with urinary incontinence at 3 months postpartum still had the problem 6 years later, despite conservative nurse-led pelvic floor and bladder training management of urinary and faecal incontinence (Glazener et al., 2005).

Neonatal Jaundice

- *Jaundice within 24 hours of birth:* admit.
- *Deep jaundice developing after 24 hours:*
  - Admit if the baby is unwell or is at risk because of prematurity, small for dates, or birth asphyxia.

- Otherwise arrange for a serum bilirubin. If the level is 290 mol/L or above, discuss with the paediatric team.
- *Jaundice still present at 2 weeks:* test the urine for bilirubin and the serum for conjugated bilirubin. If either is positive, admit. The baby may have biliary atresia. The earlier surgery is performed, the more successful it is likely to be (Mackinlay, 1993).
- *Admit if jaundice is associated with any of the following:*
  - Pale fatty stools
  - Dark yellow urine
  - Failure to thrive
  - Poor feeding
  - Tendency to bleed or bruise
  - Enlarged liver or spleen, or ascites

References

Appleby, L., Warner, R., Whitton, A., & Faragher, B. (1997). A controlled study of fluoxetine and cognitive-behavioural counselling in the treatment of postnatal depression. *British Medical Journal, 314*, 932–936.

Askie, L. M., Duley, L., Henderson-Smart, D. J., et al. (2007). Antiplatelet agents for prevention of pre-eclampsia: A meta-analysis of individual patient data. *Lancet, 369*, 1791–1798.

Bech, B. H., Obel, C., Henriksen, T. B., et al. (2007). Effect of reducing caffeine intake on birth weight and length of gestation: Randomised controlled trial. *British Medical Journal (Clinical Research Ed.), 334*, 409–412.

Best, J. B., O'Shea, S., Tipples, G., et al. (2002). Interpretation of rubella serology in pregnancy—pitfalls and problems. *British Medical Journal (Clinical Research Ed.), 325*, 147–148.

Bracken, M. B., Triche, E. W., Belanger, K., et al. (2003). Asthma symptoms, severity, and drug therapy: A prospective study of effects on 2205 pregnancies. *Obstetrics and Gynecology, 102*, 739–752.

Braig, S., Luton, D., Sibony, O., et al. (2001). Acyclovir prophylaxis in late pregnancy prevents recurrence of genital herpes and viral shedding. *European Journal of Obstetrics, Gynecology, and Reproductive Biology, 96*, 55–58.

British Association for Sexual Health and HIV and Royal College of Obstetricians and Gynaecologists. (2014). *Management of genital herpes in pregnancy.* Retrieved from www.rcog.org.uk/good_practice/clinical_green_top_guidelines.

British HIV Association. (2018). *Guidelines for the Management of HIV in Pregnancy and Postpartum 2018.*

Brocklehurst, P. (2000). Interventions aimed at decreasing the risk of mother-to-child transmission of HIV infection. *Cochrane Database of Systematic Reviews, (2)*, CD000102. Retrieved from www.nelh.nhs.uk/cochrane.asp.

Brown, S., & Lumley, J. (1998). Maternal health after childbirth: Results of an Australian population based survey. *British Journal of Obstetrics and Gynaecology, 105*, 156–161.

Caprilli, R., Gassull, M. A., Escher, J. C., et al. (2006). European evidence based consensus on the diagnosis and management of Crohn's disease: Special situations. *Gut, 55*(1), i36–i58.

Cedergren, M. I. (2007). Optimal gestational weight gain for body mass index categories. *Obstetrics and Gynecology, 110*, 759–776.

Chappell, L. C., & Shennan, A. H. (2008). Assessment of proteinuria in pregnancy. *British Medical Journal (Clinical Research Ed.), 336*, 968–969.

Crowley, P. (2002). Interventions for preventing or improving the outcome of delivery at or beyond term (Cochrane review). In *The Cochrane Library* (Issue 1). Oxford: Update Software. Retrieved from www.nelh.nhs.uk/cochrane.asp.

Crowther, C. A., Hiller, J. E., Moss, J. R., et al. (2005). Effect of treatment of gestational diabetes mellitus on pregnancy outcomes. *The New England Journal of Medicine, 352*, 2477–2486.

Douglas, K. A., & Redman, C. W. G. (1994). Eclampsia in the United Kingdom. *British Medical Journal (Clinical Research Ed.), 309*, 1395–1400.

Drug Therapy Bulletin. (1994b). Folic acid to prevent neural tube defects. *Drug and Therapeutics Bulletin, 32*, 31–32.

Drug Therapy Bulletin. (1995). The practical management of thyroid disease in pregnancy. *Drug and Therapeutics Bulletin, 33*, 75–77.

Everett, C. (1997). Incidence and outcome of bleeding before the 20th week of pregnancy: Prospective study from general practice. *British Medical Journal (Clinical Research Ed.), 315*, 32–34.

Fairgrieve, S., Jackson, M., Jonas, P., et al. (2000). Population based, prospective study of the care of women with epilepsy in pregnancy. *British Medical Journal (Clinical Research Ed.), 321*, 674–675.

Fergusson, C. B., Mahsu-Dornan, S., & Patterson, R. N. (2008). Inflammatory disease in pregnancy. *British Medical Journal (Clinical Research Ed.), 337*, 170–173.

Friedman, T. (1989). Women's experiences of general practitioners' management of miscarriage. *The Journal of the Royal College of General Practitioners, 39*, 456–458.

Gil, M. M., Quezada, M. S., Bregant, B., Ferraro, M., & Nicolaides, K. H. (2013). Implementation of maternal blood cell-free DNA testing in early screening for aneuploidies. *Ultrasound in Obstetrics and Gynecology, 42*, 34–40. doi:10.1002/uog.12504.

Glazener, C. (1997). Sexual function after childbirth: Woman's experiences, persistent morbidity and lack of professional recognition. *British Journal of Obstetrics and Gynaecology, 104*, 330–335.

Glazener, C., Herbison, P., MacArthur, C., et al. (2005). Randomised controlled trial of conservative management of postnatal urinary and faecal incontinence: Six year follow up. *British Medical Journal (Clinical Research Ed.)*, doi:10.1136/bmj.38320.613461.82.

Harris, R., Lane, B., Harris, H., et al. (1999). National confidential enquiry into counselling for genetic disorders by non-geneticists: General recommendations and specific standards for improving care. *British Journal of Obstetrics and Gynaecology, 106*, 658–663.

Holden, J. M., Sagovsky, R., & Cox, J. L. (1989). Counselling in a general practice setting: Controlled study of health visitor intervention in treatment of postnatal depression. *British Medical Journal (Clinical Research Ed.), 298*, 223–226.

Inskip, H. M., Crozier, S. R., Godfrey, K. M., et al. (2009). The Southampton Women's Survey Study Group. Women's compliance with nutrition and lifestyle recommendations before pregnancy: General population cohort study. *British Medical Journal (Clinical Research Ed.), 338*, b481.

Jewell, D., & Young, G. (2003). Interventions for nausea and vomiting in early pregnancy. *Cochrane Database of Systematic Reviews, (4)*, CD000145, doi:10.1002/14651858.CD000145.

Jones, G. (1990). Congenital rubella in great britain. *Health Trends, 22*, 73–76.

Juarez-Vazquez, J., Bonizzoni, E., & Scotti, A. (2002). Iron plus folate is more effective than iron alone in the treatment of iron deficiency anaemia in pregnancy: A randomised, double blind clinical trial. *BJOG: An International Journal of Obstetrics and Gynaecology, 109*, 1009–1014.

Lilford, R. J. (1991). The rise and fall of chorionic villus sampling. *British Medical Journal (Clinical Research Ed.), 303*, 936–937.

Luise, C., Jermy, K., May, C., et al. (2002). Outcome of expectant management of spontaneous first trimester miscarriage: Observational study. *British Medical Journal (Clinical Research Ed.), 324*, 873–875.

Lumley, J., Austin, M. P., & Mitchell, C. (2004). Intervening to reduce depression after birth: A systematic review of the randomized trials. *International Journal of Technology Assessment in Health Care, 20*, 128–144.

MacArthur, C., Bick, D., & Keighley, M. R. (1997). Faecal incontinence after childbirth. *British Journal of Obstetrics and Gynaecology, 104*, 46–50.

MacArthur, C., Winter, H., Bick, D., et al. (2002). Effects of redesigned community postnatal care on women's health 4 months after birth: A cluster randomised trial. *Lancet, 359*, 378–385.

MacGillivray, I., & Thomas, P. (1991). Recording diastolic blood pressure in pregnancy (letter). *British Medical Journal (Clinical Research Ed.), 302*, 179.

Mackinlay, G. A. (1993). Jaundice persisting beyond 14 days after birth. *British Medical Journal (Clinical Research Ed.), 306*, 1426–1427.

Martel, M. J., Rey, E., Beauchesne, M. F., et al. (2005). Use of inhaled corticosteroids during pregnancy and risk of pregnancy induced hypertension: Nested case-control study. *British Medical Journal (Clinical Research Ed.), 330*, 230.

Marx, H., Amin, P., & Lazarus, J. H. (2008). Hyperthyroidism and pregnancy. *British Medical Journal (Clinical Research Ed.), 336*, 663–667.

Milkiewicz, P., Elias, E., Williamson, C., et al. (2002). Obstetric cholestasis. *British Medical Journal (Clinical Research Ed.), 324*, 123–124.

Morgan-Capner, P., & Crowcroft, N. S. (2002). *On behalf of the PHLS Joint Working Party of the Advisory Committees of Virology and Vaccines and Immunisation Guidelines on the management of, and exposure to, rash illness in pregnancy (including consideration of relevant antibody screening programmes in pregnancy)*. Retrieved from www.hpa.org.uk.

Nachum, Z., Ben-Shlomo, I., Weiner, E., et al. (1999). Twice daily versus four times daily insulin dose regimens for diabetes in pregnancy: Randomised controlled trial. *British Medical Journal (Clinical Research Ed.), 319*, 1223–1227.

National Institute for Health and Care Excellence (2002). *Guidance on the use of routine antenatal anti-D prophylaxis for RhD-negative women*. Retrieved from www.nice.org.uk.

National Institute for Health and Care Excellence (2014). *Antenatal and postnatal mental health: Clinical management and service guidance. NICE clinical guideline 45*. Retrieved from www.nice.org.uk.

National Institute for Health and Care Excellence. (2014). *Antenatal and Postnatal mental health: Clinical Management and Service Guidance. NICE clinical guideline 192*. Updated 2018.

Oates, M. (2003). Postnatal depression and screening: Too broad a sweep? *The British Journal of General Practice, 53*, 596–597.

O'Brien, P. (2007). Head to Head: Is it all right for women to drink small amounts of alcohol in pregnancy? Yes. *British Medical Journal (Clinical Research Ed.), 335*, 856.

Olesen, C., Steffensen, F. H., Nielsen, G. L., et al. (1999). Drug use in first pregnancy and lactation: A population-based survey among Danish women. The EUROMAP group. *European Journal of Clinical Pharmacology, 55*, 139–144.

Regan, L., Braude, P. R., Trembath, P. L., et al. (1989). Influence of past reproductive performance on risk of spontaneous abortion. *British Medical Journal (Clinical Research Ed.), 299*, 541–545.

Robinson, R. (1991). Surveying rare diseases of childhood. *British Medical Journal (Clinical Research Ed.), 303*, 1091.

Royal College of Obstetricians and Gynaecologists. (2014). *Vitamin D in Pregnancy: Scientific Impact Paper No. 43*.

Royal College of Obstetricians and Gynaecologists. (2016). *Epilepsy in Pregnancy. Green Top Guideline No. 68*.

Royal College of Obstetricians and Gynaecologists. (2016). *The Management of Nausea and Vomiting of Pregnancy and Hyperemesis Gravidarum. Green Top Guideline No.69*.

Royal College of Obstetricians and Gynaecologists (2017). *Prevention of early onset neonatal Group B streptococcal disease. RCOG "Green Top" guideline 36*. Retrieved from www.rcog.org.uk/good_practice/clinical_green_top_guidelines.

Rush, D. (1994). Periconceptional folate and neural tube defect. *The American Journal of Clinical Nutrition, 59*(2), S511–S515.

Sikorski, J., Wilson, J., Clement, S., et al. (1996). A randomised controlled trial comparing two schedules of antenatal visits: The antenatal care project. *British Medical Journal (Clinical Research Ed.), 312*, 546–553.

Silverberg, M. J., Thorsen, P., Lindeberg, H., et al. (2003). Condyloma in pregnancy is strongly predictive of juvenile-onset recurrent respiratory papillomatosis. *Obstetrics and Gynecology, 101*, 645–652.

Smaill, F. (2001). Antibiotics for asymptomatic bacteriuria in pregnancy (Cochrane review). In *The Cochrane Library* (Issue 4). Oxford: Update Software. Retrieved from www.nelh.nhs.uk/cochrane.asp.

Snowden, H. M., Renfrew, M. J., & Woolridge, M. W. (2001). Treatments for breast engorgement during lactation (Cochrane review). In *The Cochrane Library* (Issue 4). Oxford: Update Software. Retrieved from www.nelh.nhs.uk/cochrane.asp.

Spigset, O., & Martensson, B. (1999). Fortnightly review: Drug treatment of depression. *British Medical Journal (Clinical Research Ed.), 318*, 1188–1191.

Steel, J. M., Johnstone, F. D., Hepburn, D. A., et al. (1990). Can prepregnancy care of diabetic women reduce the risk of abnormal babies? *British Medical Journal (Clinical Research Ed.), 301*, 1070–1074.

Stotland, N. E. (2009). Obesity and pregnancy. *British Medical Journal (Clinical Research Ed.), 338*, 107–110.

Three Centres Consensus Guidelines on Antenatal Care Project (2001). *Melbourne: Mercy Hospital for Women, southern health*. Melbourne, Australia: Women's and Children's Health.

Villar, J., Carroli, G., Khan-Neelofur, D., et al. (2001). Patterns of antenatal care for low-risk pregnancy (Cochrane review). In *The Cochrane Library* (Issue 4). Oxford: Update Software. Retrieved from www.nelh.nhs.uk/cochrane.asp.

Ward, V. B. (2008). Eating disorders in pregnancy. *British Medical Journal (Clinical Research Ed.), 336*, 96.

Watson, J., Elliot, S., Rugg, A. J., & Brough, D. (1984). Psychiatric disorder in pregnancy and the first postnatal year. *The British Journal of Psychiatry: The Journal of Mental Science, 144*, 453–462.

Weng, X., Odouli, R., & Li, D. K. (2008). Maternal caffeine consumption during pregnancy and the risk of miscarriage: A prospective cohort study. *American Journal of Obstetrics and Gynecology, 279*, e1–e8.

Wisborg, K., Kesmodel, U., Bech, B. H., et al. (2003). Maternal consumption of coffee during pregnancy and stillbirth and infant death in first year of life: Prospective study. *British Medical Journal (Clinical Research Ed.), 326*, 420–422.

Wisner, K., Perel, J., & Findling, R. L. (1996). Antidepressant treatment during breast-feeding. *The American Journal of Psychiatry, 153*, 1132–1137.

Wong, M. K. Y., Crawford, T. J., Gask, L., et al. (2003). A qualitative investigation into women's experiences after a miscarriage: Implications for a primary healthcare team. *The British Journal of General Practice, 53*, 697–702.

15

Older People's Health

IAN REEVES

CHAPTER CONTENTS

Keeping Older People Healthy

Screening and Prevention

- In general, cancer screening programmes continue until older age. There is little evidence that screening is no longer worthwhile as people age and most programmes recommend continuing to age 75 years, although in the United Kingdom some *routine* screening ends at 65. However, the benefits and risks of screening older adults should be assessed on an individual basis, taking into account the patient's estimated remaining life expectancy, comorbidities, and the action to be taken as a result of any screening results.
- If older people can tolerate their medication, then treating those with high blood pressure and high cholesterol will prolong life expectancy and reduce the risk of heart disease and stroke. The decision to initiate in older adults, and particularly those 80 years and older, should be individualized based on comorbidities and recognition of problems that may arise from polypharmacy in this population (Gueyffier et al., 1993).
- Influenza and pneumococcal vaccination are recommended in the United Kingdom and elsewhere for all persons aged 65 years and over. More than 90% of deaths from influenza are in the over-60 age group (Nichol et al., 1994).
- Herpes zoster vaccination is also now offered to those aged 70 with a catchup programme for those aged 70 to 79, based on the evidence of cost effectiveness and as this age group is likely to have the greatest benefit from vaccination (Oxman et al., 2005).

Smoking

- Advise smoking cessation for all older people. Stopping reduces mortality by 50%, regardless of the age at which a person stops. Nicotine replacement has not been specifically studied in older adults but can be used (Curb et al., 1996). Simple advice from primary care doctors is effective in smoking cessation (Abdullah & Simon, 2006).

Alcohol

- Although alcohol consumption decreases with age, 17% of men and 7% of older women exceed safe limits; 1% to 5% of older people who drink more than occasionally report that they are "problem drinkers," males more so than females (Department of Health and Social Security [DHSS], 1994).
- Simple advice from the general practitioner (GP) may be effective in reducing alcohol consumption (Anderson, 1993).
- Using brief interventions could reduce excessive drinking but there still appears to be a gap between actual practice and potential for preventive work relating to alcohol problems: Primary care doctors report little specific training and a lack of support (Wilson et al., 2011).

The National Institute for Health and Care Excellence (NICE) has specific guidance on the prevention of disease and frailty in later life as a result of excessive alcohol consumption.

Exercise

- Sustained low-level activity (e.g., walking) for 30 to 60 minutes on at least 3 days per week (Manley, 1996) will result in moderate health benefits such as reduced fatigue, weight loss, increased socialization, improved control of type 2 diabetes, and less shortness of breath on exertion (Rooney, 1993).
- Older people who exercise develop disability at a quarter of the rate of those who do not, even though the exercisers have a higher rate of fractures and resultant short-term disability. Even the very old benefit from exercise because of improvements in muscle strength, gait velocity, and the ability to climb stairs (Elon, 1996).
- Advise regular, safe, physical activity as part of daily activities. Simple advice delivered in primary care is effective in increasing activity for older patients (Elley et al., 2003; Kerse et al., 1999).
- Recommend exercise that mimics the activities of daily living (ADLs) such as repetitive sit to stand and walking. This type of exercise is more acceptable and more beneficial for older people.
- Referral to physiotherapy for specific strength and balance training will reduce falls by 40% in women over age 80 years (Campbell et al., 1997).
- Participation in group-based tai chi chuan for older people is associated with better fitness outcomes, including improvements in maximal oxygen uptake (VO_2 max), muscular strength and flexibility, and a reduced risk of falls.

Nutrition

- The National Diet and Nutrition Survey (1989–2016) in the United Kingdom indicated that in those over the age of 65:
  - average intake of vitamins and minerals was above recommended levels except for some in residential and nursing homes;
  - vitamin D status was poor in some, particularly those in residential and nursing homes;
  - poor oral health, especially a lack of natural teeth, was associated with poor diet and nutritional status;
  - average intake of sugars and saturated fatty acids exceeded recommended levels;
  - average fibre intake was lower than recommended;
  - the diet of older adults is generally better than younger peers.
- Among independent older people, 3% of men and 6% of women are underweight, and in nursing and residential care, these figures rise to 16% and 15%, respectively (Finch et al., 1998).

- Poorer households consume:
  - less of the following: fruit and vegetables, salads, whole-meal bread, whole grain and high fibre cereals, and oily fish;
  - more of the following: white bread, full-fat milk, table sugar, and processed meat products which are often high in fat.
- With regard to nutrition, a national survey of older people in private households (Department of Health, 1992) found the following:
  - Half of the women and a quarter of the men aged 85 years and over were not able to cook a main meal alone.
  - Only 1 in 10 received Meals-on-Wheels (daily hot food or weekly frozen meal deliveries).
- Assess the risk of dietary deficiencies in older patients especially those with chronic diseases, poor dentition, poor mobility, on low incomes, or who are housebound.
- Have a low threshold for checking the vitamin B_{12} status of older people especially if they develop neuropsychiatric symptoms.
- Consider checking a patient's vitamin D status. Vitamin D deficiency is common in older people as the skin decreases in capacity to synthesize the provitamin calcidol, exacerbated by their low exposure to sunlight. Deficiencies are more common in the elderly housebound. Poor muscle strength and weakness is associated with vitamin D deficiency and this weakness may contribute to the risk of falls.
- Advise patients, no matter what age, to maintain a healthy diet including at least five portions of fruit and vegetables a day. There is indirect evidence that the modified Mediterranean diet is associated with increased survival among older people (Trichopoulou, 2005). Refer to a dietician if there is concern about dietary intake. Ask the patient to do a food diary for 1 week prior to being seen.
- Advise isolated patients to contact social services and local nongovernmental organizations (e.g., Age Concern). Eating with others may offer more interaction and reduce loneliness, and there is evidence that family-style meals may improve nutrition in older people (Nijs et al., 2006).
- The involuntary loss of more than 5% to 10% of an older person's usual weight during 1 year is an important clinical sign associated with increased risk of mortality. Weight loss should thus be treated as a serious symptom and prompt a search for the cause.
- Involuntary weight loss is generally related to one or a combination of four conditions: inadequate dietary intake, appetite loss (anorexia), muscle atrophy (sarcopenia), or inflammatory effects of disease (cachexia).

Managing Frailty

- Frailty is best regarded as "a condition or syndrome which results from a multi-system reduction in reserve capacity to the extent that a number of physiological systems are close to, or passed the threshold of symptomatic clinical failure. As a consequence, the frail person is at increased risk of disability and death from minor external stresses" (Campbell & Buchner, 1997).
- General practice, as part of the primary healthcare network, is well placed to detect and treat emerging frailty and prevent further deterioration.
- The Nottingham Extended Activities of Daily Living (EADL; see Appendix 30) scale may be useful in detecting unsuspected functional decline. Electronic indexes are being developed to identify individuals with frailty, but the effectiveness of this type of case finding has not been proved.
- Comprehensive geriatric assessment is associated with improved outcomes for older people such as reducing hospital admission and readmission as well as physical and cognitive functioning (Ellis et al., 2017).
- One specific organ manifestation of frailty is the decline in renal function with age—a decline which has implications for the prescribing of drugs that are renally excreted and for the management of conditions which, in themselves, impair renal function. A rise in serum creatinine is a late sign of renal impairment; estimation of the glomerular filtration rate (GFR) is more useful.

Early Intervention

- Preventive home visits by health professionals or laypeople trained in case-finding reduce mortality and admission to residential care and may promote independence and improve quality of life for frail older people (Elkan et al., 2001).
- Effective management of minor ailments, such as painful foot problems, may halt declining mobility and improve long-term outcomes.
- Physical therapy aimed at reducing functional impairment in older people with moderate frailty will delay functional decline (i.e., in ADL score) (Gill et al., 2002).
- Maximizing the management of chronic problems and minimizing polypharmacy may halt functional decline. The UK National Service Framework recommends an annual review of medication for people aged 75 and over, with a 6-monthly review for those taking four or more medicines.

Supporting Older People at Home

- There is considerable variation in the availability of services for older people internationally and within countries, both in formal and informal provision. Generally there is a multitude of services available aimed at staying healthy, either maintaining function or providing rehabilitation.
- Services can be accessed either by direct referral or through specialist geriatric services.
- A comprehensive assessment is recommended before referring to services.
- In general, services are accessed in the United Kingdom through a social worker; in Australia by direct referral or

through geriatric assessment services; and in New Zealand through the needs assessment service coordinator.

Difficulty Maintaining Living Arrangements

- Refer to an occupational therapist for assessment of ADL function at home and provision of equipment.
- Refer to a social worker to arrange a home carer for housework.
- Refer to a social worker for Meals-on-Wheels where these are available.
- Refer to a podiatrist/chiropodist for foot care.

Isolation

- Refer to Age Concern for provision of a volunteer/befriending service.
- Refer to a social worker for day centre placement.
- Refer to Dial-a-Driver or social worker to access a subsidized taxi service.

Carer Stress

- Ask carers specifically how they are coping.
- Ascertain the source of any stress.
- Refer for access to respite services, including day and night respite, and residential home placement for short periods.
- Refer for home care for personal assistance.
- Refer to an occupational therapist, for assessment of ADL function and equipment.

Functional Deterioration at Home

Refer to:
- a geriatrician for comprehensive assessment;
- a day hospital, for multidisciplinary assessment and treatment;
- physiotherapy for musculoskeletal assessment and exercises (Gill et al., 2002);
- occupational therapy for ADL functional assessment, provision of equipment, and treatment;
- a social worker for personal home care;
- the district nurses for a bathing service;
- a speech language therapist if the condition affects communication or swallowing;
- a dietician.

Poor Recovery After an Acute Episode

* Consider referral to:
  - the appropriate hospital service;
  - the district nursing service;
  - the occupational therapist, physiotherapist for functional assessment, and provision of equipment;
  - the social worker for temporary provision of personal care and housework.

Suicide (O'Connell et al., 2004)

- Late-life depression often goes undetected and has a significant adverse impact on quality of life, outcomes of medical disease, healthcare utilization, morbidity, and mortality.
- Suicide rates are almost twice as high in the older adult compared with the general population, with the rate highest for white men over 85 years of age.
- The ratio of parasuicide to completed suicide is much lower suggesting that suicidal behaviour in older people has a much greater degree of intent.
- The main psychologic factor associated with suicide in older people is recurrent major depression.
- Poor physical health and disability seem to be associated with the wish to die.
- Consider identifying all those with a known history of depressive disorder and question directly as to whether they have considered suicide. Treat and/or refer as appropriate.

Delirium, Acute Confusion, Behavioural and Psychological Symptoms of Dementia (BPSD) Loss of Mobility

- A change in mental or physical status of usually well, independent older people should be taken seriously and treated urgently. Symptoms of serious illness are often masked and pyrexia may be lower than expected, even in overwhelming infection.
- Acute change can be due to serious disease without overt symptomatology related to that disease. Confusion can be as simple as "the patient has suddenly changed, something is wrong, the level of function has deteriorated."
- Behaviour change may occur and can be described as verbal, vocal, or motor activity that is not explained by needs. The cause of this may be subtle and may be due to undiagnosed pain, acute illness, or simply the inability to communicate needs.
- A loss of mobility or taken to bed may be due to serious illness, particularly when the deterioration is rapid.
- Establishing the onset of deterioration and prior function is essential to identify delirium characterized by a fluctuating level of consciousness, disorientation, and global cognitive deficit. This is almost always due to an organic cause, usually infection, which is hard to diagnose with confidence.

Confirmation of the Presence of an Acute Confusional State

- A formal assessment is the Confusion Assessment Method (CAM), which states that the patient has delirium if:
  - there was an acute onset with a fluctuating course;
  - there is inattention; and
  - there is either disorganized thinking or an altered level of consciousness. Consciousness may be depressed or the patient may be hyperalert.

- The CAM has a sensitivity of at least 94% and a specificity of at least 90% for the diagnosis of delirium when used by nonpsychiatrists (Inouye et al., 1990).

Diagnosis of the Cause of the Confusion

A diagnosis of acute serious illness or medication toxicity should be assumed until proven otherwise. There are many causes for acute confusion, including (O'Keefe & Sanson, 1998):

- infection, most commonly pneumonia and urinary tract infection;
- cardiovascular disorder, especially myocardial infarction and congestive heart failure;
- neurologic disorder, most commonly stroke;
- medication interaction or toxicity, particularly psychotropic or cardiovascular medications;
- acute alcohol withdrawal;
- acute psychiatric disorder, including psychosis;
- electrolyte disturbance, dehydration, hyponatraemia;
- endocrine disorder, thyroid disease, diabetes;
- acute change in hearing or vision;
- faecal impaction or retention of urine;
- neoplasia;
- acute surgical emergency, such as peritonitis from appendicitis or gallbladder disease;
- undiagnosed fracture;
- hypothermia.

Specific Evaluation

A thorough history and physical examination are necessary, including:

- history of prior functional level, social support, medications, and medical problems. Involving caregivers or family members to get a history may be necessary;
- examination of cardiovascular and neurologic systems;
- musculoskeletal examination, especially for those with reduced mobility. Suspect undiagnosed fracture after apparent minor injury with excessive disability;
- abdominal examination to exclude an acute abdomen;
- rectal examination;
- investigations will be guided by the history and physical examination.

Possible Investigations

- Full blood count (FBC) and erythrocyte sedimentation rate (ESR)
- Creatinine, estimated GFR (eGFR), and electrolytes
- Liver function tests (LFTs)
- Measurement of Vitamin B_{12} levels
- Thyroid function tests (TFTs)
- Midstream urine (MSU) or dipstick urine test
- Blood glucose
- Calcium
- Blood cultures
- Electrocardiogram (ECG)

- Chest x-ray (CXR) and other x-rays as suggested by the examination

Management

Delirium, Acute Confusion

- Refer for assessment if the diagnosis cannot be clearly identified and the patient cannot initially be managed at home, or if a diagnosis is made (e.g., pneumonia or stroke), which requires admission.

If treating the patient at home:

- Treat any infection with an appropriate antibiotic.
- Stop medications with potential toxicity, especially sedative/hypnotics if they are suspected of causing acute confusion. Check for new medication as a precipitant cause.
- Treat dehydration with fluids with attention to cardiovascular function.
- Be alert to the possibility of an acute kidney injury.
- Deal with faecal impaction in the usual way, with attention to follow-up bowel function. Fluids, exercise, and fibre are all needed for adequate bowel function in older people.

Change in Behaviour, With Stress and Distress Behaviour Evident

- Behavioural management is useful for any agitated patient, including:
  - allowing the person to wander in a safe environment;
  - relocating to alternative living arrangements if distress becomes a constant problem and cannot be managed in the current living arrangement;
  - encouraging participation in usual activities;
  - avoiding confrontation if aggression is a feature;
  - avoiding physical restraint; it worsens agitation and can cause injury.
- Treat the cause as discussed, especially undiagnosed pain.
- Refer for admission to geriatric or psychogeriatric assessment ward if the patient cannot be managed at home.
- Refer to a psychiatrist for evaluation if psychosis is suspected.
- If no cause is found and the patient has underlying dementia, see upcoming discussion.
- *Medication.* Avoid medication to sedate, as this may prolong delirium, or shift to a hypoactive delirium instead. Reserve antipsychotics, typical or atypical, for patients who are so agitated that they pose a risk to themselves or to others. They are also associated with increased mortality, especially from stroke and sudden cardiac death. Haloperidol may be associated with less risk than the atypicals. Use the smallest dose, for the shortest duration possible.
- Avoid benzodiazepines. Even short-acting benzodiazepines accumulate in the older person and worsen the confusion. They increase the risk of injury from falling, with patients on higher doses of certain drugs (e.g., oxazepam, flurazepam, and chlordiazepoxide) having the highest risk (Tamblyn et al., 2005).

Loss of Mobility

- Treat acute illness as for acute confusion earlier.
- If minor injury is the cause, and significant disability has resulted and there is no fracture:
  - give adequate pain relief;
  - mobilize as soon as possible;
  - refer to community physiotherapy or outpatient department or day hospital services for rehabilitation (Forster, Young, & Langhorne, 2002).
- Refer the patient to a day hospital, which can improve overall functional outcome and reduce service utilization when compared with no comprehensive care (Forster et al., 2002).
- Refer for comprehensive inpatient geriatric assessment and management if overall function has deteriorated without apparent cause (Stuck et al., 1993).

Deterioration Over a Longer Period Without Acute Illness, Depression, or Dementia

- Deterioration in mental or physical status can be slow and progressive and not apparently due to acute illness (i.e., not delirium).
- If the onset is slow and workup has not shown a treatable acute cause, then the differential diagnoses of dementia and depression must be considered.

Diagnosis

- The diagnosis of depression is often missed in older people as the prominence of physical symptoms compounds the diagnosis.
- Dementia is of more insidious onset than depression.
- In depression, cognitive and physical deterioration is worse in the mornings.
- In depression, insight is present; in dementia, it is rare.
- Orientation is poor in dementia and preserved in depression.
- Memory loss is characteristically worse for recent events in dementia but can be similar for recent and remote events in depression.

Specific Evaluation

- Ask about a family and personal history of depression.
- Ask about recent significant events. Bereavement and relocation predispose to social isolation and depression.
- Check functional status and independence in living activities.
- Check the patient's social and financial supports.
- Ask about driving. Specific driving assessment may be necessary later.
- The five-question geriatric depression scale is useful in diagnosing depression in those without severe dementia and works in a variety of settings (Rinaldi et al., 2003).
- Assess the patient's cognitive state formally using one or both of the following tests or use the "test your memory" (TYM) test:

- *Clock drawing* is a useful, nonthreatening test of mental function. Simply draw a circle and ask the patient to make it into a clock with the time at "10 til 2." If numbers are not spread throughout all four quadrants, then the test is suggestive of dementia, particularly if short-term recall is reduced for three words (Mini-Cog Test).
- A standardized mental test score, such as the Abbreviated Mental Test Score (see box), is only reliable if used precisely (Holmes & Gilbody, 1996). A more well-validated but time-consuming score is the Mini-Mental State Examination (MMSE; discussion to come).

ABBREVIATED MENTAL TEST SCORE

Each question scores 1. A score of 6 or less suggests dementia.

1. Age (exact number of years)
2. Time (to the nearest hour)
3. A simple address (e.g., 42 West Street, to be repeated by the patient at the end of the test)
4. Year (the current year)
5. The place (exact address or the name of the surgery or hospital)
6. Recognition of two persons present (by name or role)
7. Date of birth (correct day and month)
8. Year of the second World War (1939 or 1945 is enough)
9. Name of the monarch (must be current monarch)
10. Count backwards from 20 to 1 (with no mistakes, or with mistakes which the patient corrects without prompting)

AMT4 can be found at https://www.racgp.org.au/your-practice/guidelines/silverbook/tools/abbreviated-mental-test-score/

Management

- Treatment of dementia is outlined in the next section.
- Refer for geriatric medical or geriatric psychiatric assessment if the diagnosis is not clear.
- Treat depression, if present, with:
  - an antidepressant (Wilson et al., 2002); and/or
  - psychologic therapy, including cognitive behaviour therapy. Poor access to publicly funded counselling services may limit its availability.
- Follow-up is essential to ensure recovery of function.

Dementia

GUIDELINES

National Institute for Health and Care Excellence. (2006). *Dementia: Supporting people with dementia and their carers in health and social care. NICE clinical guideline 42, updated 2016.* Retrieved from www.nice.org.uk.

- Dementia affects 10% of those over age 65 years and 20% of those over age 80 years.
- Absolute numbers of those with dementia will increase exponentially in the next two decades as the world population ages.

- New therapies recently available and currently under investigation mean that identification of early dementia may become important in the future.
- A UK parliamentary committee report (House of Commons, 2008) criticized the whole range of dementia care:
  - Poor diagnosis: only a third receive a formal diagnosis
  - Fragmented home support
  - Untrained staff in care homes
  - Failure to recognize and manage dementia in hospitals

Diagnosis

- Suspect dementia when the patient has:
  - impairment in short- and long-term memory, abstract thinking, judgment, other higher cortical function, or personality change; and
  - the disturbance is severe enough to interfere significantly with work, social activities, or relationships; and
  - delirium is absent (American Psychiatric Association, 1987).
- * Confirm it with a formal assessment. NICE mentions:
  - six-item cognitive impairment test;
  - the General Practitioner Assessment of Cognition (GPCOG);
  - the 7-minute screen;
  - MMSE.
- A good combination is the Abbreviated Mental Test Score plus the clock drawing test (see earlier discussion). The former tests orientation and memory; the latter tests praxis and spatial perception.
- A newer test is the TYM test (Brown et al., 2009). It has three advantages over the tests currently in use. It tests many different cognitive domains; it is performed by the patient alone, taking less than a minute of the doctor's or nurse's time to score it; and it is sensitive for the detection of early Alzheimer's disease (AD). Using a score of 42 or less out of 50 as positive, it is 93% sensitive and 86% specific for AD. The original article and the test itself are available on www.tymtest.com.
- * Determine, from the history and examination, whether it is possible to decide on the cause of the dementia (see upcoming discussion). This entails examination of the patient's mental state and cognition, a neurologic and cardiovascular examination, and a screen for depression. However, many patients have atypical or nonspecific presentations.
- * Exclude the few cases of reversible cognitive impairment as detailed later in the chapter. The box lists the clinical features of the types of dementia.

Specific Evaluation

- * Take a history from a caregiver or a source other than the patient. Objective assessment of change (e.g., from the carer) may help support the diagnosis. Use the Informant Questionnaire on Cognitive Decline in the Elderly (IQCODE) or the informant component of GPCOG.
- * Screen for depression.

TYPES OF DEMENTIA LISTED IN ORDER OF PREVALENCE

Dementia—Alzheimer Type

- Accounts for the majority of dementia cases
- Insidious onset over several years
- Global deficits

Vascular Dementia

- Accounts for 10% of dementia cases, although 29%–41% of dementia cases autopsied have some vascular pathology
- Stepwise progression
- Bilateral neurological signs
- A history of cardiovascular disease suggests vascular dementia
- Risk factors, or a history of risk factors for cardiovascular disease, make vascular dementia more likely

Dementia With Lewy Bodies

Dementia plus the following:
- Balance and gait disorder
- Prominent hallucinations and delusions
- Sensitivity to antipsychotics
- Fluctuations in alertness

Frontotemporal Dementia

- Early loss of personal awareness
- Early loss of social awareness
- Hyperorality (putting inappropriate things in the mouth)
- Stereotyped, perseverative behaviours

Prion Disease (Creutzfeldt–Jakob Disease [CJD])

- Rapidly progressive symptoms
- Characteristic electroencephalogram (EEG) pattern of periodic sharp wave complexes
- Pathologic brain tissue diagnosis
- Cerebrospinal fluid (CSF) 14-3-3 protein (high sensitivity and specificity for diagnosis of CJD).

- * Examine the patient's mental state, cognition, neurological system.
- * Examine the cardiovascular system.
- * Investigations:
  - Vitamin B_{12} level
  - Thyroid function
  - FBC, creatinine, eGFR, electrolytes, LFTs, calcium, glucose, ESR
  - CXR, MSU
  - Syphilis screening may no longer be needed unless there is a specific risk factor or they are from certain parts of the United States.
- Imaging with computed tomography (CT) or magnetic resonance imaging (MRI) scan. Availability will limit access in some regions.
- Other options are not recommended or not appropriate for primary care. Imaging with single photon emission computerized tomography (SPECT) or positron emission tomography (PET) is not recommended for routine use. Genetic testing and genotyping is not currently recommended. The CSF 14-3-3 protein may become available

and has overall sensitivity of 92% and a specificity of 80% in diagnosing CJD (2012 systematic review sponsored by the American Academy of Neurology).

Management
General

- It is widely accepted that patients with dementia should be assessed by a psychogeriatrician or geriatrician.
- Cognition, function, mood, and behaviour as well as general health should be reevaluated in patients with dementia every 6 months.
- *Prognosis.* If the family wishes to know, explain that a diagnosis of AD reduces life expectancy in a way that depends on the person's age. At age 65, median survival with AD is 8 years; at 90, at is 3 years (Brookmeyer et al., 2002).
- *Driving.* Advise patients to inform the Driver and Vehicle Licensing Agency (DVLA) and their insurance company. If there is reasonable concern about public safety, the GP should inform the DVLA as well. Download and give to the patient a leaflet such as "Driving and Dementia" (available from https://www.alzheimers.org.uk/sites/default/files/migrate/downloads/driving_and_dementia_factsheet_439.pdf). Indicate that the maximum driving time allowed may be 3 years (Breen et al., 2007). Be wary of being too certain, as clinical assessment is poorly associated with driving ability. There is no evidence-based information to guide physician assessment of medical fitness to drive (Molnar, Byszewski, Marshall, & Man-Son-Hing, 2005).

Training the Carers

- Refer for intensive long-term education and support for caregivers (if available) to delay time to residential care placement. A meta-analysis has shown that interventions designed to support carers can improve their mental health and result in the patient with AD staying at home longer (Spijker et al., 2008).
- Explain the principles of reality orientation and how to cope with a person exhibiting behavioural and psychological symptoms of dementia.
- If sleep is a problem, train the carers in sleep hygiene practices: advice about exercise, sleep at regular times, and avoiding naps. This has been shown to improve sleep patterns with daytime benefits as well. To achieve these benefits the carers will need considerable support (McCurry et al., 2003).
- Refer for home support.
- Consider referral for placement in dementia-specific long-term care. This may reduce carer strain.
- Consider whether the patient might be in pain. Many older patients suffer from painful conditions. A patient with dementia may be unable to communicate that pain is a problem. Look out for signs of distress (frowning, looking frightened, aggression, agitation, or withdrawal) and give an analgesic if pain could be the cause (Scherder et al., 2005). Specific assessment and treatment of pain can reduce distress (Husebo, Ballard, Sandvik, Nilsen, & Aarsland, 2011).

For Patients in Residential Care

- Offer residential care staff education about the behavioural management of patients with AD.
- Explain that a safe wandering space is essential for the older person with dementia to avoid agitation and unnecessary restraint, although there is no direct evidence of benefit (Price et al., 2002). This is especially useful for sundowning (increased agitation in the late afternoon).
- Scheduled toileting and prompted voiding reduces urinary incontinence.
- Music therapy, simulated natural sounds, and intensive multimodality group training may improve overall function.
- Specific assessment and treatment of pain can reduce distress (Husebo et al., 2011).

Psychosocial Interventions

- The main nonpharmacologic approaches that can play a role are as follows (Gitlin, Kales, & Lyketsos, 2012):
  - Reality orientation; this is based on the belief that continual, repetitive reminders will keep the patient stimulated and better orientated. There is some evidence of improved cognition and behaviour in dementia sufferers (Spector et al., 2000).
  - Memory enhancement strategies; these include setting shorter term goals, maintaining a social circle and family role.
  - Presenting dementia as a disability that can be accommodated and emphasizing continuing abilities.

General Principles for Carers

- Treat the patient with respect and dignity and address the patient as though you expect him or her to understand.
- Recognize the patient's level of capability but do not talk down or treat the person as a child.
- Encourage all attempts at personal care and activities of daily living.
- When talking, look directly at the person and maintain eye contact.
- Use short sentences expressing one thing at a time.
- Do not use implied messages; say exactly what is meant.
- If not understood, repeat the message a different way. Do not shout and do not rush the person.
- Mention names of familiar people, the date, week, and time in all conversations.
- Reward the patient's attempts with a smile or compliment. *Reality orientation in the patient's home could include:*
- a large clock and a calendar visible at all times;
- wearing a watch with a date display;
- having stimulating materials available (e.g., newspapers and magazines);
- a reality orientation board with a schedule of daily activities and reminders (e.g., appointments, at what time to expect a carer that day, as well a reminder of the day and date).

Medications for Cognitive Symptoms

- The pharmacologic treatment of symptoms is complex and rapidly changing. Each decision should be personalized to the individual's needs rather than an improvement on a score.

Alzheimer's Disease

- NICE (2018) has issued guidance on the use of donepezil, galantamine, rivastigmine, and memantine for treatment of AD (available: https://www.nice.org.uk/guidance/ta217).
- *Cholinesterase inhibitors* have been shown to improve cognition and global functioning in patients with AD. The improvements are small and come at the cost of an increase in adverse effects. The benefits are greatest for those in whom the disease is moderate or moderately severe:
  - Donepezil, galantamine, and rivastigmine are now recommended as options for managing mild as well as moderate AD.
  - Memantine is now recommended as an option for managing moderate AD for people who cannot take cholinesterase inhibitors and as an option for managing severe AD.
- Treatment should be continued only when it is considered to be having a worthwhile effect on cognitive, global, functional, or behavioural symptoms.
- The severity of the condition may be assessed using the MMSE, where *moderate* to *moderately severe* are represented by scores of 10 to 20 points (Table 15.1). However, the MMSE should not be used if another condition makes it unreliable (e.g., learning difficulties, sensory impairment, or linguistic problems).
- The drug should be initiated by a specialist in the care of patients with dementia.
- When assessing the severity of AD and the need for treatment, healthcare professionals should not rely solely on cognition scores.
- Families may ask their GP's opinion of various drugs that can be bought over the counter, such as:
  - *vitamin E* supplementation. This might slow functional decline in men with mild to moderate AD but neither vitamin E nor memantine appears to affect cognitive function or dementia severity;
  - *Gingko biloba.* There is inconsistent evidence of benefit in cognitive function from taking gingko biloba and no evidence of increased harm. Over-the-counter preparations vary considerably in potency compared to the pure product used in randomized controlled trials (RCTs). Relatives can be advised that the chance of benefit is small.

Ischaemic Vascular Dementia and Mixed Dementia

- Evidence-based data supporting pharmacologic efficacy of agents to treat non-AD dementia are less strong than for AD.
- Some research shows that patients with vascular dementia (VaD) benefit from galantamine (Erkinjuntti et al., 2002). Galantamine 16 to 24 mg/day is associated with improved activities of daily living and cognition scores.
- Donepezil 5 to 10 mg/day is associated with small improvements in cognitive function (Malouf & Birks, 2004).
- Offer all the measures appropriate for the secondary prevention of cardiovascular disease if the patient's condition and life expectancy warrant it. Blood pressure control with perindopril and indapamide has been shown to slow cognitive decline and reduce disability (Fransen et al., 2003). Blood pressure lowering strategies have not been specifically tested for treatment or prevention of VaD and this effect is likely to be due to further stroke prevention.
- Similarly, other interventions (e.g., aspirin) may not halt cognitive decline, although they are likely to reduce the risk of other vascular disease (Rands et al., 2005).
- Based on the observed prevalence of potentially modifiable risk factors (e.g., hypertension, diabetes, inactivity), combined with their associated relative risk for dementia, it has been estimated that risk factor reductions of 10% to 25% could prevent up to half of dementia cases, if treated early.

Medication for Behavioural Symptoms

- The treatment of *delirium*, an acute change in mental status characterized by fluctuation in level of consciousness, attention, and cognitive function, is more complex than in those with the stable symptoms of dementia (Britton & Russell, 2002).
- Look for an organic cause, most commonly undiagnosed pain, infection, and cardiovascular disorder as with well older people.
- Use behavioural and environmental modification. Reality orientation (presenting orientation information based on time, place, and person related) has been shown in one systematic review of small RCTs to improve behaviour (Spector et al., 2000).
- Treat stress and distress behaviour and symptoms of psychosis as follows:
  - Psychotropic medication should be cautiously used for treatment of severe agitation or psychosis with the potential for harm (e.g., low-dose haloperidol [0.5–1.0 mg orally

TABLE 15.1	Grading of Severity in Alzheimer Disease According to the Mini-Mental State Examination	

Severity	MMSE Score
Mild	21–26
Moderate	15–20
Moderately severe	10–14
Severe	<10

MMSE, Mini-mental state examination.

or intramuscularly]). Use the smallest possible dose for the shortest periods of time. In patients with a parkinsonian disorder, use an atypical antipsychotic instead.

- Benzodiazepines should be avoided in patients with delirium, except in withdrawal syndromes or when other drugs cannot be used.
- Withdraw an antipsychotic from a patient with dementia unless the need for it is overwhelming. A UK RCT in patients with dementia on antipsychotic treatment found that those whose antipsychotic medication was switched to placebo had a better chance of surviving over 12 months than those in whom the medication was continued (Ballard et al., 2009).

Teaching the Patient to Cope With Cognitive Impairment

- In the early stages of cognitive impairment, the patient can be taught how to minimize the functional disability. A simple analogy, such as "If you had a limp you'd use a stick—but since it's your memory that's not so good, you need to learn ways to help it," may help the patient to accept the concept. Another phrase that is readily understood is "Use it or lose it."
- Family and carers should be involved in this process from the beginning. It will help to overcome their frustration at living with a cognitively impaired relative and, as the patient becomes more impaired, they can take over some of the tasks.
- Cognitive impairment is embarrassing and frustrating. The natural tendency is to cover it up. The following approach depends on the opposite: accepting it and adopting techniques to minimize its effect.
- Advise the patient to:
  - do things when most alert;
  - take rest;
  - use relaxation techniques to reduce stress;
  - keep active (e.g., household jobs, visiting, reading)
  - be involved in sports, music, and other activities that involve coordination;
  - keep a regular routine;
  - learn to live with pain and not expect all pain to be relieved but use analgesics when necessary, particularly for night pain;
  - express feelings;
  - eat well-balanced meals;
  - reduce alcohol intake;
  - consider counselling.

Memory Difficulties

- Memory involves learning, storage, and recall. There is little that can be done to improve the storage of memory, but there are techniques to improve learning and recall.
- Advise patients to:
  - avoid undermining their confidence. Remember: No one's memory is perfect! If you forget something, don't get too upset about it;
  - reduce alcohol and avoid sedatives;
  - try to concentrate in a place free of distractions;
  - try to motivate yourself to learn. Make sure you understand and remember all the information;
  - improve retention by rehearsing/repeating information and by making associations to improve retention;
  - learn one new thing at a time and try to avoid the confusion that comes with information overload;
  - when learning something, study for short periods and frequently, rather than long periods;
  - use memory aids (e.g., dry wipe boards, sticky notes, diaries, a calendar, alarms).

Anxiety, Moodiness, and Irritability

- Advise the patient to:
  - identify the sources of aggravation and try to come up with a simple solution;
  - practice talking to oneself (e.g., stay calm, relax);
  - leave the situation explaining that you will need to calm down and go back to it later;
  - use relaxation techniques (e.g., tapes, therapy, counting to 10);
  - take regular exercise;
  - get things off your chest by talking or writing.

Difficulty in Initiating Activities

- Advise the patient to:
  - improve your organizational skills (daily routines, use of a diary, avoid putting things off, priority lists, break the task into smaller tasks, use simple methods to achieve things, ask for help or delegate, take time and not to rush, if necessary, involve others in decision making);
  - involve others so they can help motivate you;
  - reward yourself when steps are completed. Do this frequently and make the goals reasonable;
  - if orientation is a problem, use maps and landmarks, plan routes, and write directions.

Reading

- Having to reread something several times is common. This may be a result of concentration or memory problems but may also result from a change in the brain's ability to handle a lot of information.
- Advise patients to:
  - move a finger under each word at a comfortable pace;
  - block off the words underneath the sentence with a sheet of paper;
  - create a window, in card, that only allows one line to be read at a time;
  - take notes to help focus and concentrate on the important parts;
  - read larger print;
  - test themselves on what they have read.

Problems in Social Situations

- Dementia sufferers may have difficulties in understanding certain social situations and jump to conclusions that are inappropriate.

- Different patterns of cognitive impairment require different specific approaches. See entries under Alzheimer Disease, Parkinson Disease, and Huntington Disease.
- Advise patients to:
  - clarify what was meant;
  - explain what they believe was said;
  - get feedback from others;
  - recognize problem situations or people and plan how to respond beforehand;
  - communicate openly and honestly; above all respect the others' position;
  - give the benefit of the doubt to others and assume they mean no harm.

Financial and Legal Aspects (UK)

- Patients may be eligible for exemption from Council tax.
- Advise that it may be appropriate for someone else to be given power of attorney.

SUPPORT GROUPS

Alzheimers New Zealand, www.alzheimers.org.nz.
   Alzheimer's Association Australia, www.alzheimers.org.au.
   Alzheimer's Society UK, www.alzheimers.org.uk.
   Details of Alzheimer Associations in other countries can be found on the website of the Alzheimer's Disease International, www.alz.co.uk.
   Age Concern New Zealand, www.ageconcern.org.nz.
   AGEUK, https://www.ageuk.org.uk/.

Falls

GUIDELINES

American Geriatrics Society/British Geriatrics Society (AGS/BGS). (2011). Clinical practice guideline on prevention of falls in older persons. *Journal of the American Geriatrics Society, 59*(1), 148.
   National Institute for Health and Care Excellence. (2017). *Falls in older people: Assessing risk and prevention.* Retrieved from https://www.nice.org.uk/guidance/qs86.

Falls are serious and common for those over age 75 years. Risk factors have been identified and specific interventions proven to reduce falls.

Risk Factors

- Age over 80 years
- Cognitive impairment
- History of fall and fall-related injury
- Arthritis
- Depression
- Use of mobility aid
- Gait and balance impairment
- Lower limb muscle weakness
- Visual deficit

- Impaired daily functioning, or a low score on the Nottingham EADL scale (see earlier discussion)
- Use of psychotropic medications
- Those with multiple risk factors are at a higher risk of falls.

Diagnosis

- Ask older people (aged 75 and older) routinely, once a year, "Have you had a fall in the last year?"
- Perform a simple gait assessment (to come).
- Distinguish between *hot* and *cold* falls.
  - Hot falls result from major medical conditions such as stroke, myocardial infarction, or seizure. Treatment of the acute illness usually entails admission to hospital.
  - Cold falls occur in the absence of serious acute illness. This part of the chapter deals with management of cold falls and those with high risk of falls.
- Refer anyone with a recent cold fall, with recurrent falls in the last year, or with an abnormality of gait or balance for falls risk assessment.
- NICE recommends a multifactorial risk assessment of older people who present for medical attention because of a fall or who report recurrent falls in the past year.

Specific Evaluation

A falls risk assessment includes:
a. history of fall circumstances;
b. medication review;
c. review of chronic medical problems, including alcohol misuse;
- examination of:
  - vision;
  - gait and balance (see upcoming discussion);
  - lower leg strength;
  - neurologic system, especially proprioceptive and coordination function and including mental status;
  - cardiovascular system, especially heart rate and rhythm, lying and standing blood pressure, and the murmurs of valvular disease.
- the environment in which the falls occurred, with attention to:
  - hazards such as loose mats, cords, and unstable furniture;
  - lighting levels.
- assessment of the person's fear of falling and the effect it is having on functional ability;
- investigations including FBC and ECG.

SIMPLE GAIT ASSESSMENT

Ask the patient to stand from a chair, without using the arms, walk 3 m, turn around and return (the Get Up and Go test) (Mathias, Nayak, & Isaacs, 1986). Unsteadiness or difficulty completing this in less than 30 sec shows a gait and balance deficit and further evaluation is needed.

Management

- Results of the evaluation will guide specific management. Most patients needing intervention will have multiple risk factors.
- Multifactorial intervention is more effective than single intervention in preventing future falls.
- Refer all with a history of unexplained syncope to a physician. Investigations such as a lying and standing blood pressure or multiday ECG may reveal a cause. Carotid sinus hypersensitivity can be detected by carotid sinus massage in controlled conditions, including cardiac monitoring.

Community-Dwelling Older People at High Risk of Recurrent Falls

- Exercise may reduce falls in community-dwelling older persons (Sherrington et al., 2008).
- Review medications and reduce psychotropics. Drugs that are especially likely to cause falls are benzodiazepines, tricyclic antidepressants, phenothiazines and butyrophenones, antihypertensives, anticholinergics, and hypoglycaemic agents (American Geriatrics Society [AGS], 2015).
- Assess vision and refer if necessary. Cataract surgery reduces the risk of fall with hip fracture (Tseng, Yu, Lum, & Coleman, 2012).
- *Home environment.* Assess whether shoes and slippers fit properly. Check for loose carpets, poor lighting, or general cluttering of furniture, as these increase the risk. Refer for modification of other environmental hazards according to the availability of occupational therapy.
- Review all medical conditions. Treat cardiovascular disorders, including postural hypotension and any cardiac arrhythmia.
- *Osteoporosis.* When patients can tolerate it, consider giving vitamin D_3 800 IU daily with calcium cosupplementation to reduce the risk of fractures. The vitamin D may, in addition, increase muscle strength, particularly for those who are deficient in vitamin D (Kahwati et al.).

Older People in Residential Care and Assisted Living Settings at High Risk of Recurrent Falls

- A systematic review of studies of fall prevention in hospitals and long-term care facilities found inconclusive evidence for the effectiveness of most approaches. These approaches appear less effective in the real world than in research studies (Coussement et al., 2008).
- Refer to physiotherapy for gait and balance training and advice on use of assistive devices. This depends on the availability of physiotherapy services in long-term care.
- Consider giving vitamin D_3 to achieve over 30 ng/mL.
- It is reasonable for clinicians to consider the use of hip protectors in patients at high risk of hip fractures who are willing to comply with their use. They are only effective if actually worn. They do not work at an institutional level (Parker, 2005).

Vestibular Rehabilitation Exercises

a. *In bed*, performed slowly initially then more rapidly:
   - *eye movements:* up and down, side to side, focusing on a finger as it moves from 1 m away to 30 cm away
   - *head movements:* moving head forward, then backward, and turning from side to side
b. *Sitting:* rotating the head; bending down and standing up with eyes open and closed
c. *Standing:* throwing a small ball from hand to hand, turning through 360 degrees
d. *Moving about:* walking across the room, up and down a slope, up and down stairs with eyes open and then closed

Lower Leg Problems

Night Cramps (Butler, Mulkerrin, & O'Keeffe, 2002)

Nocturnal leg cramps are common occurrences among older, generally healthy adults, 70% of whom experience them at some time.

Diagnosis

Most are idiopathic but they are more common in certain conditions:
- Peripheral vascular disease
- Renal failure
- Diabetes
- Thyroid disease
- Hypomagnesaemia
- Hypocalcaemia
- Hypokalaemia

Possible Investigations

- FBC and ESR
- Creatinine, eGFR, and electrolytes
- LFTs
- Blood glucose
- Calcium and magnesium
- TFTs

Management

- Treat the underlying cause when possible.
- Look for a drug cause: Diuretics, nifedipine, beta-agonists, steroids, morphine, cimetidine, penicillamine, statins, and lithium have all been implicated.
- Explain the technique to abort a cramp as it is starting: Forcibly stretch the muscle that is in spasm. Thus for cramp in the calf, the patient should stand up with the leg straight and forcibly dorsiflex the foot by pressing the ball of the foot on the floor.
- Recommend a trial of calf stretching exercises; they have been found helpful. The technique is to stand 3 feet from a wall, rest against it with the arms outstretched, then tilt toward it, keeping the heels on the floor, until the stretch is felt in the calves, holding the position for 10

seconds. Do this exercise three times a day, with three stretches each time. If after 3 days there is improvement, continue it long term.

- *Drug treatment:*
  - Quinine sulphate is not recommended. Quinine carries the risk of a severe sensitivity reaction in 1 in 1000 to 3500, of which the main manifestation is severe thrombocytopenia. Hepatitis and haemolytic uraemic syndrome have also been described. It also is very dangerous in overdose. Because of these risks the US Food and Drug Administration has banned its marketing for cramp, but it remains licensed for cramp in the United Kingdom.
  - There is limited and inconsistent evidence that calcium channel blockers, vitamins, minerals, or naftidrofuryl reduce the frequency of cramps (Blyton, Chuter et al., 2012).

Restless Legs Syndrome

> ### REVIEWS
>
> European Federation of Neurological Societies/European Neurological Society/European Sleep Research Society (EFNS/ENS/ESRS). (2012). Guideline on management of restless legs syndrome. *European Journal of Neurology,* *19*(11), 1385.
>
> Leschziner, G., & Gringras, P. (2012). Restless legs syndrome. *BMJ (Clinical Research Ed.), 344*.

- The syndrome is characterized by creepy crawly sensations in the lower limbs. These occur at rest in the evenings or at night and are temporarily relieved by moving the limbs. The minimum diagnostic criteria proposed by the International Restless Legs Syndrome Study Group (IRLSSG) and National Institutes of Health (NIH) are:
  - urge to move legs often accompanied by an unpleasant feeling;
  - onset or worsening of symptoms when at rest;
  - partial or complete relief by movement for as long as movement continues;
  - circadian pattern of symptom expression with high frequency of occurrence in evening and at night (often interferes with sleep).
- Evidence is inconsistent for association with iron deficiency, but screening is generally recommended by consensus panels.

Workup

1. FBC
2. Serum ferritin
3. Folic acid
4. B_{12}
5. Creatinine, eGFR, and electrolytes
   - Examine to exclude peripheral neuropathy.
   - Review the patient's drugs. Possible causes are neuroleptics, lithium, beta-blockers, calcium channel blockers,

tricyclic antidepressants (TCAs), phenytoin, and H_2 blockers.

- Explain what to do during an attack: walk about, stretch the legs, have a bath, do something interesting as a distraction, or massage the legs.
- Nonpharmacologic therapy options for prevention include avoidance of aggravating drugs and substances such as caffeine, mentally alerting activities, exercise, leg massage, and applied heat. In patients with mild and/or intermittent symptoms, these therapies may be sufficient for symptom relief.
- Consider drug treatment for patients with symptoms that are sufficiently severe and frequent. Be wary of treating mild and infrequent symptoms with indefinite medication duration. Options include:
  - a dopamine agonist. These classes of drugs have been shown to be effective compared with placebo, but the diagnostic uncertainty and side effects often limit their use.
  - a calcium channel ligand (e.g., gabapentin), which appears to improve symptoms in patients with moderate to severe restless legs syndrome (RLS) particularly if neuropathy is present.

> ### PATIENT SUPPORT AND INFORMATION
>
> RLS-UK: www.rls-uk.org/.
> Bandolier: www.bandolier.org.uk (search on "restless legs").

Postural Ankle Oedema

- Many patients are given diuretics inappropriately for postural oedema. Diuretics can cause paradoxic oedema.
- Assess carefully to exclude a cardiac, renal, or hepatic cause.
- Treat postural oedema by advising the patient to:
  - keep active;
  - elevate legs when sitting; and
  - use support hosiery.
- Give a diuretic only where the oedema is too severe to permit the patient to pull on a support stocking; and even then, only give it for a maximum of 3 weeks.
- Consider a trial without diuretics for those already started on them. In one study, 85% of those suitable were successfully withdrawn from diuretics (de Jonge et al., 1994). Be aware that even patients who do not need their diuretics are likely to suffer an initial increase in oedema as a rebound phenomenon, which may take 6 weeks to settle.

Elder Abuse

- A UK study has shown the prevalence of abuse in the patient's own home to be significant, with physical abuse in 2%, verbal in 5%, and financial in 2% (Ogg

& Bennett, 1992); 45% of carers of older people in respite care admitted to some form of abuse (Homer & Gilliard, 1990).

- There are no statutory guidelines or legislation; however, abuse is a crime. Intervention should always be interdisciplinary.
- Abuse may take the form of:
  - *physical:* hitting, slapping, pushing, kicking, misuse of medication, restraint, inappropriate sanctions;
  - *psychological:* emotional abuse, threats of harm or abandonment, deprivation of contact, humiliation, blaming, controlling, intimidation, coercion, harassment, verbal abuse, isolation or withdrawal from services or supportive networks;
  - *sexual:* rape and sexual assault or sexual acts to which the vulnerable adult has not consented, could not consent to, or was pressurized into consenting to;
  - *financial or material abuse:* theft, fraud, exploitation, pressure in connection with wills, property or inheritance or financial transactions, or the misuse or misappropriation of property, possession, or benefits;
  - *neglect and acts of omission:* ignoring medical or physical care needs, failure to provide access to appropriate health, social care or educational services, the withholding of the necessities of life such as medication, adequate nutrition;
  - *discriminatory abuse:* racist, sexist, based on a person's disability and other forms of harassment.
- Abuse can occur anywhere, including in:
  - someone's own home;
  - a carer's home;
  - day care;
  - a residential or nursing home;
  - hospital.
- Abuse may occur for many reasons:
  - In the home the causes include poor quality long-term relationships, a carer's inability to provide the level of care needed, a carer with mental or physical health problems.
  - In other settings it may be a symptom of a poorly run establishment, especially when staff are inadequately trained and poorly supervised.
- Suspect abuse when:
  - there is delay in seeking medical help;
  - there are differing histories from patient and carer, especially if explanations are implausible;
  - there are inconsistencies on examination;
  - there are frequent calls for visits by the GP or accident and emergency (A&E) department attendances;
  - the carer does not accompany the patient when that would be expected;
  - there is abnormal behaviour in the presence of the carer (e.g., fear or withdrawal).
- Discuss the situation with the patient, carer, and involved care agencies. Further action will depend on the wishes and competence of the patient and the nature and severity of the abuse.
- Discuss the case with Action on Elder Abuse (see box).

PROFESSIONAL AND PATIENT INFORMATION

Information leaflets are available from Action on Elder Abuse, PO Box 60001, Streatham, London SW16 9BY, tel. 020 8835 9280; helpline 080 8808 8141, www.elderabuse.org.uk.

For advice on what to do when you suspect patients are being abused in residential or nursing homes, download the Commission for Social Care Inspection leaflet "Abuse of Older People—What You Can Do to Stop It," available from http://lx.iriss.org.uk/sites/default/files/resources/Abuse%20 of%20older%20people.pdf.

Sex and the Elderly

- Sexual activity is common in the elderly with studies indicating at least 50% of 60- to 90-year-olds remain sexually active. Although coitus declines in frequency, interest is maintained in different ways (e.g., masturbation, oral sex). There is a shift from genital sex to intimacy.
- In a study looking at the secular trends in health, the sexual activity of Swedish 70-year-olds in 1971 was compared with 70-year-olds in 2001. Men and women from the latter group reported higher satisfaction with sexuality, fewer sexual dysfunctions, and more positive attitudes to sexuality in later life (Beckman et al., 2008).
- Medication may cause changes in sexual function, particularly beta-blockers, antidepressants, and antipsychotics (Montejo, 2015).
- Phosphodiesterase (PDE) 5 inhibitors are used in the treatment of erectile dysfunction. They work in older men, but less than in younger men (Müller et al., 2007).
- *For men,* explain the normal changes associated with ageing (Masters & Johnson, 1970):
  - The urgency of sexual interest declines from the late fourth decade.
  - Erection is less frequent.
  - Erection needs more stimulation, especially tactile.
  - Erection is more difficult to sustain.
  - Turgidity of the erection diminishes.
  - Ejaculation is less forceful.
  - Refractory period is longer.
  - There may be periods of difficulty establishing an erection and the frequency of these episodes increases over time. However, the pleasure derived from sex may not be significantly altered.
- *For women,* explain the normal changes associated with ageing (Masters & Johnson, 1966):
  - Arousal requires more stimulation.
  - Lining of the vaginal wall thins and vaginal lubrication decreases.
  - There is less vaginal vasocongestion and tensing.
  - Uterine contractions are fewer.
  - Clitoral detumescence is rapid.
  - The capacity to achieve orgasm remains into old age but the length of time taken to achieve it increases.

- Consider the risk of sexually transmitted infection in older people embarking on new relationships and counsel them on the importance of safe sex.
- Be willing to discuss sexual issues with all, but particularly with:
  - women undergoing gynaecologic operations;
  - men undergoing prostate treatment;
  - patients who have severe arthritis (changing position and timing of analgesia may be needed);
  - patients who have had a stroke or myocardial infarction.

Sexual Activity in Residential and Nursing Homes

- Patients in nursing or residential homes may continue to have an interest in sexual activity. Sexual behaviour is often seen as a problem rather than an expression of a need for love and intimacy. Men with dementia are more likely to exhibit inappropriate sexual behaviour.
- *Inappropriate behaviour:* Advise staff about sexuality in the elderly and advise them against unintentionally giving cues that may be misinterpreted (e.g., when washing them). In addition, consider:
  - *behavioural approaches:* for example, tell the patient that the behaviour is inappropriate, isolate the patient from residents of the sex being subjected to inappropriate behaviour, use clothing that opens at the back for a male who exposes his genitals;
  - *drug therapy:* there is little evidence but consider selective serotonin reuptake inhibitors (SSRIs) in very difficult cases.

Legal Aspects

Power of Attorney

- At an early stage of declining mental function, suggest to the family that they consult a solicitor about a lasting power of attorney (LPA) *before* the patient is incapable of signing the form.
- To sign, the patient must be capable of understanding the implications of so doing, and may be capable of this even if incapable of managing his or her affairs. If it is left too late, it is then necessary to apply to the Court of Protection to appoint a receiver, and this is much more cumbersome.
- The LPA must be registered before it can be used. Note that this is different from the registration of the older power, the enduring power of attorney (EPA), which only becomes necessary when the person who signed it is, or is becoming, incapable of managing his or her own affairs.

For more information about enduring power of attorney, lasting power of attorney, Court of Protection, and other relevant legal aspects in the England and Wales go to https://www.gov.uk/government/organisations/office-of-the-public-guardian. For Scotland, http://www.publicguardian-scotland.gov.uk/home.

Detention of an Older Person

GUIDELINE

UK: The Mental Capacity Act 2005. Retrieved from https://www.legislation.gov.uk/ukpga/2005/9/contents.

- In 2005 an amendment was made to the Mental Capacity Act, known as the Deprivation of Liberty Safeguards, which took effect in England and Wales. The use of these safeguards should be considered when someone is subject to continuous supervision or control, and whether they are free to leave a given environment.
- These safeguards make provision for the use of restrictions and restraint (including, for example, the use of locks to stop people going to different parts of a building or the use of bed rails). They apply only to hospitals and care homes but the Court of Protection can authorise the deprivation of liberty in other settings.
- They are applicable to those who lack capacity to consent to the restrictions placed upon them.
- An application for the deprivation of someone's liberty should be made to the local authority who will then appoint an assessor to adjudicate as to whether the act applies or whether other legislation (such as the Mental Health Act) may be more applicable.
- Under the act, those who lack capacity and who do not have the support of family or friends to make decisions are entitled to have access to an independent mental capacity advocate (IMCA) who can be appointed by social services.
- In Australia and New Zealand, refer to the local geriatric assessment team if there is a need for legal intervention to ensure patient safety and well-being.

References

American Geriatric Society. (2015). Updated beers criteria for potentially inappropriate medication use in older adults. *Journal of the American Geriatrics Society*, 63(11), 2227–2246.

American Psychiatric Association (1987). *Diagnostic and statistical manual of mental disorder* (3rd ed. rev.). Washington, DC: APA.

Anderson, P. (1993). Effectiveness of general practice interventions for patients with harmful alcohol consumption. *The British Journal of General Practice: The Journal of the Royal College of General Practitioners*, 43, 386–389.

Ballard, C., Hanney, M. L., Theodoulou, M., et al. (2009). The dementia antipsychotic withdrawal trial (DART-AD): Long-term follow-up of a randomised placebo-controlled trial. *Lancet Neurology*, 8, 151–157.

Bates, B., Lennox, A., Prentice, A., Bates, C., & Swan, G. (2013). *National Diet and Nutrition Survey. Department of Health and Food standards agency, 1–79.* Retrieved from https://assets.publishing.service.gov.uk/government/uploads/system/uploads/attachment_data/file/551352/NDNS_Y5_6_UK_Main_Text.pdf

Beckman, N., Waern, M., Gustafson, D., et al. (2008). Secular trends in self reported sexual activity and satisfaction in Swedish 70 year olds; cross sectional survey of four populations, 1971–2001. *British Medical Journal (Clinical Research Ed.), 337*, 151–154.

Breen, D. A., Breen, D. P., Moore, J. W., et al. (2007). Driving and dementia. *British Medical Journal (Clinical Research Ed.), 334,* 1365–1369.

Britton, A., & Russell, R. (2002). Multidisciplinary team interventions for delirium in patients with chronic cognitive impairment (Cochrane review). In *The Cochrane Library* (Issue 1). Update Software, Oxford.

Brookmeyer, R., Corrada, M. M., Curriero, F. C., et al. (2002). Survival following a diagnosis of alzheimer disease. *Archives of Neurology, 59,* 1764–1767.

Brown, J., Pengas, G., Dawson, K., et al. (2009). Self administered cognitive screening test (TYM) for detection of Alzheimer's disease: Cross sectional study. *British Medical Journal (Clinical Research Ed.), 338,* b2030.

Butler, J. V., Mulkerrin, E. C., & O'Keeffe, S. T. (2002). Nocturnal leg cramps in older people. *Postgraduate Medical Journal, 78,* 596–598.

Campbell, A., & Buchner, D. (1997). Unstable disability and the fluctuation of frailty. *Age and Ageing, 26,* 315–318.

Campbell, A., Robertson, M., Gardner, M., et al. (1997). Randomised controlled trial of a general practice programme of home based exercise to prevent falls in elderly women. *British Medical Journal (Clinical Research Ed.), 315,* 1065–1069.

Curb, J., Pressel, S., Cutler, J., et al. (1996). Effect of diuretic-based antihypertensive treatment on cardiovascular disease risk in older diabetic patients with isolated systolic hypertension. Systolic hypertension in the elderly program cooperative research group. *JAMA: The Journal of the American Medical Association, 276,* 1886–1892.

de Jonge, J., Knotternerus, J. A., van Zutphen, W. M., et al. (1994). Short term effect of withdrawal of diuretic drugs prescribed for ankle oedema. *British Medical Journal (Clinical Research Ed.), 308,* 511–513.

Department of Health (1992). *Report on health and social subjects 31–the nutrition of elderly people.* Committee on Medical Aspects of Food Policy. HMSO.

Department of Health and Social Security (1994). *Living in Britain: Results from the 1994 general household survey.* Norwich: HMSO.

Elkan, R., Kendrick, D., Dewey, M., et al. (2001). Effectiveness of home based support for older people: Systematic review and meta-analysis. Commentary: When, where, and why do preventive home visits. *British Medical Journal (Clinical Research Ed.), 323,* 719.

Elley, C. R., Kerse, N., Arroll, B., et al. (2003). Effectiveness of counselling patients on physical activity in general practice: Cluster randomised controlled trial. *British Medical Journal (Clinical Research Ed.), 326,* 793.

Elon, R. D. (1996). Geriatric medicine. *British Medical Journal (Clinical Research Ed.), 312,* 561–563.

Erkinjuntti, T., Kurz, A., Gauthier, S., et al. (2002). Efficacy of galantamine in probable vascular dementia and Alzheimer's disease combined with cerebrovascular disease: A randomised trial. *Lancet, 359,* 1283–1290.

Finch, S., Doyle, W., Lowe, C., et al. (1998). National diet and nutrition survey: People aged 65 years and over. In *Report of the diet and nutrition survey* (Vol. 1). London: The Stationery Office.

Forster, A., Young, J., & Langhorne, P. (2002). Medical day hospital care for the elderly versus alternative forms of care (Cochrane review). In *The Cochrane Library* (Issue 1). Update Software, Oxford.

Fransen, M., Anderson, C., Chalmers, J., et al. (2003). Effects of a perindopril-based blood pressure-lowering regimen on disability and dependency in 6105 patients with cerebrovascular disease: A randomized controlled trial. *Stroke; a Journal of Cerebral Circulation, 34,* 2333–2338.

Gill, T., Baker, D., Gottschalk, M., et al. (2002). A program to prevent functional decline in physically frail, elderly persons who live at home. *The New England Journal of Medicine, 347,* 1068–1074.

Holmes, J., & Gilbody, S. (1996). Differences in use of the abbreviated mental test score by geriatricians and psychiatrists. *British Medical Journal (Clinical Research Ed.), 313,* 465.

Homer, A., & Gilliard, C. (1990). Abuse of elderly people by their carers. *British Medical Journal (Clinical Research Ed.), 301,* 1359–1362.

House of Commons. (2008). *Public Select Committee. Improving services and support for people with dementia. Sixth report.* Retrieved from www.publications.parliament.uk/pa/cm200708/cmselect/cmpubacc/228/228.pdf.

Husebo, B. S., Ballard, C., Sandvik, R., Nilsen, O. B., & Aarsland, D. (2011). Efficacy of treating pain to reduce behavioural disturbances in residents of nursing homes with dementia: Cluster randomised clinical trial. *British Medical Journal (Clinical Research Ed.), 343,* doi. https://doi.org/10.1136/bmj.d4065.

Inouye, S., van Dyck, C., Alessi, C., et al. (1990). Clarifying confusion: The confusion assessment method. A new method for detection of delirium. *Annals of Internal Medicine, 113,* 941–948.

Kerse, N., Jolley, D., Arroll, B., et al. (1999). Improving health behaviours of the elderly: A randomised controlled trial of a general practice educational intervention. *British Medical Journal, 319,* 683–687.

Malouf, R., & Birks, J. (2004). Donepezil for vascular cognitive impairment (Cochrane review). In *The Cochrane Library* (Issue 1). Chichester, UK: John Wiley.

Manley, A. (1996). *Physical activity and health. A report of the surgeon general.* Pittsburgh, PA: Department of Health and Human Services.

Masters, W. H., & Johnson, V. E. (1966). *Human sexual response.* (Several different publishers since 1966.).

Masters, W. H., & Johnson, V. E. (1970). *Human sexual inadequacy.* (Several different publishers since 1970.).

Mathias, S., Nayak, U., & Isaacs, B. (1986). Balance in elderly patients: The 'get up and go' test. *Archives of Physical Medicine and Rehabilitation, 67,* 387–389.

McCurry, S. M., Gibbons, L. E., Logsdon, R. G., et al. (2003). Training caregivers to change the sleep hygiene practices of patients with dementia: The NITE-AD project. *Journal of the American Geriatrics Society, 51,* 1455–1460.

Molnar, F. J., Byszewski, A. M., Marshall, S. C., & Man-Son-Hing, M. (2005). In-office evaluation of medical fitness to drive: Practical approaches for assessing older people. *Canadian Family Physician, 51,* 372–379.

Nijs, K. A., de Graaf, C., Kok, F. J., et al. (2006). Effect of family style mealtimes on quality of life, physical performance, and body weight of nursing home residents: Cluster randomised controlled trial. *British Medical Journal (Clinical Research Ed.), 332,* 1180–1183.

O'Connell, H., Chin, A. V., Cunningham, C., et al. (2004). Suicide in older people. *British Medical Journal (Clinical Research Ed.), 329,* 895–899.

Ogg, J., & Bennett, G. (1992). Elder abuse in britain. *British Medical Journal (Clinical Research Ed.), 305,* 998–999.

O'Keefe, K., & Sanson, T. (1998). Elderly patients with altered mental status. *Emergency Medicine Clinics of North America, 16,* 701–715.

Price, J., Hermans, D., & Grimley Evans, J. (2002). Subjective barriers to prevent wandering of cognitively impaired people (Cochrane review). In *The Cochrane Library* (Issue 1). Update Software, Oxford.

Rands, G., Orrel, M., Spector, A., et al. (2005). Aspirin for vascular dementia. *Cochrane Database of Systematic Reviews, (1),* CD001296, The Cochrane Collaboration. John Wiley.

Robertson, M. C., Gardner, M. M., Devlin, N., et al. (2001). Effectiveness and economic evaluation of a nurse delivered home exercise programme to prevent falls. 2: Controlled trial in multiple centres. *British Medical Journal (Clinical Research Ed.), 322,* 701–704.

Robinson, J., & Turnock, T. (1998). *Investing in rehabilitation; review findings.* London: King's Fund.

Rooney, E. (1993). Exercise for older patients: Why it's worth the effort. *Geriatrics, 48*, 68–72.

Scherder, E., Oosterman, J., Swaab, D., et al. (2005). Recent developments in pain in dementia. *British Medical Journal (Clinical Research Ed.), 330*, 461–464.

Schneider, L. S., Dagerman, K. S., & Insel, P. (2005). Risk of death with atypical antipsychotic drug treatment for dementia. *JAMA: The Journal of the American Medical Association, 294*, 1934–1943.

Sherrington, C., et al. (2008). Effective exercise for the prevention of falls: A systematic review and meta-analysis. *Journal of the American Geriatrics Society, 56*(12), 2234–2243.

Spector, A., Orrell, M., Davies, S., et al. (2000). Reality orientation for dementia. *Cochrane Database of Systematic Reviews*, (*3*), CD001119, John Wiley.

Stuck, A. E., Sui, A., Wieland, G. D., et al. (1993). Comprehensive geriatric assessment: A meta-analysis of controlled trials. *Lancet, 342*, 1032–1036.

Tabet, N., Birks, J., Grimley Evans, J., et al. (2002). Vitamin E for Alzheimer's disease (Cochrane review). In *The Cochrane Library* (Issue 1). Update Software, Oxford.

Tamblyn, R., Abrahamowicz, M., du Berger, R., et al. (2005). A 5-year prospective assessment of the risk associated with individual benzodiazepines and doses in new elderly users. *Journal of the American Geriatrics Society, 53*, 233–241.

Trichopoulou, A., for members of the Elderly Prospective Study Group (EPIC). (2005). Modified Mediterranean diet and survival: EPIC–elderly prospective cohort study. *British Medical Journal (Clinical Research Ed.), 330*, 991–995.

Venning, G. (2005). Recent developments in vitamin D deficiency and muscle weakness among elderly people. *British Medical Journal (Clinical Research Ed.), 330*, 524–526.

Vetter, N., & Ford, D. (1990). Smoking prevention among people aged 60 and over: A randomized controlled trial. *Age and Ageing, 19*, 164–168.

Walters, A. (1995). Towards a better definition of restless legs syndrome. The international restless legs syndrome study group. *Movement Disorders, 10*, 634–642.

Warner, J., Butler, R., & Arya, P. (2005). Dementia. In *Clinical evidence* (Vol. 12). London: BMJ Publishing Group.

Wilson, K., Mottram, P., Sivanranthan, A., et al. (2002). Antidepressants versus placebo for the depressed elderly (Cochrane review). In *The Cochrane Library* (Issue 1). Update Software, Oxford.

Wolf, S., Barnhart, H., Kutner, N., et al. (1996). Reducing frailty and falls in older persons: An investigation of tai chi and computerized balance training. Atlanta FICSIT group. Frailty and injuries: Cooperative studies of intervention techniques. *Journal of the American Geriatrics Society, 44*, 489–497.

16

Contraception, Sexual Problems, and Sexually Transmitted Infections

LINDSEY POPE

CHAPTER CONTENTS

CONTRACEPTION

INFORMATION

For Professionals
Faculty of Sexual & Reproductive Healthcare, www.fsrh.org

For Patients
Family Planning Association, 23–28 Penn Street, London, N1 5DL, tel. 020 7608 5240, www.fpa.org.uk.

- When giving contraceptive advice it is good practice if this is backed up with appropriate and accessible written information. The Family Planning Association (FPA) provides a range of leaflets covering all methods, which is regularly revised and is available through the local Health Promotion Unit or from the website (see box).
- These leaflets should be used when a patient is deciding on a method, initiating a method, and from time to time as a refresher. However, leaflets are not a substitute for discussion (Jones, 2008).

- Patients wanting to go to a family planning clinic or who are being referred from general practice can get details of a convenient clinic from the FPA. Their website allows a search on a map with details right down to street level.

Hormonal Contraception

Combined Oral Contraceptive Pill

Effectiveness

With perfect use of the combined oral contraceptive (COC) failure rates are as low as 0.3% in the first year (Trussell, 2007). However, with typical use this rises to 8%.

Assessment of the Patient (Clinical Effectiveness Unit, 2006a)

The following are the essential components of the assessment before initiating the COC:

- Menstrual and obstetric history
- History of migraine—presence of aura
- Past or current illnesses that might represent contraindications

- Family history of venous thromboembolism (VTE), myocardial infarction (MI), cerebrovascular accident (CVA), hypertension, and breast cancer
- Current drug therapy (prescribed and over the counter [OTC])
- Allergies
- Blood pressure (BP) measurement (defer starting the COC until 8 weeks after delivery in women who have had preeclampsia, even if BP is normal)
- Baseline height/weight: body mass index (BMI) (important, as it is a risk factor for VTE)
- No blood tests are necessary before first prescription of a COC without specific clinical indication.
- In asymptomatic women breast and pelvic examinations are not recommended before first prescription of a COC (Stewart et al., 2001).

Contraindications

UK Medical Eligibility Criteria (UKMEC) give four categories of condition in which use of the COC is (or is not) contraindicated:

- UKMEC1 is a condition for which there is no restriction on use of the method.
- UKMEC2 is when the advantages of the method generally outweigh the theoretical or proven risks.
- UKMEC3 is when the theoretical or proven risks usually outweigh the advantages. Provision of a method requires expert clinical judgment and/or referral to a specialist contraceptive provider.
- UKMEC4 is a condition that represents an unacceptable health risk and the method should not be used.

Unacceptable Health Risk (UKMEC4) (Clinical Effectiveness Unit, 2016)

- *Breast feeding:* less than 6 weeks postpartum (Clinical Effectiveness Unit, 2009b)
- *Smoking:* aged over 35 years and smoking more than 15 cigarettes/day
- *Cardiovascular disease:* multiple risk factors for arterial cardiovascular disease such as older age, smoking, diabetes, and hypertension. Also, atrial fibrillation and cardiomyopathy with impaired cardiac function.
- *Hypertension:* high BP (≥160 systolic or ≥95 diastolic)
- *Vascular disease:* peripheral vascular disease, hypertensive retinopathy, and transient ischemic attacks (TIAs)
- *Venous thromboembolism:* current or past history
- *Major surgery with prolonged immobilization*
- *Known thrombogenic mutations:* such as factor V Leiden, prothrombin variant G20210A, protein S, protein C, and antithrombin III deficiencies
- *Ischaemic heart disease:* current or past history
- *Stroke:* history of CVA
- *Valvular heart disease:* complicated by pulmonary hypertension, atrial fibrillation, history of infective endocarditis
- *Migraine,* with aura (MacGregor, 2007): The following suggest transient ischaemia and preclude use of the COC: loss of a part of the visual field, unilateral weakness/

paraesthesiae, disturbance of speech, first ever migraine attack after starting COC, status migrainosus. Migraine without aura is relatively safe (this includes blurred vision, photophobia, phonophobia, and flashing lights affecting the whole visual field) for those who did not first develop it while on the COC.

- *Breast cancer:* current
- *Diabetes:* nephropathy, retinopathy, neuropathy, or other vascular disease
- *Viral hepatitis:* acute or flare
- *Cirrhosis:* severe (decompensated)
- *Liver tumours:* benign (hepatocellular adenoma) or malignant (hepatoma)
- *Systemic lupus erythematosus (SLE):* with positive or unknown antiphospholipid antibodies

Risks Usually Outweigh Benefits (UKMEC3) (Clinical Effectiveness Unit, 2016)

- *Breastfeeding:* between 6 weeks and 6 months postpartum and primarily breastfeeding
- *Postpartum* (in non-breastfeeding women): less than 21 days
- *Smoking:* aged 35 years and older and smoking less than 15 cigarettes/day; aged 35 years and older and stopped smoking less than 1 year ago
- *BMI:* 35 and above
- *Multiple risk factors for arterial cardiovascular disease*
- *Hypertension:* on treatment with BP adequately controlled; elevated BP 140 to 159 systolic or 90 to 94 diastolic
- *Family history of VTE:* in a first-degree relative aged 45 years and younger
- *Immobility:* wheelchair use, debilitating illness
- *Hyperlipidaemia:* familial hypercholesterolaemia, for example
- *Migraine:* past history of migraine with aura 5 or more years ago, at any age
- *Breast cancer:* past history of and no evidence of recurrence for 5 years; carriers of known mutations associated with breast cancer (e.g., BRCA1)
- *Gallbladder disease:* symptomatic medically treated or current
- *History of cholestasis:* past COC related
- *Potent enzyme-inducing drugs:* rifampicin, rifabutin, and certain antiepileptic drugs
- *Organ transplant:* complicated by graft failure

Arterial and Venous Thrombosis

- The risk factors for VTE and arterial disease should be assessed separately.
- Age is a risk factor common to both conditions. Many of the risk factors can be viewed as being on a sliding scale—for instance there is not suddenly a problem with age on the 35th birthday.
- Smoking status, weight, and immobility are the only factors that may be changed in the future and the suitability for the COC reviewed.

Choosing a Combined Pill

- Pill formulations contain one of eight progestogens.
- The initial dose of oestrogen should normally be in the range 20 to 35 µg combined with a low or standard dose of progestogen.
- A monophasic COC containing 30 µg ethinylestradiol with norethisterone or levonorgestrel is a suitable first pill.
- As from June 1999, desogestrel- and gestodene-containing pills were recommended again as first line COCs, following the pill scare of October 1995 (Anon., 1999). However, in view of the apparent increased risk of VTE with these preparations (relative risk [RR] 1.7 compared to levonorgestrel or norethisterone pills [Kemmeren, Algra, & Grobbee, 2001]) the slightly increased risk of VTE should be explained to the patient (Table 16.1) and these pills should not be used in those with a risk factor for VTE. Norgestimate-containing pills have similar rates of VTE to levonorgestrel pills (Jick, Kaye, Russmann, & Jick, 2006).
- For all COCs the risk of VTE is greatest in the first year of use. For COCs containing levonorgestrel, for instance, the RR for VTE in the first year is 6.6 compared to women not taking the pill, falling to 1.3 after 5 years of use (Brechin & Penney, 2004).
- Desogestrel- and gestodene-containing pills are probably best avoided for young first-time users. Their risk of VTE is 3.1 times the risk they would run with a levonorgestrel or norethisterone preparation (Kemmeren et al., 2001). These brands may be useful, however, for those who have side effects, for acne sufferers, or for those with cycle control problems.
- Co-cyprindiol (ethinylestradiol with cyproterone acetate) is licensed as an acne treatment but is an effective contraceptive, too. It should be used only in those with significant acne. There is a higher risk of VTE than with levonorgestrel pills: RR 3.9 (Vasilakis-Scaramozza & Jick, 2001).
- Women react individually to the pill; if side effects are experienced it is well worth trying at least one other brand before abandoning the method.

TABLE 16.1	Risks of Venous Thromboembolism	
Background rate of VTE in healthy nonpregnant women not taking a COC	5/100,000/year
Healthy women taking levonorgestrel or norethisterone COCs	15/100,000/year
Healthy women taking gestodene or desogestrel COCs	25/100,000/year
Pregnancy	60/100,000/year

COC, Combined oral contraceptive; *VTE,* venous thromboembolism.

Higher Doses of Oestrogen

Formulations containing 50 µg of ethinylestradiol should not be used unless specific individual circumstances warrant a higher dose:

- Long-term use of an enzyme-inducing drug. NICE recommends that women taking enzyme-inducing antiepileptic drugs are started on 50 µg; if breakthrough bleeding (BTB) occurs, the dose may be increased to 75 or 100 µg daily (Stokes et al., 2004).
- Persistent BTB on a standard-strength COC, provided no other cause is found.
- Past true COC method failure, suggesting unusually rapid metabolism or malabsorption (an alternative is tricycling and shortening the pill-free interval [PFI] to 4 days; see upcoming discussion).

Special Cases

- Recommend an alternative method when there has been a previous failure of COC or where pill efficacy may be reduced because the patient:
  - is on long-term hepatic enzyme-inducing drugs (e.g., for fungal infection, tuberculosis [TB], epilepsy, daytime sleepiness, or human immunodeficiency virus [HIV]) or taking OTC drugs (e.g., St John wort [consult the British National Formulary (BNF)]) (Clinical Effectiveness Unit, 2005a); or
  - has severe malabsorption.
- If an alternative method is unacceptable, consider:
  - starting a high-dose pill or two low-dose pills to give at least 50 µg of ethinylestradiol; or
  - running three packs of pills together (the *tricycle* regimen) plus reducing the 3-monthly PFI to 4 days.
- If BTB still occurs, try 75 or 100 µg per day (Stokes et al., 2004).
  Phased preparations:
- give a better bleeding pattern for a lower monthly dose (has been shown for levonorgestrel preparations) (Rosenberg & Long, 1992);
- are more expensive than fixed-dose preparations, not least because these products attract two dispensing fees (biphasics) or three dispensing fees (triphasics) in the United Kingdom;
- have a reduced margin for error, especially early in the packet;
- may cause premenstrual tension–like symptoms toward the end of the packet;
- are less flexible when a patient wants to postpone a period.

Taking the Pill: Procedure and Advice

Starting the Pill (Clinical Effectiveness Unit, 2006a)

- *Days 1 to 5 of the cycle:* If started on or before day 5, then no other precautions are necessary.
- *After day 5,* other precautions should be used for the first 7 days.
- *Changing from a hormonal method:* COC can be started immediately if the previous method has been used consistently and correctly, or if it is reasonably certain she is not pregnant (Table 16.2). There is no need to wait for the next period.
- *After childbirth:* If starting at the end of the third week postpartum, no other precautions are needed. A later start necessitates extra precautions for 7 days. Note that the earliest recorded ovulation after delivery is day 30 (Guillebaud, 1989), so waiting until a postnatal examination is not an option unless a woman is exclusively breastfeeding.
- *After miscarriage or termination of pregnancy (TOP):* Start within 7 days. If starting later, extra precautions are needed for 7 days. The earliest recorded ovulation after TOP is day 16 (Guillebaud, 1989).

Changing the Pill

- Same or higher strength oestrogen but the same progestogen. Start it after the 7-day break. No extra precautions are necessary.
- Lower strength oestrogen or a different progestogen. Omit the 7-day break. If the break is not omitted, extra precautions are needed for 7 days.

Postponing a Bleed

This is possible (see upcoming discussion).

TABLE 16.2	How a Clinician Can Be Reasonably Certain a Woman Is Not Pregnant (Anon., 2005; Clinical Effectiveness Unit, 2006a)

- There should be no symptoms or signs of pregnancy and any ONE of the following criteria should be met:
  - There has been no sex since the start of the last normal menstrual period.
  - She has been correctly and consistently using a reliable* method of contraception.
  - She is within the first 7 days of her cycle.
  - She is within the first 7 days after an abortion or miscarriage.
  - She is fully breastfeeding, amenorrhoeic, and less than 6 months postpartum.
  - She is not breastfeeding and is less than 3 weeks postpartum or has had no unprotected sex since delivery.
- A pregnancy test adds weight to the diagnosis, but only if 3 weeks have elapsed since the date of last sex.

*The author does not regard condoms, *coitus interruptus,* or fertility awareness as reliable enough to exclude the possibility of pregnancy.

Stopping the Combined Oral Contraceptive

Alternative methods of contraception are needed from the day of stopping the COC, not the end of the PFI.

Advice

Mode of Action

The main action of the pill is to suppress the normal cycle so that ovulation does not occur; the periods while on the pill are withdrawal bleeds. Within 7 days of use the ovaries are fully suppressed. Conversely, during the PFI there is no significant follicular development unless the PFI is lengthened beyond 7 days.

Risks

- *Venous thromboembolism.* The risk of VTE while using any COC is increased but is less than the risk of VTE during pregnancy (see Table 16.1) (Brechin & Penney, 2004).
- *Myocardial infarction.* The risk of MI on a COC is confined to smokers (RR 9.5 compared to nonsmokers not on COC) (Khader, Rice, John, & Abueita, 2003) and those with arterial risk factors. Women who do not smoke, who have their BP checked, and who do not have hypertension or diabetes are at no increased risk of MI on a COC, regardless of their age.
- *Ischaemic stroke.* The risk of ischaemic stroke in COC users is increased (RR 2.7) (Chan et al., 2004). Among women with no history of migraine, who do not smoke, have their BP checked, and who do not have hypertension, the risk is less.
- *Gallstones.* COCs may accelerate the presentation of cholelithiasis in those who are predisposed. Their use should be avoided in those with known gallbladder disease. They can be used after cholecystectomy (UKMEC2) but usually not after medical treatment for gallstones (UKMEC3).
- *Hypertension.* COCs can induce hypertension, particularly in the early months of use (Poulter, 1996). About 1% of COC users become clinically hypertensive with modern formulations. Pill-induced hypertension should not be treated with antihypertensive drugs, but the pill should be stopped and observation continued.
- *Cancer.* Overall the balance of risks and benefits of the COC on cancer is beneficial. There is an increased risk of cancer of the cervix; this is mitigated by a large reduction in risk of cancer of the ovary (RR 0.73) (Collaborative Group on Epidemiological Studies of Ovarian Cancer, 2008) and the endometrium (Weiderpass et al., 1999) and by a reduction in the risk of cancer of the colon (RR 0.82) (Fernandez et al., 2001). The COC probably accelerates development of cancer of the cervix caused by chronic infection with oncogenic human papillomavirus (HPV); with 5 years or more of use the RR is 1.90 (International Collaboration of Epidemiological Studies of Cervical Cancer, 2007). The literature on the COC and breast cancer is conflicting but some good quality

studies show no increased risk (Clinical Effectiveness Unit, 2010b). Both UK cohort studies show no increased risk: RRs of 1.0 (Vessey & Painter, 2006) and 0.90 (Hannaford et al., 2010), respectively. By the age of 40 to 44 however, COC use is associated with 30 extra cancers per 100,000 women.

- *Inflammatory bowel disease (IBD).* IBD may be associated with VTE, hepatobiliary disease, and osteoporosis, all of which would need to be taken into consideration when considering suitability for the COC (Clinical Effectiveness Unit, 2009b). Also the efficacy of the COC may be reduced in women with Crohn disease who have small bowel disease and malabsorption.

Side Effects

There are side effects but most wear off after the first few cycles, especially bloating, nausea, and breast tenderness. Nausea may be reduced by taking the pill at night.

Noncontraceptive Benefits

- The following have been shown to be beneficial effects of the COC:
  - Lighter, shorter bleeding (less anaemia)
  - Less dysmenorrhoea
  - Less premenstrual syndrome (PMS) symptoms
  - Less pelvic inflammatory disease (PID)
  - Fewer ectopic pregnancies
  - Less benign breast disease
  - A bone sparing effect
  - Fewer functional ovarian cysts
  - Less hospitalization for fibroids
  - Less symptomatic endometriosis
- The COC tends to improve acne. There is little to choose between COC formulations. COCs need to be taken for at least 6 months for their full effect on the skin to become apparent. Evidence for the use of co-cyprindiol, if a COC fails to improve acne, is of poor quality (Arowojolu, 2009).

Bleeding

- Withdrawal bleeds are usually lighter than periods.
- BTB may occur during the first two or three cycles.
- BTB is not a reason for stopping the pill in midpacket.

Missed Pills (Clinical Effectiveness Unit, 2006a)

- The riskiest time for pills to be forgotten is on either side of the pill-free week.
- Forgetting in the middle of a packet is less likely to give rise to breakthrough ovulation or pregnancy.
- *If more than 24 hours late*, this is classed as *missed pills* and the agreed rules are as in Fig. 16.1.

Diarrhoea or Vomiting

- This requires extra precautions for the period of illness and for 7 days afterwards, as discussed.
- If this would run into the PFI, the PFI should be omitted.

- However, it is known that diarrhoea has to be of dysenteric proportions to reduce pill absorption.

Drugs for Infections (Clinical Effectiveness Unit, 2005a, 2011)

- The Faculty of Sexual and Reproductive Healthcare (FSRH) no longer recommends the need to use barrier methods of contraception for non–enzyme-inducing antibiotics.
- Rifampicin, rifabutin, griseofulvin, and some antiretroviral drugs (notably ritonavir-boosted protease inhibitors) induce liver enzymes.
- Oral antifungal agents have also been associated with anecdotal reports of COC failure.
- Extra precautions should be taken during the treatment and for 7 days thereafter. If this runs into the PFI the next packet should be started without a break. Rifampicin and rifabutin are such powerful enzyme inducers that extra precautions should be taken for 4 weeks even after a 2-day course and elimination of PFIs during this time (Clinical Effectiveness Unit, 2006a).

Surgery

The COC should be stopped from 4 weeks before until 2 weeks after any major surgery, varicose vein surgery or sclerotherapy, or any operation likely to be followed by immobilization (e.g., leg surgery) (Clinical Effectiveness Unit, 2009). It is otherwise not necessary to stop the COC.

Postponing or Avoiding Bleeds

Monophasic Pills

Patients on a fixed-dose combined pill can postpone the next withdrawal bleed by starting the next packet immediately, omitting the PFI.

Phased Preparations

- If on Synphase, another packet can be taken immediately following the first.
- If taking other phased preparations there would be an abrupt drop in progestogen levels if the above regimen were followed, leading to a risk of bleeding. Advise:
  - tablets from the last phase of a spare packet can be taken, to give 7 (TriNovum) or 10 (Logynon, Triadene) or 14 (Binovum) days' postponement; or
  - a packet can be started of the next higher dose monophasic pill, omitting the PFI. With Qlaira, the 17 highest dose tablets should be used.
- *If postponement by a few days* is needed (e.g., to avoid a bleed at weekends), the necessary number of pills from a fresh pack should be taken and the rest of that pack thrown away. If on phased preparations, they should follow the principles stated earlier.
- *Note: Every Day (ED) preparations.* In all the above mentioned advice, the seven inactive pills in ED preparations should be discarded.
- Extended use of the COC has become widespread; running several or all packets together reduces bleeding days and

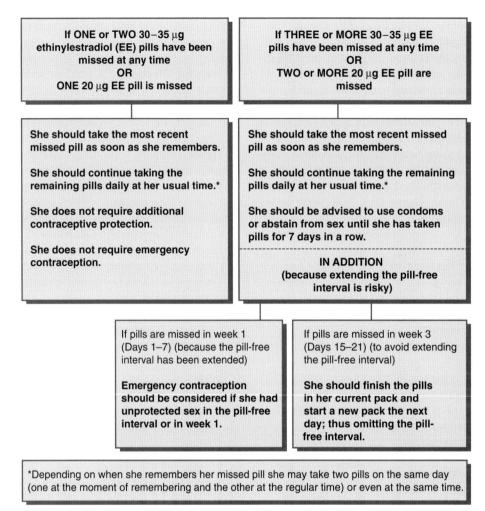

If ONE or TWO 30–35 µg ethinylestradiol (EE) pills have been missed at any time
OR
ONE 20 µg EE pill is missed

She should take the most recent missed pill as soon as she remembers.

She should continue taking the remaining pills daily at her usual time.*

She does not require additional contraceptive protection.

She does not require emergency contraception.

If THREE or MORE 30–35 µg EE pills have been missed at any time
OR
TWO or MORE 20 µg EE pill are missed

She should take the most recent missed pill as soon as she remembers.

She should continue taking the remaining pills daily at her usual time.*

She should be advised to use condoms or abstain from sex until she has taken pills for 7 days in a row.

IN ADDITION
(because extending the pill-free interval is risky)

If pills are missed in week 1 (Days 1–7) (because the pill-free interval has been extended)

Emergency contraception should be considered if she had unprotected sex in the pill-free interval or in week 1.

If pills are missed in week 3 (Days 15–21) (to avoid extending the pill-free interval)

She should finish the pills in her current pack and start a new pack the next day; thus omitting the pill-free interval.

*Depending on when she remembers her missed pill she may take two pills on the same day (one at the moment of remembering and the other at the regular time) or even at the same time.

• **Fig. 16.1** Action to be taken if pills are missed. (Faculty of Family Planning and Reproductive Health Care Clinical Effectiveness Unit. (2005). WHO selected practice recommendations for contraceptive use update. "Missed pills": New recommendations. *Journal of Family Planning and Reproductive Health Care, 31,* 153–155. Reproduced with permission.)

menstrual cycle–related symptoms (Archer, 2006). When used continuously for 1 year, 18% of women achieve amenorrhoea by 3 months of use and 88% by 10 months (Miller & Hughes, 2003). Extended use can be at the personal preference of the woman according to how often she wishes to bleed or recommended on medical grounds (e.g., for low bone density, endometriosis, PMS, or withdrawal headaches).

Follow-Up

- The patient should be seen again at 3 months, or earlier if side effects occur. Do not give repeat prescriptions without someone seeing the patient and at least checking the blood pressure.
- Once established on the pill, see the patient 6-monthly and:
  - assess whether there are any new risk factors, including migraine;
  - check whether the patient is smoking;
  - ask about side effects;

- check BP (discontinue if BP increases to and remains at 160/95 mm Hg). If the BP is satisfactory 2 years after commencement of the COC, BP checks can be extended to annually in women without risk factors or relevant diseases.

Changing the Pill Because of Side Effects

When changing a pill because of side effects, the choice lies between changing oestrogen/progestogen dominance and changing to a pill with a different progestogen (see upcoming discussion).

Breakthrough Bleeding

- BTB occurs in up to 30% of users in the first few cycles but tends to settle by the third cycle. Unless prior warning of this is given, discontinuation rates will be high, especially in the young.
- *If BTB occurs in the first 3 months*, ask whether pills have been missed; encourage the patient to persevere.

- *If BTB continues beyond 3 months*, exclude lesions of the cervix and problems with taking the pill (e.g., vomiting). Also encourage smokers to quit, as they are more likely to have BTB (Rosenberg, Waugh, & Stevens, 1996). Give a pill with a higher progestogen dose, change to a progestogen with better cycle control (e.g., gestodene), or change to a triphasic formulation of the same progestogen. If this fails, consider increasing the oestrogen content as well.
- *If BTB occurs when previous control had been good*, exclude lesions of the cervix, chlamydia infection, interacting drugs, gastrointestinal disorder, and a change to a vegetarian diet.
- *Absent withdrawal bleeds (WB):*
  - Explain that this is not unsafe and does not signify overdosage.
  - Missing one WB does not need any action. If two are missed, exclude pregnancy.
  - If the patient is concerned despite reassurance, consider a switch to a triphasic pill.

Oestrogen Withdrawal Headache During Pill-Free Interval

- Consider advising the patient to use three packets consecutively without a break, followed by a 7-day break (tricycle regimen).

Combined Transdermal Patch

> **RECOMMENDATION**
>
> Recommend the information leaflet from the Family Planning Association at www.fpa.org.uk.

- At present there is only one product in the UK, Evra. This patch releases norelgestromin 150 µg/day and ethinylestradiol 20 µg/day into the circulation. The patch is applied weekly for 21 days and the fourth week is patch free. Suitable sites are the upper outer arm, upper torso (excluding breast), buttock, or lower abdomen.
- Effectiveness is similar to the COC. The same contraindications apply as for the COC. Also, the same drug interactions as for the COC must be presumed. BTB and spotting and breast tenderness are more common than with the COC in the first two cycles.
- *If a patch is partly detached for less than 24 hours,* it should be reapplied to the same site or replaced with a new patch immediately. No additional contraception is needed and the next patch should be applied on the usual change day.
- *If a patch remains detached for more than 24 hours* or if the user is not aware when the patch became detached she should stop the current contraceptive cycle and start a new cycle by applying a new patch, giving a new day 1—additional precautions must be used concurrently for the first 7 days of the new cycle.
- *If application of a new patch at the start of a new cycle is delayed*, contraceptive protection is lost. A new patch should be applied as soon as remembered giving a new day 1—additional nonhormonal methods of contraception should be used for the first 7 days of the new cycle. If intercourse has occurred during this extended patch-free interval, a possibility of fertilization should be considered.
- If applications of a patch in the middle of the cycle is delayed (i.e., the patch is not changed on day 8 or day 15):
  - for up to 48 hours, apply a new patch immediately; next patch change day remains the same and no additional precautions are required;
  - for more than 48 hours, contraceptive protection may have been lost. Stop the current cycle and start a new 4-week cycle immediately by applying a new patch giving a new day 1. Additional precautions should be used for the first 7 days of the new cycle.
- *If the patch is not removed at the end of the cycle* (day 22), remove it as soon as possible and start the next cycle on the usual change day, after day 28. No extra precautions are required.

Combined Vaginal Ring (Clinical Effectiveness Unit, 2009c)

- NuvaRing was launched in 2009. It releases 120 µg etonogestrel and 15 µg ethinylestradiol/day from an ethylene vinyl acetate copolymer ring with an outer diameter of 54 mm. The same contraindications and drug interactions apply as for the COC.
- Tampon use has no effect on the systemic absorption of the hormones released from NuvaRing.
- A ring can be removed (e.g., for sex) for up to 3 hours.
- Prior to dispensing, NuvaRing is stored at 2° to 8°C. Once dispensed, storage is at room temperature and the shelf life is 4 months.
- Women use a ring for 3 weeks followed by a ring-free week during which time they have a withdrawal bleed. A new ring is needed for each 4-week cycle.
- NuvaRing has high effectiveness no different from the combined pill, especially when adherence is good (Ahrendt et al., 2006; Oddsson, Leifels-Fischer, de Melo, et al., 2005).
- Cycle control is better than with the combined pill (Bjarnadóttir, Tuppurainen, & Killick, 2002; Merki-Feld & Hund, 2007; Oddson, Leifels-Fischer, Wiel-Masson, et al., 2005; Roumen, op ten Berg, & Hoomans, 2006).
- The ring can cause leucorrhoea, vaginal discomfort, vaginitis, and ring-related events comprising foreign-body sensation, coital problems, and expulsion (Ahrendt et al., 2006; Oddsson, Leifels-Fischer, de Melo, et al., 2005).
- *If the ring-free interval is extended beyond 7 days*, the woman should insert a new ring as soon as she remembers. Extra precautions should be used for the next 7 days. If unprotected sex took place during the ring-free interval, the use of emergency contraception can be considered or a pregnancy test done after 3 weeks.
- *If the ring was temporarily outside the vagina*, it should be rinsed in lukewarm water and reinserted. If the ring was outside the vagina for less than 3 hours, no further

action is necessary. If the ring was outside the vagina for more than 3 hours, extra precautions should be used for the next 7 days. If the loss in continuity of use of the ring for more than 3 hours occurs in the third week of use, a new ring should be inserted without the ring-free interval.

- *If the ring is left in place for more than 3 weeks,* this is acceptable up to a total of 4 weeks, even if there is then a ring-free week. If the ring has been left in the vagina for longer than 4 weeks, pregnancy should be excluded before another ring is inserted.

Progestogen-Only Pill (Clinical Effectiveness Unit, 2008a)

There are four traditional progestogen-only pills (POPs) available. A POP containing desogestrel (Cerazette) was launched in 2002 (Clinical Effectiveness Unit, 2003b). This is much more likely than traditional POPs to inhibit ovulation, but comparative data on efficacy are lacking. Available data show that effectiveness is similar to the COC (Trussell, 2007) but traditional POPs are probably less effective than COCs.

Patients for Whom the Progestogen-Only Pill Is Particularly Indicated

- *Older women:* those over 45 years old without risk factors, and those over 35 years old who smoke
- *Those with medical contraindications to oestrogen,* including a personal history of VTE
- *Those with risk factors for arterial disease,* including hypertension, diabetes mellitus, migraine with aura, and smokers aged 35 years and older
- *Lactating mothers:* progestogen in the breast milk has no adverse effect on the baby (Clinical Effectiveness Unit, 2009b)
- *Those who choose it,* especially those aged over 25 or 30 years, and who accept that it may be less reliable than the COC

Unacceptable Health Risk (UKMEC4)
(Clinical Effectiveness Unit, 2016)

- *Breast cancer:* current

Risks Usually Outweigh Benefits (UKMEC3)
(Clinical Effectiveness Unit, 2016)

- *Ischaemic heart disease:* current or past history, if occurred when on POP
- *Stroke:* history of CVA, if occurred when on POP
- *Breast cancer:* past and no evidence of current disease for 5 years
- *Cirrhosis:* severe (decompensated)
- *Liver tumours:* benign (hepatocellular adenoma) and malignant (hepatoma)
- *SLE:* with positive or unknown antiphospholipid antibodies
- *Enzyme-inducing drugs.*

Taking the Progestogen-Only Pill: Procedure and Advice

INFORMATION FOR PATIENTS

Recommend the information leaflet from the Family Planning Association at www.fpa.org.uk.

Starting the POP:

- *Days 1 to 5 of the cycle:* If started on or before day 5 then no other precautions need be taken.
- *After day 5:* Extra precautions should be taken for the first 2 days.
- *Switch from COC:* If changing from a COC, go straight on to the POP without a 7-day break. Extra precautions are not necessary although it may be necessary to take the pill at a different time of day.
- *Postpartum:* Start at 3 weeks postpartum. Extra precautions are only needed for the next 2 days if starting later than that.

  Note: Time of day. Traditional POPs must be taken regularly at the same time each day (ideally at least 4 hours before the most frequent time of intercourse to ensure maximal mucous-thickening effect).

Advice

- *Efficacy.* Efficacy is lowest in women with no alteration in cycle activity and is greatest in those with complete suppression of cycles and consequent amenorrhoea. Roughly 40% of women continue to ovulate, in 40% there is variable interference with the follicular and luteal phase, and in 20% ovulation is inhibited completely.
- *Bleeding pattern.* From efficacy, it follows that 40% have similar cycles to their normal pattern, 40% have shorter cycles (which may gradually lengthen toward normal over time) with episodes of spotting or BTB, and 20% have long cycles or amenorrhoea.
- *Safety.* There is no evidence of increased cardiovascular risk (Heinemann, Assmann, DoMinh, & Garbe, 1999). However, there is limited evidence of an increased risk of breast cancer for use in the previous 5 years (RR 1.17), but no increase 10 or more years after stopping (Collaborative Group on Hormonal Factors in Breast Cancer, 1996).
- *Antibiotics.* The POP is not affected by antibiotics, except rifampicin, rifabutin, and griseofulvin (see Enzyme-inducing drugs [last bullet of this list]).
- *Missed pills.* If one or more pills are missed or delayed for more than 3 hours then take one pill as soon as remembered; take the next pill at the usual time (this may mean taking two pills in 1 day); continue taking pills, one daily; extra precautions need to be taken for 2 days. For Cerazette the instructions are the same, except the window is 12 hours instead of 3 hours. Emergency contraception can be considered if unprotected sex occurs during this 2-day period.

- *Diarrhoea or vomiting.* If vomiting or diarrhoea occurs, continue to take the pill regularly but take extra precautions during the attack and for the next 2 days.
- *Obesity.* There is no evidence that the efficacy of POPs is reduced in women weighing over 70 kg; the licensed use of one pill per day is recommended.
- *Enzyme-inducing drugs.* Those on enzyme-inducing drugs are best advised not to rely on POPs (Clinical Effectiveness Unit, 2005a, 2008a).

Side Effects

Non-Menstrual

These are the usual progestogenic ones such as headaches, tender breasts, acne, depression, weight gain, and loss of sexual drive. But because the dose of progestogen is so low, these side effects are not that common and often not severe.

Irregular Bleeding

- Examine to exclude a pathologic cause.
- Do not change to another POP. There is no suggestion that with traditional POPs changing brand will improve menstrual or nonmenstrual side effects.
- Suggest a change to another method.

Abdominal Pain of Gynaecologic Origin

- Consider ectopic pregnancy. If it can be excluded, then refer for ultrasound. It may be due to a functional ovarian cyst. Such a cyst usually resolves without treatment.

Amenorrhoea When Cycles Have Been Present

- Exclude pregnancy before assuming that it is due to the POP.
- Encourage the woman to persevere with the POP. She is in the group least likely to become pregnant with it.

Injectable Progestogens (Clinical Effectiveness Unit, 2008b)

> **INFORMATION FOR PATIENTS**
>
> Recommend the information leaflet from the Family Planning Association at www.fpa.org.uk.

Preparations

- Depot Medroxypogesterone acetate (DMPA) as Depo-Provera (150 mg in 1 mL) or Sayana Press (104 mg in 0.65 mL). Mix the pre-loaded syringe thoroughly before administration.
- Norethisterone enantate (NE), or Noristerat: 200 mg in 1 mL. Warm the vial close to body temperature before administration.
  Note: NE is not licensed for long-term use. When used for longer than 16 weeks, this use outside the licence must be discussed with the patient.

Indications

The indications are similar to those for the POP. Patients for whom injectable progestogens are especially indicated are women:

- *likely to forget* (or to worry about forgetting) to take daily pills;
- *for whom higher dose, long-term progestogens are beneficial* (e.g., those with fibroids or endometriosis);
- *with sickle cell disease:* DMPA improves the blood picture and reduces the number of crises (Westhoff, 2003).

Unacceptable Health Risk (UKMEC4) (Clinical Effectiveness Unit, 2016)

- *Breast cancer:* current

Risks Outweigh Benefits (WHO3) (Clinical Effectiveness Unit, 2016)

- *Vascular disease:* ischaemic heart disease, peripheral vascular disease, hypertensive retinopathy, or TIAs (Injectables have hypooestrogenic effects and reduce HDL levels.)
- *Stroke:* history of CVA
- *Unexplained vaginal bleeding:* before evaluation
- *Breast cancer:* past and no evidence of current disease for 5 years
- *Diabetes:* with nephropathy, retinopathy, neuropathy, other vascular disease
- *Cirrhosis:* severe (decompensated)
- *Liver tumours:* benign (hepatocellular adenoma) or malignant (hepatoma)
- *SLE:* with positive or unknown antiphospholipid antibodies

Before Starting

Discuss with the patient the following factors.

Advantages

- Injectables are effective and independent of coitus, with no oestrogenic side effects.
- They are invisible to others, which may be important to some women (e.g., those in controlling or abusive relationships).
- They decrease the risk of endometrial cancer, pelvic inflammatory disease, ectopic pregnancy, fibroids, and iron deficiency anaemia (Westhoff, 2003).
- They may enhance lactation and relieve premenstrual and menstrual symptoms.
- Seizure control has been reported to be improved in some epileptics.

Effectiveness

- Injectables are a very effective means of contraception: perfect use failure rates are below 0.7% for DMPA in the first year and below 1.0% for NE. Typical use failure rates are 3%.
- Blood levels of DMPA are not affected by drugs including enzyme inducers; there is no justification

for increasing the dose or reducing injection intervals for this reason (Clinical Effectiveness Unit, 2005a). With NE, care is needed with concurrent antiretroviral therapy, certain antiepileptics, and rifampicin/rifabutin (UKMEC2).

Side Effects

- *Erratic bleeding.* This will occur in most women initially. Prolonged episodes of bleeding may occur but are rarely heavy and decrease over time (World Health Organisation [WHO], 1987).
  - Examine (especially the cervix).
  - Give either:
    a. the next injection early (but not earlier than 4 weeks after the last one); or
    b. a short course of oestrogen (e.g., the COC, if no contraindication); or
    c. a course of mefenamic acid.
  - Refer if the above do not control the bleeding.
  - Alternatively, the patient may prefer to discontinue the method.
- *Amenorrhoea.* This is likely, more so the longer the method is used. The amenorrhoea rate with DMPA is around 70% at 12 months (Canto De Cetina, Canto, & Ordoñez Luna, 2001). With NE, episodes of bleeding are the more usual pattern and the amenorrhoea rate at 12 months is 25%. Explain that these methods make the lining of the womb so thin that there is no monthly shedding. Many women find the amenorrhoea a very acceptable side effect.
  - Exclude pregnancy (beware of weight gain at successive visits with nausea or breast symptoms).
  - Discuss other concerns. There is concern that injectables can lower ovarian oestradiol production; see *Reduced Bone Mineral Density* (under Risks). There is a lack of consensus on any action to be taken with continuous amenorrhoea for over 5 years. Some authorities have recommended checking serum oestradiol but this is not a useful proxy indicator for bone mineral density (BMD). Bone densitometry is the test of choice but is expensive and not always freely available.
- *Weight gain.* This is possible, through appetite stimulation, although some studies show no effect on weight (Westhoff, 2003). The weight gain is not generally the result of fluid retention. Modification of diet and behaviour will tend to counteract the weight gain. Any weight gain is less likely with NE.
- *Return of fertility.* This may be delayed, with a mean time to ovulation of 18 weeks from the expiry of the last dose of DMPA (maximum 49 weeks). Return of fertility is much faster with NE: mean of 4 weeks and maximum of 26 weeks (Fotherby & Howard, 1986).

Risks

- *Reduced BMD.* DMPA reduces BMD in many women who use it. However, so far no studies have shown an increased risk of osteoporosis or fractures. When a reduction in BMD occurs, it takes place over the first 2 or 3 years and then tends to level off. The reduction is generally less than 1 SD (i.e., not into the osteopenic range) (Curtis & Martins, 2006). After discontinuation of DMPA, BMD consistently returns toward, or to, baseline values in women of all ages (Kaunitz, Arias, & McClung, 2008). Patterns of BMD recovery are similar to those seen after cessation of lactation. Available evidence does not justify the requirement of a limit to the duration of DMPA use, even in adolescents. Care is needed in high-risk groups: smokers, BMI less than 19, thyroid disease, long-term antiepileptic therapy, and those with a family history of osteoporosis. Avoid in those on oral steroids.
- *Cancer.* There is limited evidence of an increased risk of breast cancer for use in the previous 5 years (RR 1.17), but no increase 10 or more years after stopping (Collaborative Group on Hormonal Factors in Breast Cancer, 1996). DMPA has a strong protective effect against endometrial cancer (RR 0.21) (WHO, 1991).

Initiating Treatment and Follow-Up

Schedule for the Injections

- Give the first injection within 5 days of the onset of menstruation, within 3 weeks of delivery, or 1 to 5 days after miscarriage or termination. The patient should use additional precautions for 7 days after the first injection unless it was given as mentioned earlier.
- Use the upper outer quadrant of the buttock or the lateral thigh. The deltoid is used when the patient is obese, as it is important the drug reaches muscle. Warn the patient not to massage the site as this may speed up drug release.
- Give subsequent injections: Depo-Provera 150 mg Sayana Press 13-weekly; Noristerat 200 mg 8-weekly.
- If the patient returns late for the next injection of DMPA or NE, proceed as in Table 16.3.

Etonogestrel-Releasing Implant: Nexplanon (Clinical Effectiveness Unit, 2014)

INFORMATION FOR PATIENTS

Recommend the information leaflet from the Family Planning Association at www.fpa.org.uk.

- Nexplanon releases a mean etonogestrel dose of 60–70 µg/day when first inserted, decreasing to 25–30 µ/day by the end of year 3.
- Subdermal implants should only be inserted and removed if specific practical training has been obtained and a minimum number of implants are inserted and removed to keep up the necessary skills.
- Nexplanon has the advantage that it lasts for 3 years but is reversible should the need arise. It has a high effectiveness, 0.05% in the first year, higher even than vasectomy.

TABLE 16.3 Management of Late Injections of Injectable Progestogens (Clinical Effectiveness Unit, 2008)

Timing of Injection	Has Unprotected Sex Occurred?	Can the Injection Be Given?	Is Emergency Contraception Indicated?[a]	Is Additional Contraception or Abstinence Advised?	Should a Pregnancy Test Be Performed?
Up to 14 weeks since last DMPA injection or up to 10 weeks since last NET-EN injection	Not applicable, as long as next injection is given 14 weeks since last DMPA injection or 10 weeks since last NET-EN injection or before	Yes	No	No	No
When an injection is overdue: 14 weeks + 1 day or more since last DMPA injection; or 10 weeks + 1 day or more since last NET-EN injection	No (abstained or used barrier methods)	Yes	No	Yes, for the next 7 days	No, if abstained Yes, if used barrier methods, but at least 21 days later
	Yes, but only in the last 3 days[b]	Yes	Yes, should offer Levonelle 1500 or a copper IUD	Yes, for the next 7 days	Yes, at least 21 days later
	Yes, but only in the last 4–5 days[b]	Yes	Yes, should offer a copper IUD	No, if opts for copper IUD	Yes, at least 21 days later
	Yes, more than 5 days ago[b]	No	No	Yes, for 21 days until a pregnancy test is confirmed negative and for a further 7 days after giving injection	Yes, at the initial presentation and at least 21 days later

[a]If EC is declined, decisions about ongoing use of DMPA/NET-EN should be tailored to the individual woman. Alternative methods if required should then be considered.
[b]Not applicable if unprotected sex occurred within 14 weeks of last DMPA injection or 10 weeks of last NET-EN injection.
DMPA, Depot medroxyprogesterone acetate; *EC,* emergency contraception; *IUD,* intrauterine device; *NET-EN,* norethisterone enanthate.
Reproduced with permission of the Faculty of Sexual and Reproductive Healthcare.

Pregnancies in women using a contraceptive implant are generally due to noninsertion and drug interactions (Harrison-Woolrych & Hill, 2005).

- The return of fertility after removal of Nexplanon is immediate; ovulation occurs mostly within 3 weeks of removal. Progestogen only implants have a beneficial effect on dysmenorrhoea. Nexplanon is more cost effective than the COC.
- Disadvantages are the discomfort of insertion and removal.
- *Practicalities.* If it is implanted other than on days 1 to 5 of the menstrual cycle, extra precautions are needed for the first 7 days, if there is no previous method providing cover. For postpartum women, including those who are breastfeeding, insert at up to 3 weeks postpartum. Following abortion or miscarriage, insert at up to 5 days. The patient should use additional precautions for 7 days after insertion unless timed as above.

Unacceptable Health Risk (UKMEC4)
(Clinical Effectiveness Unit, 2016)

- *Breast cancer:* current

Risks Outweigh Benefits (UKMEC3)
(Clinical Effectiveness Unit, 2016)

- *Ischaemic heart disease:* current or past history
- *Stroke:* history of CVA, if occurred when using implant
- *Unexplained vaginal bleeding:* before evaluation
- *Breast cancer:* past history and no evidence of current disease for 5 years
- *Cirrhosis:* severe (decompensated)
- *Liver tumours* benign (hepatocellular adenoma) or malignant (hepatoma)
- *SLE:* with positive or unknown antiphospholipid antibodies

Monitoring

- There is no reason to check weight and blood pressure.
- There is no reason to do any routine follow-up.

Problems With the Implant
Menstrual

- Bleeding patterns are variable even in an individual over time. Frequent irregular bleeding, spotting, and prolonged bleeding are all possible; heavy bleeding is rare.

- Amenorrhoea occurs in 21% of users.
- Those who discontinue tend to be from the groups with less favourable patterns: prolonged bleeding (17%) and frequent bleeding (6%).
- Problematic bleeding can be treated as per injectables (see page 255). Some clinicians add a progestogen such as Cerazette or norethisterone; there are no data to support this.

Non-Menstrual

Non-Menstrual problems include acne, mastalgia, headache, weight gain, abdominal pain, emotional lability, and depression.

Nonhormonal Methods of Contraception

Intrauterine Devices (Clinical Effectiveness Unit, 2015)

INFORMATION FOR PATIENTS

Recommend the information leaflet from the Family Planning Association at www.fpa.org.uk.

- Typical use failure rates for copper intrauterine devices (IUDs) are 0.8% in the first year (Trussell, 2007).
- IUDs should only be fitted if specific practical training has been obtained and a minimum number of devices are fitted to keep up the necessary skills.
- All IUDs with frames have copper on the stem and/or on the arms. GyneFix is a frameless device with six copper cylinders on a thread. Modern copper-containing IUDs are clinically effective and safe for at least 5 years. The TT380 Slimline and TCu380A QuickLoad are effective for 10 years.
- The risk of perforation associated with insertion of IUDs is 1 in 1000.
- IUDs do not offer any protection against sexually transmitted infections (STIs) but previous studies that purported to show an increased risk of pelvic inflammatory disease (PID) have now been shown to be flawed (Grimes, 2000). There is no evidence that prophylactic use of antibiotics for IUD insertion is of significant benefit in healthy women (Grimes, Lopez, Schulz, & Stanwood, 2004).
- Currently available high-load IUDs protect against ectopic pregnancy when compared to using no contraception.
- Cumulative expulsion rates at 5 years for copper IUDs are around 5%. Expulsion may occur at any time after insertion, but is most likely in the early cycles, especially during menstruation. Patients who are older and of higher parity are less likely to expel their device.

Unacceptable Health Risk (UKMEC4) (Clinical Effectiveness Unit, 2016

- Pregnancy
- Puerperal sepsis
- Immediately after septic abortion
- Insertion before evaluation of unexplained vaginal bleeding

- Gestational trophoblastic disease—with persistently elevated beta-human chorionic gonadotropin (β-hCG) levels or malignant disease
- Cervical or endometrial cancer: current
- STI (current purulent cervicitis, chlamydial infection, or gonorrhoea) or PID: current
- Pelvic TB

Risks Usually Outweigh Benefits (UKMEC3) (Clinical Effectiveness Unit, 2016)

- Postpartum insertion between 48 hours and 4 weeks postpartum—in women who are breastfeeding, not breastfeeding, or post caesarean section.
- Distortion of the uterine cavity (e.g., congenital malformation, submucous fibroids)
- Ovarian cancer

Adverse Effects

Heavier Periods, Intermenstrual Bleeding, Dysmenorrhoea

- Warn the patient that these are common in the first few cycles after insertion.
- Examine for infection or malposition of the device.
- Prescribe nonsteroidal antiinflammatory drugs (NSAIDs), which may reduce pain and bleeding.
- Remove the IUD if it appears to be associated with a change in bleeding pattern. If the pattern does not return to normal, refer for gynaecologic assessment.

Pelvic Infection

- Symptoms of infection require examination and endocervical swabs for STIs.
- Treat with antibiotics.
- If the symptoms settle, the IUD can be left in place.
- *Actinomyces-like organisms (ALOs)* may be found on a cervical smear:
  - If the patient is asymptomatic, leave the IUD in place.
  - If the patient has symptoms (i.e., pain or discharge) remove the IUD and investigate the patient for pelvic pain/STIs, treat with antibiotics as appropriate, and consider referral to genitourinary medicine (GUM) or gynaecology.

Pregnancy

- If symptoms suggest an ectopic pregnancy, admit to hospital; 6% of pregnancies that occur with an IUD in place are ectopic.
- If a scan indicates that the pregnancy is intrauterine, gently remove the IUD if the threads are visible and the pregnancy is less than 12 weeks. This will halve the miscarriage rate. If the pregnancy is beyond 12 weeks or no threads are seen, refer early for antenatal assessment.

Lost Threads

- Teach the patient to feel for the threads after each period, or on the first of the month if there is amenorrhoea with the IUD.

- If the threads are not palpable, warn the patient temporarily to use other precautions, and arrange for ultrasound scan (USS).
- If USS confirms that the device is in situ, leave in place until it is due to be changed. Repeat vaginal examination yearly, and only repeat USS if there is reason to suspect expulsion.

Timing of Insertion

- Insertion can be at any time during the menstrual cycle if it is reasonably certain a woman is not pregnant (see Table 16.2).
- Do not insert before 4 weeks postpartum.
- An IUD can be safely fitted immediately after a first trimester abortion (spontaneous or therapeutic), although this carries an increased risk of expulsion (Grimes et al., 2004).

Removal or Refit

- *Women aged 40 and over:* An IUD fitted after the age of 40 can be left as the only means of contraception until the menopause. When there has been 6 months of amenorrhoea it should be removed; later removal may be difficult because of cervical stenosis. If a woman presents more than 6 months after the menopause with a device in situ, attempt to remove it. If difficulty is encountered try again after a short course of treatment with topical oestrogen.

Timing of Removal

- *If pregnancy is desired*, the IUD may be removed at any time.
- *If pregnancy is not desired*, remove the IUD when the patient is established on a hormonal method or when barrier methods have been used carefully since the last period.
- *Emergency contraception* may be necessary if intercourse has occurred within the last 5 days and removal of the IUD is urgent.

Prophylactic Antibiotics for Cardiac Disease

For women with previous endocarditis or with a prosthetic heart valve it is no longer recommended to give antibiotic prophylaxis during IUD insertion or removal (NICE, 2008).

Follow-Up

- Review after 6 weeks. Thereafter follow-up is not necessary.
- Ask about menstrual blood loss, pelvic pain, vaginal discharge, and discomfort to the partner.
- Do a pelvic examination and check the presence of the threads.

Intrauterine System (Clinical Effectiveness Unit, 2015)

INFORMATION FOR PATIENTS

Recommend the information leaflet from the Family Planning Association at www.fpa.org.uk.

- The steroid reservoir in the Mirena IUS contains 52 mg levonorgestrel. It is licensed for contraception and menorrhagia (for 5 years) and for endometrial protection (4 years). It is more cost effective than the COC (National Collaborating Centre for Women's and Children's Health, 2005).
- The steroid reservoir in the Jaydess IUS contains 13.5 mg levonorgestrel. It is licensed for contraception (for 3 years) but not for menorrhagia although it does reduce menstrual bleeding. It is smaller in size than Mirena.
- *Protection after insertion.* The IUS takes 7 days to provide effective contraceptive protection. Unless the IUS is inserted within the first 7 days of the cycle, extra precautions are advised for the next 7 days. If there has been a risk of conception it would be inappropriate to insert an IUS that cycle.
- *The IUS in older women.* Women who have the Mirena inserted at the age of 45 or over for contraception can retain the device until the menopause is confirmed or until contraception is no longer required.

Advantages of the IUS Over IUDs

- They reduce blood loss instead of increasing it and they are a form of therapy for menorrhagia (although Jaydess is not licensed for this), even in the presence of fibroids.
- They can reduce dysmenorrhoea.
- They are more reliable as a contraceptive, with a failure rate of 0.2% in the first year compared to 0.8% for copper IUDs. The IUS approximate in effectiveness to female sterilization.
- It has a very low rate of ectopic pregnancy.

Disadvantages of the IUS

- The initial cost is much more than IUDs.
- It is slightly more difficult to insert than a copper IUD because of a wider insertion diameter (although this is less of an issue with Jaydess).
- The patient may have irregular slight bleeding in the first 3 months of use.
- Progestogenic side effects (headache, breast tenderness, nausea, mood changes, acne) are possible, especially at the start, as there is some systemic absorption; the rate of occurrence is no different from IUDs after 5 years.

Patients for Whom the IUS Is Particularly Indicated

- As an alternative to sterilization when the family is complete
- Those with menorrhagia
- Those in whom the COC is contraindicated
- Those with learning disabilities or physical disabilities needing long-term contraception

Unacceptable Health Risk (UKMEC4) (Clinical Effectiveness Unit, 2016)

In addition to the conditions listed for the IUD:

- *Breast cancer:* current

Risks Usually Outweigh Benefits (UKMEC3) (Clinical Effectiveness Unit, 2016)

In addition to conditions listed for the IUD:

- *Ischaemic heart disease:* current or past history, if developed while IUS in situ
- *Cirrhosis:* severe (decompensated)
- *Liver tumours:* benign (hepatocellular adenoma) and malignant (hepatoma)
- *SLE:* with positive or unknown antiphospholipid antibodies

Barrier Methods (Clinical Effectiveness Unit, 2007a, 2007b)

INFORMATION FOR PATIENTS

Recommend the information leaflet from the Family Planning Association at www.fpa.org.uk.

- These have the advantage of protecting against STIs and HPV, as well as pregnancy.
- However, efficacy is utterly dependent on consistent use before/during sex; there is considerable potential for user failure, especially among young people.
- Condoms and diaphragms made of latex rubber can be damaged by oil-based products such as:
  - baby oil/bath oil/body oil/Vaseline;
  - suntan oil/massage oil;
  - cream/ice cream/salad cream;
  - lipstick/hair conditioner;
  - many antithrush preparations;
  - progesterone pessaries.

Male Condoms

- Male condoms give a pregnancy rate of 2% to 15% in the first year. Non-latex condoms are now available in addition to latex rubber products; they cannot be damaged by oil-based products.
- Ensure the couple knows to use condoms bearing the CE mark and preferably also the British Standards Institution Kitemark.
- Advise the couple about use of emergency contraception in the event of a mishap.

Female Condom

- Femidom is a loose-fitting polyurethane sheath with two flexible rings, which is inserted into the vagina.
- It is prelubricated with dimeticone, an odourless, non-spermicidal lubricant.
- It lines the vagina and covers some of the vulva. It is disposable and comes in one size. Its failure rate is 5% to 21% in the first year.

Diaphragms

- Diaphragms are more effective than the condom; they have the advantage that they do not need to be inserted and removed at the time of intercourse.

- They are not as effective a protector as condoms against STIs.
- They have a failure rate of 6% to 16% in the first year.
- They come in sizes rising in steps of 5 mm and in the form of coiled spring, arcing spring, or flat spring. Coil spring and arcing diaphragms are also available in silicone. Correct size and type are determined on vaginal examination.
- *Use:*
  - The diaphragm should be inserted before sex and left in place for at least 6 hours after the last act of sex.
  - A strip of spermicide about 5 cm long should be placed on the upper side of the diaphragm before insertion. If sex takes place more than 3 hours later, more spermicide should be inserted, either as a pessary or as cream with an applicator.
  - The diaphragm must be washed in warm soapy water, dried after use, and stored in a cool place in its container to maintain its shape.
- Check the fit and comfort after 1 week and discuss again the routine for its use.
- See after 3 months and then annually, but more frequently if there are difficulties or if there is a weight change of more than 3 kg.
- Prescribe a new diaphragm annually.

Cervical Caps

- FemCap is made of silicone. Failure rates are 10% to 18% in the first year. Before starting, sizing is needed by a doctor or nurse. FemCap comes in three sizes and is reusable.
- Diaphragms and caps should not be used if the woman has a history of toxic shock syndrome (UKMEC3).
- Condoms, diaphragms, and caps should not be used in people with latex allergy (UKMEC3).

Fertility Awareness

- Fertility awareness or natural family planning (NFP) relies on avoidance of intercourse around the time of ovulation.
- Failure rates can be as low as 2.6% in the first year when multiple indicators are used to define the beginning and the end of the fertile period (European Natural Family Planning Study Groups, 1993), but this high efficacy is only achieved by highly motivated and well-trained couples.
- Expert training is essential; advise the patient to contact Fertility UK (see box) for information about local classes. Computerized thermometers and saliva testing kits are on sale but they are unevaluated and cannot be recommended.

PATIENT INFORMATION

Fertility UK, Bury Knowle Health Centre, 207 London Road, Headington, Oxford, OX3 9JA, www.fertilityuk.org.

- Recognized indicators are:
  - waking (basal) body temperature changes;
  - changes in cervical secretions;
  - cervical changes;
  - calculation based on cycle length;
  - minor changes (e.g., mittelschmerz [midcycle pain])
- Combining indicators is best; the combination of temperature and cervical secretions (*symptothermal*) is commonly used.
- *Persona* is a fertility monitor that measures estrone-3-glucuronide and luteinizing hormone (LH) in the urine and predicts fertile days for an individual by storing information on the woman's biochemistry and cycle length. It requires eight urine tests per cycle. A red light indicates fertile days and a green light indicates non-fertile days. A yellow light indicates that a urine test is required. It must be realized that when this device is used by the non-NFP fraternity without combining indicators, failure rates will be higher. Nevertheless, a failure rate of 6.2% in the first year is predicted in such a population (Bonnar et al., 1999).

Emergency Contraception (Clinical Effectiveness Unit, 2017)

Hormonal Preparations

- *The progestogen-only method* is available as levonorgestrel 1500 µg: Levonelle 1500 on prescription and as Levonelle One Step as a pharmacy item.
- Ulipristal acetate 30 mg (ellaOne), a progesterone receptor modulator is on prescription only.

Intrauterine Device Insertion

- *Insertion of a copper-IUD* can be considered if:
  - the patient presents within 5 days of unprotected intercourse; or
  - the patient presents within 5 days of the calculated time of ovulation if intercourse took place more than 5 days before presentation.
- Patients who have failed to take oral contraception correctly:
  - *COC.* Either method can be considered for a patient who misses three or more pills (see Fig. 16.1).
  - *POP.* Either method can be considered for a patient who has unprotected sex during the 48-hour window after regular pill taking has been re-established after missed pills.

Regimen for Hormonal Emergency Contraception

- One tablet of Levonelle 1500 taken within 72 hours of (the first episode of) unprotected intercourse.
- One tablet of ulipristal taken within 120 hours of (the first episode of) unprotected intercourse.

Contraindications

- Established pregnancy.
- *IUD.* Contraindications to the insertion of an IUD apply except that, in an emergency, an IUD can be inserted with antibiotic cover in a patient at risk of PID. Contraindications to the long-term use of an IUD do not apply because the IUD can be removed after the next period.
- Ulipristal should not be used in those needing oral steroids such as asthma or in those on drugs which increase gastric pH (e.g., antacids, H2-receptor antagonists, or proton pump inhibitors).

Special Situations

- *Enzyme-inducing drugs.* These may be prescribed or bought OTC. Patients taking enzyme-inducing drugs should take two Levonelle 1500 pills instead of one. Ulipristal should not be used in those taking enzyme-inducers.
- *Previous ectopic pregnancy.* Patients should understand that neither method will protect against a further ectopic pregnancy.
- The woman who wants the most reliable method or in whom there has been multiple exposure; use an IUD.
- Use of hormonal contraception is possible immediately following administration of Levonelle, with use of condoms or abstinence for 7 days (2 days for POP). When ulipristal is used, there is a possibility that it may reduce the efficacy of hormonal methods for up to a week, so advise condoms or abstinence for 2 weeks after administration.

Management

- The treatment of choice is usually Levonelle, even in low-risk situations, in view of patient anxiety and the safety of the method.
- Ulipristal can be offered for those presenting between 72 and 120 hours after unprotected intercourse. But patients should be informed about the copper IUD method and its greater effectiveness.
- Establish from the consultation:
  - date of LMP;
  - whether the LMP was normal;
  - the normal menstrual cycle length and probable date of ovulation;
  - *all* the occasions of unprotected sexual intercourse (UPSI) in the last cycle;
  - number of hours since first episode of UPSI;
  - the method of contraception normally used.
- Warn the woman that the maximum risk of pregnancy after midcycle UPSI is about 9% (Wilcox et al., 2001), but depends on the inherent fertility of the couple.
- Explain to the patient that:
  - the method is not guaranteed. The average risk of pregnancy from a single episode of coitus is 3% (Wilcox et al., 2001). The progestogen-only method

and ulipristal reduce this risk by around 85%. The IUD is more effective, reducing the risk by 99% (Liying & Bilian, 2001);

- if the hormonal method is given, barrier methods must be used until the next period, which may be a little earlier or later than expected. The COC may then be started;
- she should reattend if the next period does not come, or she has any other worries;
- if vomiting occurs within 2 hours of taking the dose she should reattend urgently.

Follow-Up

- If a normal period has not occurred, exclude pregnancy and bear in mind the possibility of ectopic pregnancy.
- Discuss the long-term need for contraception. Use the opportunity to counsel the young and inexperienced. Consider whether a supply of Levonelle 1500 in advance might be appropriate for a woman who does not wish planned contraception but who anticipates the need for occasional emergency contraception after unplanned sex. In a US study it increased the use of emergency contraception without reducing the use of routine contraception (Jackson, Bimla Schwarz, Freedman, & Darney, 2003).

Contraception in Special Cases

Contraception and Young People
(Clinical Effectiveness Unit, 2010a)

INFORMATION AND ADVICE

Brook: Free confidential counselling service for young people, at www.brook.org.uk.
  Sexwise: For under 18-year-olds with problems with sex, relationships, and contraception, at https://sexwise.fpa.org.uk.

- In England and Wales, provision of contraceptive advice and treatment by health professionals to those aged under 16 is governed by a health circular (Anon., 2004a). Advice and treatment may be given, according to the Fraser guidelines, without parental knowledge when the young person:
  - has sufficient maturity to understand the moral, social, and emotional implications of the treatment;
  - cannot be persuaded to inform the parents or allow them to be informed;
  - is very likely to begin, or to continue, sexual intercourse with or without contraception;
  - would be likely to suffer in terms of physical or mental health if no contraceptive advice or treatment were given;
  - has his or her best interests served by being given contraceptive advice or treatment without parental consent.

- Young people continue to have concerns about the possibility of breaches of confidentiality. Improving young people's trust in the confidentiality of their practice should help remove one of the main obstacles that deter some teenagers from seeking early sexual health advice (Donovan et al., 2000). Every practice should develop its own confidentiality policy.
- *Legal aspects.* Inform the patient (and, if she gives her consent, her parents) of the legal situation; it is an offence for a person to have sexual contact with a girl under the age of 16, even if the girl consents (Sexual Offences Act, 2003).
- *Smoking.* Discuss the importance of not smoking, especially if the COC is to be used.
- Discuss the risks of contracting STIs, especially chlamydia, and how condoms protect against transmission.
- Raise the advantages, both psychological and physical, of not having sex at a young age.

Combined Oral Contraceptive

- Warn the patient that BTB can occur in the first few packets, is not harmful, and to come in and discuss the problem rather than stop the pill.
- Stress the value of using the condom as well to reduce the risk of STIs, including HIV (dual protection). Young people should be shown how to use condoms.

Contraception and Older Women
(Clinical Effectiveness Unit, 2010b)

- Women over 40 are more likely to have irregular cycles, but ovulation still occurs in around 35% of these cycles and there is still need for contraception.
- Current advice is for contraception to be continued in women aged 40 to 50 until there has been 2 years of amenorrhoea, and in women over 50 until there has been 1 year of amenorrhoea.

Women on the Combined Oral Contraceptive

- *Age.* Healthy non-smokers without risk factors may continue until the age of 50.
- Advise women who have stopped the COC at 50 to use the POP, barrier methods, or spermicide until they have had 1 year of amenorrhoea. If menstruating on the POP, follow the advice given next.

Women on the Progestogen-Only Pill (Clinical Effectiveness Unit, 2010b)

- When amenorrhoea occurs in those who have been having periods, stop the POP but use other precautions for 1 year if aged over 50, for 2 years if aged 50 or less.
- Alternatively, check the follicle-stimulating hormone (FSH).
- Those women who have always had amenorrhoea on the POP can have their FSH checked after age 50.

Hormone Replacement Therapy

- Hormone replacement therapy (HRT) is not contraceptive as the natural oestrogens do not necessarily inhibit ovulation.

- *Women started on HRT before the menopause* should continue contraception (barrier or IUD, possibly the POP) until there is reason to think that they have reached the menopause (e.g., at age 50). It is impossible to assess the timing of the natural menopause in women using HRT. If a woman is unwilling to discontinue HRT for 3 to 4 months to allow accurate assessment of FSH levels, then barrier contraception, an IUD, or the POP can be used until the age of 55, at which time loss of natural fertility can be assumed.
- *Women on the COC* do not need HRT until the COC is stopped.

Contraception and Learning Disability (Cooper, 2000)

- Contraception is most likely to be considered in women with learning disability who:
  1. are entering a sexual relationship. There is a 40% chance of learning disability in children born to a couple where both parents have learning disability;
  2. are in danger of being exploited.
     - *Consent.* Consult a consultant psychiatrist if there is doubt about the ability to give consent. The majority of patients with moderate and mild learning disability are able to give consent.
     - *Sex education.* Refer to the local community learning disability team, social services department, education department, or voluntary organization.
     - *Epilepsy.* If patients are on enzyme-inducing anti-epileptics, the dose of the COC needs to be higher. Those on the POP should change the method.

Sterilization (Anon., 2004b; Brechin and Brigg, 2006)

When counselling for sterilization the following should be borne in mind:
- Both partners should ideally be seen together.
- Patients should be made aware of the high efficacy of alternative long-acting reversible contraceptive methods (National Collaborating Centre for Women's and Children's Health, 2005).
- The possibility of death of partner or child should be covered.
- The possibility of relationship breakdown should be discussed.
- The pros and cons of male versus female sterilization should be explained.

Which Partner Should Be Sterilized?

Sometimes it is not the partner who presents who is subsequently sterilized. Points to be raised here are:
- Vasectomy is more effective than tubal occlusion: 1 in 2000 lifetime pregnancy risk (when postoperative semen analysis is adhered to) compared with 1 in 200 for tubal occlusion (all varieties of technique). Effectiveness of the Filshie clip is a little more favourable, but the data are less robust.

- Vasectomy is a more minor operation.
- Vasectomy is safer as it is usually performed under local anaesthesia.
- A man has a longer reproductive span to lose.
- A man is more likely to feel threatened (fear of loss of sexual drive and sexual prowess).

Reversal

- If a patient wants a reversal of sterilization, patency rates of around 90% can be achieved with microsurgical techniques but fertility is lower: 31% to 92% in females and 9% to 82% in males (rates tend to be at the low end of this range when the vasectomy was performed more than 10 years previously).
- When counselling a patient, be aware that risk factors for subsequent regret about sterilization include:
  - age younger than 30;
  - no children;
  - not in a relationship;
  - association in time with pregnancy (full term or abortion);
  - crisis in relationship or not in mutually faithful relationship;
  - coercion by partner or health professional;
  - psychological or psychosocial issues.

Termination of Pregnancy (Anon., 2004c)

In the UK, the Abortion Act of 1967, as amended by the Human Fertilisation and Embryology Act of 1990, allows TOP if two doctors agree that:
- the continuance of the pregnancy would involve risk to the life of the pregnant woman greater than if the pregnancy were terminated; or
- the termination is necessary to prevent grave permanent injury to the physical or mental health of the pregnant woman; or
- the pregnancy has not exceeded its 24th week and the continuance of the pregnancy would involve risk, greater than if the pregnancy were terminated, of injury to the physical or mental health of the pregnant woman; or
- the pregnancy has not exceeded its 24th week and the continuance of the pregnancy would involve risk, greater than if the pregnancy were terminated, of injury to the physical or mental health of any existing child(ren) of the family of the pregnant woman; or
- there is a substantial risk that if the child were born it would suffer from such physical or mental abnormalities as to be seriously handicapped.

Note: There is no time limit for the first, second, and last grounds.
- Mortality for a TOP is 0.2 per 100,000 compared to 6 per 100,000 for death in childbirth.
- The risk of serious complications and death increases with advancing gestation, so do not be responsible for delays in referral.
- TOP is not associated with an increase in breast cancer risk.

- There are no proven associations between TOP and subsequent ectopic pregnancy, placenta praevia, or infertility.
- TOP may be associated with a small increase in the risk of subsequent miscarriage or preterm delivery.
- Higher quality studies show no higher risk of mental health sequelae in those who have TOPs compared to women with unintended pregnancies who continue (Charles, Polis, Sridhara, & Blum, 2008).
- Counsel the woman to help her come to her own informed decision about TOP that she will not regret and to lessen the risk of emotional disturbance whatever decision is reached.
- Ensure that she is aware of the alternative of continuing the pregnancy and keeping the baby or giving it up for adoption.
- Check she is not under pressure from partner or parent.
- Discuss the need for and if possible plan future contraception, including information about emergency contraception if not already known about.
- Arrange a follow-up appointment 2 weeks after the termination to check for medical and psychological sequelae.
- Medical abortions with mifepristone and misoprostol are available up to 24 weeks. Up 9 weeks the two oral tablets are usually given 1–2 days apart. Between 10 and 24 weeks the misoprostol is given as a vaginal pessary. Multiple pessaries may be required, given every three hours, until the foetus is delivered. Feticide should be carried out from 22 weeks gestation.

The Patient Under 16 Years Old
(Anon., 2004a)

- Involve the parents or guardians, with the patient's consent. They will be needed to sign the consent form as well as to support the patient before and after the termination.
- If the patient refuses to inform a parent or guardian, she has the right, under the Family Law Reform Act of 1969, to consent to treatment herself, provided she understands the nature of the procedure, including its risks and complications.
- If a competent child consents to treatment, a parent cannot override that consent.

Infertility

GUIDELINE

National Institute for Health and Care Excellence. (2013). *Fertility problems: Assessment and treatment. NICE clinical guideline 156.* Retrieved from www.nice.org.uk.

- Reassure the couple that 75% of couples achieve conception within 6 months, and 84% by 12 months. If the woman is aged 35 the success rate is 94% over 3 years. If the woman is aged 38 the success rate is 77% over 3 years.

- Start investigations as soon as the couple voices anxiety about conceiving. Explain that in 30% of cases the problem lies with the male alone, in 30% with the female alone, and that in the remainder it is mixed or unexplained.
- Aim to consider referral after 1 year, or sooner if there is good reason to predict difficulties (e.g., oligoamenorrhoea or amenorrhoea, abnormal sperm count, a history of PID, or maternal age over 36). Refer the couple directly to a tertiary centre holding the contract for the treatment of subfertility, not to a general gynaecology clinic.

Investigations
Assessment of the Woman

- History should include details of menstrual cycle, previous pregnancies, pelvic infections, or operations. Regular periods are a reliable guide to the fact that the woman is ovulating. Check that they are having intercourse at the woman's most fertile time (as well as throughout the cycle). Do not bother with temperature charts.
- Check that the woman is rubella immune and taking folic acid.
- Screen for *Chlamydia*.
- Examine for evidence of pelvic pathology.
- *Progesterone level.* Take blood 7 days before menstruation is due. A level of more than 16 nmol/L suggests ovulation, and a level of more than 30 nmol/L confirms it. Borderline levels may be due to a deficient luteal phase or to mistimed sampling. Levels less than 16 nmol/L confirm that the cycle was anovulatory.
- *Measure FSH and LH* in a woman with irregular cycles in whom it is impossible to predict when to check the blood progesterone.

Note: There is no value in measuring TFTs or prolactin in women with regular menses in the absence of galactorrhoea or symptoms of thyroid disease.

Assessment of the Man

- Medical history should include operations on or infections of the testes and operations on the prostate.
- Drug history: sulfasalazine, tetracyclines, allopurinol, anabolic steroids, cannabis, and cocaine have all been shown to interfere with male reproductive function.
- Examine him, including genitals and secondary sexual characteristics.
- Screen for *Chlamydia*.
- Arrange for semen analysis. Semen should be produced by masturbation 3 days after the last ejaculation and examined within an hour.
- If the count is low, repeat after 3 months and refer to a specialist fertility clinic if still low. However, if the count is severely low, refer after a single count.
- Warn the patient that even a normal sperm count does not mean that there is not some sperm dysfunction, which can only be detected on more sophisticated tests.

Normal Values For Semen (World Health Organization)

- Volume: ≥2 mL
- pH: ≥7.2
- Concentration: ≥20 million/mL
- Total sperm number: ≥40 million/ejaculate
- Motility: ≥50% with ≥25% showing progressive motility
- Vitality: >75% live
- Morphology: >4% normal forms
- White blood cells: <1 million/mL

Advice

Advice to the couple should routinely be:
- both should stop smoking;
- the woman should drink no more than 1 or 2 units of alcohol once or twice weekly while trying to conceive;
- men who drink heavily should cut their drinking to no more than 3 to 4 units in any day;
- women and men with a BMI greater than 30 should lose weight regardless if ovulation is a problem;
- men should avoid soaking in hot baths, wearing tight underwear, and remaining seated for many hours at a time;
- couples should have regular sex throughout the cycle, every 2 to 3 days; there is no evidence that use of temperature charts and LH detection tests to time sex improve pregnancy rates.

Use of clomifene in general cannot be justified in general practice in view of the increased risk of multiple pregnancy and ovarian cancer. An exception to this is if a woman who previously conceived using it presents again with anovulatory cycles.

The Role of the General Practitioner After Referral

- Administer the drugs for assisted conception according to a protocol agreed with the specialist clinic.
- Support the couple throughout the drawn-out process of investigation and treatment.

INFORMATION FOR PATIENTS

Infertility Network UK is a self-help organization that supplies literature and runs support networks. Tel. 01424 732361, www.infertilitynetworkuk.com.

The Human Fertilization and Embryology Authority, 10 Spring Gardens, London, SW1A 2BU, tel. 020 7291 8200, www.hfea.gov.uk, has books and videos about assisted conception.

Sexual Problems

REVIEW

Wylie, K. (Ed.), (2015). *ABC of sexual health* (3rd ed.). Malden: Blackwell.

- Sexual problems may have a physical or psychological origin, but often they are mixed.
- All patients with sexual problems develop performance anxiety, where they are not relaxed and spontaneous in love making, are alert to further failure, and become a spectator of their own sexual performance.
- In about 30% of patients, the partner also has a problem.
- In any consultation about sexual problems it is important to ascertain the following:
  - What is the real complaint?
  - Why is the problem being presented now?
  - Is the desire for change real?
  - Who is really complaining, the patient or the partner?
  - What are the expectations of the patient?
- Consider the following psychological aspects in any patient presenting with a problem:
  - *Ignorance and misunderstanding.* This includes faulty sex education and technique, inability to communicate sexual needs, and unrealistic expectations due to stereotyped views of expected behaviour and performance.
  - *Anger and resentment.* This often remains unresolved, with the couple unable to communicate their feelings to each other clearly. It often arises where the partners are unable to express their feelings as children because of excessive unresolved anger in their parents. It may occur in response to relationship difficulties, financial difficulties, children, in-laws, or stress at work.
  - *Shame, embarrassment, and guilt.* This may be due to a negative sexual attitude laid down in childhood, where the parents looked upon sexuality as bad. Traumatic sexual experiences may add to these fears.
  - *Anxiety/fear about sex.* Fear of closeness, vulnerability, letting go, and failure may lead to a self-perpetuating cycle of anxiety.
  - *Poor self-image* may contribute to lack of interest in sex and sexual response. Changes in women may occur after operations, especially mastectomy or hysterectomy, postmenopausally and after childbirth. Both sexes commonly suffer after redundancy and when depressed.

INFORMATION FOR PATIENTS

For self-help material online, go to www.netdoctor.co.uk (search "sex and relationships").

Erectile Dysfunction

- Erectile dysfunction (ED) occurs in 10% to 15% of men but varies with age, with some degree of dysfunction being experienced by 40% of men at age 40 and by 70% at age 70. ED in an otherwise asymptomatic man may be a marker for underlying cardiovascular disease. Although at least 50% of the patients referred to specialist clinics have an organic component, anxiety about the situation will make things worse (Hackett et al., 2007).

- From the history, assess particularly whether:
  - the ED has arisen suddenly, with a precipitating cause, and is variable, with erections occurring in the early morning but not during intercourse. These patients are likely to have a psychological cause for the problem; or
  - the onset was gradual, is constant, with partial or poorly sustained erections and no full early-morning erections. These patients are likely to have a physical cause, although a psychological component is frequently superimposed.
- Consider the psychological aspects discussed earlier under Sexual Problems.
- Be alert to psychiatric problems, including generalized anxiety states (excessive adrenergic constrictor tone), depression, psychosis, body dysmorphic disorder, gender identity problems, and alcoholism.
- Check for the cause being an adverse drug reaction to beta-blockers, thiazides, spironolactone, cimetidine, antidepressants, phenothiazine antipsychotics, and especially alcohol.
- Examine:
  - blood pressure, heart rate, waist circumference, and weight;
  - genitalia (including testicular size, fibrosis in the shaft of the penis, and retractibility of the foreskin).
- Further examination may sometimes be indicated by age or findings in the history especially cardiovascular, neurological, endocrine, and urinary systems.

Workup

- Fasting blood glucose and lipid.
- Testosterone (if history or examination suggests possible hypogonadism or if required to reassure patient); take blood at 9 am and not within 3 months of serious illness, which can depress the testosterone level.

ED as a Risk Factor for Cardiovascular Disease

- Observational studies show that factors associated with ED are similar to those associated with cardiovascular disease (CVD; i.e., sedentary lifestyle, obesity, smoking, hypercholesterolaemia, and the metabolic syndrome).
- ED seems to carry an independent risk for CVD of 1.46, making it as powerful a predictor of CVD as smoking.
- When a man presents with ED which appears to be vascular in origin, assess his risk of CVD.

Treatment in General Practice

- *Exercise and weight loss.* In the Massachusetts Male Aging Study (MMAS) men who started exercise in midlife had a 70% reduced risk for ED later in life. There is some evidence that exercise and weight loss, in those with established ED, leads to a significant reduction in ED.

Phosphodiesterase Type-5 Inhibitor

- These are facilitators rather than initiators of erections and require sexual stimulation to facilitate an erection;

they have a slower onset of action than injected or transurethral alprostadil (see later in chapter). Sildenafil and vardenafil are relatively short-acting phosphodiesterase type-5 (PDE5) inhibitors, having a half-life of about 4 hours (suitable for occasional use), whereas tadalafil has a longer half-life of 17.5 hours (suitable for longer periods such as over a weekend).
- In the United Kingdom, generic sildenafil is available on the National Health Service (NHS) for all men with erectile dysfunction and can now be bought over the counter. Other PDE5 inhibitors can only be prescribed at NHS expense to men who have not responded to sildenafil and who have any of the conditions approved by the Department of Health (DoH; see the BNF), marking the prescription Selected List Scheme (SLS), and giving enough (usually) for one treatment a week. A private prescription can be issued to any patient who does not come within the DoH guidelines.
- Studies have shown that patients often take PDE5 inhibitors incorrectly and that almost half of previous nonresponders respond if the drugs are taken correctly.
- Instruct the patient to:
  - take sildenafil or vardenafil 30 to 60 minutes before intercourse and tadalafil several hours before intercourse;
  - avoid excessive food or alcohol although absorption is less of a problem with tadalafil.
- Beware the drug interaction with nitrates and nicorandil in those with cardiovascular comorbidity.

Non-responders

- Patients should use the drug eight times at maximal dosage before being classified as a non-responder.
- Recheck testosterone and prolactin levels in non-responders. PDE5 inhibitors are less effective in those with low or low-normal testosterone levels and there is some evidence of improved response with testosterone replacement.
- *Counselling* may be successful in psychogenic impotence and is appropriate for couples who do not wish to be referred:
  - See the couple together.
  - Recommend a manual (e.g., *The Relate Guide to Sex in Loving Relationships* [see previous box]).
  - Instruct the couple on the sensate focus programme. Instructions can be downloaded from the web (e.g., at https://counselling-matters.org.uk/sites/counselling-matters/files/SensateFocus.pdf).
  - Set homework assignments for the couple; these can be tailored to meet specific needs.

Referral

- Refer those not responding for sex therapy via the local family planning clinic or Relate. The outcome is successful in 50% to 80% of cases.
- Refer for relationship counselling those whom you sense have larger relationship or personality problems.
- Refer to a urologist those with physical causes, those who have not responded to PDE5 inhibitors or who have

contraindications to it, and those with psychological causes that are proving intractable. Possible treatments are:

- hormone replacement therapy in those with hypogonadism;
- alprostadil, as injections into the corpus cavernosum or transurethrally;
- vacuum devices;
- penile prostheses.

DETAILS OF THERAPISTS ARE AVAILABLE FROM

British Association for Sexual and Relationship Therapy, tel. 020 8543 2707, www.basrt.org.uk.
    Institute of Psychosexual Medicine, Building 3, Chiswick Park, 566 Chiswick High Road, Chiswick, London, W4 5YA, tel. 020 7580 0631, www.ipm.org.uk.

Lack of Sexual Desire (Basson, 2006)

- This is the most common presenting female sexual dysfunction.
- A low level of sexual desire is usually accompanied by low levels of arousal and sexual excitement and infrequent orgasms, and is frequently associated with sexual dissatisfaction.
- Underlying psychological difficulties are frequent. These may relate specifically to sex (e.g., previous sexual abuse) or they may relate to a more widespread psychological disorder. Physical illness and drugs/substances are also possible causes.
- Women specifically lose sexual desire:
  - postpartum;
  - because of pain;
  - where their partner's performance repeatedly leads to frustration, as in premature ejaculation or ED.
- In general, psychological interventions and sex therapy are of greater benefit than drugs.
- Check for the presence of depression and anxiety.
- Reassure the patient that sexual desire varies at different times of life and that loss of desire is not necessarily abnormal.
- Enquire whether she wants to improve her sexual desire or whether it is her partner's wish.
- Consider factors that may be contributing (see previous discussion).
- Recommend the British Association for Sexual and Relationship Therapy website, at www.basrt.org.uk, for discussion on the problem of lack of desire.
- Offer counselling along the lines described under erectile dysfunction.

Dyspareunia (Weijmar Schultz et al., 2005)

- This may be primary, or secondary to a physical cause, and considerable skill may be needed to unravel the problem.
- Distinguish from the history and examination between:
  - lack of lubrication due to lack of interest;

- vaginismus, which usually becomes apparent at vaginal examination (see upcoming discussion);
- vulval or vaginal causes: infections, vulvar vestibulitis syndrome, lichen sclerosus, lichen planus, urethral caruncle, postmenopausal vaginitis, post-episiotomy syndrome. Those for whom there is no specific treatment may benefit from 5% lidocaine ointment applied 20 minutes before sexual intercourse; they can also be referred to specialist physiotherapists;
- pelvic causes with tenderness on rocking the cervix or palpating the fornices (e.g., endometriosis, pelvic infection, ovarian pathology); and
- psychogenic causes, where vulval burning or pain is due to somatization of other difficulties.
- Where a physical cause is not found, cognitive behavioural therapy (CBT) and selective serotonin reuptake inhibitors (SSRIs) have been found to be beneficial.

INFORMATION FOR PATIENTS AND THEIR PARTNERS

Vulval Pain Society, PO Box 7804, Nottingham NG3 5ZQ, www.vulvalpainsociety.org.

Vaginismus

- This consists of a phobia of penetration and involuntary spasm of the pubococcygeal and associated muscles surrounding the lower third of the vagina. Such women may avoid having cervical smears and sometimes present with infertility.
- Explore the root cause. It may be:
  - fear of the unknown or the patient's ignorance of her own anatomy;
  - a past history of unpleasant experiences such as rape, sexual abuse or severe emotional trauma, or previous dyspareunia;
  - a defence mechanism against growing up and becoming a woman. (A common pattern is for the patient to live close to her parents, remaining the daughter and marrying an unassertive man.)
- Desensitize simple cases by encouraging the woman to examine herself, and also encourage her partner to be confident enough to insert a finger into the vagina. Some women may prefer to use vaginal trainers.
- Refer to a sex therapist if this simple approach fails. Hypnotherapy may be helpful (McGuire & Hawton, 2003).

Disorders of Orgasm

Anxiety tends to delay a woman's orgasm, but accelerates a man's.

Premature Ejaculation (Waldinger, 2007)

- This is present when ejaculation occurs sooner than either partner would wish, usually before penetration or soon after. Interest in sex may be reduced in both partners.

- Advise the patient that, with practice, he can learn to delay ejaculation. The stop/start technique can be taught by therapists or learnt from the book cited earlier. In essence, when, during caressing or during intercourse, a man feels he is close to climax he should stop being stimulated and relax for 30 seconds. Stimulation can then recommence until he is close to climax again, when the relaxation is repeated. If this fails, the woman should squeeze the penis at the base of the glans between finger and thumb during relaxation phases.
- Clomipramine 25 mg daily or paroxetine 20 mg each evening are effective in delaying ejaculation.

Retarded Ejaculation

- This is usually a sign of longstanding sexual inhibition. Often the patient can ejaculate by masturbation, but not intravaginally.
- Explore any feelings of anxiety and guilt.
- Start a sensate focus programme (see previous discussion).
- If home therapy fails, refer for psychosexual counselling.

Orgasmic Problems in Women (Meston, Hull, Levin, & Sipski, 2004)

- A woman who has never achieved an orgasm may have deep-seated psychological reasons for being afraid to let go. She may need permission to investigate her body's own responses further, either by masturbation or vibrator. When she has learnt how to relax, she should be encouraged to tell her partner and incorporate caressing into their usual lovemaking.
- Women who have lost the ability to achieve orgasm may need counselling, especially about their current relationship or a recent loss of self-image.
- Check that she is not taking drugs that inhibit orgasm (e.g., clonidine) and that her failure to achieve orgasm is not due to neurological disease or pelvic surgery. Total hysterectomy does not impair ability to achieve orgasm (Farrell & Kieser, 2000).

Sexually Transmitted Infections and Human Immunodeficiency Virus

- Sexually transmitted infections (STIs) frequently coexist, so patients diagnosed with one STI generally need further investigation to exclude other infections.
- GUM or sexual health clinics provide full screening, immediate microscopy, and assistance for patients in the treating and informing of partners (partner notification or contact tracing). This is important in limiting the spread of disease, and patients diagnosed with an STI should be routinely referred to GUM for further management.
- Late diagnosis of HIV is a major cause of avoidable mortality in infected individuals and general practitioners (GPs) have an important role in making earlier diagnoses which improves prognosis and can limit ongoing transmission.

Patients Requiring Investigation by the General Practitioner

- Those who are eligible for a local or national screening programme (e.g., for chlamydia).
- Those who require treatment urgently and cannot attend GUM immediately (e.g., symptomatic pelvic inflammatory disease out of hours).
- Those who are unwilling or unable to attend a GUM clinic after discussion and recommendation, and require testing for STIs or HIV.
- Those presenting with a possible STI-related problem in a primary care setting which has training and experience in managing STIs, including partner notification (e.g., through Locally Enhanced Service schemes or GPs with a special interest).
- See discussion later in the chapter for other circumstances in which HIV testing should be considered.

Patients Requiring Management by the General Practitioner

- Those who have tested positive for an STI at the surgery and wish to be managed in primary care or cannot attend GUM immediately.
- Those who present as contacts of an STI and decline to attend GUM for testing, treatment, and partner notification advice, after discussion and recommendation of this course of action.

Contact Tracing (Partner Notification)

- This is usually best done by GUM, or at least with their support and advice.
- As a minimum, screening of all contacts of acute STIs over the last 3 months should be attempted. For syphilis and HIV there is no arbitrary limit, and partner notification will depend on who is contactable and the earliest likely time of infection.
- If the patient is diagnosed with nonspecific urethritis (NSU), chlamydia, syphilis, *Trichomonas vaginalis*, or gonorrhoea, the partner should be treated even if tests are negative.

Principles of Treatment

- Give appropriate antibiotics, bearing in mind any recent travel history.
- Advise complete abstinence from all sexual contact until both patient and partner are treated.
- Follow-up after completion of antibiotics for compliance and possibly retesting (which is indicated only in pregnancy or where symptoms persist).

Workup for Cases to Be Managed in Primary Care

- Take a full sexual history, focusing on the last two partners (irrespective of time interval) or all partners in the last 3 months (if more than two).

- Current practice is moving toward testing asymptomatic individuals without examination and reserving examination for those who are symptomatic.
- Where examination is indicated, examine the genitalia for discharge, ulcers, or warts (including the vagina and cervix in females); examine the mouth for ulcers; and perform proctoscopy if there are anal symptoms or a history of anal intercourse.

Diagnostic Tests in Women

- *Gonorrhoea:* cervical, urethral swabs; also oropharyngeal and rectal swabs if symptomatic at those sites, if a partner has gonorrhoea, or if suggested by the sexual history.
- *Chlamydia:* Vulvovaginal swab for nucleic acid amplification testing (NAAT) has been shown to be more sensitive than endocervical swabs (Schoeman et al, 2012). First catch urine can also be used.
- *T. vaginalis, bacterial vaginosis, and candida:* high vaginal swabs may detect candidal infection but are only useful in the diagnosis of *T. vaginalis* if inoculated into a trichomonal culture medium. Swabs without immediate microscopy are of limited use for diagnosing bacterial vaginosis.
- Check that cervical smears are up to date.

Diagnostic Tests in Men

- *Chlamydia:* Testing is by NAAT. First catch urine is the test of choice for men. If urethral swabs are taken then insert 1–4 cm into the urethra and rotate once.
- *Gonorrhoea:* Usually diagnosed by culture via urethral/rectal swab in order to identify resistant strains. It can also be diagnosed by NAAT either from swabs or first catch urine, but NAAT positive patients should also be cultured.

Tests to Be Done in All Patients Suspected of Having a Sexually Transmitted Infection

- Check syphilis serology and repeat it 3 months after exposure if there has been a significant risk.
- Check hepatitis B serology in patients who have been exposed in countries with high incidence, if a sexual partner comes from an endemic area, in homosexual men, and where the patient and partner have a history of injecting drug use. Consider the need for immediate hepatitis B immunization.
- Discuss and offer HIV testing to all patients. Where a patient does not wish to attend a GUM clinic, consideration should be given to testing in primary care.

Specific Management of Sexually Transmitted Infections

Gonorrhoea
Genital Gonorrhoea (Uncomplicated)

> **GUIDELINE**
>
> British Association for Sexual Health and HIV. (2011). *National guideline on the management of gonorrhoea in adults.* Retrieved from www.bashh.org/guidelines.

- Gonorrhoea is strongly concentrated among individuals with high-risk sexual behaviours and their partners. Referral to or, at the least, advice from GUM is therefore strongly recommended, and screening for other STIs should be routinely undertaken.
- Antibiotic resistance patterns are changing rapidly; it is advisable to check with the GUM clinic for current recommendations.
- Ceftriaxone 500 mg intramuscularly as a single dose with 1 g azithromycin as a single dose, or cefixime 400 mg oral as a single dose (if IM injection is contraindicated or not tolerated), or spectinomycin 2 g intramuscularly as a single dose. (At the time of writing, resistance patterns are changing rapidly.)
- Treat all patients for chlamydia infection. The coinfection rate is 40%.
- Seek advice for all pregnant women.
- Trace and treat contacts over the previous 3 months.
- Follow-up at least once to confirm compliance, resolution of symptoms, and partner notification.

Chlamydia Infection (Uncomplicated)

> **GUIDELINE AND REVIEW**
>
> British Association for Sexual Health and HIV. (2015). *National guideline on the management of* Chlamydia *trachomatis genital tract infections.* Retrieved from www.bashh.org/guidelines.

- Nucleic acid amplification tests (NAATs) are now standard for swab or urine samples. Their sensitivity is over 95%.
- Treatment and partner notification should be undertaken on strong suspicion (e.g., mucopurulent cervicitis or pelvic inflammatory disease) before the result is back. Endocervical swabs should be rotated firmly and male urethral swabs should be rotated 1 to 4 cm inside the urethra.
- Give:
  - azithromycin 1 g as a single oral dose; or
  - doxycycline 100 mg twice a day for 7 days; or
  - erythromycin 500 mg twice a day for 14 days (if both of the above are contraindicated).
- In pregnancy, give:
  - erythromycin 500 mg twice a day for 14 days or 500 mg four times a day for 7 days; or
  - amoxicillin 500 mg three times a day for 7 days; and
  - a test of cure performed 3 weeks after completing therapy.
- Patients should be referred to GUM to discuss partner notification with a trained health adviser. The UK chlamydia pilots suggest that this is acceptable to patients diagnosed in primary care. A cutoff for 4 weeks is used for symptomatic men; for all others, the lookback should be for 6 months or to the last partner (whichever is the longer).

Screening for Chlamydia

- A screening programme for genital chlamydia has been implemented in England aimed at covering 17% of people under 25 years of age every year (NHS, 2009).

- Screening is particularly important for:
  - women seeking TOP and their partners;
  - sexually active women and men under the age of 25, especially teenagers;
  - men and women aged 25 and over with a new sexual partner, or two or more partners in a year.
- Offer screening with a vulvovaginal swab because it is more sensitive and stable, but agree to urine testing (where available) by a NAAT if the woman prefers it.
- Repeat the screen if the woman changes her partner.

Nonspecific Urethritis

GUIDELINE AND REVIEW

British Association for Sexual Health and HIV. (2015). *National guideline on the management of non-gonococcal urethritis.* Retrieved from www.bashh.org/guidelines.

- Test all patients who have urethritis for gonorrhoea and chlamydia.
- First line treatment, if tests for chlamydia and gonorrhoea are negative, is doxycycline 100 mg twice a day for 7 days, or azithromycin 1 g orally stat. Follow-up at 2 weeks. For symptomatic patients, all partners during the past 4 weeks should be treated, and treatment of the regular partner is recommended in all cases.
- Patients should abstain from sexual intercourse until they and their sexual partner have completed treatment.
- Refer unresolving cases to GUM, and all cases where you are unable to complete partner notification. Some men have recurring urethritis due to non-infectious causes; in these cases specialist advice and diagnostics, followed by reassurance, are important.

Trichomonas vaginalis

GUIDELINE AND REVIEW

British Association for Sexual Health and HIV. (2014). *National guideline on the management of Trichomonas vaginalis.* Retrieved from www.bashh.org/guidelines.

- *Trichomonas vaginalis* (TV) infection is almost exclusively sexually transmitted through urethral or vaginal inoculation. It is sometimes diagnosed on cervical cytology, where there is a false positive rate of about 30%, so tests should be repeated.
- *Trichomonas* infection is strongly associated with other STIs, and full screening should be undertaken.
- Metronidazole 2 g orally stat, or metronidazole 400 mg twice a day for 5 to 7 days, will clear 95% of infections. The stat dose is as effective as the 7-day course but is more likely to be associated with adverse effects (Forna & Gulmezoglu, 2000). Test of cure is required only if

symptoms persist, in which case the patient should attend GUM. Alcohol should be avoided during and for 48 hours after treatment.
- Symptomatic disease in early pregnancy can be controlled with clotrimazole pessaries 100 mg daily for 7 days, or Aci-gel, before systemic treatment in the second trimester.
- Current partners should be screened for STIs.

Anogenital Warts

GUIDELINE AND REVIEW

British Association for Sexual Health and HIV. (2015). *National guideline on the management of anogenital warts.* Retrieved from www.bashh.org/HPV_guideline.

- Most anogenital warts cause minor irritation or are simply cosmetic. However, they cause a good deal of psychological distress. Patients should be given an explanation of their condition, emphasizing that the majority of anogenital warts are caused by HPV types 6 and 11, which are not associated with cervical neoplasia.
- Many carriers of HPV have no visible lesions.
- Condom use may prevent transmission of warts to uninfected partners. Their use with regular partners, however, has not been shown to affect the outcome of treatment in patients with visible warts.
- Perianal warts are associated with anal sex (although they can occur without) and should suggest the need for anorectal samples for other STIs, and GUM referral.
- None of the existing treatments is satisfactory, and all have high recurrence rates. Patients should be made aware of this. The evidence base for distinguishing first and second line treatments is weak.
- Pregnancy: pregnant women can be treated using cryotherapy, trichloroacetic acid, or other ablative therapies in a specialist setting. However, warts often worsen during pregnancy and improve afterwards. The risk of transmitting warts or laryngeal papillomata to the neonate is small, and caesarean section is indicated only in rare cases of giant vulval warts or gross cervical warts.

Soft, Nonkeratinized Warts

- Prescribe podophyllotoxin 0.5% (twice daily for 3 days, repeated weekly for up to 4 weeks). Patients using podophyllotoxin at home must take great care to follow the instructions to avoid chemical burns. It should not be used in pregnancy and is not licensed for extragenital lesions such as anal warts.
- Imiquimod 5% cream is an immune response modifier which can be used three times weekly for up to 16 weeks. It should not be used in pregnancy.

Keratinized Warts

- Use ablative therapy such as cryotherapy which is available at GUM clinics.

Herpes Genitalis

GUIDELINE AND REVIEW

British Association of Sexual Health and HIV. (2014). *National guideline on the management of genital herpes.* Retrieved from www.bashh.org/guidelines.

- New diagnoses of primary herpes may be due to herpes simplex virus (HSV) type 1 or type 2. After childhood, HSV1 is equally likely to be acquired in the genital or oral areas (Langenberg et al., 1999).
- Much genital herpes is due to orogenital contact and can therefore occur in patients who may not consider themselves as sexually active.
- Primary herpes is often asymptomatic, and patients often present many years later with symptoms which are due to recurrence.
- Autoinoculation (e.g., from labial herpes) can only occur during primary episodes. Patients who have developed herpes for the first time but had no recent sexual contact should be referred to a consultant in GUM who will be familiar with such cases, and able to advise patients at a time of considerable distress and uncertainty.
- Genital herpes can be acquired from asymptomatic partners, sometimes in a long-term relationship. Some patients never develop symptoms, although those with HSV2 will usually develop symptoms at some point (Langenberg et al., 1999).
- Initial episodes are typically far more severe, and of longer duration, than recurrences. Recurrences tend to decrease over time but are more frequent with HSV2 (Benedetti, Zeh, & Corey, 1999).
- Diagnosis is by culture or PCR testing and typing of the virus using a swab from the base of an ulcer, sent rapidly to the laboratory in special transport media.
- In primary episodes, patients can benefit from practical counselling in relation to the natural history and issues in relationships (including risk to the partner). This can be provided at the GUM clinic. Psychological stress does not increase recurrences (Green & Kocsis, 1997).
- Partner notification is guided by the individual case and history of symptoms in the partner. Health advisers in the GUM clinic are experienced in this issue and can help with this.

Management of a First Symptomatic Episode

- *Oral antiviral therapy*, commenced within 5 days of the episode or while new lesions are forming, reduces the severity and duration of that first episode. Options are acyclovir 200 mg five times daily, valacyclovir 500 mg twice a day, or famciclovir 125 mg twice a day with a duration of 5 days.
- *Offer analgesia* and recommend saline bathing. Topical anaesthetics can be used although they occasionally cause sensitization. It may be easier to pass urine in a tepid bath.

- *Admit* patients with urinary retention, meningism, or severe systemic symptoms.
- *Offer counselling*, including a discussion of the risk of asymptomatic shedding and its implications for relationships, and the need to inform healthcare workers in the case of later pregnancy. Health advisers at the GUM clinic are experienced in this area.

Management of Recurrences

- Most recurrences cause minor symptoms of a few days duration.
- Severe recurrences may be shortened by oral antiviral agents as discussed. There is no evidence that topical antiviral creams are effective. Saline bathing, petroleum jelly, or lidocaine gel may aid symptoms.
- *Suppressive therapy.* Depending on patient preference, relationship status, and severity of symptoms, it may be appropriate to offer systemic antiviral treatment to reduce the duration and severity of attacks and frequency. This can reduce anxiety, help in adjustment, and improve quality of life, usually in patients with six or more recurrences a year. Suppressive therapy should be undertaken for a defined period of time before review, and is best undertaken by or in collaboration with the GUM clinic.

PATIENT SUPPORT GROUP

The Herpes Viruses Association, 41 North Road, London N7 9DP, tel. 0845 123 2305, info@herpes.org.uk, www.herpes.org.uk.

Syphilis

- Like gonorrhoea, syphilis is concentrated among individuals at high behavioural risk and their partners, and untreated syphilis also has major long-term sequelae.
- Suspected or diagnosed syphilis must be referred to the GUM clinic, where further investigation, treatment, and partner notification will be undertaken.
- Long-term partner notification is required, and these patients may be at very high risk for other STIs and bloodborne viruses.

Human Immunodeficiency Virus and Acquired Immunodeficiency Syndrome
Prevention and Early Diagnosis

- Prevention of HIV is an essential part of contraceptive care, travel care, and well-person clinics. Testing for HIV should now be universally offered as part of antenatal care, so that women avoid vertical transmission, and access services.

Advising on Safer Sex and Avoiding High-Risk Activities

- Hugging, kissing, and mutual masturbation are safe.
- HIV has been transmitted through oral sex, but this is rare. A condom can be used for receptive oral sex, to

improve protection. Condoms can be lubricated with KY Jelly or similar lubricants but *not* oils or Vaseline, which reduce their strength by 95%.

- High-risk sexual activities include penetrative vaginal or anal sex without a condom.
- Other high-risk activities include sharing needles or syringes for intravenous drug use.
- Sex with local residents in high prevalence areas of the world (e.g., Africa, Thailand, parts of South America) or with people otherwise at high risk (e.g., men who have sex with men [MSM]) increases the risks in the event of condom breakage or unprotected sex.
- By the end of 2015, an estimated 101,200 people were living with HIV in the United Kingdom, of whom 13% remained unaware of their infection. HIV incidence is increasing among MSM. In 2015, 2800 MSM were diagnosed with HIV in the United Kingdom, of whom most probably became infected there. In 2015 there were 2360 cases of new heterosexually acquired HIV and this was the first year since the 1990s that the number of new heterosexual diagnoses of people born within the United Kingdom exceeded the number of those born outside the country.
- MSM, migrants from countries with high HIV incidence, and injecting drug users remain the populations at greatest risk of HIV infection.
- A high proportion of deaths are now avoidable and attributable to late diagnosis, and early diagnosis is now recognized as a mainstay both of transmission prevention and of clinical care.
- HIV testing is now recommended on GP registration in high prevalence areas, and for a range of indicator diseases in which HIV is much more likely than in the general population. These indicator diseases include all sexually transmitted infections, as well as many other conditions likely to present to the GP, such as severe psoriasis or seborrhoeic dermatitis, chronic diarrhoea, unexplained weight loss or lymphadenopathy, bacterial pneumonia, recurrent herpes zoster, unexplained blood dyscrasia, peripheral neuropathy, pyrexia of unknown origin, aseptic meningitis, mononucleosis–like syndrome, and dementia (British Association for HIV, British Association for Sexual Health and HIV, British Infection Society, 2008).

  Note regarding insurance reports: The British Medical Association (BMA) and Royal College of General Practitioners (RCGP) advise doctors *not* to answer the lifestyle questions on insurance reports, even with consent. These questions allocate a person to an at-risk group, which is discriminatory, while only high-risk behaviour is relevant.

The Human Immunodeficiency Virus Antibody Test

- The HIV test is 99.9% sensitive and specific 3 months after exposure to the virus (Sloand, Pitt, Chiarello, & Nemo, 1991), although the window period before becoming positive can occasionally be longer (e.g., after post-exposure antiretroviral prophylaxis).

- If HIV primary infection is suspected, P24 antigen and plasma proviral DNA or HIV RNA testing may be appropriate, as prognosis may be improved by antiretroviral therapy at this time. GUM specialist advice should be sought.
- A positive antibody test should be repeated to exclude identification errors.

Human Immunodeficiency Virus Testing

- HIV testing is now more accepted as part of good clinical care, and in the United Kingdom is offered to all pregnant women and patients with TB. Primary care practitioners are now encouraged to undertake HIV testing, particularly where this is unlikely to occur in another setting.
- Patients who do not wish to have the result recorded in their notes in primary care should be referred to the GUM clinic.
- The patient should understand that having the test is entirely voluntary.
- Written information about the test and its pros and cons is available at www.tht.org.uk (choose "HIV Testing").

Pre-Test Discussion

- Patients should have an HIV test only with their informed consent and normally need to come back in person for the result.
- Issues to be covered in pretest discussion for HIV:
  - Difference between HIV infection and acquired immunodeficiency syndrome (AIDS), how the virus is transmitted, whether the patient has any misapprehensions.
  - Latency between transmission and seroconversion. Ensure that the patient is not in the 3-month window period (occasionally longer). If so, discuss the need to postpone or repeat the test.
  - Importance of screening for other STIs and of making plans for safer sex whatever the test result.

  Advantages of the Test
  1. Effective therapies are available, which extend life expectancy to near normal.
  2. Knowing the result means that partners can be protected if it is positive or make decision to move to safer sex if negative.
  3. Decisions about pregnancy can be made.
  4. Anxiety due to uncertainty about HIV status is ended.
  5. Informed decisions about medical issues, such as live vaccines, can be made.

  Other Considerations
  1. If positive, the patient will need to cope with a difficult diagnosis. He or she will need to consider whom to tell.
  2. A positive (but not a negative) result may affect insurance, and possibly employment prospects.

Post Test Discussion
  Negative Results
- Discuss any concerns that have given rise to the test and how the patient plans to protect him or herself in the future. Discuss the window period and whether further testing will be needed for full reassurance.

Positive Results

- Ensure that you have time and there will be no interruptions to the interview. Tell the patient early in the interview, to allow time for reflection and questions.
- Establish what the patient knows and expects to happen, and ensure that he or she understands the difference between HIV infection and AIDS. Ensure the patient understands that there are now many very effective therapies that dramatically improve prognosis.
- Explain that the virus is not passed on by normal domestic or work contact.
- Refer to a specialist clinic, which may be the GUM service or the Infectious Diseases Unit, for specialist follow-up and support. Clinics will fit in a newly diagnosed patient urgently.
- Discuss and advise on concerns about transmission to others (see box "Advising on Safer Sex and Avoiding High-Risk Activities") and the need for protected sex.
- Find out what the patient's plans are for the rest of the day and ensure that he or she arranges to meet someone for support.
- Arrange to see the patient again in a few days; do not overload with information and issues at this initial interview.
- Give information on patient helplines.

PATIENT INFORMATION

Terrence Higgins Trust, 314-320 Gray's Inn Road, London, WC1X 8DP, tel. 080 8802 1221, www.tht.org.uk.

The National AIDS Helpline (NAH) on 0800 567 123 for free and confidential advice and information about HIV/AIDS, other sexually transmitted infections, or sexual health matters. A 24-hour 7-days a week telephone service, NAH can also give details about local services, including sexual health clinics and support agencies for people with HIV/AIDS, their partners, family, and friends.

Managing the Human Immunodeficiency Virus-Positive Patient in the Community

- In the last few years, communication between specialist HIV clinicians and primary care has improved, and patients are often managed in collaboration. This allows GPs to gain experience in the condition, while encouraging patients to access care for unrelated conditions and to use out of hours care and community nursing appropriately.
- Following publication of the Standards for HIV Clinical Care (BHIVA, RCP, BASHH, BIS, 2009) there has been an emphasis on provision of HIV care within a managed service network, which will be expected to support primary care and others in providing nonspecialist HIV services.

Routine Care

- Regular estimates of viral load and CD4 measurements are important in advising patients to start highly active anti-retroviral therapy (HAART) at the optimal time (usually when the CD4 count is $<350 \times 10^6/1$). These are best done through the specialist HIV services (usually GUM).
- Syphilis serology, baseline hepatitis B and C serology, FBC, and LFT should be repeated yearly, while cytomegalovirus (CMV) antibodies and toxoplasma antibodies should be assessed at baseline.
- Lipids, blood sugar, calcium/phosphate, and possibly other monitoring tests are needed if on therapy. Women should have yearly cervical smears because of the increased incidence of carcinoma.
- Advise patients which symptoms should be treated seriously, including fever, weight loss, diarrhoea, lymphadenopathy, shortness of breath or cough, paraesthesiae, headache, mouth ulceration, and visual disturbances.
- Avoid bacille Calmette-Guérin (BCG) and yellow fever vaccines; seek specialist advice for other live vaccines but otherwise vaccinate as usual. Hepatitis B vaccination should be offered if seronegative.
- Advise the patient to avoid exposure to toxoplasmosis (uncooked meat and unwashed salads), and to cryptosporidium if severely immunosuppressed (unboiled tap water).
- Encourage patients with a CD4 count less than 200 to take prophylaxis against *Pneumocystis carinii* pneumonia (PCP) in the form of co-trimoxazole 960 mg daily or thrice weekly, or dapsone 100 mg daily, or nebulized pentamidine 300 mg every 4 weeks.
- Ensure the patient has adequate psychologic support in adjusting to the diagnosis.
- The issue of pregnancy and contraception, together with safe sex, needs to be discussed with women on an ongoing basis. Effective interventions are now available which can reduce the risk of transmission to the baby to under 1%. Specialist advice should be sought at an early stage.
- Risk reduction in relation to sexual partners needs to be regularly reviewed. Transmission of HIV to uninfected partners, or transmission of resistant strains, is possible and safe sex must be practised.

Symptoms Needing Special Consideration

- *Cough*, especially dry cough with breathlessness in a patient with minimal chest signs, and (initially) a normal chest x-ray (CXR) can indicate PCP. This requires urgent specialist care. Patients are also at increased risk of community acquired pneumonia, TB, and bacterial chest infection.
- *Headaches* can suggest cerebral toxoplasmosis, non-Hodgkin lymphoma, tuberculoma, or, importantly, cryptococcal meningitis, which may *not* be accompanied by neck stiffness or headache.
- *Diarrhoea* can indicate opportunistic bowel infection, including cryptosporidium or microsporidium, although often no cause is found and symptomatic treatment is required.
- *Dysphagia* can indicate oesophageal candidiasis, treatable with fluconazole 100 mg once a day for 14 to 21 days, or (in the severely immunocompromised) CMV ulceration.
- *Visual disturbances,* including flashes and floaters, can suggest CMV retinitis. This should be referred urgently.

Venepuncture

- The same universal precautions should be taken as with patients of unknown serostatus (gloves, avoid resheathing needles, place in appropriately sealed packaging, and transport in safe containers). Avoidance of resheathing needles should be standard practice.
- Some laboratories require *high-risk* stickers depending on local policy. High risk does not require stating the diagnosis of HIV for transport purposes, which is unnecessary for routine tests and can generally be avoided in other cases. This practice is an unnecessary risk to patient confidentiality.
- Spills should be mopped up with hypochlorite (10 parts water to 1 part household bleach) or undiluted Milton.

Post-Exposure Prophylaxis for Healthcare Workers (Including Needlestick Injuries)

> **GUIDELINE**
>
> Department of Health (2008). *HIV post-exposure prophylaxis: guidance from the UK Chief Medical Officer's expert advisory group on AIDS* (rev. ed.). London: Department of Health. Retrieved from www.gov.uk/government/uploads/system/uploads/attachment_data/file/203139/HIV_post-exposure_prophylaxis.pdf.

- The risk of acquiring HIV infection following percutaneous exposure to HIV-infected blood is on average around 3 per 1000, and less than 1 in 1000 after mucocutaneous exposure.
- The risk is increased in cases of deep injury, visible blood on the device causing the injury, a needle which had entered an artery or vein, or terminal illness in the source patient.
- An 80% reduction in the transmission rate can be achieved by appropriate prophylaxis, and all districts should have an arrangement for 24-hour access to such supplies for exposed healthcare workers.
- The risk of acquiring hepatitis is, in most parts of the world, greater than that of HIV.

Management

- After *any* exposure to blood (regardless if the source patient is known to be positive for HIV or hepatitis B or C), wash the wound liberally with soap and water but do not scrub. Antiseptics should not be used.
- Telephone for advice on local arrangements for 24-hour access to HIV prophylaxis, and specialist advice on risk assessment, based on the nature of the exposure, the risk posed by the source, and the immune status of the contact. The local consultant in Communicable Disease Control (via the Public Health Department), consultant microbiologist/virologist, or consultant in GUM will be able to advise if you do not have information to hand.

Drug starter packs are usually held at the local accident and emergency department.

- Take blood for baseline HIV and hepatitis B and C serology.
- If the risk is assessed as potentially significant, antiretroviral drugs should be commenced as soon as possible, preferably within 1 hour. Medication should be continued for a total of 4 weeks if subsequent risk assessment confirms this is appropriate. The contents of starter packs are under constant review.
- Unless the source is already known to be negative for hepatitis B, or the contact known to be fully immunized, give active immunization against hepatitis B. Passive immunization with hepatitis B immunoglobulin (HBIG) can be given within 48 hours, but may still be worthwhile up to 7 days after exposure. However, HBIG is expensive, in short supply, and only available for immunocompromised/pregnant patients exposed to known hepatitis B. Patients already immunized against hepatitis B need a booster of active immunization.
- If the source patient is of unknown status, he or she should routinely be approached (by someone other than the exposed patient) to ask for consent for testing.
- Arrange follow-up by Occupational Health, the GUM department, or another appropriate department for the exposed worker, to consider testing for HIV and hepatitis B and C in confidence at a later stage.

Summary of Post-Exposure Prophylaxis

1. Clean the wound.
2. Get advice. If significant risk exists, offer:
   - antiretroviral drugs within 1 hour;
   - active immunization with hepatitis B vaccine;
   - passive immunization with hepatitis B immunoglobulin if donor is HBV positive and recipient immunocompromised or pregnant.
3. Take blood for baseline serology of contact and source (with consent).
4. Arrange follow-up.

Post-Exposure Prophylaxis Following Sexual or Other Non-Occupational Exposure

- Post-exposure prophylaxis for HIV may be required following sexual exposure. Examples may include some cases of sexual assault and condom failure between HIV discordant couples or unprotected anal sex in men who have sex with men. In these circumstances, prophylaxis against hepatitis B should also be considered.
- Policies and regimens for HIV post-exposure prophylaxis, including indications for use after sexual exposure, are to be found on the British Association for Sexual Health and HIV (BASHH) website (www.bashh.org/documents/58/58.pdf). The consultant at the local GUM clinic should be able to give immediate advice and to assist in risk assessment. Prophylaxis, if required, should be started as soon as possible and certainly within 72 hours.

Notification and Surveillance

- Microbiology laboratories voluntarily notify positive HIV results (confidentially and anonymously) to the Communicable Disease Surveillance Centre (CDSC), Centre for Infections, 61 Colindale Avenue, London NW9 5EQ, or Health Protection Scotland (www.hps.scot.nhs.uk/). These establishments then write to the clinician concerned asking for further clinical details.

- Doctors may also notify cases directly. If the patient has not been referred on for further specialist management, the GP who receives a positive test result may be invited to provide information for the voluntary, confidential, anonymized database.

- Details of HIV and AIDS surveillance, together with recent data, can be seen at www.gov.uk.

References

Ahrendt, H. J., Nisand, I., Bastianelli, C., et al. (2006). Efficacy, acceptability and tolerability of the combined contraceptive ring, nuvaring, compared with an oral contraceptive containing 30 mg ethinyl estradiol and 3 mg of drospirenone. *Contraception, 74,* 451–457.

Anon. (1999). Combined oral contraceptives containing desogestrel or gestodene and the risk of venous thromboembolism. *Current Problems in Pharmacovigilance, 25,* 12.

Anon. (2004a). *Best practice guidance for doctors and other health professionals on the provision of advice and treatment to young people under 16 on contraception, sexual and reproductive health.* London: Department of Health.

Anon. (2004b). *Male and female sterilisation. Evidence-based guideline 4* (2nd ed.). London: Royal College of Obstetricians & Gynaecologists.

Anon. (2004c). *The care of women requesting induced abortion. Evidence-based guideline 7* (2nd ed.). London: Royal College of Obstetricians & Gynaecologists.

Anon. (2005). *Selected practice recommendations for contraceptive use* (2nd ed.). Geneva: World Health Organization.

Archer, D. F. (2006). Menstrual-cycle-related symptoms: A review of the rationale for continuous use of oral contraceptives. *Contraception, 74,* 359–366.

Arowojolu, A. O., Gallo, M. F., Grimes, D. A., & Garner, S. E. (2009). Combined oral contraceptive pills for treatment of acne. *Cochrane Database of Systematic Reviews,* (3), CD004425.

Basson, R. (2006). Sexual desire and arousal disorders in women. *The New England Journal of Medicine, 354,* 1497–1506.

Benedetti, J. K., Zeh, J., & Corey, L. (1999). Clinical reactivation of genital herpes simplex infection decreases in frequency over time. *Annals of Internal Medicine, 131,* 14–20.

BHIVA, RCP, BASHH, & BIS. (2009). *Standards for HIV clinical care.* Retrieved from www.bhiva.org/cms1191535.asp.

Bjarnadóttir, R. I., Tuppurainen, M., & Killick, S. R. (2002). Comparison of cycle control with a combined contraceptive vaginal ring and oral levonorgestrel/ethinyl estradiol. *American Journal of Obstetrics and Gynecology, 186,* 389–395.

Bonnar, J., Flynn, A., Freundl, G., et al. (1999). Personal hormone monitoring for contraception. *The British Journal of Family Planning, 24,* 128–134.

Brechin, S., & Bigrigg, A. (2006). Male and female sterilisation. *Current Obstetrics & Gynaecology, 16,* 39–46.

Brechin, S., & Penney, G. C. (2004). *Venous thromboembolism and hormonal contraception.* Guideline 40, 1–13. London: Royal College of Obstetricians & Gynaecologists.

British Association for HIV, British Association for Sexual Health and HIV, & British Infection Society. (2008). *UK National Guidelines for HIV Testing.*

Canto De Cetina, T. E., Canto, P., & Ordoñez Luna, M. (2001). Effect of counselling to improve compliance in Mexican women receiving depotmedroxyprogesterone acetate. *Contraception, 63,* 143–146.

Chan, W. S., Ray, J., Wai, E. K., et al. (2004). Risk of stroke in women exposed to low-dose oral contraceptives: A critical evaluation of the evidence. *Archives of Internal Medicine, 164,* 741–747.

Charles, V. E., Polis, C. B., Sridhara, S. K., & Blum, R. W. (2008). Abortion and long-term mental health outcomes: A systematic review of the evidence. *Contraception, 78,* 436–450.

Clinical Effectiveness Unit. (2003b). Desogestrel-only pill (Cerazette). *The Journal of Family Planning and Reproductive Health Care / Faculty of Family Planning & Reproductive Health Care, Royal College of Obstetricians & Gynaecologists, 29,* 162–164.

Clinical Effectiveness Unit. (2004c). *Femcap.* London: Faculty of Family Planning & Reproductive Healthcare.

Clinical Effectiveness Unit. (2005a). Drug interactions with hormonal contraception. *The Journal of Family Planning and Reproductive Health Care / Faculty of Family Planning & Reproductive Health Care, Royal College of Obstetricians & Gynaecologists, 31,* 139–150.

Clinical Effectiveness Unit. (2006a). *First prescription of combined oral contraception.* London: Faculty of Family Planning and Reproductive Healthcare.

Clinical Effectiveness Unit. (2007a). *Male and female condoms.* London: Faculty of Family Planning & Reproductive Healthcare.

Clinical Effectiveness Unit. (2007b). *Female barrier methods.* London: Faculty of Family Planning & Reproductive Healthcare.

Clinical Effectiveness Unit. (2008a). *Progestogen-only pills.* London: Faculty of Sexual & Reproductive Healthcare.

Clinical Effectiveness Unit. (2008b). *Progestogen-only injectable contraception.* London: Faculty of Sexual & Reproductive Healthcare.

Clinical Effectiveness Unit. (2009b). *Sexual and reproductive health for individuals with inflammatory bowel disease.* London: Faculty of Sexual and Reproductive Healthcare.

Clinical Effectiveness Unit. (2009c). *Combined vaginal ring (NuvaRing).* London: Faculty of Sexual and Reproductive Healthcare.

Clinical Effectiveness Unit. (2010a). *Contraceptive choices for young people.* London: Faculty of Sexual and Reproductive Healthcare.

Clinical Effectiveness Unit. (2010b). *Contraceptive choices for women aged over 40 years.* London: Faculty of Sexual and Reproductive Healthcare.

Clinical Effectiveness Unit. (2011). *Drug interactions with hormonal contraception.* London: Faculty of Sexual and Reproductive Healthcare.

Clinical Effectiveness Unit. (2014). *Progestogen-only implants.* London: Faculty of Sexual & Reproductive Healthcare.

Clinical Effectiveness Unit. (2015). *Intrauterine contraception.* London: Faculty of Sexual & Reproductive Healthcare. Retrieved from www.fsrh.org.

Clinical Effectiveness Unit. (2016). *Postnatal sexual and reproductive health.* London: Faculty of Sexual and Reproductive Healthcare.

Clinical Effectiveness Unit. (2016). *UK medical eligibility criteria.* London: Faculty of Sexual and Reproductive Healthcare.

Clinical Effectiveness Unit. (2017). *FSRH guideline: emergency contraception*. London: Faculty of Sexual & Reproductive Healthcare. Retrieved from www.fsrh.org.

Collaborative Group on Epidemiological Studies of Ovarian Cancer. (2008). Ovarian cancer and oral contraceptives: Collaborative reanalysis of data from 45 epidemiological studies including 23 257 women with ovarian cancer and 87 303 controls. *Lancet, 371*, 303–314.

Collaborative Group on Hormonal Factors in Breast Cancer. (1996). Breast cancer and hormonal contraceptives: collaborative reanalysis of individual data on 53 297 women with breast cancer and 100 239 women without breast cancer from 54 epidemiological studies. *Lancet, 347*, 1713–1727.

Cooper, E. (2000). Couples with learning disabilities. In S. Killick (Ed.), *Contraception in practice* (pp. 229–240). London: Martin Dunitz.

Curtis, K. M., & Martins, S. L. (2006). Progestogen-only contraception and bone mineral density: A systematic review. *Contraception, 73*, 470–487.

Donovan, C., Hadley, A., Jones, M., et al. (2000). *Confidentiality and young people*. London: Royal College of General Practitioners and Brook.

European Natural Family Planning Study Groups. (1993). Prospective European multicenter study of natural family planning (1989–1992): Interim results. *Advances in Contraception, 9*, 269–283.

Farrell, S. A., & Kieser, K. (2000). Sexuality after hysterectomy. *Obstetrics and Gynecology, 95*, 1045–1051.

Fernandez, E., La Vecchia, C., Balducci, A., et al. (2001). Oral contraceptives and colorectal cancer risk: A meta-analysis. *British Journal of Cancer, 84*, 722–727.

Forna, F., & Gulmezoglu, A. M. (2000). Interventions for treating trichomonas in women (Cochrane review). In *The Cochrane Library* (Issue 3). Oxford: Update Software.

Fotherby, K., & Howard, G. (1986). Return of fertility in women discontinuing injectable contraceptives. *Journal of Obstetrics and Gynaecology, 6*, S110–S115.

Green, J., & Kocsis, A. (1997). Psychological factors in recurrent genital herpes. *Genitourinary Medicine, 73*, 253–259.

Grimes, D. (2000). Intrauterine device and upper-genital-tract infection. *Lancet, 356*, 1013–1019.

Grimes, D. A., Lopez, L. M., Schulz, K. F., & Stanwood, N. L. (2004). Immediate post-abortal insertion of intrauterine device. *Cochrane Database of Systematic Reviews*, (4), CD001777.

Guillebaud, J. (1989). Contraception and sterilization. In A. Turnbull & G. Chamberlain (Eds.), *Obstetrics* (pp. 1135–1152). Edinburgh: Churchill Livingstone.

Hackett, G., Dean, J., Kell, P., et al. (2007). *Guidelines on the management of erectile dysfunction*. Lichfield: British Society for Sexual Medicine. Retrieved from www.bssm.org.uk/downloads/BSSM_ED_Management_Guidelines_2007.pdf.

Hannaford, P. C., Iversen, L., Macfarlane, T. V., Elliott, A. M., Angus, V., & Lee, A. J. (2010). Mortality among contraceptive pill users: Cohort evidence from Royal College of General Practitioners' oral contraception study. *British Medical Journal (Clinical Research Ed.), 340*, c927.

Harrison-Woolrych, M., & Hill, R. (2005). Unintended pregnancies with the etonogestrel implant (Implanon): A case series from postmarketing experience in Australia. *Contraception, 71*, 306–308.

Heinemann, L. A. J., Assmann, A., DoMinh, T., & Garbe, E. (1999). Oral progestogen-only contraceptives and cardiovascular risk: Results from the transnational study on oral contraceptives and the health of young women. *The European Journal of Contraception*

& Reproductive Health Care: The Official Journal of the European Society of Contraception, 4, 67–73.

International Collaboration of Epidemiological Studies of Cervical Cancer. (2007). Cervical cancer and hormonal contraceptives: Collaborative reanalysis of individual data for 16 573 women with cervical cancer and 35 509 women without cervical cancer from 24 epidemiological studies. *Lancet, 370*, 1609–1621.

Jackson, R. A., Bimla Schwarz, E., Freedman, L., & Darney, P. (2003). Advance supply of emergency contraception: Effect on use and usual contraception—a randomized trial. *Obstetrics and Gynecology, 102*, 8–16.

Jick, S. S., Kaye, J. A., Russmann, S., & Jick, H. (2006). Risk of nonfatal venous thromboembolism with oral contraceptives containing norgestimate or desogestrel compared with oral contraceptives containing levonorgestrel. *Contraception, 73*, 566–570.

Jones, S. (2008). Legal aspects of family planning. In A. Glasier & A. Gebbie (Eds.), *Handbook of family planning and reproductive healthcare* (5th ed., pp. 249–267). Edinburgh: Churchill Livingstone.

Kaunitz, A. M., Arias, R., & McClung, M. (2008). Bone density recovery after depot medroxyprogesterone acetate injectable contraception use. *Contraception, 77*, 67–76.

Kemmeren, J. M., Algra, A., & Grobbee, D. E. (2001). Third generation oral contraceptives and risk of venous thrombosis: Meta-analysis. *British Medical Journal (Clinical Research Ed.), 323*, 131–134.

Khader, Y. S., Rice, J., John, L., & Abueita, O. (2003). Oral contraceptive use and risk of myocardial infarction: A meta-analysis. *Contraception, 68*, 11–17.

Langenberg, A. G., Corey, L., Ashley, R. L., et al. (1999). A prospective study of new infections with herpes simplex virus type 1 and type 2. *The New England Journal of Medicine, 341*, 1432–1438.

Liying, Z., & Bilian, X. (2001). Emergency contraception with multiload Cu-375SL IUD: A multicentre clinical trial. *Contraception, 64*, 107–112.

MacGregor, E. A. (2007). Migraine and use of combined hormonal contraceptives: A clinical review. *The Journal of Family Planning and Reproductive Health Care / Faculty of Family Planning & Reproductive Health Care, Royal College of Obstetricians & Gynaecologists, 33*, 159–169.

Mansour, D., Korver, T., Marintcheva-Petrova, M., & Fraser, I. S. (2008). The effects of Implanon® on menstrual bleeding patterns. *The European Journal of Contraception & Reproductive Health Care: The Official Journal of the European Society of Contraception, 13*(1), S13–S28.

McGuire, H., & Hawton, K. (2003). Interventions for vaginismus. *Cochrane Database of Systematic Reviews*, (1), CD001760.

Merki-Feld, G. S., & Hund, M. (2007). Clinical experience with NuvaRing in daily practice in Switzerland: Cycle control and acceptability among women of all reproductive ages. *The European Journal of Contraception & Reproductive Health Care: The Official Journal of the European Society of Contraception, 12*, 240–247.

Meston, C. M., Hull, E., Levin, R. J., & Sipski, M. (2004). Disorders of orgasm in women. *The Journal of Sexual Medicine, 1*, 66–68.

Miller, L., & Hughes, J. P. (2003). Continuous combination oral contraceptive pills to eliminate withdrawal bleeding: A randomized trial. *Obstetrics and Gynecology, 101*, 653–661.

National Collaborating Centre for Women's and Children's Health. (2005). *Long-acting reversible contraception (NICE guideline)*. London: RCOG. Retrieved from www.nice.org.uk.

National Health Service. (2009). *National Chlamydia Screening Programme*.

National Institute for Health Care and Excellence. (2008). *Prophylaxis against infective endocarditis*. London: NICE. NICE Clinical Guideline 64.

Oddsson, K., Leifels-Fischer, B., de Melo, N. R., et al. (2005). Efficacy and safety of a contraceptive vaginal ring (NuvaRing) compared with a combined oral contraceptive: A 1-year randomized trial. *Contraception, 71*, 176–182.

Oddson, K., Leifels-Fischer, B., Wiel-Masson, D., et al. (2005). Superior cycle control with a contraceptive vaginal ring compared with an oral contraceptive containing 30 mcg ethinylestradiol and 150 mcg levonorgestrel: A randomized trial. *Human Reproduction, 20*, 557–562.

Poulter, N. R. (1996). Oral contraceptives and blood pressure. In P. C. Hannaford & A. M. C. Webb (Eds.), *Evidence-guided prescribing of the pill* (pp. 77–88). Carnforth: Parthenon.

Rosenberg, M. J., & Long, S. C. (1992). Oral contraceptives and cycle control: A critical review of the literature. *Advances in Contraception, 8*(1), 35–45.

Rosenberg, M. J., Waugh, M. S., & Stevens, C. M. (1996). Smoking and cycle control among oral contraceptive users. *American Journal of Obstetrics and Gynecology, 174*, 628–632.

Roumen, F. J. M. E., op ten Berg, M. M. T., & Hoomans, E. H. M. (2006). The combined contraceptive ring (NuvaRing): First experience in daily clinical practice in The Netherlands. *The European Journal of Contraception & Reproductive Health Care: The Official Journal of the European Society of Contraception, 11*, 14–22.

Schoeman, S. A., Stewart, C. M., Booth, R. A., et al. (2012). Assessment of best single sample for finding chlamydia in women with and without symptoms: a diagnostic test study. *British Medical Journal, 12345*, e8013.

Sloand, E. M., Pitt, E., Chiarello, R. J., & Nemo, G. J. (1991). HIV testing. State of the art. *JAMA: The Journal of the American Medical Association, 266*(20), 2861–2866.

Stewart, F. H., Harper, C. C., Ellertson, C. E., et al. (2001). Clinical breast and pelvic examination requirements for hormonal contraception. *JAMA: The Journal of the American Medical Association, 285*, 2232–2239.

Stokes, T., Shaw, E. J., Juarez-Garcia, A., et al. (2004). *Clinical guidelines and evidence review for the epilepsies: Diagnosis and management in adults and children in primary and secondary care.* London: Royal College of General Practitioners.

Trussell, J. (2007). Contraceptive efficacy. In R. A. Hatcher, J. Trussell, A. L. Nelson, W. Cates, F. H. Stewart, & D. Kowal (Eds.), *Contraceptive technology* (19th ed., pp. 747–826). New York: Ardent Media.

Vasilakis-Scaramozza, C., & Jick, H. (2001). Risk of venous thromboembolism with cyproterone or levonorgestrel contraceptives. *Lancet, 358*, 1427–1429.

Vessey, M., & Painter, R. (2006). Oral contraceptive use and cancer. Findings in a large cohort study, 1968–2004. *British Journal of Cancer, 95*, 385–389.

von Hertzen, H., Piaggio, G., Ding, J., et al. (2002). Low dose mifepristone and two regimens of levonorgestrel for emergency contraception: A WHO multicentre randomised trial. *Lancet, 360*, 1803–1810.

Waldinger, M. D. (2007). Premature ejaculation: State of the art. *The Urologic Clinics of North America, 34*, 591–599.

Weiderpass, E., Adami, H., Baron, J. A., et al. (1999). Use of oral contraceptives and endometrial cancer risk. *Cancer Causes and Control, 10*, 277–284.

Weijmar Schultz, W., Basson, R., Binik, Y., et al. (2005). Women's sexual pain and its management. *The Journal of Sexual Medicine, 2*, 301–316.

Westhoff, C. (2003). Depot-medroxyprogesterone acetate injection (Depo-Provera®): A highly effective contraceptive option with proven long-term safety. *Contraception, 68*, 75–87.

Wilcox, A. J., Dunson, D. B., Weinberg, C. R., et al. (2001). Likelihood of conception with a single act of intercourse: Providing benchmark rates for assessment of post-coital contraceptives. *Contraception, 63*, 211–215.

World Health Organisation. (1987). A multicentred phase III comparative trial of depotmedroxyprogesterone acetate given three-monthly at doses of 100 mg or 150 mg: II. The comparison of bleeding patterns. *Contraception, 35*, 591–610.

World Health Organisation. (1991). Collaborative study of neoplasia and steroid contraceptives. Depot medroxyprogesterone acetate (DMPA) and risk of endometrial cancer. *International Journal of Cancer, 49*, 186–190.

17

Infectious Diseases and Vaccination

NEIL RITCHIE

CHAPTER CONTENTS

Varicella (Chickenpox) and Herpes Zoster

Varicella Vaccine and Immunoglobulin
Confirming Susceptibility
Indications (Vaccine)
Practicalities (Vaccine)
Contraindications (Vaccine)
Adverse Reactions
Indications (Immunoglobulin)
Practicalities

Shingles Vaccine
Indications
Practicalities

Treatment of Varicella

Treatment of Herpes Zoster

Pre-travel Advice

Taking Medicines Out of the United Kingdom

Travellers' Diarrhoea

Malaria

Travel-Related Vaccination
Special Considerations for Vaccines on the UK Vaccination Schedule
Cholera
Japanese Encephalitis
Rabies
Tickborne Encephalitis
Typhoid
Yellow Fever

Symptoms in Travellers Returning From Abroad

History

Fever

Malaria

Enteric Fever

Rickettsial Infection

Fever-Arthralgia-Rash Arboviruses

Viral Haemorrhagic Fever

Other Causes of Fever

Diarrhoea

Dermatologic Presentations

Eosinophilia

Screening of Immigrants and Long-Term Travellers

Schistosomiasis

Strongyloides

Tuberculosis

Sexually Transmitted Infection

Sexually Transmitted Infection and HIV

General Approach
Patients Requiring Investigation by the General Practitioner
Patients Requiring Management by the General Practitioner
Contact Tracing
Principles of Treatment
General Investigation in Primary Care
How to Take Samples

Management of Specific Sexually Transmitted Infection
Genital Gonorrhoea
Chlamydia Infection
Lymphogranuloma Venereum
Nonspecific Urethritis
Trichomonas Vaginalis
Anogenital Warts
Soft, Nonkeratinized Warts
Keratinized Warts
Herpes Genitalis
Syphilis
Human Immunodeficiency Virus Infection

Notification of Infectious Diseases

Infectious diseases requiring notification to public health authorities are outlined in Table 17.1. Notification serves two important purposes: It allows epidemiologic monitoring of infectious diseases and it allows a coordinated public health response when required. There is a long list of pathogens that the laboratory is required to notify to public health authorities. However, some of the infectious diseases require notification on reasonable clinical suspicion by the treating medical practitioner.

Note that the list of notifiable diseases varies in Scotland and Northern Ireland.

Vaccination: General Considerations

A routine schedule of immunization is provided in Table 17.2.

Organization of an Immunization Programme in Primary Care

Ensure that:
- effective call and recall systems are in place;

GUIDANCE

The Department of Health (DoH) publishes *Immunisation Against Infectious Disease* ("The Green Book"), which contains guidance on the use of vaccines. The book is regularly updated and presents detailed advice on the individual vaccines. It is an excellent reference for more complex vaccination questions (https://www.gov.uk/government/collections/immunisation-against-infectious-disease-the-green-book).

Vaccine-specific advice contained in this chapter references each specific chapter of "The Green Book"; additional references will be specified.

Advice about vaccination should also be available through the local health protection team.

- there is an effective system for the ordering and proper care of vaccines;
- there are dedicated immunization clinics at times that are feasible for the patients; and
- written material about the vaccines is available; and that parents and patients have time to study them and discuss any concerns, before giving consent.

TABLE 17.1	**Notifiable Diseases**

Acute encephalitis*	Malaria*
Acute infectious hepatitis*	Measles
Acute meningitis*	Meningococcal
Acute poliomyelitis	septicaemia
Anthrax	Mumps
Botulism	Plague
Brucellosis	Rabies
Cholera	Rubella
Diphtheria	Severe acute respiratory
Enteric fever (typhoid or	syndrome (SARS)
paratyphoid)	Scarlet fever*
Food poisoning*	Smallpox
Haemolytic uraemic	Tetanus
syndrome	Tuberculosis
Infectious bloody diarrhoea	Typhus*
(or suspected	Viral haemorrhagic fever
Escherichia coli O157	Whooping cough
in Scotland)	Yellow fever
Invasive group A	
streptococcal disease*	
Legionnaires disease	
Leprosy*,†	

*Not in Scotland, where notifiable diseases additionally include *Haemophilus influenzae* type b, necrotizing fasciitis, tularemia, West Nile fever.
†Not in Northern Ireland, where notifiable diseases additionally include chickenpox and gastroenteritis (<2 years).

TABLE 17.2	**Routine Schedule of Immunizations**

Age	Immunization
2 months	DTaP/IPV/Hib, rotavirus, MenB, and PCV
3 months	DTaP/IPV/Hib and rotavirus
4 months	DTaP/IPV/Hib, MenB, and PCV
12 months	Hib/MenC
13–15 months	MMR, MenB, and PCV
2–7 years	Annual influenza vaccine
3 years 4 months– 5 years (preschool)	DTaP/IPV or dTaP/IPV and MMR
12–13 (girls only)	HPV
13–18 years	Td/IPV and Men ACWY
18–24 years	Men C (one dose) if not already given
65 onwards	Flu annually and PCV once
70 years	Shingles

aP, acellular pertussis; *D*, diphtheria; *d*, low-dose diphtheria; *flu*, influenza; *Hib, H. influenzae* b; *HPV*, human papillomavirus; *IPV*, inactivated polio vaccine; *MenC*, meningococcal C; *MMR*, mumps, measles, and rubella; *PCV*, pneumococcal vaccine; *T*, tetanus.

Procedure When Giving an Immunization

- Establish that the immunization is needed.
- Check that the patient is fit and that there are no contraindications. Minor illness does not mean that the immunization need be postponed. More severe illness may, but only because of the difficulty of distinguishing subsequent symptoms of the illness from an adverse effect of the immunization.
- Check that consent has been obtained. In childhood immunizations this usually consists of:
  - written consent to the programme in general; and
  - verbal consent to the specific immunization at the time. Bringing a child to an immunization clinic has been viewed as giving consent, but parents may not realize which vaccines are going to be given. To be considered informed, parents must have been given information about the benefits and possible adverse effects of the vaccine and had a chance to discuss them.
- Explain how to treat the more likely adverse effects (e.g., paracetamol or ibuprofen for pain or fever).
- Explain that information about those who have been immunized will be kept and used to monitor the safety and efficacy of the vaccination programme. This is a requirement of current Data Protection guidance.
- Check that the vaccines are not out of date and that the cold chain has not been interrupted. This means you are satisfied the vaccines have not, at any stage, frozen or warmed to more than 8°C.
- Check that facilities for resuscitation are available. This includes a resuscitation pack containing adrenaline that is up to date.
- Record the date, vaccine, and batch number in each patient's medical record.
- Do not clean the limb unless it is obviously dirty.
- Use a long (25-mm, blue hub) needle (either 23 or 25 gauge). This reduces the incidence of adverse reactions, presumably because it is more likely to reach muscle than the short (16-mm, orange hub) needle (Diggle, Deeks, & Pollard, 2006).
- If more than one injection is to be given, give them into different limbs. If the same limb must be used, give injections at least 2.5 cm apart. Record the site of each vaccine given.
- Give vaccines intramuscularly unless the patient has a bleeding disorder, when deep subcutaneous injection should be used. Exceptions to this are Bacillus Calmette-Guérin (BCG), Japanese encephalitis (JE), varicella, yellow fever (YF), and some influenza vaccines.
- Use the deltoid or the anterolateral thigh. Using the buttock risks inadvertent injection into fat which may reduce the effect of the immunization.
- Consider how to reduce the trauma of the event for the child. Infants who were given 25% sucrose solution to drink 2 minutes before the injection and who continue to suck on the bottle or on a pacifier while being held by their parents while the injection was given cried significantly less (Reis, Roth, Syphan, Tarbell, & Holubkov, 2003).

- Do not insist that the patient wait in the clinic for 20 minutes after the immunization. There is no evidence in favour of this time-honoured custom. An exception to this might be the patient with a history of syncope after injections.

Prevaccination Quality Control Checks

- Check that the vaccine is in its original packaging, so that batch number and expiry date can be checked.
- Check that the vaccine is not out of date.
- Check that the vaccines have been kept in a dedicated refrigerator with a max/min thermometer whose readings have been recorded and have not gone below 2°C or above 8°C.
- If transported in a cool box to the clinic, check that the box also has a max/min thermometer which shows the correct range has been adhered to. Check that vaccine has not frozen because it was packed too close to the ice.
- Dispose of multidose vials at the end of the clinic.

Contraindications

It is important to be clear about the genuine contraindications to immunization (see under individual vaccines) and not to be deflected from immunizing children, for instance, because of:
- eczema;
- a family history of allergy;
- a personal history of allergy unrelated to the vaccine in question;
- a personal history of epilepsy or febrile convulsions;
- a minor infection, without fever or systemic upset; or
- a nonallergic reaction to a previous immunization.
  Serious concomitant infection may be grounds for postponing immunization but only because of the difficulty of distinguishing adverse effects of the vaccination from symptoms due to the infection.

Adverse Reactions

- Previous editions of "The Green Book" listed severe local or systemic reactions as relative contraindications to further immunization with that vaccine. The 2006 edition reverses this advice, pointing out that these reactions are not allergic and may not recur with subsequent doses.
- There is some evidence that antipyretic drugs can reduce the effectiveness of vaccines if given prophylactically to prevent fever but do not prevent febrile convulsions (Prymula et al., 2009). However, there is no evidence that paracetamol given once fever develops has any impact on vaccine response. Therefore prophylactic paracetamol or ibuprofen is no longer suggested following vaccination. The only exception is in the case of the 2- and 4-month doses of 4CMenB, where postvaccination fever is very common. See the section on meningococcal vaccines for details.
- Anaphylaxis is usually the only absolute contraindication. Two situations in which immunization should be deferred until the child is stable are:

- where encephalopathy or encephalitis occurred within 7 days of the previous immunization, no cause was found, and the child had not recovered after 7 days; or
- where seizures and fever occurred within 72 hours of the previous immunization, no cause was found, and the child had not recovered after 24 hours.
- This tightening of the grounds on which immunization might be refused or deferred comes from the realization that the danger of infection in an unimmunized child puts him or her at greater risk than repeating the immunization. Except in the case of anaphylaxis, repetition of most other apparent adverse effects seems to occur no more than would be expected by chance.

Vaccine Damage Payments

- Vaccine damage payments are for those suffering 60% or more disablement as a result of immunization with one of the recommended childhood vaccines administered in the United Kingdom under the age of 18. Payment can also be made for damage due to polio, rubella, and meningococcal C vaccines given after the age of 18, and for damage due to vaccines given as part of the management of an outbreak of infectious disease in the United Kingdom.
- Claim forms are available from the Vaccine Damage Payments Unit, Palatine House, Lancaster Road, Preston PR1 1HB, tel. 01772 899944, or downloaded from the government website, http://www.direct.gov.uk (search on Vaccine Damage Payments).

Live Vaccines

- There are particular issues around the use of live vaccines. This is because live vaccines contain attenuated pathogens which can cause clinically significant infection in the immunocompromised.
- Live vaccines currently on the UK vaccination schedule are as follows:
  - Measles, mumps, and rubella (MMR)
  - Rotavirus
  - Live attenuated influenza vaccine (LAIV)
  - BCG vaccine
  - Shingles
- Live vaccines in regular use but not given routinely to all are as follows:
  - Varicella
  - YF
  - Oral typhoid vaccine
- All polio vaccines currently in use in the United Kingdom are inactivated, but live vaccine may be in use elsewhere in the world.

Special Considerations for Use of Live Vaccines

- Until recently, when using multiple live vaccines, it was advised to give them on the same day or to separate them by at least 4 weeks. However, the guidance has recently changed to highlight specific instances where vaccines are known to interact (Public Health England [PHE], 2015c):

- YF and MMR: do not coadminister on the same day. Leave at least 4 weeks between the vaccines. If urgent protection is required then give at any time but consider a further dose of MMR.
- Varicella/zoster vaccines and MMR: give on the same day or leave at least 4 weeks between vaccines.
- Tuberculin skin testing and MMR: MMR increases the likelihood of a false negative skin test. Wait until the skin test has been read before giving MMR and do not commence a skin test until 4 weeks after MMR has been given.
- Other live vaccines can be given at any time before and after each other.
- Previous advice that live vaccines should not be given within 3 weeks of receiving normal human immunoglobulin now applies only to MMR. Other live vaccines can be given at any time with respect to immunoglobulin.
- Live vaccines should not be given to the following:
  - Pregnant women: In most cases the risk is theoretical only. Women inadvertently vaccinated during pregnancy should be reassured that the risk is thought to be very low.
  - The immunocompromised, including:
    a. patients who have received high-dose systemic steroids in the last 3 months. This means children who have received 2 mg/kg/day for at least 1 week or 1 mg/kg/day for at least 1 month, or adults who have received the equivalent of 40 mg prednisolone per day for more than 1 week or 20 mg/day for at least 1 month. Lower doses may suppress immunity, especially if combined with cytotoxic drugs. Discuss each case with the specialist concerned;
    b. patients on biological therapies (e.g., infliximab);
    c. patients with malignancy of the reticuloendothelial system; or
    d. patients who are immunosuppressed due to radiotherapy or chemotherapy in the last 6 months or who are in some other way immunodeficient.

This list is abbreviated and incomplete. For detailed advice on the use of live vaccines in the immunocompromised, see "The Green Book." Note that not all cases are clear cut and, if there is doubt about whether vaccination is indicated, this should be discussed with a specialist.

Special Cases

Incomplete or Uncertain Vaccination History

- A flowchart outlining action to be taken in the event of a child presenting late for vaccines is available from the Department of Health and regularly updated (PHE, n.d.b).
- If the patient is uncertain, treat as though unimmunized. With the exception of BCG, the adverse effects of repeat doses of vaccine are usually lower than the original dose and certainly lower than the risk of remaining unprotected.
- If the patient is certain but the course is incomplete, restart where the course left off.
- Usually a course started with one vaccine may be completed with another vaccine brand. Inactivated polio vaccine can be used to complete a course begun with live polio vaccine.
- Note that for some vaccines, there is a different schedule for older children. For example, four doses of *Haemophilus influenzae* type B (Hib) vaccine are given when the course is started in infancy but children 1 year or older require only a single dose.

People Living With Human Immunodeficiency Virus

- Generally speaking, inactivated vaccines can be given to those with human immunodeficiency virus (HIV) as normal. However, many vaccines are less effective in HIV positive individuals. Combination vaccines, including a hepatitis A component (Hep A/B and Hep A/typhoid) should be avoided as there is evidence of decreased efficacy.
- Some live vaccines, such as MMR, varicella, shingles, and YF, can be safely given if the CD4 count is high.
- Where there is a choice between live vaccines and a nonreplicating alternative (influenza, typhoid, polio), the nonreplicating vaccine should be selected.
- BCG is absolutely contraindicated in HIV.

Guidelines on the use of vaccines in HIV positive adults (British HIV Association, 2015) is published by the British HIV Association, available at http://www.bhiva.org (choose Guidelines).

Other Immunosuppressed Patients

- Ensure that the full course of routine immunization has been given. If further immunization is needed, discuss timing with the physician in charge. Time their administration when immunosuppression is least, in order to:
  - maximize the chance that immunity will develop; and
  - in the case of live vaccines, reduce the risk of fulminating infection.
- In addition, give influenza and pneumococcal vaccination and warn the patient to avoid contact with chickenpox and exposed shingles. If exposure does occur, consider urgent immunoglobulin (see page 293).

Contacts of Immunosuppressed Patients

- Check that the full course of routine immunizations has been given. Make good any deficiencies.
- Immunize against varicella (unless already immune) and influenza, to reduce the risk of catching the disease and passing it to the patient.

Patients Without an Active Spleen

- Give Hib, influenza, meningococcal vaccines and pneumococcal vaccine.
- Give oral phenoxymethylpenicillin prophylaxis against pneumococcal and meningococcal infection.

- The lifetime risk of overwhelming infection postsplenectomy is around 5% but the greatest risk is in the first few years following loss of splenic function. Most cases are preventable (Newland, Provan, & Myint, 2005).

Patients With Cochlear Implants or Cerebrospinal Fluid Leak

- Give pneumococcal vaccine.

Patients on Haemodialysis

- Give hepatitis B vaccine at double the normal dose for four doses.
- Patients should also receive influenza and pneumococcal vaccine.

Patients With Haemophilia

- Give hepatitis A and B vaccines.
- Note that patients with bleeding disorders may receive some vaccines by an alternative route to reduce the risk of bleeding.

Patients With Chronic Medical Conditions: Diabetes or Heart, Lung, Liver, or Renal Disease

- Give influenza and pneumococcal vaccines.

Clinical Staff

- Check that they have documented evidence of two MMR doses or of antibodies to measles and rubella.
- Consider BCG if Mantoux negative and in close contact with patients with tuberculosis.
- Give hepatitis B vaccine if working with blood or body fluids contaminated with blood, or at risk of sharps injuries, or of being bitten by a patient.

Non-Clinical Staff Who Are in Contact With Patients

- Check that they are immunized with MMR, as for clinical staff.
- If no clear history of chickenpox or shingles, check for varicella antibodies and immunize if negative.
- Give hepatitis B vaccine if they may come into contact with contaminated sharps.

Specific Infectious Diseases and Immunizations

Diphtheria, Tetanus, and Polio

- Diphtheria is very rare in the United Kingdom and almost all cases are either imported or arise in the contacts of imported cases. Tetanus is also rare but sporadic cases do occur, usually in elderly individuals whose immunity has waned. Good wound care and appropriate use of immunization is vital in prevention of such cases. Polio is also extremely rare in the United Kingdom and throughout most of the world but remains endemic in some areas, most notably Pakistan and Afghanistan.

- The vaccines to prevent these illnesses are no longer available as single component vaccines and therefore the combination vaccine should be used even if there is only an indication for one of the conditions. Four- and five-component vaccines with the addition of pertussis (and Hib) are available and are used routinely in childhood (see Table 17.2).

Indications

- As part of UK immunization schedule (five doses as shown in Table 17.2).
- Travellers to countries with outbreaks/endemic diphtheria or polio or travellers who may not be able to seek immediate medical attention for a tetanus-prone wound who have not received a dose of vaccine within the last 10 years.
- Contacts of a diphtheria case. A booster dose should be given even if previously fully vaccinated.
- Healthcare staff at risk of contact (i.e. microbiology laboratory staff) should receive a booster every 10 years.

Contraindications

- Anaphylaxis to the vaccine or a vaccine component
- Tetanus-prone wounds. A tetanus-prone wound is defined as a wound or burn:
  - that requires surgical intervention which is delayed more than 6 hours;
  - where there is a significant amount of devitalized tissue or a puncture type injury, especially with soil/manure contamination;
  - where there is the presence of a foreign body;
  - with compound fracture; or
  - in the presence of systemic sepsis.

  High-risk wounds are those that have been heavily contaminated with material thought likely to contain tetanus spores (i.e., soil) or wounds that contain extensive devitalized tissue.

Management

- Clean the wound thoroughly.
- Note that high-risk wounds (as defined) require treatment with human tetanus immunoglobulin even if the patient is fully vaccinated.
- For nonimmunized or incompletely immunized patients with a tetanus-prone wound, a detailed summary of actions for incompletely immunized patients is available in the DoH "Green Book." Give:
  - a tetanus toxoid booster (combined with low-dose diphtheria) or a primary course as appropriate; and
  - tetanus immunoglobulin. This is available from Bio Products Laboratory (020 8258 2342), or from the Scottish National Blood Transfusion Services (0131 536 5300). Give one vial (250 IU) intramuscularly or two vials if more than 24 hours have elapsed, the wound is heavily contaminated or is a burn, or the patient weighs over 90 kg.
- In patients of unknown immune status, if patients are uncertain whether a primary course has been given, assume that they will have received primary immunization only if they were born in the United Kingdom after 1960 or were in the Armed Forces in or after 1938.

Group A Streptococcal Infection

GUIDANCE

Scottish Intercollegiate Guidelines Network. (2010). Management of sore throat and indications for tonsillectomy. SIGN clinical guideline 117. http://www.sign.ac.uk/pdf/sign117.pdf.

Public Health England. (2014). Interim guidelines for the public health management of scarlet fever outbreaks in schools, nurseries and other childcare settings. https://www.gov.uk/government/uploads/system/uploads/attachment_data/file/322727/PHE_Interim_guidelines_for_scarlet_fever_outbreaks_in_schools_and_nurseriesFINAL2.pdf.

- Sore throat is a common presentation in general practice. The majority of patients require reassurance and symptom management only. Discriminating this group from those who would benefit from a therapeutic intervention is a significant challenge.
- Suspect epiglottitis in patients with stridor, respiratory difficulty, or severe systemic illness. **Do not examine the throat of such patients** as it may precipitate airway obstruction. Such patients should be admitted to hospital immediately.
- Other indications for admission to hospital are dehydration and progressive difficulty swallowing.
- Recommend ibuprofen or paracetamol for pain relief.
- Asymptomatic carriage of group A streptococci is common and there is little evidence that throat swabs or rapid antigen tests are helpful and their routine use is not recommended.
- For the majority of patients well enough to be managed in the community use the Centor criteria to guide a decision on the use of antibiotics.
- The Centor criteria suggest that patients with three or four of the following criteria are more likely to benefit from antibiotics: tonsillar exudate, tender anterior cervical lymph nodes, history of fever, and absence of cough.
- If antibiotics are prescribed, consider whether a delayed prescribing strategy is appropriate.
- Penicillin V 500 mg four times per day for 10 days is recommended for first line treatment. Macrolides are appropriate therapy for patients unable to take penicillin. Avoid amoxicillin and co-amoxiclav since these often cause a rash in patients with mononucleosis.
- There has been a recent increase in cases of scarlet fever in the United Kingdom. Scarlet fever is caused by toxin-producing strains of group A streptococci and presents with a history of current or recent pharyngitis and extensive erythematous rash.
- Consider scarlet fever in patients with a history of pharyngitis and rash. Features that increase the likelihood of scarlet fever are the presence of a sandpaper texture to the rash and a strawberry tongue. Desquamation, particularly of the fingers and toes, often occurs in convalescence.
- Patients are at risk of complications such as disseminated infection, glomerulonephritis, and rheumatic fever.
- If scarlet fever is suspected, the following actions should be taken:
  - A throat swab for culture although note that a negative swab does not exclude scarlet fever as the cause of the illness. The differential diagnosis includes measles, parvovirus (slapped cheek), and infectious mononucleosis.
  - Do not wait for the result of the throat swab before prescribing antibiotics: penicillin V 500 mg four times per day for 10 days or the age-appropriate dose for children. Use a macrolide in those unable to take penicillin.
  - Advise self-isolation for 24 hours after commencing antibiotic therapy.
  - Do not wait for the result of the throat swab before notifying the local health protection team.

Haemophilus influenzae Type B

Hib is a cause of meningitis and epiglottitis, principally in children. Since the introduction of vaccine it has become rare in the United Kingdom.

Indications

- As per national schedule (see Table 17.2). A child who misses these doses should be immunized up to the age of 10. If diphtheria, tetanus, and polio have been given, give a single dose of Hib/meningococcal C (MenC) vaccine.
- Household contacts of invasive Hib disease if aged under 10 and not already immunized.
- Non-household contacts aged under 10 at a creche, nursery, or playgroup if not already immunized.
- A patient with invasive Hib disease, regardless of age, unless subsequent serology shows that immunity has been acquired.
- High-risk patients: children and adults with a non-functioning spleen, or otherwise immunocompromised, should receive a single booster of Hib/MenC provided they have been fully immunized against Hib. If not, the primary course should be completed if under 10 or, if aged 10 or over, two doses of Hib/MenC should be given 2 months apart.

Contraindications

- Acute illness
- Confirmed anaphylactic reaction to a previous dose or to neomycin, streptomycin, or polymyxin B
- A deteriorating neurologic condition is grounds for deferring immunization, but a severe reaction to a previous dose without anaphylaxis (e.g., fever, convulsions, screaming, or a hypotonic–hyporesponsive episode) is not a contraindication.

Hepatitis (Viral)

Hepatitis A and E

- Hepatitis A and E are clinically indistinguishable infections characterized by symptoms of acute hepatitis (fever, jaundice, right upper quadrant pain, pale stools, and dark urine). Historically hepatitis A was the principle agent of acute viral hepatitis in the United Kingdom but the incidence of this infection has declined (around 400 cases per year in England and Wales) and hepatitis E has been increasingly reported (around 800 cases per year in England and Wales). Hepatitis E should be considered in any patient with evidence of acute hepatitis (Kamar, Dalton, Abravanel, & Izopet, 2014).

- Hepatitis A is readily preventable through vaccination but there is no vaccine to prevent hepatitis E licensed in the United Kingdom.
- Hepatitis A is spread by the faecal-oral route and contaminated foodstuffs such as shellfish. It does not cause chronic infection and rarely causes death.
- In the United Kingdom, hepatitis E is zoonosis spread principally through eating infected pork. Travel-associated disease is usually contracted in a similar manner to hepatitis A. Note that no vaccine for hepatitis E is available in the United Kingdom.

Hepatitis A Vaccination

Indications
- Laboratory staff working with the virus
- Haemophiliacs and any others treated with coagulation factors (give the injection subcutaneously)
- Those with chronic liver disease, including hepatitis B or C, because of the severity of hepatitis A infection in an already compromised liver
- Travellers to areas of poor sanitation, especially if travelling to areas of high or medium risk repeatedly or for more than 3 months
- Individuals who are at risk because of their sexual behaviour, including men who have sex with men (MSM)
- Injecting drug users
- *Immunization should be considered for:*
  - close contacts of those with hepatitis A or in the context of outbreaks in schools, nurseries, and closed communities. Take advice from the Consultant in Communicable Disease Control or, in Scotland, from the Consultant in Public Health Medicine (CPHM);
  - residents of institutions for those with learning difficulties; and
  - workers at risk (e.g., sewage workers, laboratory workers exposed to hepatitis A, and those working in institutions for those with severe learning disabilities).

Contraindications
- Severe febrile illness
- Anaphylactic reaction to the vaccine or, in the case of Epaxal only, to egg

Practicalities
- Give one dose of vaccine intramuscularly into the deltoid. This gives immunity for 3 years. A second dose 6 to 12 months later gives immunity for 10 to 20 years. A further dose may be given at 20 years if the risk continues. Combination vaccines

offering protection against hepatitis B or typhoid are also available and can be used where indicated.
- Human normal immunoglobulin (HNIG) to provide passive protection is now limited to high-risk contacts of those with hepatitis A. Supplies are scarce and it should be used only on expert advice.

Hepatitis B

- Hepatitis B is a common infection throughout much of the world but is relatively uncommon in the United Kingdom.
- Due to the low risk, vaccination is directed at those at risk.
- Hepatitis B can present as either an acute hepatitis clinically indistinguishable from hepatitis A or as a chronic infection with mildly abnormal (or entirely normal) liver function tests (LFTs).
- Chronic hepatitis B infection predisposes to cirrhosis and primary hepatocellular carcinoma which can be present at presentation.

Serology

Hepatitis serology is confusing due to the wide range of laboratory tests used. In brief:
- Surface antigen (HBsAg) is the best marker of active infection while surface antibody (anti-HBsAg) is the best marker of immunity (acquired naturally or through vaccination). Core antibody (anti-HBc) is not acquired through vaccination and therefore suggests previously cleared infection in HBsAg negative individuals.
- The presence of e antigen (HBeAg) usually implies high viral load and high infectivity while e antibody (anti-HBeAg) usually implies low viral load and low infectivity although there are some pitfalls.
- Any patient who has active hepatitis B infection should be referred to a specialist even if they have normal LFTs.

Vaccination

Indications
"The Green Book" lists a large number of indications for hepatitis B vaccine. The following summarize the recommendations.

Pre-exposure Prophylaxis
- All those who inject drugs, or those considered to be at risk of injecting drugs in the future. Close contacts of persons who inject drugs should also be offered vaccination
- Those who change sexual partners frequently
- Close contacts of those with hepatitis B infection
- Families adopting children from countries of high prevalence and those who may provide foster care at short notice for children with infection
- Those who may be at increased risk of infection due to medical treatment, including repeated blood product administration, and renal dialysis, including those who may require such interventions in the future

- Patients with chronic liver disease
- Prisoners
- Individuals in residential accommodation for those with learning difficulties and other persons with learning difficulties based on an individual risk assessment
- People travelling to areas with intermediate or high prevalence of hepatitis B based on an individualized risk assessment
- Those at occupational risk, including healthcare workers, laboratory staff, those working in prisons, those working in residential accommodation for those with learning difficulties, and any other occupation based on an appropriate risk assessment

Post-exposure Prophylaxis

- Infants born to mothers with chronic hepatitis B or acute hepatitis B during pregnancy (note that further management, including administration of immunoglobulin [HBIG] to the infant and treatment of the mother with antiviral drugs may be indicated based on specialist assessment)
- Those who may have been exposed to hepatitis B sexually, including victims of sexual assault (HBIG may also be indicated, seek advice)
- Persons who are accidentally inoculated with potentially infected body fluids (HBIG may also be indicated, seek advice)
- HBIG is in limited supply and should be used in post-exposure prophylaxis in genuinely high-risk cases after discussion with a specialist. Hepatitis B vaccine is effective postexposure prophylaxis and is sufficient in cases in which the risk of hepatitis B is low.
- Note that hepatitis B vaccine is frequently indicated for those who present for advice about post-exposure prophylaxis even when it can be established that the exposure does not present a risk of hepatitis B transmission (e.g., blood splashes onto intact skin) because the person has an indication for preexposure vaccination.

Contraindications

- Anaphylaxis to a previous dose of hepatitis B vaccine or a vaccine component

Practicalities

- There are a wide variety of hepatitis B vaccines available and schedules vary. It is important to refer to the product literature to ensure the appropriate vaccine and schedule are chosen. The standard schedule of hepatitis B vaccination should be used infrequently since the accelerated schedule (doses at 0, 1, and 2 months) gives similar responses and higher compliance. A further dose should be given at 12 months if the risk is ongoing.
- Where a course is interrupted and there is a high likelihood of future noncompliance, practitioners should take advantage of any opportunity to offer additional doses of vaccine with the aim of delivering three doses to persons at risk. This is particularly important for injecting drug users, who are at particularly high risk of infection.
- Only where there is no urgency and an absence of factors suggesting compliance may be poor should the standard schedule be used.

- Alternative schedules are available for use in special patient populations. Children aged 1 to 15 can be protected by two doses of adult strength vaccine at 0 and 6 months. For those with an urgent need of protection (e.g., those imminently travelling abroad), a very rapid schedule (0, 7, and 21 days) can be used with a further dose at 12 months.
- Patients with chronic renal failure respond poorly to hepatitis B vaccine and a higher dose vaccine (40 μg) is recommended.

Monitoring of Vaccine Protection

- All those who are still at risk of hepatitis B should receive a final booster dose 5 years after initial vaccination.
- Vaccine protection can be assessed by measuring anti-HBsAg levels. There is no indication to do this except in patients with occupational exposure and those receiving renal dialysis. In the case of occupational exposure do the following:
  a. Check anti-HBsAg levels 1 to 4 months after the primary course.
  b. Those with levels above 100 mIU/mL do not require further monitoring and should receive the booster at 5 years only.
  c. Those with levels 10 to 100 mIU/mL should receive an immediate further dose and the booster at 5 years. They also do not require further monitoring.
  d. Those with levels below 10 mIU/mL should receive a further primary course and further assessment of antibody levels at the end of this course. If the levels remain below 10 mIU/mL then they should be considered unprotected and would have to receive HBIG in the case of significant exposure to hepatitis B.
- Patients with renal failure on dialysis require annual monitoring of antibody levels with booster doses when antibody levels drop below 10 mIU/mL.

Hepatitis C

- Hepatitis C causes chronic hepatitis in a high proportion of those who have been infected. No vaccine is available and acute infection is usually relatively mild and commonly does not come to medical attention.
- At the time of writing, a revolution in the management of hepatitis C is in progress with treatment changing from regimes consisting of pegylated interferon-α and ribavirin to those based on directly acting antivirals. Such regimes are highly effective and it is likely that within the lifetime of this book that such treatments will be available to all patients with chronic hepatitis C.
- It is therefore important to identify patients with chronic hepatitis C (including patients previously identified but not in specialist follow-up) so that they can be offered treatment.
- Some patients do not attend clinics because they are concerned about possible side effects of treatment or previously failed therapy. They should be encouraged to attend for assessment.

Human Papillomavirus

- Human papillomavirus (HPV) is a cause of warts and premalignant/malignant conditions at a variety of sites. More than 99% of cases of cervical cancer are associated with the presence of HPV and prevention of infection is associated with a substantial reduction in the development of cervical cancer, particularly among young women.
- Several other cancers are also strongly associated with infection with HPV, including oral cancer and anogenital cancers.
- Many varieties of HPV exist but the majority of cancers are associated with types 16 and 18. The currently available vaccine protects against these types and also types 6 and 11, which are the principal cause of genital warts.

Indications

- The vaccine is offered to all young women aged between 11 and 14 as part of the UK national vaccination programme. Two doses are given at 0 and 6 to 24 months.
- Men are currently not offered vaccination on the UK routine vaccination schedule (RVS) but at the time of writing there is availability of the vaccine on a pilot for use of vaccine in sexual health clinics for men who have sex with men (PHE, n.d.a).

Contraindications

- Anaphylaxis to HPV vaccine or a vaccine component

Influenza

- That influenza is common should not reduce the importance of influenza vaccination as influenza is a common cause of death in the winter months when seasonal infection occurs. As well as direct mortality from respiratory tract infection, influenza is also associated with increased cardiovascular mortality (Clar, Oseni, Flowers, Keshtkar-Jahromi, & Rees, 1996).
- Two types of influenza vaccine are available:
  - Inactivated vaccine, which is usually given to adults and is administered intramuscularly (or occasionally intradermally)
  - Live, attenuated vaccine, which is used in children aged 2 years or older and is administered intranasally
- Both vaccines types, with the exception of specially produced vaccines for emerging strains of influenza A such as the H1N1 pandemic in 2009, contain three or four strains of influenza, including both influenza A and B. The vaccine is reformulated annually based on the strains of influenza likely to be prevalent in the winter months.

Indications

- All adults aged over 65 years should be offered annual vaccination. In addition, all those aged 6 months and over in the following risk groups should be offered vaccination:

- Patients with chronic respiratory, heart, kidney, liver, or neurologic disease
- Patients with diabetes mellitus
- Patients with significant immunosuppression, including asplenia
- Pregnant women
- Those with a BMI greater than 40
- Health and social care workers
- Residents in residential care homes
- In addition, children aged over 2 years now receive influenza vaccine as part of the routine childhood immunization programme.

Contraindications

- Anaphylaxis to a previous dose of influenza vaccine or a vaccine component
  Note that nasally administered influenza vaccines are live, attenuated, and should not be given to those with significant immunosuppression as defined in the section on live vaccines. In cases where live vaccine is contraindicated, inactivated vaccine can be given as an alternative.

Practicalities

Influenza vaccines are given as a single dose except where children in clinical risk groups are receiving influenza vaccine for the first time. In such cases, a second dose 4 weeks later may be required; refer to "The Green Book" for details.

Antivirals for Influenza

> **GUIDANCE**
>
> Detailed advice on the use of antivirals in influenza is available from Public Health England (2016c).

- Several drugs with antiviral efficacy against influenza are available but the only drugs in common clinical use are oseltamivir and zanamivir. These drugs are recommended for treatment and post-exposure prophylaxis in selected patients. Oseltamivir is prescribed in tablet form whereas zanamivir is a dried powder inhaler.
- Generally speaking, antiviral therapy is not recommended in patients who are previously fit and well and do not require admission to hospital. Patients with chronic illnesses or are 65 years or older, who are therefore at increased risk of developing complicated influenza, should be offered antivirals if they present within 48 hours of onset or later at the prescriber's discretion. The risk factors for complicated influenza are the same as those used to indicate eligibility for annual vaccination. It is not necessary to wait until the diagnosis is confirmed before prescribing antivirals.
- Most patients should receive oseltamivir for 5 days. Patients with severe immunosuppression (defined as in the section on live vaccines) may be better managed with zanamavir

because of concern about the development of resistance and such patients should be discussed with a specialist.

Lyme Disease

Lyme disease is caused by *Borrelia burgdorferi* and presents a variety of clinical difficulties. It is transmitted by tick bites. In its acute form it is relatively uncontroversial and usually straightforwardly managed successfully with antibiotics. Cases of late disease are much less common but can be far more difficult to diagnose and manage. The disease has become highly politicized, particularly in the United States, where some states have legislated on issues around diagnosis and treatment.

Presentation

- Lyme disease has a varied initial presentation. In classic early Lyme, patients present with a slowly enlarging target lesion known as *erythema chronicum migrans*. Occasionally there may be multiple lesions. Patients are often nonspecifically unwell with low grade fever, arthralgia, and lethargy. The rash may be not seen, atypical, or absent and there is often no reported history of tick bite.
- Early complications include painful radiculopathy, cranial nerve (especially facial nerve) palsies, meningoencephalitis, and carditis (typically presenting with heart block). Late complications include arthritis, peripheral neuropathy, and chronic encephalomyelitis. These complications are uncommon.

Diagnosis

- Early Lyme infection is a clinical diagnosis.
- Serologic testing is unhelpful since it is frequently negative in early infection and seropositivity among asymptomatic controls in endemic areas is relatively common. Therefore patients with a typical rash and history of a tick bite should be treated on clinical grounds without serology.
- Patients with early disease who are appropriately treated often do not develop antibodies and so convalescent serology is also unhelpful in these cases.
- Serology should be reserved for those where there is significant doubt regarding the diagnosis or those who have complicated disease, in which serology is likely to be positive.

Treatment

- First line treatment of early Lyme infection is doxycycline 100 mg twice daily or 200mg once daily for 21 days. If doxycycline is contraindicated, then amoxicillin 1g three times daily for 21 days is an alternative.
- NICE guidelines suggest that patients not responding to one course of antibiotics may be offered further treatment with one further course of an antibiotic from a different class (for example amoxicillin for patients previously treated with doxycycline. Patients with suspected late or complicated Lyme should be referred to a specialist.

Post-Lyme Syndrome

Some patients develop chronic, disabling symptoms following treatment for Lyme disease. Management is controversial and some physicians recommend intravenous or prolonged antibiotic therapy. There is no evidence of a benefit of prolonged antibiotics and such patients may require specialist assessment.

Tick Bites

- Tick bites are common, and concern about Lyme disease prompts an increasing number of patients to present for assessment.
- When a patient presents with a tick attached, this should be removed with the use of a pair of tweezers. The tick should be gripped as close to the skin surface as possible and pulled gently and smoothly away from the skin without twisting.
- Antimicrobial prophylaxis of tick bites is not usually recommended in the United Kingdom but can be considered in immunocompromised patients.
- The US Centers for Disease Control and Prevention (CDC) suggests some circumstances in which antimicrobial prophylaxis can be recommended but these circumstances are unlikely to be encountered in the United Kingdom.

Measles, Mumps, and Rubella

These infections were rare in the United Kingdom. However, following the MMR vaccine scare in the late 1990s, vaccination rates fell and were slow to recover. Thus there is a current cohort of young adults who are at increased risk of infection and cases of measles, mumps, and rubella occur in the United Kingdom. Recognition is important since public health measures are required to prevent outbreaks.

Clinical Presentation

- Measles presents as a febrile, coryzal illness followed by florid, erythematous macular rash which usually covers the whole body. Koplik spots may be seen prior to the development of the rash but are rarely clinically detected in view of the rarity of the diagnosis today. Complications include pneumonia, meningitis, and the late, devastating subacute sclerosing panencephalitis.
- Mumps presents with fever and bilateral, painful parotid swelling. Complications include meningitis, pancreatitis, and orchitis.

- Rubella is a mild illness characterized by coryza and macular rash. It is only significant because of the severe consequences of *intrauterine* infection. Rubella is detected only very rarely in the United Kingdom.

Vaccination

Indications

- All previously unvaccinated individuals born after 1970 should be vaccinated unless they give a past history of infection. Note that vaccinated individuals born in the 1970s will have received measles vaccine only and those born in the 1980s will have received a combined measles/ rubella vaccine.
- Children are vaccinated at 13 to 15 months and receive a preschool booster.
- Older children and adults should receive two doses of vaccine 1 month apart.
  Other indications for vaccination include the following:
- Women of childbearing age who are seronegative for rubella. Note that this is commonly only detected in pregnancy and, since live vaccines are contraindicated during pregnancy, should be deferred until after delivery
- Healthcare workers in regular contact with pregnant women who are seronegative
- Immunocompetent, previously unvaccinated individuals less than 3 days postcontact with a confirmed case of measles
- Immunocompromised individuals and nonimmune pregnant women can receive human normal immunoglobulin prophylaxis following measles contact. Immunoglobulin is not recommended following contact with mumps or rubella.

Contraindications

- Anaphylaxis to MMR vaccine or its components, including gelatin. Note that a gelatin-free vaccine is available as an alternative. Egg allergy, even if severe, is not a contraindication to vaccination.
- Note that MMR is a live vaccine and has the same contraindications and special precautions as other live vaccines (see section Live vaccines).

Adverse Effects

- Fever, malaise, and rash are common post vaccine and usually occur in the first week but can occur several weeks after vaccination.
- Febrile seizures occur in around 1:1000.
- Immune thrombocytopenic purpura occurs rarely and resolves spontaneously.
- The putative association between MMR and autism or inflammatory bowel disease has not been found in a large number of well-conducted studies and is not a reason to avoid vaccination.
- There is no evidence that giving individual vaccine components is safer and is not recommended.

Practicalities

- MMR is given by intramuscular injection.

Meningococcal and Pneumococcal Infection

- Encapsulated organisms continue to represent a major source of morbidity and mortality. Meningococcal disease is the principle cause of bacterial meningitis in the young while *Streptococcus pneumoniae* dominates in older patients. The pneumococcus is also the most common cause of bacterial pneumonia.
- Meningitis represents a challenging diagnosis, particularly in the early stages. While a minority of patients present with the classic triad of fever, headache, and neck stiffness, most present with less specific features. Particularly challenging is diagnosis in those at the extremes of age, who often present very nonspecifically. Rash is usually absent in pneumococcal meningitis and is absent or nonspecific in the early stages of meningococcal infection. However, a petechial rash in a patient with features of systemic illness is a very specific sign of meningococcal infection and should prompt immediate action.
- A recent UK guideline on the management of meningitis and meningococcal sepsis (McGill et al., 2016) recommends that:
  - patients with suspected meningitis or meningococcal sepsis should be referred to hospital for assessment;
  - if possible, the patient should arrive in hospital within 1 hour of initial assessment;
  - there should be clear documentation of clinical signs of meningitis (headache, altered mental status, neck stiffness, fever), presence or absence of rash, and signs of shock (hypotension, capillary refill time); and
  - Kernig and Brudzinski signs are insensitive and should not be used to exclude bacterial meningitis.
- The evidence for use of antibiotics in the community is mixed. However, early antibiotics are strongly associated with survival in bacterial meningitis and the UK guidelines recommend use of prehospital antibiotics in the following circumstances:
  - Patients with signs of meningococcal disease (i.e., rash and severe sepsis or meningism)
  - Presence of features of severe sepsis (i.e., hypotension, poor capillary refill, altered mental state)
  - Where bacterial meningitis is suspected and there will be a delay of greater than 1 hour in getting to hospital
- Recommended antibiotics are benzylpenicillin or ceftriaxone, which can both be given intramuscularly. Patients with allergy to these antibiotics should not receive antibiotics prehospital and hospital transfer should not be delayed by administration of antibiotics.

Meningococcal Vaccines

There are now a variety of meningococcal vaccines in routine use in the United Kingdom and reflect the different serotypes of meningococci. Children receive vaccines against serogroups B and C while teenagers are given a quadrivalent vaccine protecting against serogroups A, C, W, and Y. The serogroup

B vaccine was the most recently developed vaccine and at the time of writing has only recently been introduced into the UK immunization schedule.

Indications

- Infants, children, and teenagers as part of the national vaccination schedule.
- Students up to 25 years attending university for the first time who have not previously received quadrivalent meningococcal vaccine should receive MenACWY.
- Adults and children with asplenia, functional asplenia, and complement disorders, including pharmacologic complement inhibition, should receive additional doses of MenC, MenACWY, and MenB (×2) on the schedule shown in "The Green Book."
- Travellers to countries with high prevalence of meningococcal infection should receive MenACWY.
- Travellers to the Hajj pilgrimage should receive MenACWY (this is an entry requirement for pilgrims entering Saudi Arabia).
- Contacts of patients with meningococcal disease as part of a coordinated public health response.

Contraindications

- Anaphylaxis to a previous dose of a meningococcal vaccine or a vaccine component

Practicalities

- All meningococcal vaccines are given by intramuscular injection.
- Prophylactic paracetamol is suggested after the MenB vaccine at 2 and 4 months due to a high risk of fever; 60-mg doses of paracetamol are suggested immediately following vaccination and then two more at 4- to 6-hour interverals (PHE, 2015d).

Pneumococcal Vaccines

Two pneumococcal vaccines are available in the United Kingdom. Pneumococcal polysaccharide vaccine (PPV) provides protection against 23 common serotypes and is given to adults but ineffective in young children, while pneumococcal conjugate vaccine (PCV) is given to infants and children and is effective against 13 common invasive serotypes.

Indications

- Infants receive three doses as part of the national immunization schedule.
- Those aged 65 and over should be offered vaccination on the first occasion they attend for influenza vaccine.
- Those in clinical risks groups:
  - Chronic respiratory, heart, kidney, or liver disease
  - Diabetes mellitus
  - Immunosuppression, including asplenia or splenic dysfunction
  - Those with cochlear implants
  - Those with cerebrospinal fluid leaks

Contraindications

- Anaphylaxis to a previous dose of a pneumococcal vaccine or a vaccine component

Practicalities

Pneumococcal vaccines are given by intramuscular injection. Infants receive three doses but adults and children over 1 year are protected with a single dose of vaccine. Booster doses are not usually required except in cases of asplenia/splenic dysfunction or chronic renal failure where a booster should be given every 5 years.

Pertussis

Whooping cough is a toxin-mediated condition that causes chronic cough often followed by a characteristic postcough whoop or posttussive vomiting. Infants are at particular risk of complications and the majority of deaths occur in this age group. Pertussis vaccines in use in the United Kingdom are acellular and contain purified pertussis proteins.

Management of Suspected Cases

> **GUIDELINES**
>
> Public Health England (2016b) publishes "Guidelines for the Public Health Management of Pertussis in England" which includes sections on diagnosis and management in primary care.

- Pertussis should be suspected in any patient presenting with a prolonged acute cough (≥14 days) and paroxysms of coughing, whooping, or post-tussive vomiting. Apnoeic episodes in infants are another concerning feature. There should be increased vigilance in contacts of confirmed cases or in the context of a known outbreak.
- Children with suspected whooping cough should be excluded from school or nursery until they have completed 2 days of antibiotic therapy or 3 weeks from the onset of symptoms.
- There is limited evidence that antibiotics shorten the duration of cough unless given in the early stages of infection. However, antibiotics are recommended to eradicate the organism and prevent onward transmission.
- If antibiotics are given, newer macrolides such as clarithromycin or azithromycin are usually recommended. See PHE guidelines for dosing and advice in infants and pregnant women.
- Attempt to confirm the diagnosis in all patients. Anterior nasal swabs and throat swabs have low sensitivity for culture and so a posterior nasopharyngeal swab is preferred. Using a swab designed for the purpose, pass the swab along the floor of the nasal cavity into the nasopharynx and send urgently to the laboratory.
- Polymerase chain reaction (PCR) is now available from many laboratories and has higher sensitivity than culture.

Throat swabs are also useful in this group. Discuss with your local laboratory.

- Detection of antipertussis toxin IgG in saliva (children) or blood (adults) is available for those who have had symptoms for more than 2 weeks and have not been recently vaccinated. Discuss with public health.
- Prophylactic therapy may be appropriate for close contacts if any of the contacts are vulnerable or at high risk of infecting vulnerable groups (i.e., those caring for newborn babies). Public health will advise on this.

Indications for Vaccination

- Pertussis vaccine is only available in combination with other vaccine products. It is given as part of the UK national vaccination schedule. Four doses are given starting at 2 months and is completed with the preschool booster.
- Pregnant women are offered a booster, ideally between weeks 16 and 32 of gestation although the vaccine can be given later in pregnancy, even up to the time of delivery. The vaccine is given to promote passive immunity in the infant and introduction of the antenatal booster has been associated with a significant reduction in infant pertussis. Since only combination vaccines are available, women should be offered a single dose of diphtheria, tetanus, polio, and pertussis vaccine.

Contraindications

- Anaphylaxis to a previous dose of a pertussis vaccine or a vaccine component.

Staphylococcus aureus, Including MRSA

> **GUIDELINES**
>
> The British Society of Antimicrobial Chemotherapy publishes guidelines on management of MRSA infection in the community (Nathwani et al., 2008).
>
> There are also guidelines from the Royal College of Nursing (2010) which include a section on care in the community.
>
> The Department of Health has published an information sheet for patients in primary care affected by MRSA (http://mrsaactionuk.net/pdfs/MRSA_Advice.pdf).

- *S. aureus* is a common colonizing bacteria. However, it can cause serious soft tissue infections, particularly in patients with wounds or immune compromise. Complications include endocarditis and osteoarticular infection. While great strides have been made in the last 10 years to reduce the burden of disease caused by methicillin (flucloxacillin)–resistant *S. aureus* (MRSA), which is usually hospital acquired, there has been little impact on cases of community-acquired staphylococcal disease that are usually sensitive to flucloxacillin.
- Recently there has also been increased awareness of isolated cases and outbreaks of cutaneous abscesses caused by *S. aureus* expressing the Panton–Valentine leukocidin (PVL) toxin. PVL-producing *S. aureus* has also been associated with severe necrotizing pneumonias and can affect young, otherwise healthy people.
- No vaccine is currently available to protect against staphylococcal disease.

Management of Methicillin-Resistant *Staphylococcus aureus* in the Community

- MRSA colonization is more common in patients with a history of hospital treatment and those who are residents in care homes. MRSA colonization does not require systemic antibiotic therapy, although decolonization may be attempted using topical treatments but this is usually attempted only in patients who are hospitalized or considering elective hospital treatment. Such treatment should be discussed with an infection specialist.
- MRSA infection should also be suspected in patients with soft tissue infections that fail to respond to standard therapy.
- Patients known to be colonized with MRSA should be advised to:
  - continue usual social activities, as there is no need to self-isolate;
  - be particularly careful with hygiene;
  - exercise caution when in contact with people who may be particularly susceptible to infection, including those with open wounds, in-dwelling vascular devices, and dermatologic conditions. Close contacts should be advised to keep wounds and sores covered;
  - avoid sharing personal items such as towels with others; and
  - inform any treating healthcare professionals of the history of MRSA colonization.
- Patients known to have MRSA or at high risk should be discussed with an infection specialist if treatment is required. MRSA is often resistant to multiple antibiotics and a regime of treatment should be carefully chosen to suit the patient's needs:
  - Oral antibiotic therapy usually consists of a combination of oral antibiotics to reduce the risk of further resistance developing.
  - If rifampicin is used, be aware of the potential for drug interactions and seek help from a pharmacist if necessary. Rifampicin should always be used as part of a combination therapy.
  - Note that a culture positive for MRSA from a wound does not mandate treatment if the wound is not showing clinical signs of infection.
- All doctors and other healthcare professionals have a responsibility to maintain good infection control practice to protect patients from harm.
  - Ensure you are aware of the dress code for your place of work and adhere to it.
  - Wash your hands after every patient contact.
  - It is good practice to carry alcohol hand gel when conducting home visits so that the hands can be cleansed if there is no soap and water available.

Tuberculosis

GUIDELINES

National Institute for Health and Care Excellence (NICE, 2016) guidelines contain important information on the diagnosis and public health response to tuberculosis as well as recommendations for specialist clinics.

- The incidence of tuberculosis (TB) has been rising in the United Kingdom since the 1980s, although this may now be reversing. This rise has been driven by a rising number of cases among those born outside the United Kingdom.
- The highest incidence of tuberculosis is found in people born in India and Pakistan, and among black Africans. Most patients who develop TB do so after they have lived in the United Kingdom for years.
- Other risk factors for TB include ethnic minorities born in the United Kingdom; immunocompromise, including HIV infection; and a family history of TB.
- All tuberculosis in the United Kingdom should be managed in specialist clinics. All patients with suspected TB should be referred to a specialist for investigation.
- Suspect TB in any patient with a persistent productive cough, especially if there are risk factors and/or constitutional symptoms such as fever, night sweats, and weight loss.
- Many laboratories do not routinely perform microscopy and culture for TB on sputum so ensure the clinical suspicion of TB is indicated on the request.

Vaccination

BCG vaccine contains a live, attenuated strain of *Mycobacterium bovis*. Immunization is now targeted on those at highest risk as the incidence in the general population has declined. BCG offers particular protection against extrapulmonary forms of disease but only modest protection against pulmonary disease.

Indications

- All infants living in a part of the United Kingdom with an incidence of TB greater than 40/100,000 (mostly inner-city areas with large immigrant populations)
- Infants and children under age 16 born in a country or who have a parent or grandparent born in a country with an incidence of TB greater than 40/100,000
- Infants and children under age 16 who are previously unvaccinated, tuberculin negative contacts of a case of pulmonary TB; neonates should not receive BCG in this situation
- Those considered to be at occupational risk of tuberculosis
- Those under age 16 planning to live or work with local people for more than 3 months in a country with an incidence of TB greater than 40/100,000
- Tuberculin skin testing is not usually performed before vaccinating those under 6 years of age unless they are a

known contact of a case of pulmonary TB. There are intermittent shortages of BCG vaccination which mandate prioritization of BCG vaccination. The highest priority for vaccination is infants at high risk.

Contraindications

- Significant immunosuppression or immunocompromised, including HIV infection
- Previous BCG vaccination or a positive tuberculin skin test/interferon gamma release assay (If there is an uncertain vaccination history then the vaccine should only be given after a negative tuberculin skin test.)
- A personal history of TB infection
- A history of anaphylaxis to BCG
- Those with septic skin conditions and patches of eczema

Practicalities

- BCG is given by strictly intradermal injection as deeper inoculation causes significant risk of abscess formation, keloid scarring, and other local complications. BCG should only be given by staff who have been appropriately trained in its delivery.
- Axillary lymphadenitis with or without ulceration usually resolves spontaneously. Evidence of dissemination beyond the local lymph node is likely to imply immunosuppression and such patients should always be referred to a specialist.
- After BCG is given, the arm must be avoided for further vaccinations for 3 months.

Varicella (Chickenpox) and Herpes Zoster

- Chickenpox is one of the few vaccine preventable diseases that remains common in the United Kingdom. The Joint Committee on Vaccination and Immunisation (JCVI) has concluded that universal varicella vaccination would not be cost effective and there is the theoretical risk of paradoxically increasing incidence of chickenpox and shingles in adults although such an effect is not demonstrated in the United States where the vaccine has been in use for some time. However, the varicella vaccine is available for certain groups in whom protection is particularly desirable.
- The herpes zoster vaccine is unusual in that it is given to boost naturally acquired immunity to varicella to reduce the risk of virus reactivation. It is particularly effective in reducing morbidity due to postherpetic neuralgia.
- Both vaccines are live, attenuated vaccines. They differ in that the inoculum is much smaller in the varicella vaccine.

Varicella Vaccine and Immunoglobulin
Confirming Susceptibility

- Generally a clear personal history of chickenpox can be considered a reliable indicator of immunity to varicella.

- Where there is doubt those in whom therapy is being considered can be tested for varicella zoster antibodies.
- In cases where a patient has been exposed to varicella and immunoglobulin therapy is being considered, there is usually sufficient time to check serology.

Indications (Vaccine)

- Susceptible individuals undertaking healthcare or laboratory work in which exposure to infected patients or material is likely
- Susceptible close contacts of severely immunosuppressed children in whom exposure would be likely in the event of varicella infection (i.e., siblings)

Practicalities (Vaccine)

- Two different vaccines are available. Varilrix is licensed only for use in those aged 13 and over while Varivax can be used from 12 months. Both vaccines are given in two doses 4 to 8 weeks apart.
- There is evidence that recent MMR can blunt varicella vaccine immune responses. MMR should either be given simultaneously or separated by an interval of at least 4 weeks.

Contraindications (Vaccine)

- Anaphylaxis to varicella vaccine or one of its components.
- Varicella vaccine is a live vaccine and so should not be given to patients who are pregnant or immunosuppressed (see the section on live vaccines).

Adverse Reactions

Rash, which may be vesicular, is commonly associated with the vaccine (5%–10%). Otherwise the vaccine is usually well tolerated.

Indications (Immunoglobulin)

Varicella zoster immunoglobulin (VZIG) is indicated only in cases where the following four criteria are met:
- The patient has no varicella antibodies—most adults who report no clinical history of chickenpox infection have detectable varicella antibodies. Therefore every effort should be made to test before giving VZIG; however, this should not extend the wait for VZIG to more than 7 days.
- There is a history of significant exposure to varicella. This can be difficult to assess:
  - Generally persons with varicella are infectious from 48 hours prior to the appearance of rash and those with shingles are infectious from the appearance of the rash. The period of infectivity ends when the lesions are crusted over.
  - In shingles, usually contact with a person with exposed lesions is required for transmission. Exceptions include immunocompromised patients with shingles who may shed large amounts of virus.
  - A significant exposure usually requires contact for a significant period of time (e.g., sharing a room for 15 minutes).
- The patient at risk of acquiring varicella comes from a group at high risk of complications. Those at risk include pregnant woman; neonates from seronegative mothers, including in cases of maternal chickenpox within 7 days of delivery; and those with significant immunosuppression.
- The contact with varicella is in the preceding 7 days (10 days in cases where the antibody level is already known to be negative).

Practicalities

- VZIG is given by intramuscular injection at an age-dependent dose.
- Patients with bleeding disorders who cannot receive intramuscular injections can be given normal human immunoglobulin.
- Note that VZIG contains other antibodies as well and so can interfere with the development of immunity to live vaccines. Defer vaccination for 3 months or if vaccination cannot be avoided then repeat the vaccination after 3 months.

Shingles Vaccine
Indications

- Those aged 70 to 79 who have not previously received a dose of shingles vaccine

Practicalities

- The vaccine is administered intramuscularly or subcutaneously as a single dose.
- It can be given at the same time as influenza vaccine and pneumococcal vaccine if these vaccines are also indicated.

Treatment of Varicella

- Healthy children with chickenpox do not usually require treatment.
- Treatment with aciclovir can be considered for those aged 14 or older presenting with chickenpox within 48 hours of the onset of rash as this group is at increased risk of severe disease (Tunbridge, Breuer, Jeffery, & British Infection Society, 2008).
- Complications of chickenpox include pneumonitis, superadded bacterial infection, central nervous system involvement, and haemorrhagic complications.
- Pneumonitis is particularly concerning since it can be present with symptoms but no clinical signs on auscultation and can be rapidly progressive.
- Risk factors for pneumonitis include smoking, preexisting lung disease, pregnancy, and immunosuppression.
- All patients with complicated chickenpox should be admitted to hospital. Patients with immunosuppression (as defined in the section on live vaccines) and pregnant patients beyond 36 weeks of gestation should also be seen at hospital.

Treatment of Herpes Zoster

- Treatment is usually only indicated within 72 hours of the onset of rash.

- Those aged under 50 rarely have severe shingles and the risk of postherpetic neuralgia is low. They should not be routinely treated with antivirals unless they have:
  - particularly severe pain or rash;
  - non-truncal involvement; or
  - immunocompromise (consider admitting to hospital unless the patient is not severely immunocompromised, is systemically well, and the shingles rash is localized).
- Those over age 50 are at increased risk of severe pain and postherpetic neuralgia. They should usually be treated with antivirals if they present within 72 hours of the onset of rash.
- There is no risk to the foetus/neonate from maternal shingles since maternal antibodies will be present. Treatment in pregnancy is not usually recommended unless the risks outweigh the benefits of treatment and specialist advice should be sought if there is concern.
- Antiviral treatment of shingles should consist of aciclovir, valaciclovir, or famciclovir. There is some evidence that use of valaciclovir and famciclovir are more effective for early pain but evidence that they are more effective at preventing postherpetic neuralgia is lacking (Chen et al., 1996).
- Postherpetic neuralgia is common, particularly in older patients with shingles and can be very painful. Be prepared to intervene early with a drug effective against neuropathic pain.
- Recurrent shingles is a common reason for referral to infectious diseases and immunology clinics. Recurrent shingles in young patients is an important indicator of underlying immune dysfunction (e.g., HIV infection). However, it is important to consider other diagnoses such as herpes simplex virus (HSV) and dermatologic conditions. If possible, confirm the diagnosis by swabbing the lesions for PCR.

Pre-travel Advice

- Discuss the itinerary in relation to the traveller's existing health problems. Travellers often do not consider the impact of their travel plans on their health. Consider if patients are fit to travel and any changes to their treatment prior to travel.
- Explain that most countries outside the European Economic Area (EEA) do not have reciprocal health agreements with the United Kingdom. Travel insurance is needed. Within the EEA and Switzerland treatment needed while abroad is covered by the use of the European Health Insurance Card (EHIC), which should be obtained before travelling, from the website http://www.dh.gov.uk or by phoning 0300 330 1350. Applicants will need to have their NHS or National Insurance number at hand. Application may also be made by post on a form obtainable from a post office but the applicant should allow 21 days for the EHIC to arrive.
- The EHIC gives the cardholder the same right to state-provided treatment as though a resident of that country. Note that this will not necessarily cover all the costs nor extra items, such as repatriation back to the United Kingdom for which insurance is still needed. It will not cover the traveller at all if the main purpose of the trip is to obtain treatment.
- Check that the traveller has received all the routine immunizations recommended for the United Kingdom. Consider giving the following boosters if the last immunization was over 10 years ago and the planned travel poses more risk than is present in the United Kingdom: polio, tetanus, and diphtheria. The combined Td/IPV vaccine should be used even if only one or two of the immunizations is needed.
- Recommend that patients visit the Department of Health website to review current advice for travellers (http://www.nhs.uk/nhsengland/Healthcareabroad/pages/Healthcareabroad.aspx). The Foreign Office also publishes up-to-date information on a country-by-country basis with general advice about travel (https://www.gov.uk/foreign-travel-advice).
- In regard to prevention, stress the importance of preventive measures against gastroenteritis, insect bites, sunburn, accidents, and sexually transmitted diseases. Travellers should know that accidents are the greatest cause of morbidity and mortality, and that more become HIV positive than contract typhoid or malaria.
- Recommend the appropriate immunizations from an up-to-date source (see the beginning of this section). For a suggested table of how the necessary immunizations can be scheduled see Appendix 3.
- Specialist travel clinics are available throughout the country and are useful for patients with complex or unusual itineraries. Some infectious disease units run specialist travel clinics (although they will still charge for vaccines). In other parts of the country, specialist services may only be available privately. Make sure you know where specialist travel advice may be obtained in your area.
- Altitude sickness is common among travellers going above 3000 m and can occur above 2500 m. Risk factors include cardiorespiratory disease. The best way to prevent altitude sickness is to acclimatize properly and to limit the rate of ascent. Inexperienced travellers are often exposed to a significant risk of altitude illness by attempts to rapidly climb mountains such as Kilimanjaro. Climbers should be advised to stop ascending if they experience headache while climbing and should descend immediately if they are not feeling better after 6 hours of rest or develop shortness of breath or alteration of consciousness. A climber who is feeling unwell should never be left alone.
- Prophylactic treatment with acetazolamide 125 mg twice daily can be given to patients at high risk of altitude-related illness (Ritchie, Baggott, & Todd, 2012). It should be started 2 days prior to ascending above 3000 m and continued until the day after the descent is begun. Adverse effects are common but usually mild and include paresthesia in the hands and feet, urinary frequency, and alteration in taste. Acetazolamide is not a licence to ignore the advice about regulating the rate of ascent. Clinical trials of acetazolamide involve very few cases of severe altitude sickness and there is no evidence that acetazolamide is effective in preventing life-threatening illness.

- The British Moutaineering Council has an information book on travelling at high altitudes as well as information sheets about common tourist climbs (https://www.thebmc.co.uk/mountain-specific-altitude-advice-sheets).
- Advise skiers and snowboarders that the evidence is now in favour of wearing helmets in the prevention of head injuries, with a 60% reduction in risk (Sulheim et al., 2006).
- In regard to deep vein thrombosis (DVT), warn those at increased risk of DVT about the hazard posed by longhaul travel (say, >8 hours) whether by plane, bus, train, or car. Explain the need for exercises and avoidance of constricting clothing. For those at greatest risk recommend class 2 below-knee graduated compression stockings. Consider, in conjunction with a haematologist, the need for injections of low molecular weight heparin in those with a previous DVT or pulmonary embolus.

Taking Medicines Out of the United Kingdom

- Recommend that a patient who plans to take prescription drugs abroad should take them in their original, labelled bottles, as well as a copy of the prescription (or the slip for ordering repeat prescriptions). In some countries it is an offence to enter with drugs which the patient will consider harmless (e.g., codeine or a hypnotic) without such documentation.
- Controlled drugs are a special case:
  - Advise the patient that there are limits on the quantity of controlled drugs that can be taken out of the United Kingdom. To find out what these limits are and for further information see the leaflet published by HM Revenue and Customs, "Taking Medicines With You When You Go Abroad," HMRC reference notice 4, available at http://www.hmrc.gov.uk (search on Drugs Abroad).
  - Provide a letter detailing the patient's condition and drugs taken.
  - Explain that if they are within the limit then there is no need to declare these drugs to customs in the United Kingdom.
  - Advise the patient who has to carry more than the accepted limit of controlled drugs to apply for a licence from the Home Office at least 14 days before travelling. Details of how to apply can be found at http://www.hmrc.gov.uk.
  - Advise the patient to contact the relevant Embassy, High Commission, or the Home Office Drugs Branch (Room 239, 50 Queen Anne's Gate, London SW1 9AH, tel. 020 7217 8457/8446) for information about an individual country's restrictions.

Travellers' Diarrhoea

- Travellers' diarrhoea is one of the most common conditions affecting those travelling abroad.
- Among patients travelling to the tropics, a diarrhoeal illness will occur in 60% (Steffen, 2005).

- Traveller's diarrhoea is usually caused by enteroaggregative *Escherichia coli* and is a self-limiting, non-severe illness for most affected travellers.
- Advise the traveller that:
  - travellers' diarrhoea is usually mild and self-limiting;
  - rehydration is the most important treatment. Ordinary water is perfectly acceptable for mild cases but in more severe and prolonged cases there is a benefit to oral rehydration solutions;
  - loperamide can be useful to control symptoms but should not be used if there is bloody diarrhoea or high fever. It should also not be used in young children; and
  - medical attention should be sought if there is persistent blood in the stools, persistent fever, confusion, the traveller is unable to get out of bed, or is unable to maintain hydration by the oral route.
- Antibiotics can be useful in shortening the duration of symptoms. Ciprofloxacin is commonly prescribed but rising rates of ciprofloxacin resistance among campylobacter and salmonella, particularly in India and Southeast Asia, is a concern and azithromycin is a useful (unlicensed) alternative. A convenient, single dose of 1 g has been well studied and is effective. A recent American clinical practice guideline summarizes the antibiotic treatment options for acute diarrhoea (Riddle, DuPont, & Connor, 2016).
- Antibiotic resistance is a concern. One study found high rates of carriage of resistant organisms in the faeces of travellers who had taken antibiotics (Kantele et al., 2015). Antibiotics should only be prescribed for those in whom a diarrhoeal illness would be particularly troublesome and travellers should be counselled not to use them for mild symptoms.

Malaria

GUIDANCE

Public Health England (2015a) publishes guidelines for malaria prevention in travellers from the United Kingdom. The guidelines contain detailed information about all aspects of malaria prevention. However, the country-specific information is not regularly updated.

For detailed, country-specific information on malaria risk, prevention, and antimalarial resistance, see the country-specific pages and maps available through the National Travel Health Network & Centre (NaTHNaC) or Travax.

- Malaria is prevalent throughout the tropics and is capable of causing severe disease.
- As with most travel-related infections, those visiting friends and relatives are at greatest risk of acquiring malaria and are also the least likely to seek pre-travel advice.
- Those born in regions where malaria is common often do not recognize that their immunity wanes when they move to a nontropical region. They are therefore at risk of developing severe malaria when they return to visit.

- All travellers to tropical regions should receive advice about malaria and some will require pharmacologic prophylaxis.
- Malaria risk varies from country to country, and often varies from region to region within countries. Specific advice about the country to be visited will be available from NaTHNaC or Travax.
- All travellers to tropical countries should be advised about bite avoidance. Travellers should be advised about bite avoidance even if there is no risk of malaria in the region they are visiting. This is important, since other mosquito-borne diseases such as dengue, chikungunya, and Zika are common throughout the tropics and can only be prevented by effective bite avoidance:
  - Wear appropriate clothing: loose fitting clothing covering as much of the body as possible, preferably sleeves to wrists, long trousers, socks, and shoes.
  - Be aware of the peak biting period of mosquitoes. While mosquitoes may bite throughout the day, mosquitoes are most active at dawn and dusk and continue to bite through the night.
  - Ensure protection at night; if not sleeping in a properly screened room, use an insecticide-treated net. Check the net for tears before use.
  - Use insect repellent throughout the time in the tropics; 50% DEET is most effective and is known to be safe in pregnancy although it is not suitable for those younger than 2 months. Apply after sunscreen to skin and reapply frequently. Permethrin treatment of clothes is also known to be effective in reducing bites.
  - An information sheet on bite avoidance is available (https://www.gov.uk/government/uploads/system/uploads/attachment_data/file/507350/Mosquito_advice_sheet_v2.pdf).
- All travellers to areas with any risk of malaria should be advised about the need to consider malaria and seek urgent medical attention if a fever develops up to 1 year after travel.
- Malaria prophylaxis is recommended for those visiting areas with a high risk of malaria transmission:
  - No malaria prophylaxis is 100% effective, but efficacy is significantly reduced if it is not taken diligently.
  - It is important to note that chloroquine resistance is widely disseminated, and chloroquine is not recommended for malaria prophylaxis in most areas. See country-specific guidelines on NaTHNac or Travax for advice.
  - In some areas with low level resistance to chloroquine, chloroquine + proguanil is suggested.
  - In other areas where there is high level resistance to chloroquine, the recommended agents are doxycycline, atovaquone/proguanil, or mefloquine.
  - *Chloroquine* is taken weekly. It is generally well tolerated and suitable for long-term use. The dose for adults is 310 mg weekly and weight-adjusted doses are available from birth. Patients should begin treatment 1 week before arrival and continued for 4 weeks after leaving the malaria risk area.

- *Proguanil* is never taken as monotherapy but is used to enhance the efficacy of chloroquine in areas with low level resistance to chloroquine. It is taken daily and the dose for adults is 200 mg. Weight-adjusted doses are available from birth.
- *Mefloquine* is taken weekly and is highly effective malaria prophylaxis in most areas, including those with quinine resistance. There is some mefloquine resistance in Southeast Asia, particularly on the Thai/Cambodian border and this drug is not recommended for these areas. The adult dose of mefloquine is 250 mg weekly. It can be used in children weighing over 5 kg. There is significant concern about neuropsychiatric side effects and while these are uncommon, they can be severe. Mefloquine is contraindicated in those with a history of psychiatric illness or seizures. Those planning to take mefloquine should be advised to begin 3 weeks prior to travel so there is time to assess whether adverse effects will occur and an alternative agent selected. Like chloroquine, it should be taken for 4 weeks after leaving the malaria risk area.
- *Doxycycline* is taken daily and is highly effective malaria prophylaxis throughout all risk areas. Side effects include dyspepsia, vulvovaginal candidiasis, and skin photosensitivity. The dose for those 12 years and older is 100 mg daily but it is not recommended for those under 12 years. It can be commenced 2 days prior to travel and should be continued for 4 weeks after leaving the malaria risk area.
- *Atovaquone/proguanil* is also taken daily. Adverse effects include headache and gastrointestinal upset. Atovaquone/proguanil has the advantage that it only needs to be taken for 2 days prior to entering the area of malaria risk and 7 days after leaving it. This makes it particularly convenient for short periods of travel in risk areas. However, atovaquone/proguanil is the most expensive of the commonly used prophylactic regimes which limits its use for most longer term travellers. The adult dose of the fixed-dose combination is 1 tablet daily and it is suitable for children weighing more than 5 kg.
- *Pregnancy* is a difficult issue. Pregnancy is a major risk factor for severe malaria and pregnant women are at generally increased risk from tropical infection. Pregnant women should be advised not to travel to regions with malaria risk. If travel is unavoidable, malaria prophylaxis should be carefully selected. Chloroquine/proguanil is thought to be safe in all trimesters but is only suitable for a minority of destinations. It is advisable to seek expert advice about the prophylaxis of pregnant women travelling to regions with significant chloroquine resistance.
- Occasionally it may be appropriate to prescribe standby therapy for malaria for those who may have difficulty accessing prompt treatment for malaria. Atovaquone/proguanil is most commonly prescribed for this indication since it is readily available in the United Kingdom. It is important to note that standby treatment is not a

substitute for medical assessment. It should only be prescribed for those who may genuinely struggle to obtain prompt medical attention and those who begin treatment should seek medical advice as soon as possible.

Travel-Related Vaccination

Special Considerations for Vaccines on the UK Vaccination Schedule

- Ensure that travellers are up to date with standard vaccines and offer boosters as appropriate. Remember that vaccine preventable diseases now rare in the United Kingdom may be common elsewhere in the world.
- Only inactivated polio vaccine is in use in the United Kingdom. However, countries with active transmission of polio often use live, attenuated polio vaccine. Travellers without proof of their vaccination status are sometimes subject to vaccination with live, attenuated polio vaccine when visiting such countries (Afghanistan, Pakistan, and Nigeria at the time of writing). Immunosuppressed travellers should not receive live, attenuated polio vaccine and so should travel with proof of having received the vaccine within the preceeding 10 years.
- Vaccination with meningococcal ACWY is mandatory for pilgrims entering Saudi Arabia for the Hajj.

Cholera

- Cholera is a disease of extremely poor living conditions causing profuse watery diarrhoea which is rapidly disabling and commonly fatal if there is no access to treatment. If treated promptly, patients should recover fully.
- It is extremely rare in tourists and vaccination is only recommended for those whose reason for travel (usually humanitarian work) puts them at particular risk.

Indications

- Travellers planning on undertaking disaster relief or aid work who may be at risk. Note that most travellers undertaking humanitarian work among local populations are not at risk and do not require the vaccine
- Travellers to areas with active reported transmission of cholera where there may be a delay in obtaining medical assistance
- Travellers considered at significant risk of acquiring cholera for other reasons
- Laboratory staff who may be exposed to cholera for occupational reasons (usually limited to those in reference and research laboratories)

Practicalities

- Cholera vaccine is an oral vaccine delivered in two doses (three doses for children 2–6 years) 1 to 6 weeks apart. It is not recommended for children under the age of 2.
- If an interval of more than 6 weeks elapses between doses, the primary course must be restarted.
- A booster dose can be given to those at ongoing risk after 2 years (6 months for those aged 2–6). It is unclear how long immunity persists after this booster dose is given. It is reasonable to consider further boosters for those at continuing high risk.

Contraindications

- Anaphylaxis to cholera vaccine or one of its components

Japanese Encephalitis

- JE is endemic throughout most of India, Southeast Asia, and parts of China.
- Most cases of JE are asymptomatic but it occasionally causes a severe encephalitis with high mortality and frequent neurologic sequelae.
- Cases are rare in travellers and those visiting cities are unlikely to be at risk.
- Transmission is usually during the summer months in temperate areas and year-round in the tropics and subtropics. Country-specific information on transmission is available through NaTHNac and Travax.
- Vaccine is usually recommended for those visiting endemic areas for more than 1 month if travelling during the transmission season, particularly if travellers are visiting agricultural areas.

Practicalities

- The licensed JE vaccine (IXIARO) has now replaced the older unlicensed vaccine (Green Cross) which is no longer recommended.
- Two intramuscular doses of vaccine are given on days 0 and 28. Only if necessary, the course can be accelerated by 4 days.
- A booster dose can be given to those at ongoing risk 1 to 2 years following the primary course but the duration of protection following this dose is uncertain.
- Those who have previously received a primary course of JE vaccine at any time are protected by a single dose of vaccine (those who previously received Green Cross can receive IXIARO).

Contraindications

- Anaphylaxis to a dose of JE vaccine or one of its components

Rabies

- Rabies is a severe viral encephalitis that is almost universally fatal. However, it can be effectively prevented by appropriate use of pre- and postexposure prophylaxis.
- Terrestrial mammals have been the traditional reservoir for rabies infection and, globally, most infections are spread through bites and scratches from infected wild animals such as dogs, cats, raccoons, and monkeys.
- Rabies in terrestrial mammals has been eradicated from the United Kingdom for more than 100 years. However, related viruses are occasionally present in bats and a man died from rabies caused by European bat lyssavirus 2 (EBLV-2) after exposure to a bat in 2002.
- Thus there are two groups of individuals that require protection from rabies:

- Travellers to countries where rabies is endemic
- Those likely to be exposed to animals in the United Kingdom that may carry rabies or associated viruses (usually for occupational reasons)
- For most travellers making short duration itineraries to endemic countries, pre-exposure vaccination will not be recommended because the risk is small and post-exposure prophylaxis is likely to be readily available.

Rabies Vaccine

Indications for Preexposure Prophylaxis

- Those continuously exposed to rabies for occupational reasons (e.g., working in a reference or research laboratory handling rabies virus–infected materials)
- Those with ongoing risk of exposure to rabies vaccine (e.g., bat handlers, those working with imported animals, those undertaking veterinary or healthcare work in countries with endemic rabies)
- Those with infrequent periods of exposure risk (e.g., travellers to endemic areas). Country-specific risk assessments are maintained through PHE (Health Protection Scotland [HPS] in Scotland).

Practicalities

- Two rabies vaccines are available in the United Kingdom (Rabies Vaccine BP and Rabipur). They are interchangeable.
- Regardless of the indication, all groups should receive three doses of rabies vaccine on days 0, 7, and 28 (if necessary, the third dose can be given on day 21).
- Those with continuous or ongoing risk should have their protection monitored with serology and booster doses of vaccine given to maintain antibody levels in the protective range. It is anticipated that this will usually be managed by occupational health departments.
- Those with infrequent risk of exposure do not require serology but may be offered a booster at 10 years if there is ongoing infrequent risk.
- Note that even in those who have been vaccinated, further action is still required in the event of a significant exposure (see the section on postexposure prophylaxis).

Contraindications

- Anaphylaxis to rabies vaccine or one of its components
- Note that when rabies vaccine is used for postexposure prophylaxis there are no absolute contraindications and if the patient had a previous severe reaction then expert advice should be sought since the risk of rabies is usually higher than the risk of a further adverse reaction.

Post-exposure Prophylaxis

- Rabies can be transmitted by bites and scratches from infected mammals. Infrequently, transmission has also been reported following exposure of blood or saliva onto broken skin or mucous membranes. The United Kingdom has been free of rabies transmitted from the terrestrial mammal population for more than 100 years.
- Exposure to bats should be considered to carry a (small) risk of transmission of rabies wherever in the world it occurs (including the United Kingdom).

- Those with a potential exposure should be carefully assessed. Risk assessment guidance is available through PHE (HPS in Scotland).
- Management of individuals potentially exposed to rabies will include use of vaccine (including giving booster doses to those previously vaccinated) and in some cases where the risk is high, administration of human rabies immunoglobulin.
- Advice on rabies postexposure prophylaxis can be obtained through the duty doctor in Colindale (020 8200 4400). For contact information in Scotland, Wales, and Northern Ireland see "The Green Book."

Tickborne Encephalitis

Tickborne encephalitis (TBE) is an important cause of meningoencephalitis across Central and Eastern Europe, Russia and the Caucasus, and Japan. It is spread by the bite of infected Ixodes ticks and travellers at risk include those travelling to endemic areas who plan to spend time in forested areas during the tick season (spring to early autumn).

- Advise travellers about the risk from tick bites and suggest the following:
  - Tuck long trousers into socks and spray exposed skin with an insect repellent containing DEET and clothes with one containing permethrin.
  - Warn travellers to avoid unpasteurized milk; it can be caught from the milk of an infected animal.
  - Inspect the skin for ticks daily. If found, ticks should be pulled off (intact) by applying steady traction. Do not rupture the tick; mouth parts will be left in the skin.
  - Offer vaccine to those planning to walk, camp, or work in forested regions in the infected areas in spring or summer. The vaccine is effective and safe. It has been used in Austria as part of the national routine vaccination programme for over 25 years. However, there has never been a case of TBE reported in a traveller returning to the United Kingdom and travellers may reasonably decide to rely on tick-avoidance measures instead of the vaccine.

Practicalities

- TBE vaccine is given in three doses at 0, 1, and 6 months.
- A shortened course given at 0 and 2 weeks can be given if limited time is available but gives less effective protection.
- Booster doses can be given every 3 years if there is ongoing risk.

Contraindications

- Anaphylaxis to TBE vaccine or a vaccine component
- Anaphylaxis to egg

Typhoid

- Enteric fever is caused by *Salmonella typhi* and *S. paratyphi*.
- In contrast to other types of salmonella infection in humans, typhoid does not cause prominent gastrointestinal symptoms. Instead, patients present nonspecifically unwell

with fever. In severe cases, patients develop multiorgan failure.

- Typhoid is common in parts of the world with inadequate sanitation and is spread principally through consumption of contaminated food and drink.
- Typhoid vaccine offers protection against *S. typhi* but is not effective at preventing paratyphoid.

Indications
- Travellers visiting typhoid-endemic areas with plans indicating higher risk
- Travellers with frequent or prolonged exposure to poor sanitation
- Laboratory staff who may handle typhoid

Practicalities
- Two typhoid vaccines are available in the United Kingdom:
  - Vi vaccine is given by intramuscular injection in a single dose.
  - Ty21a vaccine is given as three oral capsules on days 0, 2, and 4.
- Vi vaccine is an inactivated vaccine; Ty21a is a live, attenuated vaccine.
- Injectable typhoid vaccines can be given as a combined injection with hepatitis A.
- Whatever preparation of typhoid vaccine is given, booster doses should be given to those at continuing risk every 3 years.

Contraindications
- Typhoid Vi vaccine should not be given to those who have had anaphylaxis following a previous dose of Typhoid Vi vaccine.
- Ty21a is a live vaccine and should not be given to those with immunosuppression. It should also not be given to those with a history of anaphylaxis to Ty21a or enteric-coated capsules, as these capsules contain gelatin.

Yellow Fever
- YF is an arbovirus infection spread by Aedes mosquitoes. YF is present in many countries in Africa and South America. There are also countries that have the mosquito vector present but do not report cases of YF infection.
- YF vaccine is a live attenuated vaccine that is very effective in the prevention of YF. It should be administered 10 days prior to travel.
- YF vaccine can only be given by registered centres and these centres are authorized to issue YF vaccination certificates that travellers can use to demonstrate previous vaccination.
- In a recent change, YF vaccination certificates are now valid for life and booster doses of the vaccine are no longer recommended by the World Health Organisation (WHO).
- It is important to note that travellers may require YF vaccine even if they are not at risk of YF based on their travel itinerary (e.g., if they are crossing borders at which a YF vaccination certificate will be required).

Indications
- Laboratory staff who may handle infectious material
- Travellers to countries that require evidence of vaccination on entry
- Travellers to areas with a risk of YF infection even if no certificate is required on entry

Adverse Effects
- Mild adverse effects such as headache, myalgia, and fever are common.
- Rarely serious adverse effects can occur which may be life threatening, including YF vaccine–associated neurotropic disease which causes encephalitis and YF vaccine–associated viscerotropic disease which causes multiorgan failure.
- Severe adverse reactions are rare—around four per million doses—but are more common in those older than 60 years.

Contraindications
- Those under 6 months of age
- Those with a history of anaphylaxis to YF vaccine, a vaccine component, or egg
- Those who have a disorder of the thymus
- Immunosuppressed individuals

Symptoms in Travellers Returning From Abroad

History

The assessment of patients with a history of foreign travel can be complex. At a minimum, it requires a careful history of the travel, including:
- countries and areas visited: A particularly important distinction is between urban and rural travel. Generally, rural travel is more likely to be associated with transmission of tropical disease;
- activities undertaken;
- contact with animals;
- freshwater contact;
- healthcare contact;
- sexual contact; and
- pretravel health assessment, vaccination history, whether antimalarial prophylaxis was taken.

Fever

> **GUIDANCE**
>
> The British Infection Association published recommendations for the investigation of fever in the returning traveller (Dockrell et al., 2009). However, it should be noted that acute fever in patients returned from the tropics will usually require discussion with a specialist.

- Assessment of travellers with undifferentiated fever is the mainstay of the inpatient work of any service dealing with returning travellers. Fever is a common presenting symptom and requires prompt investigation since it is the usual presenting feature of a number of life-threatening conditions.

- The initial step in the assessment of any returning traveller with fever is to conduct a viral haemorrhagic fever (VHF) risk assessment. The large outbreak of Ebola virus disease in West Africa in 2013 to 2015 raised the awareness of VHF but the concern is not limited to West Africa. In primary care, if all of the following conditions are met then the patient should be discussed with the local infection specialist prior to admission to hospital:
  - A history of fever
  - A history of travel to a country known to have endemic VHFs
  - The onset of fever was within 21 days of leaving the risk area

- Note that guidelines are regularly reviewed and that the most up-to-date advice, including the countries considered at risk, will be available through PHE (2016a) or the appropriate public health body in the devolved administrations.

- The vast majority of those meeting this definition will not be considered high risk after discussion with a specialist and will be able to be admitted to hospital in the usual way. For further information on VHFs see the respective section in this chapter.

- GeoSentinel is an ongoing collaboration between many travel centres across the world (principally in Europe and North America) collecting information on returning travellers presenting with illness. This study provides important information on the prevalence of diseases in unwell returning travellers. There are important geographical differences in the epidemiology of infections in returning travellers (Table 17.3).

- Note that surveillance of secondary care presentations will favour more serious diagnoses. It is likely that nontropical infection will predominate but high-quality data are not available.

Malaria

- Malaria represents a major risk to the health of returning travellers. It is capable of rapid progression from nonspecific and relatively mild symptoms to death within a few hours and a common finding in deaths from malaria in returning travellers is delayed recognition of the significance of symptoms by medical practitioners.

- Around 1500 cases are imported into the United Kingdom each year.

- Patients may present without fever. A history of fever is all that is required to consider the diagnosis.

- While malaria caused by *Plasmodium falciparum* is usually the most severe, all types of malaria are capable of causing severe disease and, in particular, severe disease caused by *Plasmodium vivax* is increasingly recognized.

| TABLE 17.3 | **Most Common Diagnoses in Patients Presenting to GeoSentinel Sites With Fever Stratified by Region of Travel (Leder et al., 2013)** |

Sub-Saharan Africa	Latin America/ Caribbean	Southeast Asia
Plasmodium falciparum	Dengue	Dengue
Rickettsia, spotted fever	*P. vivax*	*P. falciparum*
Dengue	Enteric fever	*P. vivax*
Plasmodium vivax	*P. falciparum*	Chikungunya
Enteric fever	Hepatitis A	Enteric fever
		Leptospirosis
South-Central Asia	**Middle East and North Africa**	**Northeast Asia**
Enteric fever	Hepatitis A	Dengue
Dengue	*P. falciparum*	Extrapulmonary tuberculosis
P. vivax	Acute brucellosis	Hepatitis E
Chikungunya	Enteric fever	Hepatitis A
Extrapulmonary tuberculosis	Dengue	Enteric fever
	Q-fever	Rickettsia, spotted fever

- It is vital to remember that while antimalarial prophylaxis is highly effective, 100% adherence to prophylaxis is not sufficient grounds on which to exclude malaria.

- *P. falciparum* usually presents within 2 to 3 months of exposure but presentations after 6 to 12 months do occur and other types of malaria can rarely present years after exposure.

- Diagnosis of malaria is made on blood films. However, most nonexpert laboratories use rapid diagnostic tests (antigen tests) as an initial screening tool. These require much less training and experience than performing blood film examination. It is important to note that no single test excludes malaria and that three separate examinations 12 to 24 hours apart are required to exclude the diagnosis.

- If malaria is considered then urgent blood tests are required. Unless there is a reliable service in primary care to ensure that same-day results will be made available, suspected malaria should be referred to secondary care.

Enteric Fever

- Approximately 300 cases of typhoid fever are confirmed in England each year although this is probably an underestimate since blood cultures are often negative.

- The majority of cases of enteric fever occur in travellers who have returned from India, Pakistan, and Bangladesh.

- A small number of cases report no travel history but this is extremely rare.

- Suspected cases should be referred to secondary care for assessment.

Rickettsial Infection

- Rickettsia are another cause of undifferentiated fever in returning travellers. Rickettsia species cause a wide range of diseases which are widely distributed throughout the world. Mortality varies widely depending on the causative organism.

- Rickettsia are zoonoses spread by insects although the vector varies from ticks to mites to fleas.
- In some cases there will be an eschar (e.g., in African tick typhus) but in others this is variable or unlikely to be seen.
- Common features include petechial rash and thrombocytopenia.
- Testing is by PCR and serology but empiric therapy with doxycycline is indicated for suspected cases who should usually be referred to hospital.

Fever-Arthralgia-Rash Arboviruses

- Arboviruses are the group of viruses spread by arthropods such as mosquitoes and ticks. They are not necessarily closely related in other respects and can cause a variety of clinical syndromes.
- One group of arboviruses causes a syndrome consisting of fever with associated maculopapular (or petechial) rash and prominent joint symptoms but only unusually cause serious disease. Until rather recently dengue fever was the only prominent member of this group but progressive globalization has led to global dissemination of dengue and emergence of previously localized viruses such as chikungunya and Zika.
- The fever-arthralgia-rash (FAR) group is not reliably clinically distinguishable and is a common cause of presentation to secondary care with fever following travel.
- These viruses are rarely life threatening (although they can be extremely unpleasant) and treatment is usually supportive. The most important diagnostic challenge is usually distinguishing these infections from others that require urgent treatment.
- At the time of writing, there is global concern about the implications of Zika virus infection during pregnancy. Recommendations about this issue are evolving rapidly and will not be addressed here.

Viral Haemorrhagic Fever

- The four most prominent VHF–causing viruses are Ebola, Lassa, Marburg, and Congo-Crimean haemorrhagic fever (CCHF). There are a number of other viruses that can also cause VHF with much more limited distributions.
- With the exception of very rare cases of healthcare workers infected in non-endemic countries, Ebola, Lassa, and Marburg are limited to parts of sub-Saharan Africa. However, CCHF has a much broader area of distribution, including Africa, Eastern Europe, Turkey, Russia, and Central Asia. In 2016, cases of CCHF were acquired in Spain representing the first cases acquired in Western Europe.
- In 2013 to 2015 there was a large outbreak of Ebola in West Africa which caused thousands of deaths. However, most outbreaks of VHF are small and sporadic.

- VHF initially presents with undifferentiated fever but a significant number of patients go on to develop haemorrhagic complications and mortality is high. Fortunately, imported cases are rare although there have been a handful of cases presenting de novo to hospitals in the United Kingdom in the last 10 years.
- For information on VHF risk assessment see the introduction to the section on fever.

Other Causes of Fever

- Viral hepatitis: Hepatitis A is unusual now that most travellers are vaccinated and acute hepatitis B is relatively uncommon in travellers. However, hepatitis E has become increasingly recognized as a cause of acute hepatitis both in the United Kingdom and among travellers. Presentation is with fever and right upper quadrant pain preceding jaundice (which is not always a feature of the infection).
- Epstein-Barr virus: Infectious mononucleosis is common in younger returning travellers. In those who have negative investigations or are older and so likely to be EBV immune consider cytomegalovirus (CMV). Always consider an HIV test in patients with a mononucleosis-like illness. Toxoplasmosis is another cause of persistent lymphadenopathy in travellers.
- Amoebic liver abscess: An abscess can present many months after travel without necessarily a history of diarrhoea. Suspect liver abscess in patients with fever and right upper quadrant pain.
- Influenza: Flu is common among travellers given the close contact involved in air travel.

Diarrhoea

- Diarrhoea is very common in returning travellers. Usually it is mild and self-limiting. Specific treatment is usually not required.
- Note that diarrhoea can be a nonspecific symptom of severe sepsis and fever, with diarrhoea a common presenting feature of malaria.
- Common causes are similar to locally acquired gastroenteritis with salmonella and campylobacter predominating. Note that antibiotic resistance is much more common in infections acquired abroad and varies depending on geographic location. Seek advice from microbiology/infectious diseases if treatment is considered.
- Malabsorptive diarrhoea is relatively common following travel. Patients present with nausea, abdominal pain and bloating, watery diarrhoea, and weight loss which may last for months:
  - A number of pathogens can be associated with this presentation but *Giardia lamblia* is the most common and can be acquired anywhere in the world.
  - Giardia can be difficult to detect on stool microscopy and serial faeces examinations are often required. If the history is typical then empiric treatment is often

necessary. Some laboratories now offer giardia antigen tests on faeces and this is more sensitive.

- First line treatment for giardia is with metronidazole or tinidazole, although community pharmacies sometimes struggle to obtain tinidazole.
- In recent years, there have been a series of large outbreaks of cyclosporiasis centered on Mexico although many cases have been seen in the United States thought to be associated with imported fruit and vegetables. Travellers have been commonly affected. Diagnosis is through faeces microscopy although this is insensitive. It is sometimes detected on duodenal biopsy. Make sure the lab is aware of any clinical suspicion and the travel history. Treatment is with co-trimoxazole. Seek advice if alternative treatment is required.
- Acute bloody diarrhoea may be caused by salmonella or campylobacter although the odds of other pathogens increase significantly.
  - Bloody diarrhoea in an afebrile patient (traveller or not) suggests *E. coli O157* infection, particularly if there is a risk factor such as livestock contact, camping on agricultural land, or eating poorly prepared red meat. Such patients should usually not receive antibiotics because of a possible increased risk of developing haemolytic uraemic syndrome, particularly in children.
  - Acute bloody diarrhoea with mucus and fever suggests dysentery. Possible causes include *Shigella dysenteriae* and *Entamoeba histolytica*. Treatment is quite different and so diagnosis is vital. Send faeces (fresh if possible) to the lab for ova, cysts, parasites examination as well as culture.
  - Shigella is diagnosed on culture but amoebae are seen on microscopy although some laboratories use antigen testing as an adjuvant. Note that not all amoebae are pathogenic and reference lab reports are not always easy to understand for the nonexpert. Detection of *Entamoeba dispar* or *Entamoeba coli* is generally considered nonpathogenic; if there is any uncertainty then seek advice.

Dermatologic Presentations

GeoSentinel collects data on dermatologic presentations to specialist travel medicine centres. The top diagnoses by region of travel are shown in Table 17.4.

- Cutaneous larva migrans (CLM) is caused by intradermal non-human hookworm larvae. The larvae are unable to penetrate through the basement membrane and so migrate with the skin causing an intense pruritic reaction with a tracking appearance. The infestation is self-limiting but is distressing, painful, and can precipitate bacterial infection. Mebendazole can be used but is inferior to other unlicensed treatments such as topical thiabendazole, albendazole, or ivermectin. Therefore, patients should usually be referred to a local infectious disease/post travel service for treatment.

TABLE 17.4	Most Common Diagnoses in Patients Presenting to GeoSentinel Sites With Dermatologic Complaints Stratified by Region of Travel (Checkley et al., 2010)

Sub-Saharan Africa	Latin America/ Caribbean	Southeast Asia
Cutaneous larva migrans	Cutaneous larva migrans	Rabies PEP
Rabies postexposure prophylactics (PEP)	Cutaneous leishmaniasis	Cutaneous larva migrans
Myiasis	Rabies PEP	Scabies
Tungiasis	Myiasis	Marine envenomation
South-Central Asia	**Middle East and North Africa**	**Northeast Asia**
Rabies PEP	Rabies PEP	Rabies PEP
Cutaneous leishmaniasis	Cutaneous leishmaniasis	Other diagnoses from this area were very unusual
Scabies	Cutaneous larva migrans	
Cutaneous larva migrans	Marine envenomation	

- Myiasis is caused by the intradermal inoculation of fly eggs. A painful swelling develops at the site of inoculation which can be distinguished from a furuncle by the presence of a central breathing pore. A variety of treatment strategies can be tried but surgical removal is often necessary. Referral to an expert is usually appropriate.
- Tungiasis is caused by the invasion of the skin by a gravid flea. A firm, pruritic swelling develops, usually in the feet. The lesions eventually resolve spontaneously but can be surgically removed.
- Cutaneous leishmaniasis is a relatively common condition affecting travellers with an extensive distribution across South/Central America, the Mediterranean, and Central/South Asia. It is spread by the bite of the sandfly. There are important geographic differences with Old World cutaneous leishmaniasis rarely becoming complicated (although it may cause scarring) but New World cutaneous leishmaniasis can be life threatening and usually requires systemic treatment. Patients usually present with slowly developing ulcerating lesion on an exposed area. There are often multiple lesions. Diagnosis can be confirmed on biopsy but is often made clinically. If suspected, patients should be referred to an infectious disease/post travel specialist.
- Scabies is another common skin condition presenting in travellers. Patients complain of pruritis and may have extensive excoriation. The diagnosis is made by finding skin burrows, which are usually present in the finger webs.

Eosinophilia

- Asymptomatic eosinophilia is common in those who have travelled in the tropics. It may be present in up to 5%

of tropical travellers. However, significant eosinophilia, with an eosinophil percentage greater than 15%, is likely to be associated with an underlying diagnosis.

- Remember that a variety of non-infectious conditions can be associated with eosinophilia. Consider whether atopic conditions may be the cause; other conditions associated with eosinophilia include drugs, vasculitis, and haematologic malignancy.
- Eosinophilia in tropical travellers should always be investigated as some causes are associated with significant long-term consequences. Common causes include:
  - intestinal helminths. These are a diverse group and many carriers are asymptomatic. Passing a worm is often very distressing for patients. If possible it should be retained and sent to a laboratory for identification;
  - strongyloides. This may be asymptomatic but patients often have nonspecific abdominal symptoms. Worms migrating through the skin may be visible as a slowly moving pruritic rash. If carries become immuno-suppressed, it can cause hyperinfestation syndrome which presents with paralytic ileus and sepsis, and is often fatal;
  - schistosomiasis. This is very commonly acquired by travellers and is covered in the next section;
  - toxocariasis. Hydatid is often asymptomatic but causes the development of cysts which can develop in most of the internal organs. If these become large, they can cause significant local symptoms; or
  - filariasis: There are a number of different types of filarial infection which cause a diverse range of symptoms, including dermatologic reactions, elephantiasis, and visual problems.
- A reasonable initial approach is to send faeces for microscopy on three occasions and ask the lab to arrange serology for strongyloides (for all travellers who have visited the tropics) and schistosomiasis (for those who have visited Africa). Regardless if a cause is found, it is reasonable to refer all patients to a specialist clinic since it is unlikely that treatment will be available outside specialist centres.
- Note that serology can be difficult to interpret since there is often cross reactivity between different parasite serologies.

Screening of Immigrants and Long-Term Travellers

Returning travellers from the tropics often request screening for acquired infections, particularly parasitic infection. Unfortunately, with only a couple of exceptions, such testing is usually unhelpful and may expose travellers to needless worry and

treatment. Returning travellers with intestinal parasites could not be distinguished from those without on the basis of symptoms in a questionnaire study (Forna & Gulmezoglu, 2000). Most tropical intestinal helminths cannot complete their life cycle in the developed world and so there is neither a clinical nor a public health benefit to testing asymptomatic travellers.

Schistosomiasis

Schistosomiasis is very common in travellers returning home after visiting Africa. In this context it is usually asymptomatic. Travellers are often advised to seek testing to check if they have been infected and may attend their general practitioner (GP).

- Symptoms of schistosomiasis include lower urinary symptoms and haematuria.
- Early infection with schistosomiasis sometimes causes a syndrome of acute fever, abdominal pain, splenomegaly, and marked eosinophila (known as Katayama fever).
- In symptomatic cases, serology and urine/faeces microscopy should be undertaken. Note that these investigations are usually negative in Katayama fever.
- In asymptomatic cases, serology alone is sufficient and should be delayed until 12 weeks after the last possible time of exposure to avoid false negatives.
- Treatment is with praziquantel, which is usually only available from specialist centres.

Strongyloides

Strongyloides is unusual among intestinal nematodes in that it can complete its life cycle within a single host. This allows for lifelong infection within tropical travellers. Strongyloides hyperinfestation syndrome is a risk for those who have lived within the tropics who become immunosuppressed. However, strongyloides is relatively uncommon among short-term travellers. A pragmatic approach is to test asymptomatic individuals with prolonged tropical travel if they have been living in areas of particular deprivation or immunosuppression is planned.

Tuberculosis

- As discussed in this chapter, the United Kingdom has a significant burden of tuberculosis among immigrant populations. Most tuberculosis is diagnosed years after the initial entry to the United Kingdom.
- All entrants to the United Kingdom from high incidence countries are screened for active pulmonary TB prior to being issued with a long stay visa.
- Screening for latent TB in those aged 16 to 35 arriving from high incidence countries is about to be introduced in England. Identification of selected individuals with latent TB allows treatment to reduce the burden of symptomatic TB infection in the future (NICE, 2016).
- Screening for latent TB involves the use of either tuberculin skin testing (Mantoux) or interferon gamma release assays (IGRA) blood tests. A positive test should prompt a search

for evidence of active TB. If no active disease is found, selected groups may be offered treatment for latent TB.

- Note that while immunologic testing can support a clinical suspicion of active TB, negative testing does not exclude the diagnosis and must not be interpreted in this way.

Sexually Transmitted Infection

Travellers who have been sexually active should be offered a sexual health screen (see next section).

Sexually Transmitted Infection and HIV

GUIDANCE

Guidelines on the diagnosis and management of sexually transmitted infection are available through the British Association of Sexual Health and HIV (BASHH). Individual guidelines are available for each disease mentioned over the next few pages. To see individual guidelines, visit https://www.bashh.org/guidelines.

General Approach

- Sexually transmitted infection is common and not limited to conventional risk groups. It is important to consider **sexually transmitted infection (STI)** in any patient and not allow preconceived ideas about a patient's lifestyle to influence the approach. That is not to say that one should not be aware of risk factors and recognize that certain groups are at increased risk of infection.
- Questions should be open and not make unwarranted assumptions about a person's sexuality. Be self-critical in ensuring that a nonjudgmental approach is taken at all times.
- Genitourinary medicine (GUM) clinics provide a variety of services, including screening, symptom-based assessment, counselling, and contact tracing. Those with a diagnosis of STI should be routinely referred to a GUM clinic for assessment and management.
- Testing for HIV should be a routine part of practice in primary care. Primary care studies have found a missed opportunity for HIV testing in up to 60% of patients presenting with advanced HIV in the United Kingdom.

Patients Requiring Investigation by the General Practitioner

- Those who are eligible for a local or national screening programme (e.g., for chlamydia)
- Those who require treatment urgently and cannot attend GUM immediately (e.g., symptomatic pelvic inflammatory disease out of hours)
- Those who are unwilling or unable to attend a GUM clinic after discussion/recommendation and require testing for STIs or HIV
- Those presenting with a possible STI-related problem in a primary care setting which has training and experience

in managing STIs, including partner notification (e.g., through either Locally Enhanced Service schemes or GPs with a special interest)

Patients Requiring Management by the General Practitioner

- Those who have tested positive for an STI at the surgery and wish to be managed in primary care or cannot attend GUM immediately
- Those who present as contacts of an STI and decline to attend GUM for testing, treatment, and partner notification advice after discussion and recommendation of this course of action

Contact Tracing

- This is usually best done by GUM, or at least with their support and advice.
- As a minimum, screening of all contacts of acute STIs over the last 3 months should be attempted. For syphilis and HIV there is no arbitrary limit, and partner notification will depend on who is contactable, and the earliest likely time of infection.
- If the patient is diagnosed with nonspecific urethritis (NSU), chlamydia, syphilis, *Trichomonas vaginalis*, or gonorrhoea, the partner should be treated even if tests are negative.

Principles of Treatment

- Give appropriate antibiotics, bearing in mind any recent travel history.
- Advise complete abstinence from all sexual contact until both patient and partner are treated.
- Follow up after completion of antibiotics for compliance and possibly retesting (which is indicated only in pregnancy or where symptoms persist).

General Investigation in Primary Care

- GUM clinics offer testing services for asymptomatic individuals. When an asymptomatic person presents to primary care seeking investigation, the local testing clinic should be suggested. However, some may be unable to attend GUM services and investigations should be offered in primary care.
- Take a sexual history focusing on the last two partners and all partners in the last 3 months.
- Asymptomatic individuals do not require clinical examination.
- A basic asymptomatic screen includes the following investigations:
  - An appropriate genital sample for chlamydia and gonorrhoea
    Men: first pass urine for PCR
    Women: self-taken vulvovaginal swab for PCR
    Microscopy and culture are not required for asymptomatic patients
  - Serology for HIV and syphilis
- Additional testing should be offered for those requiring additional investigation:

- MSM and women reporting receptive oral intercourse should have a pharyngeal swab for chlamydia and gonorrhoea PCR.
- Those reporting receptive anal intercourse should have a rectal swab for chlamydia and gonorrhoea PCR.
- Consider testing for hepatitis B and C for those at risk.

How to Take Samples

Samples for chlamydia and gonorrhoea are usually analysed using PCR as these organisms are difficult to grow in routine culture. Specialist sample collection containers exist and should be used for these samples. Most laboratories will not accept samples except in the recommended collection containers. Ensure to check what is needed locally.

First pass urine	• Ask patient to urinate into a plain collection bottle; this may need to be transferred into a PCR collection container depending on local laboratory requirements.
Self-taken vulvovaginal	• Ask the patient to insert the swab about 2 inches (5 cm) into the vagina and gently rotate it for 10–30 s.
Pharyngeal swab	• Swab the tonsils and posterior pharynx and remove the swab without touching the mouth.
Rectal swab	• Insert the swab about 2 inches (5 cm) into the rectum. Rotate the swab at least three times against the rectal wall before removing.

Management of Specific Sexually Transmitted Infection

See also Chapter 13, *Women's Health*.

Genital Gonorrhoea

- Gonorrhoea represents a major public health threat. Laboratory diagnoses of gonorrhoea have increased markedly over the last 10 years. This has been accompanied by a steep rise in antibiotic resistance; and 2016 marked the first reported case of treatment failure with combined ceftriaxone and azithromycin therapy due to resistance in a patient in the United Kingdom. This is particularly frightening since there is no clear alternative treatment strategy if such multidrug-resistant organisms become widespread.
- Gonorrhoea presents with genital discharge and is an important cause of pelvic inflammatory disease.
- Pharyngeal colonization is rarely symptomatic but is more difficult to treat and is an important reservoir of infection.
- PCR is the mainstay of diagnosis although microscopy and culture are available in specialist clinics.
- Current treatment recommendation is to use ceftriaxone 500 mg intramuscularly and azithromycin 1 g orally.

Monotherapy treatment should not be given as it is associated with the development of resistance, and quinolones should not be used.
- Partner notification, testing, and treatment are important to prevent reinfection and onward transmission.
- Follow-up with test of cure is important in view of reports of treatment failure.

Chlamydia Infection

- The majority of infections with *Chlamydia trachomatis* are clinically inapparent. When symptoms do exist they are often mild. However, infection can cause severe symptoms and impacts on female fertility. Therefore, it is important to diagnose and treat whenever possible.
- Of sexually active young people 3% to 7% are infected.
- Two-thirds of partners of cases will also be infected.
- Symptoms when they occur:
  - Men: dysuria and urethral discharge
  - Complications: reactive arthritis and epididymoorchitis
  - Women: vaginal discharge, postcoital bleeding and dyspareunia, abdominal pain
  - Complications: pelvis inflammatory disease (PID), infertility, reactive arthritis, and perihepatitis
- Since patients are usually asymptomatic, screening is the most important method of case acquisition. Rectal and pharyngeal infection also occur and are usually asymptomatic.
- Screening should be conducted when patients present for sexual health screening and annually or on change of partner for all sexually active people under the age of 25.
- Urethral and endocervical swabs are not required for diagnosis of chlamydia. First pass urine in men and self-taken vulvovaginal swabs in women are much more acceptable to patients and just as sensitive.
- Treatment is with azithromycin 1 g stat or doxycycline 100 mg twice daily for 7 days.
- Note that doxycycline is contraindicated in pregnancy. Azithromycin will be the best option for the majority of patients in pregnancy but off licence (consult guidelines).
- Seek expert advice for extragenital infection.
- Refer to GUM for partner notification unless this can be appropriately managed within primary care. Ensure that an explanation of the importance of attendance at GUM is given to patients who receive treatment within primary care.

Lymphogranuloma Venereum

- Lymphogranuloma Venereum (LGV) has emerged as an increasingly common infection affecting almost exclusively MSM. It is caused by invasive serovars of *Chlamydia trachomatis*. It causes severe proctitis in those with rectal infection which can scar and mimic inflammatory bowel disease. It is important to consider the diagnosis in those with risk factors.

Nonspecific Urethritis

- Urethritis in the absence of chlamydia and gonorrhoea is relatively common. It is best assessed in a GUM clinic where microscopy of a urethral swab can be carried out.

- Common causes of NSU include *Mycoplasma genitalium*, *Trichomonas vaginalis*, *Candida* sp., HSV, adenovirus.
- Consider treatment with azithromycin 1 g stat or doxycycline 100 mg twice daily.
- Partner notification and treatment is required. Both patient and partner should abstain from sex until treatment.

Trichomonas Vaginalis

- *Trichomonas vaginalis* (TV) infection is almost exclusively sexually transmitted, through urethral or vaginal inoculation. It is sometimes diagnosed on cervical cytology, where there is a false positive rate of about 30%, so tests should be repeated.
- Symptoms are of vaginal discharge in women and urethritis in men.
- Diagnosis is usually made on culture or vaginal or urethral swabs although PCR is available in some areas.
- *Trichomonas* infection is associated with other STIs, and full screening should be undertaken.
- Metronidazole 2 g orally stat, or metronidazole 400 mg twice daily for 5 to 7 days, will clear 95% of infections. The stat dose is as effective as the 7-day course but is more likely to be associated with adverse effects (Smith et al., 2014). Test of cure is required only if symptoms persist, in which case the patient should attend GUM. Alcohol should be avoided during and for 48 hours after treatment.
- Recent and current partners should be treated for TV and screened for STIs.

Anogenital Warts

- The majority of patients with anogenital warts have mild symptoms or cosmetic concerns only. However, the psychological impact should not be underestimated.
- Since 2012 the vaccine used to prevent HPV-associated cancers has included components that give protection against the common viral causes of anogenital warts. However, this vaccine is usually only available to women.
- Many carriers of HPV have no visible lesions.
- Condom use may reduce transmission of warts to uninfected partners. Their use with regular partners, however, has not been shown to affect the outcome of treatment in patients with visible warts.
- Perianal warts are associated with anal sex (although they can occur without) and should suggest the need for anorectal samples for other STIs, and GUM referral.
- None of the existing treatments is satisfactory, and all have high recurrence rates. Patients should be made aware of this. The evidence base for distinguishing first and second line treatments is weak.

Soft, Nonkeratinized Warts

- Prescribe podophyllotoxin 0.5% (twice daily for 3 days, repeated weekly for up to 4 weeks). Patients using podophyllotoxin at home must take great care to follow the instructions, to avoid chemical burns. It should not be used in pregnancy, and is not licensed for extragenital lesions, such as anal warts.

- Imiquimod 5% cream is an immune response modifier which can be used three times weekly for up to 16 weeks. It should not be used in pregnancy.

Keratinized Warts

- Use ablative therapy such as cryotherapy which is available at GUM clinics.

Herpes Genitalis

- Genital herpes may be due to infection with either HSV-1 or HSV-2.
- Many patients who carry HSV are asymptomatic but shedding of virus can result in infection of sexual partners even in the absence of visible lesions.
- A significant proportion of genital HSV is thought to be acquired through orogenital contact and so patients may not consider themselves sexually active.
- Autoinnoculation of the genital area from another site (e.g., the lips) may also occur during primary episodes.
- It is useful to confirm the diagnosis, even in clinically certain cases by sending a swab to virology for PCR. This can also provide the HSV type causing infection which has implications for prognosis.
- Partner notification can be tricky, since HSV is very common and may present many years after initial infection. Seek advice from GUM.

First Symptomatic Episode
- Note that the first symptomatic episode does not occur at the time of primary infection in the majority of cases. This is important since source of infection is an important concern for many patients.
- Analgesia is the most important treatment modality. Topical local analgesics (5% lidocaine ointment) occasionally cause sensitization but can be useful. Saline bathing is also useful for some, particularly if there is significant difficulty passing urine.
- Antiviral therapy with aciclovir 200 mg five times daily, valaciclovir 500 mg twice daily, or famciclovir 125 mg twice daily for 5 days should be offered if:
  - within 5 days of onset of symptoms; or
  - new lesions are continuing to form; or
  - there are significant systemic symptoms.
- Patients with urinary retention, meningism, or severe systemic symptoms should be admitted to hospital.
- Discuss with patients:
  - asymptomatic shedding and implications for relationships; and
  - the importance of informing obstetric team in case of future pregnancy.

Recurrences
- In most patients recurrences cause minor, short-lived symptoms.
- Recurrences should be managed using one of three strategies:
  - Supportive: Use the symptom management strategies outlined in this chapter.

- Standby treatment: Prescribe patients antivirals to store at home and take as soon as possible after onset of symptoms (aciclovir 800 mg three times daily for 2 days, famciclovir 1 g twice daily for 1 day, valaciclovir 500 mg twice daily for 3 days, note the shorter duration of therapy).
- Suppressive therapy: Usually considered when the patient is experiencing six or more recurrences per year. Treat with aciclovir 400 mg twice daily, aciclovir 200 mg four times daily, famciclovir 250 mg twice daily, or valaciclovir 500 mg once daily. Treatment should be discontinued after a year to reassess ongoing need for treatment.

Syphilis

- Like other STIs, syphilis is becoming increasingly common in the United Kingdom. Cases have risen steadily over the last 10 years principally among MSM although cases are also seen outside traditional risk groups. Early syphilis presents with a painless ulcer at the site of initial infection. Secondary syphilis presents with rash while late stage syphilis may be asymptomatic or present with a wide variety of nonspecific symptoms which make diagnosis difficult.
- Genital ulcers should be swabbed for syphilis PCR. Ground-glass microscopy is a point-of-care test that can immediately confirm the diagnosis but is limited to specialist clinics.
- All patients presenting for a sexual health screen should have syphilis serology carried out. It should be noted that serology can take up to 3 months after infection to become positive and so it should be repeated if appropriate.
- Management of syphilis requires specialist expertise and should be managed through GUM clinics.

Human Immunodeficiency Virus Infection

- Advances in the treatment of HIV have revolutionized prognosis and quality of life for patients over the last 20 years.
- Highly active antiretroviral therapy (HAART), which involves the use of drug combinations to control viral replication, has proved effective in generating prolonged viral suppression in the vast majority of patients. Most patients are now able to take one of a number of fixed-dose combinations involving one tablet taken once per day.
- Viral suppression allows recovery of the immune system and even patients who have presented with advanced disease are usually returned to good health.
- Life expectancy has dramatically improved and cause of death in developed countries has evolved with acquired immunodeficiency syndrome (AIDS) accounting for only one in five deaths (BASHH/EAGA, 2014). Important causes of non-AIDS deaths are similar to the general population with non-AIDS cancers and cardiovascular diseases dominating. There remains a significant excess of liver disease–related deaths among people living with HIV.
- There are two principle roles for primary care in the management of HIV infection:
  - Identifying people living with undiagnosed HIV infection through appropriate use of HIV testing

- Working with local HIV services to deliver care to people living with HIV (e.g., when a patient known to have HIV attends primary care with a symptom that would normally be dealt with within primary care)

Human Immunodeficiency Virus Testing

> **GUIDANCE**
>
> British HIV Association testing guidelines provide a comprehensive guide to HIV testing in the United Kingdom (http://www.bhiva.org/HIV-testing-guidelines.aspx). Note, however, that recommendations on the *window period* (PHE, 2015b) have been updated since these guidelines (also see upcoming discussion).

- In 2015, around 103,700 people were estimated to be living with HIV infection with 18,100 unaware of their infection (British HIV Association, 2008).
- Among those already infected with HIV, those without apparent risk factors—especially men—are most likely to be undiagnosed.
- Early diagnosis of HIV has two principle benefits:
  - Permitting early treatment, since early treatment of asymptomatic patients has been associated with long-term health benefits and those who are diagnosed with advanced disease are much more likely to die and suffer chronic ill health than those diagnosed with early stage disease.
  - Preventing further infections, as people are much less likely to transmit infection to others once they are aware of their infection.
- HIV testing should not be limited to specialists. All GPs should feel comfortable offering an HIV test.
- Modern fourth generation HIV tests are able to detect both HIV antigen and antibody. This means that it is rare for a patient with symptoms of HIV seroconversion to have a negative HIV test although testing should be repeated after 7 days in those in whom HIV seroconversion is strongly suspected who test negative. However, the window period is still important for asymptomatic patients who require repeat testing.
  - Antigen/antibody (fourth generation) testing should be offered by all laboratories performing testing on whole blood samples.
  - Other tests (e.g., point-of-care tests or dried blood spots) are not as sensitive and are therefore more likely to yield a false negative result in early HIV.
- If a fourth generation test is used then a negative test 4 weeks after the potential exposure is highly likely to exclude HIV infection. A further test at 8 weeks following exposure is only required if the risk of HIV transmission is thought to be particularly high.
- Note that the window period quoted is shorter than previously advised in the 2008 guidelines.
- Patients should not be asked to wait 4 weeks after an exposure to test for HIV if they are concerned. Patients

should always be offered an HIV test if they are concerned.

- Note that this advice regarding the window period only applies to HIV. The window period in hepatitis B and C is longer (6 months).
- HIV testing should be offered to the following people:
  - Those attending specialist services in which universal testing is appropriate (e.g., drug dependency services, antenatal services, blood donors)
  - Those registering with a GP in areas where the HIV prevalence in the local population is relatively high (>2/1000) as part of a locally arranged policy
  - Asymptomatic individuals who have a risk factor for HIV infection (people at ongoing risk should be tested annually or more frequently if appropriate):
    i. Those diagnosed with a STI
    ii. Sexual partners of those living with HIV
    iii. Men who have sex with men and female sexual contacts of MSM
    iv. People who inject drugs
    v. Those from a country of high HIV prevalence (>1%) and anyone reporting sexual contact with a person from such a country.
  - Those with indicator illnesses, suggesting an increased chance of HIV infection, including all those with symptoms which may be directly attributable to HIV infection (Table 17.4)

Practicalities of Testing

- In the past, HIV testing has been regarded as *different* from other blood tests for serious medical conditions. However, the prognosis in HIV infection is now very much improved and testing should be normalized.
- Written consent is not required in the United Kingdom and a prolonged pretest discussion is not necessary for the majority of patients.
- Pretest discussion should involve three key features:
  - An explanation of why the test is being offered (e.g., that HIV is a possible cause of unexplained lymphadenopathy or that HIV is more common among people who inject drugs).
  - An explanation of the benefits of testing. This will usually involve a brief discussion of the excellent prognosis with modern treatment and advantages of early treatment.
  - Discussion of how the test results will be delivered. This will depend on the clinical context and the outcome of the discussion with the patient. It is not always necessary to communicate the result face to face but this should be the preferred option if there is a high pretest probability.
- Some patients may have concerns about the consequences of HIV testing:
  - HIV testing should be entirely voluntary and those being tested should have a reasonable assurance of confidentiality. While those testing positive may choose to disclose their diagnosis to others, they are under no obligation to do so. Counselling relating to these issues is undertaken sensitively in the HIV clinic.

TABLE 17.4	Conditions Encountered in Primary Care Which Should Prompt the Offer of a Human Immunodeficiency Virus Test (Whittle, 2008; DoH, 2008)
Respiratory	**Bacterial pneumonia**
Neurology	Peripheral neuropathy Dementia
Dermatology	Severe or difficult to treat seborrheic dermatitis or psoriasis **Severe or recurrent herpes zoster**
Gastroenterology	**Oral candida** or hairy leukoplakia **Chronic, unexplained diarrhoea** **Unexplained weight loss** Salmonella, shigella, or campylobacter Hepatitis B or C infection
Gynaecology	Cervical intraepithelial neoplasia or invasive cancer Vaginal intraepithelial neoplasia
Haematology	**Any unexplained blood dyscrasia**
ENT	**Unexplained lymphadenopathy** Chronic parotitis
Other	Mononucleosis-like syndrome Pyrexia of unknown cause **Unexplained lymphadenopathy** Any sexually transmitted infection

Conditions highlighted in bold are those commonly identified as missed opportunities for testing in patients who subsequently were diagnosed with advanced infection.

- A negative test has no implications for insurance since the industry code of practice prohibits asking about this information. However, a positive test would have implications for insurance like any other chronic medical condition.
- There have been a number of prosecutions in the United Kingdom relating to the transmission of HIV and some people are concerned about the possible forensic implications of a positive test. Such concerns should not be a barrier to testing but should be dealt with sensitively. In general, it is very unlikely that persons who have no reason to believe they were infected with HIV would be prosecuted for passing on the infection to a sexual partner; however, the law is incredibly complex and varies depending on which UK legal jurisdiction is in force. Unless such concerns can be readily dealt with, expert advice should be sought.
- Post test discussion following a negative test should involve two principal objectives:
  - Offering health promotion advice: For individuals at ongoing risk this is often best achieved by referral to specialist services.
  - Advising on the need for repeat testing in some cases (e.g., those who remain within the window period

following a defined exposure [see discussion in this chapter] or those who are ongoing risk who should be retested periodically).

- Post test discussion following a positive test:
  - If unsure, speak to specialist services about the appropriate onward referral so that the plan is clear during the discussion.
  - Approach the discussion like any other consultation involving the breaking of bad news. Avoid interruptions and give consideration to issues such as the need for a translator.
  - Non-specialists should acknowledge their lack of detailed clinical knowledge and make clear that more detailed counselling will be provided in the specialist clinic.
  - Patients should not be pressured to disclose their status to sexual partners although clearly many will choose to do so at this stage. Partner notification requires experience and will be undertaken through specialist services.
  - Advice should be given about how HIV is transmitted and patients should be advised to abstain from sex until reviewed in specialist services
- If a person does not attend to receive a positive result, attempts should be made to recall the patient. Where these attempts fail, local specialist services should be contacted for advice and support.

Primary Human Immunodeficiency Virus Infection

- HIV seroconversion illness usually occurs a few weeks following infection and occurs in the majority of cases. Symptoms are nonspecific and therefore diagnosis is often not considered. However, detection at this stage allows early treatment and intervention to prevent onward transmission.
- Symptoms of HIV seroconversion illness include:
  - fever and myalgia;
  - pharyngitis and lymphadenopathy;
  - oral ulceration;
  - headache; and
  - maculopapular rash.
- Symptoms are often mild and may include a minority of the symptoms listed. They resolve spontaneously after a few weeks.
- It is important that HIV is added to the differential diagnosis of any mononucleosis-like illness and HIV testing considered. This is particularly important if the Monospot is negative but cases of Monospot positive HIV seroconversion have been occasionally reported.
- Occasionally, a fourth generation HIV test is negative shortly after the onset of symptoms. If acute HIV infection is strongly suspected, this should be discussed with a specialist as repeat testing or testing for HIV RNA may be considered.

Management of Patients Living With Human Immunodeficiency Virus

- As the management of HIV has developed and the illness has evolved from one which dramatically shortens life to a chronic manageable condition, there has been an increasing role for primary care in the management of those with HIV infection. A small minority of patients now die of the complications of AIDS and the focus in stable, treated patients has shifted to regarding HIV as a risk factor for illnesses such cardiovascular disease and non-AIDS related cancers. As life expectancy has improved, the HIV-infected cohort has grown older and many patients now have HIV as one of a number of chronic medical conditions.
- The key clinical parameters for assessment of patients known to have HIV are the $CD4^+$ lymphocyte count and HIV viral load.
- $CD4^+$ count is highly correlated with the risk of developing opportunistic infections. Patients with a $CD4^+$ count greater than 250 are unlikely to develop opportunistic infections although some infections, such as pneumococcal disease and tuberculosis, are significantly increased regardless of $CD4^+$ count.
- HIV viral load is an important parameter for those on antiretroviral therapy. Treatment guidelines now recommend considering treatment in all patients regardless of $CD4^+$ count and the goal of treatment is to suppress viral replication so that the viral load in blood becomes undetectable (this is usually reported as a viral load less than the limit of detection of the assay—i.e., <40 copies/mL).
- Long-term follow-up studies have demonstrated that HIV does not progress in patients with a suppressed viral load and, indeed, the $CD4^+$ count usually rises back toward the normal range on therapy.
- It follows that a patient known to have HIV infection who attends primary care and is on treatment with a $CD4^+$ count above 250 and an undetectable viral load is very unlikely to be presenting with an HIV-related illness.
- Antiretroviral therapy has improved significantly since the early days of HAART. Most patients are now managed with one fixed-dose combination tablet per day. However, adverse effects occur and drug interactions remain a significant concern:
  - Some common drugs have critical interactions with some antiretrovirals. It is the responsibility of the prescriber of any new drug to check whether significant interactions exist.
  - Interactions can be life threatening and involve everyday drugs (e.g., the interaction of some corticosteroids, including inhaled corticosteroids, with protease inhibitors resulting in iatrogenic Cushing syndrome).
  - The University of Liverpool operates an online service to check for drug interactions and is regularly updated (http://www.hiv-druginteractions.org; a smartphone app is also available).
  - Most HIV clinics have a specialist pharmacist who may be consulted for advice.

Routine Care

- Those with HIV should be encouraged to attend routine cancer screening. Cervical cancer screening should be offered annually.

- Inactivated vaccines can be given as usual, although vaccines may be less effective when given to those with HIV, particularly if the CD4+ count is low. Hepatitis B vaccine is indicated for all with HIV.
- Live vaccines, including YF, can often be given to those with a high CD4+ count but this should only be done following expert advice.
- Family planning should be actively undertaken and women who seek advice about pregnancy should be advised to discuss this with the HIV clinic prior to conception. Effective treatment has reduced the risk of mother to child transmission to less than 1%.
- Risk reduction in relation to sexual partners needs to be regularly reviewed. Transmission of HIV to uninfected partners, or transmission of resistant strains, is possible and safe sex should be advised. However, the risk of transmission is thought to be extremely low when on treatment with a persistently suppressed HIV viral load. Some couples may make an informed decision to have unprotected sex—they should be advised to seek specialist advice from the HIV clinic.

Patients With Low CD4+ Counts

- Patients with CD4+ counts below 250 cells/mm³ are at increased risk of opportunistic infections and AIDS-related cancers such as lymphoma, Kaposi sarcoma, and cervical cancer.
- The risk of complications increases as the CD4+ falls further and patients with a CD4+ count below 50 cells/mm³ are at very high risk.
- Patients with a CD4+ count below 200 cells/mm³ are offered prophylaxis against pneumocystis pneumonia (PCP), usually with co-trimoxazole if tolerated. Those with a CD4+ count below 50 cells/mm³ are offered prophylaxis against *Mycobacterium avium*, usually with weekly azithromycin.
- Management of patients with a low CD4+ count is very complex and a specialist should be consulted for advice on management.
- Particular symptoms to be aware of are as follows:
  - *Oral candida* is common and may be accompanied by oesophageal candida. Systemic antifungal therapy is usually required and fluconazole is the usual first choice. High doses of fluconazole (≥100 mg) may be required, particularly for oesophagitis. Patients not responding to treatment within a few days should have an oral swab sent to the laboratory for resistance testing and be discussed with a specialist.
  - *Cough/shortness of breath*: PCP is a particular concern and may present with a clear chest and normal chest x-ray (CXR). Exercise desaturation is a helpful sign. Suspected PCP requires urgent specialist assessment. Patients are also at increased risk of community acquired pneumonia and tuberculosis.
  - *Headaches* or other neurologic symptoms: Immuno-suppressed patients with a low CD4+ count are at risk of a range of neurologic complications, including

toxoplasmosis, tuberculosis, lymphoma, and cryptococcal meningitis. Note that meningism is often absent in these cases.
- *Diarrhoea* and weight loss are common and may occur in the absence of infection. Possible causes include bacterial, protozoal, or viral infection. Send faeces for culture and discuss with a specialist if not improving.

Possible Exposure to Bloodborne Viruses

There are two ways in which people may present concerned about having acquired HIV or other bloodborne viruses.
- Following percutaneous or mucosal exposure to potentially infected body fluids: Most such exposures are occupational but members of the public will occasionally be exposed (e.g., through a needlestick from a discarded needle) (British Association for Sexual Health and HIV, 2015) but see the subsequent notifications online.
  - After any exposure to blood (whether the source patient is known to be HIV or hepatitis B or C positive), wash the wound liberally with soap and water, but do not scrub. Antiseptics should not be used.
  - The Department of Health advises that all healthcare staff, including those in primary care, should be educated on the risks from possible exposures and be made aware of how to report an injury. A local policy on how to obtain advice will be available and will provide information on how to obtain advice.
  - HIV post-exposure prophylaxis starter packs are usually available through the emergency department.
  - Take baseline blood for storage from the injured party unless immediate testing for bloodborne viruses is indicated.
  - If the risk is assessed as potentially significant, antiretroviral drugs should be commenced as soon as possible, preferably within 1 hour. Medication should be continued for a total of 4 weeks if subsequent risk assessment confirms this is appropriate. The contents of starter packs are under constant review.
  - See the section on hepatitis B for information on post-exposure prophylaxis.
  - If the source patient is of unknown status, he or she should routinely be approached (by someone other than the exposed patient) to ask for consent for testing.
  - Arrange follow-up by Occupational Health, the GUM department, or another appropriate department, for the exposed party, to consider testing for HIV and hepatitis B and C in confidence at a later stage.
  - Generally speaking, incidents involving members of the public injured by a discarded needle in a public place should not receive HIV post-exposure prophylaxis or hepatitis B immunoglobulin as the risk of transmission is extremely low. They should be offered hepatitis B vaccination and follow-up. It is, however, reasonable to discuss such cases with a specialist.
- Following sexual exposure: it is important to be aware that postexposure prophylaxis is available to those who may have been exposed through sexual contact. HIV

postexposure prophylaxis is available up to 72 hours after exposure (British Association for Sexual Health and HIV, 2015).

- There should be clear local protocols to seek urgent assessment for those who have been sexually assaulted and victims of sexual assault should receive specialist assessment.
- Other cases should be discussed urgently with the local sexual health clinic. Such cases should still be referred to GUM even if there is no indication for post-exposure prophylaxis as a sexual health screen and health promotion intervention will be indicated.
- There is evidence that pre-exposure prophylaxis of individuals at risk with daily antiretrovirals reduces the risk of HIV acquisition. At the time of writing, such treatment is not available on the National Health Service, but some people obtain it privately.

References

BASHH/EAGA. (2014). *Statement on HIV window period*. Retrieved from https://www.gov.uk/government/publications/time-period-for-hiv-testing-position-statement.

British Association for Sexual Health and HIV. (2015). *UK guideline for the use of HIV post-exposure prophylaxis following sexual exposure (PEPSE)*. Retrieved from https://www.bashh.org/documents/PEPSE%202015%20guideline%20final_NICE.pdf.

British HIV Association (2008). *UK national guidelines for HIV testing 2008*. Retrieved from http://www.bhiva.org/HIV-testing-guidelines.aspx.

British HIV Association. (2015). *Guidelines on the use of vaccines in HIV-positive adults*. Retrieved from http://bhiva.org/vaccination-guidelines.aspx.

British Infection Association. (2011). The epidemiology, prevention, investigation and treatment of Lyme borreliosis in United Kingdom patients: A position statement by the British Infection Association. *Journal of Infection, 62,* 329–338.

Checkley, A. M., Chiodini, P. L., Dockrell, D. H., et al. (2010). Eosinophilia in returning travellers and migrants from the tropics: UK recommendations for investigation and initial management. *Journal of Infection, 60,* 1–20.

Chen, N., Li, Q., Yang, J., Zhou, M., Zhou, D., & He, L. (1996). *Antiviral treatment for preventing postherpetic neuralgia*. Chichester, UK: John Wiley & Sons, Ltd. doi:10.1002/14651858.CD006866.pub3.

Clar, C., Oseni, Z., Flowers, N., Keshtkar-Jahromi, M., & Rees, K. (1996). Influenza vaccines for preventing cardiovascular disease. PubMed—NCBI. *The Cochrane Database of Systematic Reviews*, 2015 May 5;(5):CD005050. doi: 10.1002/14651858.CD005050.pub3.

Department of Health. (2008). *EAGA guidance on HIV post-exposure prophylaxis*. Retrieved from https://www.gov.uk/government/uploads/system/uploads/attachment_data/file/203139/HIV_post-exposure_prophylaxis.pdf.

Diggle, L., Deeks, J. J., & Pollard, A. J. (2006). Effect of needle size on immunogenicity and reactogenicity of vaccines in infants: Randomised controlled trial. *British Medical Journal, 333,* 571.

Dockrell, D. H., Johnston, V., Stockley, J. M., et al. (2009). Fever in returned travellers presenting in the United Kingdom: Recommendations for investigation and initial management. *Journal of Infection, 59,* 1–18.

Forna & Gulmezoglu (2000).

Kamar, N., Dalton, H. R., Abravanel, F., & Izopet, J. (2014). Hepatitis E virus infection. *Clinical Microbiology Reviews, 27,* 116–138.

Kantele, A., Lääveri, T., Mero, S., et al. (2015). Antimicrobials increase travelers' risk of colonization by extended-spectrum betalactamase-producing Enterobacteriaceae. *Clinical Infectious Diseases: An Official Publication of the Infectious Diseases Society of America, 60,* 837–846.

Leder, K., Torresi, J., Libman, M. D., et al. (2013). GeoSentinel surveillance of illness in returned travelers, 2007–2011. *Annals of Internal Medicine, 158,* 456–468.

McGill, F., Heyderman, R. S., Michael, B. D., et al. (2016). The UK Joint Specialists Societies guideline on the diagnosis and management of acute meningitis and meningococcal sepsis in immunocompetent adults. *Journal of Infection, 72,* 405–438.

Nathwani, D., Morgan, M., Masterton, R. G., et al. (2008). Guidelines for UK practice for the diagnosis and management of methicillin-resistant *Staphylococcus aureus* (MRSA) infections presenting in the community. *The Journal of Antimicrobial Chemotherapy, 61,* 976–994.

National Institute for Health and Care Excellence. (2016). *Tuberculosis | Guidance and guidelines*. Retrieved from https://www.nice.org.uk/guidance/ng33.

Newland, A., Provan, D., & Myint, S. (2005). Preventing severe infection after splenectomy. *British Medical Journal, 331,* 417–418.

Prymula, R., Siegrist, C.-A., Chlibek, R., et al. (2009). Effect of prophylactic paracetamol administration at time of vaccination on febrile reactions and antibody responses in children: Two open-label, randomised controlled trials. *Lancet, 374,* 1339–1350.

Public Health England. (n.d.a). *HPV vaccination pilot for men who have sex with men (MSM)*. Retrieved from https://www.gov.uk/government/publications/hpv-vaccination-pilot-for-men-who-have-sex-with-men-msm.

Public Health England. (n.d.b). *Vaccination of individuals with uncertain or incomplete immunisation status*. Retrieved from https://www.gov.uk/government/publications/vaccination-of-individuals-with-uncertain-or-incomplete-immunisation-status.

Public Health England (2015a). *Guidelines for malaria prevention in travellers from the UK*. Retrieved from https://www.gov.uk/government/publications/malaria-prevention-guidelines-for-travellers-from-the-uk.

Public Health England. (2015b). *HIV in the UK—situation report 2015. Incidence, prevalence and prevention*. Retrieved from https://www.gov.uk/government/uploads/system/uploads/attachment_data/file/477702/HIV_in_the_UK_2015_report.pdf.

Public Health England. (2015c). *Revised recommendations for the administration of more than one live vaccine*. Retrieved from https://www.gov.uk/government/uploads/system/uploads/attachment_data/file/422798/PHE_recommendations_for_administering_more_than_one_live_vaccine_April_2015FINAL_.pdf.

Public Health England. (2015d). *Supply or administration of paracetamol oral suspension 120 mg/5 mL to infants under 12 months of age receiving primary doses of MenB vaccination*. Retrieved from https://www.gov.uk/government/uploads/system/uploads/attachment_data/file/453782/20150811PHEParacetamolProtocolFinalv01_00.pdf.

Public Health England. (2016a). *Advisory Committee on Dangerous Pathogens. Viral haemorrhagic fever: ACDP algorithm and guidance on management of patients*. Retrieved from https://www.gov.uk/government/publications/viral-haemorrhagic-fever-algorithm-and-guidance-on-management-of-patients.

Public Health England. (2016b). *Guidelines for the public health management of pertussis in England*. Retrieved from https://www.gov.uk/government/uploads/system/uploads/attachment_data/file/541694/

Guidelines_for_the_Public_Health_Management_of_Pertussis_in_England.pdf.

Public Health England. (2016c). *PHE guidance on use of antiviral agents for the treatment and prophylaxis of seasonal influenza.* Retrieved from https://www.gov.uk/government/uploads/system/uploads/attachment_data/file/563029/PHE_guidance_antivirals_influenza_2016_to_2017_FINAL.pdf.

Reis, E. C., Roth, E. K., Syphan, J. L., Tarbell, S. E., & Holubkov, R. (2003). Effective pain reduction for multiple immunization injections in young infants. *Archives of Pediatrics and Adolescent Medicine, 157,* 1115–1120.

Riddle, M. S., DuPont, H. L., & Connor, B. A. (2016). ACG clinical guideline: Diagnosis, treatment, and prevention of acute diarrheal infections in adults. *American Journal of Gastroenterology, 111,* 602–622.

Ritchie, N. D., Baggott, A. V., & Todd, W. T. A. (2012). Acetazolamide for the prevention of acute mountain sickness—a systematic review and meta-analysis. *Journal of Travel Medicine, 19,* 298–307.

Royal College of Nursing. (2010). *Methicillin-resistant* Staphylococcus aureus *(MRSA) guidance for nursing staff.* Retrieved from https://www.nhs.uk/Conditions/MRSA/Documents/RCN%20MRSA%20guidelines.pdf.

Smith, C. J., Ryom, L., Weber, R., et al. (2014). Trends in underlying causes of death in people with HIV from 1999 to 2011 (D:A:D): A multicohort collaboration. *Lancet, 384,* 241–248.

Soonawala, D., van Lieshout, L., den Boer, M. A. M., et al. (2014). Post-travel screening of asymptomatic long-term travelers to the tropics for intestinal parasites using molecular diagnostics. *The American Journal of Tropical Medicine and Hygiene, 90,* 835–839.

Steffen, R. (2005). Epidemiology of traveler's diarrhea. *Clinical Infectious Diseases: An Official Publication of the Infectious Diseases Society of America, 41*(8), S536–S540.

Sulheim, Holme, Ekeland, et al. (2006).

Tunbridge, A. J., Breuer, J., Jeffery, K. J. M., & British Infection Society. (2008). Chickenpox in adults—clinical management. *Journal of Infection, 57,* 95–102.

Whittle, A. (2008). *Increasing opportunities for HIV diagnosis in primary care.* BHIVA Annual Conference.

18

Psychiatric Problems

DOMINIQUE THOMPSON

CHAPTER CONTENTS

Depression

- About 25% to 40% of general practitioner (GP) consultations have a significant psychological component (Goldberg & Lecrubier, 1995). Of these only about 5% are referred to specialist services.
- Recent research has shown how specific questions help to elicit crucial information about the patient's mental state.
- Qualitative research has shown the importance of the patient's relationship with the GP in such situations. Patients value an empathetic, interested doctor with whom they have a continuing relationship (Buszewicz et al, 2006).

> ### GUIDELINES
>
> National Institute for Health and Care Excellence. (2016). *Depression in adults: Recognition and management. NICE clincial guideline 90.* www.nice.org.uk.
>   Anderson, I. M., Ferrier, I. N., Baldwin, R. C., et al. (2008). Evidence-based guidelines for treating depressive disorders with antidepressants: A revision of the 2000 British Association for Psychopharmacology guidelines. *Journal of Psychopharmacology / British Association for Psychopharmacology, 22,* 343–396.

- GPs fail to diagnose up to half of their patients with a major depressive illness, and often fail to treat adequately those whom they do recognize (Anderson, Nutt, & Deakin, 2000; Freeling et al., 1985).
- Depression in people from the African–Caribbean, Asian, refugee, and asylum-seeking communities is often overlooked, although the prevalence is 60% higher than in the white population (Department of Health, 1999). People from black and minority ethnic communities are much less likely to be referred to psychological therapies (Department of Health, 1999).
- Those patients whose depression is most likely to be missed are those with somatic complaints or with physical illness, those with long-standing depression, those who do not look depressed, and those who do not realize they are depressed (Freeling et al., 1985; Gill & Hatcher, 2002).
- Depression is often accompanied and masked by anxiety (Goldberg & Bridges, 1987), yet treatment of the anxiety alone is insufficient and may appear to worsen the depression.

Presenting Complaints

- Screen for depression in patients with low mood, or with a past history, or who are at risk because of physical illness or other mental illnesses such as anxiety or dementia. Ask two specific questions: During the past month have you felt:
  - low, depressed, or hopeless?
  - little interest or pleasure in doing things? (Whooley et al., 1997)

- If the answer to either question is yes, confirm the diagnosis of depression using the DSM-V criteria as follows. Used by GPs this is highly specific (Van Weel-Baumgarten et al., 2000). However, if the score conflicts with clinical judgment, treat it as a checklist only and act on your clinical judgment.
- A *major depressive illness* exists if the patient has low mood or diminished interest or pleasure for at least 2 weeks, occurring most of the day or nearly every day, and a positive score on at least five of the following:
  - Depressed mood
  - Loss of interest or pleasure
  - Change in weight or altered appetite almost every day
  - Disturbed sleep
  - Agitation or slowing of movement or speech
  - Fatigue or loss of self-energy
  - Guilt or low esteem
  - Poor concentration
  - Recurrent suicidal thoughts or acts
- *Minor depression* is characterized by three or four of the above. The evidence that it responds to antidepressant drugs is poor, unless it lasts for at least 2 years, when it may be called *dysthymia*, which may respond to drugs (Barrett et al., 2001).

Cautions

- The scoring system cannot be used in patients reacting appropriately to a life crisis or who are schizophrenic.
- To score as positive, the symptoms should indicate significant distress or impairment in functioning.
- No scoring system can be totally accurate. Modify the result in light of the patient's circumstances. A past or family history of major depression, for instance, would increase the chance of major depression in a patient whose score does not reach that threshold.
- The distinction between major and minor depression on the DSM-V criteria should not be confused with mild, moderate, and severe depression on the ICD-10 criteria (World Health Organisation [WHO], 2003), where the scoring is out of 10, not 9, and includes an assessment of functioning rather than a more rigid count of symptoms. This leads to the imperfect correlation between the two scores shown in Table 18.1.

Differential Diagnosis

- *Schizophrenia.* Look for evidence of schizophrenia, which may present with depression. If delusions or hallucinations are also present, depression should not be the initial diagnosis.
- *Bipolar affective disorder.* Ask about a past history of a manic episode or hypomania. The management of bipolar affective disorder is different (see page 333). A study in US primary care looked at the prevalence of a current diagnosis of depression plus a positive screen for bipolar affective disorder. In the adult primary care population, 4% had both but the GPs who were managing the depression did not detect concurrent

TABLE 18.1 Depression: Definitions and Scoring		
ICD-10 Definition	**ICD-10 Scores**	**Equivalent DSM-V Definition**
Mild depression	2–3. The patient is distressed but able to continue functioning	Minor depression
Moderate depression	4 or more. The patient is likely to have great difficulty in continuing with normal activities	Minor or major depression
Severe depression	Several symptoms are marked and distressing, typically loss of self-esteem and ideas of worthlessness and guilt. Suicidal thoughts are common and a number of somatic symptoms are usually present. Hallucinations or delusions also mean that the episode is severe, regardless of other symptoms	Major depression

bipolar affective disorder in any of these patients (Das et al., 2005).

- *Iatrogenic cause.* Check for drugs that can cause depression (e.g., antihypertensives, histamine type-2 [H_2] blockers, steroids, and beta-blockers).
- *Life events.* Ask about recent life events such as recent childbirth, bereavement, termination of pregnancy, loss of job, work stress, family illness, or divorce. They may have triggered the depression.

Management of Depression

- The GP will manage 90% of depressed patients without referral to a specialized mental health service. The following steps are common to almost all severities of depression.
- *Life events:* Identify relevant life events which may have precipitated the illness and focus on small steps that might be taken to reduce their impact.
- Explore the impact of the depression on behaviour and relationships at home and work.
- Explain the nature of the illness, its treatment. and good prognosis.
- Discuss the link between physical symptoms and mood.
- Encourage the patient not to make major or irreversible decisions about work or family until their mental state improves.
- *Exercise:* Recommend exercise, to the same extent as for cardiovascular fitness, for at least 10 weeks, even (or especially) on days when the patient feels like staying in bed (Dunn et al, 2005). High-dose exercise 3 days a week is likely to lead to remission in one in five depressed patients compared to controls. The depressed patient will have little motivation and will need supervision. Refer to an exercise referral scheme if one is available.
- *Light therapy:* Recommend it for seasonal affective disorder. However, if using artificial lights, exposure to a bank of lights is needed for 1 hour a day, preferably in the morning. Similar benefit is seen with exposure to natural light, even if the sky is cloudy (Jorm, Christensen, Griffiths, & Rodgers, 2002). Exposure to daylight could usefully be combined with exercise.
- *Discuss drug therapy and counselling* (see upcoming discussion).

- *Follow-up:* Explain the need for and frequency of follow-up.
- *Patient information:* Provide one of the leaflets listed in the box on page 318 and give the patient details of sources of information and support.

Referral

Refer to a specialist mental health service if:
- psychotic features are present or the depression is severe;
- the history suggests a bipolar illness;
- there is a significant risk of suicide or severe neglect;
- other forms of treatment are needed (e.g., cognitive behavioural therapy) if they are not available in primary care;
- the patient is a child or adolescent with major depressive illness;
- there has been a poor response to an appropriate antidepressant in maximum dosage, with good compliance, taken for an adequate period of time;
- there is social isolation, little family support, or poor compliance.

Specific Treatment of Minor Depression (or Mild Depression on the ICD-10 Criteria)

- Explain the possible options:
  - Watchful waiting. The patient may choose to return in, say, 2 weeks without treatment other than the general measures described previously.
  - Guided self-help. The patient works through a written or computer programme which is usually designed along cognitive behavioural lines (see upcoming Information for Patients box). National Institute for Health and Care Excellence (NICE) has approved a computerized cognitive behavioural therapy (CBT) programme, "Beating the Blues," for mild to moderate depression, suitable for those with no computer experience. If the GP is unable to offer access to it using National Health System (NHS) funding, the patient can access it, for a considerable fee, at www.beatingtheblues.co.uk.
  - Counselling or psychotherapy. There is evidence that brief CBT, problem-solving therapy, and other forms of counselling are beneficial.
- Explain that antidepressants are usually ineffective in minor depression unless it has lasted for 2 years (i.e., dysthymia).

Any possible benefit is likely to be outweighed by the adverse effects. However, a patient with a past history of major depression who presents with minor depression may choose to take an antidepressant at this stage.

Specific Treatment of Major Depression (or Moderate-Severe Depression on the ICD-10 Criteria)

- *Offer an antidepressant.* The NICE guideline recommends a selective serotonin reuptake inhibitor (SSRI) because they are as effective as tricyclics but with a 10% less chance of being discontinued because of adverse effects. Cost-effectiveness studies, in which doctors' time is costed as well as drug expenditure, favour SSRIs or are at least neutral (Simon et al., 1999; Stewart, 1998). However, both types of drug have considerable but different adverse effects. Attempt to make a choice that is the best for that patient (see upcoming discussion).
- Explain to patients that:
  - even if their depression is a reaction to life events, they are as likely to benefit from an antidepressant as if it was endogenous;
  - they will not notice any improvement for the first 10 days to 3 weeks but that adverse effects are most likely to occur in this period and then lessen;
  - antidepressants are not addictive. They will not develop craving or tolerance, but there is the possibility of a discontinuation reaction especially if stopped abruptly;
  - stopping the drug early increases the risk of relapse. All patients should take the drug for 6 months after recovery. Anyone with a recent previous episode of major depression should take it for 2 years, as should other people at high risk of relapse (e.g., the elderly) (see upcoming discussion).
- *Prescribe a generic preparation.* There is some evidence that venlafaxine is more effective than other antidepressants (Smith et al., 2002) but adverse effects may also be greater (Cipriani, Geddes, & Barbui, 2007). One study suggests that the risk-benefit profile from 117 randomized controlled trials (RCTs) favours sertraline (Cipriani et al., 2009).
- *Drug dosage:*
  - If choosing a tricyclic, start at the equivalent of amitriptyline 75 mg daily and expect to increase to 150 mg daily. A much-criticized meta-analysis (Furukawa, McGuire, & Barbui, 2002) has suggested that the lower doses may be adequate. Such studies, and their critics, inevitably examine the mean response of a large number of patients. In clinical practice what matters is the response of that individual. Assess the effect of the lower dose and increase the dose monthly if the response is inadequate.
  - If choosing an SSRI start at the standard dose. Evidence that subsequent dose increases are beneficial is poor (although higher doses are effective in other conditions).
- *Follow-up.* See the patient 1 week after starting a drug, to discuss any adverse effects (e.g., agitation or akathisia on an SSRI) and to check on compliance. A quarter of patients either never cash in their prescription or only do so once (Boardman & Walters, 2009). If an SSRI is causing agitation, a 2-week course of a benzodiazepine is an alternative to stopping the drug. Slowly increase the time between consultations as the patient responds.
- *Response.* Do not be disappointed by a partial response. Studies of published and unpublished studies combined show that the effect size of all antidepressants is small (number needed to treat [NNT] = 6) (Boardman & Walters, 2009) and certainly less than the claims of manufacturers, based on published studies alone (Turner & Rosenthal, 2008).
- *Maintenance.* Continue the drug for at least 6 months after remission. This reduces the relapse rate from 50% to 20%. A reduction in dose should only be made if side effects are a problem. Consider treatment for 1 to 2 years if there has been a previous episode in the recent past or the patient is at high risk because of age, family history, or other features (see upcoming discussion).

Factors That Will Influence the Choice of an Antidepressant

- *The elderly:* Avoid highly anticholinergic drugs (e.g., amitriptyline, clomipramine, doxepin, imipramine, and maprotiline).
- *Young people:* The Committee on Safety of Medicines (CSM) has concluded that the majority of SSRIs are contraindicated in children and adolescents up to the age of 18 because of poor efficacy and a possible increase in the risk of self-harm and suicide. Fluoxetine seems to be an exception to this. The CSM also cautions that very young adults may be at similar risk, even though such a risk has not been detected in trials (CSM Expert Working Group, 2004).
- *Pregnancy:* Treat only if the benefit outweighs the risks. Consider seeking specialist advice before starting antidepressants or switching the antidepressant of a woman who is already being treated for depression when she falls pregnant. Evidence about the relative risks and benefits of antidepressant use in pregnancy is inadequate making informed decision making difficult (McDonagh et al, 2014). Between 3–8% of pregnant women in Europe currently take an antidepressant so experience of antidepressant use in pregnancy is rapidly growing and untreated depression is associated with the risks of preterm birth and low birth weight (Jarde et al, 2016). NICE clinical knowledge summaries advise use of a tricyclic antidepressant, SSRI, or SNRI after discussion of risks and benefits (NICE, 2018). Use tricyclics with caution; neonatal irritability has been reported with imipramine.
- *Prostatism or glaucoma:* Avoid all anticholinergic drugs.
- *Cardiac disease:* Avoid tricyclics and venlafaxine; the best evidence for use in ischaemic heart disease is for sertraline.
- *Suicide risk:* There is no evidence that one class of drugs poses a greater risk of suicide (Cipriani, Barbui, & Geddes, 2005) but intuitively doctors will avoid the more toxic tricyclics.

- *Lethargy:* Avoid sedative drugs (e.g., amitriptyline, clomipramine, dosulepin, doxepin, maprotiline, mianserin, trazodone, and trimipramine).
- *Anxiety or insomnia:* Use a sedative drug.
- *Obesity:* Use an SSRI.
- *Epilepsy:* Avoid SSRIs.
- *Other drugs:* All classes of antidepressants show considerable interaction with other drugs, but any one interaction rarely applies to all classes and may not be seen with all members of one class. Choose an antidepressant tailored to the patient's other medication.

Management of a Poor Response to Drug Therapy

- Check that the patient was taking the drug correctly. An apparent relapse could be due to a discontinuation reaction in a patient who has omitted one or more doses.
- Where there is evidence that an increased dose may be associated with an improved response, and there are no adverse effects, consider increasing the dose gradually, waiting 4 weeks each time before deciding that the response is inadequate.
- If dosage increase is not a possibility, assess whether referral is needed or whether the patient's condition allows the trial of another drug. Make a choice, according to any adverse effects experienced with the first drug, between another SSRI, a tricyclic (but not dosulepin), and a member of a different class (e.g., moclobemide, mirtazapine, or reboxetine). Because it is a Reversible Inhibitor of Monoamine Oxidase A (RIMA), moclobemide cannot be started until the previous antidepressant has washed out of the system. For a tricyclic this is 1 week but for fluoxetine it is 5 weeks. The STAR* D study found that putting non-responders through four steps of antidepressant treatment (either increased dosage or a change of drug) increased the rate of remission from 37% with step 1 to 67% by step 4, in those who adhered to treatment (Rush et al., 2006). Against these impressive-sounding results is the fact that dropout rates were high and the percentage remitting fell with each step.
- Consider combining psychotherapy with drug treatment. Response is greater than with either alone, even if this is just because patients who also receive psychotherapy are more likely to take their drugs (Pampallona, Bollini, & Tibaldi, 2004).

Stopping Maintenance Therapy and Managing Discontinuation Reactions

- Tail off, over 4 weeks, any antidepressant that has been given for 8 weeks or more, to reduce the risk of a discontinuation reaction (Haddad, Lejoyeux, & Young, 1998). A long-acting drug (e.g., fluoxetine or sertraline) may be given at the same dose but every other day, then every third day. A short-acting drug (e.g., paroxetine or citalopram) should be given daily at decreasing dosage. Tablets may be cut in half or a liquid form prescribed.
- Warn the patient that a discontinuation reaction is possible on stopping an antidepressant. The incidence is unclear. Estimates based on reports of adverse drug reactions suggest that it is uncommon (5% with paroxetine, <1% with other SSRIs) (Price et al., 1996) but such reports rely on the reporting doctor making the diagnosis. A retrospective analysis of patients discontinuing antidepressants found that a reaction occurred in 31% who had taken clomipramine, in 17% who had taken a short-acting SSRI (paroxetine or fluvoxamine), and in only 1.5% who had taken a long-acting SSRI (fluoxetine or sertraline) (Coupland, Bell, & Potokar, 1996). Even if half of these are due to a placebo effect (Haddad et al., 1998), the study suggests that the reaction is more common with the shorter acting drugs.
- Explain that a discontinuation reaction is unlikely to feel like a recurrence of depression. Dizziness, paraesthesia, tremor, anxiety, nausea, and palpitations are the most common symptoms. They occur within days of stopping the drug and last for 10 days on average.
- If a discontinuation reaction occurs:
  - A mild reaction: Explain what is happening and continue the planned reduction, if the patient agrees.
  - A more severe reaction, either:
    a. increase the dose to the last dose that gave no reaction; or
    b. change the patient to a longer acting drug of the same class; and
    c. prepare to tail off over a longer period (e.g., 3–6 months).
- Review patients 4 weeks after finally stopping the drug to ensure they remain well. Advise them to return at the earliest sign of a recurrence.

How to Distinguish an Antidepressant Discontinuation Reaction From a Return of the Underlying Disorder

- Its onset is within days (against weeks for a recurrence of depression).
- It resolves with 24 hours of restarting the antidepressant.
- Although the patient may report mood disturbance (low mood, irritability, anxiety) there are likely to be somatic symptoms as well (numbness, paraesthesia, dizziness, headache, myalgia, fatigue, insomnia with vivid dreams).

Cognitive Behavioural Therapy/Counselling/Other Psychotherapies

- In patients at the mild to moderate end of the spectrum of major depression, cognitive and interpersonal therapies can be as effective as antidepressants and may prevent relapse (Gloaguen et al., 1998). In a meta-analysis, antidepressants and psychotherapy both resulted in remission at a mean of 16 weeks in 46% of patients against 24% of controls (Casacalenda, Perry, & Looper, 2002).
- More patients would choose counselling than drugs if given the choice (Chilvers et al., 2001).
- In major depression, a combination of antidepressants and cognitive behavioural therapy can be more effective than either alone (Timonen & Liukkonen, 2008). Other

psychotherapies have not shown a benefit from being combined with drugs.

- Most of the evidence for the benefit of psychological therapies in depression lies with certain techniques only, mainly cognitive behavioural, interpersonal, and problem-solving ones (Mynors-Wallis et al., 2000) and cannot be assumed to exist for all forms of counselling (Department of Health, 2001).
- A 6-year follow-up study suggests that a course of cognitive behavioural therapy, in addition to drug therapy, leads to fewer subsequent relapses than drug therapy alone (40% vs. 90% in a study of 40 patients) (Fava, Ruini, & Rafanelli, 2004).

Prevention of Recurrence

- The continuing nature of the condition and the benefit to be gained from early intervention argue strongly for depression to be managed as a chronic disease, with a systematic approach to follow-up by a dedicated team following agreed protocols (Scott, 2006).
- Of patients with a first episode of major depression, 75% have a recurrence within the next 10 years (Angst, 1997). A second episode during the next 4 years requires full initial treatment, followed by psychiatric referral to consider prophylaxis with long-term antidepressant medication. In the first 3 years this will reduce the rate of recurrence from 41% to 18%. Only slightly more patients withdraw from treatment on an antidepressant than on placebo (odds ratio [OR] 1.3) (95% confidence interval [CI] 1.07–1.59) (Geddes et al., 2003).
- Long-term prophylaxis after a single episode may be appropriate in the following because their risk of recurrence is even higher:
  - The elderly
  - Those with a first-degree relative with bipolar disorder or recurrent major depression
- As a minimum, consider a 3-monthly telephone review by a doctor or nurse over the 2 years after treatment is stopped. In a US study it increased remission over 2 years by 33% (95%CI 7–46) (Rost et al., 2002).

Postnatal Depression

GUIDELINES

Scottish Intercollegiate Guidelines Network. (2012). *Management of perinatal mood disorders. SIGN guideline 127, 2002*. www.sign.ac.uk.

National Institute of Health and Care Excellence. (2014). *Antenatal and postnatal mental health: Clinical management and service guidance. NICE clincial guideline 192*, updated 2017. www.nice.org.uk.

- Postnatal depression occurs in 10% to 15% of women in the first year after delivery, usually in the first 6 months. The symptoms are almost always present at 6 weeks. It is distinct from the transient blues of the first 10 days, and from a puerperal psychosis which is likely to need admission.
- Most at risk are those with:
  - previous psychological disturbance in pregnancy;
  - poor social support;
  - a poor marital relationship;
  - recent stressful events;
  - an episode of the baby blues.
- The strongest risk factors for puerperal psychosis are a personal or family history of an affective psychosis. A woman who has one episode of puerperal psychosis has a 25% to 57% risk of a recurrence in a subsequent pregnancy. The risk of non-puerperal affective psychosis at some stage is even greater.
- Every practice should be aware of the need to identify at-risk patients during the antenatal period and should ensure that they receive more intensive help after birth. Risk factors should be identified during pregnancy and the primary care team needs to decide:
  - what extra care this group should receive; and
  - who is responsible for identifying this condition as early as possible.
- Patients often do not realize that they are depressed, and doctors recognize it even less frequently. Women often present with a feeling of not coping rather than with classic symptoms of depression.
- The Scottish Intercollegiate Guidelines Network (SIGN) guideline recommends that every woman should be screened for depression at 6 weeks and 3 months postpartum. The Edinburgh Postnatal Depression Scale (EPDS) (Cox, Holden, & Sagovsky, 1987) may be administered by a trained professional (see Appendix 20) as part of that screening process but with the understanding that it is a screening, not a diagnostic, tool. Clinical assessment is needed to establish the diagnosis.
- If the EPDS is not available, ask four simple questions:
  - How are you feeling?
  - How are you sleeping?

- How are you eating?
- Are you enjoying the baby?

If Depression Is Found

- Check thyroid function tests (TFTs) in those complaining mainly of tiredness.
- *Counsel.* Simple, nondirective counselling by health visitors, weekly for 8 weeks, doubles the recovery rate (Holden, Sagovsky, & Cox, 1989).
- Explain to the patient that she is ill: it is not her fault and does not mean that she is a poor mother.
- *Literature.* Recommend one of the sources of information in the box Patient Organisations or print the information for the patient.
- *Antidepressants.* Offer drug treatment on the same basis that you would offer it to a non-puerperal patient (i.e., if major depressive illness is present). SIGN recommends that tricyclics (other than doxepin) or SSRIs (although avoid fluoxetine, escitalopram, and citalopram if possible) may be used and the patient may continue to breastfeed. This goes beyond the manufacturers' advice and indeed a mother should be told that the SSRIs, especially, will be excreted in the breast milk but that there is no evidence that this is harmful to the baby. However, the baby may experience a discontinuation reaction. Use a long-acting drug and tail off breastfeeding (or the drug if still breastfeeding) slowly.
- Consider referral if a multidisciplinary mental health team is able to offer more than the primary healthcare team.
- Refer immediately for urgent psychiatric assessment any woman with ideas of suicide or of harming the baby or with symptoms of puerperal psychosis.

PATIENT ORGANIZATIONS

Association for Post Natal Illness, 145 Dawes Road, Fulham, London SW6 7EB, tel. 020 7386 0868, www.apni.org
Mental Health Foundation; www.mentalhealth.org.uk.
National Childbirth Trust, Alexandra House, Oldham Terrace, London W3 6NH, tel. 0300 330 0700, www.nct.org.uk (search on "depression").

Suicide and Suicidal Risk

- Two-thirds of successful suicides are mentally ill (Owens, Lloyd, & Campbell, 2004), mostly with undiagnosed depression. In the elderly the prevalence of mental illness in suicides rises to up to 95% (O'Connell, Chin, Cunningham, & Lawlor, 2004).
- The risk of completed suicide in the first 9 days of drug treatment is 38 times that of the risk in a patient who has been on treatment for at least 3 months (Jick, Kaye, & Jick, 2004). This is independent of the type of antidepressant used.

- There is no evidence that SSRIs increase the risk of suicide in adults, though they appear to do so in children and adolescents. On the contrary, it seems likely that effective treatment of depression offers the most hope of reducing the risk of suicide. Even in adolescents the risk of suicide is greater in the month before starting antidepressants than in the first month on therapy (Brent, 2007).
- Suicide is uncommon even in major depressive illness. One study found that only 4% of patients admitted because of depression killed themselves (Bostwick & Pankratz, 2000). Furthermore, that 4% is hard to detect, though an attempt should be made.
- In all patients with depression, assess the risk. For instance, ask a series of questions, only stopping when the answer is no:
  - Have you thought how nice it would be if you did not wake up one morning?
  - Have you thought of killing yourself?
  - Have you decided how to do it?
  - Have you decided when to do it?
- Judge the risk according to the following risk factors:
  - History of previous attempts, especially if determined or violent methods were used, or if a suicide note was left
  - Intense feelings of hopelessness and worthlessness
  - Major mental illness, including depression
  - Suicidal ideation or evidence of planning (e.g., if the patient has decided when to do it, and if a sudden and infallible method has been chosen) (Boardman & Walters, 2009)
  - Chronic physical illness or in much pain
  - Recent bereavement or other significant loss, including job
  - Males. The male to female ratio for suicide is 4 : 1
  - Old age; the risk age over 75 is three times that of ages 15 to 24
  - Alcohol or other substance misuse
  - Previous inpatient psychiatric treatment
  - Family history of mental illness, suicide, or alcoholism
  - Positive for aquired immunodeficiency syndrome (AIDS) or HIV
  - Unmarried, separated, or divorced, especially if living alone

Management of Suicidal Patients

Low Risk

- Manage at home patients who have thoughts of suicide but who have:
  - no clear suicidal plans or past history of a serious suicidal attempt;
  - good rapport with their GP or local psychiatric services;
  - 24-hour home support;
  - a stable personality;
  - no psychotic illness, chronic physical illness, or drug or alcohol misuse
- *Drugs.* If prescribing, give small quantities of medication, initially.

High Risk

- Refer urgently to the mental health team. Check that the patient meets the previously agreed local criteria for same-day referral. A domiciliary visit by a psychiatrist may be indicated (even if a patient refuses all offers of help).
- If the GP and psychiatrist cannot visit together, make sure that the GP is notified immediately of the outcome of the visit.
- Ensure that the carers can provide observation for 24 hours a day, until the risk diminishes. The family may need help to provide this level of care. If drug treatment is started, a relative or carer ought to be asked to supervise the medication.

Follow-Up After Attempted Suicide

Often the first time a GP hears about a suicidal patient is when a hospital discharge report is received. When this occurs, the doctor should:

- review the records to see if the patient has recently attended;
- discuss the management with the mental healthcare team, if the patient has a severe longstanding mental illness;
- identify anything that might indicate the patient was a suicide risk;
- enter suicide attempt on the notes;
- ask the patient to make an appointment to see the GP for review;
- follow-up to:
  - identify depression or other precipitating life events;
  - assess the need for treatment, including counselling;
  - make a care plan to review outcome and prevent recurrence.
- start treatment if indicated, as discussed next.

SUPPORT ORGANIZATIONS

The Samaritans. Tel. 116 123; email: jo@samaritans.org; website: www.samaritans.org.

PAPYRUS (prevention of young suicide). Helpline 08000 684141; www.papyrus-uk.org.

Helping Those Bereaved by Suicide

- Grief after suicide seems to be particularly intense and often associated with shame and guilt. On average six people have intense grief for every suicide (Hawton, 2003). Identify the people most likely to be affected and give them a chance to talk about their feelings.
- If their grief is intense, refer for counselling or recommend self-help literature or self-help groups, according to its severity.

Stress Reactions

SUPPORT ORGANIZATIONS

Survivors of Bereavement by Suicide (SOBS). National helpline 0300 111 5065; www.uk-sobs.org.uk.

Winston's Wish is specifically for children bereaved by suicide. Helpline 08088 020 021; www.winstonswish.org.uk.

CRUSE offers support to all those who are bereaved. Day by Day helpline 0844 4779400, Young Person's helpline 0808 808 1677; www.crusebereavementcare.org.uk.

The Compassionate Friends helps parents and siblings who have lost a child, including from suicide. Helpline 0345 123 2304; www.tcf.org.uk.

- Stress reactions may be:
  - acute and brief;
  - an adjustment reaction which may last a few months; or
  - posttraumatic stress disorder (PTSD), with a delay between the stress and the onset of symptoms.
- Stress may be a reaction to loss or trauma. Symptoms may be those of anxiety, depression, abnormal behaviour, or inability to cope with normal events. Symptoms may have been present for a long time before help is sought.
- Stressful events include:
  - crime or accidents involving psychological and/or physical trauma;
  - bereavement, including siblings in a family where a child has died;
  - termination of pregnancy, miscarriage;
  - redundancy, loss of job, occupational stress;
  - divorce, separation, relationship difficulties;
  - housing or financial problems;
  - surviving a disaster;
  - having to perform in front of an audience, or having a work appraisal;
  - seeking asylum;
  - drug or alcohol withdrawal.

Management

- Identify underlying precipitating events and the steps taken by the patient to modify or cope with the situation.
- Exclude a physical or drug cause for the symptoms (drug or alcohol withdrawal, sudden stopping of a beta-blocker, hyperthyroidism).
- Identify others who might help (e.g., Relate, Citizens' Advice Bureau, Victim Support, union representative, local police domestic violence unit).
- Review what support can be obtained from family, friends, work colleagues, and sources of community support.
- Discuss coping strategies.
- Assess the need for counselling.
- Decide if short-term time off work might be helpful.
- Consider prescribing a beta-blocker if somatic symptoms (shaking and tachycardia) are prominent. Avoid anxiolytic drugs but if the symptoms are very severe give them for a maximum of 2 weeks.

Posttraumatic Stress Disorder

- The risk of developing PTSD varies according to the nature of the trauma and the susceptibility of the patient, ranging from 10% following a road traffic accident, to 32% following a myocardial infarct (Jones et al., 2007), to 57% following rape (Hull, 2004).
- A study from the Netherlands suggests that non-traumatic life events (e.g., divorce or unemployment) may be more frequently the cause of PTSD than trauma (Mol et al., 2005).
- Presentation may be delayed for several months after the event. In the United States the lifetime prevalence is 8% (American Psychiatric Association, 2000a). An Israeli study found that only 2.4% of patients with PTSD had been detected by their GPs (Munro, Freeman, & Law, 2004).
- Look for PTSD specifically in patients who have had an extremely traumatic incident in their lives. The cues to the diagnosis are when, at least 1 month after the event, the patient's life is disturbed by:
  - intrusive symptoms; memories, flashbacks, and nightmares;
  - avoidance of thoughts, activities, situations associated with the event; emotional numbing;
  - symptoms of autonomic arousal (e.g., hypervigilance, insomnia, irritability, excessive anger, and impaired concentration and/or memory).
- Check whether the patient has taken refuge in drug or alcohol misuse.
- In severe cases assess the risk of suicide.

Management

- *Debriefing.* Do not routinely offer debriefing after a traumatic event. It appears to be useless and may be harmful (Bisson, 2004). A follow-up appointment 1 to 2 months after the event is more likely to be useful. Even then, beware of overdiagnosing it in a patient who is recovering spontaneously from a traumatic event.
- Provide information for patient and family (see box).
- Encourage discussion of the precipitator event once PTSD has developed.
- Encourage the patient to discuss his or her feelings and fears.
- Explain how avoiding things that remind the patient of the trauma prolongs the syndrome.
- Draw up a gradual plan to face avoided activities and situations.
- *Alcohol.* Warn about the need to avoid excess use of alcohol. If the patient is already misusing alcohol or other drugs, treatment of the misuse must come before treatment of the PTSD.
- *Psychological therapy.* Refer for trauma-focused CBT if symptoms are present 3 months after the event. Refer at 1 month if symptoms are severe (NICE, 2005a).
- *Antidepressants.* SSRIs reduce all symptoms of PTSD as well as treating any associated anxiety and depression. Sertraline has been shown to increase the response rate from one-third (with placebo) to half, although the reduction in symptoms was small (Jick et al., 2004). It may take 8 weeks before effects are seen; and high doses may be needed. If effective, continue for at least 6 months in total, or at least 12 months if the PTSD has lasted more than 3 months, to avoid relapse. There is an impression that patients do better if the drugs are started early in the course of the condition. NICE recommends paroxetine and mirtazapine for general use and other antidepressants for use by mental health specialists (NICE, 2005b).
- *Other drugs.* Consider a beta-blocker for a patient disabled by startle and hyperarousal symptoms. The evidence for benzodiazepines is poor. However, consider a nighttime short-acting benzodiazepine for a patient exhausted by poor sleep. Explain the disadvantages (dependence and tolerance) and obtain the patient's agreement that it will only be used, at the most, twice a week while waiting for the SSRI to take effect.
- Inform the patient about the resources listed in the box.

PATIENT ORGANIZATIONS

Victim Support provides emotional and practical support for victims of crime. Support line: 0808 1689 111; email: support@victimsupport.org.uk; website: www.victimsupport.org.uk.

The Refugee Council. Tel. 020 7346 6700; www.refugeecouncil.org.uk.

Combat Stress (Ex-Services Mental Welfare Society) supports ex-service people with PTSD. Tel. 0800 138 1619; email: contactus@combatstress.org.uk; website: www.combatstress.org.uk.

MIND has excellent information. Call the Mindinfoline 0845 766 0163 or download it from www.mind.org.uk (search "post-traumatic stress disorder").

Insomnia

- Insomnia may be primary, or secondary to another mental or physical disorder or to medication. Common causes of insomnia are depression, anxiety, menopausal symptoms, restless legs syndrome, pain, and drugs. Half of patients with insomnia have a specific mental disorder and an overlapping half have a physical disorder (NICE, 2004a).
- Patients with secondary insomnia need treatment both of the underlying condition and of the insomnia. A study of patients with rheumatoid arthritis found that treating insomnia with a short-acting benzodiazepine improved morning stiffness as well as sleep (Walsh et al., 1996).
- Sedatives significantly increase sleep duration and quality but at the risk of adverse effects, especially cognitive impairment next day and daytime sleepiness (Glass et al., 2005). They also have addictive potential.
- Check that the insomnia is not due to an underlying disorder which needs treatment in its own right. Drugs which can cause insomnia include SSRIs and venlafaxine, and high-dose steroids.

- Explain that failing to sleep is a natural part of a reaction to stress and not harmful; and that worrying about not sleeping makes sleep harder to achieve.
- Check that the patient is not using alcohol to sleep. In non-dependent drinkers it does improve sleep in the first part of the night but at the expense of early-morning rebound awakening. Dependent drinkers lose even this early benefit.
- Explain that simple rules will help (see discussion to come) and offer a leaflet (e.g., www.patient.co.uk (search on "insomnia"). Behavioural techniques can be more effective than drug treatment, with longer-lasting benefit, but they take longer to administer (Sivertsen et al., 2006).
- Offer medication only if the patient's functioning is affected by the lack of sleep and the reason for the insomnia is temporary (e.g., jet lag or changing shifts). Obtain the patient's agreement that the course will not extend beyond 14 days because of the dangers of dependence, tolerance, and difficulties on withdrawal. Use a short-acting benzodiazepine. NICE (2004a) has assessed the Z drugs (zaleplon, zolpidem, and zopiclone) and found insufficient evidence to recommend them over the cheaper benzodiazepines.
- Be aware that some specialists in sleep disorders think that the approach set out in the British National Formulary (BNF) and repeated earlier is too draconian; and that the evidence of tolerance and dependence, when short-acting benzodiazepines are used for true primary insomnia, is poor (Wilson & Nutt, 2003). A compromise position is to prescribe a short-acting benzodiazepine for, say, 14 nights, to be repeated every 2 months, allowing the patient to use them when the need is greatest.
- Consider a tricyclic antidepressant in those for whom all other approaches have failed or are inappropriate. Dependence is not a problem but daytime drowsiness and other adverse effects are. Consider it an option of last resort. An early resort to drugs will distract the patient from the changes in lifestyle, and in their mental attitude to insomnia, that are necessary.
- Do not prescribe melatonin for most types of insomnia. A meta-analysis has shown that it is ineffective both in secondary insomnia and in jet lag (Buscemi et al., 2006). It may be useful in people with delayed sleep phase syndrome (in which the patient's circadian rhythm is off kilter) (Buscemi et al., 2004).
- Consider referral for cognitive behavioural therapy if the patient is sufficiently troubled by the problem. Even long-term users of hypnotics can benefit, with improved sleep, improved quality of life, and reduction in use of hypnotics (Morgan et al., 2003).

Simple Rules to Reduce Insomnia

- Go to bed and get up at the same time, even on weekends. It helps set your internal clock.
- Prepare for sleep by doing something restful in the half hour before bed. Avoid exercise in the 3 hours before bed. Refuse to discuss exciting or worrying things in bed; keep the bed for sleep and sex.
- Make sure the room is dark and quiet. Use earplugs if necessary.
- Avoid caffeine from about 4 pm. This may include chocolate and tea as well as coffee and cola.
- If you find yourself worrying, write down what the problem is and when you are going to think about it properly. Worrying about something at night magnifies a problem that may seem perfectly solvable in the day.
- Distract yourself with thoughts of something pleasant: gardening, sex, an imaginary dinner party in which you light a candle in front of each of your friends and visualize their faces in detail. You need something more interesting than counting sheep.
- If you still can't sleep, don't lie there fretting. Get up, sit somewhere warm, do something restful, and go back to bed when you feel sleepy.
- However tired you feel in the day, don't nap. It will mean you sleep even less well at night.
- If you've slept badly, accept it and lead a full day. Most people can function on less sleep than they think they need.

INFORMATION FOR PATIENTS

The Royal College of Psychiatrists has leaflets and audio tapes at www.rcpsych.ac.uk (search on "sleep problems").

Anxiety Disorders

- Anxiety disorders (Table 18.2) are more common than depression, rarely present as pure anxiety, are even less frequently diagnosed, yet the majority of patients will respond to treatment: usually an SSRI or cognitive behavioural therapy.
- Detection of an anxiety disorder is improved if the GP uses a few screening questions (Katon & Roy-Byrne, 2007).
- There are few conditions in which a positive, persistent, and supportive stance by the doctor is more important. The patient's instincts will be to avoid facing up to situations that provoke anxiety while treatment relies on facing up to them.
- Almost all anxiety disorders can be managed in primary care, especially if a member of the team is trained in cognitive behavioural therapy. However, any patient sufficiently distressed by an anxiety disorder who has not responded to primary care management should be offered referral to a specialist mental health service.
- Individual SSRIs and related drugs are licensed in the United Kingdom for one or more types of anxiety but not for all types. There is every reason to think that this is a quirk of licensing and that the benefits are common to all drugs of that class.
- Do not lead the patient to expect a cure; they are likely to be disappointed. Most however can expect significant improvement with treatment.

TABLE 18.2	Prevalences of the Anxiety Disorders in the General Population (American Psychiatric Association, 2000b; Ballenger & Tylee 2003)	
Condition	**Lifetime Prevalence**	
Generalized anxiety disorder	5%	
PD	2%–3%	
Panic attacks without reaching the criteria for PD	10%	
Agoraphobia	6%	
Social anxiety	13%	
Specific phobias	7%–11%	
OCD	2%–3%	
Obsessive or compulsive symptoms without reaching the criteria for OCD	8%	

Note that most patients suffer from more than one condition.
Note that the prevalence in a primary care population will be higher, since patients with anxiety present more frequently, usually with somatic complaints.
OCD, Obsessive-compulsive disorder; *PD*, panic disorder.

- Anxiety disorders rarely start in midlife or later. Such a presentation suggests another underlying disorder, especially depression or alcohol misuse.

Generalized Anxiety

GUIDELINE

National Institute for Health and Care Excellence. (2011). *Generalised anxiety disorder and panic disorder in adults: Management. NICE clincial guideline 113.*

- Check whether the patient also suffers from other mental conditions which need treatment in their own right (e.g., panic disorder, obsessive-compulsive disorder [OCD], phobia, depression, PTSD, or the misuse of alcohol or drugs).
- Check that there is no physical condition mimicking the symptoms of anxiety (e.g., thyrotoxicosis or asthma).

Management of a Crisis

- It may take a crisis to bring the patient to seek help. Immediate treatment is needed to tide the patient over and gain the confidence of patient and family.
- Give a brief but clear explanation of what is happening and that effective help is available.
- Consider prescribing anxiolytics for 2 to 4 weeks with the clear understanding that this is crisis management only. Use a benzodiazepine although, in a patient who has misused a benzodiazepine in the past, a sedating antihistamine or an antipsychotic may be preferred, though

NICE does not recommend this in primary care. Warn of the risks of dependence, sedation, industrial accidents, and road traffic accidents (Gale & Oakley-Browne, 2004a). Outside the United Kingdom a longer term role for benzodiazepines is accepted, with the view that dependence and tolerance is rare when prescribed for anxiety (Ballenger & Tylee, 2003).
- Arrange an early appointment to begin definitive treatment for the condition.

Long-Term Treatment

- Explain how anxiety causes physical symptoms and how they in turn increase anxiety. Offer a leaflet (see Information for Patients box).
- Assess the patient's disability. How does it affect family relationships, sex, work, and physical and mental state? Is a job at risk? Is alcohol or caffeine intake excessive?
- Explain the options:
  - *Cognitive behavioural therapy (CBT).* CBT has the strongest evidence of benefit (Gale & Oakley-Browne, 2004b). A 1- to 2-hour weekly session will be needed for a total of 8 to 20 hours with a trained professional. Briefly, it involves training the patient to act and think differently from his or her usual manner until a new response to life becomes natural. However, do not oversell CBT to the patient. Even in randomized controlled trials only half have recovered at 6-month follow-up (Fisher & Durham, 1999). Those who do show some response continue to improve for at least 2 years after treatment has ended (Dugas, Ladouceur, & Leger, 2003). Anxiety management, without cognitive restructuring, can achieve similar benefit (Gale & Davidson, 2007).
  - *An SSRI.* Almost half of patients show significant improvement with follow-up periods of up to 6 months. However, this yields an NNT of only 5 (because several improve on placebo) (Kapczinski, Lima, & Souza, 2003). Although this seems an easier option than CBT there are disadvantages: benefit may not be seen for some weeks and maximum benefit not for 6 months; anxiety may worsen in the first few weeks; at least 6 months of treatment will be needed; and, while not addictive, there is the possibility that the patient will notice a discontinuation reaction, especially if the drug is stopped suddenly. NICE recommends sertraline first line. In patients who cannot take an SSRI use a tricyclic antidepressant.
  - *Self-help,* using a written approach with supportive visits to the doctor or nurse. This is also CBT but without a personal therapist; the patient needs to find the motivation to succeed and be comfortable with reading and with acting on the written word.
- *Recommend a self-help group,* whichever treatment the patient chooses. Some can assist the patient in a CBT approach, but all will provide support and help the patient realize that he or she is not the only one with this problem.
- *Follow-up.* Unless the patient will be seeing a therapist within 2 weeks, arrange for follow-up along the following lines: at 2, 4, and 6 weeks; then at 3 and 6 months. This

applies whether the patient decides on an SSRI or self-help or is waiting to see a CBT therapist.

Practical Details When Prescribing SSRI for Anxiety

1. Start with a low dose to minimize the increase in anxiety seen with standard doses. For instance, start with paroxetine 5 mg daily for 2 weeks and double the dose every fortnight until reaching 20 mg daily. This means cutting up tablets or prescribing it in liquid form.
2. If the response at 8 weeks is inadequate, increase slowly to the maximum recommended dose.
3. Treat for a minimum of 6 months after a response is achieved. Patients who show some response at 2 months may continue to improve over the subsequent 6 months.
4. Decide, with the patient, how long to continue to prevent relapse. Treatment for 1 to 2 years is likely to be needed if the condition is longstanding.
5. With prolonged use, sexual dysfunction becomes the most significant adverse effect. For men with erectile dysfunction, sildenafil and related drugs can be used.
6. When stopping the drug, tail it off in fortnightly steps over 1 to 2 months according to what dose was used. If a discontinuation reaction occurs, go back a step and tail off more slowly.

Special Situations

- *The patient who fails to respond to an SSRI* or in whom it is contraindicated or not tolerated: Consider a tricyclic antidepressant in the same doses as for depression. An alternative is pregabalin, originally used in partial seizure epilepsy. Give it twice daily (Pohl et al., 2005) with a maximum dose of 200 mg/day; further dosage increases are of no benefit.
- *The patient whose anxiety returns when the SSRI is stopped:* It can be hard to distinguish a discontinuation reaction from the return of anxiety. The symptoms (dizziness, numbness, tingling, nausea, headache, sweating, insomnia, and feeling anxious) are common to both. Sometimes the patient is clear that the symptoms feel different from the original anxiety. If in doubt, restart the SSRI and taper the dose more slowly.
- *The patient whose physical symptoms of anxiety are crippling:* Consider a beta-blocker, although there is a dearth of evidence (Gale & Oakley-Browne, 2004c). A long-acting preparation will be needed.

Panic Disorder

- Follow the management outlined under Generalized Anxiety, but without the offer of a benzodiazepine. It is even more important to explain the link between the feeling of panic and the physical symptoms it produces, since patients often see it as a physical illness.
- Offer the same triad of behavioural therapy or CBT, an SSRI, or self-help. In addition, NICE has approved the use of computer-assisted CBT (NICE, 2006). *Fearfighter* is an 8- to 12-week computer course of treatment accessed

online by the patient. The patient needs a password to access the programme, for which Clinical Commissioning Group (CCG) approval is needed.

- If there has been no response after 12 weeks of an SSRI, consider a tricyclic antidepressant.
- The details in the box Information for Patients are the same as for generalized anxiety.
- Teach the patient first aid for a panic attack (see next section).
- Do not offer a benzodiazepine or another anxiolytic. They are less effective than SSRIs and they are inappropriate in a disorder that usually lasts over 4 weeks and where dependence can occur. They do not treat the depression that is often coexistent or which may emerge as the panic disorder is treated.
- Consider a long-acting beta-blocker. It will abolish some of the somatic symptoms of panic and may help the subjective terror as well (Mol et al., 2005). However, it will not lead to a lasting cure and may distract the patient from the need to enter more definitive therapy (i.e., CBT).
- Monitor progress with two questions:
  - How many panic attacks have you had since I last saw you?
  - How severe were they, on a scale of 1 to 5, where 1 is very mild and 5 is extremely severe?
- Prepare yourself, if not the patient, for a relatively poor response to treatment. A Cochrane review (Furukawa, Watanabe, & Churchill, 2007) found that 2 years after the start of treatment, 60% of patients had not achieved a sustained response. Combining psychotherapy with an antidepressant was more likely to achieve a response in the short term than either alone, with a NNT of 10. In other words, if 10 patients are treated with both treatments one more will respond than if treated with one *or* the other. However, follow-up of 1 or 2 years found that the combination of psychotherapy and antidepressant was better than antidepressant alone (NNT 6) but no better than psychotherapy alone.

First Aid for a Panic Attack—Instructions for the Patient

- Panic always subsides, even if it can take an hour.
- If some situation has triggered the attack, try to stay in the situation. Leaving can make it harder to go back later.
- Breathe slowly but not deeply. Deep breathing can mean you hyperventilate and develop more symptoms.
- Check your watch. What seems like an hour may only be 5 minutes.
- Distract yourself (e.g., read every detail of the label on something on the supermarket shelf).
- Have something you say to yourself during the attack (e.g., "It's only a panic attack. I'm not going to faint or vomit [or whatever you most fear]—and so what if I do?").
- Don't use alcohol. Attacks are more likely as the alcohol wears off.
- Check whether caffeine has played a part in triggering the attack.

Social Anxiety/Social Phobia

- Patients with social anxiety often think they are excessively shy, rather than suffering from a treatable mental disorder.
- Take even more care than usual to explain the nature of the condition. The concept of *an overactive circuit deep in the brain* may be acceptable to a patient who already understands the concept of, for instance, an overactive thyroid.
- Follow the management outlined under *generalized anxiety*, but without the offer of a benzodiazepine. An SSRI, exposure therapy, and a combination of the two are all effective during treatment. A large study suggests that those treated with exposure therapy alone continue to improve in the 6 months after treatment, whereas those treated with sertraline, with or without exposure, show some loss of benefit (Haug et al., 2003). If the SSRI is continued long term, the benefit is sustained and a treatment course of a minimum of 6 months, following remission, is needed (Schneier, 2003).
- Offer a beta-blocker to a patient with a circumscribed social anxiety which is disabling and where the somatic symptoms (tremor, palpitations) are preventing the patient from functioning. Performing musicians are the prime example. Warn the patient that they will find it hard not to become psychologically reliant on the drug. However, they may prefer this to the loss of their chosen career.

Phobias

- Phobias require energetic management if they present early, to prevent them from becoming fixed. Even those presenting late are amenable to treatment if the patient is willing to undergo therapy. All patients with phobias need treatment.
- Many patients who are phobic do not present with the phobia but with a consequence of it: alcohol or drug misuse, truancy, failure to attend appointments at the surgery, anxiety, or depression. Failure to discover the underlying phobia will result in a failure of treatment.
- Offer referral for CBT, an SSRI, or a self-help programme along CBT lines (see Generalized Anxiety).
- In those patients who choose to be treated without referral, use the following programme, with or without treatment with an SSRI:
  - Urge the patient not to avoid the phobic situation. Avoidance increases the strength of the phobia.
  - Teach the patient the rules of first aid during an attack of panic (see previous section).
  - Plan a programme of gently increasing exposure to the phobia. Do this with imaginary exposure if real exposure is not possible. Exposure must be daily, and the patient must stay in the phobic situation until the panic has subsided. Ask the patient to keep a diary to discuss at each appointment.
  - Ask what would be the worst possible scenario. Often it turns out to be unpleasant but acceptable. Usually it is that other people will see that the patient is being phobic. Being prepared to own up to a phobia is often a great step forward.
- Recommend *Manage Your Mind: The Mental Fitness Guide* by Gillian Butler and Tony Hope for details of strategies that patients can use for themselves.
- *Drug treatment at the time of the phobic event:* Avoid giving benzodiazepines for a phobia that poses a problem more than occasionally. The patient is likely to become even less able to face the situation without drugs than before treatment began. Consider a beta-blocker (e.g., propranolol 40 mg) 1 to 2 hours before exposure to the phobic situation in those who cannot tolerate the physical symptoms of panic.

Specific Phobias

- *Fear of flying.* Exposure therapy, either using a computer stimulation or just sitting in an aircraft and imagining that it is flying, shows marked short-term benefits with over half of patients who previously refused to fly now managing to fly. However, the effect does not last and is almost completely lost after 6 months (Maltby et al., 2002). It is therefore most suitable for someone who has to make a one-off flight. Several organizations offer exposure therapy. For instance, Virgin Atlantic offers "Flying Without Fear" courses (tel: 01423 714900; www.flying withoutfear.info/).
- *Fear of medical or dental procedures.* Cognitive behavioural therapy is the most effective treatment, but most patients present too late, when the need for help is urgent. Diazepam 10 mg 1 to 2 hours before the event has been shown to reduce anxiety significantly more than placebo, although the placebo effect is also marked (Wilner et al., 2002).
- *Patients with agoraphobia* are likely to find themselves unable to attend a primary care clinic and even more likely to have difficulty attending a specialist centre. Treatment in primary care, using an SSRI and a simple CBT

approach (see previous discussion) will be successful in some and allow others to improve enough to participate in more definitive therapy.

Obsessive-Compulsive Disorder

- Be on the alert for the diagnosis, as patients are often reluctant to admit to the disorder. In patients whose symptoms raise the possibility of OCD ask specific questions: "Do you find yourself doing things repeatedly in a way you can't control?" and "Do you find yourself bothered by certain thoughts that you can't get out of your mind?" Conditions that raise the possibility of OCD include depression, anxiety, eating disorders, fear of illness, fear of causing others harm, and skin disorders that suggest repeated hand washing.
- Once OCD is diagnosed, check for depression. One-third with OCD are currently depressed and two-thirds will become depressed at some stage (Ballenger & Tylee, 2003).
- Assess the risk of self-harm and suicide.
- The NICE (2005b) guideline suggests a stepped-care approach, with the starting point being the recognition of the disorder and the offer of information about the condition and the support groups that are available (see box). Later steps involve the provision of self-help material, referral for CBT, and the offer of an SSRI (see upcoming discussion).
- Involve the family or carers in the process of finding out about the disease and its treatment.
- When functional impairment is at least moderate, offer an SSRI as described under Generalized Anxiety. Expect the response to take even longer (up to 12 weeks) than with other forms of anxiety. Expect to continue it for at least 1 year.
- If the patient cannot take an SSRI, consider clomipramine (Ballenger & Tylee, 2003). NICE advises against other tricyclic antidepressants.
- Offer CBT if it is available. It involves gradual exposure of the patient to situations that provoke anxiety while not allowing the patient the relief of using a ritual to relieve that anxiety. At the same time the therapist retrains the patient in different patterns of thought. Patients who

refuse CBT at first because it sounds too threatening may accept it after partial remission with drug treatment. CBT appears to offer most hope for lasting remission.
- If the patient responds then relapses after discharge, refer back urgently before the pattern of behaviour becomes firmly established.

Self-Harm

- In the United Kingdom 1 in 10 teenagers deliberately self-harms. In 2015–2016 in England and Wales nearly 19,000 required admission to hospital (National Society for the Prevention of Cruelty to Children [NSPCC], 2016). Seven of eight are female.
- It is the strongest single predictor of successful suicide, being found in 40% to 60% of suicides (Hawton, Zahl, & Weatherall, 2003). However, that does not make it a useful predictor of suicide. Of self-harmers in the United Kingdom, only 0.7% kill themselves within a year and 3% in 15 years.
- Two of three self-harmers consult their GP in the subsequent 3 months (Bennewith et al., 2002). One in six will self-harm again within a year. However, attempting to assess the risk of repeated self-harm is unlikely to be successful (Kapur et al., 2005).
- A large study of an intervention in which patients were sent an invitation to consult following an episode of self-harm failed to show any benefit in terms of reducing repeated episodes (Bennewith et al., 2002). Indeed, systematic review has failed to identify benefit from any treatment (Soomro, 2004).

- Ask what the patient did, what precipitated it, and whether the problem is still present. Assume it is evidence of serious emotional distress.
- Assess the current mental state and the suicidal risk.
- Look for other problems: medical illness, social problems, past or present physical or sexual abuse.
- Manage according to what is found. The underlying problem may be trivial (an impulsive act, immediately regretted) or grave (a psychotic illness). Among those who are not mentally ill, being unclear about the reason for the self-harm is a bad prognostic sign, as is male sex and being an older rather than a younger adolescent (Royal College of Psychiatrists, 1998). Self-harm in people over 65 years of age is especially associated with depression and suicide (NICE, 2004b).
- Teach the patient ways of reducing the risk of serious harm, while the underlying problem is being attended to (Mental Health Foundation, 2004):
  - *Harm minimization:* for example, make a small cut rather than a large one, or take aspirin rather than paracetamol and never more than four at once.
  - *Distraction:* have a plan of something to do once the urge to self-harm starts to build up (e.g., go for a run or play music very loudly).
  - *Identify someone* you can talk to when you feel in danger.

> **PATIENT INFORMATION**
>
> The Basement Project. www.basementproject.co.uk.
>   Royal College of Psychiatrists. *Self harm.* www.rcpsych.ac.uk (search on "self harm").

Acute Psychotic Disorders

The possibility of acute psychosis is raised by the following:
- Hallucinations
- Delusions
- Disorganized or strange speech
- Agitation or bizarre behaviour
- Extreme and labile emotional states
- Family concern about recent changes in personality, behaviour, or function

Initial Assessment

- Obtain a careful history from family or friends of recent events and changes in the patient's behaviour.
- Ask about drug or alcohol misuse.
- Assess the mental state including the risk of suicide and of harm to others.
- Make a differential diagnosis if this is a first episode. Consider the possibilities of acute confusional state, drug-induced psychosis, and epilepsy. An episode that is related to cannabis use probably signifies an underlying psychosis triggered by the cannabis.

- If this is a relapse, review past management and outcomes.
- Decide if admission or referral is necessary.
- Explain to the family what you think is wrong and what action is needed. If feasible, give the patient the same information and obtain consent.

When There Is a Risk of Violence

> **GUIDELINES**
>
> National Institute of Heath and Care Excellence. (2015). *Violence and agression: Short-term management in mental health, health and community settings.* NICE clincial guideline 10.
>   National Institute of Heath and Care Excellence. (2014). *Psychosis and schizophrenia in adults: Prevention and management.* NICE clincial guideline 178. www.nice.org.uk.

- First, try to calm the patient (see previous guidance).
- Appoint one member of staff to relate to the patient. Others should move away.
- Encourage the patient to move to a safe place.
- If there is a weapon, ask the patient to put it in a neutral place, not to hand it over.
- Explain to the patient throughout, in a calm manner, what you are doing.
- Ask the patient open questions (e.g., "Tell me what's going on.").

Drug Treatment

- NICE advises against starting antipsychotics in primary care, particularly for a first episode. Treatment decisions should be made in conjunction with local mental health services.
- For relapses follow the treatment care plan, if one is available, and refer to specialist mental health services for further management. Treatment decisions should be based on patient preference, previous response to medications, and medical history.
- *If a patient initially refuses medication that is urgently needed,* spending time, in a calm manner, can often win the patient's confidence. Do not deny the patient's delusions or hallucinations but say something like: "I can see you are pretty upset about all this and I can help with that."
- *Rarely, an agitated or aggressive patient needs rapid tranquilization.* Tranquilization makes subsequent assessment difficult, it is traumatic for the patient, and sedated patients need observation, which may not be possible. If there is no alternative to forcible tranquilization do it only when sufficient police, or mental health staff, have arrived. For a strong patient, four male officers are likely to be needed.
- *Options for rapid tranquilization:*
  - lorazepam 2 to 4 mg orally or, preferably, sublingually; or
  - haloperidol 5 to 10 mg orally; or, if refused,

- lorazepam 1 to 2 mg intramuscularly; have flumazenil available for use if oversedated; or haloperidol 5 to 10 mg intramuscularly combined with promethazine 25 mg intramuscularly.

  If two drugs are needed combine lorazepam and haloperidol (with promethazine).
- After rapid tranquillization, check pulse, blood pressure, and respiratory rate while waiting for the ambulance to arrive. Ask the crew to continue monitoring with pulse oximetry in the ambulance.

Precautions When Visiting a Disturbed Patient at Home

- Ensure there is no past history of violence or delusions focused on the GP.
- If necessary, organize support and do not go alone.
- Try to ensure that a relative or friend is present.
- Tell someone in the practice whom you are visiting and when.
- Arrange for the practice staff to phone you after a specified time.
- Have an action plan if you do not respond to the phone call.

Referral and Admission

- *Refer all patients suffering from acute psychosis to the psychiatrist or specialist mental health team.* The specialist services will usually decide whether the patient needs admission or can be managed at home.
- *Admission* is usually required in acute psychosis especially if:
  - it is the first episode;
  - there is a significant risk of suicide, violence, or neglect;
  - the patient is non-compliant or has serious side effects; or
  - there is coexisting alcohol or drug misuse.
- *Management at home can be considered* in a patient who is suffering from a relapse of a known mental illness with a previous good response to treatment, where the patient agrees to restart treatment, is at low risk, where home care is safe, and community support is available.
- *Driving.* A patient suffering from an acute psychosis or relapse of bipolar affective disorder should not drive and the Driver and Vehicle Licensing Agency (DVLA) must be informed.

Compulsory Admission

Indications for Use of the Mental Health Act (England and Wales) 1983

This account includes amendments made to the Mental Health Act up to 2015. It focuses on sections of the act most relevant to general practice.
- The Mental Health Act can only be used if the following conditions are met:

- The patient is suffering from a mental disorder of a nature or degree that warrants detention in a hospital for assessment (or assessment followed by medical treatment) for at least a limited period.
- The patient ought to be detained in the interests of his or her own health or safety, or with a view to the protection of others.
- There is no alternative management other than compulsory admission to hospital.
- *Mental disorders* are mental illness, psychopathic disorder, mental impairment, and severe mental impairment. The latter two disorders refer to patients with learning difficulties associated with abnormally aggressive or seriously irresponsible conduct.
- Although often called by relatives or neighbours, the doctor's role is to safeguard the patient's welfare and not that of the relatives or neighbours, unless they are in danger.
- A patient can be admitted compulsorily even when posing no danger provided that he or she is sufficiently ill (e.g., acutely psychotic) to need compulsory admission, because treatment is urgently needed for the sake of the patient's health.
- An approved mental health professional (AMHP) is responsible for making the application for compulsory admission, coordinating the medical assessment of the patient, providing the forms, and arranging for the transport of the patient to hospital.
- Every practice, and CCG, should have agreed on a procedure for the management of psychiatric crises. Appendix 21 is an example.

The Assessment Under the Act

- Obtain all available information, from the patient's records and from available friends and family. Try to find out who is the nearest relative (note that this is not necessarily the same person as the next of kin): They have the right to be informed, to object to detention, and to insist that a detained patient be discharged, unless that patient poses a danger.
- Telephone the AMHP and agree on a plan. This should include whether to involve a second doctor or the police at this stage.
- If admission looks likely, contact the duty psychiatrist to discuss the availability of a bed and the need for his or her attendance.
- If the decision is made not to admit the patient, work out a care plan. Essential features are that family members know whom to call in an emergency and that intensive follow-up arrangements are put in place.

Which Section of the Act Should Be Used?
How Desperate Is the Situation?

- *The patient is about to injure others or self.* The doctor may restrain the patient or give emergency treatment knowing that under common law such action is defensible if done in good faith. Such action would normally be followed by an admission under the act using Section 2 (28 days) although if the emergency continues Section 4 (72 hours) might be needed.

- *Admission is needed and is so urgent that:*
  - the doctor cannot leave the patient; and
  - waiting for an approved clinician (usually an approved psychiatrist) would cause undesirable delay.

Use Section 4 (detention for 72 hours). This requires assessment by a doctor and an AMHP. Admission must take place within 24 hours of the assessment or the application, whichever is earlier. The fact that attendance by the approved clinician is inconvenient is not grounds for the use of this section.

- *Admission is needed but there is time to wait for an approved clinician.* Use Section 2 (28 days). This is the preferred section and will be used in almost all cases. It requires assessment by a mental health professional approved under Section 12 of the act (the "first" doctor) and by a doctor with previous knowledge of the patient (the "second" doctor) and an AMHP. Admission must take place within 5 days or the application is void. Arrange to see the patient together if possible, although the act allows the two doctors to examine the patient up to 5 days apart.

Further Clarifications

- The *second* doctor should be one with previous knowledge of the patient. However, if no such doctor is available, any doctor may sign provided he or she does not work in the same hospital as the *first* doctor.
- In theory the application for compulsory admission may be made by the nearest relative. In practice this is rarely wise: An AMHP is needed to ensure that the formalities are observed, that a full assessment is made, and to avoid later recriminations within the family if the nearest relative made such a decision.
- It is occasionally possible to commit a patient to hospital under the act even if he or she agrees to informal admission. A psychiatrist may recommend this course of action if, from previous knowledge of the patient, a judgment is made that an apparent agreement to informal admission is not likely to be sustained. If taking this line of action, the reasons for doing so must be stated on the form.
- Once an application has been signed, decide how to escort the patient into an ambulance. Given time and patience it is usually possible to achieve it without force. If force is needed it is the role of the police rather than the ambulance crew.
- Drug or alcohol dependency is not in itself grounds for compulsory admission. This is only possible if the person also suffers from a mental disorder as defined in the act. If a patient is under the influence of drugs or alcohol so that a proper assessment cannot be made, it should be postponed until such assessment is possible.

- Learning difficulty is not grounds for compulsory admission under Sections 3 or 4 unless associated with "abnormally aggressive or seriously irresponsible conduct." However, the other relevant sections, including Section 2, can be used.
- Psychopathic disorder is defined as "a persistent disorder or disability of mind (whether or not including significant impairment of intelligence) that results in abnormally aggressive or seriously irresponsible conduct on the part of the person concerned." It is grounds for compulsory admission, regardless of whether it is treatable, provided that the other criteria are met. Only in using Section 3 is it necessary that the psychopathy should be "treatable"; that is, treatment should be necessary to alleviate or prevent deterioration in the patient's condition.

Other Sections of Value

- *Section 3* allows for detention for 6 months. It is occasionally used in the community instead of Section 4 if the patient is already known to the psychiatric services. In practice it is almost always used once the patient is in hospital and before a Section 2 or 4 has expired.
- *Section 7* allows the appointment of a guardian for up to 6 months. The guardian has the power to insist that the patient live at a specified place and attend for work, training, or medical appointments.
- *Section 136* allows the police to remove a person from a public place to a hospital or police station, for a maximum period of 72 hours, if the person is:
  - suffering from a mental disorder; and
  - in immediate need of care and control.
- *Section 135* allows a magistrate to authorize a police officer (with a doctor and AMHP) to enter any premises to which access has been denied, and remove the patient to a place of safety if there is reasonable cause to suspect that the person is:
  - suffering from a mental disorder;
  - being ill-treated or neglected or not kept under proper control;
  - unable to care for oneself and lives alone.

The GP can usually gain entry legally without using Section 135, for instance by asking the neighbours to open the door or by using his or her relationship with the patient to get the door open.

- *A Community Treatment Order (CTO)* ensures that assessment and treatment are carried out in the community with the responsible clinician having the power to recall the patient to hospital if necessary.

Regulations for Scotland and Northern Ireland

These follow similar principles to those for England and Wales, but the brief details of the acts are as follows (Tables 18.3 and 18.4):

TABLE 18.3	Mental Health (Care and Treatment) (Scotland) Act 2003 (see www.nes.scot.nhs.uk/mha/)		
Type of Compulsion	**Professionals**	**Duration**	
Emergency detention	GP, and MHO if practicable	72 hours	
Short-term detention	GP and MHO	28 days	
Compulsory treatment order	MHO, AMP, and patient's GP or another AMP	6 months	
Power of entry	MHO obtains from sheriff or JP	Single event	

AMP, Approved medical practitioner; *GP,* general practitioner; *MHO,* mental health officer.

TABLE 18.4	Mental Health (Northern Ireland) Order 1986		
Situation	**Section**	**Professionals**	**Duration**
Emergency	4	GP and ASW or relative	7 days
Power of entry	129	ASW obtains from JP, GP and police enter	Single event

AMP, Approved medical practitioner; *ASW,* approved social worker; *GP,* general practitioner; *JP,* justice of the peace; *MHO,* mental health officer. For more details, see www.psychiatry.ox.ac.uk/cebmh/whoguidemhpcuk/mha.html.

- *For emergency detention the following must apply:*
  - The person has a mental disorder that causes his or her decision making to be significantly impaired.
  - It is necessary as a matter of urgency to detain the person for assessment.
  - The person's health, safety, or welfare or the safety of another person would be at significant risk if he or she was not detained.
  - Making arrangements for the possible granting of a short-term detention certificate (see below) would involve undesirable delay.
- *For short-term detention* the same four criteria must apply except that it need not be a matter of urgency, and detention is for assessment or treatment.
- *For a compulsory treatment* order, the following must apply:
  - The patient has a mental disorder.
  - Medical treatment is available which would be likely to prevent the disorder worsening, or would be likely to alleviate the symptoms or effects of the disorder.
  - There would be a significant risk to the patient or to any other person if the patient was not provided with such treatment.

- The patient's ability to make decisions about the provision of medical treatment is significantly impaired because of his or her mental disorder.
- The making of the compulsory treatment order is necessary.

A compulsory treatment order may authorize detention in hospital or impose certain requirements on the patient in the community (a community-based compulsory treatment order).

- The act also allows for the removal to a place of safety of a person who is exposed to ill treatment or neglect, or who is unable to look after oneself or property/financial affairs. It further allows for a person to be removed from a public place to one of safety where it is in the interests of that person or where it is necessary to protect other people (NHS Education for Scotland, 2004).

ADVICE FOR PATIENTS AND PROFESSIONALS

MIND provides a leaflet on the act at www.mind.org.uk (search on "Mental Health Act").
  Royal College of Psychiatrists, www.rcpsych.ac.uk (search on "Mental Health Act").

Chronic Schizophrenia

GUIDELINE

National Institute of Heath and Care Excellence. (2014). *Psychosis and schizophrenia in adults: Prevention and management. NICE clincial guideline 178.* www.nice.org.uk.

- About 1% of a practice population will suffer from schizophrenia at some time in their life, more in cities and in immigrant communities.
- Structured care offers a chance of improving the management of such patients.
- In the United Kingdom the average GP will look after 12 patients with schizophrenia, half of them without current involvement of the specialist mental health services (Picchioni & Murray, 2007).

Structured Care

This entails:
- establishing a register of patients with severe and enduring mental illness. This can be done from existing clinical codes, from repeat prescriptions for psychotropic drugs, from addresses of hostels and homes catering for the mentally ill, and opportunistically;
- using the register to ensure that patients are seen at least anually and actively seeking out patients who default from follow-up. See upcoming discussion for details of the annual review;
- developing a care plan that is individualized for patients taking into account psychiatric, medical, social, and

occupational or educational issues. Ideally this care plan should be shared with carers;

- working with local mental health teams to identify agreed policies and guidelines for treatment, referral, and the management of relapse;
- adapting existing computer templates to record long-term follow-up and undertaking practice audit of these goals.

Referral

- Arrange for urgent assessment of the following:
  - Those presenting for the first time
  - Those posing a risk to themselves or to others
  - Those relapsing, or showing the prodrome of a relapse
  - Those at risk of relapse because of:
    a. a deterioration in their home circumstances;
    b. poor compliance; or
    c. abuse of drugs or alcohol.
  - Those suffering from side effects of medication or who are not taking it.

Such an assessment is better done at home than in the outpatient department if possible.

- Patients will also need to be referred, although not necessarily urgently, if:
  - they are becoming increasingly disabled by their illness;
  - a care plan needs to be drawn up, as when a patient moves to a new area; or
  - the patient or family request referral or the therapeutic relationship has broken down.

General Management

- *Education.* The patient and the family need to know:
  - that 85% to 90% recover from the first episode in the following 2 years (WHO, 1979). In the 5 years following the first episode, half do not relapse, or relapse but recover completely between episodes; 20% will never have another episode (Picchioni & Murray 2007);
  - how to identify early signs of relapse. Looking for early warning signs can prevent relapse or reduce its severity (Falloon, Laporta, Fadden, & Graham-Hole, 1993). The Early Warning Signs Form (see Appendix 22) can be used to help with this;
  - how to obtain early treatment;
  - that avoiding extremes of expressed emotion by family members, whether hostility or overprotectiveness, can reduce the risk of relapse.
- *Advance directives.* Discuss the use of advance directives with patient and family. These indicate what the patient wants to happen if a relapse occurs. If one is drawn up, the patient, and primary and secondary care, all need copies.
- Check that the patient has been offered the benefits of case management. In the United Kingdom this takes the form of the care programme approach, in which a specialist team assists the patient with daily living, in the understanding of the condition and in its management.
- If fit for sheltered work, liaise with the mental health team or the disablement resettlement officer.
- Assess the patient's housing needs.
- Help the patient to claim the disability living allowance if eligible.

Drug Treatment

- Early drug treatment seems to lead to better medium- and long-term outcomes (Loebel et al., 1992).
- Without drugs, 60% of patients relapse in the 9 months after an acute attack. Maintenance with antipsychotics reduces this by over one-half.
- Atypical antipsychotics are now first line drugs in the United Kingdom, although if a patient is successfully treated with a conventional antipsychotic it should not be changed. Atypical antipsychotics are chosen because of the lower incidence of extrapyramidal adverse effects and possibly greater effect on cognition and on negative symptoms. However, they are no more effective than typical antipsychotics and overall they have as many, but different, adverse effects (Picchioni & Murray, 2007). The exceptions to this are clozapine and olanzapine, which may be more effective than other drugs (Citrone & Stroup, 2006).
- The choice of long-term medication should be made by the psychiatrist and patient together. It will be needed for at least 1 to 2 years after a relapse and monitoring will be needed for 2 years after that.
- All antipsychotics are associated with an increased risk of sudden cardiac death as well as of stroke. A baseline electrocardiogram (ECG) is recommended if the manufacturer advises one is necessary, if the patient has a personal history of cardiovascular disease, if physical exam identifies a cardiovascular risk factor (such as high blood pressure), or if the patient is being admitted (NICE, 2014).

Relapse

Ascertain whether the relapse is due to the patient discontinuing medication. If it is then:

- assess the reason for stopping treatment (e.g., the presence of side effects, failure to obtain a prescription);
- decide if restarting previous medication is appropriate and acceptable;
- review the need for urgent psychiatric assessment;
- if assessment is needed but will be delayed, and there is concern about medication, phone for advice from the psychiatrist;
- inform the patient's care coordinator or the lead clinician identified in the care plan if this is available.

Medication Review

- Patients need a medication review at least annually (NICE, 2014). The repeat prescription slip should indicate when a medication review is due.
- Someone in the practice needs to be responsible for ensuring such patients have attended for this review, and to know what action to take if the patient defaults. The medication review will include:
  - assessment of mental state and compliance;
  - presence of adverse effects or drug interactions. Adverse effects with conventional antipsychotics are likely to

be extrapyramidal; with atypical antipsychotics they are likely to be weight gain and hyperprolactinaemia;
- existence of drug or alcohol problems;
- whether the patient has been admitted in the past 6 months;
- patients on clozapine need monitoring for agranulocytosis, weekly for 6 months then monthly in the United Kingdom. Organizing this is the responsibility of the prescriber. If delegated to primary care a written protocol is needed.

Side Effects of Medication

Conventional Antipsychotics
- *Extrapyramidal adverse effects.* If they occur, discuss management with the specialist. The main options are:
  - reduce the dose of the antipsychotic;
  - add an anticholinergic drug (e.g., orphenadrine 50 mg three times a day). Avoid procyclidine, which is a stimulant and can be abused. Try to withdraw an anticholinergic after 3 months without symptoms. Tetrabenazine may help in tardive dyskinesia;
  - change to an atypical antipsychotic. Clozapine is the treatment of choice.
- *Neuroleptic malignant syndrome* occurs in 0.5%.

Atypical Antipsychotics
- Weight gain
- Dizziness and postural hypotension in the early stages
- Diabetes
- Extrapyramidal adverse effects, but they are uncommon and usually respond to dose reduction

All Antipsychotics
- *Palpitations.* Repeat the ECG. If the QT interval is prolonged but is less than or 500 ms, reduce the dose. If it is over 500 ms, stop the drug (Medicine and Healthcare Products Regulatory Agency [MHRA], 2006).

Psychotherapy

Good evidence exists for both cognitive behavioural therapy and family therapy and NICE recommends that both forms of therapy be offered to patients and their families suffering with psychosis. A minimum course of 6 months of either is needed. If they are available they should be offered as well as medication.

Annual Review

The annual review is likely to be more comprehensive if a checklist or computer template is used. Topics to cover are:
- current mental state, including the presence of depression, delusional thoughts, anxiety, hallucinations, and signs of self-neglect. Half of patients with schizophrenia develop depression at some stage. It carries a higher risk of suicide than depression in other patients (Jones & Buckley, 2003);
- problems, crises, or admissions since last seen;

- daily activities, employment, training, income, and disability benefits;
- substance misuse, which is likely in half of patients;
- accommodation needs;
- carers, relationships, dependants (children), home support;
- assessment of physical health, including weight, blood pressure, cervical screening, smoking status, family planning needs, fasting sugar, Hba1C, lipids, and assessment of cardiovascular disease (CVD) risk. Smoking cessation should be offered where appropriate and coexisting cardiovascular disease and diabetes should be treated. In the United States an annual ECG is recommended in those on an antipsychotic because it can prolong the QT interval;
- medication review and monitoring blood tests if necessary;
- whether care is GP only or shared with psychiatrist, community psychiatric nurse (CPN), or social worker;
- assessment of carer's needs.

Carers' Needs
- People who care for someone with severe and enduring mental illness should have:
  - a needs assessment at regular intervals;
  - a care plan which is reviewed annually;
  - links with local carer support groups.
- Carers need to be identified and this information should be put on their summary card or computer problem list. The practice should have a carers' register and a practice policy on whom to assess, when, and by whom. Social services should record each carer's needs and draw up an agreed care plan that includes:
  - information about the mental health needs of the patient;
  - how to identify a relapse and what action to take;
  - advice on benefits, housing, and employment;
  - arrangements for short-term breaks;
  - social support including access to carers' support groups;
  - information about appeals or complaints procedures.
- The plan should be confirmed in writing and communicated to the primary care team. The GP is the professional most likely to identify signs of stress or deteriorating health of a carer. The plan will indicate who should review the carer's needs at such times, which the GP can initiate.

PATIENT ORGANIZATIONS

Rethink Severe Mental Illness, 89 Albert Embankment, London SE1 7TP. General enquiries tel. 0121 522 7007; national advice line 0300 5000 927; www.rethink.org.
 MIND, Mind Infoline 0300 123 3393; www.mind.org.uk.
 SANE, Saneline tel. 0300 304 7000; email support via the website: www.sane.org.uk.

Patient Information

The Royal College of Psychiatrists, www.rcpsych.ac.uk (search on "schizophrenia").

Bipolar Affective Disorder

GUIDELINE

National Institute of Health and Care Excellence. (2014). *Bipolar disorder: Assessment and management. NICE clincial guideline 185*, updated 2016. www.nice.org.uk.

General Management

- Check that the patient has had a recent assessment by a specialist and that everyone is clear who the key worker is, in case of difficulties.
- Explain the nature of the condition to the patient and family.
- Agree on what the warning signs of relapse are for that individual (see Appendix 22).
- Draw up a plan of action for when relapse occurs. This will depend on the form the relapse takes; in hypomania it may mean removing cheques, debit cards, and credit cards from the patient; in depression it may mean intensifying social support. In mania it may involve supplying medication (an antipsychotic or a benzodiazepine) to be taken at the first sign of relapse.
- Explore whether stressors seem to trigger a relapse: irregular hours, lack of sleep, use of alcohol or drugs.
- Enter the patient on the practice register of patients with severe mental illness.
- Ensure recall for annual reviews.
- Offer information about the local and national support that is available (see box).

During Episodes of Depression

- Arrange for specialist assessment and discuss any medication changes with the specialist prior to assessment if there will be a delay.
- NICE recommends fluoxetine combined with olanzapine as first line. Lamotrigine on its own is an alternative as are olanzapine or quetiapine which can both be used on their own.
- If the patient is already on lithium then check lithium levels and titrate to the therapeutic range. Fluoxetine and olanzapine can be added to lithium and, if this fails, then lamotrigine can be added to lithium in place of fluoxetine with olanzapine.
- Similarly, if the patient is on valproate then titrate this to the maximum tolerated dose and then fluoxetine with olanzapine can be added.

During Episodes of Mania or Hypomania

- Avoid unnecessary confrontation.
- Check if there was a trigger for the relapse and whether it can be rectified.
- Assess the risk of impulsive behaviour (e.g., financial or business recklessness).

- Assess the need for admission, including compulsory admission, or for referral to the community mental health team.
- Tell the family who to contact if the patient becomes very agitated or severely disruptive.
- Identify the carer's needs. In chronic illness consider respite care.

Medication

- Discuss the options with the patient's specialist. They are likely to involve:
  - an oral antipsychotic (usually haloperidol, olanzapine, quetiapine, or risperidone);
  - increasing lithium while keeping the blood level within the therapeutic range;
  - short-term use of a benzodiazepine for night sedation;
  - tailing off an antidepressant if one is being taken.
- Do not expect dramatic improvement. Even in the ideal setting of clinical trials only about half the patients have a 50% improvement of symptoms over 3 to 4 weeks (Keck, 2003).
- Prepare to taper off the antipsychotic over at least 2 weeks once in full remission. Continued use can precipitate depression.

Prevention of Relapse

- The choice of medication to prevent relapse should be based on patient preference and what has previously been effective.
- Lithium is the first line drug as it is most effective.
- Alternatives are valproate (which can also be added to lithium if lithium alone is ineffective) or olanzapine. Quetiapine can also be used especially if this has been effective in previous relapses.

Lithium

The GP needs to:
- ensure clear agreement on who is responsible for monitoring lithium treatment;
- have an agreed protocol for monitoring blood levels, identifying side effects, and taking appropriate action. Put the patient on the recall register for monitoring blood levels;
- provide the patient with a written description of drug side effects and what to do if these develop (e.g., see *Lithium: Your Medicine* available at www.rcpsych.ac.uk);
- check the patient knows to maintain adequate fluid intake and avoid dehydration and nonsteroidal antiinflammatory drugs (NSAIDs);
- check that the patient understands that the lithium should not be stopped unless toxicity occurs, as relapse may occur.
- check *lithium levels* every 3 months. Take blood 12 hours after the last dose. Levels of 0.4 to 0.8 mmol/L are adequate for maintenance but in acute mania a level of 0.8 to 1 mmol/L is necessary;
- check for *change in dose*. If the dose is changed, check levels weekly for 4 weeks, then monthly for 3 months and then 3-monthly.

- Check thyroid and renal function annually.
- Warn women of reproductive age that lithium is an enzyme inducer, which reduces the efficacy of the combined oral contraceptive, and that it carries a risk of teratogenicity.

Management of Suspected Lithium Toxicity

- Symptoms of toxicity include muscle weakness, shaking, trembling, fasciculation, nausea, vomiting or diarrhoea, ataxia, confusion, slurred speech, toxic psychosis, convulsions, coma, and cardiac arrhythmias.
- Check the lithium level and urea and electrolytes (U&Es).
- Stop lithium. Levels usually fall to safety within 24 hours. If the lithium level is more than 1.5 mmol/L, or there is diarrhoea and vomiting, stop lithium immediately and seek urgent specialist advice.
- Identify the cause of the toxicity before restarting lithium.
- If no cause is found, restart at a lower dose.
- Monitor levels monthly for 3 months after toxicity for which there was no obvious reason.

SUPPORT AND ADVICE FOR PATIENTS AND FAMILIES

Bipolar UK. Tel. 0333 323 3880, www.bipolaruk.org.
The Mental Health Foundation. They do not offer advice or support and there is no helpline, but the website has useful information: www.mentalhealth.org.uk.

Dealing With Violence

Every practice needs a policy for dealing with violent patients. Many of these patients have a past history of violent or threatening behaviour. A typical policy would include:

- a notice in the waiting room stating that physical or verbal abuse, racism, threats, or violence to staff will result in removal from the practice;
- panic buttons in consulting rooms and a clear procedure to follow if one is set off;
- clear guidelines on who should deal with an aggressive, abusive, or violent patient in the waiting room;
- how risks will be assessed and what action will be taken;
- a protocol for the management of a patient whose delusions are focused on a specific doctor or nurse;
- written indications on when to call the police and who should do so;
- guidance on how to deal with home visit requests to a potentially violent patient;
- sympathetic support for staff exposed to violent situations;
- a policy of informing local GPs that a violent patient who has been removed from the practice list may want to register with them;
- a record kept of all such incidents;
- a way to report these incidents as significant events so that lessons can be learnt by others.

Eating Disorders

GUIDELINES

National Institute for Health and Care Excellence. (2017). *Eating disorders: Recognition and treatment. NICE clincial guideline 69*. www.nice.org.uk.
King's College London. (n.d.). *A GP's guide to eating disorders.* www.kcl.ac.uk (search on "GP guide eating disorders").
King's College London. (2009). *Guide to the medical risk assessment for eating disorders.* www.kcl.ac.uk (search on "eating disorders").

- Approximately 1.25 million people are thought to have eating disorders in the United Kingdom, according to B-eat, a national eating disorders charity.
- It is estimated that 10% have anorexia nervosa, 40% have bulimia nervosa, and the rest fall into the category of other specified feeding and eating disorders (OSFED), including binge eating disorder (BED) (B-Eat).
- Although eating disorders can develop at any age, the risk is highest for young men and women between 13 and 17 years of age.
- Of sufferers, 20% die prematurely from their illness, either by suicide or from physical complications (Herzog et al., 2000).
- Anorexia nervosa has the highest mortality of all the mental health conditions, with one in five anorexia patients dying by suicide (Arcelus, 2011).
- In 2007 it was estimated through the Adult Psychiatric Morbidity Survey that 6.4% of all adults (>16 years) in England showed signs of an eating disorder, up to 25% of whom were male (NHS Information Centre for Health and Social Care, 2007).
- Anorexia is characterized by low weight, a fear of gaining weight, a desire to be thin, and a distorted body image; patients believe themselves to be overweight when often they are underweight. BMI is usually lower end of normal or below normal.
- Bulimia is characterized by episodes of binge eating (described as eating a significant amount at one time to the point of being uncomfortably overfull), followed by episodes of compensatory behaviour such as vomiting (purging) or excessive exercise, use of laxatives or diuretics. Body mass index (BMI) may be normal or slightly above normal.
- Binge eating disorder is similar to bulimia without the compensatory behaviours, and BMI is usually high.

Assessment in Primary Care

- The following should be asked about, or noted, during history-taking for eating disorders, or when deciding how urgently to refer people:
  - An unusually low or high BMI or body weight for their age

- Rapid weight loss
- Dieting or restrictive eating practices (such as dieting when they are underweight) that are worrying them, their family members or carers, or professionals
- Family members or carers reporting a change in eating behaviour
- Social withdrawal, particularly from situations that involve food
- Other mental health problems, including depression, anxiety, self-harm, obsessive-compulsive disorder, as well as suicidal ideation
- The possibility of alcohol or substance misuse
- A disproportionate concern about their weight or shape (e.g., concerns about weight gain as a side effect of contraceptive medication)
- Problems managing a chronic illness that affects diet, such as diabetes or coeliac disease
- Menstrual or other endocrine disturbances, or unexplained gastrointestinal symptoms
- Physical signs of:
  - malnutrition, including poor circulation, dizziness, palpitations, fainting, or pallor;
  - fractures;
  - compensatory behaviours, including laxative or diet pill misuse, vomiting, or excessive exercise.
- Abdominal pain that is associated with vomiting or restrictions in diet, and that cannot be fully explained by a medical condition
- Unexplained electrolyte imbalance or hypoglycaemia
- Atypical dental wear (such as erosion)
- Whether they take part in activities associated with a high risk of eating disorders (e.g., professional sport, fashion, dance, modelling)
- Risk factors for boys and men include non-hetreosexuality, previous dieting, previous obesity, and participation in sports that emphasize thinness, or body building (Thompson, 2017).
- Be aware that children and young people with an eating disorder may also present with faltering growth (e.g., a low weight or height for their age) or delayed puberty.
- Do not use single measures such as BMI or duration of illness to determine whether to offer referral or treatment for an eating disorder.
- Do not use screening tools (e.g., SCOFF) as the sole method to determine whether people have an eating disorder.
- Good questions to screen for eating disorders (Cotton, Ball, & Robinson, 2003) include:
  - Do you worry that you have lost control over how much you eat?
  - Do you make yourself sick when you feel uncomfortably full?
  - Do you ever eat in secret?
  - Does your weight affect the way you feel about yourself?
  - Are you satisfied with your eating patterns? (If the answer is no and yes, respectively, to the latter two questions, then an eating disorder is much less likely.)

Investigation and Monitoring

- When first assessing a person with an eating disorder it is likely that blood monitoring will be required, at least once, but possibly more frequently if BMI is low or there is ongoing purging, laxative or diuretic use. Recommended tests include FBC, renal function, liver function, glucose, creatine kinase (and thyroid function and C-reactive protein [CRP] at the first appointment only, to rule out other causes of weight change).
- Other investigations should include blood pressure, pulse, BMI, muscle strength using the sit up/squat test (see box), and skin condition.

TESTS FOR MUSCLE STRENGTH

1. Squat Test. The patient is asked to squat down on haunches and is asked to stand up without using the arms as levers if at all possible.
2. Sit-Up Test. The patient lies flat on a firm surface such as the floor and has to sit up without using the hands.

- The King's College Guide to Medical Risk Assessment also contains a handy summary of *when to refer* because of *concern* (appropriate within 2 weeks) and when to *alert* (red flag/same-day assessment likely required). For example, if weight loss is below 0.5 kg a week, in a person with a low BMI, that would be a concern, but more than 1 kg a week would be an alert. Similar guidance is included for all blood results (Treasure J, 2018).
- It is important to obtain a BMI, but this can be challenging as many patients are reluctant to be weighed. It may require building of trust before they will agree to stepping onto the scales, but a potential option can be to ask them to step onto the scales *backwards* so that they cannot see the result, but you can note it discreetly. With time, they may then agree to step on forwards, as you will have demonstrated sensitivity to their concerns and anxieties.
- Assess whether ECG monitoring is needed in people with an eating disorder, based on the following risk factors:
  - Rapid weight loss
  - Excessive exercise
  - Severe purging behaviours, such as laxative or diuretic use or vomiting
  - Bradycardia
  - Hypotension
  - Excessive caffeine (including from energy drinks)
  - Prescribed or nonprescribed medications
  - Muscular weakness
  - Electrolyte imbalance
  - Previous abnormal heart rhythm
- Advise those who are taking laxatives or diuretics that these will not help weight loss and should be stopped gradually.

- Advise those who are exercising excessively, or obsessively, to stop doing so.
- Advise those who are vomiting regularly to have regular dental checkups and avoid brushing their teeth immediately after purging.
- GPs should offer a physical and mental health review at least annually to people with anorexia nervosa who are not receiving ongoing secondary care treatment for their eating disorder. The review should include:
  - weight or BMI (adjusted for age if appropriate);
  - blood pressure;
  - relevant blood tests;
  - any problems with daily functioning;
  - assessment of risk (related to both physical and mental health);
  - an ECG, for people with purging behaviours and/or significant weight changes;
  - a discussion of treatment options.
- Monitor growth and development in children and young people with anorexia nervosa who have not completed puberty (e.g., not reached menarche or final height).
- Consider a bone mineral density scan after:
  - after 1 year of underweight in children and young people, or earlier if they have bone pain or recurrent fractures;
  - after 2 years of underweight in adults, or earlier if they have bone pain or recurrent fractures.
- Do not routinely offer oral or transdermal oestrogen therapy to treat low bone mineral density in children or young people with anorexia nervosa.
- Seek specialist paediatric or endocrinologist advice before starting any hormonal treatment for low bone mineral density. Coordinate any treatment with the eating disorders team.

Medication

- Medication should never be the sole treatment for eating disorders but antidepressants or anti-anxiety medication may be helpful if there are comorbidities.
- Encourage people with anorexia nervosa to take an age-appropriate oral multivitamin and multimineral supplement until their diet includes enough to meet their dietary reference values.
- When prescribing medication for people with an eating disorder and comorbid mental or physical health conditions, take into account the impact malnutrition and compensatory behaviours (e.g., vomiting) can have on medication effectiveness and the risk of side effects.
- When prescribing for people with an eating disorder and a comorbidity, assess how the eating disorder will affect medication adherence (e.g., for medication that can affect body weight). Patients may decline to take any medication they are concerned may cause them to gain weight, for example.
- When prescribing for people with an eating disorder take into account the risks of medication that can compromise physical health due to preexisting medical complications (e.g., hypokalaemia secondary to vomiting).
- Offer ECG monitoring for people with an eating disorder who are taking medication that could compromise cardiac functioning (including medication that could cause electrolyte imbalance, bradycardia <40 beats/min, hypokalaemia, or a prolonged QT interval).

Referral

- If an eating disorder is suspected after an initial assessment, refer immediately to a community-based, age-appropriate (specialist) eating disorder service for further assessment or treatment.
- The aim of treatment is to reach a healthy weight/BMI and psychological well-being.
- It is vital not to delay referral because recent evidence shows that people have on average already had symptoms of an eating disorder for almost 3 years (B-eat, 2017) before they seek help, and then wait up to 6 months between first GP visit and starting treatment. It takes on average 21 months for people to recognize that they have an eating disorder, and then another year before they seek help from a healthcare professional. This leads to a cycle of relapse and recovery of, on average, 6 years in duration. The same report showed that boys and men had to wait over twice as long as girls and women before being referred by their GP. In other words, GPs are not yet recognizing eating disorders rapidly enough in males.
- It is important to take patient and family/carer concerns seriously and to avoid potentially dismissive comments implying that the behaviour is a phase or that they will grow out of it.
- Dietary advice (and dietician referral) should only be offered as part of a multidisciplinary approach.
- The mainstay of all eating disorders treatment is psychologic therapy. This should be provided by a specialist trained in the appropriate evidence-based modalities.
- For those with an eating disorder who have another condition such as diabetes, the secondary care teams will need to collaborate closely to minimize risk and optimize monitoring and treatment.
- Pregnant women with an eating disorder will require coordinated care from both obstetric and eating disorders specialist teams.
- Admit people with an eating disorder whose physical health is severely compromised to a medical inpatient or day patient service for medical stabilization and to initiate refeeding, if these cannot be done in an outpatient setting.
- For people with an eating disorder and acute mental health risk (such as significant suicide risk), consider psychiatric crisis care or psychiatric inpatient care.
- If people's physical health is at serious risk due to an eating disorder, they do not consent to treatment, and they can only be treated safely in an inpatient setting, follow the legal framework for compulsory treatment in the Mental Health Act of 1983.

References

American Psychiatric Association. (2000a). Posttraumatic stress disorder. In *Diagnostic and statistical manual of mental disorders* (4th ed.). Washington, DC: American Psychiatric Association.

American Psychiatric Association. (2000b). *Diagnostic and statistical manual of mental disorders* (4th ed.). Washington, DC: American Psychiatric Association.

Anderson, I., Nutt, D., & Deakin, J. (2000). Evidence-based guidelines for treating depressive disorders with antidepressants: A revision of the 1993 British association for psychopharmacology guidelines. *Journal of Psychopharmacology / British Association for Psychopharmacology, 14*, 3–20.

Angst, J. (1997). A regular review of the long-term follow-up of depression. *British Medical Journal (Clinical Research Ed.), 315*, 1143–1146.

Arcelus, J. (2011). Mortality rates in patients with anorexia nervosa and other eating disorders. *Archives of General Psychiatry, 68*(7), 724.

B-eat. (2017). *Delaying for years, denied for months*. Retrieved from www.beateatingdisorders.org.uk/uploads/documents/2017/11/delaying-for-years-denied-for-months.pdf.

Ballenger, J., & Tylee, A. (2003). *Anxiety*. St. Louis, MO: Mosby.

Barrett, J., Williams, J., Oxman, T., et al. (2001). Treatment of dysthymia and minor depression in primary care. *The Journal of family practice, 50*, 405–412.

Bennewith, O., Stocks, N., Gunnell, D., et al. (2002). General practice-based intervention to prevent repeat episodes of deliberate self harm: Cluster randomised controlled trial. *British Medical Journal (Clinical Research Ed.), 324*, 1254–1257.

Bisson, J. (2004). Post-traumatic stress disorder: What are the effects of preventive psychological interventions? *Clinical Evidence*. Retrieved from www.clinicalevidence.com.

Boardman, J., & Walters, P. (2009). Managing depression in primary care: It's not only what you do it's the way that you do it. *The British Journal of General Practice: The Journal of the Royal College of General Practitioners, 59*, 76–78.

Bostwick, J., & Pankratz, V. (2000). Affective disorders and suicide risk: A reexamination. *The American Journal of Psychiatry, 157*, 1925–1932.

Brent, D. (2007). Antidepressants and suicidal behavior: Cause or cure? *The American Journal of Psychiatry, 164*, 989–991.

Buscemi, N., Vandermeer, B., Hooton, N., et al. (2004). Melatonin for treatment of sleep disorders. In *Evidence report/technology assessment no. 108*. Rockville, MD: Agency for Healthcare Research and Quality.

Buscemi, N., Vandermeer, B., Hooton, N., et al. (2006). Efficacy and safety of exogenous melatonin for secondary sleep disorders and sleep disorders accompanying sleep restriction: Meta-analysis. *British Medical Journal (Clinical Research Ed.), 332*, 385–388.

Buszewicz, M., Pistrang, N., Barker, C., et al. (2006). Patients experiences of GP consultations for psychological problems: A qualitative study. *The British Journal of General Practice: The Journal of the Royal College of General Practitioners, 56*, 496–503.

Casacalenda, N., Perry, J., & Looper, K. (2002). Remission in major depressive disorder: A comparison of pharmacotherapy, psychotherapy, and control conditions. *The American Journal of Psychiatry, 159*, 1354–1360.

Chilvers, C., Dewey, M., Fielding, K., et al. (2001). Antidepressant drugs and generic counselling for treatment of major depression in primary care: Randomised trial with patient preference arms. *British Medical Journal (Clinical Research Ed.), 322*, 772–775.

Cipriani, A., Barbui, C., & Geddes, J. (2005). Suicide, depression, and antidepressants. *British Medical Journal (Clinical Research Ed.), 330*, 373–374.

Cipriani, A., Furukawa, T., Salanti, G., et al. (2009). Comparative efficacy and acceptability of 12 new-generation antidepressants: A multiple-treatments meta-analysis. *Lancet, 373*, 746–758.

Cipriani, A., Geddes, J., & Barbui, C. (2007). Venlafaxine for major depression. *British Medical Journal (Clinical Research Ed.), 334*, 215–216.

Citrone, L., & Stroup, T. (2006). Schizophrenia, clinical antipsychotic trials of intervention effectiveness (CATIE) and number needed to treat: How can CATIE inform clinicians? *International Journal of Clinical Practice, 60*, 933–940.

Cotton, M., Ball, C., & Robinson, P. (2003). Four simple questions can help screen for eating disorders. *Journal of General Internal Medicine, 18*(1), 53–56.

Coupland, N., Bell, C., & Potokar, J. (1996). Serotonin reuptake inhibitor withdrawal. *Journal of Clinical Psychopharmacology, 16*, 356–362.

Cox, J. L., Holden, J. M., & Sagovsky, R. (1987). Detection of postnatal depression. *The British Journal of Psychiatry, 150*, 782–786.

CSM Expert Working Group. (2004). *Safety of selective serotonin reuptake inhibitor antidepressants*. London: Committee on Safety of Medicines. Retrieved from www.mca.gov.uk/aboutagency/regframework/csm/csmhome.htm.

Das, A., Olfson, M., Gameroff, M., et al. (2005). Screening for bipolar disorder in a primary care practice. *JAMA: The Journal of the American Medical Association, 293*, 956–963.

Department of Health. (1999). *National service framework for mental health*. London: The Stationery Office. www.dh.gov.uk.

Department of Health. (2001). *Treatment choice in psychological therapies and counselling: evidence based clinical practice guideline*. DoHealth: London. www.dh.gov.uk.

Dugas, M., Ladouceur, R., & Leger, E. (2003). Group cognitive-behavioral therapy for generalized anxiety disorder: Treatment outcome and long-term follow-up. *Journal of Consulting and Clinical Psychology, 71*, 821–825.

Dunn, A., Trivedi, M., Kampert, J., et al. (2005). Exercise treatment for depression: Efficacy and dose response. *American Journal of Preventive Medicine, 28*, 1–8.

Falloon, I., Laporta, M., Fadden, G., & Graham-Hole, V. (1993). *Managing stress in families: Cognitive and behavioural strategies for enhancing coping skills*. London: Routledge.

Fava, G., Ruini, C., & Rafanelli, C. (2004). Six-year outcome of cognitive behavior therapy for prevention of recurrent depression. *The American Journal of Psychiatry, 161*, 1872–1876.

Fisher, P., & Durham, R. (1999). Recovery rates in generalized anxiety disorder following psychological therapy: An analysis of clinically significant change in the STAI-T across outcome studies since 1990. *Psychological Medicine, 29,* 1425–1434.

Freeling, P., Rao, B., Paykel, E., et al. (1985). Unrecognised depression in general practice. *British Medical Journal (Clinical Research Ed.), 290,* 1880–1883.

Furukawa, T., McGuire, H., & Barbui, C. (2002). Meta-analysis of effects and side effects of low dosage tricyclic antidepressants in depression: Systematic review. *British Medical Journal (Clinical Research Ed.), 325,* 991–995.

Furukawa, T., Watanabe, N., & Churchill, R. (2007). Combined psychotherapy plus antidepressants for panic disorder with or without agoraphobia. *Cochrane Database of Systematic Reviews, 1,* CD004364.

Gale, C., & Davidson, O. (2007). Generalised anxiety disorder. *British Medical Journal (Clinical Research Ed.), 334,* 579–581.

Gale, C., & Oakley-Browne, M. (2004a). Generalised anxiety disorder: What are the effects of drug treatments? Benzodiazepines. *Clinical Evidence.* www.clinicalevidence.com.

Gale, C., & Oakley-Browne, M. (2004b). Generalised anxiety disorder: What are the effects of cognitive therapy? *Clinical Evidence.* www.clinicalevidence.com.

Gale, C., & Oakley-Browne, M. (2004c). Generalised anxiety disorder: What are the effects of drug treatments? Beta-blockers. *Clinical Evidence.* www.clinicalevidence.com.

Geddes, J., Carney, S., Davies, C., et al. (2003). Relapse prevention with antidepressant drug treatment in depressive disorders: A systematic review. *Lancet, 361,* 653–661.

Gill, D., & Hatcher, S. (2002). Antidepressants for depression in medical illness (Cochrane review). In *The Cochrane library* (Issue 1). Oxford: Update Software.

Glass, J., Lanctot, K., Herrmann, N., et al. (2005). Sedative hypnotics in older people with insomnia: Meta-analysis of risks and benefits. *British Medical Journal (Clinical Research Ed.), 331,* 1169–1173.

Gloaguen, V., Cottraux, J., Cucherat, M., et al. (1998). A meta-analysis of the effects of cognitive therapy in depressed patients. *Journal of Affective Disorders, 49,* 59–72.

Goldberg, D., & Bridges, K. (1987). Screening for psychiatric illness in general practice: The general practitioner versus the screening questionnaire. *The Journal of the Royal College of General Practitioners, 37,* 15–18.

Goldberg, D., & Lecrubier, Y. (1995). Form and frequency of mental disorders across centres. In B. Ustun & N. Sartorius (Eds.), *Mental illness in general health care: An international study* (pp. 323–334). Chichester: WHO, John Wiley.

Haddad, P., Lejoyeux, M., & Young, A. (1998). Antidepressant discontinuation reactions. *British Medical Journal (Clinical Research Ed.), 316,* 1105–1106.

Haug, T., Blomhoff, S., Hellstrom, K., et al. (2003). Exposure therapy and sertraline in social phobia: 1 year follow-up of a randomised controlled trial. *The British Journal of Psychiatry, 182,* 312–318.

Hawton, K. (2003). Helping people bereaved by suicide. *British Medical Journal (Clinical Research Ed.), 327,* 177–178.

Hawton, K., Zahl, D., & Weatherall, R. (2003). Suicide following deliberate self-harm: Long-term follow-up of patients who presented to a general hospital. *The British Journal of Psychiatry, 182,* 537–542.

Herzog, D., Greenwood, D., Dorer, D., Flores, A., Ekeblad, E., Richards, A., et al. (2000). Mortality in eating disorders: A descriptive study. *The International Journal of Eating Disorders, 28*(1), 20–26.

Holden, J., Sagovsky, R., & Cox, J. (1989). Counselling in a general practice setting: Controlled study of health visitor intervention in treatment of postnatal depression. *British Medical Journal (Clinical Research Ed.), 298,* 223–226.

Hull, A. (2004). Primary care management of post-traumatic stress disorder. *Prescriber,* 1940–1948.

Jarde, A., Morais, M., Kingston, D., et al. (2016). Neonatal outcomes in women with untreated antenatal depression compared with women without depression: A systematic review and meta-analysis. *JAMA Psychiatry, 73*(8), 826–837. doi:10.1001/jamapsychiatry.2016.093.

Jick, H., Kaye, J., & Jick, S. (2004). Antidepressants and the risk of suicidal behaviors. *JAMA: The Journal of the American Medical Association, 292,* 338–343.

Jones, P., & Buckley, P. (2003). *Schizophrenia.* St. Louis, MO: Mosby.

Jones, R., Chung, M., Berger, Z., et al. (2007). Prevalence of post-traumatic stress disorder in patients with previous myocardial infarction consulting in general practice. *The British Journal of General Practice: The Journal of the Royal College of General Practitioners, 57,* 808–810.

Jorm, A., Christensen, H., Griffiths, K., & Rodgers, B. (2002). Effectiveness of complementary and self-help treatments for depression. *The Medical Journal of Australia, 176,* S84–S96.

Kapczinski, F., Lima, M., & Souza, J. (2003). Antidepressants for generalized anxiety disorder. *Cochrane Database of Systematic Reviews, 2.*

Kapur, N., Cooper, J., Rodway, C., et al. (2005). Predicting the risk of repetition of self harm: Cohort study. *British Medical Journal (Clinical Research Ed.), 330,* 394–395.

Katon, W., & Roy-Byrne, P. (2007). Anxiety disorders: Efficient screening is the first step in improving outcomes. *Annals of Internal Medicine, 146,* 390–392.

Keck, P. (2003). The management of acute mania. *British Medical Journal (Clinical Research Ed.), 327,* 1002–1003.

Loebel, A., Lieberman, J., Alvir, J., et al. (1992). Duration of psychosis and outcome in first-episode schizophrenia. *The American Journal of Psychiatry, 149,* 1183–1188.

Maltby, N., Kirsch, I., Mayers, M., et al. (2002). Virtual reality exposure therapy for the treatment of fear of flying: A controlled investigation. *Journal of Consulting and Clinical Psychology, 70,* 1112–1118.

McDonagh, M., Matthews, A., Phillipi, C., Romm, J., Peterson, K., Thakurta, S., et al. (2014). Depression drug treatment outcomes in pregnancy and the postpartum period: A systematic review and meta-analysis. *Obstetrics and Gynecology, 124*(3), 526–534.

Medicines and Healthcare Products Regulatory Agency. (2006). Cardiac arrhythmias associated with antipsychotic drugs. *Current Problems in Pharmacovigilance, 31,* 9.

Mental Health Foundation. (2004). Self harm. *Mental Health Foundation.* www.mentalhealth.org.uk.

Mol, S., Arntz, A., Metsemakers, J., et al. (2005). Symptoms of post-traumatic stress disorder after non-traumatic events: Evidence from an open population study. *The British Journal of Psychiatry, 186,* 494–499.

Morgan, K., Dixon, S., Mathers, N., et al. (2003). Psychological treatment for insomnia in the management of long-term hypnotic drug use: A pragmatic randomised controlled trial. *The British Journal of General Practice: The Journal of the Royal College of General Practitioners, 53,* 923–928.

Munro, C., Freeman, C., & Law, R. (2004). General practitioners' knowledge of post-traumatic stress disorder: A controlled study. *The British Journal of General Practice: The Journal of the Royal College of General Practitioners, 54,* 843–847.

Mynors-Wallis, L., Gath, D., Day, A., et al. (2000). Controlled trial of problem solving treatment, antidepressant medication, and combined treatment for major depression in primary care. *British Medical Journal (Clinical Research Ed.), 320,* 26–30.

NHS Education for Scotland. (2004). Education for frontline staff. *Mental Health (Care and Treatment) (Scotland) Act.* www.nes.scot.nhs.uk/mha.

NHS Information Centre for Health and Social Care. (2007). *Adult psychiatric morbidity in England, 2007: Results of a household survey.* Retrieved from https://digital.nhs.uk/catalogue/PUB02931.

National Institute for Health, & Care Excellence. (2004a). *Zaleplon, zolpidem and zopiclone for the short-term management of insomnia. NICE technology appraisal guidance 77.* Retrieved from www.nice.org.uk.

National Institute for Health and Care Excellence. (2004b). *Self-harm: The short-term physical and psychological management and secondary prevention of self-harm in primary and secondary care. NICE clincial guideline 16.* Retrieved from www.nice.org.uk.

National Institute for Health and Care Excellence. (2005a). *Post-traumatic stress disorder: The management of PTSD in adults and children in primary and secondary care. NICE clincial guideline 26.* Retrieved from www.nice.org.uk.

National Institute for Health and Care Excellence. (2005b). *Obsessive-compulsive disorder: Core interventions in the treatment of obsessive-compulsive disorder and body dysmorphic disorder. NICE clincial guideline 31.* Retrieved from www.nice.org.uk.

National Institute for Health and Care Excellence. (2006). *TA97. Depression and anxiety—computerised cognitive behavioural therapy (CCBT).* Retrieved from www.nice.org.uk.

National Institute for Health and Care Excellence. (2014). *Psychosis and schizophrenia in adults: Prevention and management. NICE clincial guideline 178.*

National Institute for Health and Care Excellence. (2014). *Antenatal and postnatal mental health: Clinical management and service guidance. NICE clincial guideline 192, updated 2017.* Retrieved from www.nice.org.uk.

National Institute for Health and Care Excellence. (2015). *Violence and agression: Short-term management in mental health, health and community settings. NICE clincial guideline 10.*

National Institute for Health and Care Excellence. (2017). *Eating disorders: Recognition and treatment.* London: NICE.

National Institute for Health and Care Excellence. (2018). *Clinical Knowledge Summaries: Depression—antenatal and postnatal.* Retrieved from cks.nice.org.uk.

National Society for the Prevention of Cruelty to Children. (2016). *Rise in children hospitalised for self-harm as thousands contact Childline.* Retrieved from www.nspcc.org.uk/what-we-do/news-opinion/rise-children-hospitalised-self-harm-thousands-contact-childline/.

O'Connell, H., Chin, A. V., Cunningham, C., & Lawlor, B. (2004). Recent developments: Suicide in older people. *British Medical Journal (Clinical Research Ed.), 329,* 895–899.

Owens, C., Lloyd, K., & Campbell, J. (2004). Access to health care prior to suicide: Findings from a psychological autopsy study. *The British Journal of General Practice: The Journal of the Royal College of General Practitioners, 54,* 279–281.

Pampallona, S., Bollini, P., & Tibaldi, G. (2004). Combined pharmacotherapy and psychological treatment for depression: A systematic review. *Archives of General Psychiatry, 61,* 714–719.

Picchioni, M., & Murray, R. (2007). Schizophrenia. *British Medical Journal (Clinical Research Ed.), 335,* 91–95.

Pohl, R., Feltner, D., Fieve, R., et al. (2005). Efficacy of pregabalin in the treatment of generalized anxiety disorder: Double-blind, placebo-controlled comparison of BD versus TID dosing. *Journal of Clinical Psychopharmacology, 25,* 151–158.

Price, J., Waller, P., Wood, S., et al. (1996). A comparison of the postmarketing safety of four selective serotonin re-uptake inhibitors including the investigation of symptoms occurring on withdrawal. *British Journal of Clinical Pharmacology, 42,* 757–763.

Rost, K., Nutting, P., Smith, J., et al. (2002). Managing depression as a chronic disease: A randomised trial of ongoing treatment in primary care. *British Medical Journal (Clinical Research Ed.), 325,* 934–937.

Royal College of Psychiatrists. (1998). Managing deliberate self-harm in young people. In *Council report CR64.* London: Royal College of Psychiatrists.

Rush, A., Trivedi, M., Wisniewski, S., et al. (2006). Acute and longer-term outcomes in depressed outpatients requiring one or several treatment steps: A STAR* D report. *The American Journal of Psychiatry, 163,* 1905–1917.

Schneier, F. (2003). Social anxiety disorder. *British Medical Journal (Clinical Research Ed.), 327,* 515–516.

Scott, J. (2006). Depression should be managed like a chronic disease. *British Medical Journal (Clinical Research Ed.), 332,* 985–986.

Simon, G., Heiligenstein, J., Revicki, D., et al. (1999). Long-term outcomes of initial antidepressant drug choice in a 'real world' randomized trial. *Archives of Family Medicine, 8,* 319–325.

Sivertsen, B., Omvik, S., Pallesen, S., et al. (2006). Cognitive behavioral therapy vs zopiclone for treatment of chronic primary insomnia in older adults: A randomized controlled trial. *JAMA: The Journal of the American Medical Association, 295,* 2851–2858.

Smith, D., Dempster, C., Glanville, J., et al. (2002). Efficacy and tolerability of venlafaxine compared with selective serotonin reuptake inhibitors and other antidepressants: A meta-analysis. *The British Journal of Psychiatry, 180,* 396–404.

Soomro, G. (2004). Deliberate self-harm. In *Clinical evidence.* London: BMJ Publishing Group.

Stewart, A. (1998). Choosing an anti-depressant: Effectiveness based pharmacoeconomics. *Journal of Affective Disorders, 48,* 125–133.

Thompson, D. (2017). Boys and men get eating disorders too. *Trends in Urology & Men's Health, 8*(2), 9–12.

Timonen, M., & Liukkonen, T. (2008). Management of depression in adults. *British Medical Journal (Clinical Research Ed.), 336,* 435–439.

Treasure, J. (2018). *Cite a website—cite this for me.* Retrieved from www.kcl.ac.uk/ioppn/depts/pm/research/eatingdisorders/resources/GUIDETOMEDICALRISKASSESSMENT.pdf.

Turner, E., & Rosenthal, R. (2008). Efficacy of antidepressants. *British Medical Journal (Clinical Research Ed.), 336,* 516–517.

Van Weel-Baumgarten, E., Van Den Bosch, W., Van Den Hoogen, H., et al. (2000). The validity of the diagnosis of depression in general practice: Is using criteria for diagnosis as a routine the answer? *The British Journal of General Practice: The Journal of the Royal College of General Practitioners, 50,* 284–287.

Walsh, J., Muehlbach, M., Lauter, S., et al. (1996). Effects of triazolam on sleep, daytime sleepiness, and morning stiffness in patients with rheumatoid arthritis. *The Journal of Rheumatology, 23,* 245–252.

Whooley, M. A., Avins, A. L., Miranda, J., et al. (1997). Case-finding instruments for depression: Two questions are as good as many. *Journal of General Internal Medicine, 12,* 439–445.

Wilner, K., Anziano, R., Johnson, A., et al. (2002). The anxiolytic effect of the novel antipsychotic ziprasidone compared with diazepam in subjects anxious before dental surgery. *Journal of Clinical Psychopharmacology, 22,* 206–210.

Wilson, S., & Nutt, D. (2003). Insomnia: Recommended practice management. *Prescriber, 45,* 57.

World Health Organiztion. (1979). *Schizophrenia: An international follow-up study.* Chichester: John Wiley & Sons.

World Health Organization. (2003). *International statistical classification of diseases and related health problems* (10th ed.). Retrieved from www.who.int.en (search on "ICD 10").

19

Urinary and Renal Problems

LINDSEY POPE

CHAPTER CONTENTS

Urinary Tract Infections

Uncomplicated Lower Urinary Tract Infection in Nonpregnant Women of Childbearing Age

Cystitis/Uncomplicated Lower Urinary Tract Infection

- Half of women who present with frequency and dysuria do not have bacterial infection. Half of those with bacterial infections resolve within 3 days without antibiotics (Brumfitt et al., 1994). The key to management is in distinguishing an uncomplicated from a complicated urinary tract infection (UTI) (acute pyelonephritis, unusual organism, structural predisposition, refractory, recurrent, or systemic symptoms) and in avoiding unnecessary antibiotics in those without infection or in the elderly with asymptomatic bacteriuria.
- The management of uncomplicated lower UTI in women can be as effective *over the telephone* as if the patients are seen in person, although this must be done with caution, given General Medical Council (GMC) advice on prescribing antibiotics in this manner. Women with moderate or severe typical cystitis symptoms can be treated based on history alone but where there is doubt or if the symptoms are mild, refractory or relapse, then it is better to do a urine dipstick test and consider the need for a midstream specimen of urine (MSU) test.
  - If *positive for nitrites and/or leukocytes*, assume that this is infection and treat with antibiotics without sending an MSU. Where positive for leukocytes but not nitrites, remember that the symptoms may represent urethral syndrome (see upcoming discussion).
  - If *positive for protein and/or blood only*, then consider the diagnosis and differentials further.
  - If *negative for all four tests*, send an MSU for microscopy and culture without starting antibiotics; 95% will have a negative MSU and do not require antibiotics at this stage (MeReC, 1995). Urethral syndrome is still possible with these results.
- If *treating, give antibiotics for 3 days.* This is as effective as a 7-day course. Seven days are, however, appropriate when treating the elderly, men, pregnant women and catheterized patients. A single dose is less effective than a 3-day course but may be justified when compliance is likely to be a problem. Follow local guidelines where available. When not available, for the 3-day course use trimethoprim 200 mg twice a day, although resistance can be above 25% in some areas. Nitrofurantoin 50 mg four times a day, or 100 mg modified release twice daily, is an alternative where renal function is normal.
- Patients with resistant organisms may need a change of antibiotics. Women who are infected with unusual organisms (e.g., *Proteus* or *Pseudomonas*) need a repeat MSU and further investigation if still present.
- Explain to the patient that symptoms should clear within 7 days (i.e., may persist after the 3 days of antibiotics). Advise the patient to return if symptoms are still severe after 3 days or persist after 7 days.
- *Prevention.* In women with recurrent infection offer self-help advice, as discussed later in the chapter.

Which Midstream Specimen of Urine Results Are Abnormal?

- Bacterial counts of 10^5/mL are significant and reported on MSU results, but lower counts may be found with organisms that are difficult to culture (e.g., *Staphylococcus saprophyticus, Chlamydia, Gardnerella*). Counts of 10^3 and 10^4/mL should be repeated if the symptoms suggest infection.
- Organisms without cells can be ignored, except in pregnant women and young children. Cells without organisms need further investigation, unless the MSU was taken after antibiotics had been started.
- Repeat the MSU and refer if cells are still present.
- Females aged over 40 years old with a refractory UTI with haematuria or recurrent UTIs with haematuria need a referral to a urologist.

Recurrence of Symptoms
- Repeat the MSU, or do one for the first time, and assess whether the patient is suffering from:
  - relapse—the organism is the same;
  - reinfection—a different organism is present; or
  - the urethral syndrome (see upcoming discussion).

Relapse
- Treat, with an antibiotic to which the original organism was sensitive, for 7 days.
- Look for a reason for the failure to clear the original infection. Consider stones and chronic retention. Repeat the dipstick test for protein and haematuria.

Reinfection(s)
- Consider using a different antibiotic; the new organisms are likely to be resistant to the one originally used.

Frequent Reinfection
- *Investigations.* After more than three infections in a short period of time, consider an ultrasound scan (USS); an abdominal x-ray of the urinary tract; and urea, electrolytes, and creatinine to rule out underlying abnormalities. If

normal, there is no need for specialist referral, but consider prophylaxis.

- *Prophylaxis.* Consider low-dose prophylaxis in those with at least four attacks per year. Use nitrofurantoin (immediate-release) 50 to 100 mg at night or trimethoprim 100 mg at night for 6 months in the first instance. They will more than halve the number of attacks. If an infection occurs while on prophylaxis, use a different drug as treatment. A Cochrane review in 2012 failed to show significant benefit from cranberry products for preventing UTIs and therefore did not recommend its use (Jepson, Williams & Craig, 2012).

Infections Occurring After Intercourse

- Advise emptying the bladder after intercourse.
- Give a single dose of antibiotics to be taken within 2 hours of intercourse (e.g., trimethoprim 200 mg, off-licence use).

Asymptomatic Bacteriuria

- Asymptomatic bacteriuria in the elderly requires no treatment but does in pregnancy.

Self-Help

- Recommend that patients:
  - increase fluids;
  - increase the frequency of micturition (practise double voiding, i.e., attempting to pass urine a second time immediately after the first);
  - empty the bladder before sleep and after sexual intercourse;
  - wear loose-fitting cotton underwear and avoid tights;
  - avoid external sanitary towels;
  - make sure a diaphragm, if worn, fits comfortably (or change contraceptive method);
  - use a lubricant (e.g., K-Y jelly) if vaginal dryness makes intercourse painful;
  - wipe from front to back (should be routine) and wash the vulva with soapy water.

Urethral Syndrome aka Abacterial Cystitis

- The diagnosis will have been made on the basis of repeated attacks of frequency and dysuria with repeatedly sterile MSUs. There are no clear diagnostic criteria and it overlaps with other diagnoses such as interstitial cystitis.
- Examine to exclude:
  - vaginal infection, especially *Candida, Chlamydia, Trichomonas, Gardnerella*, or gonorrhoea;
  - urethral herpes or warts;
  - significant anterior prolapse;
  - atrophic vaginitis.
- Ask the patient to keep a diary of input, output, and symptoms for 1 week, and consider managing as for detrusor instability (see Urge Incontinence, to come).
- *Self-help.* Patients should:
  - alkalinize the urine (e.g., with potassium citrate mixture);
  - avoid coloured toilet paper, scented soaps, bubble baths, douches, antiseptics, talcum powder, vaginal deodorants, and deodorized tampons;

- ensure that sexual intercourse is not traumatic because, for instance, of lack of lubrication.
- Do not treat with antibiotics, as overgrowth with lactobacilli and candida may be encouraged.
- *If symptoms are disabling,* refer to a urologist. Urethral dilatation is now only used when true urethral stenosis is found due to little evidence for its effectiveness otherwise and potential for dilatation to cause periurethral fibrosis leading to strictures.

Lower Urinary Tract Infection in Men
Initial Assessment and Management

- Consider possible causes: prostate problems, congenital urinary tract problems, phimosis, previous urinary tract surgery, immunodeficiency, or anal intercourse.
- Examine the abdomen (for a palpable bladder), the testes and epididymis to assess the extent of infection, the prostate, and the urethral meatus for discharge.
- Exclude diabetes with a fasting glucose.
- Arrange for an MSU before, and 7 to 14 days after finishing, antibiotics.
- Treat with antibiotics for 7 days in the first instance (trimethoprim or nitrofurantoin) and review the MSU results.
- If ill, admit.

Further Management

- Consider USS and an abdominal x-ray to look for abnormalities of the urinary tract. This has been shown to detect all pathology that would have been detected on intravenous pyelogram (IVP) as well as some that would have been missed.
- If infection recurs, refer and consider low-dose prophylaxis until seen by a urologist.
- Consider the possibility of a urinary tract cancer in men with recurrent or persistent UTIs.

Note: Most episodes of dysuria in young men will be due to urethritis. Consider referral to a genitourinary medicine (GUM) clinic.

Acute Prostatitis

- Send an MSU, plus urethral swabs if there is any suggestion of a sexually transmitted infection.
- Start treatment with a quinolone antibiotic (ciprofloxacin 500 mg twice a day or ofloxacin 200 mg twice a day) for 28 days. If these cannot be taken then trimethoprim 200 mg twice a day for 28 days is recommended.
- Give analgesics (e.g., paracetamol) or a nonsteroidal anti-inflammatory drug (NSAID) for symptomatic relief.
- If defecation is painful, offer a stool softener such as lactulose.
- Reassess after 48 hours.
- Admit patients who are ill or in whom rectal examination suggests a prostatic abscess.
- Following recovery, refer for investigation to exclude underlying urinary tract abnormality.

Chronic Prostatitis

GUIDELINE

National Institute for Health and Care Excellence. (2015). *Prostatitis—chronic. NICE clinical knowledge summaries.* Available at https://cks.nice.org.uk/prostatitis-chronic.

- Patients present with at least a 3-month history of pain in the perineum or pelvic floor and lower urinary tract symptoms. This diagnosis is made once other conditions have been excluded (e.g., UTI; benign prostatic hyperplasia [BPH]; cancer of prostate, bladder, or colon; urethral stricture; calculus; pudendal neuralgia). Only 5% to 10% of patients with this symptom complex (perineal pain, lower urinary tract symptoms, variable dipstick, and MSU results) have bacterial infection.
- Establish the diagnosis: Order microscopy and culture on the *first part of the stream of the first urine passed in the morning.* Threads of white cells suggest prostatitis. Prostatic massage is not usually done in primary care.
- *If culture is positive:* Treat with a quinolone (e.g., ciprofloxacin 500 mg twice a day for 4 to 8 weeks). Repeat the MSU at 4 weeks and advise an early review if symptoms return. If a sexual infection was implicated, check that the partner has been adequately assessed and treated.
- *If culture is negative:* No treatment has been clearly shown to aid resolution. Offer a trial of NSAIDs for symptomatic relief and referral to a urologist if symptoms are not resolving. The value of referral is to confirm the diagnosis and assist in explaining it to the patient.
- If there are significant lower urinary tract symptoms then consider a 4–6 week trial of an alpha blocker (e.g. Tamsulosin). NICE advise not to prescribe an alpha blocker and an antibiotic concurrently (NICE, 2015).

Lower Urinary Tract Infection in Other Situations

Children

See Chapter 6, Children's Health.

Pregnancy

- All women are screened for bacteriuria at the first antenatal visit.
- If asymptomatic bacteriuria is found then a second urine sample should be sent for culture.
- If the second sample confirms asymptomatic bacteriuria then treat for 7 days with an antibiotic to which the organism is sensitive.
- If local guidelines are not available, options when sensitivities are known (in order of preference):
  - Nitrofurantoin 50 mg four times a day or 100 mg (modified release) twice a day

- Trimethoprim 200 mg twice a day (off-label use). Give a folic acid supplement if first trimester and do not give if folate deficient, taking a folate antagonist, or have been treated with trimethoprim in the past year.
- Cefalexin 500 mg twice a day or 250 mg four times a day.
- Repeat an MSU 7 days after completion of treatment, and then at every antenatal visit until delivery.
- *Acute pyelonephritis:* Admit.
- *Second UTI during pregnancy:* Refer to an obstetrician.

Postmenopausal Women

- Recurrent UTIs are common after the menopause, affecting more than 10% of women. This is in addition to symptoms due to urogenital atrophy.
- *Oestrogen therapy.* Prescribe low-dose oestrogen therapy in those with no contraindications. It has been shown to change the colonization of the vagina and decrease infections. Topical treatment may be sufficient.
- *Culture-negative cystitis.* Organize a further culture if symptoms persist, asking specifically for *Ureaplasma urealyticum* and *Mycoplasma hominis.* Consider treating with tetracycline or erythromycin for 3 months, if present.
- Refer for urodynamic investigation women not responding to the above measures or unsuitable for oestrogen.
- *Interstitial cystitis.* Treatment is palliative and should be decided by the urologist. The options are:
  - oral therapy with, for example, a tricyclic antidepressant; or
  - intravesicular with, for example, botulinum toxin injections.

PATIENT SUPPORT

The Cystitis and Overactive Bladder Foundation, www.cobfoundation.org.

Catheterized Patients

- Of patients with an indwelling catheter, 90% have bacteriuria after 17 days (Drug Therapy Bulletin [DTB], 1998). Dipsticks are of little value when catheterized, and asymptomatic bacteriuria does not usually need treatment.
- Infection cannot be prevented by topical antimicrobials applied to the meatus, nor by irrigation with antimicrobials or antiseptics. The best defence against infection is to open the closed drainage system as infrequently as possible.
- *Give antibiotics* for 7 days only if the patient is clearly symptomatic, if the infection is systemic (i.e., the patient is febrile), or if the causative organism is *Proteus. Proteus* may give rise to triple-phosphate stones and is worth eradicating with antibiotics.

- *If giving antibiotics,* remove the catheter if the patient can manage without it for a few days. Insert a new one once the urine is sterile.
- Consider whether intermittent catheterization by the patient, or a suprapubic catheter, might be a better option.
- Wash the meatus daily with soap and water.
- Only give antibiotics prophylactically if they are needed to prevent endocarditis or if patients do badly with UTIs (e.g., many patients catheterized with multiple sclerosis).

Acute Pyelonephritis

- Admit if too ill to take oral fluids and medication, if the patient shows signs of sepsis, or if the patient is pregnant. Otherwise:
  - arrange an MSU;
  - prescribe a broad spectrum antibiotic (e.g. ciprofloxacin 500 mg twice daily for 7 days, or co-amoxiclav 625 mg three times daily for 14 days);
  - consider the need for analgesics;
  - review the patient and the MSU result and confirm that the antibiotic was appropriate;
  - repeat the MSU 7 days after the antibiotics are finished;
  - *follow-up:* Consider a USS and an abdominal x-ray of the urinary tract.

Urinary Incontinence

> **GUIDELINE**
>
> National Institute for Health and Care Excellence. (2013, updated 2015). *Urinary incontinence in women: Management. NICE clinical guideline 71.* www.nice.org.uk.

- Urinary incontinence effects both men and women across the spectrum of ages and can have a significant physical and psychological impact on sufferers.
- Many patients will not volunteer the problem to their GP.

History

- Be ready to ask anyone about incontinence if they have a condition which puts them at risk. A question such as, "Do you ever have trouble holding your water?" is less threatening than using the word *incontinence.*
- Check, from the history, for other urinary symptoms. Incontinence is usually part of a larger problem. Consider benign prostatic hypertrophy (BPH) in older men and perform an International Prostate Symptom (IPS) score if indicated (see Appendix 24).
- Identify the type of incontinence from the history: stress, urge, overflow, or continuous, or a mixture. Many sufferers have at least two types.
- Ask about precipitating events: excess fluids or alcohol, behavioural or cognitive problems, and poor mobility or access to a toilet.

- Check for other underlying conditions. Constipation and UTIs are leading causes of incontinence in the elderly. Neurogenic incontinence may present with a mixture of symptoms. Cauda equina syndrome is a surgical emergency, where results are poor when surgery is undertaken more than 48 hours after first presentation (Markham, 2004).

Examination

- Examine the abdomen, the genitals, and prostate in men, with a pelvic examination in women, and a rectal examination in both sexes for constipation and for the integrity of the anal reflex.
- Proceed to the BPH guidance for further evaluation (discussion to come) in men where this is the suspected cause of the incontinence, as well as performing the upcoming investigations.

Investigations

- Dip the urine for sugar and evidence of infection. Consider an MSU.
- Frequency/volume diary.
- Consider the use of a validated questionnaire for incontinence severity and quality of life (such as the King's Health Questionnaire).
- Consider a urinary USS to assess residual volume, especially if there is a possibility that overflow incontinence is present or if the patient does not respond promptly to the upcoming measures. A residual volume of 200 mL or more is abnormal. In men a residual volume above 100 mL is associated with other problems relating to BPH.
- Consider referral for urodynamic studies if the type of incontinence is not clear or if a trial of treatment fails.
- *Refer to a urologist or gynaecologist,* as appropriate, at this stage if there is:
  - a severe vaginal or uterine prolapse;
  - a pelvic mass (to be seen within 2 weeks in the United Kingdom as a suspected cancer);
  - a vesical fistula;
  - persistent or recurrent infection;
  - evidence of bladder outflow obstruction;
  - evidence of a large residual urine.
- Refer to a neurologist if there appears to be a neurological cause. The possibility of cauda equina syndrome or myelopathy needs urgent discussion with the neurosurgeons (or orthopaedic surgeons).

Management of Primarily Stress Incontinence (Men and Women)

- *Reduce intraabdominal pressure* by weight loss, the avoidance of constipation, and reducing cough by stopping smoking.
- Increase external sphincter tone (87% cured or improved) (US Department of Health and Human Services, 1992):
  - by pelvic floor exercises for men and women. Teach the patient to practice stopping the flow of urine momentarily midstream and then continue tensing

those same muscles for 4 seconds at a time with 4 seconds rest, for a total of 1 hour a day in 10 tightening bursts. Short, repeated bouts of exercises are the most useful. Continue for 3 months before deciding that exercises have not helped;

a. by using intravaginal weighted cones for women (available through urologists or local chemists). The patient inserts the lowest weight cone, with the pointed end downwards, and learns to retain the cone. The weight of the cones is steadily increased to 100 g;

b. by referral to an appropriate physiotherapist for electrical stimulation therapy.

- *Postmenopausal women with an atrophic vagina.* The Women's Health Initiative has shown that oral oestrogen, with or without progestogen, significantly *worsened* continence, both in those troubled by incontinence at the start of the trial and in those who had no incontinence at the start of the trial (Hendrix et al., 2005). No clearcut evidence exists for local oestrogen.
- *Referral.* Refer those with troublesome symptoms that do not respond to the measures above. Surgery cures or improves 85% of those operated on. Operations include the older open abdominal retropubic suspension procedures as well as the newer and less invasive suburethral sling procedures (including those using transvaginal tape).
- *Consider prescribing duloxetine in addition to pelvic floor exercises.* It has an NNT for reduction of stress incontinence by over 50% of 5.7 (95%CI 4.5–7.8). However, most women report adverse effects, with nausea the most common, and one in five women in trials stop the drug (Anon., 2004).

Management of Primarily Urger Incontinence (Men and Women)

- Reduce excessive fluid intake and try avoiding caffeine.
- *Bladder retraining* results in up to 87% cured or improved (US Department of Health and Human Services, 1992).
- Instruct the patient to:
  - keep a frequency/volume chart for 1 week;
  - return for discussion of the pattern the diary reveals. In addition, check that the total volume of urine passed does not suggest that the patient is drinking too much;
  - practise holding the urine when the urge to pass it is there; and
  - slowly increase the interval between voiding up to 2 to 3 hours.
- *Anticholinergic drugs* are helpful in up to 83% (Malone-Lee et al., 2001) but are limited by side effects. Undertake a trial for 6 weeks and, if working, review again after 6 months. Use oxybutynin, tolterodine, trospium, or propiverine; the last three are more expensive than oxybutynin but may have fewer adverse effects (Anon, 2001). Sixty percent show marked improvement or cure in the presence of detrusor instability (Haeusler et al., 2002).
- *Desmopressin* given as a single evening dose can be considered when nocturia is a particular problem (off label use).

- *Oestrogen* given orally does not help incontinence in postmenopausal women (see earlier discussion), in contrast to the conclusions of a Cochrane review based on smaller earlier studies (Moehrer, Hextall, & Jackson, 2003). The case for local oestrogen is unclear.
- *Referral.* Refer to a urologist for consideration of augmentation cystoplasty for those still sufficiently troubled by symptoms despite treatment and who might be candidates for surgery.

> **PATIENT SUPPORT**
>
> The Cystitis and Overactive Bladder Foundation, www.cobfoundation.org.

Management of Primarily Overflow Incontinence

- Refer for assessment by a urologist, neurologist, or other specialist, according to the cause.

Management of Incontinence in the Frail Elderly or Cognitively Impaired

- Assess:
  - *is it due to infection?* Older people often do not experience the typical symptoms of urinary infection. Send an MSU where possible;
  - *is it a symptom of another physical illness or of dementia?*
  - *are drugs causing or exacerbating the situation?* Diuretics, sedatives, for example;
  - *are there issues of practicality and mobility?* How easy is it to get to the toilet? Can mobility be improved? Can clothing be made easier to unfasten?
- Encourage the patient to pass urine regularly to try to pre-empt the incontinence.

Coping With Incontinence: Conservative Containment Advice for All

- Where the situation does not respond to any of the above measures, a continence adviser will be able to advise the patient on appliances, some of which are prescribable. Others may be available through the social services (including bath and laundry allowance).

Bedding Protection

- *Plastic mattress covers and one-way sheets* can be bought if not available from the community nursing service. They not only increase comfort but also reduce bedsores.

Pads and Appliances

- *Inco pads* may be available from the community nursing service.
- *Cellulose wadding* can be prescribed.

- *Body-worn pads and waterproof pants* usually have to be bought (e.g., Urocare, Kanga, and Kanga pouch).
- *Collecting devices* such as commodes, pans, and urinals can be bought from pharmacists or hired from the Red Cross or may be obtained via Social Services in the UK.
- *Penile sheaths* are available on prescription. Conveen provides a free sizing kit and sheaths from 17 to 35 mm.

Urinary Drainage Bags

- Assess the patient's requirements: the length of tubing (short for wearing on the thigh or long on the calf); the type of tap (selection should depend on the patient's dexterity); the capacity needed (350, 500, 750 mL).
- Night bags hold 2 L and should only be used for bed-bound patients or overnight.

Urinary Catheters and Problem Solving

> **GUIDELINE**
>
> National Institute for Clinical Excellence. (2012). *Healthcare-associated infections: Prevention and control in primary and community care. NICE clinical guideline 139,* updated 2017. www.nice.org.uk.

- Infection makes catheterization an unattractive solution but one that is likely to be necessary in those with retention or neurogenic bladder dysfunction, with severe pressure ulcers, who are terminally ill, or who cannot cope with less invasive appliances.
- Choose intermittent catheterization over an indwelling catheter if it is feasible.
- *Catheters* for long-term use should always be silicone with a 10-mL balloon.
- *Catheter insertion* should be performed using a no-touch technique and clean, but not necessarily sterile, gloves.
- *Catheter changes* should only be done when there is malfunction or contamination or according to the manufacturers' recommendations.
- *Urine samples* should be taken from a sampling port, not by disconnecting the bag, nor from the bag drainage outlet.
- *Debris* may be reduced by acidification of the urine with ascorbic acid. Encrustation ends up affecting half of all long-term catheters and is associated with infection by *Proteus.* When a patient starts to develop encrustation, plan a regular catheter change before the encrustation becomes troublesome.

Infection

- See page 343. Inflammation around the urethral meatus may be related to encrustation of the catheter and/or infection.

Bypass

- This is caused by obstruction of the catheter or by detrusor instability, not by the catheter being too small.

- Check that the bag is lower than the bladder; change the catheter and see if the old one was blocked; use a small bulb size (e.g., 5 mL); exclude and, if necessary, treat bladder stones and infection; and if there is no improvement use anticholinergic drugs (e.g., oxybutynin) (Foster, Upsdell, & O'Reilly, 1990).

Catheterizing a Patient in Chronic Retention

- *Haematuria* is inevitable if the bladder has been distended for some time. Clamping to release the urine in stages does not prevent this.
- *Diuresis* may occur after the obstruction is relieved. Diuretic doses may need to be reduced. Admit patients whose diuresis is severe.

> **PATIENT INFORMATION**
>
> The Bladder and Bowel Foundation provides a continence nurse helpline for medical advice: 0800 031 5412; www.bladderandbowelfoundation.org.
>
> Incontinence Advisory Service, Disabled Living Foundation, 34 Chatfield Road, Wandsworth, London SW11 3SE, tel. 020 7289 6111; helpline 0300 999 004; www.dlf.org.uk.
>
> ERIC (Enuresis Resource and Information Centre for children and young adults). 36 Old School House, Britannia Road, Kingswood, Bristol BS15 8DB; helpline 0845 970 8008; www.eric.org.uk.

Difficulty Voiding

Bladder Outflow Problems in Men and Benign Prostatic Hypertrophy

> **GUIDELINES**
>
> National Institute for Health and Care Excellence. (2010). *Lower urinary tract symptoms in men: Management. NICE clinical guideline 97,* updated 2015. Available at: www.nice.org.uk.
>
> National Institute for Health and Care Excellence. (2015). *Suspected cancer: Recognition and referral. NICE clinical guideline 12.* www.nice.org.uk.

- BPH is the most common cause of bladder outflow problems in men and occurs with increasing age and with variable symptoms.
- Once symptoms are present, the *rule of thirds* applies with one-third deteriorating, one-third remaining stable, and one-third improving over time (Ball, Feneley, & Abrams, 1981).

History

- Take a history for relevant symptoms and score them (see Appendix 24). BPH is very common, with 41% of men over 50 years old reporting moderate or severe symptoms.
- Consider differential diagnoses: UTI, diabetes, prostatitis, medications, or lifestyle factors such as fluid and alcohol intake.

- Identify whether the patient has:
  - voiding/obstructive symptoms (poor flow, hesitancy, terminal dribbling, and incomplete emptying);
  - filling/overactive bladder symptoms (frequency, urgency, urge incontinence, small volume urinating, and nocturia).
- Is there nocturia out of proportion to other lower urinary tract symptoms (LUTS)? Nocturia three or more times a night raises the possibility of nocturnal polyuria, which can be defined as a nocturnal urine volume greater than 35% of the total 24-hour urine volume (Marinkovic, Gillen, & Stanton, 2004). This suggests a disturbance of the normal diurnal excretory rhythm. It can occur in chronic renal disease, diabetes mellitus, diabetes insipidus, right-sided heart failure, or can be an adverse effect of phenytoin, digoxin, lithium, diuretics, and excess vitamin D. Any of these would need treatment followed by reassessment of the LUTS. In the absence of a treatable cause it may respond to restriction of fluid at night, diuretics in the morning, compression stockings for those with oedema, or desmopressin at night.
- Are there filling symptoms with no evidence of obstruction? Manage as for urge incontinence (see page 344).

Examination

- Examine the abdomen for signs of chronic retention and pelvic or renal masses.
- Consider performing a digital rectal examination to examine for prostate size, to exclude sinister features, and as an aid to management decisions.

Investigations

- Perform a dipstick urinalysis.
- Test the blood for urea, creatinine and electrolytes, fasting glucose and consider (with informed consent) a PSA, though men with BPH are no more likely than others to have prostate cancer.
- Consider ordering an ultrasound scan (with post void residual volume) where there is a suspicion of chronic retention or an obstructive uropathy (e.g., palpable bladder, raised creatinine, overflow incontinence); uroflowmetry may also be available locally. Refer if the postvoiding residual volume is greater than 100 mL.

Immediate Management

- Admit those with acute urinary retention or acute kidney failure.
- Refer to be seen urgently (in the United Kingdom within 2 weeks) those with macroscopic haematuria (in the absence of infection, or persisting after treatment of infection), a nodular or firm or irregular prostate, a raised PSA for the patient's age, or abnormal urinary cytology, where done.
- Refer to be seen urgently (in the United Kingdom within 2 weeks) those over 45 with persistent microscopic haematuria.
- Consider a non-urgent referral for men over 60 with recurrent or persistent UTIs.

- Refer, at a timescale appropriate to the individual, those with chronic kidney disease (CKD) or with refractory symptoms affecting the quality of life.

The Management of Those Not Needing/Wanting Referral After Viewing Investigation Results

- Offer the patient a choice from the following options according to how bothered he is by his symptoms and whether he is at increased risk of progression of the obstruction. Explain that surgery is by no means inevitable. In one study only 7% required surgery over the next 3 years (Wasson et al., 1995).
  1. *Lifestyle advice and consider watchful waiting.* This is a key first line approach to management. Advice includes advising a fluid intake reduced to 2 liters per day and avoiding caffeine. Recommend bladder training to those with filling symptoms. Briefly, this means gradually lengthening the time between passing urine. Explain that avoiding excess fluid or alcohol intake, and avoiding constipation, will help to reduce the risk of acute retention. Review medications that might predispose to retention (especially anticholinergics).
  2. *Drugs:*
     - *Use an alpha-blocker* in those with mild symptoms without risk factors for progression and where a quick symptomatic response is required. They are generally the first line drugs for BPH. If there is benefit, it is felt within 4 to 6 weeks and lasts for at least 3 years. A trial in the individual patient is therefore feasible, using the IPS score to follow a trend (see Appendix 24). All alpha-blockers share this effect; a considerable saving can be made by choosing the least expensive. A reduction in BP from the less selective alpha-blockers such as doxazosin might be beneficial in hypertensive patients.
     - *Use a 5-α reductase inhibitor* (finasteride, dutasteride) in those at higher risk of progression. Given to men with a large prostate or raised PSA, it will reduce the risk of acute retention and the likelihood of prostatectomy by 50% to 60%. Use the other risk factors to sway the decision in cases of doubt (Lepor et al., 1996). No symptomatic benefit may be seen for 3 to 6 months. If there is benefit, it is sustained while the drug is continued. Libido and erection problems occur in 9%, and there are risks of gynaecomastia, reduced ejaculate volume, and presence of the drug in semen (such that condoms are advised). PSA rates are, on average, halved, to be remembered when performing future PSAs.
     - *Use a combination of the two* in those more troubled by their symptoms. A study of 3047 men with at least moderately symptomatic BPH found that clinical progression of symptoms over 4 years occurred in 17% on placebo, in 10% on either finasteride or doxazosin, and in only 5% on both drugs (McConnell et al., 2003).

- *Antimuscarinics:* Where BPH has caused a predominantly overactive bladder presentation consider these drugs in addition to bladder training. There is little evidence to suggest that they can precipitate acute urinary retention even in the presence of severe BPH.
- *Saw palmetto:* has only weak and conflicting evidence for efficacy in treating BPH symptoms.
3. *Surgery* (usually transurethral resection of prostate, TURP) is much more effective than drugs in improving symptoms and flow rates, but only in two-thirds of those who undergo it. It is most likely to be successful in those most bothered by their symptoms (Wasson et al., 1995). It does, however, carry not only the short-term risks of any operation but also, in the case of TURP (Brookes et al., 2002), the risk of incontinence in one-third although only 6% are bothered by it. After TURP, 9% need reoperation within 5 years. The rates for sexual dysfunction vary according to the type of surgery but the main techniques all worsen ejaculatory dysfunction (Emberton et al., 1996).

Review Patients at 6 to 12 Weeks if on an Alpha-Blocker; Otherwise at 3 to 6 Months

- Consider whether medications are working and tolerated, whether further medications need to be used in combination, whether lifestyle advice should be repeated, and whether a referral to a urologist is now indicated.
- Check creatinine and PSA annually.

Risk Factors for Progression of Bladder Outflow Problems in Men

- Large prostate (>30 cc)
- PSA >1.4 ng/mL regardless of age
- Age >70 years
- IPS score >7 (at least *moderate* severity)
- A low flow rate (<12 mL/sec)
- A postvoiding residual volume >100 mL on ultrasound

Carcinoma of the Prostate

GUIDELINES

National Institute for Health and Care Excellence. (2015). *Suspected cancer: Recognition and referral. NICE clinical guideline 12.* www.nice.org.uk.
National Institute for Health and Care Excellence. (2014). *Prostate cancer: Diagnosis and management. NICE clinical guideline 175.* www.nice.org.uk.

- Prostate cancer raises difficult issues relating to screening and the question of the value of treatment in the asymptomatic man in whom carcinoma is discovered incidentally. Symptomatic patients will benefit from referral.
- Nearly 10,000 die annually in the United Kingdom from prostate cancer.

PSA Counselling and Interpretation (Public Health England, 2016)

- Population screening for cancer of the prostate is not recommended in the United Kingdom, but should be available for a man who requests it and is able to give informed consent.
- A number of high profile campaigns have raised public awareness of prostate cancer and PSA testing and GPs should be prepared to discuss the risks and benefits of testing.

Risk Factors for Cancer of the Prostate

- *Age.* Half of men aged over 80 years have prostate cancer but most are asymptomatic and will die of other causes. Guidance suggests that PSA screening should not be offered to an asymptomatic man over 75 years with less than 10 years life expectancy.
- *Family history.* A family history of cancers of the prostate, breast, ovary, bladder, and kidney increase the risk.
- *Race.* Men of black ethnic origin have a rate that is double that of whites. Asian and Oriental men have the lowest rates.

Counselling for the Patient Who Requests PSA Screening

- Explain the following points:
  - A rectal examination is considered as well as the blood test.
  - If screening is positive, a biopsy may be needed. The biopsy itself is uncomfortable, risks infection, and is followed by haematuria or haematospermia for up to 3 weeks in a third of patients. The mortality is 1 : 10,000.
  - Only about 25% of men who have a positive PSA turn out to have cancer. About 15% of men with a normal PSA may have cancer. Even biopsy will miss up to 20% of cancers.
  - It is not clear that early treatment saves lives or improves other outcomes; and the treatments that may be offered can have potentially severe adverse effects including effects on sexual functioning and continence. Studies are conflicting on the benefits of screening, and the chief medical officer (CMO) of England has advised to continue to screen asymptomatic men if they ask for it and are appropriately informed. Where the patient has symptoms or signs suggestive of prostate cancer (see NICE guidance on referring suspected cancer, earlier), PSA testing is more likely to be useful. Consider performing a digital rectal examination (DRE) and a PSA where there is unexplained haematuria, lower urinary tract symptoms, erectile dysfunction, bone pain, low back pain, or weight loss. Refer urgently patients with an abnormal DRE or where the PSA is rising or above the age-specific thresholds (see upcoming discussion). Repeat the PSA after 1 to 3 months if borderline and refer urgently if rising.

- The stress and anxiety of knowing that you have or might have cancer is considerable and will affect life insurance applications.

PSA Interpretation

1. The upper limit of normal rises with age and was revised in the BAUS BPH 2004 guideline (see earlier):
   - Age <50: 2.5 ng/mL
   - Age 50–59: 3.0 ng/mL
   - Age 60–69: 4.0 ng/mL
   - Age 70+: 5.0 ng/mL
2. Probability of cancer at different levels of PSA:
   - PSA 4–10: 25%
   - PSA ≥11: 66%
   - PSA >60: usually indicates metastatic prostate cancer
3. Repeat a borderline level in 2 weeks (or according to local guidance); the result can alter by up to 30%.
4. Double the result if the patient has been taking finasteride or dutasteride for 6 months or more. Conversely, an enlarged prostate due to BPH can double the PSA level without indicating cancer.
5. Rectal examination does not raise the PSA but more invasive manoeuvres (even catheterization) can, as can UTI, prostatitis, and benign prostatic hypertrophy.

Treatment Options

This remains controversial. NICE guidance has been issued (see earlier, NICE CG175) and there are various options:

- Active surveillance. Especially appropriate for men whose life expectancy is less than 10 years and those reluctant to face radical treatment.
- Radical (potentially curative) therapy. Surgery carries a risk of incontinence that is mild in 4% to 21% and total in up to 7%. Erectile dysfunction varies between 20% and 80%.
- Hormone therapy or orchidectomy (androgen deprivation) is indicated for noncurable disease that is not organ-confined. Early treatment in the form of androgen deprivation prolongs survival in advanced local and in metastatic disease. Hormone escape disease refers to a rising PSA despite hormonal measures. The life expectancy is about 6 months. Drug options are:
  - LHRH analogues (e.g., goserelin and leuprorelin), which can improve quality of life but not life expectancy. They may also cause hot flushes, reduced libido, erectile dysfunction, gynaecomastia, and an initial tumour flare;
  - nonsteroidal antiandrogens (e.g., flutamide and bicalutamide), which can be used as adjunctive therapy for total androgen blockade.

Urinary Stones

> **REVIEW**
>
> Holdgate, A., & Pollock, T. (2004). Nonsteroidal anti-inflammatory drugs (NSAIDs) versus opioids for acute renal colic. *The Cochrane Database of Systematic Reviews*, (2), CD004137.

> **GUIDELINE**
>
> National Institute for Health and Care Excellence. (2015). Renal or Ureteric Colic - Acute. NICE CKS. Available https://cks.nice.org.uk

- *Consider:* a family history of urinary stones, dehydration, urinary infection (especially by *Proteus*), hypercalcaemia, hyperuricaemia, and a chronic obstructive uropathy.
- *Analgesia.* Use an NSAID parenterally (e.g., diclofenac 75 mg intramuscularly). Opioids may be necessary if that fails; use morphine not pethidine.
- Check for microscopic haematuria with a dipstick. The presence of haematuria supports the diagnosis but its absence does to exclude it (NICE, 2015). The presence of nitrites suggests possible infection. Check MSU and serum urea, electrolytes, and creatinine.
- Arrange, usually by urgent referral to urology within 7 days, urgent computed tomography of kidneys, urethra, bladder (CT KUB) or USS according to local guidelines:
  - to establish the diagnosis;
  - to assess the size, position, and number of stones;
  - to look for obstruction.
- *Admit* for:
  - uncontrolled pain;
  - inability to drink adequate liquids;
  - infection;
  - complete unilateral or bilateral obstruction on intravenous urogram (IVU);
  - known renal insufficiency;
  - known to have a single kidney.
- *Refer to outpatients* all those not requiring admission.
- Instruct the patient to save any stone passed by passing urine through a filter (e.g., a woman's stocking). Send it for analysis.

Once the Patient Is Discharged From Follow-Up

- If conservative management has been chosen, support the patient with the information that 90% of small stones (<5 mm) pass spontaneously and that 50% of stones that are 5 to 10 mm in diameter also pass. Although dehydration is a risk factor for developing stones, a Cochrane review in 2012 found that no recommendations could be made with regards to water intake and prevention of urinary tract stones based on current evidence (Bao & Wei, 2012).
- Check that an attempt has been made to find a cause (i.e., serum calcium and uric acid and a 24-hour urinary calcium). If there is a family history or the patient has recurrent stones, the following should also be checked:
  - 24-hour urine for pH, oxalate, phosphate, and uric acid
  - random urine for cystine
- If an abnormality is found:
  - Treat *hypercalciuria* and calcium phosphate calculi with a low calcium diet and consider the use of bendroflumethiazide or potassium citrate.
  - Treat *hyperuricaemia* and urate calculi with allopurinol.

- Explain the importance of avoiding dehydration.
- Give dietary advice for oxalate stones (avoid chocolate, tea, rhubarb, spinach) and calcium stones (reduce amount of dairy products).

Asymptomatic Proteinuria in Men and Non Pregnant Women

> **GUIDELINE**
>
> Renal Unit, Royal Infirmary of Edinburgh (EdREN). (2010). *GP info: Proteinuria.* www.edren.org (search on "proteinuria").

Protein + or more on dipstick is likely to be significant, but false positives (40%) and negatives (<20%) for urinary tract disease occur. False positives can result from a sample being highly concentrated or alkaline, or taken after exercise, during a fever, during menstruation, or in the presence of vaginal or urethral discharge. False negatives occur in dilute or acidic urine or in non-albuminuric proteinuria.

Interpretation

- Proteinuria which is absent on waking suggests orthostatic proteinuria (but beware of diagnosing this in patients >30 years old).
- Proteinuria that disappears on repeat testing may have been idiopathic transient proteinuria, which is found particularly below the age of 20 years, or may have been associated with another medical condition (e.g., UTI or heart failure). Repeat after a further 6 months.
- Proteinuria that is intermittent but not showing one of the patterns above: investigate as for persistent proteinuria and, if no grounds for referral are found, repeat the dipstick test, blood pressure, and serum creatinine 6- to 12-monthly.
- Persistent proteinuria: investigation is needed.

Investigative Strategy if a Dipstick Shows Persistent Proteinuria + or ++

- History, including urinary tract symptoms, family history of renal disease, and medications.
- Examination, including abdomen and loins, blood pressure, weight, and oedema.
- Investigations:
  - MSU and check the dipstick for haematuria (1+ is significant)
  - Urine for albumin/creatinine ratio (ACR) to quantify the degree of proteinuria (see Appendix 26)
  - Serum urea, creatinine and electrolytes, and estimated glomerular filtration rate (eGFR)
  - Fasting blood sugar
  - Serum protein electrophoresis and urinary Bence Jones protein if other features (anaemia, bone pain) suggest myeloma or the patient is over 50 years old

Management

- *Protein +++ or more: refer promptly that day* (by telephone discussion with the nephrologists). The protein loss is likely to be heavy enough to lead to nephrotic syndrome (proteinuria >3.5 g/day or urinary albumin/creatinine ratio >300 mg/mmol).
- *Protein + or ++:* Take an MSU and confirm that there is *persisting* proteinuria with a second and a third sample 1 week apart, at least one taken on waking.
- Refer less urgently to nephrology outpatients those:
  - with a protein excretion of more than 1 g/day (consider sending a request-for-advice letter if proteinuria is between 150 mg and 1 g/day), or an albumin/creatinine ratio of greater than 120 mg/mmol, even if they have a primary condition which is likely to be the cause (e.g., diabetes);
  - with a protein excretion of 250 mg/L or an albumin/creatinine ratio of over 30 mg/mmol if they *also* have a raised creatinine or hypertension. Refer with more urgency if the creatinine is clearly rising over weeks;
  - with a decreased creatinine clearance;
  - with any proteinuria and a family history of renal disease.
- If proteinuria is present but does not meet the above criteria for referral, repeat the investigations 6-monthly until it resolves or meets those criteria. Continue to check the BP, serum creatinine, and a dipstick for haematuria.

Asymptomatic Haematuria

Visible Haematuria

- Check that it is not due to menstruation or other bleeding.
- Check the urine with a dipstick, send MSU for culture and blood for urea, creatinine, and electrolytes.
- Where the MSU is negative for red blood cells consider beeturia, obstructive jaundice, and (rarely) porphyria. However, if these are not present and repeat dipstick is still positive, believe the dipstick. Red cells may have lysed on the journey to the laboratory.
- Refer any patient with painless macroscopic haematuria urgently (via the 2-week pathway in the United Kingdom) to a urologist. The exception is haematuria during a proven UTI, which does not need further investigation provided a test for haematuria 7 days after completing antibiotics is clear. However, women aged over 40 with recurrent haematuria with UTIs, or refractory haematuria despite treating a UTI successfully, need an urgent urology referral, and men with a first UTI may also need referring even if the haematuria resolves (National Collaborating Centre for Primary Care, 2004).

Non-Visible Haematuria

- Screening is not routinely recommended (poor specificity).
- Aspirin, warfarin, etc., are not an *excuse* for haematuria.

GUIDELINE

National Institute of Health and Care Excellence (2015). Suspected Cancer: Recognition and Referral. NICE Guideline 12. Available: www.nice.org.uk

- The patient should collect an early-morning urine sample in a plain white bottle for dipstick analysis. False positives occur after exercise, during menstruation or a UTI.
- An MSU is usually not necessary in primary care to confirm the non-visible haematuria.
- A finding of 1+ or more is significant when persistent in two of three early-morning urines over 4 to 6 weeks. Almost half of these patients will have glomerular disease, the proportion rising in the younger patient (Topham et al., 1994).
- Common causes are:
  - *urologic:* BPH, prostatitis, urologic cancers (especially >40 years old) or calculi;
  - *renal:* glomerular disease is relatively more common in those under 40 years old, especially IgA nephropathy; polycystic kidney disease.

Investigative Strategy if Persistent Unexplained Microscopic Haematuria

- Always consider the history and examination. Is the patient ill or have red flags for urologic cancer? Urologic symptoms + haematuria makes a urology referral to exclude underlying pathology appropriate.
- Consider age, BP, and the presence of significant proteinuria. A renal cause is more likely if the patient is under 40 years old, is unwell, or there is proteinuria, a raised BP, or ankle oedema. Quantify the proteinuria. An albumin:creatinine ratio (ACR) over 30 mg/mmol or a protein:creatinine ratio (PCR) over 50 mg/mmol is significant.
- Assess renal function by measuring serum urea, electrolytes, creatinine, and an eGFR.
- Referral:
  - *If the patient is 60 years or older* consider urgent referral to exclude cancer if there is persistent non-visible haematuria and either dysuria or a raised white cell count on blood test.
  - If cancer is excluded, consider nephrology referral if the eGFR is persistently below 60, or the ACR is 30 mg/mmol or more, or the PCR is 50 mg/mmol or more, or the BO is 140/90 mm Hg or more.
  - If the patient is under 40 years old, consider nephrology referral with appropriate urgency if necessary if any of the factors listed are present.
- Where no cause is found after referral, monitor annually with BP, creatinine, eGFR, and an albumin:creatinine ratio (ACR) or protein:creatinine ratio (PCR) urine test. Consider urology re-referral if haematuria becomes symptomatic or macroscopic. Consider nephrology re-referral if the ACR or PCR deteriorate as above, or if the eGFR falls persistently to under 30 or falls by more than 5 per year or more than 10 per 5 years (NICE CKD clinical guideline, reference ahead).

Chronic Kidney Disease

GUIDELINES

National Institute for Health and Care Excellence. (2014). *Chronic kidney disease in adults: Assessment and management. NICE clinical guideline 182.* www.nice.org.uk.

- The incidence of CKD is rising due to an ageing population and increases in the incidence of the main causes (e.g., diabetes). There is an accompanying growing incidence of the need for renal replacement therapy (RRT) for end-stage CKD.
- Most patients with CKD are asymptomatic. Nearly half of all patients with CKD are in the stage 3A/B area, with much smaller numbers for stages 4 and 5.
- The principal causes of CKD in the United Kingdom are (from common to uncommon): diabetes mellitus, hypertension (these two cause three quarters of all CKD), vasculitis and glomerulonephritis, pyelonephritis, renovascular disease, and obstructive uropathies. Adult polycystic kidney disease (APKD), medications, and amyloidosis are less common. CKD, diabetes, and proteinuria are interlinked and are strong, independent risk factors for cardiovascular disease and increased mortality.
- Management should be based on an eGFR. The serum creatinine alone is an insensitive measurement of renal function, only becoming abnormal after considerable renal function decline. A study in primary care showed that using the eGFR increased the detection of CKD from 22% to 85% (Akbari et al., 2004). NICE guidance aims to increase the detection of CKD in at-risk groups and thus assist in reducing the rates of associated cardiovascular disease and mortality, and in identifying and referring those at risk of progression to end-stage CKD requiring RRT.
- Calculating eGFRs (mL/min/1.73 m^2):

  Use the modification of diet in renal disease (MDRD) formula based on values for creatinine, urea, and albumin; and the patient's age, race, and gender. UK labs are now routinely providing eGFRs.

  Age is never an excuse for a low eGFR. Consider the whole picture, trend, and comorbidity when considering further assessment and management.

Assessment and Management of Chronic Kidney Disease

Patients at Risk of Developing Chronic Kidney Disease

- Screen those with predisposing factors for CKD (e.g., hypertension, diabetes, cardiovascular disease, persistent haematuria or proteinuria, nephrotoxic drugs, structural renal problems or calculi, BPH, a family history of CKD stage 5, or multisystem disease [e.g., systemic lupus erythematosus (SLE)]).
- Perform annual serum creatinine, eGFR, and a PCR or ACR. NICE supports the ACR over PCR.

Action to Be Taken on Finding an eGFR Under 60 or a Normal eGFR With Other Signs of Kidney Damage

- Consider if the patient is ill, raising the suspicion of glomerulonephritis. If so, act according to the clinical picture, not just the laboratory results.
- Consider a repeat creatinine and eGFR with the patient fasted and well hydrated, off oral NSAIDs. Consider past creatinine levels to assess the stability of the result. Note that the eGFR may fall by 25% as a result of taking an angiotensin-converting enzyme (ACE) inhibitor. If giving an ACE inhibitor, monitor closely, stop if over 25% deterioration in eGFR or over 30% rise in creatinine. Such deterioration raises the possibility of renal artery stenosis.
- Beware of misinterpreting the eGFR because of the fact that serum creatinine is dependent on muscle mass. In those with high muscle mass the eGFR will be underestimated whilst in those with low muscle mass (including amputees and paraplegics) it will be overestimated. Equally, significant oedema and pregnancy cause problems with using the eGFR.
- Beware of overinterpreting eGFR changes where values are greater than 60. Look instead for a greater than 20% rise in the creatinine.
- Repeat a new finding of eGFR less than 60 in 2 weeks and ensure three eGFRs are assessed over 3 months. At least two under 60 suggest a true reduced eGFR and CKD. Consider the rate of progression and whether this is likely to be a problem, based on the patient's age and comorbidity. Significant progression is more likely if there is also significant proteinuria.
- NICE now recommends using a cystatin C-based estimation of eGFR on those who have an eGFR persistently between 45 and 59 who have no other markers of renal disease. If there are no other markers of renal disease and eGFR cystatin C is over 60, do not diagnose CKD.

- Consider renal ultrasound if there is a family history of APKD, or there are obstructive urinary symptoms, persistent haematuria, significant progression of eGFR decline, or possibly in CKD stages 4/5.
- Monitor blood and urine tests according to the CKD stage identified and in discussion with the patient (Table 19.1). Plan future monitoring to identify progression early. Most complications occur at eGFRs less than 60. Check urea, creatinine, electrolytes, eGFR, BP, and ACR or PCR at least annually. Check the calcium and phosphate in CKD stages 4/5; check the haemoglobin (Hb) in CKD stages 3B/4/5.
- Be aware that for many people CKD will not progress.

Further Management

- *Consider referral:* CKD stages 4/5 (for consideration of RRT), ACR over 70 mg/mmol or PCR over 100 mg/mmol (heavy proteinuria suggests progression and/or underlying disease), ACR over 30 mg/mmol or PCR over 50 mg/mmol with persistent haematuria (1+ on dipstick), significant eGFR deterioration (>5/year, >10/5 years), suspected renal artery stenosis or genetic kidney disease, or uncontrolled hypertension despite four antihypertensives.
- *Medications review:* Consider drugs that may be causing a reduced eGFR, and those whose dosage is affected by reduced renal function.
- Consider the need for smoking cessation and healthy lifestyle advice.
- Control hypertension to 120 to 139/<90 mm Hg (120–129/<80 mm Hg with diabetes or ACR >70 mg/mmol). Use an ACE inhibitor first line.
- Give an ACE inhibitor (or angiotensin-2 receptor antagonist) to maximal dosage if the patient has diabetes and significant microalbuminuria; or ACR over 70 mg/mmol; or CKD and hypertension and ACR over 30 mg/mmol.

TABLE 19.1 **Classification and Key Actions for Chronic Kidney Disease**

Stage of Kidney Disease	GFR (mL/min/1.73 m²)	Action
Stage 1. Evidence of kidney damage* but normal GFR	≥90	Address CVD risk factors, treat comorbidity. Monitor annually
Stage 2. Evidence of kidney damage* and mildly reduced GFR	60–89	As above. Monitor annually
Stage 3A. Moderately reduced GFR	45–59	Closer monitoring 6-monthly
Stage 3B. Moderately reduced GFR	30–44	Check for complications; treat/refer. 6-monthly monitoring
Stage 4. Severely reduced GFR	15–29	Refer to a nephrologist to consider RRT. 3-monthly monitoring
Stage 5. Established kidney failure	<15	RRT possibly indicated (haemodialysis, peritoneal dialysis, transplantation). 6-weekly monitoring

Cardiac risk can be calculated over 10 years using a validated tool such as QRisk.
*Kidney damage: persistent proteinuria, haematuria, anatomic abnormalities (e.g., polycystic or scarred), shrunken kidneys, biopsy-proven glomerulonephritis.
CVD, Chronic kidney disease; *GFR,* glomerular filtration rate; *RRT,* renal replacement therapy.
Adapted From NICE Guidance.

- Optimize the management of risk factors for CKD progression: CVD, significant proteinuria, hypertension, diabetes, smoking, chronic use of oral NSAIDs, and urinary outflow obstruction. Asian and black ethnicity are also risk factors for progression.
- Anaemia (Hb <11 g/dL), acidosis, and metabolic bone disease are all complications increasingly prevalent from CKD stage 3B downward and may require referral or primary care-initiated assessment, dependent upon local guidance. In CKD stages 3/4/5 iron deficiency anaemia is likely at ferritin levels below 100 µg/L. NICE has published guidance on anaemia in CKD, and after excluding other causes iron can be given to get the ferritin to above 200 µg/L. If this fails refer for consideration of erythropoietin therapy aiming in adults for a Hb of 10.5 to 12.5 g/dL.
- If monitoring shows an ACR over 70 mg/mmol or PCR over 100 mg/mmol no repeat is needed; this is heavy proteinuria requiring referral. However, an ACR 30 to 70 mg/mmol needs to be repeated on the first-morning sample to confirm the proteinuria. Haematuria is also grounds for referral when persistent. In diabetes an ACR over 2.5 mg/mmol in men and over 3.5 mg/mmol in women is significant and needs repeat confirmation on an early-morning ACR.

Note: The above plan assumes that the patient is not suffering from another condition that makes an active approach inappropriate.

References

Abrams, P. (1995). Managing lower urinary tract symptoms in older men. *British Medical Journal (Clinical Research Ed.), 310,* 1113–1117.

Akbari, A., Swedko, P. J., Clark, H. D., et al. (2004). Detection of chronic kidney disease with laboratory reporting of estimated glomerular filtration rate and an educational program. *Archive of Internal Medicine, 164,* 1788–1792.

Anon. (2001). Managing incontinence due to detrusor instability. *Drug and Therapeutics Bulletin, 39,* 59–64.

Anon. (2004). Duloxetine for female stress urinary incontinence. *Bandolier, 129,* 4–5. www.jr2.ox.ac.uk/bandolier.

Ball, A. J., Feneley, R. C., & Abrams, P. H. (1981). The natural history of untreated "prostatism". *British Journal of Urology, 53,* 613–616.

Bao, Y., & Wei, Q. (2012). Water for preventing urinary stones. *The Cochrane Database of Systematic Reviews,* (6), CD004292.

Brookes, S. T., Donovan, J. L., Peters, T. J., et al. (2002). Sexual dysfunction in men after treatment for lower urinary tract symptoms: Evidence from randomised controlled trial. *British Medical Journal (Clinical Research Ed.), 324,* 1059–1061.

Brumfitt, W., & Hamilton-Miller, J. M. T. (1994). Consensus viewpoint on management of urinary infections. *Journal of Antimicrobial Chemotherapy, 33,* S147–S153.

Drug Therapy Bulletin. (1998). Managing urinary tract infection in women. *Drug and Therapeutics Bulletin, 36,* 30–32.

Emberton, M., Neal, D. E., Black, N., et al. (1996). The effect of prostatectomy on symptom severity and quality of life. *British Journal of Urology, 77,* 233–247.

Foster, M. C., Upsdell, S. M., & O'Reilly, P. H. (1990). Urological myths. *British Medical Journal (Clinical Research Ed.), 301,* 1421–1423.

Haeusler, G., Leitich, H., van Trotsenburg, M., et al. (2002). Drug therapy of urinary urge incontinence: A systematic review. *Obstetrics and Gynaecology, 100,* 1003–1016.

Hendrix, S. L., Cochrane, B. B., Nygaard, I. E., et al. (2005). Effects of estrogen with and without progestin on urinary incontinence. *JAMA: The Journal of the American Medical Association, 293,* 998–1001.

Jepson, R.G., Williams, G, & Craig, J.C. (2012). Cranberries for Treating Urinary Tract Infections. *The Cochrane Database of Systematic Reviews,* (10), CD001321.

Lepor, H., Williford, W. O., Barry, M. J., et al. (1996). The efficacy of terazosin, finasteride, or both in benign prostatic hyperplasia. Veterans Affairs Cooperative Studies Benign Prostatic Hyperplasia Study Group. *The New England Journal of Medicine, 335,* 533–539.

Malone-Lee, J. G., Walsh, J. B., Maugourd, M. F., et al. (2001). Tolterodine: A safe and effective treatment for older patients with overactive bladder. *Journal of the American Geriatric Society, 49,* 700–705.

Marinkovic, S. P., Gillen, L. M., & Stanton, S. L. (2004). Managing nocturia. *British Medical Journal (Clinical Research Ed.), 328,* 1063–1066.

Markham, D. E. (2004). Cauda equina syndrome: Diagnosis, delay and litigation risk. *MDU, 20*(1), 12–15.

McConnell, J. D., Roehrborn, C. G., Bautista, O. M., et al. (2003). The long-term effects of doxazosin, finasteride, and combination therapy on clinical progression of benign prostatic hypertrophy. *The New England Journal of Medicine, 349,* 2387–2398.

MeReC. (1995). Urinary tract infection. *MeReC Bulletin, 6*(8), 29–32. (See also the *Health Protection Agency* guideline referenced at the top of Urinary Tract Infections section).

Moehrer, B., Hextall, A., & Jackson, S. (2003). Oestrogens for urinary incontinence in women. *Cochrane Database of Systematic Reviews,* (2), CD001405.

National Collaborating Centre for Primary Care. (2004). *Referral guidelines for suspected cancer; draft for second consultation.* Retrieved from www.nice.org.uk/pdf/RSC_2ndcons_Full_version.pdf.

National Institute for Health and Care Excellence. (2015). *Suspected cancer: Recognition and referral. NICE clinical guideline 12.* Retrieved from www.nice.org.uk.

O'Brian, J., & Long, H. (1995). Urinary incontinence: Long-term effectiveness of nursing intervention in primary care. *British Medical Journal (Clinical Research Ed.), 311,* 1208.

Public Health England. (2016). *PSA testing and prostate cancer: Advice for well men aged 50 and over.*

Stothers, L. (2002). A randomized trial to evaluate effectiveness and cost effectiveness of naturopathic cranberry products as prophylaxis against urinary tract infection in women. *The Canadian Journal of Urology, 9,* 1558–1562.

Topham, P. S., Harper, S. J., Furness, P. N., et al. (1994). Glomerular disease as a cause of isolated microscopic haematuria. *The Quarterly Journal of Medicine, 87,* 329–335.

US Department of Health and Human Services (1992). *Urinary incontinence in adults.* Rockville, MF: Agency for Health Care and Policy Research (AHCPR).

Wasson, J. H., Reda, D. J., Bruskewitz, R. C., et al. (1995). A comparison of transurethral surgery with watchful waiting for moderate symptoms of benign prostatic hyperplasia. The Veterans Affairs Cooperative Study Group on Transurethral Resection of the Prostate. *The New England Journal of Medicine, 332,* 75–79.

20

Ear, Nose, and Throat Problems

ADAM STATEN

CHAPTER CONTENTS

The Ear

Pain in the Ear

- Examine the external canal and drum. If these are normal then the pain is very unlikely to be due to ear disease.
- *Consider:*
  - temporomandibular (TM) joint pain;
  - dental causes;
  - cervical lymphadenopathy;
  - sinus pain;
  - mumps;
  - cervical spine pain;
  - pharyngeal tumour, oral cancer, tonsil cancer. Any unilateral ear pain with normal ear drum in a smoker should be suspicious for tonsil carcinoma.

Acute Otitis Media (AOM)

Diagnosis

- Much commoner in children, especially less than 10 years of age.
- Usually presents with acute onset of otalgia.
- Younger children may present with pyrexia, crying, irritability, and rubbing the ear.
- The tympanic membrane is red and bulging.
- There may be discharge if the tympanic membrane perforates, when the pain becomes less.
- Acute otitis media (also known as serous otitis media) should be distinguished otitis media with effusion and myringitis (rare).

Management

- Eighty-five percent of children with acute otitis media (AOM) and otalgia are free of pain within 24 hours, without antibiotics (van Buchem, Dunk, & Van't Hof, 1981).
- It can be caused by viruses or bacteria.
- Most patients do not need antibiotics as symptoms usually resolve within a few days.
- Antibiotics reduce pain and fever at 3 to 7 days in infants and children under 2 years old and in those with bilateral AOM (Rovers et al., 2006). They reduce the risk of developing contralateral AOM but have no effect on pain in the first 2 days, and no effect on the incidence of deafness at 1 month.
- If an antibiotic is required, the recommended first line is amoxicillin for 5 days. If there is penicillin allergy then use erythromycin or clarithromycin.
- Writing a prescription for antibiotics but suggesting to the parents that they only use it if the otitis media has not resolved in 3 days can reduce the number taking antibiotics to a quarter with only minor delay in the resolution of symptoms. Parents given a delayed prescription are less likely to believe that they need to consult a doctor in future episodes (Little et al., 2001).
- Pain and fever should be managed with paracetamol or a nonsteroidal anti-inflammatory drug (NSAID; e.g., ibuprofen).

- Antibiotics should be considered in patients who are systemically unwell, those whose symptoms are not improving after 4 days, children under 2 years of age with bilateral AOM, and children with perforation and/or discharge in the canal.
- In older children discuss with the parents the question of whether to prescribe an antibiotic. Explain that the evidence suggests that it is unlikely to be of benefit unless the AOM is bilateral or there is otorrhoea. Recommend watchful waiting or prescribe amoxicillin, suggesting that they only use it if symptoms persist after 3 days.
- If a tympanostomy tube is in place, give antibiotics more readily. They can more than halve the duration of the illness (from 8 to 3 days) with an number needed to treat (NNT) of 3 for freedom from discharge at 1 week (Ruohola et al., 2003). Use a topical drop such as ciprofloxacin first rather than oral antibiotics and if no help use a topical drop and oral antibiotics for 1 week before considering referral to ENT emergency clinic for review.
- Review in 4 to 6 weeks for deafness and/or effusion. Half of all children will have an effusion at 1 month and 10% will have an effusion at 3 months. Persistent fluid is not an indication for further antibiotic treatment (van Buchem et al., 1981).

Referral to ENT

- Children younger than 3 months with a temperature of 38°C or more.
- Suspected complications such as mastoiditis or meningitis or facial nerve palsy.
- The patient has five or more attacks of AOM in one winter, or six or more in 1 year.

Acute Otitis Media Prevention

- Avoid cigarette smoke exposure (Strachan & Cook, 1998).
- Encourage breastfeeding.
- Feed upright where possible.

Mastoiditis

- Admit any patient with:
  - tenderness, redness, or oedema over the mastoid, or a new onset of a protruding ear;
  - vertigo, vomiting, increasing deafness, and nystagmus; or
  - acute otitis media with continuing fever despite antibiotics.

Acute Furunculosis of the External Canal

- Early cases respond to antibiotic/corticosteroid drops.
- Surrounding cellulitis needs oral antibiotics as well (e.g., flucloxacillin or erythromycin).
- Exclude diabetes.

Bloody Discharge (Bullous Myringitis)

The patient usually suffers severe pain followed by bleeding. A number of serosanguinous bullae appear on the tympanic membrane or surrounding skin.

- Prescribe adequate analgesia and advise the patient to keep the canal dry.

- Reserve broad-spectrum antibiotics for patients with middle ear effusions (Marais & Dale, 1997).
- Consider topical drops containing steroids to reduce inflammation & therefore pain.
- Refer if the patient suffers persisting pain or hearing loss (Biedlingmaier, 1994).

Herpes Zoster (Ramsay Hunt Syndrome)

As well as a vesicular eruption of the auricle or external auditory meatus, the patient may develop facial palsy or hearing loss and vertigo.

- Treat as for shingles anywhere, with oral acyclovir and adequate analgesia.
- Arrange urgent (on-call) review by ENT for consideration of IV anti-virals particularly if their is any VII or VIII nerve dysfunction.

Discharge From the Ear

Otitis Externa

- Otitis externa is inflammation of the skin of the external auditory canal. Itch is a common presenting symptom.
- Common predisposing factors are abuse of the ear with cotton buds and any scaling skin disorder (e.g., eczema, psoriasis).
- Discharge may be purulent but not mucopurulent. Muco-purulent discharge orignates in the middle ear, not the external ear.
- The principles of management:
  - Correct predisposing factors.
  - Topical steroids are effective in dermatitis from cotton bud abuse. Hydrocortisone cream applied by the tip of a finger is often effective and can be reused inter-mittently if symptoms recur.
  - If there is profuse discharge, prescribe ear drops con-taining antibacterial agents and steroid (van Balen et al., 2003). If treatment is still needed after 1 week, change to steroid drops alone.
  - Tell the patient that recurrence is likely if the ear canal is scratched, cotton buds are used, or water enters the canal. When contact with water is unavoidable (e.g., showering), the meatus should be plugged with cotton wool impregnated with petroleum jelly.
  - Make sure that patients prone to recurrent attacks have appropriate medication at home to use at the onset of symptoms.
- If the canal is severely swollen:
  - Refer for the insertion of an antibiotic/corticosteroid wick or insert 0.5-inch ribbon gauze soaked in steroid cream. Change it every 24–48 hours.
  - Give oral antibiotics if there is cellulitis of the sur-rounding tissues.

Refractory Otitis Externa

- This is more likely if there is a history of eczema or sebor-rhoeic dermatitis. It is usually due to undiagnosed *Candida* or *Aspergillus* infection and may follow prolonged use of topical antibiotics. The canal is filled with blackish spots or brownish-cream deposits.
- Swab for bacteria and fungi.
- Consider the need for microsuction and referral to ENT.
- Treat with clotrimazole solution 1% instilled three times a day and continued for 14 days after the disappearance of obvious infection.

Malignant Otitis Externa

- This is an uncommon condition where infection spreads into the bone of the mastoid and base of skull.
- Patients present with pain more severe than expected from examination.
- It is most commonly presents in older diabetics or immu-nocomprimised, and pseudomonas is the most common pathogen.
- Suspected cases should be referred urgently as it is poten-tially fatal and requires specialist management.

Chronic Otitis Media (COM)

- Chronic otitis media (COM) can be active or inactive:
  - Active COM has inflammation and mucopurulent discharge.
  - Inactive COM has a perforation or a retraction pocket with no discharge.
- There are two main types of chronic otitis media: mucosal and squamous.

Mucosal Chronic Otitis Media

- There is a perforation of the tympanic membrane.
- If active, ideally the discharge should be cleaned by micro-suction or by mopping with cotton wool.
- Topical antibiotics are more effective than systemic anti-biotics in the management of active COM (Macfadyen, Acuin, & Gamble, 2006).
- Although manufacturers advise against using topical prepa-rations containing aminoglycosides in the presence of a perforation, the consensus opinion of ENT-UK is that antibiotics such as gentamicin can be used in active COM but for a maximum of 2 weeks (Phillips et al., 2007).
- Cases where otorrhoea does not settle and cases where there is recurrence of otorrhoea should be referred to a specialist. Surgery to close the perforation (*tympanoplasty*) is often very effective management.

Squamous Chronic Otitis Media—Cholesteatoma

- In squamous chronic otitis media there is a retraction pocket into the middle ear and mastoid with collection of squamous debris. In simple terms, this is skin growing into the middle ear with the accumulation of dead skin cells. The debris gets infected, which causes inflammation and erosion of surrounding tissues.
- The potential complications are hearing loss, facial palsy, meningitis, and intracranial abscess.
- The only effective treatment for active squamous chronic otitis media is surgery. This usually entails some form of mastoid surgery.

- All cases of suspected cholesteatoma should be referred to a specialist.

Hearing Loss

- At least one-third of patients over 70 and half of patients over 80 have hearing loss severe enough to be helped by a hearing aid (i.e., roughly a 35-decibel [dB] hearing loss at speech frequencies).
- All hearing-impaired people, particularly the elderly, may become isolated, depressed, and difficult to live with (Hickish, 1989).
- Hearing loss is:
  - sensorineural (lesion of the inner ear or of cranial nerve VIII); or
  - conductive (middle or outer ear).
- The appearance of the ear is an effective guide to the type of hearing loss.

Sensorineural Hearing Loss

- Examine the drum and remove any wax that may be contributing.
- Refer patients with:
  - *unilateral hearing loss of acute onset.* If the patient is seen within 3 days of onset, arrange for outpatient assessment within 24 hours. All patients with sudden sensorineural hearing loss should receive steroids (under specialist guidance).
  - *unilateral hearing loss with a longer history.* Referral is less urgent, but the patient may have a treatable cause (e.g., acoustic neuroma).
- Be active in detecting hearing loss and encourage patients to consider a hearing aid.
- All patients who have noticeable hearing difficulty during consultation should be referred to audiology.
- The whispered voice test is useful for assessing the significance of hearing impairment, particularly in those who think their hearing is fine (Swan & Browning, 1985).
- Refer patients for a hearing aid early rather than late, and encourage them to persevere with it once supplied. Hearing-impaired patients lose the ability to discriminate between sounds and so have to relearn this skill. They may take some time to get the full benefit from an aid. One follow-up in the United Kingdom at between 8 and 16 years found that fewer than half were still using an aid (Gianopoulos, Stephens, & Davis, 2002).

Conductive Hearing Loss

- Assume that all conductive deafness is treatable. This is true whether the drum looks normal, as in otosclerosis, or abnormal, as in middle ear effusion or COM.
- Examine the ear canal and tympanic membrane.
- *If wax is present and occluding the ear canal* it may be contributing to the hearing loss, although removal of wax only raises the hearing threshold by more than 10 dB in one-third (Memel et al., 2002):

- Syringe if the wax is soft.
- Disimpact hard wax with a wax hook, then syringe the rest if necessary.
- Instill drops (tap water is as effective as anything) and syringe after waiting for at least 15 minutes (Browning, 2005; Hand & Harvey, 2004).
- Suggest that the patient instills ear drops into the ear canal for 3 to 7 nights and then re-attends for syringing. Instillation of either an oil-based or a water-based solvent for 1 week will clear wax in 20% of patients (Keane et al., 1995) and facilitate syringing in the others. There is no evidence of the superiority of commercial drops over water or sodium bicarbonate (Burton & Doree, 2009).
- Refer all patients with conductive hearing loss not due to wax.

Otitis Media With Effusion (OME)

Fluid in the middle ear without signs or symptoms of inflammation can result in hearing loss.

Children

- This is also known as secretory otitis media, or glue ear.
- Half of affected children resolve spontaneously within 3 months (American Academy of Pediatrics, 1997). However, 2% to 3% of children under 7 have a more prolonged hearing loss due to OME and need specialist assessment.
- A period of 3 months of watchful waiting is appropriate.
- Even those having specialist assessment are unlikely to be helped by surgery, the benefits of which are only temporary. Watchful waiting and immediate pre-surgery testing may reduce inappropriate surgery (NHS Centre for Reviews and Dissemination, 1994). For instance, ventilation tubes (grommets) improve hearing 6 months after insertion but very little after 12 months. Adenoidectomy is recommended with the second set of ventilation tubes and has been shown to prolong the disease free time period before recurrence. Adenoidectomy improves hearing, but for only up to 2 years. Tonsillectomy and/or myringotomy does not help hearing.
- OME is more common in children whose parents smoke in the same room.
- *Antibiotics.* There may be some benefit from antibiotics in the short term but the effect is small, not maintained, and outweighed by side effects (Scottish Intercollegiate Guidelines Network [SIGN], 2003).
- Antihistamines and decongestants, orally or topically, are of no value and may cause harm (Griffin & Flynn, 2011).
- *Steroids.* They are not recommended. There is evidence that oral steroids lead to quicker resolution of OME in the short term but there is no evidence of longer term benefit (Simpson et al., 2010). There is no evidence of benefit from topical intranasal steroids (Simpson et al., 2010).

- Refer to the community audiology service to determine:
  - severity;
  - that the hearing loss is conductive;
  - the overall disability.
- Refer direct to ENT outpatients if hearing loss is:
  - persistent (i.e., more than 3 months); or
  - severe (i.e., a hearing loss >25 dB or the child is having difficulties with hearing, speech, learning, or social functioning because of it); and
  - associated with persistent pain.
- If a child has other disabilities, refer if there is any degree of hearing loss because normal hearing is crucial.

Adults

- OME may follow an upper respiratory tract infection (URTI) or barotrauma.
- Prescribe ephedrine nose drops to be instilled into the nasopharynx twice daily for 5 days and followed by auto-inflation with a Valsalva manoeuvre after 15 minutes.
- Prescribe a steroid nasal spray if there is generalized rhinitis.
- Refer if the effusion persists for more than 6 weeks. A nasopharyngeal tumour must be excluded, especially in Chinese patients.

Ventilation Tubes (Grommets)

- The majority of ventilation tubes are extruded in 3 to 9 months, and only need to be reinserted if hearing loss recurs.
- Discharge should be treated by aural toilet and antibiotic/corticosteroid drops (see mucosal chronic otitis media).
- Swimming and bathing pose no significant risk but diving should be banned.

Hearing Tests

The Whispered Voice Test

This is a good screening test and is easily performed (Eekhof et al., 1996) with 90% to 100% sensitivity and 70% to 87% specificity in adults. In children the sensitivity is slightly less but the specificity is higher (Pirozzo, Papinczak, & Glasziou, 2003).

1. Cover one of the patient's ears with a finger in the meatus. Move it gently to and fro to mask the whisper in that ear.
2. Stand at arms' length with your head behind the patient's other ear.
3. Two correct responses are required to pass. Whisper, then ask the patient to repeat what he or she has heard: for children under 6 years old use familiar terms (e.g., "bread and butter" or "Father Christmas"); for children over 6 years old use multisyllabic numbers (e.g., "362").

Dizziness

Diagnosis in dizziness comes mainly from history. Examination is mainly to support diagnosis. Investigations are usually not necessary. It is important to distinguish between vertigo, unsteadiness, and the sensation of lightheadedness.

Vertigo

Vertigo is the illusion of movement of the subject or of their surroundings, most commonly rotatory.

Episodic

- *Vertigo lasting only a few seconds or minutes* indicates a short-lived depression or stimulation of the labyrinth or central connections. It is present on sudden changes in posture commonly due to benign paroxysmal positional vertigo (BPPV; see upcoming discussion).
- *Vertigo lasting a few minutes to a few hours* indicates a physiological or metabolic disturbance of the labyrinth. It occurs in Ménière disease.

Prolonged

Vertigo lasting more than 24 hours. The clinical picture is of severe incapacitating vertigo associated with nausea and vomiting, and is due to:

- peripheral vestibular pathology or deficit, usually vestibular neuronitis, in which there is no hearing loss (Cooper, 1993) or Ménière's;
- a central cause usually associated with other signs, as in multiple sclerosis, stroke, a posterior fossa tumour, or secondary deposits in the brain stem.

Examination

The following should be included when relevant:

- Taking the patient's temperature and testing for neck stiffness in the acute attack
- Inspection of the ear drums for acute or chronic otitis media
- Testing for (or at least enquiring about) hearing loss in acute vertigo or possible vestibular schwannoma
- Looking for nystagmus (In peripheral lesions the nystagmus will be horizontal with the fast phase toward the healthy side. Looking toward that side will increase the amplitude of the nystagmus. In central lesions the nystagmus may be horizontal, vertical, or rotatory.)
- Looking for other neurological signs, especially cerebellar and cranial nerve signs and papilloedema, as in vestibular schwannoma or other central lesions. Rhomberg and Unterberger tests should be performed.

Treatment

Acute Vertigo

- Give prochlorperazine 12.5 mg intramuscularly followed by 25 mg suppositories 8-hourly until the vomiting stops. Continue with prochlorperazine 5 to 10 mg three times a day orally for a few days only. Longer term use delays recovery in acute vertigo.

Recurrent Vertigo

Treatment should be directed at encouraging central compensation.

- *Labyrinthine sedatives* such as prochlorperazine delay central compensation so should only be used as required for symptom relief.
- Compensation may occur naturally, especially in younger people, but can be accelerated by vestibular rehabilitation exercises. One study in primary care found that two 30-minute sessions tripled the number of patients who improved (Yardley et al., 1998).

Vestibular Rehabilitation Exercises

- *In bed*, performed slowly initially then more rapidly:
  - *eye movements*—up and down, side to side, focusing on a finger as it moves from 1 m away to 30 cm away;
  - *head movements*—moving head forward then backward and turning from side to side.
- *Sitting:* rotating the head; bending down and standing up with eyes open and closed.
- *Standing:* throwing a small ball from hand to hand, turning through 360 degrees.
- *Moving about:* walking across the room, up and down a slope, up and down stairs with eyes open and then closed.

PATIENT INFORMATION

Dizziness and Balance Problems is available from British Brain & Spine Foundation, Lincoln House, Kennington Park, 1-3 Brixton Road, London SW9 6DE, helpline 0808 808 1000, www.brainandspine.org.uk.

Ménière's Disease

- It is often confused with vertiginous migraine (which should be treated as per normal migraine guidelines). Patients with migraine have no hearing loss and the vertigo usually lasts hours. It is often associated with other symptoms of migraine but these may be absent.
- This is characterized by episodic vertigo associated with hearing loss, tinnitus, and often a feeling of aural fullness. Symptoms are usually unilateral and vary in severity. In the early years hearing improves between attacks, but in the long term, hearing loss becomes permanent. Some people develop bilateral disease.
- A patient with the condition who drives must inform the Driver and Vehicle Licensing Agency (DVLA). Driving will be permitted once symptoms are controlled.

Refer to an ENT Consultant

- To confirm diagnosis
- To exclude a vestibular schwannoma in patients with persistent unilateral symptoms

Medical Treatment: Acute

- No randomized controlled trials (RCTs) exist for acute management with betahistine, benzodiazepines, or anticholinergics.

- Betahistine is commonly used but a Cochrane review concluded that there was no evidence that it is effective or ineffective in patients with Ménière's disease or syndrome (James & Burton, 2001), and a more recent RCT showed betahistine to be no better than placebo (Adrion et al., 2016).
- *Acute attacks:* Give a labyrinthine sedative (e.g., prochlorperazine 5 mg three times a day or cinnarizine 30 mg three times a day). Buccastem is useful in patients with vomiting.
- *Recurrent attacks:* Betahistine 16 mg three times a day is often given but the evidence shows that it is no better than placebo (Adrion et al., 2016).
- *Poor response:* Consider referral to ENT. Treatment in unresponsive cases is intratympanic therapy:
  - intratympanic gentamicin: usually effective but risk to remaining hearing (Pullens & van Benthem, 2011); or
  - intratympanic steroids: unproven but no risk to hearing.

Prophylactic

- There is no evidence for prophylactic management of Ménière's disease or syndrome (James & Thorp, 2001). Reducing dietary salt and caffeine is often recommended; there is no scientific evidence, but it is sensible medical advice nowadays in the Western world. There is no evidence that use of diuretics is effective (Burgess & Kundu, 2006).

PATIENTS' ORGANIZATION

The Ménière's Society, The Rookery, Surrey Hills Business Park, Wotton, Dorking, Surrey, RH5 6QT, UK, helpline 01306876883, www.menieres.org.uk.

Benign Paroxysmal Positional Vertigo (BPPV)

GUIDELINE

Strickland, C., & Russell, R. (2003). What is the best way to manage benign paroxysmal positional vertigo? *Journal of Family Practice, 52*, 971–973.

- The vertigo lasts 5 to 10 seconds, though patients commonly think it lasts much longer.
- The vertigo is brought on by head movement, typically turning to one side in bed.
- This condition is diagnosed from the history and by performing the Hallpike test (Lempert, Gresty, & Bronstein, 1995).
- It is thought to be caused by debris in the semicircular canals, most commonly in the posterior canal (95%).

The Hallpike Test

Before performing the Hallpike Test check for back or neck problems and advise that the patient should not drive home afterwards.

1. Sit the patient on a couch, hold the patient's head in both hands, and turn it 45 degrees toward the test ear. Support the neck and, maintaining torsion along with fixed gaze, move head rapidly backward to a head-hanging position, 30 degrees (optimally) below the horizontal.
2. Maintain the head-hanging position for 30 seconds and observe the patient's eyes. Typically nystagmus is rotatory with the upper pole going to the downmost ear.
3. Return the patient to the upright position.
4. Test the opposite side if no nystagmus is seen on the first side or when the patient has settled from the first test. *Note:* The nystagmus may only last a few seconds and will not occur at all in some patients, in whom the diagnosis must be made on the history alone. Note also that the patient will experience vertigo at the same time as the nystagmus.

Management of BPPV

- Do not give labyrinthine sedatives.
- Teach the patient to minimize the vertigo by sitting up or lying down in stages.
- The Epley (canalith repositioning) manoeuvre is a safe and effective treatment for BPPV (Hilton & Pinder, 2004). It involves a brief series of exercises to reposition debris out of the posterior canal.
- The Epley manoeuvre can be completed in less than 5 minutes and does not require specialist training. Explanatory videos are available on YouTube (e.g., www.youtube .com/watch?v=ZqokxZRbJfw).
- Explain that many patients (about 35%) have recurrence of symptoms.
- Patients should not drive for 24 hours afterwards.

Instructions for Performance of the Modified Epley Manoeuvre

These instructions are for a patient whose left ear is affected. If it is the right ear that is affected, for left read right and for right read left.

1. Sit up on the bed with your head turned 45 degrees to the left, having placed a pillow on the bed so that it will be under your shoulders, not your head, when you lie down.
2. Lie back quickly, keeping your head turned as before. Wait 30 seconds.
3. Turn your head to the other side. Wait 30 seconds.
4. Roll on to your right side. Wait 30 seconds.
5. Sit up without rolling over on to your back (i.e., still facing right).
6. Repeat this three times a day until the symptoms have ceased.

Unsteadiness

Episodic

- Unsteadiness lasting a few seconds indicates a physiological overload of the vestibular or central systems. It occurs most frequently on rapid movement, associated with a minor inadequacy of the proprioceptive or labyrinthine systems. In young people it occurs in the later stages of recovery after head injury, and in the elderly after standing or turning rapidly.
- Unsteadiness lasting hours or days is due to temporary impairment of the central connections or decompensation of the vestibular system. It commonly occurs with alcohol or drug overdose, normal doses of tranquillizers or sedatives, and hyperventilation.

Prolonged

Unsteadiness lasting weeks or months is usually due to central or vestibular inadequacy, and is common in the elderly.

Lightheadedness

Patients with lightheadedness often report a momentary sensation of spinning; this does not mean that the vestibular system is the cause of their symptoms.

Tinnitus

> **GUIDELINES**
>
> Guidelines are available from the British Tinnitus Association, www.tinnitus.org.uk.

- Generally 1% to 2% of the population has tinnitus that severely affects the quality of life.
- Reassure the patient that 15% of people experience tinnitus. For most, it improves with time. Worry about it can lead to a vicious circle of increasing distress and more intrusive tinnitus.
- Exclude a drug cause (e.g., aspirin, NSAIDs, quinine, loop diuretics, tricyclics, aminoglycosides).
- Perform a hearing test. Hearing loss is often a cause of tinnitus.
- Refer patients with:
  - tinnitus associated with hearing loss. Hearing aids are often helpful;
  - unilateral tinnitus, for exclusion of cerebellopontine angle tumours, especially if there is hearing loss on the same side;
  - neck and skull bruits (carotid artery stenosis or arteriovenous [AV] fistula);
  - tinnitus severe enough to need specialist help;
  - tinnitus associated with systemic or neurological disease.

Treatment

- Non-specific support and counselling are very helpful.
- Look for depression associated with tinnitus and treat it in its own right. Suicide is known as a consequence of depression and tinnitus. There is no evidence that antidepressants are helpful in the treatment of tinnitus (Baldo et al., 2012).
- *Amplification:* A hearing aid may be used to amplify ordinary background noise.
- Encourage the patient to mask the tinnitus with background noise such as TV, radio, music.

- *Tinnitus retraining therapy* (TRT): This combines directive counselling with sound therapy to reduce the attention that the patient pays to the tinnitus. There is evidence that this is more effective than tinnitus maskers (Phillips & McFerran, 2010).
- *Cognitive behavioural therapy* (CBT) does not change the subjective loudness of tinnitus but has a significant improvement in depression scores and quality of life (Martinez Devesa, Perera, Theodoulou, & Waddell, 2010). Refer if this is available locally, with a careful explanation that this does not mean you think the tinnitus is imaginary.

Facial Palsy (Lower Motor Neurone)

Refer urgently if there is evidence of:
- middle ear disease, especially cholesteatoma;
- parotid tumour;
- cerebellopontine angle tumour (i.e., hearing loss, loss of facial sensation, diplopia, or cerebellar signs);
- trauma;
- Ramsay Hunt syndrome (look for herpetic vesicles on the pinna or in the external auditory canal).

Bell's Palsy

OVERVIEW

Davenport, R.J., McKinstry, B., Morrison, J.M., et al. (2009). Bell's palsy: New evidence provides a definitive drug therapy strategy. *British Journal of General Practitioner*, 59, 569–570.

- Characterized by a unilateral facial weakness. The weakness may be associated with mild pain behind the ear. The onset is typically hours. It is more common in pregnant women, in those with diabetes, and following a recent upper respiratory infection.
- The majority recover without treatment.

Referral

- If loss of power is complete, refer to an ophthalmic surgeon to be seen that day. Tarsorrhaphy is likely to be needed.
- If the eyelid, when closed, does not cover the cornea. Refer to an ophthalmic surgeon.
- If recovery has not started at 6 weeks. Refer to an ENT surgeon to look for an underlying cause.
- If recovery at 9 months is incomplete. The patient may benefit from cosmetic surgery.

Management in Primary Care

- *Protect the eye* with a patch and/or artificial tears. Warn the patient that the eye is not protected by reflex blinking and must be safeguarded. This is especially true in windy, dry conditions and during sleep.
- *Give oral prednisolone.* Early treatment with prednisolone significantly improves the chance of complete recovery at 3 and 9 months (Sullivan et al., 2007). Give 50 mg/day for 10 days provided it can be started within 72 hours of the onset of the palsy.
- *Antiviral treatment:* There is low-quality evidence that antivirals used in addition to steroids might further improve the recovery rate (Gagyor et al., 2015). Antivirals alone are not helpful.
- *Physiotherapy* has no benefit (Teixeira, Valbuza, & Prado, 2011).
- *Surgical decompression* of the nerve is not indicated. There is insufficient evidence that it is beneficial (McAllister et al., 2013).

The Nose

Rhinosinusitis

GUIDELINES AND REVIEWS

Fokkens, W. J., Lund, V. J., Mullol, J., Bachert, C., et al. (2012). European Position Paper on rhinosinusitis and nasal polyps. *Rhinology*, 50 (23), 1–299.

- Diagnosis is usually clinical.
- X-rays are not recommended. CT is investigation of choice.

Management of Acute Rhinosinusitis

- Most cases are viral.
- *Decongestants* (topical or oral) are used widely but there are no studies to support their use.
- *Antibiotics.* A Cochrane review concluded that there is no place for antibiotics in uncomplicated acute rhinosinusitis as the incidence of side effects of treatment outweighed the minimal benefits (Lemiengre et al., 2012). The *Drug Therapy Bulletin* (2009) recommends a policy of no routine antibiotics or of delayed prescribing. Immediate antibiotics should be reserved for those who are systemically very unwell or are at risk of complications.
- Advise the patient to:
  - take simple analgesics;
  - use steam inhalations;
  - nasal douche;

- While there is no evidence for decongestants, they may aide symptomatic relief in short term. Only use for 7 days.
- Consider an antibiotic in those with (Fokkens et al., 2012):
  - pyrexia above 38°C;
  - severe local pain, mainly on one side;
  - worsening discomfort with purulent discharge.
- *Refer urgently:*
  - patients with orbital or facial cellulitis;
  - patients who are severely ill.

Management of Chronic Rhinosinusitis

- Examine the anterior nasal cavity. Refer any unilateral obstruction as suspicious for malignancy.
- Intranasal steroids give some improvement in the symptoms in chronic rhinosinusitis (Chong et al., 2016).
- Start treatment with intranasal steroids. Treat any underlying cause or allergy. Maintain treatment for at least 2 months and assess efficacy.
- Consider referral in patients with recurrent symptoms.
- A single course of antibiotics may be warranted but repeated courses of antibiotics are not indicated (Royal College of Surgeons, 2016).

Nasal Polyps

> **GUIDELINE**
>
> Scadding, G. K., Durham, S. R., Mirakian, R., et al. (2008). British Society for Allergy and Clinical Immunology guidelines for the management of rhinosinusitis and nasal polyposis. *Clinical & Experimental Allergy, 38*, 260–275.

- Nasal polyps may be associated with asthma and aspirin sensitivity, but if they occur in the presence of rhinitis it is probably coincidental.
- The initial treatment should be medical.
- Cystic fibrosis should be considered in any child under 16 with nasal polyps.
- Stop aspirin and consider stopping other NSAIDs; there is some cross-reaction.
- *Steroids.* Give betamethasone drops 0.1%, 2 drops per nostril three times a day using the head upside down position (see patient leaflet), alone or with oral prednisolone (0.5 mg/kg for 5–10 days). Significant improvement may occur within 48 hours. Some patients need indefinite prophylaxis with intranasal mometasone or fluticasone, which have lower bioavailability than betamethasone drops. The evidence for oral steroids comes from a single small trial of poor quality (Patiar & Reece, 2009).
- Give antibiotics if nasal discharge is purulent. Thick, green-brown secretions may indicate fungal infection. This is more likely to be detected on microscopy than by culture.
- The British Society for Allergy and Clinical Immunology (BSACI) guidelines (above) recommend that all new presentations be referred to ENT.

Malignancy

A polyp that does not have the typical smooth, pale, or slightly reddened appearance may be malignant, especially if unilateral. Refer urgently.

> **PATIENT LEAFLET**
>
> Nasal polyps. Available at www.patient.co.uk (search on "nasal polyps").

The Common Cold

- A consultation about the common cold is an opportunity for the education of the patient in self-treatment as well as discussion of any underlying issues.
- There is some evidence that oral over-the-counter medications containing antihistamines, decongestants, analgesics, or a combination help with recovery (De Sutter et al., 2012).
- Oral first-generation antihistamines will slightly reduce rhinorrhoea and sneezing in the first 1 to 2 days but with anticholinergic adverse effects, especially sedation (De Sutter, Saraswat, & van Driel, 2015).
- Ipratropium bromide nasal spray will probably reduce rhinorrhoea (AlBalawi, Othman, & AlFaleh, 2013).
- Steam inhalations give subjective benefit but there is no evidence of objective benefit (Singh & Singh, 2013).
- Regular use of oral vitamin C appears to reduce the duration and severity of symptoms (Hemilä & Chalker, 2013).
- There is no good evidence that echinacea improves symptoms (Karsch-Völk, 2014).
- There is no evidence that antibiotics are of benefit for purulent nasal discharge (Kenealy & Arroll, 2013).

Rhinitis

> **GUIDANCE**
>
> Bousquet, J., Reid, J., van Weel, C., et al. (2008). Allergic rhinitis management pocket reference. *Allergy, 63*, 990–996.
>   Scadding, G. K., Durham, S. R., Mirakian, R., et al. (2008). British Society for Allergy and Clinical Immunology guidelines for the management of allergic and non-allergic rhinitis. *Clinical and Experimental Allergy, 38*, 19–42.

Seasonal and Perennial Rhinitis

- Affects 15% to 20% of the population; 3% of general practitioner (GP) consultations are for allergic rhinitis.
- Treatment is best tailored to the individual's symptoms; where possible identify the underlying cause.
- Allergens should be avoided where possible (e.g., by reducing the dust in the house or driving with windows and air vents closed). However, measures to reduce exposure to the house dust mite have been disappointing (Terreehorst et al., 2003).

Intermittent Mild Symptoms or Acute Response to Allergen

- Antihistamines reduce the nasal itching, watery hypersecretion, and sneezing but do little for nasal blockage (Pearlman et al., 1995). Intermittent use may be enough.
- Use an antihistamine nasal spray for rapid relief (Ratner et al., 1998).
- Use an oral, minimally sedating H_1-selective antihistamine with a rapid onset (e.g., loratadine) for nasal and non-nasal symptoms.

Regular Symptoms

- Antihistamines may be taken regularly, and for some people are all that is necessary.
- Intranasal steroid sprays are the most effective prophylactic treatment. There is a delayed onset of action of at least 1 week. Combining them with an antihistamine adds no further benefit (Weiner, Abramson, & Puy, 1998).
- Instruct the patient on their proper use:
  - Use once or twice a day, according to manufacturers' instructions.
  - In seasonal rhinitis, start 2 weeks before the beginning of the season.
  - They should be continued until the rhinitis is likely to have subsided.
- Consider an ipratropium nasal spray, in addition to steroids, where rhinorrhoea is dominant (Sheikh, Panesar, & Dhami, 2005).
- *Use sodium cromoglycate eye drops* regularly in patients with allergic conjunctivitis.
- Consider referral to an allergy specialist.

Nasal Blockage

- Use a topical decongestant (e.g., ephedrine nasal drops or xylometazoline spray for 5 days) to open the airway enough for the steroid spray to penetrate. Longer use is likely to lead to rebound congestion on stopping.
- Use betamethasone nasal drops 0.1%. For greatest effect the patient should use these in the head-down position (for more information see leaflet on nasal polyps, earlier). Insert 2 drops two to three times a day for no more than 1 month. More prolonged use can lead to systemic side effects. Do not give more than six courses a year. Try to maintain improvement after each course with a steroid spray.

Severe Symptoms

- Oral steroids can be given if symptoms warrant them (e.g., at the time of an examination), but courses should not be repeated frequently. Give oral prednisolone 5 to 10 mg daily, or 30 to 40 mg daily for 1 week in dire situations. Intramuscular depot injections of steroids (e.g., Kenalog) last for 3 months, with the inevitable pituitary adrenal suppression, and are not recommended for use in rhinitis.
- Referral is needed for continuing severe symptoms. Nasal endoscopy may reveal pathology (e.g., a polyp), which was not otherwise visible. In addition, patients with nasal deformity may benefit from surgery.

Snoring and Obstructive Sleep Apnoea (OSA)

GUIDELINES

Scottish Intercollegiate Guidelines Network. (2003). *Management of obstructive sleep apnoea/hypopnoea syndrome in adults. SIGN guideline 73.* www.sign.ac.uk.
    National Institute for Health and Care Excellence. (2008). *Continuous positive airway pressure for the treatment of obstructive sleep apnoea/hypopnoea syndrome.* www.nice.org.uk.

- Of middle-age men, 25% are snorers; 10% of middle-aged women snore; 4% of middle-aged men and 2% of middle-aged women suffer from OSA, with at least five episodes of apnoea/hypopnoea an hour at night plus daytime sleepiness (Young et al., 1993).
- Men under 65 who admit to both snoring and daytime sleepiness are twice as likely to die as men with just one of these symptoms and men without either symptom. The excess deaths are mainly due to cardiovascular disease (Lindberg et al., 1998).
- Those with moderate to severe obstructive sleep apnoea (OSA) hypopnoea syndrome (OSAHS) or with mild OSAHS and daytime sleepiness are likely to be offered continuous positive airways pressure (CPAP) as therapy of first choice.
- Assess daytime sleepiness with the Epworth Sleepiness Scale. Alternatively, patients can score themselves on the British Snoring and Sleep Apnoea Association website (see upcoming information) (Table 20.1).
- Refer to a sleep study centre (or possibly directly to ENT) patients:
  - with excessive daytime sleepiness;
  - where a partner reports apnoeic or choking episodes or restless sleep;
  - where loud snoring is causing relationship problems; or
  - where curable pathology in the nose could be contributing (e.g., polyps or a deviated septum).

TABLE 20.1   Symptoms and Signs in Obstructive Sleep Apnoea

Symptoms	Signs
Loud snoring	Obesity
Restless sleep with recurrent wakening; nightmares	Sinusitis
Daytime fatigue or poor concentration; sleepiness; irritability	Nasal or nasopharyngeal obstruction
Family history of OSA	Large tonsils Large tongue Small chin

- Be especially ready to refer urgently patients:
  - with obstructive sleep apnoea/hypopnoea and COPD;
  - with evidence of ventilatory failure;
  - who are symptomatic and drive or operate machinery.

Driving

- When OSA is only suspected, warn the patient not to drive when feeling sleepy and not to embark on a drive if very prone to feeling sleepy.
- If the diagnosis is confirmed, the patient should inform the DVLA and insurance company. Driving will only be permitted once a doctor has confirmed that the condition is controlled.

Snoring Without Apnoea

- Advise patients to make the following lifestyle changes:
  - Lose weight if obese, especially if the neck circumference is over 43 cm (17 inches).
  - Avoid alcohol before bedtime.
  - Stop smoking.
  - Discontinue nighttime sedation.
  - Sleep on the side; a golf ball sewn into the back of the pyjamas may help this.
  - Lift the head of the bed up.
  - Dilate the nostrils using a Nozovent (available from www.britishsnoring.co.uk).
- Examine for nasal obstruction and consider a trial of intranasal steroids.
- Consider whether the patient could be hypothyroid.
- Recommend ear plugs for the partner.
- Refer to ENT in dire cases.

PATIENT INFORMATION

The British Snoring and Sleep Apnoea Association (BSSAA), Castle Court, 41 London Road, Reigate, RH2 9RJ, tel. 01737 245638, www.britishsnoring.co.uk.
   SATA (The Sleep Apnoea Trust), PO Box 60, Chinnor, OX39 4XE, tel. 0800 025 3500, www.sleep-apnoea-trust.org.

The Throat and Mouth

Sore Throat

GUIDELINE

Scottish Intercollegiate Guidelines Network. (2010). *Management of sore throat and indications for tonsillectomy. SIGN guideline 117.* www.sign.ac.uk.

SYSTEMATIC REVIEW

Spinks, A., Glasziou, P. P., & Del Mar, C. B. (2013). Antibiotics for sore throat. *Cochrane Database of Systematic Reviews, 11.*

The following evidence demonstrates the limited value of throat swabs and of antibiotics in the management of sore throat:

- Approximately 20% of sore throats are bacterial, namely beta-haemolytic streptococci group A (GABHS) and groups C and G.
- The incidence is dependent on age. Only 15% are bacterial under the age of 3, while 50% are bacterial between the ages of 4 and 13 (DTB, 1995) and 10% in adults (Cooper et al., 2001).
- The sensitivity and specificity of the throat swab are low, at most 30% and 80%, respectively. Up to 40% of adults are carriers of GABHS. A positive swab is therefore not proof of infection.
- Streptococcal tonsillitis cannot reliably be diagnosed clinically, although it is more likely if the patient is under 11 years old with:
  - myalgia;
  - tender or swollen cervical lymph glands;
  - history of fever;
  - tonsillar exudates; and
  - is less likely if there is cough or earache (Dobbs, 1996).
- Even if all 4 of the CENTOR criteria are met (tonsillar exudate, history of fever, tender anterior chain cervical lymph nodes, absence of cough) the likelihood of the infection being due to GABHS is still only 25–86%.
- Penicillin speeds up recovery only slightly in patients with streptococcal tonsillitis (7 days after the start of treatment penicillin shows no advantage over placebo in relief of symptoms). It does not get patients back to school or work more quickly (Dagnelie, van der Graaf, & De Melker, 1996).
- Antibiotics do not protect against the rare non-suppurative complications in patients with streptococcal tonsillitis, namely rheumatic fever (Howie & Foggo, 1985) and acute glomerulonephritis (Glasziou & Del Mar, 2000; Taylor & Howie, 1983) or, if they do, the incidence of those complications in developed countries is so rare that it should not influence management (Spinks, Glasziou, & Del Mar, 2013).
- Antibiotics *do* protect against the suppurative complications of sore throat, reducing the incidence of acute otitis media by two-thirds and of acute sinusitis by a half. However, these complications are uncommon. It would be necessary to treat 200 cases to prevent one case of acute otitis media (Spinks et al., 2013).
- Antibiotics have no effect on the incidence of URTI, whether bacterial or viral, in the subsequent 6 months. The early use of antibiotics may even increase the chance of recurrence (El-Daher et al., 1991).
- Patients given penicillin for immediate use are more likely to reattend than those not given antibiotics or given a prescription only to be used 3 days later if symptoms have not resolved (Little, Gould, et al., 1997; Little, Williamson, et al., 1997).
- If penicillin is used, a 10-day course is more successful than a 5-day course in eradicating streptococci from the throat. However, this seems to be of no clinical

importance, since it does not alter the number of sore throats over the following 6 months (Zwart et al., 2003).

- Patients who are more satisfied with the consultation get better more quickly (Little, Williamson, et al., 1997).

Management

The aim is to:

1. avoid unnecessarily widespread use of antibiotics, with its disadvantages: the dependence on the GP that it encourages, the possibility of antibiotic resistance, and the adverse effects of the drugs;
2. give the ill patient the possible benefit of early penicillin.
   - Antibiotics should not be used for symptomatic relief in sore throat (SIGN, 2010).
   - Recommend analgesics and antipyretics (Snow et al., 2001). Ibuprofen 400 mg three times a day is the drug of choice (SIGN, 2010).
   - Check what concerns the patient. Explain the probable viral nature of the condition, and how the patient can self-manage subsequent attacks at home (Little, Williamson, et al., 1997).
   - If giving a prescription for antibiotics when the indication is arguable, consider recommending that it only be used if there has been no improvement after 3 days. This can reduce antibiotic use by two-thirds (Arroll et al., 2003).
   - Instruct patients to return in 1 week, if still unwell, for a throat swab, full blood count (FBC), and glandular fever antibodies.
   - Be alert to the possibility that the sore throat is really an excuse to consult about some more difficult issue.

Special Cases

The modest benefit of penicillin, even in proven GABHS, makes a decision not to prescribe reasonable in almost all cases.

- *Ill patients* (e.g., with high fever, dysphagia, marked cervical lymphadenopathy, and severe pharyngitis):
  - Take a throat swab or a rapid antigen test.
  - Give phenoxymethylpenicillin 500 mg four times a day for 5 days; or consider giving a cephalosporin. Give erythromycin if the patient is allergic to penicillin.
  - Instruct the patient to telephone for the result.
  - If pathogenic streptococci are grown, urge the patient to complete the 10-day course.
- Sore throat associated with stridor or breathing difficulty: admit immediately (SIGN, 2010).
- Patients with sore throat who are members of a closed community where there is an outbreak of streptococcal pharyngitis. Treat as ill patients (earlier).
- Patients in severe pain: Consider giving oral prednisolone 60 mg daily for 2 days. It reduces pain at 12 and 24 hours with 57% pain free at 2 days compared to 33% on placebo. The benefit is more marked in sore throat due to streptococcal infection (Kiderman et al., 2005).
- Patients with prolonged tonsillitis:
  - With negative investigations:
    1. repeat glandular fever antibodies weekly for 2 more weeks;
    2. take blood for an ASO titre. The throat swab may be a false negative.
  - With persistent streptococcal infection:
    1. give a cephalosporin or co-amoxiclav. Beta-lactamase–producing organisms may be destroying the penicillin.
- *Patients with a past history of rheumatic fever* should already be taking prophylactic penicillin V 250 mg twice a day. If they develop a sore throat they should be given a cephalosporin or co-amoxiclav, in case they have beta-lactamase-producing organisms in the pharynx that are destroying the penicillin.
- *Patients on chemotherapy, immunosuppressive drugs, or carbimazole:* Check the white blood cell (WBC) count.
- *Patients with a past history of quinsy:* Treat as ill patients (earlier).

Vincent's Angina

This is an ulcerative gingivostomatitis, which can spread to the tonsils. It is due to an infection with fusiform bacilli and spirochetes.

- Give metronidazole 400 mg twice a day for 3 days.

Infectious Mononucleosis

- Consider prednisolone 40 mg daily orally for 5 days in patients with severe tonsillitis, to enable them to swallow and avoid airway obstruction.
- Consider a high-dose NSAID to improve the general well-being of patients at an important time of their lives (e.g., when taking examinations).
- Avoid ampicillin-based antibiotics, including co-amoxiclav.

Oral Thrush

- Confirm with a mouth swab.
- Treat with an oral antifungal without waiting for the swab result.
- Consider a predisposing cause (e.g., diabetes, the use of broad spectrum antibiotics or inhaled steroids, human immunodeficiency virus [HIV] infection, or other causes of immunosuppression).

Sore Throat Due to Postnasal Drip

Treat with intranasal steroids.

Tonsillectomy

- Not all sore throats are due to tonsillitis.
- In children with recurrent severe tonsillitis, surgery offers the chance of avoiding two moderate or severe throat infections in the next 2 years. Children with a history that is less severe benefit less (Marshall, 1998).
- There is no convincing evidence for tonsillectomy in adults.

Indications for Referral

- *Recurrent acute tonsillitis,* five or more episodes a year. Attacks should be severe enough to interfere with the child's normal functioning.
- *Airway obstruction,* especially if there is sleep apnoea.
- *Chronic tonsillitis,* for over 3 months, especially if associated with halitosis.
- *Quinsy or peritonsillar cellulitis,* after recovery, in patients under age 25 with a history of recurrent tonsillitis.
- *Bacterial carriers who have not responded to antibiotics* (e.g., the diphtheria carrier and the carrier of haemolytic streptococcus group A who has had rheumatic fever).
- *Unilateral tonsillar enlargement or ulceration* suggestive of a serious underlying disorder (e.g., malignancy).
- *Guttate psoriasis* that is exacerbated by recurrent throat infections.
- Less severely affected children are unlikely to benefit. One RCT found that in moderately affected children, the modest benefit was outweighed by the 7.9% who had surgery-related complications (Paradise et al., 2002).

Dysphagia

- Check haemoglobin (Hb) and refer urgently to an ENT or a general surgeon to exclude a local cause.
- If the appointment is not imminent, order a barium swallow. This is the one situation where a barium study should precede endoscopy.

Hoarseness

- Refer urgently anyone suffering from hoarseness for more than 3 weeks, especially smokers. Early tumours confined to the vocal cord treated by radiotherapy have an 80% to 90% chance of 5-year survival.
- Consider re-referring a patient with persistent constant hoarseness, even after a normal laryngoscopy performed in the early stages. A previously undetected nodule or carcinoma may now be visible.
- Do not diagnose chronic laryngitis in smokers without laryngoscopy. It is they who are most at risk of laryngeal carcinoma.
- If laryngoscopy is normal, refer to a speech therapist or voice teacher. Voice abuse is common in teachers, mothers of young children, and anyone who shouts.
- Distinguish hoarseness from functional dysphonia, in which the patient adopts a whisper for psychological reasons. These patients need laryngoscopy to exclude a pathological cause before urgent referral to a speech therapist, psychiatrist, or psychologist.

Post Laryngectomy

- Treat all respiratory infections vigorously and admit patients early if they are failing to expectorate their secretions.
- Check that the patient:

REVIEW

Gleeson, M., & Jani, P. (1994). Long-term care of patients who have had a laryngectomy. *British Medical Journal, 308,* 1452–1453.

- is attending speech therapy;
- is eating enough. The sense of smell diminishes because the nose is not being used to sniff. Patients can be taught to sniff by speech therapists;
- has been referred to the National Association of Laryngectomee Clubs, Suite 16, Tempo House, 15 Falcon Road, London, SW11 2PJ, tel. 020 7730 8585, www.laryngectomy.org.uk. Information for laryngectomees, carers, and professionals can be found at the website.

The Feeling of a Lump in the Throat

When diagnostic clues are absent:
- treat as oesophagitis for 2 weeks with antacids or a PPI;
- refer non-responders to the ENT department to exclude a physical cause;
- counsel those with negative findings to try to uncover the cause for their probable globus hystericus.

Sore Mouth
Red or White Patches in the Mouth

* Refer all as erythroplakia or leukoplakia unless the typical skin lesions show that it is lichen planus. The risk of malignancy over 10 years is 3% to 6% with leukoplakia, and far higher with erythroplakia.

Ulcerated Sore Mouth

- Be aware that ulcers may be associated with skin, genital, or eye lesions as part of a larger syndrome.

Primary Herpes Stomatitis or Labialis

SYSTEMATIC REVIEW

Chi, C. (2015). Herpes labialis. Systematic review 1704. *Clinical Evidence.* London: BMJ Publishing Group. http://clinicalevidence.bmj.com.

- *First attack:* If seen within the first 48 hours give an oral antiviral agent (e.g., acyclovir), unless mild. It can halve the time to healing, at least in children.
- *Recurrent attacks:* Use an oral antiviral agent. There is a lack of evidence of benefit for topical agents.
- *Prevention of recurrent attacks:*
  - Sunblock will dramatically reduce the rate of recurrence in those in whom sun is a factor.

- Prophylactic oral antivirals probably do reduce the number of attacks and the size and duration of lesions. Either in the prodromal stage or before a high-risk activity such as skiing, give oral acyclovir for 4 days.

Aphthous Ulcers

GUIDANCE

Scully, C., Gorsky, M., & Lozada-Nur, F. (2003). The diagnosis and management of recurrent aphthous stomatitis: A consensus approach. *Journal of the American Dental Association, 134,* 200–207.
   Scully, C. (2006). Aphthous ulceration. *New England Journal of Medicine, 355,* 165–172.

- These may be associated with stress, menstruation, poor overall health, or occasionally coeliac disease. Large single ulcers can reach 1 to 2 cm in diameter and take 6 weeks to heal, but at 3 weeks some improvement should already be seen.
- Check FBC, iron, B_{12}, and folate levels; 20% of patients with recurrent ulcers have low iron, B_{12}, or folate levels. Where ulceration is recurrent, check HIV status and antibodies for coeliac disease.
- In milder cases give:
  - triamcinalone in cellulose paste (Adcortyl in Orabase), thinly applied two to four times a day;
  - hydrocortisone pellets: dissolve one pellet slowly in contact with the ulcer, three to four times a day;
  - topical anaesthetic rinse or gel, or antimicrobial mouthwash;
  - pressurized steroids (asthma inhalers) sprayed directly onto ulcer (an unlicensed use).
- *In more severe cases* consider oral steroids.
- *In recurrent cases* use chlorhexidine mouthwash to reduce the frequency of relapse (Porter & Scully, 2007).
- Refer if there are other symptoms (e.g., uveitis, genital ulceration, arthritis) suggestive of a systemic disease.
- *Continuous aphthous ulceration or severe ulceration:* Refer to an oral medicine specialist. They may benefit from higher strength steroids or immunosuppressants, including thalidomide (an unlicensed use).

Traumatic Ulcers
- Treat the cause.
- Try a local anti-inflammatory agent, such as salicylate cream, applied three to four times a day.
- Refer for biopsy any ulcer that has not healed within 3 weeks after the removal of any local cause. It may be a squamous cell carcinoma.

Sore Mouth Without Ulceration
- Dry mouth may be due to anxiety, drugs, dehydration, or Sjögren syndrome.

- Prescribe an artificial saliva product. Do not encourage the sucking of sweets unless they are sugar free. Caries is already a hazard for patients with dry mouth.
- *Oral thrush in a patient wearing dentures:* Sterilize the dentures by soaking them overnight in dilute hypochlorite solution, then apply miconazole oral gel four times a day to the part of the denture in contact with the gum.
- *Workup where diagnosis is not clear:* Swab for candida and check FBC, B_{12}, folate, and serum iron.

Dental Problems

- Current guidance from the British Medical Association is that GPs should not treat dental problems, as they are not qualified to do so.
- Staff in GP practices are advised to be aware of local provision for emergency dental care both in and out of hours.
- GPs retain an ethical responsibility to treat patients in emergency situations but treatment for dental problems should only be given in exceptional circumstances.

Toothache
- Sensitive to hot, cold, and sweet stimuli: This is probably due to exposed dentine. Advise the patient to see a dentist.
- Severe pain, touch sensitivity, gingival swelling with or without local lymphadenopathy, and fever: This is a dental abscess. Refer for drainage. If there is likely to be delay, prescribe:
  - penicillin V 500 mg four times a day, or erythromycin 500 mg twice a day, or metronidazole 400 mg twice a day; and
  - adequate analgesia. Try an NSAID first.

Loss of a Tooth Through Trauma
- Reimplantation of a secondary tooth within 12 hours is likely to succeed, and is worth attempting after an even longer time.
  1. Pick the tooth up by its crown, not by the root.
  2. If dirty, wash it in cold water.
  3. Push it back into its socket or under the patient's tongue, or store it in a cup of milk or in the patient's saliva.
  4. Send the patient immediately to a dentist or accident and emergency department for reimplantation.

Complications After Extraction
Haemorrhage
1. Allow the patient to rinse the mouth out.
2. Place a damp gauze swab over the socket and ask the patient to bite hard for 10 to 15 minutes.
3. If this fails, either suture across the socket with 3.0 silk or refer to a dentist or oral surgeon.

Painful Socket, Bad Taste, Halitosis
- This usually occurs 4 to 5 days after an extraction and is due to the clot not forming or being removed and the socket filling with debris that gets infected.

- Refer to a dentist.
- Give strong analgesics.
- Advise the patient to wash the mouth out with warm saline.
- Start antibiotics: penicillin V 500 mg four times a day or erythromycin 500 mg twice a day and metronidazole 400 mg twice a day.

Halitosis

> **OVERVIEW**
>
> Scully, C., Porter, S., & Greenman, J. (1994). What to do about halitosis. *British Medical Journal, 308,* 217–218.

- Ninety percent of halitosis is due to bacterial putrefaction in the mouth (Tessier & Kulkarni, 1991).
- Encourage mouth hygiene. Trapped food is a common cause of halitosis, especially in denture wearers.
- Treat any local infection. This may be tonsillitis, gingivitis, sinusitis, or even bronchiectasis. A dental check is worthwhile even if there is no obvious pathology.
- Look for a furry tongue, although treatment is difficult. Stopping smoking and scrubbing the tongue with a toothbrush may help.
- Check whether the patient suffers from dry mouth. This may be due to drugs, or Sjögren syndrome, or to mouth breathing. Sugar-free mints or gum will aid salivation.
- Ask whether the halitosis only occurs when the patient is hungry. Hunger halitosis is well recognized, although the cause is not clear.
- Consider certain foods as the cause. Patients usually recognize for themselves the connection with garlic or onions but may not notice the connection with a diet high in dairy products, especially yoghurt.
- If there is no specific pointer to the cause of the trouble, consider an empirical trial of toothbrushing and flossing after every meal with an antiseptic mouthwash night and morning for 2 weeks at a time. Longer courses put the patient at risk of fungal overgrowth.
- If the above fails, then consider investigating for rare causes such as:
  - metabolic disorders; uraemia, ketosis, and liver failure;
  - small bowel pathology where bacterial overgrowth may be the cause of the halitosis (e.g., blind loop syndrome). Evidence for this may be haematological (anaemia; iron deficiency; low serum B_{12}; and a raised red cell folate) or radiological (barium meal and follow-through);
  - nasopharyngeal malignancy.
- If small bowel pathology is not suspected, try a 2-week course of antibiotics (amoxicillin or tetracycline). Chronic bacterial overgrowth of the gut may still be the cause. If the condition improves, consider long-term intermittent use of antibiotics.

- Delusional halitosis may be the only complaint of a patient with a hypochondriacal depression. Refer to a psychiatrist.

References

Adrion, C., Fischer, C., Wagner, J., Gürkov, R., Mansmann, U., & Strupp, M. (2016). Efficacy and safety of betahistine treatment in patients with Meniere's disease: Primary results of a long term, multicentre, double blind, randomised, placebo controlled, dose defining trial (BEMED trial). *British Medical Journal (Clinical Research Ed.), 352,* h6816.

AlBalawi, Z. H., Othman, S. S., & AlFaleh, K. (2013). Intranasal ipratropium bromide for the common cold. *Cochrane Database of Systematic Reviews,* (6), CD008231.

American Academy of Pediatrics. (1997). *Managing otitis media with effusion in young children.* Retrieved from www.ngc.gov.

Arroll, B., Kenealy, T., Goodyear-Smith, F., et al. (2003). Delayed prescriptions. *British Medical Journal (Clinical Research Ed.), 327,* 1361–1362.

Baldo, P., Doree, C., Molin, P., McFerran, D., & Cecco, S. (2012). Antidepressants for patients with tinnitus. *Cochrane Database of Systematic Reviews,* (9), CD.

Biedlingmaier, J. F. (1994). Two ear problems you may not need to refer. Otitis externa and bullous myringitis. *Postgraduate Medicine, 96*(5), 141–145.

Browning, R. (2005). Ear wax. *BMJ Clinical Evidence.* London: BMJ Publishing Group.

Burgess, A., & Kundu, S. (2006). Diuretics for Ménière's disease or syndrome. *Cochrane Database of Systematic Reviews,* (3), CD003599.

Burton, M. J., & Doree, C. (2009). Ear drops for the removal of ear wax. *Cochrane Database of Systematic Reviews,* (1), CD004326.

Chong, L. Y., Head, K., Hopkins, C., Philpott, C., Schilder, A. G. M., & Burton, M. J. (2016). Intranasal steroids versus placebo or no intervention for chronic rhinosinusitis. *Cochrane Database of Systematic Reviews,* (4), CD011996.

Cooper, C. W. (1993). Vestibular neuronitis: A review of a common cause of vertigo in general practice. *British Journal of General Practitioners, 43,* 164–167.

Cooper, R. J., Hoffman, J. R., Bartlett, J. G., et al. (2001). Principles of appropriate antibiotic use for acute pharyngitis in adults: Background. *Annals of Internal Medicine, 134,* 509–517.

Dagnelie, C. F., van der Graaf, Y., & De Melker, R. A. (1996). Do patients with sore throats benefit from penicillin? *British Journal of General Practitioners, 46,* 589–593.

De Sutter, A. I. M., Saraswat, A., & van Driel, M. L. (2015). Antihistamines for the common cold. *Cochrane Database of Systematic Reviews,* (11), CD009345.

De Sutter, A. I. M., van Driel, M. L., Kumar, A. A., Lesslar, O., & Skrt, A. (2012). Oral antihistamine-decongestant-analgesic combinations for the common cold. *Cochrane Database of Systematic Reviews,* (2), CD004976.

Dobbs, F. (1996). A scoring system for predicting group A streptococcal throat infection. *British Journal of General Practitioners, 46,* 461–464.

Drug Therapy Bulletin. (1995). Diagnosis and treatment of streptococcal sore throat. *Drug Ther Bull, 33,* 9–12.

Drug Therapy Bulletin. (2009). Managing acute sinusitis. *Drug Ther Bull, 47.*

Eekhof, J. A. H., de Bock, G. H., de Laat, J. A., et al. (1996). The whispered voice: The best test for screening for hearing impairment in general practice. *British Journal of General Practitioners, 46,* 473–474.

El-Daher, N. T., Hijazi, S. S., Rawashdeh, N. M., et al. (1991). Immediate versus delayed treatment of group A haemolytic streptococcal pharyngitis with penicillin V. *Pediatric Infectious Disease Journal, 10*, 126–130.

Fokkens, W. J., Lund, V. J., Mullol, J., Bachert, C., et al. (2012). European position paper on rhinosinusitis and nasal polyps. *Rhinology, 50*(23), 1–299.

Gagyor, I., Madhok, V. B., Daly, F., Somasundara, D., Sullivan, M., Gammie, F., et al. (2015). Antiviral treatment for Bell's palsy (idiopathic facial paralysis). *Cochrane Database of Systematic Reviews*, (11), CD001869.

Gianopoulos, I., Stephens, D., & Davis, A. (2002). Follow up of people fitted with hearing aids after adult hearing screening: The need for support after fitting. *British Medical Journal (Clinical Research Ed.), 325*, 471.

Glasziou, P., & Del Mar, C. (2000). Upper respiratory tract infection: Antibiotics. *BMJ Clinical Evidence* (Vol. 4). London: BMJ Publishing Group. Retrieved from www.clinicalevidence.org.

Griffin, G., & Flynn, C. A. (2011). Antihistamines and/or decongestants for otitis media with effusion (OME) in children. *Cochrane Database of Systematic Reviews*, (9), CD003423.

Hand, C., & Harvey, I. (2004). The effectiveness of topical preparations for the treatment of earwax: A systematic review. *British Journal of General Practitioners, 54*, 862–867.

Hemilä, H., & Chalker, E. (2013). Vitamin C for preventing and treating the common cold. *Cochrane Database of Systematic Reviews*, (1), CD000980.

Hickish, G. (1989). Hearing problems of elderly people. *British Medical Journal (Clinical Research Ed.), 299*, 1415–1416.

Hilton, M., & Pinder, D. (2004). The Epley (canalith repositioning) manoeuvre for benign paroxysmal positional vertigo. *Cochrane Database of Systematic Reviews*, (2), CD003162, doi:10.1002/14651858.CD003162.pub2.

Howie, J., & Foggo, B. (1985). Antibiotics, sore throat and rheumatic fever. *Journal of the Royal College of General Practitioners, 35*, 223–224.

James, A., & Thorp, M. (2001). Ménière's disease. *BMJ Clinical Evidence* (Vol. 5). London: BMJ Publishing Group. Retrieved from www.clinicalevidence.org.

James, A. L., & Burton, M. J. (2001). Betahistine for Ménière's disease or syndrome (Cochrane review). In *The Cochrane Library* (Issue 2). Update Software, Oxford.

Karsch-Völk, M., Barrett, B., Kiefer, D., Bauer, R., Ardjomand-Woelkart, K., & Linde, K. (2014). Echinacea for preventing and treating the common cold. *Cochrane Database of Systematic Reviews*, (2), CD000530.

Keane, E. M., Wilson, H., McGrane, D., et al. (1995). Use of solvents to disperse ear wax. *British Journal of Clinical Practice, 49*(2), 71–72.

Kenealy, T., & Arroll, B. (2013). Antibiotics for the common cold and acute purulent rhinitis. *Cochrane Database of Systematic Reviews*, (6), CD000247.

Kiderman, A., Yaphe, J., Bregman, J., et al. (2005). Adjuvant prednisolone therapy in pharyngitis: A randomised controlled trial from general practice. *British Journal of General Practitioners, 55*, 218–221.

Lemiengre, M. B., van Driel, M. L., Merenstein, D., Young, J., & De Sutter, A. I. M. (2012). Antibiotics for clinically diagnosed acute rhinosinusitis in adults. *Cochrane Database of Systematic Reviews*, (10), CD006089.

Lempert, T., Gresty, M. A., & Bronstein, A. M. (1995). Benign positional vertigo: Recognition and treatment. *British Medical Journal (Clinical Research Ed.), 311*, 489–491.

Lindberg, E., Janson, C., Svardsudd, K., et al. (1998). Increased mortality among sleepy snorers: A prospective population based study. *Thorax, 53*, 631–637.

Little, P., Gould, C., Williamson, I., et al. (1997). Re-attendance and complications in a randomised trial of prescribing strategies for sore throat: The medicalising effect of prescribing antibiotics. *British Medical Journal (Clinical Research Ed.), 315*, 350–352.

Little, P., Gould, C., Williamson, I., et al. (2001). Pragmatic randomised controlled trial of two prescribing strategies for childhood acute otitis media. *British Medical Journal (Clinical Research Ed.), 322*, 336–342.

Little, P., Williamson, I., Warner, G., et al. (1997). Open randomized trial of prescribing strategies in managing sore throat. *British Medical Journal (Clinical Research Ed.), 314*, 722–727.

Macfadyen, C. A., Acuin, J. M., & Gamble, C. L. (2006). Systemic antibiotics versus topical treatments for chronically discharging ears with underlying eardrum perforations. *Cochrane Database of Systematic Reviews*, (1), CD005608.

Marais, J., & Dale, B. A. B. (1997). Bullous myringitis: A review. *Clinical Otolaryngology, 22*, 497–499.

Marshall, T. (1998). A review of tonsillectomy for recurrent throat infection. *British Journal of General Practitioners, 48*, 1331–1335.

Martinez-Devesa, P., Perera, R., Theodoulou, M., & Waddell, A. (2010). Cognitive behavioural therapy for tinnitus. *Cochrane Database of Systematic Reviews*, (9), CD005233.

McAllister, K., Walker, D., Donnan, P. T., & Swan, I. (2013). Surgical interventions for the early management of Bell's palsy. *Cochrane Database of Systematic Reviews*, (10), CD007468.

Memel, D., Langley, C., Watkins, C., et al. (2002). Effectiveness of ear syringing in general practice: A randomised controlled trial and patients' experiences. *British Journal of General Practitioners, 52*, 906–911.

NHS Centre for Reviews and Dissemination. (1994/1996). The treatment of persistent glue ear in children. *Effective Health Care, 1*(4), University of York.

Paradise, J. L., Bluestone, C. D., Colborn, D. K., et al. (2002). Tonsillectomy and adenotonsillectomy for recurrent throat infection in moderately affected children. *Pediatrics, 110*, 7–15.

Patiar, S., & Reece, P. (2009). Oral steroids for nasal polyps. *Cochrane Database of Systematic Reviews*, (2), CD005232, doi:10.1002/14651858.CD005232.pub2.

Pearlman, D. S., Lumry, W. R., Winder, J. A., et al. (1995). Once daily cetirizine effective in the treatment of seasonal allergic rhinitis in children aged 6–11 years: A randomized double-blind placebo-controlled study. *Clinical Pediatrics, 36*, 209–215.

Phillips, J. S., & McFerran, D. (2010). Tinnitus retraining rtherapy (TRT) for tinnitus. *Cochrane Database of Systematic Reviews*, (3), CD007330.

Phillips, J. S., Yung, M. W., Burton, M. J., & Swan, I. R. C. (2007). Evidence review and ENT-UK consensus report for the use of aminoglycoside-containing ear drops in the presence of an open middle ear. *Clinical Otolaryngology, 32*, 330–336.

Pirozzo, S., Papinczak, T., & Glasziou, P. (2003). Whispered voice test for screening for hearing impairment in adults and children: Systematic review. *British Medical Journal (Clinical Research Ed.), 327*, 967–970.

Porter, S., & Scully, C. (2007). Aphthous ulcers (recurrent). *BMJ Clinical Evidence*. http://clinicalevidence.bmj.com.

Pullens, B., & van Benthem, P. P. (2011). Intratympanic gentamicin for Ménière's disease or syndrome. *Cochrane Database of Systematic Reviews*, (3), CD008234.

Ratner, P. H., van Bavel, J. H., Martin, B. G., et al. (1998). A comparison of the efficacy of fluticasone proprionate aqueous nasal spray and loratadine, alone and in combination, for the treatment of seasonal allergic rhinitis. *Journal of Family Practice, 47*, 118–125.

Rovers, M. M., Glasziou, P., Appelman, C. I., et al. (2006). Antibiotics for acute otitis media: A meta-analysis with individual patient data. *Lancet, 368*, 1429–1435.

Royal College of Surgeons. (2016). *Commissioning Guide: Chronic Rhinosinusitis.*

Ruohola, A., Heikkinen, T., Meurman, O., et al. (2003). Antibiotic treatment of acute otorrhea through tympanostomy tube: Randomized double-blind placebo-controlled study with daily follow-up. *Pediatrics, 111*, 1061–1067.

Sheikh, A., Panesar, S. S., & Dhami, S. (2005). Seasonal allergic rhinitis. *BMJ Clinical Evidence* (Vol. 12). London: BMJ Publishing Group.

Scottish Intercollegiate Guidelines Network. (2003). *Diagnosis and management of childhood otitis media in primary care.* Retrieved from www.sign.ac.uk.

Scottish Intercollegiate Guidelines Network. (2010). *Management of sore throat and indications for tonsillectomy. SIGN guideline 117.* Retrieved from www.sign.ac.uk.

Simpson, S. A., Lewis, R., van der Voort, J., & Butler, C. C. (2010). Oral or topical nasal steroids for hearing loss associated with otitis media with effusion in children. *Cochrane Database of Systematic Reviews,* (5), CD001935.

Singh, M., & Singh, M. (2013). Heated, humidified air for the common cold. *Cochrane Database of Systematic Reviews,* (6), CD001728.

Snow, V., Mottur-Pilson, C., Cooper, R. J., et al. (2001). Principles of appropriate antibiotic use for acute pharyngitis in adults. *Annals of Internal Medicine, 134*, 506–508.

Spinks, A., Glasziou, P. P., & Del Mar, C. B. (2013). Antibiotics for sore throat. *Cochrane Database of Systematic Reviews,* (11), CD000023.

Strachan, D. P., & Cook, D. G. (1998). Parental smoking, middle ear disease and adenotonsillectomy in children. *Thorax, 53*, 50–56.

Sullivan, F. M., Swan, I. R. C., Donnan, P., et al. (2007). Early treatment with prednisolone or acyclovir in Bell's palsy. *New England Journal of Medicine, 357*, 1598–1607.

Swan, I. R. C., & Browning, G. G. (1985). The whispered voice as a screening test for hearing impairment. *Journal of the Royal College of General Practitioners, 35*, 19.

Taylor, J. L., & Howie, J. (1983). Antibiotics, sore throat and acute nephritis. *Journal of the Royal College of General Practitioners, 33*, 783–786.

Teixeira, L. J., Valbuza, J. S., & Prado, G. F. (2011). Physical therapy for Bell's palsy (idiopathic facial paralysis). *Cochrane Database of Systematic Reviews,* (12), CD006283.

Terreehorst, I., Hak, E., Oosting, A. J., et al. (2003). Evaluation of impermeable covers for bedding in patients with allergic rhinitis. *New England Journal of Medicine, 349*, 237–246.

Tessier, J. F., & Kulkarni, G. V. (1991). Bad breath: Etiology, diagnosis and treatment. *Oral Health, 81*, 9–24.

van Balen, F. A. M., Smit, W. M., Zuithoff, N. P. A., et al. (2003). Clinical efficacy of three common treatments in acute otitis externa in primary care: Randomised controlled trial. *British Medical Journal (Clinical Research Ed.), 327*, 1201–1205.

van Buchem, F. L., Dunk, J. H., Van't Hof, M. A., et al. (1981). Therapy of acute otitis media: Myringotomy, antibiotics, or neither? A double-blind study in children. *Lancet, ii*, 883–887.

Weiner, J. M., Abramson, M. J., & Puy, R. M. (1998). Intranasal corticosteroids versus oral H_1 receptor antagonists in allergic rhinitis: Systematic review of randomised controlled trials. *British Medical Journal (Clinical Research Ed.), 317*, 1624–1629.

Yardley, L., Beech, S., Zander, L., et al. (1998). A randomised controlled trial of exercise therapy for dizziness and vertigo in primary care. *British Journal of General Practitioners, 48*, 1136–1140.

Young, T., Palta, M., Dempsey, J., et al. (1993). The occurrence of sleep-disordered breathing among middle-aged adults. *New England Journal of Medicine, 328*, 1230–1235.

Zwart, S., Rovers, M. M., de Melker, R. A., et al. (2003). Penicillin for acute sore throat in children: Randomised double blind trial. *British Medical Journal (Clinical Research Ed.), 327*, 1324–1327.

21

Eye Problems

SUZANNAH DRUMMOND

CHAPTER CONTENTS

General Points

PATIENT INFORMATION

Patient information leaflets for a number of eye conditions are available from Moorfields Eye Hospital at www.moorfields.nhs.uk/listing/conditions.

Visual Acuity Testing

- Tests of visual acuity have a reliability of 98% and provide essential referral information but only if the following steps are taken:

- The Snellen chart should be the recommended distance from the patient for the size of chart used. The distance should be marked and the patient should stand behind the mark.
- The chart should be illuminated with 480 lux (e.g., a spotlight).
- One study found that few practices fulfilled these criteria (Pandit, 1994). Mobile technology developments now allow distance visual acuity testing with iPad/iPhone. These show a high level of agreement of visual acuity results with Snellen charts suggesting this technology can be used with confidence in the primary care setting. (O'Neill 2016)

Instilling Drops Into the Eye

- *Instilling drops:* Pull the lower lid down with the patient looking up. Squeeze one drop onto the lower fornix.
- *Instilling ointments or gels:* As above but squeeze 1 cm onto the inner surface of the lid. Warn the patient it will blur the vision for a short while.

The Gritty Irritable Red Eye

Acute Infective Conjunctivitis

In an adult or child:
- the history and examination traditionally give grounds for distinguishing between bacterial and viral infections but there is no evidence to support this (Rietveld et al., 2003);
- even in proven bacterial conjunctivitis, antibiotics only modestly improve the rate of resolution. Over half will resolve without treatment in 2 to 5 days (Sheikh & Hurwitz, 2005);
- individual meta-analysis showed that acute conjunctivitis in primary care can be thought of as a self-limiting condition. Patients with a purulent discharge or a mild severity of red eye may have a small benefit from antibiotics (Au Jefferies, Perera, & Evert, 2011).

If the visual acuity is normal and the cornea is clear, advise the patient to:
- wipe away discharge;
- wash hands after touching the eyes;
- use separate towels.
  Inform patients they are highly infectious.
- It seems logical to recommend that children should stay away from school even though this is not the recommendation of the Health Protection Agency (Guidelines on the Management of Communicable Diseases in Schools and Nurseries, 2008).
- Treat only if purulent discharge with mild red eye. It may be appropriate to advise the patient to return in 3 days to collect a prescription for antibiotic drops if symptoms are not resolving (Everitt, Little, & Smith, 2006). Prescribe chloramphenicol eye drops 2-hourly for 2 days, then four times a day for a further 5 days. Gentamicin is only indicated if there is gram-negative infection.
- If symptoms are still present at 1 week but there are no complications, stop all treatment and review weekly. Adenoviral infection typically takes 2 to 3 weeks to resolve.
- Povidone-iodine is becoming increasingly used in the treatment of refractory conjunctivitis and including adeno-conjunctivitis. (Pepose, J, 2018).
- Refer to eye casualty at any stage if the visual acuity is reduced or the cornea is involved.
- *Orbital cellulitis:* Admit immediately.

In a neonate:
- The likelihood and the dangers of sexually transmissible disease are greater.
- If the eye is mildly sticky, take a swab and review.
- If the discharge is purulent, take swabs for viral, bacterial, and chlamydial infection and a smear for gonococci. Then start chloramphenicol eye drops hourly and refer for an ophthalmic opinion the same day.
- Admit for intensive antibiotic therapy if:
  - herpes simplex, chlamydia, or gonococcus is grown; or
  - the clinical situation worsens, with a red eye, cloudy cornea, blepharitis, marked preauricular lymphadenopathy, or an unwell child.
- Notify as ophthalmia neonatorum.

Allergic Conjunctivitis

Acute

- Reassure the patient that the eye will not be harmed and that the problem will settle soon.
- Advise patients not to rub their eyes.
- Discontinue contact lens use while symptomatic.
- Apply cool compresses +/− refrigerate artificial tears.
- If patients require further short-term treatment, use antihistamines +/− vasoconstrictors (e.g., olopatadine or antazoline with xylometazoline).

N.B. Vasoconstrictors cause rebound hyperaemia if taken for over 2 weeks.

Chronic or Recurrent Allergic Eye Disease

- Establish, if possible, what the allergen is and reduce or avoid contact.
- Preferred use is for an antihistamine with mast cell stabilizing properties (e.g., olopatadine), and instruct the patient to use for at least 2 weeks. If there is concurrent rhinitis, consider using a steroid nasal spray (e.g., Nasonex spray twice a day) rather than an oral antihistamine.
- *Prophylaxis:* Give sodium cromoglicate, nedocromil sodium, or lodoxamide drops four times a day. Benefit may not be seen for 2 weeks. Where symptoms are seasonal, start treatment before the season starts.
- Consider giving an oral nonsedating antihistamine if symptoms are still not controlled.

N.B. Not in dry eye patients as this can exacerbate symptoms.

- *Severe cases not responding to the above:* Refer to ophthalmology for consideration of weak topical steroid (e.g., prednisolone).
- If a patient worsens dramatically after starting to use drops consider contact sensitivity. The usual cause is the preservative in the drops.

Blepharitis

- The mainstay of treatment is patient education and counselling.
- Emphasize that this is a chronic disease with intermittent exacerbations.

- Reassure the patient that the condition will not threaten sight. Explain that it results from either colonization of eyelashes or Meibomian gland dysfunction. Treatment is long term.
- *Lid hygiene comprises three stages:*
  1. Compresses: Heat the area with a hot washcloth (not scalding) for 5 to 10 minutes.
  2. Massage: Directly after compresses, massage lids toward lid margin to empty ducts.
  3. Wash: Using dilute (1:3) baby shampoo and a cotton bud, gently scrub eyelid margins, initially twice a day then twice weekly thereafter.
- Treat patients as if they have dry eyes, as the tears evaporate more rapidly. See upcoming discussion for treatment regimen but do not continue if there is no benefit.
- If there is no improvement, give chloramphenicol ointment to be applied to the lid margins twice daily for 1 month.
- Consider topical azithromycin 1% solution for 4/52 (Luchs, 2008).
- Treat those still not responding and those with acne rosacea with long courses (three months) of oral antibiotics (e.g., oxytetracycline 250 mg twice daily or lymecycline 408 mg twice daily for fewer gastrointestinal [GI] side effects). A short course of Azithromycin 500 mg OD for three days may also be tried.
- Consider referral to an ophthalmologist for those:
  - remaining symptomatic despite treatment for a few months particularly if unilateral (masquerade syndrome of sebaceous cell carcinoma);
  - who have associated skin disease;
  - where there is suspicion of corneal involvement. The inflammation is secondary to hypersensitivity to the cell wall protein of staphylococcus and may require topical steroid and antibiotic drops for a short period. Encourage the patient to continue lid hygiene.

Dry Eye

- Early detection and treatment may help prevent corneal ulcers and scarring.
- Treat any blepharitis (see earlier).
- Check that the patient is not taking any drugs that might exacerbate the condition (e.g., antihistamines).
- Encourage the patient to alter his or her environment by minimizing air conditioning and heating and to try to increase the humidity, if appropriate.
- Advise the intake of omega 3/6 fatty acids.
- Lubrication is the mainstay of treatment.
- *Artificial tears:* Encourage the patient to use as often as necessary. First line, start with Poly-vinyl Alcohol (PVA) or Carbomer. Start at four times a day and increase. If using more than six times daily, drops should be preservative free. Second line, use Carmellose or Hyaluronate.
- If Meibomiam gland disease (MGD) is identified use Systane balance or Optive Plus (preservative free) (Argrawal, A et al., 2018). Ointments. Prescribe paraffin-containing ointments (e.g., Lacri-Lube) for use at night only, as they create a greasy tear film that is difficult to see through.
- Refer:
  - urgently if there is a sudden increase in discomfort, redness, or deterioration in vision. These patients are at increased risk of microbial keratitis;
  - routinely patients who are having to instill drops very frequently. Many other treatments may be appropriate: topical glucocorticoids or cyclosporine, autologous serum, vitamin A or oral antioxidants, punctual plugs, or lid surgery.

Trauma

- Check the visual acuity. Refer if this is diminished or has decreased when next seen.

Foreign Body

- Suspect a foreign body in any unilateral red eye with or without a history of "something going into the eye."
- Always fully evert the upper eyelid when looking for a foreign body. If a foreign body is seen, it can usually be removed from the conjunctiva without difficulty.
- If there is a history of pain while hammering metal or of exposure to glass splinters, refer to exclude an intraocular foreign body.

Corneal Foreign Body

1. Insert local anaesthetic. Start with proxymetacaine and when the stinging has stopped, deepen the anaesthesia with amethocaine 1% drops. Continue until the drops feel cold but do not sting.
2. Remove the foreign body with a cotton wool bud or the tip of a sterile needle. Do not dig into the cornea; at its centre it is only 1 mm thick.
3. After removal, prescribe antibiotic eye ointment twice a day for 2 days as prophylaxis.
4. Give a cycloplegic (e.g., cyclopentolate 1% drops four times a day) if pain continues.
5. Do not apply an eye pad (Easty, 1993).
6. Examine after 24 hours:
   - with fluorescein to be sure the epithelium has healed;
   - to exclude a rust ring if the foreign body was metallic. If present, refer to an ophthalmologist urgently for it to be removed.

Chemical Burns

- These are acid or alkali burns (usually in the form of cement, lime, caustic soda, or ammonia).
- Acid burns cause coagulation necrosis whereas alkali burns are the more serious, causing saponification of phospholipid membranes leading to rapid epithelial cell death and caustic penetration. Ammonia can cause severe injury in 2 minutes.
- Irrigate with tap water or normal saline for 20 minutes or with alkali burns until the pH is normal (pH 6.5–7.5).
- Examine the cornea with fluorescein and send to eye casualty if it is not clear.

- *Cement.* Look for cement adhering to the eye, under the lids, or in the conjunctival fornices. If found, give local anaesthetic drops (e.g., benoxinate) and remove it, however distressing this is to the patient. Refer immediately following this.
- *Detergent.* If the conjunctiva shows punctate epithelial loss (staining with fluorescein), treat with chloramphenicol and review in 3 days.

Ultraviolet Light Burns

- *Arc eye* is usually due to exposure to ultraviolet C (UVC) light through welding or using a sunbed without eye protection. Patients are usually unaware until 6 to 12 hours after exposure.
- Treatment is supportive with anticipation that damaged epithelium will regenerate within 24 to 72 hours.
- Give local anaesthetic drops (e.g., benoxinate) *once*, but do not repeat them; they retard corneal healing.
- Treat with chloramphenicol ointment for lubrication and prevention of superinfection four times a day for 2 to 3 days.
- The worst of the two eyes can be padded if it offers some relief.
- Give sufficient sedatives and analgesics to ensure a night's sleep. Opioids are likely to be needed. Cessation of blinking during sleep enables the corneal epithelium to heal.
- Review patient in 2 to 3 days.

Corneal Abrasion

- Use topical anaesthetic once for examination purposes only.
- Confirm the abrasion with fluorescein dye after examining the eye and excluding other injuries (e.g., hyphaema and open globe).
- In a contact lens wearer, use a penlight to look for an infiltrate.
- Treat with chloramphenicol ointment four times a day for 24 hours and then twice a day for a further week.
- For a large abrasion, give a cycloplegic (e.g., cyclopentolate 1% drops) twice a day if pain continues. Warn patient about driving and difficulty reading. Consider oral nonsteroidal antiinflammatory drugs (NSAIDs; e.g., ibuprofen) or topical ophthalmic NSAID drops (e.g., diclofenac sodium) (Weaver & Terrell, 2003).
- Do not apply an eye pad (Easty, 1993).
- Give oral analgesia if the pain is severe.
- Refer if:
  - there is a decrease in acuity of greater than two lines of the Snellen chart;
  - there is a large defect (>50% of the epithelium);
  - there is a purulent discharge/white infiltrate;
  - the epithelium has not healed after 3 days.
- *Recurrent abrasions (erosions).* Recurrences tend to occur in the early morning during opening of that eye, when tear secretion is less. Give long-term (3/12) artificial tears during the day and ointment at night (see Dry Eye). Explain that recurrences can continue for months or years. Refer to an ophthalmologist if not improving. Laser ablation may be needed.

Blunt Injuries

Refer all patients who receive blunt injuries (e.g., from a squash ball) as this may give rise to bleeding into the anterior chamber of the eye (hyphaema) and the pressure may rise.

Problems With Contact Lenses
Conjunctivitis

- Advise the patient to remove the lens and leave it out until recovered.

  N.B. Keep the lens and its container, in case it is needed for culture.

- Check that the patient is cleaning and disinfecting the lenses every night (or using disposable single-use lenses).
- Prescribe antibiotic eye drops.
- Arrange for slit-lamp examination to exclude keratitis, either by the lens provider or the local ophthalmology emergency department.
- *Corneal abrasion:* see earlier.
- *Microbial keratitis:* A white infiltrate viewed with a penlight needs to be referred to the ophthalmology emergency department immediately. There is a risk of perforation and endophthalmitis.
- *Other problems* need slit-lamp examination to distinguish them. Advise the patient to leave the lenses out and contact the lens prescriber or refer the patient to an ophthalmologist. National Health Service (NHS) facilities are available to lens wearers if pathologic problems have arisen.

The Painful Red Eye That Is Not Gritty

- Most need referral to eye casualty:
  - keratitis, ocular herpes simplex, corneal ulcer, scleritis, and uveitis the same day;
  - acute glaucoma immediately.
- The GP may treat:
  - *Episcleritis* with an oral NSAID if there is discomfort (e.g., diclofenac or flurbiprofen for 2 weeks). Topical NSAIDs (e.g., diclofenac four times a day) are also appropriate. Refer if not improved within a month.
  - *Recurrent uveitis.* Treatment with topical steroids can be started, provided:
    1. their use has been previously sanctioned by a consultant;
    2. the visual acuity is normal;
    3. a dendritic ulcer is excluded with fluorescein and magnified examination of the cornea; but arrange for specialist assessment;
    4. Ophthalmic supervision is always necessary because intensive topical steroids may be needed. Treat with topical antivirals if the history is suggestive of herpes, while awaiting assessment.

Ophthalmic Herpes Zoster

- Give a high-dose antiviral drug at the first sign of zoster in the ophthalmic division of the trigeminal nerve (i.e., when the rash appears on the forehead, usually before any involvement of the eye). Untreated, about half would develop eye involvement.
- Refer to an ophthalmologist if there is:
  - Hutchinson sign (involvement of the nasociliary nerve which supplies the side of the nose and the skin of the inner corner of the eye);
  - a red eye; or
  - visual complaints (Opstelten & Zall, 2005).

  This referral is for an early but not immediate appointment. The complications for which ophthalmic expertise is needed (e.g., keratitis or uveitis) tend to occur a week or more after the onset of the rash.
- Be alert to the long-term complications of eye involvement:
  - Loss of corneal sensation may make the eye vulnerable to neuropathic ulceration or exposure keratopathy.
  - Scarring of the eyelid by an extensive periorbital vesicular rash may lead to incomplete closure, putting the cornea at risk.

  Patients with either of these problems will need to use lubricating eye ointments long term with or without surgery.

Lash, Lids, and Lacrimal Problems

Acute Dacrocystitis

- Treat aggressively for presumed staphylococcal or streptococcal infection (e.g., with flucloxacillin and amoxicillin) for 1 week.
- Review after 24 hours. If the symptoms are worse, refer for an ophthalmologic opinion that day.
- Refer once recovered for an ophthalmologic opinion and possible surgery.

Chalazion

- Advise the patient to use a warm compress (e.g., face flannel) over the lump and massage toward the lid margin. Antibiotic ointments or drops are traditionally given (onto the eye, in the hope that they will penetrate the chalazion through the conjunctival surface) despite the lack of evidence of benefit.
- Treat secondary infection with oral antibiotics (see Dacrocystitis).
- Review the patient, once recovered, and treat any blepharitis present (see earlier).
- Refer if a hard lump has failed to resolve after 3 months or is particularly troublesome, for incision and curettage.
- *Prevention of recurrence.* Encourage lid hygiene (see above).

Styes

- Treat the infected eyelash follicle with topical antibiotics.
- If there is marked swelling of the lid consider oral antibiotics.

Twitching

- *Myokymia.* Reassure the patient that twitching of a small area of the orbicularis muscle is common and is not sinister. It is often exacerbated by tiredness.
- *Facial twitching.* Refer to a neurologist or paediatrician.
- *Blepharospasm.* Forcible contractions of the entire orbicularis muscle should be referred to an ophthalmologist. Further investigation may be necessary (e.g., magnetic resonance imaging [MRI] scan) and botulinum toxin injections can give short-term relief.

Watery Eye

- This may result from inflammation or stenosis of the nasolacrimal duct or malposition of the lid.
- Treat any infection with topical antibiotics.
- Consider a trial of artificial tears (e.g., carbomer). The patient's natural basal secretion of tears may be deficient causing reflexive overwatering as compensation.
- Refer patients who are bothered by it to an ophthalmologist. They may benefit from exploration of the nasolacrimal duct or lid surgery. Massage of the lacrimal sac does not help unless there is a mucocoele.

Acute Disturbance of Vision

- Establish that the loss is acute and not just sudden awareness of a preexisting field loss or cataract.
- Distinguish transient from continuing visual losses and treat as appropriate. For migraine, see Chapter 12; for transient ischemic attack (TIA), see Chapter 12.

Acute Painless Loss of Vision
Central Retinal Artery Occlusion

- Central retinal artery occlusion is an ouclar emergency and is the ocular analogue of cerebral stroke. It results in profound, usually monocular vision loss and is associated with significant functional morbidity. The risk factors for CRAO are the same atherosclerotic risk factors as for stroke and heart disease. As such, individuals with CRAO may be at risk of ischemic end organ damage such as cerebral stroke. Management is not only to restore vision but at the same time to manage risk factors that may lead to other vascular conditions (Cugati, S et al., 2013).

If seen within 24 hours:
- Arrange for the patient to be seen immediately in eye casualty. Restoration of blood flow within 90 to 100 minutes leads to no retinal injury. If any delay is anticipated then give aspirin 300 mg (unless contraindicated).

If seen after 24 hours:

- There is no treatment for the eye and the object is to try to prevent retinal artery occlusion of the other eye.
- Refer to an ophthalmologist but less urgently.
- Give aspirin 75 mg daily.
- Take blood for erythrocyte sedimentation rate (ESR). If the clinical picture suggests temporal arteritis, give steroids while awaiting the result.
- Look for evidence of more widespread cardiovascular disease, especially a carotid bruit. Check blood pressure, pulse fasting blood sugar, and lipids.
- Ensure the patient has been referred to the stroke team for full systemic workup.
- Ensure that referral has been made to the stroke team for definitive work up.
- The patient should be followed up at 1–4 weeks by the ophthalmology team for assessment and treatment of ischaemic neovascular changes.

Central or Branch Retinal Vein Occlusion

- Workup:
  - Blood pressure (BP)
  - Full blood count (FBC) for polycythaemia and leukacmia
  - Serum lipids
  - Blood sugar
- Refer to eye casualty. The patient may need photocoagulation for chronic macular oedema and ischaemia following a branch vein occlusion. Various treatment options now exist in the form of intravitreal antivascular endothelial growth factor (anti-VEGF) injections for branch or central vein occlusion with macula oedema. Monitoring by an ophthalmologist in the absence of macular oedema is required for 2 years postocclusion to assess for neovascularization. Complications can develop early; 50% develop neovascular glaucoma within 3 months.

Decreased Vision With Pain

Acute Closed Angle Glaucoma

- Suspect it when:
  - the patient is unwell, with vomiting and eye or head pain; and
  - the eye is red and tender, the cornea hazy, and the pupil semidilated;
  - there may be a past history of episodes of blurred vision, associated with halos round lights, that have been aborted by exposure to a bright light or by going to sleep. In these situations, the pupil constricts, pulling the pupillary iris out of the angle.
- Refer suspected cases urgently to eye casualty or admit. If treatment is delayed irreversible damage to the optic nerve may occur in addition to adhesions between the iris and cornea requiring surgical drainage.
- If it is not possible to get the patient to hospital immediately give acetazolamide 500 mg intravenously or two 250-mg

tablets orally and instill 2% pilocarpine, 0.5% timoptol, and 1% apraclonidine into the eye 1 minute apart.
- Treat nausea and vomiting with prochlorperazine 12.5 mg intramuscularly.
- Do not attempt to dilate the pupil of anyone with suspected acute angle glaucoma.

Optic Neuritis

- Progressive reduction in vision over a few days with the nadir at 1 to 2 weeks, with pain on eye movements. Colours appear washed out. Symptoms may be worse after a hot shower or bath.
- A third of the patients have papillitis, the remainder have retrobulbar inflammation.
- Improvement occurs within 2 weeks and full recovery is usual within 3 months.
- Of individuals aged 20 to 40 years with retrobulbar neuritis in the United Kingdom, 50% to 70% will develop multiple sclerosis (MS), almost all of them within 5 years. A second episode increases that risk fourfold (Kanski, 1989).
- Refer urgently patients having their first attack to ophthalmology. Gadolinium-enhanced MRI provides confirmation of optic neuritis and aids prognosis and treatment decisions. Arrange for the patient to be seen again if symptoms are not improving after 2 weeks.
- Refer patients with a second attack to a neurologist (if not already done) because of the chance that this is multiple sclerosis.
- In younger patients consider infectious/postinfectious causes of optic neuritis. In older patients (>50 years) consider ischaemic optic neuropathy.
- Ophthalmology/neurology may advocate intravenous steroids in severe/bilateral visual loss as they speed recovery (and decrease short-term risk of MS development) but they give no benefit to long-term visual outcome or MS development. Oral steroids are contraindicated as they cause an increased rate of recurrence of optic neuritis.

Acute Distortion of Vision

- Refer urgently. Older patients may have acute wet age-related macular degeneration (AMD), especially if that diagnosis has already been made in the other eye. Typically, they report that straight lines appear crooked.
- If vision is still better than 6/96 they may benefit from intraocular injections of an anti-VEGF approved by National Institute of Health and Care Excellence (NICE) provided they fit the criteria (Royal College of Ophthalmologists Guidelines, 2015).

Floaters and Flashes

- Refer urgently patients who report:
  - multiple floaters, especially if associated with flashing lights. They may have a posterior vitreous detachment, which carries a 5% chance of causing a retinal tear;

- the appearance of a single large blob, which then fragments. They may have a vitreous haemorrhage.
- Be readier to refer if:
  - there is a family history of retinal tear or detachment;
  - the other eye has already suffered a detachment. Almost a quarter of patients develop a detachment in the second eye;
  - the patient has high myopia;
  - there is a history of cataract surgery, which increases the risk of retinal detachment ninefold.
- Refer immediately if there is a field loss or decrease in acuity. These imply that retinal detachment has occurred. It may be visible ophthalmoscopically. Instruct the patient to lie with the face on the side of the detachment (i.e., the side opposite the field defect) on the pillow, while waiting for the ambulance.

Note: Retinal tears are unlikely to be detected by conventional ophthalmoscopy. A normal fundus is therefore no grounds for inaction.

INFORMATION FOR PATIENTS WITH RETINAL DETACHMENT

Understanding Retinal Detachment. Available online from the Royal College of Ophthalmologists; www.rcophth.ac.uk; search on "information booklets."

Information for Doctors

Kang, H. K., & Luff, A. J. (2008). Management of retinal detachment: a guide for non-ophthalmologists. *British Medical Journal, 336,* 1235–1240.

Gradual Loss of Vision

- Refer to the optometrist who can ascertain whether there is refractive error (normally acuity will improve with a pinhole) and provide spectacles or perform a more thorough examination as to any other causes and refer appropriately.
- Suggest the following to all patients with visual difficulty:
  - Use adequate lighting (e.g., an angle-poise lamp), especially for reading and close work.
  - Rearrange the room to sit with the main window behind the patient and the television away from the window.
  - If visual acuity is 6/18 or worse, refer routinely as they may be eligible for partial sight registration.
- Recommend the patient information leaflets available from the Royal National Institute of Blind People (RNIB) at www.rnib.org.uk (search for "leaflets").

Cataracts

SYSTEMATIC REVIEWS

Snellingen, T., Evans, J. R., Ravilla, T., & Foster, A. (2004). Surgical interventions for age-related cataract (Cochrane review). In *The Cochrane Library* (Issue 2). Chichester, UK: John Wiley & Sons, Ltd.

- *In a child,* refer as a matter of urgency. Any opacity of the ocular media can have a catastrophic effect on the development of vision and should be diagnosed and treated promptly.
- *In a young adult,* refer but also investigate for diabetes or any other systemic disease that a clinical history might lead you to suspect.
- *In the elderly:*
  - exclude diabetes;
  - *refer to an optometrist all patients* who have not had a recent refraction, as a myopic shift often accompanies the onset of cataract and a change in spectacle lenses can often postpone the need for cataract surgery;
  - they should be able to *refer directly to an ophthalmologist* if no improvement in vision is possible with refraction and:
    1. the patient is having significant visual problems affecting quality of vision, or activities such as driving or reading; and
    2. the patient is willing to undergo surgery. There is little point in referring those that are happy with their current level of vision and would not accept an invitation for surgery.
- There is no absolute Snellen acuity below which surgery is indicated. It depends on the patient's individual needs and circumstances. Many patients are content with vision that is 6/18 or better unless they drive or do fine work.
- Some patients find their cataract is more disabling than would be predicted from the level of Snellen acuity. This happens particularly in posterior subcapsular cataract when localized opacities scatter light, causing difficulty with reading and with glare when driving. After surgery 85% to 90% will achieve vision that is adequate for driving (Allen & Vasavada, 2006).

Problems After Cataract Surgery

- *A red eye following surgery* in 0.1% to 0.5%, is due to postoperative endophthalmitis. It would therefore be prudent to refer immediately any postoperative patient with a red eye especially if there is reduced vision and pain. More commonly however it is caused by an allergy to the antibiotic and steroid drops given postoperatively.
- *More long-term deterioration of vision after surgery:* Refer the patient back; 20% develop opacification of the posterior capsule within 2 years of operation, requiring laser treatment.

Age-Related Macular Degeneration

- This occurs in elderly patients who present with progressive loss of central vision and, frequently, distortion effects. When looking at straight lines they appear wavy. The vision is best in dim light. The eye appears normal except for the choroidoretinal changes.
- Refer all patients for optometric assessment unless there is a sudden deterioration suggestive of wet AMD (see

above, section on Acute Distortion of Vision) to confirm diagnosis and to refer to ophthalmology if appropriate.

- Reassure patients that, although they have lost some of their central reading vision, they will never be completely blind and that further deterioration will be slow. The average time it takes for vision to deteriorate to below 3/60 (eligible for blind registration) is 5 to 10 years.

- Encourage the patient to stop smoking. Smokers carry a three- to fourfold increased risk of age-related macular degeneration. There is evidence that stopping smoking reduces the incidence and progression of the disease (Kelly et al., 2004). A diet rich in carotenoids (green leafy vegetables), regular exercise and control of blood pressure and cholesterol are also beneficial in prevention.

- Following diagnosis, there is now evidence to show that nutritional supplements, including antioxidant vitamins and lutein and zeaxanthin, are beneficial in slowing the progression of AMD (AREDS2 Research Group, 2013).

PATIENT INFORMATION

Macular Disease Society. Crown Chambers, South St, Andover, Hampshire, SP10 2BN, tel. 0300 3030 111, www.macularsociety.org.
Understanding Age-Related Macular Degeneration. Available online from the Royal College of Ophthalmologists at www.rcophth.ac.uk (search on "information booklets").

Chronic Simple Glaucoma

- Treatment to lower intraocular pressure has been shown to slow the progression of the disease (Wormald, 2003).

- Loss of visual acuity is a late sign of chronic glaucoma. By this stage, disc cupping and field loss are likely to be advanced and irreversible.

- The incidence rises with age. In the United Kingdom it is 1 in 5000 at age 40 to 49 years, and only really rises over age 60. Over 85, it is 1 in 10.

- The risk increases:
  - with a family history (×10);
  - in high myopes (×3);
  - in diabetics (×3);
  - in African Caribbeans;
  - in users of topical steroid drops for over 5 days.

Screening and Referral

- Eye tests are advised every 2 years or more frequently if in a high-risk group.

- Screening for glaucoma should be completed by the optometrist who will perform tonometry (pressure measurement), visual field analysis, and fundoscopy as well as possibly gonioscopy and pachymetry (angle and corneal thickness analysis).

- Testing is free in Scotland and elsewhere for children and adults over 60 years of age. Many of those in the high-risk groups are also eligible for free testing, including:
  - age over 40 with a family history of glaucoma;
  - having glaucoma or diabetes.

PATIENT INFORMATION

International Glaucoma Association. Woodcote House, 15 Highpoint Business Village, Henwood, Ashford, Kent, TN24 8DH, tel. 01233 64 81 70, www.glaucoma-association.com. *Understanding Glaucoma* is available online from the Royal College of Ophthalmologists at www.rcophth.ac.uk (search on "information booklets").

- *Driving.* Advise the patient to notify the Driver and Vehicle Licensing Agency (DVLA) if there is significant bilateral visual field loss (Potamitis et al., 1994).

- Treatment is managed by the hospital eye department. It is helpful to know that the aim is to keep the pressure around 15 mm Hg, using:
  - *prostaglandin analogues* (latanoprost, travoprost, and bimatoprost), which increase aqueous outflow through the uveoscleral pathway and can reduce intraocular pressure by 30% to 35%. Systemic side effects are minimal; eyelashes may lengthen and darken and light irises may permanently darken;
  - *beta blockers* (timolol, carteolol, betaxolol, levobunolol, and metipranolol), which reduce the secretion of aqueous. They can cause systemic symptoms and may unmask latent and previously undiagnosed heart failure and airway obstruction (Kirwan et al., 2002). Systemic effects can be reduced by finger pressure on the caruncle or by shutting the eyes for several minutes after instilling the drops. This approach may also increase ocular absorption of the drug;
  - *carbonic anhydrase inhibitors* (dorzolamide, brinzolamide, or oral acetazolamide), which reduce the secretion of aqueous humour. Oral acetazolamide is the most effective but has significant side effects. Topical forms have few side effects. Neither should be used in patients with sulphonamide allergy.
  - *parasympathomimetic drugs* (e.g., pilocarpine) are now used only infrequently. They constrict the pupil and pull on the trabecular meshwork increasing the flow. Pilocarpine eye drops frequently cause headaches, but they tend to disappear after the first few weeks of use. Pilocarpine constricts the pupil and may cause blurred vision if central lens opacities are present.

Allergy to Drops

This may present with intense itching and irritation of the eyes and eyelids, which is exacerbated by instillation of the drops. The allergy may be to the active drug or preservative (usually benzalkonium chloride). Stopping treatment (with monitoring of the pressure) should result in rapid improvement. Some topical agents are available in a preservative-free form.

Laser Treatment

Trabeculoplasty or even ciliary body ablation may be appropriate in certain circumstances—usually as an adjunct to drops:

- *Trabeculoplasty:* Argon or diode burns are applied to the trabecular meshwork. It is used only where the drainage angle is open and is effective for a short term; hence it is used more for elderly patients.
- *Ciliary body ablation:* Usually done with a diode laser to burn the ciliary body and reduce production of aqueous humour. The process may need to be repeated to keep the pressure low and patients normally need to continue drug treatment.

Other laser methods (iridotomy and iridoplasty) are used in angle closure glaucoma.

Surgical Treatment

Trabeculectomy is the most effective glaucoma filtration procedure when medical or laser treatment has failed. A channel is created to allow flow from the anterior chamber. Once it has been performed, bacterial conjunctivitis can develop more readily into endophthalmitis.

Visual Handicap

- Over two-thirds of people who are eligible are not registered as blind or partially sighted. The majority of these receive no social care services whatsoever.
- Two-thirds of all people with visual impairment have an additional disability or serious health problem.
- Over 50% of visually impaired people live alone yet few have been offered any training in daily living skills. Almost half of all visually impaired people cannot cook for themselves because of hazards in the kitchen (Royal National Institute for the Blind, 2002).

Certification and Registration

- Certification is by a consultant ophthalmologist on form CV1.
- *Blind certification* is for those with a visual acuity (VA) below 3/60, or with a VA of up to and including 6/60 but with gross visual field restriction.
- *Certification as partially sighted* is not defined by statute. It is appropriate for patients with VA of 6/60 or worse with full visual fields, or those with a VA better than that but with restriction of visual fields. A patient with a homonymous hemianopia, for instance, is likely to be eligible.
- *Registration* is voluntary and would normally be offered at the time of certification. Registration entitles a person to a range of benefits and concessions as well as help from some local voluntary groups. The receipt of a certificate of vision impairment (CVI) by the social services department entitles that person to have his or her name added to the register. This also acts as a trigger for social services to arrange an assessment of the person's social care needs.
- Patients with low vision but not certified as blind or partially sighted should be encouraged to self-refer to social services using the "Low Vision Leaflet" (LVL) available from high street opticians. They are also likely to benefit from a low visual aid referral which is normally through the ophthalmology department.

Benefits

- Registration means that a social worker will contact the patient and provide:
  - access to a mobility officer, a teacher of braille, and daily living courses;
  - free radio and cassette aids;
  - details of the RNIB talking-book service.
- In addition, the registered blind (but not necessarily the partially sighted) are eligible for:
  - a slightly higher rate of income support;
  - extra Housing Benefit, Income Support, and Council Tax Benefit;
  - increased income tax allowance;
  - reduced fares and a Blue Parking Badge;
  - free sight tests; and
  - reduction in the TV licence fee.

> **The Royal National Institute for the Blind** (RNIB) provides information, support, and advice for anyone with a serious sight problem. Website: www.rnib.org.uk; helpline 0303 123 9999 (interpreters are available); email: helpline@rnib.org.uk.

Prescribing for Patients With Contact Lenses
(Mitchell & Edwards, 2001)

Topical Applications

Avoid:
- eye ointments;
- eye drops containing preservatives (in soft lenses);
- topical steroids;
- coloured drops: fluorescein and rose bengal;
- sympathomimetics.

Systemic Drugs

Avoid drugs that:
- reduce or alter tear secretion: oral contraceptives, hormone replacement therapy (HRT), drugs with anticholinergic activity (e.g., tricyclic antidepressants), beta blockers, diuretics, isotretinoin;
- reduce blinking: benzodiazepines;
- stain the lens: nitrofurantoin, rifampicin, sulfasalazine;
- are concentrated in the lens and can irritate the eye: aspirin.

PATIENT INFORMATION

The British Contact Lens Association; www.bcla.org.uk (search on "do's and don'ts").

Corrective Surgery for Myopia

- This remains a service provided by the private sector that is not regulated.
- While legally in the United Kingdom any registered medical practitioner may perform refractive surgery, the

Royal College of Ophthalmologists recommends that it should only be performed by a fully trained ophthalmologist who has undergone additional specialist training in refractive surgery. He or she may or may not also be an NHS consultant.

• Advise patients to download the leaflet "Refractive Surgery" from the Royal College of Ophthalmologists at www. rcophth.ac.uk/ (search on "refractive surgery").

References

Allen, D., & Vasavada, A. (2006). Cataract and surgery for cataract. *British Medical Journal, 333,* 128–132.

AREDS2 Research Group. (2013). Lutein/zeaxanthin and omega-3 fatty acids for age-related macular degeneration. The Age-Related Eye Disease Study 2 (AREDS2) controlled randomized clinical trial. *JAMA.*

Argrawal, A., Bruce, G., Cowie, A., et al. (2018). *Scottish Dry Eye Guidelines version 1.1 (2018) NHS Scotland.*

Au Jefferies, J., Perera, R., & Evert, H. (2011). Acute infective conjunctivitis in primary care: Who needs antibiotics? Individual patient data meta-analysis. *British Journal of General Practitioner, 61*(590).

Crick, R. P., & Tuck, M. W. (1995). How can we improve the detection of glaucoma? *British Medical Journal (Clinical Research Ed.), 310,* 546–547.

Cugati, S., et al. (2013). Treatment options for central retinal aftery occlusion. *Current Treatment Options in Neurology, 15,* 63–67.

Easty, D. L. (1993). Is an eye pad needed in cases of corneal abrasion? *British Medical Journal (Clinical Research Ed.), 307,* 1022.

Everitt, H. A., Little, P. S., & Smith, P. W. F. (2006). A randomised controlled trial of management strategies for acute infective conjunctivitis in general practice. *British Medical Journal (Clinical Research Ed.), 333,* 321–324.

Guidelines on the Management of Communicable Diseases in Schools and Nurseries. (2008). *Health Protection Agency.* www.hpa.org.uk/schools.

Kanski, J. J. (1989). *Clinical ophthalmology* (2nd ed.). London: Butterworths.

Kelly, S., Thornton, J., Lyratzopoulos, G., et al. (2004). Smoking and blindness. *British Medical Journal (Clinical Research Ed.), 328,* 537–538.

Kirwan, J. F., Nightingale, J. A., Bunce, C., et al. (2002). β blockers for glaucoma and excess risk of airways obstruction: Population based cohort study. *British Medical Journal (Clinical Research Ed.), 325,* 1396–1397.

Luchs, J. (2008). Efficacy of topical azithromycin ophthalmic solution 1% in the treatment of posterior blepharitis. *Advanced Therapy, 25*(9), 858.

Mitchell, R., & Edwards, R. (2001). Prescribing for patients who wear contact lenses. *Prescriber,* 40–44.

O'Neill, S., & McAndrew, D. (2016). The validity of visual acuity assessment using mobile technology devices in the primary care setting. *Australian Family Physician, 45,* 212–215.

Opstelten, W., & Zall, M. J. W. (2005). Managing ophthalmic herpes zoster in primary care. *British Medical Journal (Clinical Research Ed.), 331,* 147–151.

Pandit, J. C. (1994). Testing acuity of vision in general practice: Reaching recommended standard. *British Medical Journal (Clinical Research Ed.), 309,* 1408.

Pepose, J. S., Ahuja, A., Liu, W., Narvekar, A., & Haque, R. (2018). Randomiszed, controlled, phase 2 trial of Povidone-Iodine/Dexamethasone Ophthalmic Suspension for Treatment of Adenoviral Conjunctivitis. *American Journal of Ophthalmology, 194,* 7–15.

Potamitis, T., Aggarwal, R. K., Tsaloumas, M., et al. (1994). Driving, glaucoma and the law. *British Medical Journal (Clinical Research Ed.), 309,* 1057–1058.

Rietveld, R. P., van Weert, H. C., ter Riet, G., et al. (2003). Diagnostic impact of signs and symptoms in acute infectious conjunctivitis: Systematic literature search. *British Medical Journal (Clinical Research Ed.), 327,* 789.

Royal College of Ophthalmologists Guidelines (2015). *Age-related macular degeneration: Guidelines for management.* London: RCOphth.

Royal National Institute for the Blind. (2002). *Progress in sight: National standards of social care for visually impaired adults.* www.rnib.org.uk/social_services.

Sheikh, A., & Hurwitz, B. (2005). Topical antibiotics for bacterial conjunctivitis: Cochrane systematic review and meta-analysis update. *British Journal of General Practitioners, 55,* 962–964.

Weaver, C. S., & Terrell, K. M. (2003). Do ophthalmic nonsteroidal anti-inflammatory drugs reduce the pain associated with simple corneal abrasion without delaying healing? *Annals of Emergency Medicine, 41,* 134–140.

Wormald, R. (2003). Treatment of raised intraocular pressure and prevention of glaucoma. *British Medical Journal (Clinical Research Ed.), 326,* 723–724.

22

Skin Problems

KIERAN DINWOODIE, ANCHAL GOYAL, CATRIONA NISBETT, JANE COLGAN

CHAPTER CONTENTS

Atopic Eczema

- Atopic eczema is a chronic, relapsing, itchy skin condition. If it's not itchy it's not eczema.
- It is typically an episodic disease of flares and remissions.
- There is a tendency for it to improve in adult life.
- There is some evidence that the prognosis of atopic eczema is worse when the onset is early and in children with associated asthma.
- There is no known single cause for atopic eczema; it occurs in genetically susceptible individuals when exposed to environmental irritants or allergens.
- It may be exacerbated but not caused by trigger factors such as stress or hormonal changes (premenstrual flares occur in 30% of women and pregnancy can adversely affect eczema in up to 50%).
- A specific genetic cause has not been identified but it is present in 80% of children where both parents are affected with eczema and in 60% where one parent is affected with eczema.
- Environmental factors have an important role, particularly exposure to pets, house dust mites, pollen, and food allergens (particularly cow milk or egg).

- Atopic eczema accounts for 30% of all dermatological consultations in primary care and the prevalence is increasing.
- Eighty percent of cases occur before the age of 5 years.
- The person's age affects the distribution:
  - Infancy: Eczema primarily involves the face, the scalp, and the extensor surfaces of the limbs. The nappy area is usually spared.
  - Children: Localization to the flexures of the limbs is more likely.
  - Adults: Flexural involvement. Eczema on the hands can be the primary manifestation.

Complications of Eczema

- *Infection:*
  - Bacterial infection with *Staphylococcus aureus* may present as typical impetigo or worsening of eczema with increased redness, oozing, and crusting.
  - Herpes simplex infection presents with grouped vesicles and punched out erosions.
  - Superficial fungal infections are also more common.
- *Psychological:*
  - Causes considerable distress.
  - In preschool children it increases the rate of behavioural problems, fearfulness, and dependence on parents.
  - In schoolchildren there can be problems with time off school, impaired performance, teasing, and bullying.
  - Sleep disturbance is an important problem for sufferers and their families.
- *Erythroderma* usually occurs in people with worsening or unstable eczema.
- *Eye abnormalities:*
  - Conjunctival irritation can occur.
  - Cataracts can also occur in people with severe atopic eczema aged 15 to 25 years.
  - Retinal detachment is rarely associated with atopic eczema.
- *Failure to thrive* and growth restriction can occur in children with severe atopic eczema.

General Advice

- In children, reassure parents that eczema often improves with time.

- In adults, explain that eczema is a chronic illness characterized by flares that can usually be controlled with appropriate treatment.
- Advise the person/carer to avoid scratching (keep nails short: use baby scratch mitts).
- Advise the person to avoid trigger factors (e.g., clothing, soap, detergents, animals, heat).
- Do not offer advice about complementary therapies other than that they are generally not recommended.
- Diet should not be altered unless there is a known allergy to specific foods and exclusion diet has been recommended by a health care professional.
- Advise the person to bath daily, using a bath additive (e.g., Hydromol Bath or Dermol) for no longer than 10 minutes, to then pat dry and apply emollient.

General Advice for Bottle and Breastfed Infants

- The mothers of breastfed infants in whom allergy is suspected to be the cause of moderate or severe eczema may require referral for dietary advice.
- A 6- to 8-week trial of hydrolysed protein formula milk or amino acid formula milk may be tried in bottle-fed infants less than 6 months of age in whom eczema is not controlled by emollients or mild topical steroids.
- Children who then respond well to a change in their formula milk will require referral to a dietician.
- Children who do not respond should have cow milk restarted with monitoring of their eczema.

Emollients

- Emollients are the mainstay of treatment for patients with eczema.
- Most emollients are plain but some contain active ingredients. These are generally best avoided. Active ingredients include urea (Balneum Plus and Eucerin Intensive) and lanolin (E45 and Oilatum Bath Formula).
- Ointments are usually poorly tolerated compared to creams, which affects their compliance.
- There is no evidence from controlled trials to support the use of one emollient over another: The correct emollient is the one the person will use.
- It may be more convenient to use better tolerated products (creams and lotions) during day and use ointments at night. Application of an emollient every 2 to 3 hours should be considered normal. Patients often underestimate the amount they should be using.
- Advise the patient that it is particularly important to use emollients during or after bathing (within 3 minutes).
- Advise the patient that soap can be very damaging to people with eczema and therefore a soap substitute should also be used.
- Do not prescribe aqueous cream as it can cause skin reactions.
- Where possible prescribe an emollient with a pump dispenser to minimize risk of bacterial contamination.

- Prescribe emollients in large quantities: 600 g/week for an adult; 250 g/week for a child.
- Emollients should be applied by smoothing them into the skin along the line of hair growth.

Steroids

- Topical steroids are safe and effective antiinflammatory skin preparations that are used to control eczema (and many other skin conditions).
- They are available in different strengths.
- Side effects are rare if used appropriately but they can cause skin thinning, telangiectasia, stretch marks, easy bruising, and hypertrichosis.
- Topical steroids should be used cautiously on eyelid skin as excessive use over weeks to months can cause glaucoma.
- Fingertip units guide the amount of steroid to be applied to a body site:
  - One hand: 1 fingertip unit
  - One arm: 3 fingertip units
  - One foot: 3 fingertip units
  - One leg: 6 fingertip units
  - Face and neck: 2.5 fingertip units
  - Trunk (front and back): 14 fingertip units
  - Entire body: ~40 fingertip units
- Table 22.1 details commonly prescribeable topical steroids.

Treatment of Mild Flares

- In addition to emollients consider prescribing a mild topical hydrocortisone cream or ointment for areas of red skin.
- Treatment should continue for 48 hours after the flare has been controlled.

Treatment of Moderate Flares

- Prescribe intensive treatment until the flare is controlled.
- Prescribe a generous amount of emollient and advise frequent and liberal use.
- Prescribe a moderately potent topical steroid to be used on inflamed areas (e.g., betamethasone valerate 0.025%; clobetasone butyrate).

TABLE 22.1	Commonly used Topical Steroids
Potency	Examples of Commonly Prescribed Treatments Available
Mild	Hydrocortisone (0.5%, 1%, 2.5%)
Moderate	Clobetasone butyrate (Eumovate) Betamethasone valerate 0.025% (Betnovate RD)
Potent	Betamethasone valerate 0.1% (Betnovate) Mometasone furoate (Elocon) Fluocinolone acetonide (Synalar)
Very potent	Clobetasone proprionate (Dermovate)

- Treatment should be continued for 48 hours after the flare has settled.
- Steroids should be applied once a day and only increased to twice a day if skin does not improve.
- For delicate areas such as the face and flexures consider starting with a mild potency topical steroid and increase to moderately potent corticosteroid only if necessary.
- If there are areas of infected skin treat with a topical antibiotic. These should not be used for longer than 1 week due to the risk of antibiotic resistance.
- Between flares encourage the frequent and liberal use of emollients even when skin appears clear.
- Consider maintenance topical steroids to control areas of skin prone to frequent flares. Consider one of the following maintenance regimens:
  - *Stepdown approach:* prescribing the lowest potency and amount of topical steroid to control the condition
  - *Intermittent treatment:* weekend therapy on Saturdays and Sundays only (probably the preferred option based on the evidence of risks vs benefits)
  - *Topical calcineurin inhibitors* (tacrolimus and pimecrolimus) are a second line option. However, they should only be prescribed by a specialist (including general practitioners [GPs] with a specialist interest in dermatology). They have evidence similar to that of moderately potent steroids. They do not cause skin atrophy, but long-term side effects are unknown and there is a theoretic long-term risk of malignancy.
- If there is severe itch consider prescribing a 1-month trial of a nonsedating antihistamine.

Treatment of Severe Flares

- Prescribe a generous amount of emollients and advise frequent and liberal use.
- Prescribe a potent topical steroid (e.g., betamethasone valerate 0.1%). Aim for a maximum 5-day use. Again steroids should be prescribed once a day and only increased to twice daily if skin does not improve.
- For delicate areas such as the face and flexures, use a moderately potent topical steroid (e.g., betamethasone valerate 0.025%, clobetasone butyrate 0.05%). Aim for a maximum 5-day use.
- If itching is severe and affecting sleep prescribe a sedating antihistamine (e.g., chlorphenamine) for adults and children aged 6 months or over.
- If there is severe, extensive eczema causing psychologic distress consider a short course of oral corticosteroids (30 mg prednisolone for 7 days).
- If there are signs of infection consider an oral antibiotic.
- Consider maintenance steroid therapy as per treatment of moderate flares.

Referral

- Admit to hospital if eczema herpeticum or erythrodermic eczema.
- Refer for routine dermatology appointment if:
  - diagnosis has become uncertain;
  - current management does not control eczema satisfactorily (person having one to two flares/month or person is reacting adversely to many emollients);
  - facial eczema has not responded to appropriate treatment;
  - contact allergic dermatitis is suspected;
  - there is recurrent secondary infection;
  - eczema is associated with significant social or psychologic problems.
- Refer people in whom food allergy is suspected to either immunology or paediatrics (children <6 months who have widespread eczema that has not responded to emollients or mild topical steroids).

Irritant and Allergic Contact Dermatitis (Including Hand Dermatitis)

GUIDELINES

National Institute for Health and Care Excellence. (2013). *Dermatitis—contact. NICE clinical knowledge summaries.* Retrieved from https://cks.nice.org.uk.
   Primary Care Dermatology Society. (2014). *Eczema: Contact allergic dermatitis. Clinical guidance.* Retrieved from www.pcds.org.uk/contact_dermatitis.

- Contact dermatitis is an inflammatory skin reaction that occurs in response to an external agent acting as an irritant or allergen.
- Allergic contact dermatitis is a type IV hypersensitivity reaction that occurs after sensitization and subsequent reexposure to an allergen.
- Irritant contact dermatitis is an inflammatory response that occurs after damage to the skin, usually by chemicals.
- In practice the two often coexist.
- Atopic eczema is strongly associated with irritant contact dermatitis. The hands and face being affected in preference to other body parts helps to distinguish contact dermatitis from other forms of dermatitis.
- Pompholyx eczema is a specific type of hand and foot eczema characterized by vesicles. It is thought to be multifactorial and related to sweating as flares occur in hot weather/humid conditions. However, there is a strong association with irritant and allergic contact dermatitis.
- Physical conditions such as heat, cold, repeated frictional exposure, and low humidity can also increase the likelihood and severity of contact dermatitis.
- *Common irritants:*
  - Water
  - Detergents and soaps
  - Solvents and abrasives
  - Machining oils
  - Acids and alkalis, including cements
  - Powders, dusts, and soils

- *Common allergens:*
  - Cosmetics: particularly fragrances, hair dyes, and nail varnish
  - Metals (e.g., nickel/cobalt in jewelery)
  - Topical medications, including rare allergy to topical corticosteroids
  - Rubber additives
  - Textiles particularly from dyes and formaldehyde resins
  - Plants: composite group (chrysanthemum and sunflowers), daffodils, tulips, primula the most common
- Some occupations particularly associated with contact dermatitis are:
  - agricultural workers;
  - beauticians;
  - chemical workers;
  - cleaners;
  - construction workers;
  - cooks and caterers;
  - electronic workers;
  - hairdressers;
  - health and social care workers;
  - machine operators;
  - mechanics;
  - metal workers.

Diagnostic Investigations

- A subgroup of people with contact dermatitis will need further investigations to identify the causative stimuli and to obtain treatments not available in primary care.
- The gold standard investigation is patch testing. This needs expert knowledge as interpretation is complex.
- Consider referral to a dermatologist if:
  - the person has chronic, recurring dermatitis despite appropriate avoidance measures and appropriate strength corticosteroid treatment;
  - there is suspicion of contact dermatitis but no clear history of exposure;
  - there is a suspicion of occupational contact dermatitis that does not respond to corticosteroid therapy.

Management

- Identify the stimulus with a full occupational and recreational history. Identification and subsequent avoidance of the stimulus is an essential part of management.
- There should be frequent and liberal use of emollient.
- A soap substitute should be used instead of normal soap.
- Gloves should be used for all house/occupational work. Patients can use either cotton gloves, vinyl gloves, or rubber gloves. Vinyl or rubber gloves should be used for wet work.
- Treat localized acute dermatitis with a topical steroid appropriate to the severity and location of the dermatitis (more information available in the atopic eczema section). It is worth remembering that affected skin on the hands and feet may need a potent or very potent topical steroid (e.g., betnovate or dermovate).

- Consider short-term use of a systemic corticosteroid if there is:
  - significant impairment of function (e.g., eczema in the hands);
  - extensive acute dermatitis (>20% of body affected).
- Evidence would suggest antihistamines are not helpful in this condition although in practice they are commonly prescribed.
- You may need to consider referral to an occupational health physician.

Seborrheic Dermatitis

GUIDELINE

National Institute for Health and Care Excellence. (2013). *Seborrheic dermatitis. NICE Clinical Knowledge Summaries.* Retrieved from https://cks.nice.org.uk.

- Seborrheic dermatitis is a common inflammation of the skin, occurring in areas rich in sebaceous glands (scalp, nasolabial folds, ears, eyebrows, and chest). Blepharitis is also commonly associated.
- It is estimated to affect 3% to 5% of the population.
- It presents as erythematous plaques or patches that can vary from mild dandruff to dense, diffuse adherent scale. Dandruff is the precursor of seborrheic dermatitis.
- The exact cause of seborrheic dermatitis is unknown. It is thought to be associated with the presence of *Malassezia* yeasts.
- It is more common in men than women and commonly occurs in infants younger than 3 months of age and in adults 30 to 60 years of age. It is more common in people with Parkinson disease than the general population and it has a greater prevalence in immunocompromised people than in healthy adults. It has been established as a possible marker for early human immunodeficiency virus (HIV) infection and this should be considered particularly where there is severe disease.
- Seborrheic dermatitis in infants (commonly called cradle cap) usually appears within the first 6 weeks of life and most commonly affects the scalp. In infants it usually gets better over a few weeks with only some cases persisting past 8 to 9 months.

Management
Infants

- Parents should be reassured it is not a serious condition, it does not bother the baby, and it spontaneously resolves over 6 to 12 months.
- Advise parents to regularly wash the scalp with a baby shampoo and then use a gentle brush to loosen scales.
- Softening the scales with baby oil first can help remove the scales; and if particularly thick, soaking them overnight

in olive oil and then washing off in the morning can help.

- If the above simple measures are not effective prescribe a topical imidazole cream (clotrimazole or miconazole). Treat until symptoms resolve but ideally not for more than 4 weeks.

Seborrheic Dermatitis in the Scalp and Beard

- Reassure the person that seborrheic dermatitis is not caused by lack of cleanliness or excessive dryness of the skin and is not transferable.
- Explain that treatment cannot cure seborrheic dermatitis but can control it. Symptoms often recur after treatment is stopped.
- Remove thick crusts or scales on the scalp before using an antifungal shampoo. This can be done by applying warm olive oil to the scalp for several hours, then washing with a coal tar shampoo.
- Prescribe ketoconazole 2% shampoo for adolescents and adults (selenium sulfide shampoo is an alternative). Shampoos should be used twice a week for at least 1 month. Once symptoms are under control their use can then be reduced to once a week. Shampoos can also be applied to the beard area.
- If the patient has severe itching of the scalp consider coprescribing 4 weeks of treatment with a potent topical steroid scalp application (e.g., Bettamousse or Elocon scalp). These are not appropriate for the beard area as they may cause thinning of skin on the face.
- Topical steroids are not appropriate for long-term use and their use as maintenance treatment is not recommended.
- Consider dermatology referral if symptoms have not resolved after 4 weeks.

Seborrheic Dermatitis of the Face and Body

- Prescribe ketoconazole 2% cream twice daily for 4 weeks (clotrimazole or miconazole can also be used).
- Consider adding a mildly potent topical corticosteroid (e.g., hydrocortisone 1%) to help settle inflammation. Corticosteroids should only be used short term (1–2 weeks).
- Ketoconazole shampoo can also be used as a body wash.

Severe or Recalcitrant Symptoms

- A systemic itraconazole 100 mg/day for 14 days can be considered along with dermatology referral.
- HIV testing should be considered.

Management of Ocular Symptoms

- Lid hygiene with cotton wool soaked in cool boiled water may be enough.
- Artificial tears should be applied liberally if eyes are dry or sore.
- As with acne rosacea, systemic treatment with a tetracycline can be used for 6 to 8 weeks if symptoms are particularly troublesome. Erythromycin is an alternative if patient is unable to take tetracycline.

Acne Vulgaris

- Acne vulgaris is one of the most common skin disorders affecting the adolescent population. It can cause great psychological distress in teenagers and young people.
- It usually starts at puberty, peaks at around 16 to 20 years of age, and tends to self-resolve in most people by the third decade. In about 7% of patients it persists into the fourth and fifth decades or may resolve and recur in later life.
- There are four aetiological factors:
  1. Excessive sebum production, leading to seborrhoea; it is androgen mediated
  2. Comedone (blackhead/whitehead) formation, due to excessive proliferation of keratinocytes in intrafollicular ducts
  3. Ductal colonization with *Propionibacterium acnes*
  4. Inflammation leading to papule, pustule, and nodule formation
- Acne can be graded in various ways. The simplest way to grade it is as follows:
  1. Noninflammatory acne/comedonal acne
  2. Inflammatory acne subdivided into mild, moderate, and severe acne

Presentation

- It has usually been present for months. It tends to be worse in autumn and winter due to lack of sunlight. Patients can present with painful lesions; however, most times it is the psychological distress caused by the lesions that brings patients to seek medical advice. Lesions usually develop on the face, neck, upper limbs, chest, and upper back.
- *Mild inflammatory acne* usually presents with inflamed comedones (open or closed), papules, and pustules.
- *Moderate inflammatory acne* usually presents with inflamed papules and pustules.
- *Severe inflammatory acne* usually presents with nodules and cysts, which can be painful.
- Some special subtypes of acne are:
  - *acne conglobata:* severe nodulocystic acne which is more prominent on the trunk than on the face and tends to lead to ulceration;
  - *acne fulminans:* acute presentation with cystic ulcerating acne, typically seen in teenage boys. Commonly associated with systemic illness such as myalgia, arthralgia, fever, fatigue, leukocytosis, and raised erythrocyte sedimentation rate (ESR);
  - *drug- or chemical-induced acne:* usually presents in atypical sites and in the wrong age group. Common triggers are systemic steroids, isoniazid and adrenocorticotropic hormone (ACTH), chlorinated hydrocarbons (in insecticides, fungicides), and cosmetics;
  - *infantile acne:* rare, seen in neonates and may be self-limiting and transient. Only seen in boys in the first 2 years of life. Presentation is with comedones, papules, pustules. Treatment is usually required with oral erythromycin or co-trimoxazole.

Diagnosis

- Diagnosis is clinical and does not usually require any investigations.
- Differential diagnoses include:
  - *perioral dermatitis:* perioral non comedonal erythematous papules that tend to worsen with topical steroids but respond to oral tetracycline;
  - *seborrhoeic eczema:* dry, scaly, erythematous, itchy skin on scalp and upper trunk;
  - *rosacea:* non comedonal erythema or telangiectasia with flushing that is seen in older people. Truncal involvement is rare. May be associated with rhinophyma.

Management

- Irrespective of treatment the following should be discussed with all patients:
  - Acne can be chronic and take a long time to respond to treatment.
  - No response to treatment may be seen in the first 6 to 8 weeks.
  - Continuing treatment for at least 6 to 8 months if responding to treatment is important.
  - Stress-induced and premenstrual flare may be seen and sunlight usually causes temporary improvement but not recommended due to high risk of skin cancer.
- Treatment should be based on severity of acne and aetiology or pathogenesis.

Topical Treatment

- Indicated on its own in mild inflammatory acne, in conjunction with oral treatment in moderate acne, and as maintenance after oral treatment.
- The choice of treatment can be broken down based on mode of action, as follows:
  - *Comedolytic and anti inflammatory therapies:* milder forms such as benzoyl peroxide and azelaic acid to stronger treatments such as topical retinoids (e.g., adapalene, all-trans retinoic acid, isotretinoin)
  - *Antibiotics:* clindamycin, erythromycin, tetracycline
  - *Combination therapies:* Duac, Isotrex, Zineryt, and Epiduo, which include a comedolytic therapy and antibiotic

Systemic Therapy

- *Oral antibiotics* should be considered in acne not responding to topical treatment or where acne is difficult to reach (e.g., on the back). Common regimes include:
  - oxytetracycline 500 mg twice a day. Not used in children under 12 years of age. Warn patients regarding photosensitivity;
  - lymecycline 408 mg daily. Side effects are the same as tetracycline;
  - doxycycline 100 mg daily or, if not tolerated, 50 mg daily. Side effects include photosensitivity;
  - erythromycin 500 mg twice daily. Common side effects are gastrointestinal (GI).

Treatment should be reviewed for efficacy and tolerability after 8 to 12 weeks.
- *Hormonal contraceptives* such as co-cyprindiol can be considered in women. It is not licensed as a contraceptive in the UK but used in moderate to severe acne in women. Patients should be informed about side effects such as increased risk of venous thromboembolism.
- *Oral retinoids* should not be prescribed or managed in primary care.

Referral

- Refer to a dermatologist:
  - severe inflammatory acne;
  - patients with any grade of acne with scarring;
  - patients who have failed to respond to two or more oral antibiotic courses of at least 12 weeks duration each;
  - diagnostic uncertainty.
- All patients who have had treatment for acne can be referred to plastic surgery for scar revision; however, they should be allowed a period of 12 to 18 months post treatment to see if the skin remodels itself.

Acne Rosacea

> **GUIDELINE**
>
> Primary Care Dermatology Society. (2018). *Rosacea. Clinical guidance.* Retrieved from www.pcds.org.uk/rosacea.

- Clinical appearance is similar to acne vulgaris; however, there is marked erythema and telangiectasia. There are associated papules and pustules but no comedones (helps differentiate from acne vulgaris).
- Usually presents on face, particularly on cheeks, nose, chin, forehead, and tip of nose and most commonly presents in those aged over 40.
- *Complications* include blepharitis, conjunctivitis, keratitis, lymphoedema of face, and rhinophyma.
- *Differential diagnoses* include:
  - *acne vulgaris:* usually have comedones and earlier age of presentation;
  - *seborrhoeic eczema:* usually scaly, around nasolabial areas and scalp. Can be itchy. No pustules;
  - *perioral dermatitis:* usually in younger people and restricted to around the mouth;
  - *systemic lupus erythematosus (SLE):* usually differentiated by lack of papules and pustules and patients are often systemically unwell.

Management

- *Oral antibiotics* are the mainstay of treatment. Usually oxytetracycline 250–500 mg twice daily for 2 to 3 months. If there is no response then a further course should be prescribed. Sometimes long-term treatment may be required. Alternative regimes include doxycycline 100 mg daily, erythromycin 250–500 mg twice daily, lymecycline 408 mg once daily, minocycline 100 mg daily.

- *Topical treatment* with 0.75% metronidazole gel or cream (Rozex/Metrogel) twice a day. Consider topical ivermectin daily for 16 weeks. Repeat course if effective. Discontinue if no response after 12 weeks.
- *Treatment of telangiectasia* includes brimonidine gel/Mirvaso. Warn patient regarding hypopigmentation and the possible bleaching effect which is temporary and settles once treatment is stopped.

Psoriasis

GUIDELINES

Scottish Intercollegiate Guidance Network. (2010). *Diagnosis and management of psoriasis and psoriatic arthritis in adults. SIGN guideline 121.* Retrieved from www.sign.ac.uk.
National Institute for Health and Care Excellence. (2012). *Psoriasis: Assessment and management. NICE clinical guideline 153,* updated 2017. Retrieved from www.nice.org.uk.

- Psoriasis is a chronic inflammatory multisystem disease with predominantly skin and joint manifestations. It is characterized by scaly skin lesions which can be in the form of patches, papules, or plaques. Although it is usually chronic, the guttate form typically resolves within 3 to 4 months of onset.
- Forms of psoriasis include:
  - chronic plaque psoriasis (80%–90%): this includes flexural, scalp, and facial psoriasis;
  - localized pustular psoriasis of the palms and soles;
  - nail psoriasis;
  - guttate psoriasis;
  - erythrodermic psoriasis;
  - generalized pustular psoriasis.
- Around 1% to 3% of the population has psoriasis; it is more common in white people and, although presentation can be at any age, psoriasis most commonly presents between 15 and 30 years. Men and women are equally affected.
- Factors that may influence the onset or cause an exacerbation of preexisting psoriasis include:
  - streptococcal infection (strongly associated with guttate psoriasis but association may also apply to plaque psoriasis);
  - drugs (lithium, antimalarials, beta blockers, nonsteroidal antiinflammatory drugs [NSAIDs], angiotensin-converting enzyme [ACE] inhibitors, trazodone);
  - sunlight (usually beneficial but may exacerbate psoriasis in small number of people);
  - trauma (the Koebner phenomenon);
  - postpartum hormonal change;
  - psychologic stress;
  - excessive alcohol intake;
  - smoking;

- HIV infection/acquired immunodeficiency syndrome (AIDS).
- Psoriasis is associated with several other conditions:
  - Psoriatic arthritis
  - Traditional cardiovascular (CV) risk factors (hypertension, hyperlipidaemia, diabetes)
  - Inflammatory bowel disease
  - Obesity
  - Venous thromboembolism (VTE)
  - Nonmelanoma skin cancer

Management

General points to consider:
- Be aware of the possibility of joint involvement and refer to rheumatology if psoriatic arthropathy is affected.
- Psoriasis can be associated with mood disturbance and therefore this should be enquired about at review.
- Psoriasis is often thought of as a nonitchy skin condition; however, patients often do find itch a problem and antihistamines can help.
- All patients with psoriasis should have yearly follow-up to address cardiovascular risk factors. Despite being associated with an increased risk of CV disease it is not included in most CV risk assessment tools.
- Compliance with treatment is improved by good patient understanding of the condition. Signposting to online web resources and patient information leaflets should be considered.

Chronic Plaque Psoriasis

- Offer topical treatments first line. National Institute for Health and Care Excellence (NICE, 2012) advises prescribing a potent topical steroid (e.g., betnovate 0.1% in morning) and a topical vitamin D preparation separately (e.g., Dovonex) and avoiding using combination products (NICE, 2012). However, many general practitioners (GPs), dermatologists, and general practitioners with a special interest (GPwSIs) routinely use a combination product (e.g., Dovobet) to improve compliance and bring about rapid control of symptoms. The Primary Care Dermatology Society (PCDS) and British Association of Dermatologists (BAD) recognize this variation and their guidelines differ from NICE.
- Topical corticosteroids are only suitable for treating localized psoriasis and repeat prescriptions should be monitored as there is a risk of destabilizing disease. They should not be applied for more than 8 weeks. Treatment can be restarted after a 4-week treatment break if needed.
- Emollients should be offered to reduce scale and help with itch.
- If scale is a particular problem, preparations containing salicylic acid may be useful.
- Review the patient after 4 weeks. Continue treatment until skin is clear/nearly clear (i.e., skin is smooth but can still be red/pink).

- Topical vitamin D preparations alone can be used as maintenance treatment for chronic plaque psoriasis.
- If the patient has a poor response to 8 weeks of potent topical steroid advise the patient to stop this and apply vitamin D alone for 12 weeks twice daily.
- If there is still a poor response after this try a coal tar preparation (e.g., Exorex or Carbo-Dome) once or twice daily.
- For people with treatment-resistant psoriasis consider dithranol. Evidence for dithranol is very good but its use is limited by patient acceptance (it causes stinging sensation; stains clothes, furniture, and skin). It should only be used for large focal plaques of psoriasis. The lowest strength (0.1%) should be titrated slowly and only if tolerated. It should be applied once daily.
- Refer to secondary care for consideration of light treatment or systemic therapy if topical treatment does not control disease, if disease is widespread at onset, or if there is psychologic distress due to disease.

Scalp Psoriasis

- Initial treatment should be with a potent topical corticosteroid in a scalp application form (e.g., Elocon scalp). Advise the patient to stop the corticosteroid once the skin is clear.
- Coal tar shampoos can be considered but should not be used alone for people with severe scalp psoriasis.
- Review the patient at 4 weeks. If there is poor response check compliance and offer the topical steroid in a different form such as shampoo or mousse (e.g., Bettamouse) and consider a scalp treatment (e.g., salicylic acid, olive oil, coconut oil) to remove scale before further corticosteroid.
- If there is still a poor response to treatment after another 4 weeks consider a combined topical steroid and vitamin D preparation (Dovobet scalp).
- If the above treatments do not control scalp dermatitis consider a very potent topical steroid twice a day for 2 weeks and referral to a dermatologist.

Genital, Facial, and Flexural Psoriasis

- Emollients should be offered to all patients.
- A short-term mild or moderate topical steroid preparation should be used for up to 2 weeks.
- If there is a good response to treatment repeated short courses of topical corticosteroids may be used to maintain disease control. They should only be used for 1 to 2 weeks/month.
- Maintenance treatment for those with chronic disease should be with a topical vitamin D preparation alone. Dovonex is quite irritating to sensitive areas so a preparation such as Silkis may be better.
- Potent or very potent topical steroids should not be used on the face, flexures, or genitals.
- Antifungals should not be used unless there is evidence of fungal infection.

- Refer to dermatology if there is a poor response to topical steroid or continuous topical treatment is required to maintain disease control.

Guttate Psoriasis

- If lesions are widespread (>10% body surface area) refer to dermatology urgently for consideration of phototherapy.
- If lesions are not widespread reassure the person that guttate psoriasis is self-limiting and usually resolves within 3 to 4 months.
- No treatment may be an option.
- If topical treatment is required consider topical treatment as discussed for plaque psoriasis.
- Do not use antibiotics to treat guttate psoriasis triggered by a sore throat.

Pustular Psoriasis

- If the person has generalized pustular psoriasis refer for same-day specialist assessment and treatment.
- Even pustular psoriasis that is localized to hands and feet is difficult to control and usually requires systemic treatment. It is probably advisable to refer to dermatology at presentation and obtain same-day advice on treatment in interim.

Erythrodermic Psoriasis

- Refer for same-day specialist assessment and treatment. Erythroderma is associated with life-threatening complications.

Nail Psoriasis

- Treatment of nail psoriasis is very difficult. There is no evidence for topical or systemic treatments.
- Advise patients to keep nails short, avoid manicures which can exacerbate onychomycosis, and use nail polish to disguise appearance.

Lichen Planus

- Lichen planus is usually distributed in the flexural aspects of wrists, ankles, and the lumbar region of the back. Mouth, hair, nails, and genital areas can also be affected.
- It is recognizable by the "6Ps": purple, polygonic, planar (flat-topped) papules, and pruritic plaques.
- Wickham striae (white lines over lesions) are also present.

Investigations

- Diagnosis is usually clinical but when uncertain biopsy should be arranged to confirm.
- Patients should be screened for hepatitis C as an association is recognized.
- Exclude causative medications such as thiazide diuretics, spironolactone, beta blockers, and NSAIDs.

Management

- Give the patient an information leaflet and inform that 85% will improve by 18 months but it can be a relapsing condition.
- Offer antipruritic management such as antihistamines and/or menthol cream.
- Treat itchy active area with potent or superpotent topical steroids until lesions improve and explain to patient that treatment may take weeks. Do not apply steroids to skin which has postinflammatory changes (i.e., when lesions change from purple to grey-brown).
- *For facial lesions* tacrolimus ointment or pimecrolimus cream may be an alternative to steroid.
- *For scalp lesions* offer a topical steroid scalp preparation.
- *Mucosal areas* are difficult to manage. Inform patient to see dentist 6 monthly to monitor for oral cancer.

Referral

- *Refer if:*
  - there is clinical uncertainty;
  - it is refractory to treatment; or
  - there is scarring alopecia, ulceration, nail involvement, aggressive disease, or any suspicion of squamous cell carcinoma (SCC).

PATIENT SUPPORT ORGANIZATION

UK Lichen Planus. www.uklp.org.uk/.

Infection and Infestation

Infection manifests itself in most medical specialities but is of particular importance in dermatology. This chapter is by no means a comprehensive listing; instead it is designed to refresh knowledge and is an attempt to look systematically at skin infection groupings and to remind busy general practitioners of the most common skin infections and infestations.

Viral Infections

Warts

- Human papillomavirus (HPV) and warts are common. Most clear by 2 years but they can last up to 10 years in adults.
- Diagnosis is usually clinical and can be aided by paring down the wart which will often reveal small black dots which represent coagulated capillaries.
- Malignant change is rare except in immunocompromised individuals.
- They are categorized as:
  - *common wart:* firm and raised, resembles cauliflower, on hands and feet;
  - *plane wart:* round, flat topped, found on back of hands;
  - *filiform wart:* long and slender, found on face and neck;
  - *palmar and planter (verrucae):* central dark dots in middle and may be painful;
  - *mosaic:* when warts coalesce.
- Differentials to consider:
  - Actinic keratosis
  - Seborrheic keratosis
  - Lichen planus
  - Knuckle pads
  - SCC (rare but increased on sun-exposed sites or in immunocompromised patients)
  - Palmoplantar keratoderma

Management

- Advise the patient that warts are not harmful and most resolve spontaneously. To reduce risk of transmission wear a waterproof plaster when swimming and flip-flops in the shower and avoid sharing shoes, socks, and towels. To avoid autoinoculation do not scratch, bite, or suck warts.
- No medical therapy is often most appropriate. Only consider treatment if unsightly, painful, or if the patient requests treatment for a persisting wart.
- *Salicylic acid* topical preparations of 10% to 26% applied daily after paring with occlusion if possible. Apply for 3 months. The main complication is irritation and they are contraindicated in areas of poor healing and the face.
- *Cryotherapy.* Keep the wart frozen for 5 to 30 seconds repeating every 2 to 4 weeks for at least 3 months (six treatments). Advise about risks of pain, blistering, and hypopigmentation.
- Combination of salicylic acid and cryotherapy can be used.
- Children with verruca do not need to be banned from swimming but can instead wear verruca socks.

Specific Wart Treatment Options

- *Plantar.* Paring of the skin then salicylic acid up to 50% or 2-weekly cryotherapy for up to 4 months. Another option for painful plantar warts is to treat with corn plasters.
- *Plane.* Await self-resolution, use 2% to 10% salicylic acid cream or mild cryotherapy. Apply topical retinoic acid if they are persistent.
- *Facial wart.* Do not use salicylic acid. Mild cryotherapy (5–10 seconds to the wart but avoid surrounding skin) is an option and repeat every 2 to 3 weeks. Make sure patients are consented for risks associated with cryotherapy.
- *Warts in children.* Await self-resolution as much faster spontaneous clearing than in adults; salicylic acid is an option, cryotherapy is often poorly tolerated.

Referral

- Consider referral if:
  - symptomatic warts present for at least 2 years that are unresponsive to topical treatment and cryotherapy;
  - uncertain diagnosis;

- immunocompromised patient;
- extensive mosaic warts;
- anogenital warts, which should be referred to genito-urinary medicine (GUM).

Herpes Simplex

- Acquired by direct contact.
- Eruption may be preceded by itching, burning, tingling; and lesions, when they appear, can be very painful.
- Provide patients with written information.
- Consider the option of no treatment for herpes simplex infections that are mild and uncomplicated as episodes will self-resolve.
- See specific treatments in the sections covering herpes simplex subtypes (to come).
- Advise patients to reduce the chances of transmission to others by not kissing, participating in oral sex, or sharing cups while symptomatic.
- Advise caution to contact lens wearers during an episode to reduce the chance of herpes keratoconjunctivitis.
- *Admission* may be required for those who:
  - are immunocompromised;
  - are systemically unwell;
  - are unable to swallow and are at risk of dehydration;
  - have suspected herpes keratoconjunctivitis; or
  - have suspected eczema herpeticum (to come).
- *Consider referral if:*
  - frequent, persistent, or severe herpes simplex virus (HSV);
  - in third trimester of pregnancy with genital herpes;
  - lesions are refractory to oral treatment; or
  - diagnosis is uncertain.

Herpetic Gingivostomatitis

- Presents with white vesicles on the tongue, buccal mucosa, palate, and lips.
- Usually resolves by 2 weeks.
- Treatment is acyclovir 200 mg five times a day for 5 days.

Herpes Labialis

- Presents as grouped vesicles on the lips and perioral skin.
- Usually resolves by 10 days.
- Advise on appropriate ultraviolet (UV) protection as sunlight is a trigger.
- Use topical acyclovir (available over the counter) as soon as symptoms occur.
- If recurrent consider long-term acyclovir 200 to 400 mg twice daily.

Genital Herpes

- May cause dysuria mimicking features of urinary tract infection (UTI).
- Treatment is with acyclovir 500 mg five times a day for 5 days.
- Both the patient and partner(s) need a full sexually transmitted infection (STI) screen which may best be undertaken by the GUM clinic.

Eczema Herpeticum

- Occurs in those with atopic eczema. The lesions occur on the eczematous skin and are punched out erosions or vesicles and are often widespread. There may be systemic upset including fever and lethargy, and there may be enlarged inguinal or axillary lymph nodes.
- Treat with systemic acyclovir, which usually requires admission for treatment with intravenous acyclovir, particularly if there is systemic upset.
- Consider giving antibiotics for superadded bacterial infection which may occur.

Neonatal Herpes Simplex Virus

- High risk if mother has genital herpes at the time of delivery, particularly if it is a primary episode. It can range from localized to disseminated.
- Have a low threshold for seeking advice from a paediatrician.

Disseminated Herpes Simplex Virus Can Be Life Threatening—Early Recognition and Urgent Referral Are Required. Herpes Zoster

- Patients over 70 (who are not immunocompromised) in the United Kingdom are now entitled to a shingles vaccine which is expected to reduce the burden of shingles in this vulnerable group.
- The first manifestation of an attack is usually pain which may be severe and can be accompanied by fever, headache, and malaise. The rash onset usually follows within 3 days of pain and follows a typical dermatomal distribution. If the rash crosses the midline then consider alternative diagnoses.
- Patients are infectious until all lesions are crusted over (day 5–7 from rash onset) and should avoid contact with those who have never had chickenpox or who are immunocompromised.
- School or work need only be avoided if the rash is weeping or cannot be covered.
- *Treatment* is with acyclovir 800 mg five times a day for 7 days (alternatively valaciclovir or famciclovir can be used). Ideally this should be initiated within 72 hours of the rash developing but consider starting it up to 1 week after onset of rash particularly in those at high risk of complications.
- *Consider referral or admission:*
  - under ophthalmology if there is ophthalmic involvement with a red eye or visual complaints. If there is ophthalmic shingles with no eye involvement then start treatment and review in 1 week;
  - under otorhinolaryngology (ears, nose, throat [ENT]) if the Ramsay Hunt syndrome is present. This may present with deep ear pain, rash in the ear canal or on the auricle, and there may be associated facial droop, tinnitus, ipsilateral hearing loss, and vertigo;
  - under medics if the patient is immunocompromised and the rash is widespread.

Postherpetic Neuralgia

- The pain of postherpetic neuralgia can be severe and debilitating although it is usually self-limiting, lasting around 3 to 5 weeks. It can last for months or years. It occurs in one in five people after shingles and is more common in the elderly, in females, in the immunocompromised, and in those who have had a severe attack of shingles.
- Offer the patient an information leaflet.
- Step 1 management is paracetamol, codeine, or NSAID.
- Step 2 management is neuropathic analgesics, usually amitriptyline or gabapentin.
- Topical treatments, including capsaicin or lidocaine plasters, may be effective if oral medications have failed.
- Consider referral for pain management in those with refractory symptoms.

PATIENT SUPPORT ORGANIZATION

Herpes Viruses Association. 41 North Road, London, N7 9DP; helpline: 0845 123 2305; email: info@herpes.org.uk; website: www.herpes.org.uk.

Bacterial Infection

- It is worth remembering that skin infection can be either a primary disease process or a consequence of underlying skin disease.

Staphylococci and Streptococci

- Both these organisms account for some of the most common encounters, often causing significant morbidity and, potentially, mortality.

Impetigo

- Superficial infection of the upper layers of the skin most commonly encountered in children.
- Usually highly contagious, the child is systemically well, with classic honey-coloured crusting lesions on the face or digits and readily spreadable locally. Rarely presents as bullous lesions.
- Usually caused by *Staphylococcus aureus* but occasionally *Streptococcus pyogenes.*
- *Treatment* for localized lesions can be with topical mupirocin. Give oral antibiotics (such as flucloxacillin or erythromycin) for more widespread or severe cases.
- Provide education to patients about how it is transmitted and how to prevent transmission.

Ecthyma

- Presentation is similar to impetigo but deeper layers of skin are involved leading to ulceration on lower legs, buttocks, thighs, ankles, and feet. Patients tend to give a history of previous trauma such as insect bites. It is caused by *S. pyogenes.*
- Lesions are painful and tend to start with vesicles or pustules on inflamed skin which deepens to form ulcers

(≤3 cm in size) with an overlying greyish thick crust. Removal of crust reveals a punched-out ulcer. It tends to heal slowly with scarring. Regional lymphadenopathy can be seen.

- It is more common in diabetic patients or elderly neglected skin and more common in tropical climates.
- Complications include cellulitis, gangrene, bacteraemia, staphylococcal scalded skin syndrome, and toxic shock syndrome.
- Differential diagnosis includes:
  - *ecthyma gangrenosum.* Appearance similar but caused by pseudomonas species. Associated with significant mortality;
  - *orf/ecthyma contagiosum.* Consider diagnosis if there is relevant history of exposure to sheep or goats;
  - *pyoderma gangrenosum.* Tends to have similar appearance but usually a typical purplish appearance on edges of the ulcer;
  - *arterial ulcers.* Especially if history of arterial disease.
- *Investigations* should include blood test to rule out neutropenia and diabetes, and wound swabs.
- *Treatment* depends on extent of lesions. If localized, antibacterial washes such as Hibiscrub and topical mupirocin/ fusidic acid can be used. More extensive infections require oral flucloxacillin or phenoxymethylpenicillin if group A strep isolated. Treatment may be required for several weeks. If there are clinical concerns or doubt about diagnosis or management then refer to secondary care as surgical debridement may be necessary for extensive infection.

Folliculitis

- Present with multiple small papules or pustules on an erythematous base with or without hair follicle visible in the centre. Sometimes it can present with deeper lesions as painful nodules that may result in scarring and permanent hair loss. Usually caused by *S. aureus* (very occasionally caused by gram-negative organisms).
- Common subtypes are based on distribution:
  - Beard: folliculitis barbae
  - Lower legs: pseudofolliculitis (secondary to hair removal or shaving)
  - Trunk or buttocks: *Malassezia* or pseudomonas folliculitis
  - Scalp: folliculitis decalvans
  - Eosinophilic folliculitis
- *Treatment:*
  - Avoid or treat the causative factor. Antibacterial washes include chlorhexidine or Hibiscrub.
  - Topical or oral antistaph antibiotic again depending on disease extent; may require 4 to 6 weeks of treatment.
  - If *Malassezia* infestation then consider ketoconazole cream/shampoo regularly until clear then once or twice weekly for maintenance.
- *Refer if:*
  - diagnostic doubt;
  - there is poor response to treatment as patients can be considered for isotretinoin or phototherapy.

Furuncles, Carbuncles, and Abscesses

- A furuncle or a boil is a deeper infection of the hair follicle with subcutaneous tissue involvement leading to abscess formation. A carbuncle is when multiple inflamed hair follicles coalesce to form a single lump which discharges pus.
- *Treatment* is with an oral antistaph antibiotic (e.g., flucloxacillin) if infection is caught early but it may require surgical incision and drainage.

Erysipelas

- Erysipelas is the name given to a more superficial form of cellulitis that is usually seen following a breach in skin. Common sites are the face and legs, and can present bilaterally.
- It is caused by group A streptococcus (*S. pyogenes*), occasionally by Staphylococcus. Other pathogens may be causative in immunocompromised patients.
- Patients present with well-demarcated erythema, oedema which is hot and tender to touch.
- The patient is usually systemically well unless septic.
- *Treatment* is with oral flucloxacillin 500 mg to 1 g four times daily or clarithromycin 500 mg twice daily. If there is facial involvement, consider co-amoxiclav. Treatment may need to be prolonged for 10 to 14 days.
- *Refer if* the patient is systemically unwell or not responding to oral treatment.

Cellulitis

- Cellulitis is commonly encountered in primary care. It is usually caused by *S. aureus* but can be *S. pyogenes* and, uncommonly, *Haemophilus influenza*.
- Cellulitis involves the deep dermis and the patient is systemically unwell; the area will be red, hot, painful, and generally swollen with an ill-defined border and may have an obvious point of entry for infection.
- Risk factors include:
  - gravitational eczema;
  - leg ulcers;
  - tinea infection;
  - trauma;
  - lymphoedema;
  - high body mass index (BMI);
  - diabetes; and
  - immunocompromised patients.
  It is highly unusual to encounter bilateral lower leg cellulitis; often chronic venous stasis with red legs will be wrongly labelled as bilateral cellulitis, leading to incorrect treatment.
- Differential diagnosis:
  - Chronic venous insufficiency. Usually bilateral. No associated tenderness or heat. Patient is systemically well. Follows a more chronic history.
  - Allergic contact dermatitis. Usually there is a history of contact with an allergen. Presents acutely with associated blisters and itching.
- *Treatment,* if infection is limited, is with oral flucloxacillin, otherwise the patient will require intravenous flucloxacillin or penicillin with the addition of clindamycin if severe.

- Always treat underlying causes such as tinea or ulcers; advise weight management.
- Advise rest, elevation, analgesia.
- Mark the area and observe for tracking.
- *Refer* if the patient is systemically unwell or not responding to oral treatment.

Recurrent Cellulitis

- Cellulitis is recurrent if the patient suffers with two or more episodes of cellulitis per year.
- *Treatment* is with prophylactic antibiotics such as:
  - penicillin V 250 mg twice daily for 1 year then 250 mg once daily;
  - for penicillin-allergic patients clarithromycin 250 mg once daily or erythromycin 250 mg twice daily.
- Stop treatment after 2 years. If symptoms recur after 2 years restart prophylaxis and continue long term.

Necrotizing Fasciitis

- This is a rare but an important surgical emergency and must be referred for immediate management. It is often a polymicrobial infection involving the deep planes of the skin including fascia. Although often numerous bacteria may be involved including anaerobes, *S. pyogenes* is the most rapid, often being termed *flesh eating* and the patient is moribund within a couple of hours.
- *Presentation:*
  - Level of pain is out of proportion to clinical presentation
  - Greyish violaceous area with erythema
  - Crepitus
  - Patient develops blisters that become necrotic
  - Systemically unwell
- *Treatment* involves pattern recognition in a septic deteriorating patient with emergency onward referral for debridement, intensive support, and antibiotics. It requires multidisciplinary input.

Erythrasma

- Presents with macerated areas that are often patchy and involving either the interdigital or intertriginous areas or may also appear as reddish-brown plaques in the axillary areas. Caused by *Corynebacterium minuttissimi*.
- *Treatment* is either topical clindamycin or topical erythromycin.

Gram-Negative Bacilii

- Most commonly Pseudomonas, usually aeruginosa. Infection generally develops on skin which is already damaged, for example in severe tinea infection. Skin becomes macerated, develops a foul small, and may appear with a greenish tinge because of pigment production from the bacteria.
- *Treatment* is aimed at treating the underlying skin condition.

Lyme Disease

- Lyme disease is caused by the spirochaete organism Borrelia, transmitted by the Ixodes tick. The type of Borrelia is dependent on which continent the tick is encountered.

- Ticks removed before 24 hours of attachment are unlikely to be problematic; however, cutaneous lesions developing within a month of tick removal should be considered for evaluation of early Lyme disease.
- A history of being in woodland areas and of tick bites is useful. It is usually seen in spring and summer seasons.
- The most common presentation is that of *erythema chronicum migrans,* a distinctive rash which starts as an erythematous papule expanding to an annular erythema with central clearing. It can be seen between 1 and 33 days after exposure and fades over 3 to 4 weeks but only 70% to 80% cases develop the typical rash.
- There may be a mild flulike illness and about two-thirds of untreated patients will develop symptoms, including:
  - arthritis;
  - neuroborreliosis;
  - Bell palsy or other cranial nerve involvement; and
  - cardiac borreliosis; peri/myocarditis leading to conduction defects.
- Long-term sequelae include chronic arthritis and neurological problems.
- Advise patients travelling to at-risk areas to:
  - wear white (for easy spotting of ticks), long-sleeved clothes, long trousers tucked into socks, long boots;
  - use pesticides/repellents;
  - check whole body for ticks closely when home and repeat the following day;
  - if a tick is seen use tweezers and firmly remove it in whole and disinfect the skin.
- The presence of typical rash merits immediate treatment.
- Serology for antibodies to *Borrelia burgdorferi,* although these may be negative in the first few weeks postinfection.
- *Treatment* is with doxycycline (100 mg two or three times a day), amoxicillin, or erythromycin (less effective) for 2 to 3 weeks.

Fungal Infections

Tinea

- Consider it if there is an asymmetrical rash with scale and a leading edge.
- Take skin scrapings from the advancing edge of the rash.
- False negatives are not uncommon and samples should be repeated with treatment given if strong clinical suspicion of tinea.
- For mild tinea use topical agents but if widespread or severe then oral therapies are indicated.
- Terbinafine is first line oral agent but alternatives are imidazole preparations. If using terbinafine then get baseline liver function tests before initiation and repeat after 6 weeks of treatment.
- Advise patients not to share towels or hats and to disinfect combs, scissors, pillows, and bed covers.

Scalp Infection

- Features are hair loss and scaling.
- Take skin scrapings and hair follicles for mycology.
- Offer patient information leaflet.

- Topical management with terbinafine/imidazoles for 2 to 4 weeks can be considered for limited infection.
- Systemic treatment with terbinafine/imidazoles for 2 to 4 weeks should be given if infection is extensive or the rash is very inflamed.
- If a kerion present refer dermatology:
  - Due to risk of scarring oral therapy is offered and this is usually terbinafine although itraconazole can also be used.
  - For children griseofulvin is first line.
  - Also use antifungal shampoo for the first 2 weeks of therapy.
  - Treat family members with antifungal shampoo for 2 weeks.

Hands

- White discolouration in skin folds is often present.
- Always examine feet, hands, and nails as spread is common.

Feet

- Interdigital skin gets broken down and is a common cause of secondary cellulitis.
- Give topical treatment unless there is coexistent nail involvement in which case systemic therapy is indicated.
- Advise the patient to wear breathable footwear to reduce chance of recurrence.

Nails

- Presents with subungual hyperkeratosis and yellow or white discolouration of nails.
- Offer patient information leaflet. Self-care is often appropriate if the patient is not bothered by the nail or is concerned about side effects of treatment.
- For nail clippings first cut the nail back then remove the friable debris to be sent for mycology. This will reduce false negative results.
- Explain that cure rates are often 60% to 80%.
- *Topical treatment* is only for isolated superficial infections. Preparations such as tioconazole or Loceryl can be used.
- *Systemic treatment* is with terbinafine 250 mg once daily and should be for 6 weeks for fingernails and 3 months for toenails. Alternatively, pulsed therapy of itraconazole can be used giving 400 mg once daily for 1 week every month. Two cycles are needed for fingernails and four cycles are required for toenails. Get baseline liver function tests (LFTs) before starting oral treatment.
- Inform the patient that even with successful treatment it can take months for the toenail to grow out and look healthy again.
- In children weight-adjusted terbinafine or griseofulvin can be used.
- If recurrent infection then long-term twice weekly topical antifungal (terbinafine or imidazoles) can be used.

Candidiasis

Oral

- In healthy adults candidiasis may be the symptoms of underlying immunodeficiency so think about risk factors for diabetes, malnutrition, cancer, and HIV.

- Review known triggers if present such as poor denture hygiene, inhaler technique, and diabetic control.
- First line treatment is miconazole gel or nystatin but if extensive then offer oral fluconazole.

Skin

- Advise the patient to avoid tight-fitting clothes and keep the area as dry as possible to avoid reinfection.
- If obese give lifestyle counselling on weight loss.
- For localized infection use topical imidazole creams or terbinafine. If the rash is very inflamed or itchy consider adding topical steroid to the antifungal cream.
- Creams should be used for 7 days and if no improvement then review the diagnosis and treatment.

Pityriasis Versicolour

- Most commonly presents in children and teenagers as round or oval macules and papules that have a fine scale and may coalesce. Usually it is asymptomatic but is occasionally mildly itchy. Typically occurs on the chest, back, and upper arms. It is caused by yeasts of the genus *Malassezia*.
- Explain that it is a self-limiting, noncontagious condition that is usually easily treated though skin change back to normal can take months.
- Ketoconazole shampoo or selenium sulfide (contraindicated in pregnancy) shampoos can be used if extensive.
- Topical imidazoles can be applied if localized. Use for 2 weeks.
- If treatment fails then take skin scrapings to confirm diagnosis and consider using systemic therapy such as itraconazole or fluconazole.
- Consider referral if:
  - diagnosis is uncertain and scrapings are negative;
  - there is extensive disease;
  - immunocompromised, pregnant, or under 12 years old requiring systemic therapy.

Parasitic Infections

Scabies

- Typically presents with widespread itching and a rash that may exhibit papules, vesicles, or nodules and linear burrows that classically affect the interdigital web spaces and flexor aspects of wrists, elbows, groin, and axillae.
- Treat the patient and all household and sexual contacts with permethrin 5% Dermol cream (or malathion as alternative) immediately and after 1 week.
- Advise patients to machine wash clothes and bed linen at 50°C.
- Treat itch and concurrent bacterial infection if present.
- If crusted scabies is present then consider underlying immunodeficiency.
- Inform patients that itch may last up to 4 weeks posttreatment.
- Consider urea or crotamiton emollients to treat ongoing itch.
- Consider referral if:
  - crusted scabies or diagnosis is in doubt;

- ongoing active infection despite two courses of treatment.
- Contact Health Protection Agency if there is an outbreak in an institution such as a school or nursing home.

Head Lice

- Affected children can still attend school.
- Treat all affected family members on the same day; options include dimeticone, malathion, or wet combing.
- Insecticide preparations should be used twice (repeated again at 7 days) and detection combing should be undertaken 3 days posttreatment to make sure lice are eradicated.

Pubic Lice

- If transmitted via sexual contact then refer to GUM clinic for further STI screening and contact tracing. Alternatively screen for chlamydia and other STIs, inform patient to avoid sexual contacts until both have been treated, and undertake contact tracing for sexual contacts over the past 3 months.
- Treat with topical malathion 0.5% or permethrin 5% to be used twice 7 days apart.
- If present in a child then, although nonsexual contact is most common, consider the possibility of sexual abuse.

Skin Lesions and Malignancies

- There are many different types of skin lesions and malignancies. Discussing them all would be beyond the remit of this book. Some of the common skin lesions and malignancies that are seen in General Practice are described in this section.
- Common terminologies used when describing skin lesions:
  - *Macule:* pigmented or nonpigmented flat lesion which is not palpable
  - *Papule:* raised pigmented or nonpigmented lesion which is palpable and less than 1 cm in diameter
  - *Nodule:* raised pigmented or nonpigmented lesion which is palpable and greater than 1 cm in diameter
  - *Plaque:* a plateau-like elevation above the skin surface where the diameter is greater than the thickness of the lesion

Benign Skin Lesions (Du Vivierk, 2013; Wolff and Johnson, 2009)

Seborrhoeic Keratosis

- It is the most common of the benign epithelial lesions. Commonly seen after the age of 30. Can range from a few scattered lesions to hundreds in some elderly patients. Usually asymptomatic but they can be itchy or become inflamed.
- Lesions range from small, barely elevated papules to plaques with a warty surface and a typical stuck-on appearance. They can be nonpigmented or pigmented.
- Patients usually present worried as they think they have a melanoma. They give a history of a longstanding

pigmented mole that has grown in size or become itchy or inflamed. The presence of multiple similar lesions on further general skin examination is often reassuring.

- *Differential diagnoses* include:
  - *solar lentigo:* generally macular and lacks the warty appearance;
  - *actinic keratosis:* scaly rough appearance. Seen on sun-exposed areas;
  - *pigmented basal cell carcinoma (BCC):* appears more pearlescent and nodular;
  - *melanoma:* uneven pigmentation, irregular border.
- *Management* is with reassurance. If inflamed curettage or cryotherapy can be offered.
- *Refer* if there is diagnostic uncertainty.

Dermatofibroma/Histiocytoma

- This is a common, probably reactive benign skin tumour more frequently seen on extremities. Often seen in adults, it can be asymptomatic but unsightly. Occasionally it can be tender.
- Presents as a papule or nodule with a smooth surface. Firm in consistency and the characteristic feature is the dimple or pinch sign (the tumour indents on lateral pressure with the fingers as it is adherent to overlying skin but free from underlying structures).
- Reassure the patient.
- Refer if there is diagnostic uncertainty or if it is causing troublesome symptoms.

Sebaceous Hyperplasia

- These are common benign lesions that are often mistaken for BCC. They are usually secondary to enlarged sebaceous glands around a single hair follicle often on the face. Seen in older people and patients who have had solid organ transplant and are on ciclosporin.
- Present as small papules, 2 to 5 mm in diameter, flesh or yellow coloured with telangiectasia and central punctum. Usually there are multiple lesions in one area.
- Differential diagnosis is a small BCC which is usually solitary.
- *Management* is with reassurance. Excision or removal by light electrocautery under local anaesthetic can considered if there is diagnostic uncertainty.

Keratoacanthoma

- These are rapidly growing benign tumours which tend to simulate SCC but usually self-resolve in 4 to 6 months. They tend to rapidly grow for 3 months and reach up to 3 cm in diameter before regressing spontaneously over the next 3 months. They are most commonly seen in older age groups, patients who have had chronic sun exposure, and also in transplant recipients on immunosuppressants.
- Presents as a small spot that rapidly grows in size causing alarm. They are erythematous or flesh-coloured, well-defined nodules with a central keratin-filled crater. The appearance mimics an erupting volcano. Commonly seen

in sun-exposed areas such as the face, nose, ears, cheeks, dorsum of hands, and forearms. Usually solitary, very occasionally they can be multiple.

- Differential diagnoses include SCC (difficult to clinically differentiate) and hypertrophic solar keratosis.
- *Refer* for surgical excision or curettage and cautery depending on site as they cannot be clinically distinguished from SCCs. Multiple lesions may require systemic retinoids or methotrexate.

Precancerous Skin Lesions

Actinic (Solar) Keratosis

- Occur predominantly on chronically sun-exposed skin. Rough, occasionally sore or itchy spots. They may be single or multiple, dry, rough, adherent scaly yellowish-brown lesions. They are more easily felt than seen due to the roughness. Surrounding skin can be normal or erythematous.
- They are commonly seen on face, bald scalp, dorsum of hands, and forearms of patients over the age of 50.
- Differential diagnoses include:
  - Bowen disease: flat scaly lesions commonly seen on the shin;
  - seborrhoeic keratosis: warty stuck-on appearance;
  - superficial BCC: pearlescent appearance and telangiectasia.
- If left untreated some can progress into squamous cell carcinoma.
- *Advise prevention* or further worsening by recommending a high factor UVB/UVA sunscreen (usually >30 factor).
- *Treatment* options:
  - *Cryotherapy:* Usually freeze for 5 to 10 seconds after the white halo has appeared.
  - *5% fluorouracil/Efudex:* Usually apply twice daily for 4 weeks on and then 4 weeks off. If a vast area is involved then best to divide into quarters or sections and apply treatment in cycles. Warn the patient regarding erythema and erosions. If the reaction is too intense it can be applied once daily or 5 days per week.
  - *5% imiquimod/Aldara:* Highly effective but can cause intense reaction which may discourage patients. Treatment regime is 3 days per week for 4 weeks.
  - *Zyclara (3.75% imiquimod):* Can be used for facial lesions. Treatment regime is to apply for 2 weeks then discontinue for 2 weeks.
  - *3% diclofenac/Solaraze Gel:* Used twice daily for 3 months. Better tolerated but not as effective as imiquimod or fluorouracil.
  - *Picato gel:* Treatment is for 3 days which allows for better compliance.
  - Other treatments not commonly used are laser treatment, photodynamic therapy, and facial peels.
- If patients are finding the reactions secondary to topical treatment too intense then advise to use for 5 days per week and use topical steroids on the other 2 days to help skin recover.

- Refer if not responding to treatment or patient not tolerating treatment.

Bowen Disease (Squamous Cell Carcinoma In Situ) (Ashton & Leppard, 2009)

- This is described as an intraepidermal carcinoma of the skin that can occasionally progress to squamous cell carcinoma. Usually asymptomatic, patients usually present with a persistent solitary rough patch.
- It is a well-defined solitary plaque which may be slightly raised, scaly, and erythematous. Similar but non scaly lesions on the glans or vulva are called *erythroplasia*. HPV-induced Bowenoid changes in the vulval or penile area are called *Bowenoid papulosis*. It carries premalignant potential and hence should be treated. Common sites are sun-exposed areas such as the face, dorsum of hands, forearms, and shins.
- *Management* options include:
  - cryotherapy;
  - 5% fluorouracil/Efudex twice daily for 4 weeks;
  - Imiquimod/Aldara three times per week for 12 weeks;
  - referral for surgical treatment such as curettage and cautery, excision.
- Treat lesions on shins with care as can lead to leg ulceration due to poor healing.

Cutaneous Horn

- Horny outgrowths from the skin. These are of importance as at the base of these lesions there could be an underlying actinic keratosis, Bowen disease, or SCC.
- Refer to Secondary Care.

Atypical/Dysplastic Naevus

- Although not malignant it is considered as a precursor to melanoma. It occurs due to dysfunctional proliferation of atypical melanocytes. They can arise from preexisting moles or de novo.
- Sometimes patients present with a mole that looks different from their other moles or has been gradually evolving. However, sometimes these are picked up coincidentally when the patient presents for other pathology (e.g., when examining chest for a cough).
- Usually differentiated from benign naevi by their large, variegate appearance with irregular borders and tendency to stand out among other moles.
- Differential diagnosis is malignant melanoma. They are difficult to distinguish.
- Refer for excision due to malignant potential.

Malignant Skin Lesions

GUIDELINE

National Institute for Health and Care Excellence. (2015). *Suspected cancer: Recognition and referral. NICE clinical guideline 12.* Retrieved from www.nice.org.uk.

Basal Cell Carcinoma (Rodent Ulcer)

- This is the most common type of skin cancer. It is usually secondary to chronic sun exposure although genetic mutations are a known cause. It is locally invasive, erodes gradually through the skin, but is rarely known to metastasize, hence the name *rodent ulcer*
- *Key features:*
  - Pearly margins
  - Telangiectasia
  - Usually firm but can be cystic
  - Tends to bleed when excoriated
  - Commonly seen in middle-aged or elderly fair-skinned individuals with history of chronic sun exposure (e.g., gardeners, sailors, people who have worked abroad in tropical areas)
  - Commonly seen on the face but can be present anywhere on the body
- There are various subtypes (Table 22.2):
  - *Superficial BCC:* most common subtype. Appear as thin plaques with a fine border and telangiectasia. Best seen with use of a hand lens.
  - *Nodular BCC:* can present as well-defined nodules or papules, classically described as pearly (i.e., skin-coloured smooth surface with telangiectasia).
  - *Ulcerated BCC:* some nodular BCCs can progress to form a central ulcer covered with crust and rolled out borders and telangiectasia.
  - *Pigmented BCC:* some BCCs can be pigmented and mimic a nodular or superficial spreading melanoma.
  - *Morphoeic or sclerosing BCC:* difficult to diagnose but fortunately not very common. Presents as a macular scarlike area. Often ill defined, hypopigmented, and sclerosed appearance. Can progress to ulcerated or nodular BCC. More aggressive in nature.
- Refer for excision on a routine basis.

Squamous Cell Carcinoma

- SCC is a malignant metastasizing tumour that arises from the keratinocytes within the epidermis. It can arise de novo or evolve from preexisting precancerous skin conditions such as Bowen disease or an actinic keratosis. It can also be an underlying pathology in chronic nonhealing ulcers.
- Main risk factor is chronic sun exposure; therefore it is most commonly seen in outdoor workers and people who live in or travel to tropical countries. It is also more common in the immunosuppressed. Other risks are phototherapy and sunbeds, exposure to polycyclic hydrocarbons (tar, mineral oils), arsenic ingestion, and human papillomavirus.
- Patients usually present with a solitary keratotic papule/nodule that has either persisted for months or has been gradually growing in size. Usually there are no associated symptoms such as pain, bleeding, or itching. Appearance can be of a scaly plaque to indurated plaque or nodule. It can have an ulcerated or crusted surface. Commonly seen in sun-exposed areas such as the face, forearms, bald scalp, ears, and lower legs.

TABLE 22.2	BCC Subtypes		
BCC Subtype	**Presentation**	**Differential Diagnosis**	**Management**
Superficial	Thin plaques with a fine border, telangiectasia Often bleeds on minimal excoriation	*Fungal infection:* usually very itchy and does not bleed *Bowen disease:* scaly patch *Eczema:* especially if multiple; usually there is a history of eczema and good response to topical steroids	Cryotherapy Topical imiquimod or Aldara Refer to dermatology
Nodular BCC	Pearly appearance, nodule or papule with telangiectasia	Dermatofibroma (firm, pinch sign positive)	Usually surgical Refer to dermatology If surgery is not an option then radiotherapy or hedgehog inhibitors are considered
Ulcerated	Crust-covered ulcer with a rolled border, telangiectasia	Squamous cell carcinoma Primary chancre of syphilis (history would help)	Usually surgical Refer to dermatology If surgery is not an option then radiotherapy or hedgehog inhibitors are considered
Pigmented	Pigmented well-defined nodules, can be ulcerated	Seborrhoeic keratosis: typical stuck-on warty appearance Malignant melanoma: usually without preexisting mole	Surgical Refer to dermatology
Morphoeic	Appears as sclerosed yellowish ill-defined plaques. More aggressive	Scar tissue Scleroderma: difficult to differentiate and sometimes diagnostic biopsy is only option	Surgical: most require Moh surgery, which is highly specialized

BCC, Basal cell carcinoma.

- A history of a nodule developing on a background of a scaly or plaquelike area should also raise suspicion of SCC.
- Differential diagnoses:
  - *Bowen disease:* Usually scaly plaque with no induration.
  - *Keratoacanthoma:* Short history, rapid growth, and tends to self-resolve in 4 to 6 months. However, clinically difficult to differentiate from SCC, hence best to treat as SCC until proven otherwise.
  - *BCC:* Especially the early stages and the well-differentiated ones; however, BCCs are pearlier in appearance with telangiectasia and tend to be less indurated.
  - *Chondrodermatitis nodularis helicis (CNH):* On the free border of helix of ear. Usually develop spontaneously, grow rapidly, tend to be less than 1 cm in size, and are tender, unlike SCCs.
- Refer for excision which has to be complete (both peripheral and deep margins). This should be along a 2-week suspected cancer pathway.
- Patients with recurrent SCCs are offered systemic treatment such as Acitretin to reduce the incidence of further lesions developing.

Malignant Melanoma (National Institute for Health and Care Excellence, 2015)

- Malignant melanoma (MM) is one of the most malignant neoplasms of the skin. They are tumours that arise from the pigmented cells within the dermoepidermal junction called melanocytes. Two-thirds arise de novo and only one-third arise from preexisting moles.
- High-risk factors:
  - Fair-skinned people with red hair (i.e., skin type 1)
  - History of severe sun burns in younger years
  - People with multiple moles (>50)
  - People with dysplastic naevi
  - Use of sunbeds
  - Family history or personal history of melanoma.
- There are four main subtypes:
  1. *Lentigo maligna melanoma (LMM):* Malignant cells are limited to epidermis. The growth of this tumour is usually in the horizontal plane rather than the vertical. Presentation is usually as a 1- to 3-cm macular pigmented lesion on sun-exposed areas, usually in an elderly patient. Can evolve into superficial spreading or nodular melanoma.
  2. *Superficial spreading melanoma (SSM):* Malignant cells usually lie along the dermoepidermal junction. Again the growth is more in the horizontal plane. Presentation is usually of an enlarging macular irregularly pigmented lesion with irregular borders. Surrounding skin may show inflammation.
  3. *Nodular melanoma (NM):* The growth is mostly in the vertical plane rather than the horizontal. Presentation is usually of a darkly pigmented dome-shaped nodule. The surface tends to break down and bleed or ooze and crust over. Sometimes lesions are not darkly

This is a good and simple way to assess a mole for superficial spreading melanoma:

A: Asymmetry in shape; one half is different from the other
B: Borders: irregular borders
C: Colour: more than one shade of pigment to the lesion
D: Diameter >6 mm or also *ugly duckling* appearance, meaning it stands out as an odd-looking mole among others
E: Enlargement: history of increase in size; Expert—seek expert advice

pigmented and can be flesh coloured or erythematous; these are termed *amelanotic melanoma.*

4. *Acral melanoma:* These tend to occur on palms, soles, and nail beds. Any nontraumatic de novo pigmentation or change in mole in these areas should be referred for further assessment to rule out malignant potential.

- *Any patient that presents with a change (shape, size, colour) or itch and/or bleeding in a longstanding mole or history of developing new moles after the age of 30 should be referred to rule out a malignant melanoma* (Box 22.1).
- Referral should be urgent under the suspicion of cancer pathway for assessment and excision. The primary excision is usually carried out with a 2-mm margin and once histologically confirmed wide local excision is carried out ranging from 5 mm to 2 cm based on the type of melanoma.

Venous/Varicose Eczema

GUIDELINES

National Institute for Health and Care Excellence. (2012). *Venous eczema and lipodermatosclerosis. NICE clinical knowledge summaries.* Retrieved from https://cks.nice.org.uk.
Raju, S., Hollis, K., & Neglen, P. (2007). Use of compression stockings in chronic venous disease: Patient compliance and efficacy. *Annals of Vascular Surgery, 21*(6), 790–795.

- This ranges from haemosiderin deposits to active eczema then to lipodermatosclerosis, atrophe blanche, and the increasing chance of active ulceration.
- Give patients general advice, including:
  - avoid prolonged sitting with legs down or standing;
  - stay physically active;
  - give advice on avoidance of skin injury;
  - spend 1 hour a day in bed with legs raised; and
  - use regular emollients.
- *Topical steroids* can be used for a flare of eczema; in lipodermatosclerosis very potent steroids may be required. For persistent venous eczema consider a trial of potent topical steroid ointment under medicated bandages such as zip socks which are changed once or twice a week.

- *Treat infections* with antibiotics according to swab sensitivities.
- *Treat itch* with topical steroids moderately potent (e.g., Eumovate) to potent (e.g. Betnovate) for around 1 week at a time to avoid skin atrophy.
- Consider compression stockings for resistant cases. If compression stockings are being considered then check ankle-brachial pressure index (ABPI) first and use below-knee compression stockings if there is no evidence of arterial insufficiency (class 2 are suitable for most people or class 1 if these are not tolerated):
  - ABPI less than 0.3 or greater than 1.3: avoid compression stockings
  - ABPI greater than 0.3 but less than 0.8: use only class 1 (mild) stockings
  - ABPI greater than 0.8 but less than 1.3: use any up to class 3 stockings
- Consider the differential of allergic contact dermatitis in spreading eczema.
- Consider referral:
  - for patch testing if suspected allergic contact dermatitis;
  - if inability to control condition despite full primary care intervention;
  - if evidence of fibrosis or evidence of ulceration;
  - if ABPI is less than 0.8 then refer to vascular.

PATIENT SUPPORT ORGANIZATION

National Eczema Society. 11 Murray Street, London, NW1 9RE; helpline: 0800 089 1122; website: www.eczema.org.

Leg Ulcers

GUIDELINE

Scottish Intercollegiate Guidelines Network. (2010). *Management of chronic venous leg ulcers. SIGN guideline 120.* Retrieved from www.sign.ac.uk.

- Of leg ulcers, 70% are venous, 10% are arterial, and the rest include neuropathic, BCC, pressure ulcers, and autoimmune conditions.
- Involve nursing colleagues with experience in wound management early in the presentation.
- It is important to remember to treat associated conditions such as pain, eczema, oedema and to inform patients with regard to signs of infection.
- *Pain management.* Remember to take a history to determine if the cause is arterial, neuropathic, or cellulitic.
- Give healthy lifestyle advice as this promotes healing and reduces risk of recurrence especially smoking cessation, weight control, diet, and alcohol advice.
- Ensure the ulcer is cleaned and dressed at least weekly.

General Advice

- Give advice on exercise, as mobility keeps the calf muscle pump active and helps reduce oedema.
- Tight-fitting footwear is to be avoided and patients need to remain vigilant about avoiding trauma to the legs.
- Advise patients to elevate legs when immobile; elevation should be to the level of the heart if possible so this means advising patients that they should put pillows under their feet when in bed and not rely on footstools.

Management

- Use an emollient frequently.
- Moderately potent topical steroid can be used to improve surrounding skin venous dermatitis.
- Antibiotics are only indicated if there is clinical suspicion of infection and should not be initiated on swab results without clinical suspicion.
- Compression stockings are effective in reducing recurrent ulcers and chronic lower leg swelling but check ABPI via Doppler. Only use compression therapy if ABPI is above 0.8, it is not a diabetic ulcer or neuropathy, there is no phlebitis, no deep vein thrombosis (DVT), and no cellulitis. Discontinue compression therapy if features of arterial insufficiency or infection occur.
- Compression bandaging should be applied as follows:
  - For people who are immobile, four- or three-layer bandaging is more suitable.
  - For people who are mobile, two-layer bandaging is more practical.
  - For most patients below-knee compression stockings are most suitable; remember to prescribe two at a time and for patients to get a new prescription every 4 months as they lose elasticity.
- To aid ulcer healing pentoxifylline 400 mg three times daily can be prescribed for up to 6 months with or without compression bandages as this improves microcirculation, although check local guidelines as this is usually initiated in secondary care.
- If an ulcer is failing to heal then screen for iron deficiency and diabetes. Also consider the differential diagnosis which can include basal cell cancer.
- It is common for ulcers to recur, so support stockings are needed long term.

Referral

- *Refer routinely* to the vascular surgeons if the ABPI is below 0.8 or if there are significant varicosities.
- *Refer urgently* to vascular if the ABPI is below 0.5 or if ischaemic changes occur due to compression stockings.
- *Refer to dermatology* if there is no improvement despite primary care therapy or if there is deterioration, if malignancy is suspected, or if there is an atypical pattern of ulceration which may signify an underlying disease process (e.g., pyoderma gangrenosum, vasculitis, contact dermatitis, BCC).
- Consider referral if there is no improvement after 3 months.

Hyperhidrosis

GUIDELINES

National Institute for Health and Care Excellence. (2013). *Hyperhidrosis. NICE clinical knowledge summaries.* Retrieved from https://cks.nice.org.uk.
Primary Care Dermatology Society. (2014). *Hyperhidrosis.* Retrieved from www.pcds.org.uk/clinical-guidance/hyperhidrosis.

Primary Hyperhidrosis

- Affects scalp, face, axillae, hands, or feet.
- No apparent cause.
- Has lasted at least 6 months.
- Has at least two of the following characteristics:
  1. Bilateral
  2. Impairs activity of daily living
  3. At least one episode per week
  4. Does not occur during sleep
  5. Onset before 25 years of age
  6. Other family members affected

Generalized Hyperhidrosis

- Generalized hyperhidrosis affects the entire skin surface area and is usually secondary to other medical conditions or induced by drugs.
- Many cases are idiopathic.
- Common drugs include antidepressants, alcohol, substance abuse.
- Clinical features include asymmetrical sweating, generalized sweating, sweating during sleep, clinical features of systemic illness.
- Medical conditions include but not limited to anxiety, pregnancy, infections, malignancy, menopause, hyperthyroidism, and hyperpituitarism.

Investigations

In obvious primary hyperhidrosis these are not indicated. If generalized hyperhidrosis is a differential then further investigation is required and often includes FBC, urea and electrolytes (U&E), LFT, ESR/C-reactive protein (CRP), fasting blood glucose (FBG), thyroid function test (TFT)—if clinically indicated then chest x-ray (CXR) (neoplasm) and HIV serology.

Management

- Provide patient information leaflet.
- Advice: avoid caffeine and spicy foods, avoid tight-fitting clothes.
- Use 20% aluminum chloride hexahydrate roll-on at night. Use this at night on dry skin and wash it off in the morning until symptoms controlled. Do not apply within 12 hours of shaving. Once control achieved then use weekly.
- If feet are most affected then aluminum dusting powder.
- For skin irritation caused by aluminum 1% hydrocortisone ointment can be used for up to 2 weeks.
- Pro-Banthine can be used as second line medication.
- If anxiety is an issue then offer cognitive behavioural therapy (CBT) as alternative to propranolol or antidepressants which can worsen sweating.
- Review in 1 to 2 months to reassess.
- If not controlled then consider referral to dermatologist.

Management of Generalized Hyperhidrosis

This is targeted at finding the cause and treating it. If aetiology remains unclear and ongoing sweating occurs then consider referral to dermatology.

> **PATIENT SUPPORT ORGANIZATION**
>
> Hyperhidrosis UK. www.hyperhidrosisuk.org.

Hidradenitis Suppurativa

> **GUIDELINES**
>
> Primary Care Dermatology Society. (2014). *Hidradenitis suppurativa. Clinical guidance,* updated 2017. Retrieved from www.pcds.org.uk/hidradenitis_suppurativa.

- Hidradenitis effects about 1% of the population and ranges from mild papules, pustules, and nodules to fluctuant abscesses, draining sinuses, and severe scarring.
- It is a clinical diagnosis but consider performing FBC (for possible coexisting anaemia) and swabs of lesions prior to antibiotic therapy.
- Start treatment early to reduce the chance of future scarring.
- Advise weight loss in obese patients, which is essential, and smoking cessation.
- Advise the patient on loose-fitting clothes, antiperspirants, and good hygiene.
- Wash with Dermol or chlorhexidine to reduce future infections.
- *For acute flares* then a 2-week course of antibiotics based on local protocol and swab microbiology results.
- *For chronic disease* then at least 3 months of oral antibiotics is needed as these have an antiinflammatory effect and

first choice is lymecycline. If this is not controlling it then the dose can be doubled to 1 tablet twice daily. While off license there is no evidence of harm by using this approach. Alternative antibiotics include doxycycline, metronidazole, or macrolides.

- If no improvement after 3 months or in severe disease, then a combination approach of clindamycin 300 mg twice daily and rifampicin 300 mg twice daily should be used for 3 months. LFTs should be checked before starting and soon after initiation as rifampicin can cause hepatotoxicity.
- Combined oral contraceptive pill (COCP) may be helpful in women without contraindications.
- Antiandrogens: Dianette can be effective; however, it is contraindicated in the obese and patients at risk from clots. If eligible, and symptoms are worse between periods, then consider giving with extra 50 to 100 mg cyproterone acetate on days 5 to 14 of the cycle.
- Spironolactone 100 to 200 mg may be effective.
- *Refer:*
  - to dermatology if medical therapies are ineffective or if widespread scarring disease is present;
  - to surgery if large abscesses need incised and drained.

> **PATIENT SUPPORT ORGANIZATION**
>
> The Hidradenitis Suppurativa Trust. Cliffe House, Anthonys Way, Rochester, ME2 4DY; email: enquiries@hstrust.org; website: www.hstrust.org.

Urticaria

- Urticaria can be divided into the following subtypes:
  - Idiopathic: most common
  - Immunologic: IgE related (food allergy, infections, reactions to external agents on body), C1 esterase inhibitor deficiency, and vasculitic
  - Non-immunological: physical stimuli (heat, cold, sweat, water, pressure, solar rays, dermographism) or medication related
- The outlook is that most patients with chronic urticaria get better by 1 year.
- *Investigations.* For acute idiopathic urticaria (lasting <6 weeks) no investigations are usually indicated. In chronic or recurrent cases where a secondary cause is suspected the following can be considered:
  - FBC, ESR/CRP, Thyroid Peroxidase antibodies (TPO)
  - *Helicobacter pylori* testing
  - Exclusion of suspected medication (e.g., aspirin, NSAIDs, ACE inhibitors, opioids, penicillin)
  - Dietary changes
  - Hot/cold challenge
  - Check for dermographism
  - Investigate for autoimmune condition if associated joint pain or malaise

- IgE tests are rarely necessary and only to confirm specific triggers.
- Differentiate ordinary urticaria from physical and contact urticaria as the management in the last two is about avoiding the stimulus.
- Give lifestyle advice including avoidance of overheating such as taking hot baths, alcohol, spicy foods, and caffeine.
- First line management is a nonsedating antihistamine (initially cetirizine or loratadine but can be increased to fexofenadine if there is no improvement).
- If urticarial is severe add a short course of prednisolone (30 mg for 3 days).
- If an antihistamine is not effective then the dose can be increased to four times the licensed dose (so twice up to four times daily) unless the patient has a history of long QT syndrome or severe renal or liver problems.
- If this is not effective then try an alternative nonsedating antihistamine and/or add a sedating antihistamine such as chlorphenamine or hydroxyzine to help sleep at night.
- Try soothing agents such as 1% menthol in aqueous cream or calamine.
- *Refer:*
  - urgently to dermatology if suspected urticarial vasculitis (this is tender urticaria, associated joint pains, bruising, or static weals that are present >24 hours or contact urticaria);
  - if persistent urticaria is unresponsive to three different antihistamines each for 4 to 6 weeks;
  - in rare case to immunologist for radioallergosorbent test (RAST) or skin prick testing if thought due to food, drug, or latex allergy;
  - in rare case to dermatology for patch testing if suspected contact urticarial.

Alopecia

GUIDELINES

British Association of Dermatologists. (2012). *Guidelines for the management of alopecia areata.* www.bad.org.uk/alopecia.

- Alopecia may be either:
  1. nonscarring (no inflammation, follicular openings present, atrophy absent); or
  2. scarring (inflammation usually present, no follicular openings, atrophy present).
- Causes of nonscarring alopecia include:
  - *alopecia areata:* scalp looks normal, exclamation hairs at edges, pull test positive;
  - *tinea capitis:* subtle scale may be seen;
  - *trichotillosis* (compulsive hair pulling): different length hairs;
  - *traction alopecia:* from hair styling.
- Causes of scarring alopecia include:
  - infection (bacterial or fungal);
  - lichen planus;
  - SLE.
- *Investigations:*
  - FBC, ferritin, and TFT (consider syphilis if diffuse alopecia)
  - Enquire about childbirth, recent surgery, causative medications
  - Fungal culture
  - Consider serology for SLE

Treatment Alopecia Areata

- Provide patient information leaflet and consider counselling and psychologic support.
- Advise sunblock on bald patches.
- Nonextensive (<50% hair affected): no treatment is often indicated as spontaneous remission occurs in up to 80% of patients.
- Extensive alopecia (>50% hair affected) areata: wigs.
- Trial of potent or very potent steroids for 3 months (in nonpregnant patients who do not want referral). If referring consider a trial of this treatment while awaiting review.
- Intralesional steroid injection such as triamcinolone may be tried but warn about the possibility of atrophy.
- *Refer:*
  - if there is more than 50% hair loss or no regrowth;
  - patient preference.

PATIENT SUPPORT ORGANIZATION

Alopecia Online. www.alopeciaonline.org.uk.

References

Ashton, R., & Leppard, B. (2009). *Differential diagnosis in dermatology* (3rd ed., p. 186). Boca Raton, FL: CRC Press.

Du Vivier, A. (2013). *Atlas of clinical dermatology* (4th ed., pp. 150–152). Philadelphia, PA: Saunders.

National Institute for Health and Care Excellence (2015). *Melanoma overview.* London: NICE.

National Institute of Health and Care Excellence. (2012). *Plaque Psoriasis: Assessment and Management. Clinical Guideline 153.* Available: www.nice.org.uk.

Wolff, K., & Johnson, R. A. (2009). *Fitzpatrick's color atlas and synopsis of clinical dermatology* (6th ed., pp. 215–216). New York: McGraw-Hill.

23

Allergic Problems

AZIZ SHEIKH

CHAPTER CONTENTS

Food Allergies

GUIDELINES/SYSTEMATIC REVIEWS

National Institute for Health and Care Excellence. (2011). *Food allergy in children and young people. Diagnosis and assessment of food allergy in children and young people in primary care and community settings. NICE clinical guideline 116.*

Boyce, J. A., Assa'ad, A., Burks, A. W., et al. (2010). Guidelines for the diagnosis and management of food allergy in the United States: Summary of the NIAID-Sponsored Expert Panel Report. *Journal of Allergy and Clinical Immunology, 126,* 1105–1118.

de Silva, D., Geromi, M., Panesar, S. S., et al. with the EAACI Food Allergy and Anaphylaxis Group. (2014). Acute and long-term management of food allergy: Systematic review. *Allergy, 69*(2), 159–167.

de Silva, D., Geromi, M., Halken, S., et al. with the EAACI Food Allergy and Anaphylaxis Group. (2014). Primary prevention of food allergy in children and adults: Systematic review. *Allergy, 69,* 581–589.

- The UK incidence of severe food allergic reactions leading to hospitalization has increased in recent years (Gupta, Sheikh, Strachan, & Anderson, 2007).

- Adverse reactions to food may result from allergy (hypersensitivity)—either IgE or non-IgE mediated—or intolerance (reactions that are not clearly immunologically mediated) (National Institute for Health and Care Excellence [NICE], 2011; Sampson, 2004).

- The severity of allergic reactions is highly variable, with symptoms ranging from mild cutaneous symptoms (e.g., exacerbation of atopic eczema/dermatitis and urticaria) predominantly experienced in those with non-IgE-mediated food allergy to systemic life-threatening anaphylaxis that may be seen in those with IgE-mediated food allergy.

- Patients will often use the term *allergy* to refer to any of a number of food-related adverse reactions; double-blind, placebo-controlled studies, however, show that only a minority of these reactions have an allergic basis (Rona et al., 2007; Sampson, 2005).

- In addition to the immediate effects of allergic reactions, food allergies can have a significant impact on patients' everyday lives (Primeau et al., 2000). Activities such as food shopping, eating outside the home, and travelling abroad can become challenging. Accurate diagnosis and good long-term management are therefore crucial in maintaining quality of life and minimizing anxiety (Munoz-Furlong, 2003).

- Evidence-based guidelines for the diagnosis and management of food allergies are available (Boyce et al., 2010; NICE, 2011). Note that data from randomized controlled trials are limited in the area of food allergies (de Silva et al., 2014); these guidelines are therefore based on a systematic review of the best available evidence.

Diagnosis

- Differentiating food allergy from intolerance is important because the former will typically require meticulous avoidance of the food(s) in question; continued exposure to the triggering food(s) in those with IgE-mediated food allergy increases the risks of major systemic allergic reactions such as anaphylaxis (Sheikh & Walker, 2002; Wood, 1999).

- Attempt to differentiate food allergy from intolerance by the following features of the history and examination:
  - *Family history:* Food allergy usually occurs in those with a personal and/or family history of allergic disorders (e.g., atopic eczema, hay fever, asthma).

TABLE 23.1	Foods Commonly Responsible for Triggering Allergic Reactions	
Children	**Adults**	
Milk	Fish and seafood	
Egg white	Tree nuts	
Peanuts	Peanuts	
Wheat	Additives	
Soya beans	Fruits	

- *Type of food:* Although almost any protein-based food may provoke allergic symptoms in sensitized individuals, most reactions occur in relation to exposure to a small group of foods (Table 23.1) (Teuber, Beyer, Comstock, & Wallowitz, 2006).
- *Speed of onset:* Symptoms soon after food intake (usually <1 hour and often within minutes) are suggestive of IgE-mediated allergy.
- *Effect of re-exposure:* Re-exposure to the same food(s) will tend to produce similar reactions in those with food allergy; the picture is often much more variable in those with intolerance.
- *Pollen-food allergy syndrome* (known until recently as oral allergy syndrome) is an IgE-mediated hypersensitivity to raw fruits, root vegetables, and some nuts. It is most likely to occur in patients with tree pollen allergy (i.e., those with spring hay fever). Contact urticaria and/or angioedema of the lips and oropharynx occur through a cross-reactivity between specific epitopes in pollens and fresh fruit/vegetables, manifesting as an itchy oropharynx and swelling of the lips and tongue. More severe reactions may occur, but are unusual (Perry, Scurlock, & Jones, 2006).
- *The clinical picture:* Food allergy will typically trigger symptoms indicative of inflammation in one or more organ systems: These include features of angioedema (particularly of the lips and tongue), urticaria, conjunctivitis, rhinitis, bronchospasm, gastrointestinal oedema (cramps, vomiting, and diarrhoea), and anaphylaxis (Perry et al., 2006). Food-related symptoms of tiredness, joint and muscle pains, sleep disturbance, and emotional upset are all more suggestive of a diagnosis of food intolerance.

Management

Symptomatic Treatment
- Treat symptomatically with H_1-antihistamines; if life-threatening features are present (respiratory difficulty or symptoms suggestive of hypotension) then treat as for anaphylaxis (see below).

Further Management
- Attempt to unequivocally identify the food(s) responsible for triggering reactions. Take a detailed history of reactions from the patient/carer and, if necessary, refer to the list of the most common trigger foods to deduce likely culprits (see Table 23.1). Confirm clinical suspicion with objective allergy test if IgE-mediated disease is suspected (skin-prick test and/or serum-specific IgE) or a trial of dietary exclusion if non-IgE-mediated food allergy is suspected.
- Refer to an allergist if provision for suitable testing is unavailable, in the event of diagnostic uncertainty, and/or if the patient has experienced a life-threatening reaction (Durham & Church, 2006).
- Recommend the avoidance of food(s) found to trigger symptoms. Advise careful checking of food ingredients (e.g., by reading food labels, asking waiting staff and caterers when eating outside the home).
- Encourage patients to be proactive in seeking relevant information. For example, organizations such as Allergy UK and the Anaphylaxis Campaign (see Useful Contacts), as well as many larger food manufacturers and catering chains, now publish allergen information online.
- Recommend that patients with pollen-food allergy syndrome avoid the offending fruits and/or vegetables in their raw form; in most cases, the allergen is removed by peeling or destroyed by heating and the peeled/cooked fruits and/or vegetables can then be safely consumed.
- Enlist the help of a dietician to ensure that patients fully understand about the foods that they need to avoid, to help them manage avoidance when eating in and outside the home, and to ensure their diet is nutritionally adequate.
- Issue self-injectable adrenaline to those with a history of anaphylaxis and recommend a medical identity bracelet/necklace.
- Refer patients with severe food intolerance(s) to a gastroenterologist. Any long-term exclusion diet should be supervised by a dietician (Grimshaw, 2006).
- Review patient periodically to ensure long-term management is effective.

Reintroducing Foods After a Period of Avoidance
- Children with allergy to milk and eggs will commonly develop tolerance to these foods as they grow older. In those with a history of reactions that are not considered to be life threatening, the careful reintroduction of these foods at a later date may be appropriate.
- Consider reintroducing:
  - *milk* at the age of 3 years (by which time 85% of children with a history of milk allergy will be tolerant); and
  - *eggs* at the age of 6 to 10 years (by which time 55%–80% of children with a history of egg allergy will be tolerant) (Teuber et al., 2006).
- *Persistent symptoms.* Refer to specialist services.

Note: Peanut and fish/seafood allergy is, in the majority of individuals, lifelong (Teuber et al., 2006), and attempts at reintroduction are not normally recommended although research in reintroducing peanut proteins as part of a carefully supervised programme is ongoing.

Pregnancy, Lactation and Prevention of Allergy

- Pregnant and breastfeeding women do not need to change their diet or take supplements in an attempt to prevent allergies in infants.
- Although those with a family history of allergic disorders have been advised to avoid peanuts during pregnancy, lactation, weaning, and until the age of at least 3 years (Fiocchi, Assa'ad, & Bahna, 2006; Friedman & Zieger, 2005), there is concern that this may actually be increasing the risk of peanut allergy through preventing the development of immunologic tolerance (Du Toit et al., 2008; McLean & Sheikh, 2010). This is therefore no longer recommended.
- Encourage lactating mothers of infants with a parent or sibling with an atopic disease to exclusively breastfeed for 4 to 6 months (Friedman & Zieger, 2005).
- Encourage mothers of infants with a parent or sibling with an atopic allergic disease who are unable to exclusively breastfeed for the first 4 months of life to use a hydrolysed cow's milk formula (Friedman & Zieger, 2005).

Useful Contacts

For Patients

The Anaphylaxis Campaign, 1 Alexandra Road, Farnborough, Hampshire GU14 6SX. Tel.: 01252 546100; helpline: 01252 542029 (Monday–Friday 9 am–5 pm); fax: 01252 377140; email: info@anaphylaxis.org.uk; website: www.anaphylaxis.org.uk

Allergy UK, Planwell House, LEFA Business Park, Edgington Way, Sidcup, Kent, DA14 5BH. Helpline: 01322 619898; email: info@allergyuk.org; website: www.allergyuk.org

MedicAlert Foundation, 327 Upper Fourth Street, Milton Keynes, MK9 1EH. Tel.: 01908 951045 (Monday–Friday 9 am–5 pm, Saturday 9 am–3 pm); email: info@medicalert.org.uk; website: www.medicalert.org.uk

Supermarkets can provide information on products that are "free from" certain ingredients.

For Professionals

British Society for Allergy and Clinical Immunology, Studio 16, Cloisters House, 8 Battersea Park Road, London SW8 4BG. Tel.: 0207 501 3910; fax: 0207 627 2599; website: www.bsaci.org

Education for Health, The Athenaeum, 10 Church Street, Warwick CV34 4AB. Tel.: 01926 493313; email: info@education forhealth.org; website: www.educationforhealth.org

Skills for Health has developed competences to describe what health professionals need to do, what they need to know, and which skills they need to carry out activities related to the diagnosis and management of allergy. These are available on their website: http://tools.skillsforhealth.org.uk/suite/show/id/69

Anaphylaxis

> **GUIDELINES**
>
> Joint Task Force on Practice Parameters; American Academy of Allergy, Asthma and Immunology; American College of Allergy, Asthma and Immunology; and Joint Council of Allergy, Asthma, and Immunology. (2005). The diagnosis and management of anaphylaxis: An updated practice parameter. *Journal of Allergy and Clinical Immunology, 115,* S483–S523.
>   Soar, J., Pumphrey, R., Cant, A., et al. (2008). Working Group of the Resuscitation Council (UK) 2008. Emergency treatment of anaphylactic reactions—guidelines for healthcare providers. *Resuscitation, 77,* 157–169.
>   Simons, F. E. R., Ardusso, L. R. F., Dimov, V., et al., for the World Allergy Organization. (2013). World Allergy Organization Anaphylaxis Guidelines: 2013 update of the evidence base. *Internal Archives of Allergy and Immunology, 162,* 193–204. www.worldallergy.org/anaphylaxix.
>   Dhami, S., Panesar, S. S., Roberts, G., et al., for the EAACI Food Allergy and Anaphylaxis Guidelines Group. (2014). Management of anaphylaxis: A systematic review. *Allergy, 69*(2), 168–175.

- Anaphylaxis is a severe, life-threatening generalized or systemic hypersensitivity reaction (Johannson et al., 2004). It is rapid in onset and may cause death (Sampson et al., 2006).
- Anaphylaxis is commonly triggered by foods, drugs, and the venom of stinging insects. It may also be induced by exercise, latex, among a number of other triggers. Some cases are idiopathic.
- The UK incidence of anaphylaxis is believed to be increasing (Department of Health, 2006; Gupta et al., 2007).
- It is estimated that there are between 10 and 30 deaths from anaphylaxis in the United Kingdom each year, many of which are potentially preventable (Newton, 2006; Pumphrey & Gowland, 2007).
- The classification of reactions into anaphylactic (IgE-mediated hypersensitivity reactions) and anaphylactoid (non-IgE-mediated mast cell degranulation) is of little practical relevance to the management of anaphylaxis and is now largely avoided.
- Evidence-based guidelines for the management of anaphylaxis are available, though note that randomized controlled trials of commonly recommended treatments have not been conducted (Sheikh, Shehata, Brown, & Simons, 2008; Sheikh, Simons, & Choo, 2009; Sheikh, ten Broek, Brown, & Simons, 2007). Guidelines are based on the best available evidence.
- Anaphylaxis can have a significant long-term impact on a patient's everyday life beyond the immediate ill effects of a reaction. Managing an unfamiliar set of risks may be challenging for patients, particularly immediately after diagnosis. The possibility of further reactions can lead to increased anxiety. Allergen avoidance requires careful vigilance and may adversely affect the patient's family and social life. Good long-term management is therefore essential in maintaining quality of life (Akeson, Worth,

& Sheikh, 2007; Avery, King, Knight, & Hourihane, 2003; Mandell, Curtis, Gold, & Hardie, 2002; Panesar, Walker, & Sheikh, 2003).

Diagnosis

- Anaphylaxis presents a range of signs and symptoms, which can sometimes result in diagnostic difficulties. A diagnosis is likely when all three of the following criteria are met:
  - Sudden onset and rapid progression of symptoms
  - Life-threatening airway and/or breathing and/or circulation problems
  - Skin and/or mucosal changes (flushing, urticaria, angioedema)
- There may also be gastrointestinal symptoms such as vomiting.
- Exposure to a known allergen for the patient supports the diagnosis (Working Group of the Resuscitation Council [UK], 2008).
- Isolated skin and/or mucosal changes do not indicate anaphylaxis.
- Diagnosis of anaphylaxis should always be followed up by specialist-led investigation into the underlying cause.

Management

- Management is best considered in two stages: treatment of the acute attack and follow-up care (Dhami, 2014; Muraro et al., 2007; Simons, 2006; Simons, 2011; Simons, 2012; Simons, 2013; Soar, 2008).

Acute Management (Table 23.2)

The key steps for the treatment of an anaphylactic reaction are shown in the algorithm (see Appendix 27).

TABLE 23.2	Route of Administration and Drug Dosage for Agents Used in the Emergency Treatment of Anaphylaxis	
Drug (Route of Administration)	**Age-Related Dosage**
Adrenaline 1:1000 (IM)	<6 years: 150 µg (0.15 mL) 6–12 years: 300 µg (0.3 mL) >12 years (small or prepubertal child): 300 µg (0.3 mL) >12 years: 500 µg (0.5 mL)
Chlorphenamine (IM or slow IV)	<6 months: 250 µg/kg 6 months–6 years: 2.5 mg 6–12 years: 5 mg >12 years 10 mg
Hydrocortisone (IM or slow !V)	<6 months: 25 mg 6 months–6 years: 50 mg 6–12 years: 100 mg >12 years: 200 mg
Crystalloid fluid (IV)	Children: 20 mL/kg Adults: 500–1000 mL

IM, intramuscular; *IV,* intravenous.

1. Commence life support (basic and advanced) if indicated.
2. Give oxygen.
3. Give adrenaline (epinephrine) 1:1000 solution (intramuscular [IM] injected into the anterolateral aspect of the middle third of the thigh) if not already administered (many patients with a history of anaphylaxis will have been issued with adrenaline for self-injection). The Resuscitation Council cautions against the use of the intravenous (IV) route except by experienced practitioners treating profound shock (Working Group of the Resuscitation Council [UK], 2008).
4. Give inhaled beta$_2$-agonist if there is severe bronchospasm.
5. Repeat adrenaline 5 to 10 minutes after first dose if there is no clinical improvement.
6. Give IV crystalloid fluid infusion if symptoms of hypotension persist (a repeat dose may be necessary) (Working Group of the Resuscitation Council [UK], 2008).
7. Consider the use of antihistamines and/or glucocorticosteroids.
8. Following treatment, the patient should be observed for a minimum of 6 hours in a clinical area suitable for resuscitation if necessary (Working Group of the Resuscitation Council [UK], 2008).

- *Trigger.* Refer to an allergist to identify the trigger objectively and for consideration of desensitization therapy in those with venom-triggered reactions (Muraro et al., 2007; Working Group of the Resuscitation Council [UK], 2008). This will involve a detailed history and subsequent investigations, which may include skin-prick testing, serum-specific IgE tests, and allergen challenge.
- *Allergen avoidance.* Reinforce any allergen advice issued to patients and families, tailored to individual age and circumstances; dietetic referral may be indicated in cases of food allergy. Encourage patient/parent to be proactive in seeking relevant information (e.g., checking product labels on foods, pharmaceuticals, and cosmetic products). Advise avoidance, where possible, of products carrying "may contain" allergen labels.
- *Adrenaline.* Issue adrenaline autoinjector for self-administration (and educate the patient on when and how to use it). Delayed use of adrenaline can lead to fatality (Pumphrey & Gowland, 2007), so advise patients not to hesitate in self-administering. In addition to verbal explanation, use a trainer autoinjector and ask the patient to demonstrate its correct use. Ensure autoinjector dosage is correct. Advise patients to take note of their autoinjector expiry date and make arrangements for repeat prescription. Note that adrenaline autoinjector users can subscribe to an expiry alert service by letter, email, or SMS text message (see Useful Contacts). Multiple autoinjectors may need to be prescribed to cover different sites, such as one for home and one for school or the workplace.
- *Alert bracelet.* Recommend purchase of a medical identity bracelet/necklace or smart card documenting history of anaphylaxis and that adrenaline is carried.

- *Asthma control.* Optimize asthma management in those with a history of asthma, as the risk of fatality is increased in this group (Pumphrey & Gowland, 2007).
- Liaise with nursery/school/school nurse/work as appropriate (Vickers, Maynard, & Ewan, 1997).
- Review the patient 6 months after diagnosis, and thereafter every year, and following any subsequent reactions. Reviews should be used to support patients' self-management as appropriate: for example, reinforcing allergen avoidance advice, encouraging carrying adrenaline autoinjector, retraining in autoinjector use, or referring to specialist for retesting. A management plan incorporating training in adrenaline use, support, and follow-up may prove useful (Choo & Sheikh, 2007; Hourihane, 2001; Muraro et al., 2007; Nurmatov, Worth, & Sheikh, 2008).

Useful Contacts

For Patients

The Anaphylaxis Campaign, 1 Alexandra Road, Farnborough, Hampshire GU14 6SX. Tel.: 01252 546100; helpline: 01252 542029 (Monday–Friday 9 am–5 pm); fax: 01252 377140; email: info@anaphylaxis.org.uk; website: www.anaphylaxis.org.uk

Allergy UK, Planwell House, LEFA Business Park, Edgington Way, Sidcup, Kent, DA14 5BH. Helpline: 01322 619898; fax: 01322 470330; email: info@allergyuk.org; website: www.allergyuk.org

The MedicAlert Foundation, 327 Upper Fourth Street, Milton Keynes, MK9 1EH. Tel.: 01908 951045; email: info@medicalert.org.uk; website: www.medicalert.org.uk

Supermarkets can provide information on products that are "free from" certain ingredients.

For Professionals

British Society for Allergy and Clinical Immunology, Studio 16, Cloisters House, 8 Battersea Park Road, London SW8 4BG. Tel.: 0207 501 3910; fax: 0207 627 2599; website: www.bsaci.org

Education for Health, The Athenaeum, 10 Church Street, Warwick CV34 4AB. Tel.: 01926 493313; email: info@educationforhealth.org; website: www.educationforhealth.org

Adrenaline prescribing information. Includes autoinjector demonstration and details of expiry alert system; websites: http://www.epipen.com, www.jext.co.uk

References

Akeson, N., Worth, A., & Sheikh, A. (2007). The psychological impact of anaphylaxis on young people and their parents. *Clinical and Experimental Allergy, 37,* 1213–1220.

Avery, N. J., King, R. M., Knight, S., & Hourihane, J. O. B. (2003). Assessment of quality of life in children with peanut allergy. *Pediatric Allergy and Immunology, 14,* 378–382.

Boyce, J. A., Assa'ad, A., Burks, J. A., et al. (2010). NIAID-sponsored expert panel. Guidelines for the diagnosis and management of food allergy in the United States: Summary of the NIAID-Sponsored Expert Panel report. *Journal of Allergy and Clinical Immunology, 126,* 1105–1118.

Choo, K., & Sheikh, A. (2007). Action plans for the long-term management of anaphylaxis: A systematic review of effectiveness. *Clinical and Experiment Allergy, 37,* 1090–1094.

Department of Health (2006). *A review of services for allergy.* London: Author.

de Silva, D., Geromi, M., Halken, S., et al. with the EAACI Food Allergy and Anaphylaxis Group. (2014). Primary prevention of food allergy in children and adults: Systematic review. *Allergy, 69*(5), 581–589.

de Silva, D., Geromi, M., Panesar, S. S., et al. with the EAACI Food Allergy and Anaphylaxis Group. (2014). Acute and long-term management of food allergy: Systematic review. *Allergy, 69*(2), 159–167.

Dhami, S., Panesar, S. S., Roberts, G., et al. with the EAACI Food Allergy and Anaphylaxis Guidelines Group. (2014). Management of anaphylaxis: A systematic review. *Allergy, 69*(2), 168–175.

Durham, S. R., & Church, M. K. (2006). Principles of allergy diagnosis. In S. T. Holgate, M. K. Church, & L. M. Lichtenstein (Eds.), *Allergy* (3rd ed., pp. 3–16). Philadelphia, PA: Mosby Elsevier.

Du Toit, G., Katz, Y., Sasieni, P., et al. (2008). Early consumption of peanuts in infancy is associated with a low prevalence of peanut allergy. *Journal of Allergy and Clinical Immunology, 122,* 984–991.

Fiocchi, A., Assa'ad, A., & Bahna, S. (2006). Food allergy and the introduction of solid foods to infants: A consensus document. *Annals of Allergy and Asthma Immunology, 97,* 10–21.

Friedman, N. J., & Zieger, R. S. (2005). The role of breast-feeding in the development of allergies and asthma. *Journal of Allergy and Clinical Immunology, 115,* 1238–1248.

Grimshaw, K. E. C. (2006). Dietary management of food allergy in children. *Proceedings of the Nutrition Society, 65,* 412–417.

Gupta, R., Sheikh, A., Strachan, D. P., & Anderson, H. R. (2007). Time trends in allergic disorders in the UK. *Thorax, 62,* 91–96.

Hourihane, J. (2001). Community management of severe allergies must be integrated and comprehensive, and must consist of more than just epinephrine. *Allergy, 56,* 1023–1025.

Johannson, S. G. O., Bieber, T., Dahl, R., et al. (2004). Revised nomenclature for allergy for global use: Report of the Nomenclature Review Committee of the World Allergy Organization, October 2003. *Journal of Allergy and Clinical Immunology, 113,* 832–836.

Mandell, D., Curtis, R., Gold, M., & Hardie, S. (2002). Families coping with a diagnosis of anaphylaxis in a child. *Allergy & Clinical Immunology International, 14,* 96–101.

McLean, S., & Sheikh, A. (2010). Does avoidance of peanuts in early life reduce the risk of peanut allergy? *British Medical Journal (Clinical Research Ed.), 340,* c424. doi:10.1136/bmj.c424.

Munoz-Furlong, A. (2003). Daily coping strategies for patients and their families. *Pediatrics, 111,* 1654–1661.

Muraro, A., Roberts, G., Clark, A., et al. (2007). The management of anaphylaxis in childhood: Position paper of the European Academy of Allergology and Clinical Immunology. *Allergy, 62,* 857–871.

National Institute for Health and Care Excellence. (2011). *Food allergy in children and young people. Diagnosis and assessment of food allergy in children and young people in primary care and community settings.* NICE clinical guideline 116.

Newton, J. (2006). *An epidemiological report for the department of Health's review of services for allergy.* London: Department of Health.

Nurmatov, U., Worth, A., & Sheikh, A. (2008). Anaphylaxis management plans for the acute and long-term management of anaphylaxis:

A systematic review. *Journal of Allergy and Clinical Immunology*, *122*, 353–361.

Panesar, S., Walker, S., & Sheikh, A. (2003). Primary care management of anaphylaxis. *Primary Care Respiratory Journal*, *12*, 124–126.

Perry, T. T., Scurlock, A. M., & Jones, S. M. (2006). Clinical manifestations of food allergic disease. In S. J. Malecki, A. W. Burks, & R. M. Helm (Eds.), *Food allergy* (pp. 3–17). Washington, DC: ASM Press.

Primeau, M. N., Kagan, R., Joseph, L., et al. (2000). The psychological burden of peanut allergy as perceived by adults with peanut allergy and the parents of peanut-allergic children. *Clinical and Experimental Allergy*, *30*, 1135–1143.

Pumphrey, R. S. H., & Gowland, M. H. (2007). Further fatal allergic reactions to food in the United Kingdom, 1999–2006. *Journal of Allergy and Clinical Immunology*, *119*, 1018–1019.

Rona, R. J., Keil, T., Summers, C., et al. (2007). The prevalence of food allergy: A meta-analysis. *Journal of Allergy and Clinical Immunology*, *120*, 638–646.

Sampson, H. A. (2004). Update of food allergy. *Journal of Allergy and Clinical Immunology*, *113*, 805–819.

Sampson, H. A. (2005). Food allergy: Accurately identifying clinical reactivity. *Allergy*, *60*, S19–S24.

Sampson, H. A., Munoz-Furlong, A., Campbell, R. L., et al. (2006). Second symposium on the definition and management of anaphylaxis: Summary report. *Journal of Allergy and Clinical Immunology*, *117*, 391–397.

Sheikh, A., & Walker, S. (2002). Ten-minute consultation: Food allergy. *British Medical Journal (Clinical Research Ed.)*, *325*, 1337.

Sheikh, A., Shehata, Y. A., Brown, S. G. A., & Simons, F. E. R. (2008). Adrenaline (epinephrine) for the treatment of anaphylaxis with and without shock. *Cochrane Database of Systematic Reviews*, (4), CD006312, doi:10.1002/14651858.CD006312.pub2.

Sheikh, A., Simons, F. E. R., & Choo, K. J. L. (2009). Glucocorticoids for the treatment of anaphylaxis (Protocol). *Cochrane Database of Systematic Reviews*, (1), CD007596, doi:10.1002/14651858.CD007596.

Sheikh, A., ten Broek, V. M., Brown, S. G. A., & Simons, F. E. R. (2007). H$_1$-Antihistamines for the treatment of anaphylaxis with and without shock. *Cochrane Database of Systematic Reviews*, (1), CD006160, doi:10.1002/14651858.CD006160.pub2.

Simons, F. E. R. (2006). Anaphylaxis, killer allergy: Long-term management in the community. *Journal of Allergy and Clinical Immunology*, *117*, 367–377.

Simons, E. F. R., Ardusso, L. R. F., Bilo, M. B., et al. (2011). World allergy organization anaphylaxis guidelines: Summary. *Journal of Allergy and Clinical Immunology*, *127*, 587–593.

Simons, E. F. R., Ardusso, L. R. F., Bilo, M. B., et al. for the World Allergy Organization. (2012). Guidelines for the assessment and management of anaphylaxis. *Current Opinion in Allergy and Clinical Immunology*, *12*, 389–399.

Simons, F. E. R., Ardusso, L. R. F., Dimov, V., et al. for the World Allergy Organization. (2013). Anaphylaxis guidelines: 2013 update of the evidence base. *Internal Archives of Allergy and Immunology*, *162*, 193–204.

Soar, J., Pumphrey, R., Cant, A., et al. for the Working Group of the Resuscitation Council (UK). (2008). Emergency treatment of anaphylactic reactions—guidelines for healthcare providers. *Resuscitation*, *77*, 157–169.

Teuber, S. S., Beyer, K., Comstock, S., & Wallowitz, M. (2006). The big eight foods: Clinical and epidemiological overview. In S. J. Malecki, A. W. Burks, & R. M. Helm (Eds.), *Food allergy* (pp. 49–79). Washington, DC: ASM Press.

Vickers, D. W., Maynard, L., & Ewan, P. W. (1997). Management of children with potential anaphylactic reactions in the community: A training package and proposal for good practice. *Clinical and Experimental Allergy*, *27*, 898–903.

Wood, S. F. (1999). *GP guide to the diagnosis and management of allergic disorders in children*. London: Mosby.

Working Group of the Resuscitation Council (UK) (2008). *Emergency treatment of anaphylactic reactions. Guidelines for healthcare providers*. London: Resuscitation Council (UK). www.resus.org.uk/pages/reaction.pdf.

24

Diabetes and Endocrinology

RUSSELL DRUMMOND, FRANCES MCMANUS,
KATE HUGHES, SHARON MACKIN, DAVID CARTY

CHAPTER CONTENTS

Type 2 Diabetes Mellitus

GUIDELINES

Scottish Intercollegiate Guidelines Network. (2013). *Management of diabetes. SIGN guideline 116.* www.sign. ac.uk.
National Institute for Health and Care Excellence. (2015). *Type 1 diabetes in adults: diagnosis and management. NICE clinical guideline 17.* www.nice.org.uk.
National Institute for Health and Care Excellence. (2015). *Type 2 diabetes in adults: Management. NICE clinical guideline 28.* www.nice.org.uk.
National Institute for Health and Care Excellence. (2012). *Type 2 diabetes: Prevention in people at high risk. NICE clinical guideline 38.* www.nice.org.uk.
National Institute for Health and Care Excellence. (2015). *Diabetic foot problems: Prevention & management. NICE clinical guideline 19.* www.nice.org.uk.

- Diabetes mellitus has become a global epidemic with a rapidly expanding prevalence exceeding predictions. Recent UK data suggest:
  - almost 3.5 million people are diagnosed with diabetes in United Kingdom;
  - an estimated 500,000+ are undiagnosed;
  - more than 6% of the total population are affected;
  - current National Health Service (NHS) expenditure for diabetes care is in the region of 10% of the total budget;
  - approximately 90% type 2, 10% type 1 with small subgroups secondary/other diabetes;
  - an alarming increase in numbers of children with type 2 diabetes, a previously unknown entity.
- The key roles in primary care management of diabetes are:
  - prompt recognition and diagnosis;
  - identification of at-risk individuals and intervention to prevent type 2 diabetes;
  - identification of all patients with diabetes in practice within a registry and a means for recall that enables annual review;
  - prevention of microvascular and macrovascular complications through management of glycaemia and cardiovascular risk factors; with appropriate management/referral for established complications;
  - encourage patient self-management;
  - optimize pregnancy outcomes for woman with diabetes;
  - appropriate liaison/referral to secondary care.

Diagnosis

- The World Health Organisation (WHO) criteria is the internationally accepted diagnostic criteria for diabetes. It is defined as:
  a. the presence of symptoms of hyperglycaemia (polyuria, polydipsia, and weight loss) with:
    - random plasma glucose of >11.1 mmol/L; or
    - fasting plasma glucose (FPG) of >7 mmol/L; or
    - 2-hour plasma glucose of >11.1 mmol/L after 75-g oral glucose tolerance test (OGTT);
    - glycated haemoglobin A1c (HbA1c) >48 mmol/mol (6.5%).
  b. In the absence of hyperglycaemic symptoms, a further glucose test on a separate day should be performed.
    - *Impaired fasting glucose:* FPG of 6.1 to 6.9 mmol/L and a 2-hour OGTT <7.8 mmol/L
    - *Impaired glucose tolerance:* FPG <7 mmol/L and a 2-hour OGTT 7.8 to 11 mmol/L

Glycated Haemoglobin A1c

- The role of HbA1c in diagnosis of diabetes has been recognized. However, it is less sensitive than a FPG measurement and an HbA1c less than 48 mmol/mol (6.5%) does not exclude diabetes.
- It should NOT be used in:
  - suspected type 1 diabetes;
  - children;
  - short duration of osmotic symptoms (i.e., <3 months);
  - pregnancy;
  - suspected medication-induced secondary diabetes (e.g., steroids, antipsychotics);
  - suspected pancreatic diabetes;
  - those with haemoglobinopathies/known factors that affect red cell turnover.

What Type of Diabetes?

- This question can sometimes be challenging, but some clues can make a diagnosis more likely (Table 24.1).
- Other subtypes of diabetes may have features of either type 1 or type 2:

TABLE 24.1 Typical Features of Type 1 and 2 Diabetes

Type 1 Diabetes	Type 2 Diabetes
Young age (<40 years)	Older generally
Presentation in childhood	More indolent presentation
Presence of ketones	Metabolic syndrome
Acute osmotic symptoms	Obesity
Normal BMI	South Asian predisposition at lower BMI
Approx. 1 in 25 chance of developing condition if first-degree relative affected	Stronger genetic predisposition
Autoantibodies present	Absence of autoantibodies
C-peptide low and eventually undetectable	C-peptide raised unless significantly advanced disease with beta cell destruction

BMI, Body mass index.

TABLE 24.2	HbA1c in Relation to Mean Blood Glucose Levels	
HbA1c (mmol/mol)	**HbA1c (%)**	**Mean Blood Glucose (mmol/L)**
31	5	5.4
42	6	7.0
53	7	8.6
64	8	10.1
75	9	11.7
86	10	13.3
97	11	14.9
108	12	16.5
119	13	18.1
130	14	19.6

1. Pancreatic diabetes:
   - Known pancreatic pathology
   - Features of pancreatic exocrine dysfunction
2. Secondary diabetes:
   - Associated causative agent (e.g., steroids, antipsychotics)
   - Features of endocrinopathy (e.g., acromegalic or cushingoid appearances)
3. Latent autoimmune diabetes in adults (LADA):
   - Slow and delayed presentation of type 1 diabetes
   - Autoantibodies present
   - Low and declining levels of C-peptide
   - Often misdiagnosed as type 2 particularly in patients not phenotypically type 2 diabetes
   - Quicker progression to insulin therapy than type 2
4. Genetic diabetes (e.g., maturity onset diabetes of the young [MODY]):
   - Strong family history
   - Age less than 40 years and not requiring insulin

Primary Care Investigations

- Make the diagnosis using WHO criteria.
- Assess need for emergency treatment:
  a. Hyperglycaemia with ketones
  b. Children with glycosuria:
     - Do a point-of-care glucose test and discuss if hyperglycaemia.
     - **DO NOT** wait on labs to come back and do NOT arrange for child to come back for a second lab test to confirm diagnosis, regardless of symptoms.
  c. Suspicion of type 1 diabetes
  d. Blood glucose above 30 mmol/L
  e. Acutely unwell and hyperglycaemic
- Other tests are limited to secondary care:
  a. C-peptide
  b. Auto-antibodies (Anti-GAD)
  c. Genetics

Referral

- Those with type 2 diabetes are generally managed in primary care, unless:
  - significant micro-/macrovascular complications;
  - failure to reach glycaemic and blood pressure targets despite maximal therapy;
  - unclear diagnosis;
  - younger than 40 years of age.
- Women with gestational diabetes or preexisting diabetes in pregnancy should be referred immediately to a combined diabetes and obstetrics team.

Screening for Undiagnosed Type 2 Diabetes and Those at Risk

- Around 500,000 people in the United Kingdom are thought to have undiagnosed type 2 diabetes. Many patients have disease for 7 to 10 years preceding diagnosis and present with established complications. Despite this, there is a lack of evidence to suggest population screening for type 2 diabetes is cost effective or that it would improve population health. However, high-risk individuals should be screened, including:
  - all adults aged 40 years or above, unless pregnant;
  - people aged 25 to 39 of South Asian, Chinese, black African, African-Caribbean, or other high-risk ethnicity;
  - those with a condition known to increase risk of type 2 diabetes (e.g., polycystic ovarian syndrome).
- National Institute of Health and Care Excellence (NICE) has published guidance on preventing type 2 diabetes in those at high risk (NICE, 2012).
- The first priority is to identify high-risk patients using a validated risk assessment tool (e.g., the Diabetes Risk Score Assessment tool, available at the Diabetes UK website: www.diabetes.org.uk):
  1. Low or intermediate risk:
     a. Advice on lifestyle intervention
     b. Reassurance whilst stressing that the result doesn't mean no risk
     c. Reassess in 5 years
  2. High risk score:
     a. Perform FPG or HbA1c.
     b. FBG below 5.5 mmol/L or HbA1c below 42 mmol/mol = moderate risk
        - Inform patient of increased risk of developing type 2 diabetes.
        - Discuss risk factor modification.
        - Direct to appropriate local weight-loss or fitness programmes.
        - Reassess in 3 years.
     c. FBG 5.5 to 6.9 mmol/L or HbA1c 43 to 47 mmol/mol = high risk
        - Inform patient that he or she is high risk for developing type 2 diabetes but still preventable.
        - Offer referral to intensive lifestyle-change programme with emphasis on increasing physical

activity to at least 150 minutes moderate activity per week, weight loss, and dietary advice to increase wholegrain food and vegetables with reduction in fatty foods and simple carbohydrates.

- Review progress and biochemistry on a minimum annual basis.

d. FBG at or above 7 mmol/L or HbA1c at or above 48 mmol/mol:

- If asymptomatic, retest on another day as per WHO guidelines for overt diabetes.
- If not diagnostic of diabetes, then intervention as per high risk.

Pharmacologic Therapies in Preventing Type 2 Diabetes

- NICE suggests metformin can be used to prevent progression to type 2 diabetes in patients whose FBG/HbA1c are deteriorating despite best efforts in lifestyle intervention, or in those where such intervention is inappropriate.
- Orlistat can also be considered in those progressing biochemically to type 2 diabetes with obesity where intensive lifestyle intervention has failed. It needs to be used alongside a lowfat (<30%) diet, and weight-loss goals should be reviewed regularly to monitor effectiveness.

Management of Type 2 Diabetes

- The focus of type 2 diabetes management is ultimately to prevent development of microvascular (retinopathy, neuropathy, nephropathy) and macrovascular (coronary artery, cerebrovascular and peripheral vascular disease) complications associated with it. This is achieved by targeting glycaemia and controlling cardiovascular risk factors.
- At diagnosis and annual review, patients should have the following:
  - Explanation of type 2 diabetes, complications, and means of reducing risk
  - Weight and height
  - Blood pressure
  - Cardiovascular examination, including peripheral pulses
  - Examination of feet for neuropathy and ulcers
  - Visual acuity
  - Referral to national retinal screening programme
  - Smoking status documented and advice given
  - Ask men about erectile dysfunction
  - Mood assessed
  - Driving status and advice with regard to Driver and Vehicle Licensing Agency (DVLA) regulations
  - Referral to dietician and diabetes specialist nurse for education on lifestyle intervention
  - Referral to a locally available type 2 diabetes education programme
  - Discussion about contraception for women of childbearing age
- Laboratory tests should be sent for:
  - urea and electrolytes;
  - glucose and HbA1c; Table 24.2 defines HbA1c units and corresponding average blood glucose levels;

- liver function tests;
- lipids;
- urine for albuminuria (urinary albumin-to-creatinine ratio [ACR] convenient and widely available).
- Patients on medication for treatment of diabetes qualify for a medical exemption certificate allowing them free prescriptions, therefore form FP92A should be completed.

Glycaemic Control

- The United Kingdom Prospective Diabetes Study (UKPDS) was a randomized control study from 1977 to 1997 that showed a 25% reduction in microvascular complications with intensive glycaemic control versus conventional targets (HbA1c 7% versus 7.9%). These risk reductions were largely seen in retinopathy and nephropathy. There was no impact on macrovascular disease outcomes from improvements in glycaemic control.
- Current guidelines advise glycaemic targets that are individualized to each patient.
- Scottish Intercollegiate Guidelines Network (SIGN) suggests aiming for an HbA1c below 53 mmol/mol (<48 mmol/mol early in the diagnosis) whilst NICE suggests below 48 mmol/mol if no risk of hypoglycaemia.
- Sometimes relaxed targets are appropriate (e.g., severe hypoglycaemia risk, end-of-life care).

Treatments

- Lifestyle intervention with education on diet and physical activity should be trialled for 3 to 6 months.
- If HbA1c remains above target, then consider pharmacotherapy.
- Treatment of type 2 diabetes is becoming more complex, and less algorithm based with new evidence emerging on the newer hypoglycaemic agents and potential cardiovascular benefits they confer.
- Optimization of therapy takes time and the urge to intensify therapy needs to be balanced with time to achieve desired effect. This can lead to treatment inertia, meaning patients remain suboptimally controlled for months, and in some cases years, despite further options for treatment intensification. To minimize this, at least 3-monthly review of therapy is suggested until HbA1c is within target.

Metformin and First Intensification of Treatment
- Remains the first line oral agent for glycaemic control in type 2 diabetes.
- Cost effective and has data showing cardiovascular benefits (UKPDS).
- Biguanide: Mechanism of action not entirely understood but decreases hepatic gluconeogenesis and improves insulin sensitivity.
- Start with 500 mg daily and titrate to a maximum tolerated dose of 2 g daily (standard release).
- Patients may experience gastrointestinal (GI) side effects and should be reassured that these are often mild and should settle. A modified-release preparation may be helpful.

- Theoretic risk of lactic acidosis may require a break from therapy during acute illness.
- Contraindications: severe liver failure, kidney injury with estimated glomerular filtration rate (eGFR) less than 30 mL/min (with dose reduction at higher eGFR).
- If after 3 to 6 months of lifestyle intervention and metformin, HbA1c is above 58 mmol/mol, then the first treatment intensification should take place. Treatment should be individualized but options include:
  - metformin + sulphonylurea
  - metformin + dipeptidyl peptidase-4 (DPP-IV) inhibitor
  - metformin + sodium-glucose cotransporter 2 (SGLT-2) inhibitor
  - metformin + pioglitazone
- The target HbA1c should be less than 53 mmol/mol.

Sulphonylurea

- Gliclazide most commonly used. Works by stimulating pancreas insulin secretion. Side effects include hypoglycaemia and weight gain. Contraindications include eGFR below 30 mL/min due to risk of severe hypoglycaemia.
- Typical starting dose of 80 mg once daily and titrated to a maximum of 160 mg twice daily. Lower dose of 40 mg daily if concern of hypoglycaemia.
- Patients should be made aware of the symptoms of hypoglycaemia and be trained to check their own blood sugars at relevant times.
- DVLA restrictions should be discussed (see p. 416).

Dipeptidyl Peptidase-4 Inhibitors

- Options include saxagliptin, sitagliptin, linagliptin, alogliptin, vildagliptin; and the choice between these should be based on local policy.
- Incretin-based therapy. Blocks DPP-IV, preventing inactivation of GLP-1 and subsequent inhibition of glucagon release, increased insulin secretion from pancreas, and decreased gastric emptying. These events lead to reduced blood glucose levels.
- Expected to reduce HbA1c by approximately 0.5%.
- *Benefits:* weight neutral, low risk of hypoglycaemia unless used with insulin or sulphonylurea.
- *Side effects:* GI side effects, nasopharyngitis, pancreatitis. Dose adjustment needed for renal impairment with exception of linagliptin. While there are no data to suggest increase in cardiovascular (CV) death associated with DPP-IV use, given current conflicting data, they should be used with caution in those at high risk of heart failure.

Pioglitazone

- Thiazolidinedione, PPAR-γ agonist decreasing peripheral insulin resistance.
- Decreases triglycerides but increases high-density lipoprotein (HDL) and low-density lipoprotein (LDL) cholesterol.
- Dose 15 to 45 mg once daily.
- Risk of hypoglycaemia if used alongside a sulphonylurea or insulin.

- *Side effects:* fluid retention, weight gain, increased risk of heart failure, small increased risk of bladder cancer, increased risk of bone fractures, and liver dysfunction.
- *Contraindications:* pre-existing heart failure or high risk for heart failure, previous or active bladder cancer or significant family history of bladder cancer, hepatic impairment, haematuria of unknown aetiology.
- Use with caution in those at risk of falls or at increased risk of bone fracture (e.g., osteoporosis).
- Monitor liver function before treatment, after 2 months, and periodically thereafter.

Sodium-Glucose Cotransporter 2 Inhibitors

- These include empagliflozin, dapagliflozin, and canagliflozin. The choice of agent will depend on local policy.
- Act by blocking the SGLT2 receptor in the proximal tubule of kidney, preventing reabsorption of glucose and water resulting in glycosuria.
- *Benefits:* weight loss, reduction in blood pressure, absence of hypoglycaemia unless used with other hypoglycaemic agents.
- *Side effects:* volume depletion, hypotension, electrolyte disturbance, genitourinary infections, ketoacidosis.
- Ketoacidosis has been reported in patients with type 2 diabetes taking an SGLT2 inhibitor, even at near-normal glucose levels. Patients need to be counselled on symptoms of ketoacidosis (nausea, vomiting, abdominal pain, anorexia) and advised to seek medical attention if they develop these.
- *Contraindications:* renal impairment with eGFR below 60 mL/min, concomitant use with loop diuretic, ketoacidosis, recurrent genitourinary sepsis.
- Use with caution in patients at increased risk of volume depletion.
- Cardiovascular outcome studies:
  - Empagliflozin, Cardiovascular Outcomes and Mortality in Type 2 Diabetes (EMPA-REG) study showed patients with type 2 diabetes and established cardiovascular disease taking empagliflozin had a significant reduction in major adverse cardiovascular events (cardiovascular death, nonfatal myocardial infarction [MI], and nonfatal stroke) and all-cause mortality. These results were driven by a 38% relative risk reduction in heart failure admissions.
  - The Canagliflozin and Cardiovascular and Renal Events in Type 2 Diabetes (CANVAS) study also showed cardiovascular benefit of Canagliflozin in high-risk cardiovascular patients. There was however an increase in toe and metatarsal amputations.

Further study results in this group are awaited.

Second Intensification

- If HbA1c remains above 58 mmol/mol after 3 to 6 months on two agents, a second intensification of therapy should take place. Options include:
  - metformin, DPP-IV inhibitor + sulphonylurea;
  - metformin, pioglitazone + sulphonylurea;
  - metformin, pioglitazone or sulphonylurea + SGLT-2 inhibitor;

- metformin, sulphonylurea + glucagon-like peptide 1 (GLP-1) agonist (only if BMI >35 kg/m² in England and Wales, or >30 kg/m² in Scotland);
- insulin therapy.

Glucagon-Like Peptide 1 Agonists

- These include liraglutide, exenatide, lixisenatide, semaglutide—all of which are injectable. They work by enhancing pancreatic insulin secretion in a glucose-dependent manner, inhibit glucagon release, and delay gastric emptying thus promoting satiety.
- There are various regimes from twice-daily injection to once weekly.
- *Benefits:* promotes weight loss whilst reducing hyperglycaemia, low risk of hypoglycaemia if not used alongside insulin or sulphonylureas.
- *Side effects:* GI side effects often intolerable, skin reactions at injection sites, pancreatitis, theoretical risk of increased pancreatic and medullary thyroid cancer but not proven.
- *Contraindications:* gastroparesis, pancreatic pathology, previous or pre-existing thyroid cancer, chronic kidney disease (CKD) with eGFR below 30 mL/min, hepatic impairment.
- They are expensive:
  - Most health boards will have specific criteria to monitor effectiveness of treatment before funding for more than 6 months.
  - NICE suggests a minimum HbA1c reduction of 1% AND weight loss of 3% or more be achieved within 6 months of starting treatment or therapy should be discontinued.
  - Cardiovascular outcome trials have also shown signifcant cardiovascular benefit of GLP-1 agonist therapy in the LEADER (Liraglutide) and SUSTAIN-6 (Semaglutide) trials.

Insulin

- Once-daily NPH insulin is usually sufficient for initiation of insulin in patients with type 2 diabetes.
- A total daily dose of 0.3 to 0.5 units/kg is a reasonable starting dose (maximum first dose of 10 units).
- Metformin should continue.
- Other hypoglycaemic agents should be reviewed for continuation, stopping, or dose adjustment.
- Insulin analogues such as detemir and glargine may be preferred for those at risk of overnight or severe hypoglycaemia.
- If NPH insulin is insufficient, twice-daily mixed preparations can be tried.
- Before starting insulin, the patient must:
  - have education on insulin administration and blood glucose monitoring from a diabetes educator;
  - have open access to a clinician capable of advising on dose adjustments during initiation;
  - know how to recognize and treat hypoglycaemia;
  - discuss driving regulations and occupational hazards.

Other Therapies

- *Meglitinides* can be used for patients intolerant to sulphonylurea.
  - Similar to sulphonylureas
  - More expensive
- *Acarbose:*
  - Blocks intestinal alpha glucosidase preventing starchy compounds being broken down to simple sugars.
  - Not as effective, and intolerable GI side effects.

Home Glucose Monitoring

- Required for ALL patients on insulin, and in those on sulphonylurea who drive or are at risk of hypoglycaemia.
- Not generally required for patients with type 2 diabetes on other regimes.

Hypoglycaemia

- All patients on insulin or sulphonylurea should be educated on the symptoms of hypoglycaemia and how to treat it.
- They should be advised to check blood glucose to confirm hypoglycaemia (<4 mmol/L) if they have symptoms.
- If conscious and swallow safe, then they should take 15 to 20 g of oral glucose:
  - 200 mL fresh fruit juice
  - 120 mL Lucozade
  - 4 jelly babies
  - 4 to 5 dextrose tablets
- Blood glucose should be rechecked 15 minutes later and treatment repeated if needed.
- Once resolved, the patient should eat some complex carbohydrate (e.g., sandwich).
- If unconscious or swallow not safe, caregiver should give intramuscular (IM) glucagon 1 mg and call ambulance.
- Medically trained staff will be able to administer intravenous (IV) glucose (150 mL 10% glucose or 75 mL 20% glucose).
- Identify and correct cause for hypoglycaemia.

Sickday Rules for Patients on Insulin Therapy

- If possible, patients should keep up dietary intake.
- If unable, oral fluids are important to prevent dehydration.
- A trial of easily digested foods (soup, jelly) may be effective.
- Check blood glucose at least 4-hourly.
- **DO NOT** omit insulin therapy.
- If hypoglycaemia occurs, treat with sugary drinks.
- If refractory hypoglycaemia, seek medical advice.
- If blood glucose above 15 mmol/L, check for ketones.
- If ketones positive, administer 10% of total daily insulin dose in short-acting insulin and repeat blood glucose and ketones after 2 hours. If not resolving, repeat step but if worsening seek medical help.
- If hyperglycaemia but no ketones, patient can give a correction dose of short-acting insulin. A correction dose can be calculated as 100/total daily insulin dose. For example, a patient on 50 units of insulin per day would

have a correction dose assuming that 1 unit of insulin will correct blood glucose by 2 mmol/L.

- This can be repeated after 2 hours also, but if worsening seek medical advice.

Blood Pressure Management

- *Targets:*
  - SIGN suggests targeted blood pressure below 130/80 mmHg for all patients with diabetes.
  - NICE suggests targets of below 140/80 mmHg (or <130/80 mmHg if nephropathy, retinopathy, or cerebrovascular disease).
  - The UKPDS study showed every 10-mmHg reduction in systolic blood pressure (SBP) reduced 10-year risk of CV death by 15%.
  - Intensive blood pressure control to these targets reduces the development of microvascular complications.
  - Further intensification to below these values is not recommended (ACCORD).
- *Treatments:*
  - An angiotensin-converting enzyme (ACE) inhibitor is first line therapy, in addition to intensive lifestyle intervention:
    a. If intolerant, an angiotensin receptor blocker should be used instead.
    b. If of black origin, a calcium channel blocker is more appropriate.
  - Beta blockers and alpha blockers are not first line in patients with diabetes and hypertension, but can be used for intensification of therapy or other therapeutic reasons.
  - BP should be monitored once or twice monthly until consistently within target.

Other Cardiovascular Risk Factors

Lipids

- Statin therapy should be offered to all patients with diabetes whose 10-year CV risk is 10% or more, regardless of cholesterol.
- This generally includes all patients with diabetes aged over 40 years, and younger patients with microvascular complications.
- Primary prevention doses are:
  - atorvastatin 20 mg (NICE);
  - simvastatin 40 mg or atorvastatin 10 mg (SIGN).
- Secondary prevention doses are higher with atorvastatin 80 mg recommended.
- Fibrates may be considered for those intolerant of statin but there is a lack of evidence of efficacy.

Antiplatelet Therapy

- Not recommended for primary prevention.

Smoking

- All patients should be advised to stop and referred to smoking cessation services.

- Nicotine replacement therapies are recommended but vapours are not, in view of a lack of safety data.

Diabetic Nephropathy

- Microalbuminuria is the first sign of diabetic kidney disease, and is associated with increased cardiovascular morbidity and mortality.
- It is defined as:
  - 24-hour urinary albumin of 30 to 300 mg;
  - urinary ACR above 2.5 mg/mmol in men (3.5 mg/mmol in women).
- Overt diabetic nephropathy is defined by an ACR above 30 mg/mmol and is a strong indicator of cardiovascular risk and progression to end-stage renal failure.
- Urinary ACR and eGFR should be monitored at least annually in patients aged 12 years and older with diabetes.
- If microalbuminuria present, ACE inhibitor should be started irrespective of blood pressure as it will slow progression to overt nephropathy and can reverse microalbuminuria.
- Intensive glycaemic and blood pressure control is vital to preventing progression.

Diabetic Retinopathy and Maculopathy

- Up to 40% of patients with type 2 diabetes have retinopathy at diagnosis.
- All patients with type 2 diabetes should undergo retinal screening at diagnosis, and at least annually thereafter.
- Retinal screening is best performed as part of the national screening programme using digital photography.
- Fundoscopy is not reliable.
- Retinopathy is defined as:
  - background retinopathy;
  - preproliferative retinopathy;
  - proliferative retinopathy.
- Proliferative or referable preproliferative retinopathy should be referred to ophthalmology for consideration of laser photocoagulation therapy.
- Urgent referral if neovascularization is near the macula or associated vitreous haemorrhage.
- Macular oedema should also be referred urgently.
- Intensive blood pressure and glycaemic control should be targeted to prevent progression, and patients must stop smoking.

Diabetic Foot Disease and Neuropathy

- The principal risk factors for the development of foot ulceration in patients with diabetes are neuropathy and peripheral vascular disease.
- All patients with diabetes should have their feet screened at diagnosis, then at least annually and if any foot problems occur. Assessment must include the peripheral circulation (pulses), sensation (with a 10-g monofilament), the presence of structural abnormalities, and any history of previous ulceration. The feet should be risk stratified

(low, moderate, high, or active foot disease) and management plan discussed.

- Foot care education should be given to all patients with diabetes. Importantly, the person's current risk of developing foot problems and who to contact if a foot emergency should arise. Moderate- and high-risk feet should have input from the foot protection service.
- All patients with active ulceration and signs of sepsis, ulceration with critical limb ischaemia, gangrene, or deep-seated soft tissue/bone infection should be referred urgently to the acute hospital and the multidisciplinary foot care service informed.
- For all other active foot problems and suspected Charcot (swelling, redness, and warmth of a foot with or without pain, especially if the skin is intact), refer urgently to the multidisciplinary foot care service.
- For the management of neuropathic pain NICE (2013) recommends offering a choice of amitriptyline, duloxetine, gabapentin, or pregabalin initially. If one is not effective or tolerated then one of the remaining three agents should be offered.

Erectile Dysfunction

- Erectile dysfunction is common and a marker of underlying cardiovascular disease.
- Ask about symptoms at annual review and offer a phosphodiesterase type-5 inhibitor if no contraindications.
- If pharmacologic therapy is unhelpful, refer to a local erectile dysfunction service.
- Testosterone therapy is controversial and should not be commenced without consulting endocrinology.

Driving Regulations

- Patients treated with insulin may hold a Group 1 (car or motorcycle) or a Group 2 (lorry or bus) licence; however, the DVLA must be informed. Their licence will be reviewed every 3 years, or sooner in the context of any of these events:
  - More than one severe hypoglycaemic attack (requiring third-party assistance) in the preceding 12 months whilst awake for group 1 licence holders. or
  - Any severe hypoglycaemic attack whilst driving
  - Impaired hypoglycaemic awareness
  - Retinopathy requiring laser treatment
  - Loss of vision in one eye
  - Unable to read a car number plate (with glasses if needed) at 20 m in daylight or have reduced visual acuity of less than 6/12 (with glasses)
  - Neuropathy or peripheral vascular disease that impacts on their ability to drive a standard manual car
- Requirements for patients holding a Group 2 licence are tighter and in addition to the above, the DVLA needs to be informed if:
  - the patient is taking any medication for diabetes, regardless of perceived hypoglycaemic risk;
  - even only one severe hypoglycaemic has occurred in a 12-month period, which must be reported immediately.

- Proof of blood glucose monitoring to demonstrate acceptable control and at times appropriate to driving must be available. Three months of such monitoring (on a glucometer with date and time function) is reviewed by the patient's doctor prior to renewal of licence.

General Advice for Driving With Diabetes

- Check blood glucose immediately before driving.
- Aim to be above 5 mmol/L before commencing journey.
- Check blood glucose every 2 hours as a minimum on long journeys, but sooner if symptoms of hypoglycaemia.
- Keep quick-acting carbohydrate in the car at all times to enable prompt treatment.
- Follow-up treatment of hypoglycaemia with complex carbohydrate (e.g., sandwich).
- If blood glucose is below 4 mmol/L at any point, treat the hypoglycaemia and do not resume driving until at least 45 minutes of a blood glucose above 5 mmol/L has been achieved, and patient feels well enough to continue safely.

Gestational Diabetes

> **GUIDELINES**
>
> National Institute for Health and Care Excellence. (2015). *Diabetes in pregnancy: Management from pre-conception to the postnatal period. NICE clinical guideline 3.* www.nice.org.uk.
> Scottish Intercollegiate Guidelines Network. (2013). *Management of diabetes. SIGN guideline 116.* www.sign.ac.uk.

- Gestational diabetes mellitus (GDM) is defined as glucose intolerance with onset or first recognition during pregnancy. Maternal risk factors for GDM are shown in Table 24.3; women should be assessed for these factors in early pregnancy, and if present should be offered screening with a 75-g oral glucose tolerance test at 24 to 28 weeks of gestation, or earlier if they have a history of GDM in a previous pregnancy.

Screening and Diagnosis

- Current treatment of GDM is influenced by a number of large clinical trials, showing that treatment of GDM

TABLE 24.3	**Risk Factors for Gestational Diabetes (NICE, 2015)**
Body mass index (BMI) >30 kg/m²	
Previous macrosomic baby weighing ≥4.5 kg	
Previous gestational diabetes mellitus	
Family history of diabetes (first-degree relative with diabetes)	
Minority ethnic family origin with a high prevalence of diabetes	

TABLE 24.4	Diagnostic Criteria for Gestational Diabetes Mellitus	
	IADPSG	**NICE (2015)**
Fasting plasma glucose (mmol/L)	≥5.1	≥5.6
1-hour glucose (mmol/L)	≥10	
2-hour glucose (mmol/L)	≥8.5	≥7.8

IADPSG, International Association of the Diabetes and Pregnancy Study Groups; *NICE*, National Institute of Health and Care Excellence.

with insulin improves pregnancy outcomes, including birthweight and macrosomia, and demonstrating a continuum of risk for maternal glucose levels and adverse pregnancy outcomes.

- The optimal way to diagnose GDM, however, remains controversial. The most widely adopted diagnostic criteria were developed by the International Association of the Diabetes and Pregnancy Study Groups (IADPSG) and these criteria have been endorsed by various other bodies including the American Diabetes Association (ADA). In 2015 NICE updated their guidelines with diagnostic criteria as outlined in Table 24.4.
- The majority of centres in the United Kingdom will use these criteria; other centres, particularly in the United States, will use alternative criteria, including two-step approaches using a 50-g then 100-g oral glucose tolerance test.

Treatment

- Once diagnosed with GDM, women should be taught to undertake blood sugar monitoring to assess fasting and postprandial glycaemia and to guide treatment. Dietary modification is the mainstay of treatment, and all women should be seen by a dietician as soon as possible after diagnosis. Other lifestyle advice, including advice on smoking and exercise, should be offered.
- Metformin is used in the majority of women who fail to reach their glycaemic targets with diet alone. Although it crosses the placenta, it is thought to be safe for use in pregnancy, with no significant effect on perinatal development. Approximately 50% of women treated with metformin will require additional therapy with insulin.
- Glibenclamide, a sulphonylurea, does not cross the placenta in significant amounts and has been used in a number of studies in pregnancy, although there has been limited data on long-term pregnancy outcomes.
- Insulin therapy is used in women who fail to reach glycaemic targets with dietary measures or with metformin, or in those for whom metformin is not tolerated. Undiagnosed type 2 diabetes should be considered in women with a fasting glucose of 7 mmol/L and above; these women should be treated initially with insulin, with or without metformin.

Issues Postpregnancy

- Following pregnancy the majority of women with GDM will no longer require any treatment.
- Women should be advised of the risk of GDM in any subsequent pregnancy, and to seek medical advice if further pregnancy is desired.
- Women should be offered testing at 6 weeks postpartum, and annual testing thereafter to assess for underlying type 2 diabetes.

Type 1 Diabetes in Pregnancy

- Type 1 diabetes is associated with a number of adverse foetal and maternal outcomes, including congenital malformations, preeclampsia, miscarriage, and macrosomia.
- Women with type 1 diabetes should be referred for prepregnancy counselling and have regular checks of HbA1c, aiming for HbA1c below 48 mmol/mol (6.5%) prior to conception. Women with HbA1c of greater than 86 mmol/mol (10%) should be advised against pregnancy. Women with type 1 diabetes should be treated with high-dose folic acid, medications such as statins, and ACE inhibitors should be stopped prior to considering pregnancy.
- To help reduce the risk of preeclampsia, women should be treated with aspirin from 12 weeks of gestation.

Type 2 Diabetes in Pregnancy

- Increasing numbers of women are entering pregnancy in recent times with type 2 diabetes. The safety of modern medications such as DPP-4 inhibitors, SGLT-2 inhibitors, and GLP-1 analogues has not been studied extensively in pregnancy and these medications should be stopped prior to pregnancy.
- Women with type 2 diabetes should be referred for prepregnancy planning; the majority will require to be switched to insulin therapy prior to conception.

Thyroid Disease

GUIDELINES

Okosieme, O., Gilbert, J., Abraham, P., et al. (2015). Management of primary hypothyroidism: Statement by the British Thyroid Association Executive Committee. *Clinical Endocrinology, 84*, 799–808.

Pearce, S. H. S., Brabant, G., Duntas, L. H., Monzani, F., Peeters, R. P., Razvi, S., & Wemeau, J. L. (2013). ETA guideline: Management of subclinical hypothyroidism. *European Thyroid Journal, 2*, 215–228.

Ross, D. S., Burch, H. B., Cooper, D. S., et al. (2016). American Thyroid Association guidelines for diagnosis and management of hyperthyroidism and other causes of thyrotoxicosis. *Thyroid* (online).

Perros, P., Colley, S., Boelaert, K., et al. (2014). British Thyroid Association guidelines for the management of thyroid cancer. *Clinical Endocrinology, 81*, 1–122.

- Thyroid disease is common. Thyroid function tests (TFTs) are among the most frequently requested tests in primary care, and an understanding of how to interpret them and what to do next is essential for daily working as a general practitioner (GP).
- Most laboratories will report thyroid-stimulating hormone (TSH) and free T4 as standard, but some will include total T4 and T3. T4 and to a lesser extent T3 are bound in plasma by thyroid binding globulin, and it is the unbound component that is physiologically active. T3 is more active than T4.

Hypothyroidism

- Symptoms include lethargy, weight gain, cold intolerance, muscle cramps, slowed cognition, constipation, dry hair and skin, hoarse voice, and fluid retention.
- Severely hypothyroid patients may present with:
  - myxoedematous appearance—periorbital puffiness, macroglossia, thin hair;
  - cardiac failure;
  - hypothermia;
  - peripheral neuropathy;
  - encephalopathy;
  - coma.

Primary Hypothyroidism

- Primary hypothyroidism is most common and results from the failure of the thyroid to produce adequate thyroid hormone. Typically causes high TSH, low T4.
- Causes include:
  - autoimmune (Hashimoto): thyroid peroxidase (TPO) antibody positive, usually with goitre;
  - postradioiodine therapy or thyroid surgery;
  - iodine deficiency (endemic goitre);
  - postradiotherapy to head/neck;
  - congenital;
  - drugs: lithium, amiodarone, chemotherapy agents.

Secondary Hypothyroidism

- Secondary hypothyroidism is due to failure of the pituitary to produce TSH. Results in low TSH, low T4. Usually associated with other pituitary hormone deficiencies.
- Causes:
  - Pituitary tumours
  - Postpituitary surgery or radiotherapy
  - Postcranial irradiation
  - Empty sella
  - Rarer pituitary disorders (e.g., infiltrative, infarction/haemorrhage)
- In secondary hypothyroidism exclude cortisol deficiency as a matter of urgency. Do not initiate thyroid replacement until glucocorticoid deficiency is excluded.

Investigations in Primary Care
- TFTs
- TPO antibodies for primary hypothyroid

- Urgent 9 am cortisol if secondary hypothyroid, or refer for URGENT short synacthen test if high suspicion of glucocorticoid deficiency
- Full blood count (FBC) for associated anaemia and macrocytosis
- Urea and electrolytes (U&Es) for hyponatraemia

Treatment
- Give levothyroxine. In younger patients without cardiac disease, 50 μg daily is a typical starting dose. For older, comorbid patients and those with heart disease, 25 μg should be started.
- Repeat TFTs 6 weeks following initiation, and titrate dose in 25- to 50-μg increments. Repeat testing and dose escalation should not occur before this. Aim for normal TSH and T4.
- T3 therapy is controversial and there is little evidence to suggest greater benefit than T4, but a small number of patients report improved symptoms.
- Despite normalization of TFTs, patients may complain of symptoms. Levothyroxine should not be increased.
- Review medications as some drugs can affect absorption of thyroxine (antacids, proton pump inhibitors [PPIs], iron).

Referral
- Most primary hypothyroidism is managed in primary care.
- Refer:
  a. all secondary hypothyroid;
  b. primary hypothyroid:
    - Young patients
    - High doses (i.e., >200 μg daily) where compliance is good
    - Large goitre causing obstructive symptoms
    - Severe hypothyroidism
    - Cardiac disease
    - Pregnancy or within 6 months postpartum

Subclinical Hypothyroidism

- High TSH but normal T4.
- Treatment still debated but generally accepted if:
  - TSH is above 10 mU/L;
  - repeated testing trending toward overt hypothyroidism;
  - consider if significant cardiac disease.
- More likely to adopt a wait and see approach in extreme elderly patients as TSH rises with age.

Hyperthyroidism

- Symptoms: flushes, anxiety, tremor, palpitations, heat intolerance, loose stools, oligomenorrhoea, hair loss, eye symptoms in Graves disease.

Primary Hyperthyroidism

- Suppressed TSH, high T4, and/or high T3
- Causes:

- Graves disease: positive TSH-receptor antibodies (TRAB) usually. TRAB-negative variant also with typical features on thyroid imaging
- Autoimmune (TPO antibodies)
- Toxic multinodular goitre
- Toxic nodule
- Thyroiditis: subacute de Quervain, postpartum
- Drug induced: amiodarone
- Factitious: thyroxine abuse
- Very rarely thyroid cancer

Secondary Hyperthyroidism

- Secondary is very rare
- Causes:
  - TSH-oma
  - Thyroid hormone resistance
- Results in high TSH, high T4/T3

Graves Disease

- Autoimmune thyrotoxicosis with diffuse goitre
- Associated with TRAB antibodies
- Associated eye symptoms:
  - Gritty, dry eyes
  - Pain
  - Proptosis and lid lag
  - Periorbital oedema
  - Diplopia/ophthalmoplegia
  - Altered colour vision
  - Visual loss

Investigations in Primary Care

- TFTs
- TRAB and TPO antibodies

Treatment

- Nonselective beta blockers can be used for symptom management.
- Do not start antithyroid treatment unless discussed with endocrinologist.
- Thyroiditis does not usually require antithyroid treatment and prescribing it may precipitate profound hypothyroidism.

Antithyroid Drugs

- Usually first line in autoimmune disease. Patients typically receive 12 to 18 months of antithyroid therapy before a trial off it. Less effective in other disease but may be used as a holding bridge to other therapy.
- *Carbimazole:*
  - Varying doses from 10 to 40 mg daily depending on severity of thyrotoxicosis and response to treatment
  - Counsel patients about the risk of agranulocytosis:
    a. Should stop therapy and seek urgent medical attention if severe sore throat, mouth ulcers, and fever.
    b. Full blood count should be taken to ensure white cell count normal, and if so can recommence treatment.

- *Propylthiouracil (PTU):*
  - Used in first trimester of pregnancy or if intolerant to carbimazole.
  - Dose 200 to 400 mg daily in divided doses initially.
  - Lower risk of agranulocytosis than carbimazole.
  - Hepatitis more common.
  - Check LFTs 4 to 6 weeks after initiating treatment and periodically thereafter. Discontinue and seek advice if abnormal.
  - Monitor TFTs every 6 to 8 weeks until euthyroid and 3-monthly thereafter on maintenance therapy.

Radioactive Iodine

- Given to those who relapse or show resistance to antithyroid medication.
- Likely required in toxic nodular disease.
- Risk of hypothyroidism post-treatment.
- Not suitable for carers of young children or in pregnancy due to radiation risks.

Thyroid Surgery

- Rarely required.
- Likely to need levothyroxine post-surgery.
- Other risks include recurrent laryngeal nerve damage, hypoparathyroidism, haemorrhage, and infection.

Referral

- All hyperthyroidism should be referred.
- Treatment should be discussed with endocrinologist before initiating.
- Patients with Graves disease who become pregnant should be referred to endocrinology and obstetrics as early as possible.
- Sight-threatening Graves eye disease should be referred as an emergency to ophthalmology:
  - Globe subluxation
  - Symptoms of corneal ulceration
  - Visual loss
  - Impaired colour vision

Thyroid Nodules

- Thyroid cancer is rare (<1% of all cancers).
- TFTs are usually (but not always) normal in thyroid cancer.
- Increasing concern if:
  - rapid growth;
  - larger than 1 cm;
  - lymphadenopathy.
- All thyroid nodules should be referred.
- Followed up at least annually by endocrinology:
  - for papillary and follicular cancers, treatment aims to suppress TSH lifelong.

Sick Euthyroid

- Ideally, TFTs should not be checked in acute/subacute illness.
- Typically inappropriately normal or suppressed TSH with low T3/T4 but various patterns seen.
- Any decision to commence treatment in such cases needs monitoring closely.

Thyroid Disease in Pregnancy

- Woman with hypo- and hyperthyroidism should be referred to endocrinology as soon as pregnancy confirmed.
- Woman with hypothyroidism should increase levothyroxine dose by 25% to 30% as soon as pregnancy confirmed:
  - Target TSH <2.5 mU/L in first trimester.
  - TSH levels are normally lower in the first trimester due to biochemical similarities to human chorionic gonadotropin (hCG).
  - Diagnosis and treatment of subclinical hypothyroidism in pregnancy is controversial.
- Woman with hyperthyroidism will usually require smaller doses of antithyroid medication and may be able to stop it in pregnancy.
  - PTU is preferred in the first trimester due to risk of teratogenicity associated with carbimazole.
  - TRAB antibodies should be checked in pregnancy in women with a history of Graves; if positive there is a risk of neonatal Graves disease.
  - Women with Graves disease are at risk of recurrence in the postnatal period; TFTs should be checked 4 to 6 weeks after delivery.

Hypoadrenalism

REVIEWS AND GUIDANCE

Charmandari, E., Nicolaides, N. C., & Chrousos, G. P. (2014). Adrenal insufficiency. *GP Lancet, 383,* 2152–2167.
   Husebye, E. S., Allolio, B., Arlt, W., et al. (2014). Consensus statement on the diagnosis, treatment and follow-up of patients with primary adrenal insufficiency. *Journal of Internal Medicine, 275,* 104–115.

- Hypoadrenalism can be primary (most commonly autoimmune or Addison disease), secondary (most commonly hypopituitarism due to pituitary adenoma), or tertiary (most commonly exogenous glucocorticoid administration).
- Fatigue is a presenting feature common to all aetiologies. Patients with primary hypoadrenalism may demonstrate skin pigmentation (increased ACTH levels) and symptoms of mineralocorticoid deficiency. In secondary and tertiary hypoadrenalism, mineralocorticoid secretion is normal; therefore plasma potassium levels are normal.
- All aetiologies can present with a hypoadrenal crisis; symptoms consist of abdominal pain, vomiting, dehydration, and hypotension. This is a medical emergency.
- *Primary hypoadrenalism:*
  - Prevalence increased in recent years, likely due to rise in autoimmune hypoadrenalism.
  - More common in women than men.
  - Incidence peaks between 30 and 50 years.
- *Secondary hypoadrenalism:*
  - More common than primary hypoadrenalism.
  - Tends to present at a later age, around 60 years.

- *Tertiary hypoadrenalism:*
  - Patients receiving oral glucocorticoid treatment more than 2 to 3 weeks are at risk; therapy should not be stopped abruptly.
  - Inhaled, topical, intramuscular, and intraarticular steroids may also cause tertiary hypoadrenalism.

Diagnosis

- Measure serum cortisol levels before and after stimulation with synthetic ACTH (synacthen). Patients should not be taking exogenous steroids. False negative results can occur in acute secondary or tertiary hypoadrenalism (the adrenal glands take time to atrophy and response to ACTH is preserved in the short term). The cutoff for diagnosis varies according to the assay used and should be confirmed locally.
- Differentiating between primary, secondary, and tertiary hypoadrenalism is based on history (drug history, presence of other autoimmune conditions, family history) and further investigations, including plasma ACTH levels, aldosterone and renin measurements, adrenal androgens, adrenal autoantibodies, and, depending on clinical suspicion, pituitary function tests or adrenal/pituitary imaging. These would be undertaken by the specialist endocrine team.

Treatment

- Glucocorticoid replacement, most commonly hydrocortisone (complete form FP92A to exempt prescription charges) in divided doses mimicking diurnal rhythm (e.g., 10 mg, 5 mg, 5 mg).
- Mineralocorticoid replacement only required in primary adrenal insufficiency and is not needed if daily dose of hydrocortisone is over 50 mg.
- Adrenal androgen replacement is not currently recommended in the United Kingdom due to a lack of evidence regarding efficacy.
- All patients should be educated in sickday rules:
  - Double or triple hydrocortisone dose during intercurrent illnesses. Need to reduce slowly if illness persists for more than a few days.
  - Seek medical assistance if vomiting or unable to tolerate oral hydrocortisone treatment and wear medic alert bracelet/carry steroid card.
  - IM hydrocortisone (100 mg) for self-administration in case of emergencies and patients should be familiar in how and when to use this.
  - Inform medical staff promptly of steroid dependence if they are unwell or undergoing invasive procedures so that timely replacement treatment can be initiated.
- Abrupt cessation of steroids can precipitate adrenal crisis; patients should always be prescribed and dispensed adequate amounts of hydrocortisone to cover holiday periods and sickdays.
- Monitoring of treatment is usually undertaken by specialist endocrine team and involves assessing adequacy of replacement while minimizing risks of overreplacement

(hypertension, diabetes, reduced bone mineral density).

- Adrenal crisis is a life-threatening emergency that requires prompt treatment.
  - Give 100 mg hydrocortisone IM or IV and urgent referral to hospital.

Hypercalcaemia

GUIDELINE

Bilezikian, J. P., Brandi, M. L., Eastell, R., et al. (2014). Primary hyperparathyroidism: Management guidelines. *Journal of Clinical Endocrinology and Metabolism, 99,* 3561–3569.

- Calcium is the most abundant mineral and has vital roles in cellular function, cardiovascular stability, and bone health. It is under homeostatic control of parathyroid hormone (PTH), with lesser roles for vitamin D and magnesium. Approximately half is bound to albumin in blood, and it is the unbound component that is physiologically active. Levels need to be corrected to albumin concentration as a result.
- Corrected calcium = measured calcium + (0.02 × [40 – albumin])
- Normal levels of corrected calcium are 2.2 to 2.6 mmol/L
- Severe hypercalcaemia is generally considered at 3 mmol/L and above, but severe symptoms and/or end-organ damage at lower levels can occur.

Symptoms

- Thirst
- Frequent urination
- Bony pain
- Nausea and vomiting
- Constipation
- Renal colic
- Lethargy
- Confusion
- Altered mood

Causes

Parathyroid Hormone Dependent (High Parathyroid Hormone or Inappropriately Normal Parathyroid Hormone)

- Primary hyperparathyroidism (PHPT; common)
- Tertiary hyperparathyroidism:
  - Occurs following prolonged period of hypocalcaemia
  - Seen in end-stage renal disease and malabsorptive conditions
- Chronic vitamin D deficiency
- Familial hypocalciuric hypercalcaemia (FHH):
  - Rare defect of the calcium sensing receptor gene
  - Autosomal dominant
  - Mild hypercalcaemia of no important sequelae
- Lithium

Parathyroid Hormone Independent (Low Parathyroid Hormone)

- Drugs: calcium supplements, thiazide diuretics, high dose vitamin A and D
- Humoral hypercalcaemia of malignancy:
  - PTH-related peptide secretion by tumours, particularly breast and squamous cell lung cancers
- Bony metastases
- Multiple myeloma
- Renal failure

Initial Tests

- Serum corrected calcium above 2.6 mmol/L
- Urea and electrolytes
- PTH
- Vitamin D
- Urinary calcium to creatinine ratio (<0.01 suggestive of FHH)
- Serum protein electrophoresis and urinary Bence Jones protein
- Further tests guided by results

Primary Hyperparathyroidism

- Of PHPT, 85% caused by single adenoma. Remainder due to parathyroid hyperplasia; less than 1% parathyroid carcinoma.
- Common in postmenopausal woman.
- Many patients have mild to moderate hypercalcaemia and are asymptomatic.
- Consider multiple endocrine neoplasia (MEN) 1 if:
  - younger than 40 years;
  - parathyroid hyperplasia;
  - strong family history of PHPT;
  - other endocrine tumours.

Treatment

- *Rehydration.* Advise patient to drink 3 L of water per day unless contraindicated.
- Loop diuretics are not indicated and may increase risk of nephrocalcinosis.
- Stop offending drugs.
- Parathyroidectomy if:
  - younger than 50 years;
  - serum calcium above 2.9 mmol/L;
  - confirmed nephrolithiasis/nephrocalcinosis;
  - kidney injury as a result of hypercalcaemia;
  - osteoporosis.
- Many patients are too frail or do not meet criteria for surgery.
  - Observe symptoms and calcium levels.
  - Bone density scan every 2 to 3 years and advise weight-bearing exercise and bisphosphonate therapy where appropriate.
  - Cinacalcet 30 mg twice a day may be suggested off-licence.

TABLE 24.5	Causes of Hirsutism and Clinical Features
Cause of Hirsutism	Associated Clinical Features
Polycystic ovary syndrome	Menstrual disturbance Long duration of symptoms Obesity/features of insulin resistance
Congenital adrenal hyperplasia	Family history of congenital adrenal hyperplasia Ethnicity: Ashkenazi Jewish, Hispanic
Virilizing tumour (ovarian or adrenal)	Rapid onset Other signs of virilization (clitoromegaly, voice change) Abdominal mass Significantly elevated serum androgens
Ovarian hyperthecosis	Postmenopausal onset. Often gradual but can have virilization and significantly elevated androgens
Iatrogenic	Drug history (e.g., androgens, including DHEA, cyclosporine, minoxidil, dexamethasone, some anticonvulsants, antipsychotics, and antidepressants). Transfer of testosterone from gels
Endocrinopathy	Other relevant features of Cushing syndrome, acromegaly, thyroid dysfunction, prolactinoma Uncommon for hirsutism to be presenting feature
Idiopathic hyperandrogenism	Hirsutism with no other clinical features and elevated serum androgens
Idiopathic hirsutism	Hirsutism with no other clinical features and normal serum androgens

Hirsutism

GUIDELINES

Martin, K. A., Chang, J., Ehrmann, D. A., et al. (2008). Evaluation and treatment of hirsutism in premenopausal women: An Endocrine Society clinical practice guideline. *Journal of Clinical Endocrinology and Metabolism*, 93, 1105–1120.

Arslanian, S. A., Ehrmann, D. A., et al. (2013). Diagnosis and treatment of polycystic ovary syndrome: An Endocrine Society clinical practice guideline. *Legro Journal of Clinical Endocrinology and Metabolism*, 98, 4565–4592.

Escobar-Morreale, H. F., Carmina, E., Dewailly, D., et al. (2012). Epidemiology, diagnosis and management of hirsutism: A consensus statement by the Androgen Excess and Polycystic Ovary Syndrome Society. *Human Reproduction Update*, 18, 146–170.

- Hirsutism (an excess of terminal hair growth) is common. Most women have either no physiological abnormality or benign pathology (most commonly polycystic ovary syndrome); however, there are a number of rare but important conditions to consider and exclude.
- Caused by elevated androgens, originating from adrenal or ovarian source and peripheral conversion of testosterone to the more active compound dihydrotestosterone. This peripheral conversion may explain why many women are symptomatic despite a serum testosterone within the normal range.
- Investigation of mild hirsutism with no associated clinical features has a low probability of detecting underlying disease and a significant risk of false positives, and is not recommended.
- Serum testosterone is usually significantly elevated (twice the normal) in malignant disease.
- The laboratory measurement of testosterone is challenging, partly due to variation in the sex hormone binding globulin (SHBG) seen in a number of conditions, including obesity and diabetes. Measurement of the free androgen index (which takes account of SHBG) is useful, as is measurement of testosterone in specialist laboratories using tandem mass spectroscopy rather than immunoassays. Liaising with local services for the interpretation of difficult cases is advised.

Table 24.5 lists the common causes of hirsutism and associated clinical features.

- PCOS is the most common diagnosis. Diagnosis depends of finding two of the following three features:
  - Androgen excess
  - Ovulatory dysfunction
  - Polycystic ovaries
- TFTs, prolactin, and 17-hydroxyprogesterone (17OHP) should be checked to screen for mimics. Synacthen-stimulated 17OHP is the diagnostic test for congenital adrenal hyperplasia.

Treatment

- *Lifestyle:*
  - Weight loss and improved insulin sensitivity will improve many features of PCOS, including unwanted hair growth.

- Metformin can be used as an insulin sensitizing agent; however, effect on hirsutism is minimal.
- *Hair removal:*
  - Plucking, waxing, and shaving are effective and cheap although they must be performed frequently.
  - The illusion of thicker hair is caused by the shaved tip of hair having a blunt edge.
  - Laser and electrolysis treatment is more expensive but can be effective for up to 6 months, is most effective in light-skinned women with dark hair, and is not suitable for use on extensive areas of skin.
  - Warn those planning to seek either of the last two options to check that the practitioner is a member of the appropriate professional body (e.g., the Institute of Electrolysis, British Medical Laser Association).
- *Pharmacological treatment:*
  - Pharmacological treatment should not be evaluated for efficacy before 6 months.
  - The OCP is the first line treatment. An OCP which contains a progestin with antiandrogenic properties may be more effective (e.g., drospirenone/Marvelon or cyproterone acetate/Dianette).
  - If no improvement is seen, an antiandrogen (spironolactone or cyproterone acetate) can be added but OCP must be prescribed concurrently due to risk of female foetal virilization.
  - Spironolactone (50–200 mg) can be used; may cause hyperkalaemia, diuresis, and hypotension.
  - Cyproterone acetate is generally well tolerated but there is a risk of hepatotoxicity; LFTs should be monitored. Combination treatment in the form of Dianette carries a higher risk of venous thromboembolism (VTE) than other forms of low-dose OCP.
  - Finasteride inhibits 5α-reductase activity. It is generally well tolerated.
  - Topical treatment (i.e., eflornithine cream) is only effective in reducing hair regrowth and should only be used in combination with hair removal methods.

Referral

Rapid virilization and/or significantly elevated testosterone levels should be referred to endocrinology. In addition, if the diagnosis is unclear or there is no response to treatment, endocrine referral is warranted.

Gynaecomastia

- Gynaecomastia is benign proliferation (>0.5 cm) of glandular breast tissue as distinct from a discrete breast mass (when carcinoma must be excluded) or diffuse enlargement due to adiposity and obesity.
- Usually bilateral but can be unilateral.
- Normal physiological phenomenon in many boys during the neonatal period and adolescence. It is also a common finding in older, middle-aged men without underlying pathology.
- Can be associated with a number of endocrine and non-endocrine conditions as well as many drugs (Table 24.6).

TABLE 24.6 Aetiology of Gynaecomastia

Nondrug Causes	Drugs
Physiological (neonatal, adolescence, old age) Hypogonadism hCG-producing tumours (testis, lung) Liver disease Renal disease Hyperthyroidism	Digoxin Spironolactone Cannabis Acid suppression: ranitidine, cimetidine, omeprazole Opiates Oestrogens Androgen deprivation therapy (e.g., bicalutamide; prostate cancer) Anabolic steroids Antiretrovirals Metoclopramide, domperidone

Clinical Evaluation

- Assess for thyroid status, signs of chronic liver disease, or associated features of hypogonadism (loss of body hair, female pattern of fat distribution, loss of muscle mass).
- Testicular and abdominal examination for the presence of a palpable mass.
- Take a full drug history including any herbal remedies and recreational drugs.

Biochemical Tests

- Testosterone (early morning sample, repeat at least once if low), luteinizing hormone (LH), hCG, alpha fetoprotein (AFP), oestrogen, and LFTs particularly if rapid onset with pain.
- Elevated hCG or oestrogen suggests possible neoplasm and testicular ultrasound is indicated, proceeding to imaging of adrenals if negative.
- Most will have normal investigations and cause is idiopathic.

Management

- Majority of adolescent gynaecomastia will resolve without intervention. In most adult cases removal of any contributing medication, reassurance, and observation is sufficient.
- Tamoxifen can be used in some cases but is rarely required.

Hypogonadism in Adult Men

GUIDELINE

Bhasin, S., Cunningham, G. R., Hayes, F. J., et al. (2010). Testosterone therapy in men with androgen deficiency syndrome: An Endocrine Society clinical practice guideline. *Journal of Clinical Endocrinology and Metabolism*, 95, 2536–2559.

- The term *hypogonadism* refers to a reduction in sperm or testosterone production. Table 24.7 lists its classifications.

TABLE 24.7	Classification of Hypogonadism			
	LH/FSH	**Testosterone**	**Prolactin**	**Aetiology**
Primary hypogonadism	Elevated	Low	Normal	Testicular failure
Secondary hypogonadism	Inappropriately normal or low	Low	Normal or elevated	Hypothalamic or pituitary disease

FSH, Follicle-stimulating hormone; *LH,* luteinizing hormone.

- Symptoms suggestive of androgen deficiency in men are loss of libido, erectile dysfunction, hot flashes/sweats (if severe and of rapid onset), and breast discomfort. Less specific symptoms include reduced energy levels, low mood, poor concentration, sleep disturbance, reduced muscle bulk, and increased body fat.
- *Enquire* about illnesses (e.g., mumps) or trauma that could have affected the testicles and drugs that interfere with testicular function/testosterone metabolism (e.g., glucocorticoids, opioids, and alcohol).
- *Examination* should include testicular size and the development of secondary sexual characteristics. Other physical findings include a reduction in facial/body hair, small/shrinking testes, incomplete/delayed sexual development, inability to conceive, and height loss/low trauma fractures.
- *Biochemical assessment* consists of a fasting venous serum sample for total testosterone between 8 and 10 am along with gonadotrophins (LH, FSH) in patients with symptoms. A repeat sample should be taken to confirm the diagnosis along with prolactin and thyroid function tests in secondary hypogonadism. Assessment should not be made during acute or subacute illness.
- *Refer* to an endocrinologist patients with symptoms, with osteopenia or osteoporosis, with evidence of pituitary disease, or with markedly low testosterone levels from primary testicular failure for further investigation and a decision about testosterone replacement therapy. Recent research suggests that raising testosterone in hypogonadal symptomatic men older than 65 years of age may provide some benefit in sexual function and mood but not in respect of vitality or walking distance (Snyder et al., 2016).
- Conditions in which testosterone administration is associated with a high risk of adverse outcome include prostate cancer, an unevaluated prostate nodule or raised PSA, breast cancer, a haematocrit over 50%, severe lower urinary tract symptoms, and poorly controlled congestive heart failure.

References

Bhasin, S., Cunningham, G. R., Hayes, F. J., et al. (2010). Testosterone therapy in men with androgen deficiency syndrome: An Endocrine Society clinical practice guideline. *Journal of Clinical Endocrinology and Metabolism, 95,* 2536–2559.

Bilezikian, J. P., Brandi, M. L., Eastell, R., et al. (2014). Primary hyperparathyroidism: Management guidelines. *Journal of Clinical Endocrinology and Metabolism, 99,* 3561–3569.

Charmandari, E., Nicolaides, N. C., & Chrousos, G. P. (2014). Adrenal insufficiency. *GP Lancet, 383,* 2152–2167.

Diabetes Improvement Plan. (2014). *Scottish government publications.* Retrieved from www.gov.scot/Publications/2014/11/6742/downloads.

Diabetes UK. (2015). *Facts and stats.* Retrieved from www.diabetes.org.uk.

Diabetes UK. (n.d.). *Diabetes risk score assessment tool.* Retrieved from www.diabetes.org.uk.

Escobar-Morreale, H. F., Carmina, E., Dewailly, D., et al. (2012). Epidemiology, diagnosis and management of hirsutism: A consensus statement by the Androgen Excess and Polycystic Ovary Syndrome Society. *Human Reproduction Update, 18,* 146–170.

Green, J. B., Bethel, M. A., Armstrong, P. W., with the TECOS Study Group. (2015). Effect of sitagliptin on cardiovascular outcomes in type 2 diabetes. *The New England Journal of Medicine, 373,* 232–242.

Husebye, E. S., Allolio, B., Arlt, W., et al. (2014). Consensus statement on the diagnosis, treatment and follow-up of patients with primary adrenal insufficiency. *Journal of Internal Medicine, 275,* 104–115.

Legro, R. S., Arslanian, S. A., Ehrmann, D. A., et al. (2013). Diagnosis and treatment of polycystic ovary syndrome: An Endocrine Society clinical practice guideline. *Journal of Clinical Endocrinology and Metabolism, 98,* 4565–4592.

Marso, S. P., Bain, S. C., Consoli, A., et al. (SUSTAIN-6 investigators). (2016). Semaglutide and cardiovascular outcomes in patients with type 2 diabetes. *The New England Journal of Medicine.* doi:10.1056/NEJMoa1607141

Marso, S. P., Daniels, G. H., Brown-Frandsen, K., et al (LEADER trial investigators). (2016). Liraglutide and cardiovascular outcomes in type 2 diabetes. *The New England Journal of Medicine, 375,* 311–322.

Martin, K. A., Chang, J., Ehrmann, D. A., et al. (2008). Evaluation and treatment of hirsutism in premenopausal women: An Endocrine Society clinical practice guideline. *Journal of Clinical Endocrinology and Metabolism, 93,* 1105–1120.

Metzger, B. E., Lowe, L. P., Dyer, A. R., et al. (HAPO Study Cooperative Research Group). (2008). Hyperglycaemia and adverse pregnancy outcome. *The New England Journal of Medicine, 358,* 1991–2002.

National Institute for Health and Care Excellence. (2012). *Type 2 diabetes: Prevention in people at high risk. NICE clinical guideline 38.* Retrieved from www.nice.org.uk.

National Institute for Health and Care Excellence. (2015a). *Diabetes in pregnancy: Management from pre-conception to the postnatal period. NICE clinical guideline 3.* Retrieved from www.nice.org.uk.

National Institute for Health and Care Excellence. (2015b). *Diabetic foot problems: Prevention and management. NICE clinical guideline 19.* Retrieved from www.nice.org.uk.

National Institute for Health and Care Excellence. (2015c). *Type 2 diabetes in adults: Management. NICE clinical guideline 28*. Retrieved from www.nice.org.uk.

Okosieme, O., Gilbert, J., Abraham, P., et al. (2015). Management of primary hypothyroidism: Statement by the British Thyroid Association Executive Committee. *Clinical Endocrinology, 84*, 799–808.

Pearce, S. H. S., Brabant, G., Duntas, L. H., Monzani, F., Peeters, R. P., Razvi, S., & Wemeau, J. L.. (2013). ETA guideline: Management of subclinical hypothyroidism. *European Thyroid Journal, 2*, 215–228.

Perros, P., Colley, S., Boelaert, K., et al. (2014). British Thyroid Association guidelines for the management of thyroid cancer. *Clinical Endocrinology, 81*, 1–122.

Ross, D. S., Burch, H. B., Cooper, D. S., et al. (2016). American Thyroid Association guidelines for diagnosis and management of hyperthyroidism and other causes of thyrotoxicosis. *Thyroid* (online).

Scirica, B. M., Bhatt, D. L., Braunwald, E., et al. (SAVOR-TIMI 53 Steering Committee). (2013). Saxagliptin and cardiovascular outcomes in patients with type 2 diabetes. *The New England Journal of Medicine, 369*, 1317–1326.

Scottish Intercollegiate Guidelines Network. (2013). *Management of diabetes. SIGN guideline 116*. Retrieved from www.sign.ac.uk.

The Action to Control Cardiovascular Risk in Diabetes (ACCORD) Study Group. (2010). Effects of intensive blood pressure control in type 2 diabetes. *The New England Journal of Medicine, 362*, 1575–1585.

UK Prospective Diabetes Study Group. (1990). UKPDS 6. Complications in newly diagnosed type 2 diabetic patients and their association with different clinical and biochemical risk factors. *Diabetes Research, 13*, 1–11.

UK Prospective Diabetes Study Group. (1998a). Effect of intensive blood-glucose control with metformin on complications in overweight patients with type 2 diabetes (UKPDS 34). *Lancet, 352*, 854–865.

UK Prospective Diabetes Study Group. (1998b). Intensive blood-glucose control with sulphonylureas or insulin compared with conventional treatment and risk of complications in patients with type 2 diabetes (UKPDS 33). *Lancet, 352*, 837–853.

UK Prospective Diabetes Study Group. (1998c). Tight blood pressure control and risk of macrovascular and microvascular complications in type 2 diabetes (UKPDS 38). *British Medical Journal (Clinical Research Ed.), 317*, 703–713.

White, W. B., Cannon, C. P., Heller, S. R., et al. (EXAMINE investigators). (2013). Alogliptin after acute coronary syndrome in patients with type 2 diabetes. *The New England Journal of Medicine, 369*, 1327–1335.

Zinman, B., Wanner, C., Lachin, J. M., et al. (2015). Empagliflozin, cardiovascular outcomes and mortality in type 2 diabetes. *The New England Journal of Medicine, 373*, 2117–2128.

25

Persistent Physical Symptoms and Symptoms Without Apparent Disease

CHRISTOPHER BURTON

CHAPTER CONTENTS

- This chapter considers the common problem of physical symptoms which cannot be fully explained by current conceptualisations of organ disease. This includes persistent physical symptoms which appear disproportionate to evident organic disease processes and clusters of symptoms in syndromes such as fibromyalgia and irritable bowel syndrome.

- These physical symptoms are sometime termed "functional somatic symptoms" (because they are characterised by changes in function rather than structure) or problems of "central sensitisation". The term medically unexplained symptoms is still in common usage but is discouraged: it implies that such symptoms cannot be understood or are in some way different from other symptoms. Neither of these is true. If used at all, the term medically unexplained symptoms (MUS) should be reserved for symptoms of relatively recent onset in which there is no immediately apparent organic cause. Even then it may be better to think of them as "symptoms without apparent disease".

- Symptoms can be understood as having both peripheral and central components. Peripheral components include tissue damage or inflammation and altered function (e.g. smooth muscle spasm). Central components include changes in the way the brain processes sensory information and changes in the way the mind interprets symptoms. While in recent years, attention has focused on the mind's interpretation of symptoms (the cognitive approach), recent research suggests increasing evidence for altered (and pre-conscious) brain processing of body signals.

- This peripheral – central combination is most easily understood through the example of pain. An initial injury can trigger symptoms through peripheral mechanisms (nociceptive pain). However in some patients the pain persists or can spread to affect areas unrelated to the original injury. This occurs through central sensitisation. Many persistent physical symptoms have both peripheral and central processes.

- In some of the functional syndromes such as irritable bowel syndrome it is clear that for a substantial number of patients there are clear peripheral factors - such as dietary intake of FODMAPs (Staudacher & Whelan 2017) and it is likely that additional peripheral features will be identified over time in other syndromes. It may be helpful to think of them as disorders of brain-body communication. It is not appropriate to think of symptoms and syndromes as mental problems just because currently known physical disease has been ruled out.

- Persistent physical symptoms and emotional distress (low mood and anxiety) often co-occur (Henningsen, Zimmerman & Sattel 2003). However it is clear that emotional distress is neither necessary nor sufficient to cause persistent physical symptoms.

- There are many reasons for the interaction between symptoms and emotional distress. Symptoms are inherently distressing and physical symptoms predispose patients to anxiety and depression. In a reciprocal way, susceptibility to anxiety or depression also predisposes patients to develop persistent physical symptoms. Despite the fact that these interactions are common, many patients with symptoms will not have anxiety or depressive disorders.

- Persistent physical symptoms may occur as a single symptoms (e.g. dizziness), as one or more defined syndromes (e.g. tension type headache, fibromyalgia or irritable bowel syndrome) or in a less specific pattern of multiple symptoms, in multiple body systems on multiple occasions. The syndromes are sometimes referred to as Functional Somatic Syndromes. There are a number of classifications of multiple symptoms and systems although none is widely used in general practice. These include Somatic Symptom Disorder in DSM5 (which emphasises the presence of psychological or social features in addition to physical symptoms) and Bodily Distress Disorder which emphasises the diversity of symptoms and body systems involved.

- Table 25.1 lists a range of disorders currently considered broadly within the spectrum of functional somatic syndromes

- Two situations arise in which patients may deliberately present nonorganic symptoms:
  - Malingering, in which symptoms are fabricated for personal gain
  - Factitious disorder, in which the symptoms appear to have no direct gain other than access to health care (formerly known as Munchausen syndrome)

  These two conditions will not be considered here.

Prevalence

- In patients seeing a GP between 15 and 30% will have at least one symptom without apparent disease. Patients with only an occasional consultation for such symptoms have a low risk of the symptoms becoming persistent (Verhaak, Meijer, Visser & Wolters, 2006). However when symptoms have been present for many months, persistence - or the resolution of one symptom but the occurrence of another - is more common.

TABLE 25.1	Common Symptom Disorders by Specialty

Cardiology: chest pain with normal coronary arteries, palpitations

Ear, nose, throat: dizziness, globus pharyngis, functional dysphonia

Gastroenterology: functional dyspepsia, irritable bowel syndrome, proctalgia fugax

Gynaecology: chronic pelvic pain

Maxillofacial: facial pain, temporomandibular joint dysfunction

Musculoskeletal: chronic widespread pain, fibromyalgia

Neurology: nonepileptic attacks, functional weakness, tension-type headache

Respiratory: unexplained breathlessness/hyperventilation

Urology: chronic genital/prostatic pain

Generalized: chronic fatigue syndrome, multiple chemical sensitivity

- Around half of patients referred to specialists because of symptoms turn out to have no organic disease (Nimnuan, Hotopf, & Wessely, 2001). Many meet the criteria for one of the functional somatic syndromes.

- At least 2% of adults have persistent physical symptoms (McGorm, Burton, Weller, Murray & Sharpe 2010). Patients generally seek care in an episodic rather than continuous fashion but often end up with a number of different investigations or specialist referrals as each symptom is taken seriously and appropriately worked up. Most patients with persistent physical symptom are not immediately identified by general practice teams. As a prompt, it may be useful to think of patients presenting multiple symptoms in multiple body systems on multiple occasions.

- A small number of patients (around 2 per thousand) have severely disabling persistent physical symptoms. They are often high users of healthcare and some will be known to every General Practice. They may have had extensive specialist referrals with negative results and may be seen as facing, and presenting, multiple challenges.

- It is important to remember that some symptoms without apparent disease are actually early or subtle symptoms of a disease which becomes apparent over time. Occasionally this includes serious conditions such as cancer. Where a specialist has made an appropriate assessment of symptoms which have been present for several months, this is uncommon (occurring in 1-5% of patients). However with recent symptoms in primary care it may be more common and so GPs should always consider the possibility of organic disease alongside the probability of a functional symptom.

Principles of Management Medically Unexplained Symptoms

- Symptoms without apparent disease are common and when first presented it may be difficult to rule out physical disease. They may occur in isolation, as part of a picture of persistent physical symptoms, or as a feature of a functional somatic syndrome.

- Principles of assessment are broadly similar across the spectrum of severity, although strategies for each severity group will differ. The approach outlined here can be used consistently across different symptoms, although the specific questions, examinations, and investigations will vary by symptom.

Clinical Assessment

History

- Take a careful history, actively listen:
  - Many functional symptoms have characteristic patterns: the unchanging nature of tension-type headache, the bloating and relation to meals of irritable bowel syndrome (IBS). The absence of typical features of functional syndromes should raise concern.

- Sometimes patients will volunteer a symptom which is much more suggestive of pathology, so check for red flags but try to listen first.
- Many patients with new or persistent symptoms will have specific concerns about cause: Active listening encourages patients that disclosing concerns or distress is part of a normal consultation. In contrast, "Do you think stress could be causing this?" is often seen as threatening (Peters et al., 2009) and is best avoided.
- By actively listening and responding to the story, for instance "That must have felt terrible," you convey empathy and give the patient the legitimate opportunity to describe the emotional aspect of his or her symptoms.
- You earn yourself the opportunity to make a judgment or recommendations based on having collected sufficient information—you can demonstrate this by summarising the history back to the patient and ensuring that what he or she has described and you have heard matches up.

Examination

- A new symptom or a change in an old one usually warrants examination.
- Introduce the examination positively: "I would like to properly examine your…" rather than "… take a quick look at… ." The patient has to believe you when you find nothing abnormal.
- Consider anticipating normal findings: "I think this is X, in which case the examination will be normal, but I need to check that." Then when you find nothing, that is no surprise.
- Use the break in the consultation between history and examination to ask the patient if he or she has any ideas or concerns about what might be causing the symptoms. You won't have eye contact so it is a less threatening point in the consultation, and you can specifically direct the examination to areas of concern.
- Talk the patient through key points of your examination, either in advance ("I'm going to check your abdomen for any lumps or swellings") or afterwards ("The backs of your eyes look perfect, I was checking to see if the pressure in your brain is normal, and it is").
- Use tests that indicate functional signs as explanation rather than to prove there's nothing wrong. (If you can identify pain on light touch [allodynia] or increased sensitivity to pain [hyperalgesia] by pinching the skin of the abdominal wall, then demonstrate them as part of the "proof" of your explanation.) Similarly, if you can demonstrate normal movement in one situation and not in another (and you don't think the patient is malingering) then use that to point out that the body can do this, but the brain is sometimes inhibiting it.

Investigation

- Investigations have an important role in patients with new or changing symptoms. Doctors find them reassuring and if anxious patients lead to anxious doctors, it is understandable that we turn to them.

- In making the decision whether to investigate further, the following principles can be useful:
  - Functional symptoms do not cause abnormal results on screening tests—if these occur and are nontrivial, then follow them up with more tests or referral.
  - Normal results of diagnostic tests produce an immediate sense of relief in patients but this is only temporary. Repeated testing and relief may lead to an escalating cycle of reassurance seeking.
  - Patient satisfaction and symptom resolution isn't altered by whether investigations are conducted immediately or deferred.
  - If a plausible (non-pathological) explanation for symptoms is given before the investigation, a negative result is likely to lead to greater reassurance than if it is withheld until after (or not given at all).
  - GPs request more investigations than patients actually want. Sometimes tests are ordered as the only thing one can offer; often patients don't want more tests so much as either a reasonable explanation of what is causing their symptoms (rather than what they don't have) or some understanding of and support for their attempts to cope.

Beware of Overassessing

- It usually doesn't make sense to repeat investigations where nothing much has changed.
- When tests have all been normal and a reasonable specialist opinion (sometimes more than one) has concluded there is no serious cause, it is unlikely that a new one will find the missing problem.
- It is essential to remember that incidental and clinically unimportant findings are common (e.g., unexpected and clinically irrelevant lesions will be found on 5%–10% of cranial MRI scans).

Referral

- Specialists are good at recognizing disease but most have no more skills in managing functional symptoms than their GP colleagues. Multidisciplinary pain services are of value for some patients.
- Specialist teams for managing functional symptoms are currently rare; liaison psychiatry and psychology services may be able to assess and offer cognitive behavioural therapy (CBT) or other psychologic therapies.
- Outcomes for patients with complex persistent physical symptoms who engage in treatment can be good, though not all patients benefit.

Management

- There is no specific medical treatments for persistent physical symptoms so most management is generic and may include explanation, (e.g. low dose tricyclic for chronic pain) selective prescribing, and the use of simple cognitive or behavioural techniques.
- None of these have been formally tested in primary care, but they are in keeping with more general principles of

management and also on recognition that the previously recommended approach of reattribution is unlikely to be beneficial.

Explanation

- Brief interventions in primary care to reattribute physical symptoms to emotional states are unlikely to be effective and are actively resisted by patients (Rosendal et al., 2013).
- Many doctors tell patients what they don't have, but then fail to provide an explanation for what is (or could be) causing their symptoms.
- Studies indicate that effective explanations should make sense to both the patient and doctor, should not convey blame, and should lead to therapeutic action (Dowrick, Ring, Humphris, & Salmon, 2004).
- Explanations may be brief, but also need to be flexible; and explanation for a relatively new symptom can be straightforward, for a simplistic explanation for a symptom that has been going on for a long time may be counterproductive.
- Box 25.1 contains two examples of explanations. Both include a plausible explanation, are blame free, and outline therapeutic action and partnership.
- Neither of these explanations in Box 25.1 include questions about stress, anxiety, or depression. However, if the patient raised them, they could certainly be fit in. If issues or concerns have been handled gently during the consultation, sometimes a plausible positive explanation gives the patient the opportunity to volunteer his or her own concern (for instance, with the dizziness explanation: "That's a relief, and there was me worrying I had a brain tumour") in a lightly self-deprecating fashion.
- Care for patients with persistent physical symptoms includes management of depressive and anxiety disorders where these are identified, but should be as part of a wider formulation.

Specific Syndromes

Several clinical syndromes are currently thought to involve problems with the generation and persistence of symptoms more than primary peripheral pathology. These include fibromyalgia, Irritable Bowel Syndrome and ME/CFS (Myalgic Encephalomyelitis /Chronic Fatigue Syndrome). A fuller list is provided in Table 25.1.

These are increasingly recognised as complex disorders with multiple body and brain processes. In each syndrome the balance of importance of different processes (e.g. inflammatory, endocrine, perceptual) is currently still being resolved – and it is likely that it varies between individuals and subtypes. Classification of these syndromes continues to evolve. In some cases this can become an emotive topic, and it is important to discuss the complex nature of these syndromes with patients (who may otherwise surmise that you think that they are imagining their symptoms or bringing them on by faulty thinking).

> ● **BOX 25.1** **Explanations**

Example 1: Functional Dyspepsia

You keep describing these stomach cramps but the endoscopy was normal. That tells me there is nothing wrong with the structure of your stomach, no disease, or ulcer, or infection.... We often find this, that from time to time the stomach doesn't work properly, it churns around or cramps up, giving the sort of symptoms you describe. This is a problem with the way your stomach functions (called functional dyspepsia) rather than a sign of any disease. Treatment often helps to smooth that function out, but it's important for you to know that even if this functional dyspepsia happens it can't cause you further harm.

Example 2: Dizziness

We have tested your balance and it works fine (this might have included Dix Hallpyke test and a stepping test) but when we did those tests, even though your balance performed normally, your brain told you things weren't okay. This condition is called functional dizziness (or disequilibrium).

What it means is that although your brain is getting the right signals from your inner ears, these signals are then setting off false alarms. False alarms are quite common and normal; sometimes they occur after an episode of illness and sometimes for no good reason at all. Unfortunately, what happens is that the more they bother you, the more your brain looks out for them, and then the more they happen... . What is important here is that you find a way to trust your own balance more (we have seen that it works) and rely on these unsteadiness alarms in your brain less (because they're false alarms).

There are some techniques called vestibular rehabilitation which help and they are available from (... a range of websites or in the United Kingdom from the Meniere's Disease Foundation). I want you to look at these and start practicing them, and I will see you again in 4 weeks to see how you are starting to recover.

GPs can become confident in making these diagnoses, following appropriate diagnostic criteria (see chapter 11 for Fibromyalgia and chapter 9 for IBS). In the case of Chronic Fatigue there are a number of different sets of criteria, however all include persistent and disabling fatigue for more than 6 months. The presence of severe fatigue following effort (for instance on the next day) is seen as particularly important by some groups. Further details about diagnosis and recommendations for treatment are to be found in the NICE Clinical Guideline 53, although GPs should be aware that the guidelines are contested by some patient groups. The current edition of the guideline was published in 2007 and at the time of writing (2019) it is in revision.

References

Dowrick, C. F., Ring, A., Humphris, G. M., & Salmon, P. (2004). *Normalisation of unexplained symptoms by general practitioners: A functional typology.*

Henningsen, P., Zimmermann, T., & Sattel, H. (2003). *Medically unexplained physical symptoms, anxiety, and depression: A meta-analytic review.*

McGorm, K., Burton, C., Weller, D., Murray, G., & Sharpe, M. (2010). *Patients repeatedly referred to secondary care with symptoms unexplained by organic disease: Prevalence, characteristics and referral pattern.*

Nimnuan, C., Hotopf, M., & Wessely, S. (2001). *Medically unexplained symptoms: An epidemiological study in seven specialities.*

Peters, S., Rogers, A., Salmon, P., Gask, L., Dowrick, C., Towey, M., et al. (2009). *What do patients choose to tell their doctors? Qualitative analysis of potential barriers to reattributing medically unexplained symptoms.*

Rosendal, M., Blankenstein, A. H., Fink, P., Sharpe, M., Morriss, R., & Burton, C. (2013). Enhanced care by generalists for functional somatic symptoms and disorders in primary care. *Cochrane Database of Systematic Reviews.* Accepted for Publication.

Staudacher, & Whelan 2017, *The low FODMAP diet: recent advances in understanding its mechanisms and efficacy in IBS.*

Verhaak, P. F., Meijer, S. A., Visser, A. P., & Wolters, G. (2006). *Persistent presentation of medically unexplained symptoms in general practice.*

26

Palliative Care and Care of the Dying Patient

BEN DIETSCH

CHAPTER CONTENTS

Basic Principles

GUIDELINES

Scottish Palliative Care Guidelines. www.palliativecareguidelines.scot.nhs.uk/.

R Twycross, A Wilcock, P Howard. (2017). *Palliative care formulary* (6th ed.). City: Publisher. www.palliativedrugs.com Ltd.

M Watson, C Lucas, A Hoy, I Back. (2009). *Oxford handbook of palliative care*. Cambridge: Oxford University Press.

- Palliative care seeks to optimize the quality of living for those with advanced, incurable life-limiting illness (LLI). As such, the approach addresses physical, psychological, social, and spiritual needs as identified by the patient.
- National Institute for Health and Care Excellence (NICE) defined *end-of-life care* as that provided in the last year of life; but palliative care can encompass a much longer period spent living with life-limiting illness.
- When referring to care of the dying patient, the author has in mind those with a likely prognosis of days to a week.
- Good management and decision making in palliative and end-of-life care require careful assessment of the

presenting problem or symptom, an appreciation of the context of the person's underlying life-limiting illness, an understanding of the person's wishes, and considered communication to draw these strands together.

- Planning for symptom control and end-of-life care needs is crucial to the patient with life-limiting illness.
- The outcome of any discussions and decisions should be recorded clearly and in ways which make it readily accessible to other healthcare professionals that may be involved in the person's care (e.g., on the patient's summary care record).
- Patients with capacity should be fully involved in decisions about treatment and encouraged to consider and document Advance Care Plans (ACP), including:
  - Advance Decisions to Refuse Treatment (ADRT), Do Not Attempt Cardiopulmonary Resuscitation (DNACPR) orders and Treatment Escalation Plans (TEPs);
  - Advance Statements describing what they would ideally like to happen at the end of life (e.g., preferred place of care or death, wishes around hospital admission or care at home);
  - what should happen if they develop an intercurrent illness;
  - who they would want included in any communication or decisions involving their treatment and care, including Lasting Power of Attorney (LPA).
- If or when capacity to make specific decisions is lost, any information recorded in advance will assist best interest decision making.
- Recognizing the context of the presenting problems helps to determine appropriate management options (i.e., what is likely to be successful or not). For instance, some problems may be the natural mode of death: respiratory failure (in the context of advanced motor neurone disease), neutropenic sepsis (in advanced myelosuppression/neutropenia due to extensive bone metastases or refractory haematological malignancy), lower respiratory tract infection (in the context of advanced respiratory disease), anorexia/cachexia (in the context of advanced dementia).

Emergencies

Metastatic Spinal Cord Compression (MSCC) and Cauda Equina Syndrome

> **GUIDELINE**
>
> National Institute for Health and Care Excellence. (2008). *Metastatic spinal cord compression in adults: Risk assessment, diagnosis and management. NICE clinical guideline 75.* www.nice.org.uk/guidance/cg75.

Presenting Features

- Consider metastatic spinal cord and cauda equina Compression (MSCC) in any patient with advanced metastatic malignancy and the following signs and symptoms:

  - Symptoms suggestive of spinal metastases (spinal pain which is severe and unremitting, aggravated by straining, local spinal tenderness, nocturnal spinal pain preventing sleep) AND neurological symptoms including radicular pain, weakness in any limb, difficulty in walking, sensory loss, or bladder or bowel dysfunction.
- Consider cauda equina compression in any patient with advanced malignancy and the following neurological signs and symptoms:
  - Symptoms suggestive of spinal metastases in the lower spine AND low back pain, saddle anaesthesia/paraesthesia, bowel or bladder dysfunction, and weakness in one or both legs.

Management

- *Patients unlikely to benefit from further investigation/treatment.* Circumstances in which further imaging/treatment may not be appropriate include:
  - patients whose spinal metastases have previously been deemed untreatable; or
  - those who are in the last days to week(s) of life (i.e., whose overall clinical condition means they are unsuitable for surgical intervention and not likely to live long enough to benefit from radiotherapy); and/or
  - those who have capacity to refuse investigation.
    a. Patients in these circumstances should not be admitted to hospital.
    b. Management of these patients may include a trial of dexamethasone 16 mg orally (daily dose; usually administered as 8 mg twice daily), provision of adequate analgesia, and provision for care needs and equipment.
- *Patients with potential to benefit from investigation and treatment.* This is anyone not fulfilling the above criteria, including those with established MSCC for whom intervention may be appropriate for pain relief, if not to improve function.
  - Contact the local MSCC coordinator to arrange assessment and further management (surgery or radiotherapy):
    a. immediately (often via acute oncology hospital service) if the patient has neurological signs and symptoms suggestive of MSCC;
    b. urgently (within 24 hours) to discuss the care of patients with cancer and any symptoms suggestive of spinal metastases.
  - In practice, when MSCC is suspected and further imaging desired/appropriate:
    1. then urgent hospital admission for whole spine MRI will be required; and
    2. dexamethasone 16 mg daily PO should be commenced.

Superior Vena Cava Obstruction

Presenting Features

- Patients with known diagnosis of malignancy and lymphadenopathy.

GUIDELINE

Scottish Palliative Care Guidelines. (n.d.). *SVCO*. www.palliativecareguidelines.scot.nhs.uk/guidelines/palliative-emergencies/Superior-Vena-Cava-Obsturction.aspx.

- SVCO is most frequently due to extrinsic compression by carcinoma of the lung, lymphoma, and other cancers or thrombosis formation.
- Signs and symptoms:
  - Breathlessness, headache, dizziness, feeling of fullness in head are common symptoms.
  - Signs include oedema of conjunctivae, face, hands, and/or arm(s); dilated veins in the neck; dilated collateral veins in the arms and chest wall; stridor and cyanosis.
- Onset may be acute (often when due to thrombosis) or chronic.

Management

- Dexamethasone 16 mg daily, orally to reduce peritumour oedema
- Oxygen if available
- Urgent hospital admission: for radiological investigation; definitive management is often anticancer therapy (including radiotherapy/chemotherapy), thrombolysis, or endovascular stent.
- In patients with advanced malignancy, supportive symptomatic management with opioids and benzodiazepines should also be given (see "Symptom Management Guidelines > Respiratory > Breathlessness").
- When hospital admission for further investigation/management is not appropriate or desired, dexamethasone and oxygen can be tried for symptom benefit (as above) and focus should be on pharmacologic management of associated symptoms/distress.

Hypercalcaemia of Malignancy

GUIDELINE

Scottish Palliative Care Guidelines. *Hypercalcaemia*. www.palliativecareguidelines.scot.nhs.uk/guidelines/palliative-emergencies/Hypercalcaemia.aspx.

Presenting Features

- Patients may have known (lytic) bone metastases, but not always.
- Malignancies most often associated with malignant hypercalcaemia are: myeloma, lung, breast, renal, and thyroid.
- Signs and symptoms (often worsen over days):
  - Common: malaise, weakness, nausea, constipation, polyuria
  - Severe: delirium, vomiting, seizure, coma
  - Corrected calcium (adjusted for albumin) often needs to be greater than 3 mmol/L to be symptomatic but

some patients can be symptomatic with a rise of anything above normal.

Management

- Confirm corrected calcium and renal function.
- In the palliative setting where treatment of underlying malignancy is no longer appropriate, intravenous (IV) rehydration and bisphosphonates (most usually pamidronate 90 mg or zoledronic acid 4 mg) are the mainstay of treatment:
  - Pamidronate can be given subcutaneously via hyperdermacolysis (e.g., 90 mg pamidronate in 1 L normal saline over 12 to 24 hours).
- Hypercalcaemia can become refractory to treatment and may be a mode of death. In a moribund patient with other biochemical abnormalities/irreversible pathologies, not treating may be appropriate.

Seizures/Status Epilepticus

GUIDELINE

R Twycross, A Wilcock, P Howard. (2017). *Palliative care formulary* (6th ed.). City: Publisher. www.palliativedrugs.com Ltd.

Presenting Features

- Seizures can result in patients with primary or secondary brain tumour(s): they may be the initial presentation of these pathologies.
- They may also be a consequence of preexisting epilepsy (especially when a person becomes unable to take oral antiepileptic medication), other structural brain lesions (e.g., multiple sclerosis), metabolic abnormalities arising in advanced incurable disease, or alcohol withdrawal.
- Seizures may be of any type but in patients with intracerebral malignancy they are often focal with subsequent secondary generalization.

Management

- *Acute emergency where further hospital management is considered appropriate/desirable.*
  - a. Exclude hypoglycaemia.
  - b. Hospitalization for further investigation may be indicated especially if this is the first seizure from an unknown cause or when seizure becomes prolonged.
  - c. Diazepam 10 mg per rectum or midazolam 10 mg buccal/subcutaneous (SC)/intramuscular (IM) (repeated after 30 minutes if necessary).
- *When hospital admission is not appropriate* (e.g., at end-of-life or terminal event):
  - Control acute seizure
    - a. Diazepam 10 mg per rectum or midazolam 10 mg buccal/SC/IM.
      This can be repeated every 20 to 30 minutes until seizure activity is controlled.
    - b. If ineffective, consider phenobarbital IM, up to 10 mg/kg (seek specialist advice).

- Prevent further seizures—ensure regular antiseizure medication.
  a. Continuous subcutaneous infusion (CSCI) midazolam 20 to 30 mg/24 h. Plus as needed (PRN) midazolam 5 to 10 mg SC/IM 1-hourly. CSCI dose can be titrated every 24 hours according to PRN midazolam use; OR
  b. CSCI phenobarbital 200 mg CSCI/24 h. CSCI dose can be titrated every 24 hours according to PRN use (see below).
- If seizures remain poorly controlled despite 50 mg or more of midazolam CSCI, add phenobarbital 200 mg CSCI/24 h. This can be titrated by 100 mg daily to 400 mg CSCI/24 h.
- Longer term prevention: see "Symptom Management Guidelines > Neurological Symptoms > Seizures."

Opioid Toxicity

GUIDELINE

Electronic Medicines Compendium. www.medicines.org.uk/emc/medicine/21095.

Presenting Features

- Signs and symptoms: Consider opioid toxicity if the patient has experienced:
  - a drug error (e.g., inadvertent dose increase) or rapid escalation of opioid;
  - unexplained drowsiness or deterioration in any patient receiving an opioid;
  - confusion/hallucinations, myoclonic jerks, drowsiness, pinpoint pupils;
  - reduced respiratory rate.
- Important considerations include:
  - management is dictated by level of respiratory depression;
  - full reversal is not always necessary and can precipitate acute withdrawal reaction and pain;
  - normal oxygen saturation does not exclude respiratory depression—reduced respiratory rate occurs first, resulting in raised carbon dioxide levels. Low O_2 saturations (SaO_2) are a late sign;
  - if the drug has been given recently, the patient's condition may continue to deteriorate as the drug is absorbed;
  - naloxone is removed from the body more quickly than many opioids. Repeat doses or hospitalization may be required.

Management

- *Is there imminently life-threatening respiratory depression?*
  Respiratory rate less than 4 breaths/min AND semiconscious or unconscious.
  1. Give full reversal. Naxalone 400 µg (IV: dilute to 4 mL with 0.9% NaCl OR SC: use undiluted).
  2. Repeat every 2 minutes until respiration restored.
  3. Consider transfer to acute hospital, call 999 as assisting ventilation via bag-valve-mask may be required.
  4. If SaO_2 less than 90% give supplemental oxygen and attempt bag-valve-mask ventilation.
  5. If no response to 2 to 4 mg naloxone consider alternative diagnosis (e.g., other sedative, neurologic event, sepsis).
  6. NB buprenorphine will require higher doses.
- *Is there respiratory depression?*
  Respiratory rate less than 8 breaths/min.
  1. Titrate partial reversal. Naloxone 100 µg (IV/SC: dilute to 4 mL with 0.9% NaCl). Give 1 mL (100 µg).
  2. Repeat every 2 minutes until respiration restored to avoid complete reversal of analgesia.
  3. Try other conservative methods to stimulate respiratory rate (i.e., oxygen, bag-valve-mask).
  4. Administer 100 µg (1 mL) every 2 minutes until the patient's respiratory status is satisfactory and sustained above 8.
  5. It is important to titrate against respiratory rate, not level of consciousness, as total antagonism will cause return of severe pain with hyperalgesia and physical withdrawal/agitation.
  6. Further boluses may be necessary if respiratory rate drops below 8 because naloxone is shorter acting than many opioids; consider continuous SC infusion.
  7. If SaO_2 is less than 90% give supplemental oxygen, consider bag-valve-mask.
  8. Consider if transfer to hospital may be appropriate.
- *NO respiratory depression:*
  - Monitor respiratory rate, level of consciousness, oxygen saturation, blood pressure (BP), pulse initially every 15 to 30 minutes.

Haemorrhage (Massive)
Risk Factors

- Tumour adjacent to/invading large blood vessels (e.g., head and neck cancers, bronchogenic carcinoma)
- Disorders of coagulation (e.g., thrombocytopenia, disseminated intravascular coagulation [DIC])
- Sometimes (but not always), the patient will experience warning bleeding (e.g., minor haemoptysis)

Management

- Preparing the patient/family for this possibility is important.
- Midazolam 10 mg PRN should be available to administer in the event of distress caused by massive haemorrhage. This can be given as IM injection as cutaneous circulation will often be reduced.

Irreversible Airway Obstruction/Acute Respiratory Distress
Risk Factors/Causes

- Patients with tumour encasing or involving a large airway (e.g., trachea or bronchus):
  - Tumour may be overgrowing a tracheostomy or causing intrinsic/extrinsic pressure on a large airway such as a thyroid malignancy or bronchial carcinoma.
- Massive pulmonary embolism (PE)

- Advanced respiratory disease (e.g., COPD, pulmonary fibrosis)
- Advanced heart failure
- Motor neurone disease

Management

- High-dose benzodiazepines are often required to manage respiratory and psychological distress (e.g., midazolam 5–10 mg SC/IM).
- Opioids may also be helpful (morphine 2.5–10 mg SC if opioid naïve or an appropriate PRN dose if already taking opioids—see "Symptom Management Guidelines > Respiratory > Breathlessness").
- Both benzodiazepines and opioids may be required CSCI if obstruction happens over the course of hours/days.

Agitation (Terminal Agitation)

Presenting Features

- See also "Symptom Management Guidelines > Neurological Symptoms > Delirium."
- Agitation at the end of life is often a combination of delirium, extreme physiological symptoms, and psychological distress in response to an irreversible problem that is leading to death.
- Terminal agitation is often a diagnosis made in retrospect, but can be heralded by:
  - rapid escalation in physical symptoms which is not responding to management (e.g., intractable pain or breathlessness);
  - rapid escalation in psychological distress;
  - worsening delirium.

Management

- It is crucial to recognize and manage agitation as quickly as possible: sedation may be most appropriate management in this situation.
- The patient and those important to him/her will require support and explanation.
- Sedatives/anxiolytics should be administered PRN as frequently as is necessary until the patient is settled, and continued CSCI.
- Sedative/anxiolytics choice should be titrated in proportion to distress/agitation:
  a. Patient anxious/frightened but lucid:
     - explore fears
     - PRN: lorazepam 0.5 mg PO 4-hourly OR midazolam 2.5 to 5 mg half-hourly SC
  b. Patient has continuous/worsening anxiety:
     - Regular: diazepam 2 mg twice daily (titrated to 5 mg twice daily) OR midazolam 10 mg CSCI/24 h
     - Increase midazolam CSCI in steps of 30% to 50% (up to 100 mg); continue midazolam PRN
  c. Patient confused/agitated/hallucinating:
     - PRN and regular: haloperidol 2.5 mg SC stat + 5 mg CSCI/24 h + haloperidol PRN
  d. If worsening confusion/agitation:
     - Increase haloperidol to 10 mg CSCI/24 h + haloperidol PRN
     - Consider adding midazolam, as above

e. If agitation/distress persist despite the above:
   - PRN: levomepromazine 12.5 to 25 mg 4-hourly PRN SC
   - Regular: switch CSCI to a combination of levomepromazine (25–150 mg CSCI) and midazolam (20–100 mg CSCI)
f. If above ineffective, seek specialist advice.

Symptom Management Guidelines

Pain—General Considerations

GUIDELINES

National Institute for Health and Care Excellence. (n.d.). *Opioids for pain relief in palliative care. NICE pathways.* https://pathways.nice.org.uk/pathways/opioids-for-pain-relief-in-palliative-care.
    British Pain Society. For various professional and patient information/guidelines and pain scale, see www.britishpainsociety.org/british-pain-society-publications/patient-publications/.
World Health Organisation. (n.d.). *WHO's cancer pain ladder for adults.* www.who.int/cancer/palliative/painladder/en/
    Medications and Healthcare Products Regulatory Agency. (2009). *Off label or unlicensed use of medication: Prescribers' responsibilities.* www.gov.uk/drug-safety-update/off-label-or-unlicensed-use-of-medicines-prescribers-responsibilities.

Assessment of Pain

- Pain is a common problem in advanced Life Limiting Illness (LLI): Its presence should be identified and its management reviewed regularly.
- Pain may be due to:
  - underlying LLI;
  - treatment for disease (e.g., radiotherapy);
  - comorbidities and debility (e.g., arthritis, ulcers).
- Various means of scoring pain are available. Patients able to communicate can often provide a vivid description and rating using a visual analogue scale.
- For those unable to articulate or verbalize (e.g., in severe learning disability or advanced dementia), other pain scales are helpful such as the Abbey Pain Scale.
- Breakthrough and incident pain:
  - Breakthrough pain is a spontaneous and unpredictable increase in pain in a patient whose background pain is otherwise well controlled.
  - Incident pain is an increase in pain associated with an identifiable trigger such as movement.

Management—General Principles

- Consideration of the underlying aetiology (e.g., nociceptive, neuropathic, mixed, acute/chronic) will guide initial management. Start at the lowest effective analgesic dose and titrate gradually.
- In addition to pains caused directly by the LLI, pain may be functional or due to concurrent problems. As such, approaches other than those used palliatively may be required.

- The most appropriate analgesia should be given:
  - regularly, at the right dose, by the right route, at the right time/frequency; and
  - a suitable analgesic should be available PRN to treat breakthrough or incident pain.
- The World Health Organisation's pain ladder has been used for many years to guide management of cancer pain.
- If the nature of the pain is unclear, try simple analgesia and non-pharmacological approaches before moving on to opioids and adjuvant analgesia.
- Consider patient ability to take and self-administer medication. Various preparations of analgesia are available to enable administration by mouth, TD patch, enteral tube, or CSCI.
- Review the efficacy of analgesia frequently (daily if necessary) and consider giving patients scope to escalate their own analgesia. If analgesia proves ineffective after escalation or has burdensome side effects, be prepared to stop it.
- Consider underlying causes which might be treatable:
  - Management of constipation or urinary retention
  - Spinal metastases/impending metastatic spinal cord compression
  - Painful bone metastases that may respond to radiotherapy
  - Surgical fixation of pathologic fractures
  - Infection around tumour (often increases pain in head and neck tumours)
- If the source of pain has been managed/treated, be prepared to reduce analgesia (e.g. metastasis treated with palliative radiotherapy).
- See sections on end-stage neurological disease, renal and heart failure for specific guidance on analgesia in these contexts.

Use of Medications Off Label

- In palliative care, many medications are used off label (i.e., outside the terms of the license/marketing authorization, such as amitriptyline for neuropathic pain).
- This should be explained to patients when starting these medications.

Opioid Side Effects

- When starting a regular opioid, anticipate common side effects such as constipation, dry mouth, drowsiness/sedation, and nausea.
- Consider starting:
  - a regular laxative (docusate sodium 100–200 mg twice daily +/– senna 7.5 mg at night);
  - an antiemetic (haloperidol 1 mg at night/cyclizine 50 mg three times daily). This may only be required for a week or so, and can then be stopped.
- Explain to patient that tolerance to any drowsiness/sedation normally develops.
- To combat dry mouth, ensure good oral hygiene, encourage sips of fluid to keep mouth moist, and/or use saliva replacements.

Tolerance, Dependence, Addiction in Patients Taking Opioids

- Increasing pain in patients with LLI is often due to disease progression; however, there is increasing recognition of tolerance, dependence, and even addiction.
- This may be due to the ongoing use of opioids in patients with increasing life expectancy made possible by newer palliative therapies in oncology, for example.
- Consider potential for these problems in patients with LLI but prognosis of months to years.
- Tolerance (requiring increasing doses of analgesia to achieve the same reduction in pain) may respond to switching between opioids; for example, switch from morphine to oxycodone.
- Dependence is seen in patients taking long-term opioids, but is rarely a problem so long as they have sufficient prescribed medication.
- Addiction is rare, but may be preexisting: if so, it deserves consideration when making prescribing arrangements for strong opioids (and other addictive medication). It may lead to tolerance of opioids.

Patient Information

- Provide information to patients when starting strong opioids, including information on potential side effects and who to speak with for further advice.
- Ensure they are confident with how/when/why to take their analgesia, dosing, what they should take regularly, and when required (PRN). Local palliative care services will often have patient information leaflets, or these can be found online.

Legal Implications—Drugs and Driving, Travel Abroad

Drugs and Driving

- Patients driving while taking strong medication should be made aware that:
  - side effects from prescribed medications may affect their ability to drive;
  - ultimately, patients themselves are responsible for making the assessment on their ability to drive safely: they should not drive if they feel there may be any impairment in their ability to do so;
  - the law on drugs and driving (see www.gov.uk/drug-driving-law) states that it is illegal to drive if either:
    a. you're unfit to do so because you're on legal or illegal drugs; OR
    b. you have certain levels of illegal drugs in your blood (even if they haven't affected your driving).

    For this second point, there is a statutory "medical defence" to protect those patients who may test positive for certain specified drugs taken in accordance with the advice of a healthcare professional. They must also be fit to drive when taking these medications. It may therefore be helpful for patients to keep some suitable documentation with them when they are driving that provides evidence that they are taking the controlled drug as a medicine prescribed or supplied by a healthcare professional.

Travelling Abroad

- When travelling abroad, patients taking prescribed medications (in particular controlled drugs) will need to consider any laws governing their use, import, and export in the country from which they are leaving and any country(ies) to/through which they are travelling.
- The UK Home Office recommends patients carry a covering letter from their doctor/prescriber as supporting evidence that the medication they are carrying was prescribed for their use. This is sufficient for up to a 3-month supply of Schedule 2, 3, or 4 (parts I & II) controlled drugs for personal use. It will also permit them to take more than 100 mL of liquid medication and essential medical equipment in their hand luggage. The letter should state:
  - patient name, date of birth, and address;
  - the intended destination(s) and dates of outward/return travel;
  - names, forms, doses, strengths, and total amounts of medications being carried.
- Medication should be kept in original packaging.
- If travelling for 3 months or more and carrying 3 months or more of Schedule 2, 3, or 4 controlled drugs for personal use into/out of the United Kingdom, a personal import/export license is required (available at gov.uk).
- The requirements for prescriptions and controlled drug import/export for all countries in which the patient will pass through customs must also be fulfilled. Patients should be advised to check requirements with the relevant embassies or consulates and customs procedures before travelling.

Pain—Nociceptive

> ### GUIDELINES
>
> National Institute for Health and Care Excellence. (n.d.). *NICE pathways: Opioids for pain relief in palliative care.* https://pathways.nice.org.uk/pathways/opioids-for-pain-relief-in-palliative-care.
> World Health Organization. (n.d.). *WHO's cancer pain ladder.* www.who.int/cancer/palliative/painladder/en/.

Presenting Features

- Nociceptive pain is associated with tissue damage. It is often well localized and described as sharp or dull in nature. Synonyms include *physiological* or *inflammatory pain.*
- It will normally correlate with an area of known physical injury or disease.

Management—Nonopioids

- Simple analgesia such as paracetamol and nonsteroidal antiinflammatory drugs (NSAIDs) can be effective.
- When using NSAIDs:
  - chose those with fewest side effects and consider gastric protection in the form of a proton pump inhibitor

(PPI) or ranitidine (see notes on NSAIDs in renal and cardiac disease).
- Naproxen 250 to 500 mg PO twice daily is often the NSAID of first choice.
- Topical NSAIDs are proven to be effective in gel formulation.

Management—Opioids

- Opioids remain the mainstay of managing acute nociceptive pain in patients with life-limiting illness.
- Strong opioids in small doses are often preferred to weak opioids, as they come in various preparations; dosing is flexible; they provide scope for titration without having to switch opioid; they may have fewer side effects.
- When using opioids, as with any analgesia, consider:
  - *right analgesia:* Most people tolerate morphine so it is appropriate to begin with this;
  - *right dose:* Start with lowest possible dose in an opioid-naïve individual;
  - *route:* If possible, begin with oral opioid to allow more accurate dose titration. If oral route unavailable, consider low-dose TD or CSCI;
  - *right frequency:* Oral opioids are prescribed on a regular basis, with additional PRN dose available for breakthrough pain;
  - *review:* Be prepared to increase dose if analgesia is suboptimal or stop if no benefit.
- Anticipate common side effects (see previous discussion).
- When possible, use only one opioid at a time; there is no benefit in combining weak and strong opioids or two strong opioids.
- When given by injection, subcutaneous (SC) is preferred to intramuscular (IM) or intravenous (IV).
- Prescribers should be aware of the potential for *opioid-induced hyperalgesia.* This manifests where (often rapid) opioid escalation leads to increasing pain which is often more diffuse and less well defined than the presenting pain. Patients will exhibit hypersensitivity in the form of hyperalgesia and/or allodynia. Management requires reduction in opioid dose or switching to an alternative (and reduction in equivalent dose).
- See Appendix 33 for comparative doses of different opioids.
- The following opioids are used most often:
  - Codeine
    - a. Most often used for moderate pain, often in combination formulation with paracetamol.
    - b. Starting dose: 30 mg four times daily to 60 mg four times daily.
    - c. Maximum dose 240 mg daily is equivalent to approximately 20 mg oral morphine in 24 hours.
  - Tramadol
    - a. Use for moderate to severe pain.
    - b. Has additional nonopioid analgesic effects.
    - c. Starting dose: 50 to 100 mg four times daily.
    - d. Maximum dose 400 mg daily is equivalent to approximately 40 to 80 mg oral morphine in 24 hours.

- Morphine
  a. First choice strong opioid for moderate or severe pain.
  b. Preparations include immediate release (tablets, oral solution, injection) and modified release (tablets, capsules, granules - normally 12-hourly modified release) formulations.
  c. Can be given CSCI when patients are unable to swallow. Morphine PO:SC potency ratio is 1:2, so starting dose CSCI should be half the total 24-hour oral morphine dose.
  d. PRN oral dose for breakthrough pain should be 1/6 of the 24-hour oral dose; PRN dose for SC injection should be 1/6 of the total 24-hour CSCI dose. PRN dose is normally prescribed 4-hourly.
  e. Starting dose:
     1. Opioid naïve patient: morphine immediate release 2.5 to 5 mg PO 4-hourly regularly and PRN, OR morphine 12-hourly modified release 10 mg twice daily plus morphine immediate release 2.5 to 5 mg PO 4-hourly PRN
     2. Patient on weak opioid (e.g., codeine 240 mg daily): morphine immediate release 5 mg 4-hourly and PRN, OR morphine 12-hourly modified release 10 mg twice daily plus 5 mg immediate release PO 4-hourly PRN
  f. Titration: Aim to establish lowest effective regular (modified release dose) as soon as possible to provide even analgesia over 24 hours.
     1. Ask patient to complete daily record of all morphine used.
     2. After 2 to 3 days calculate average daily (24-hour) total morphine dose required.
     3. Divided total 24-hour dose by 2 and give this as a twice daily 12-hourly modified-release preparation.
     4. Provide PO PRN dose for breakthrough pain, equivalent to 1/6 of the oral 24-hour dose.
        For example, patient uses 6 × 5 mg immediate release morphine doses in 24 hours. Total 24 hours oral morphine dose = 30 mg.
        12-hourly modified-release morphine dose = 15 mg twice daily.
        Oral PRN dose = 5 mg immediate release morphine PO 4-hourly.
        For example, patient taking 30-mg modified-release morphine twice daily. In addition, uses four 10-mg PRN doses every day for a week. Total 24-hour oral morphine dose = 30 mg + 30 mg + 40 mg = 100 mg.
        Increase 12-hourly modified-release morphine to 50 mg twice daily.
        Increase oral PRN dose to 15 mg immediate release morphine PO 4-hourly.
- Oxycodone
  a. Indications:
     1. Useful for moderate to severe pain.
     2. Used if morphine is contraindicated or not tolerated.
     3. Most often used second line for patients taking morphine who experience opioid neurotoxicity and suboptimal analgesia.
  b. PRN oral dose for breakthrough pain should be 1/6 of the 24-hour oral dose; PRN dose for SC injection should be 1/6 of the total 24-hour CSCI dose.
  c. Starting dose:
     1. Estimates of potencies vary, but safe to consider it twice as potent as morphine (i.e., oral morphine to oral oxycodone potency ratio is 1:2.)
     2. Based on this, it is usual practice to halve the previous morphine dose when switching to oxycodone. e.g. morphine PO 30 mg in 24 hrs = oxycodone PO 15 mg in 24 hrs.
     3. If oxycodone is the first opioid used, start with 1 to 2 mg 4-hourly and PRN PO.
  d. Titration:
     1. Use same principle as for morphine.
  e. As with morphine, it comes in a variety of formulations and oxycodone PO:SC potency ratio is approximately 1:2.
- Diamorphine
  a. Indications:
     1. Useful for moderate to severe pain if SC/CSCI administration is required.
  b. Available as powder for solution for injection in ampoules—it can be reconstituted to the desired volume. This is helpful in minimizing volume of SC injections (or CSCI infusion) for patients requiring large doses of opioid.
  c. Oral morphine: SC diamorphine potency ratio is 1:3. E.g., morphine 30 mg PO in 24 hrs = diamorphine 10 mg CSCI/24 h
  d. Diamorphine PRN dose (SC) should be 1/6 of the total daily diamorphine CSCI dose.
- Fentanyl (TD patch)
  a. Indicated for chronic pain management in:
     1. patients who are unable to swallow or prefer not to take oral medications;
     2. patients experiencing intolerable side effects from morphine (especially constipation, nausea/vomiting, hallucinations);
     3. situations where there is risk of tablet diversion/misuse;
     4. situations where it is safer, in severe renal impairment/failure (glomerular filtration rate [GFR] <30%).
  b. For patients with prognosis of months (due to time required for titration).
  c. Considered less constipating than morphine or oxycodone—reduce laxative dose if switching from these opioids.
  d. TD dose is expressed in micrograms per hour. Smallest dose is 12 µg/h. This is equivalent to at least 30 mg oral morphine in 24 hours.
  e. Equivalences to morphine/potencies vary, but Appendix 33 draws on several sources when estimating

equivalence. TD absorption may be influenced by skin temperature, circulation, and patch adherence.

f. Starting dose:
1. Should not be used on opioid naïve patients given strength of dose.
2. Often more practical to titrate patient on alternative PO/CSCI strong opioid first, and when satisfactory analgesia achieved, to convert this to equivalent fentanyl TD patch.
3. NB: When switching patient from morphine or oxycodone to fentanyl, a temporary partial opioid withdrawal reaction can occur as fentanyl is predominantly centrally acting: Gastric flulike signs of opioid withdrawal can occur (e.g., shivering, sweating, diarrhoea). These can be managed by giving a PRN dose of the previous opioid.

g. Titration:
1. Patches are reapplied to a fresh site every 3 days and may take 3 days or so to reach steady-state plasma concentrations and maximum therapeutic benefit.
2. Morphine or oxycodone PRN should be prescribed for breakthrough pain if the patient does not have severe renal failure.
3. If three or more PRN doses of breakthrough opioid analgesia are required every day, the strength of the next patch applied can be increased by between 12 and 25 μg/h.
4. Increase TD patch no more often than every 3 days (preferably weekly), giving patch time to reach maximum therapeutic benefit between increases. It is therefore unsuitable for acute pain requiring rapid titration of analgesia.

- Buprenorphine (transdermal patch)
a. Indications:
Patch helpful in same patient groups as fentanyl.
b. Given partial agonist and antagonist action of buprenorphine on opioid receptors, there may be less tendency toward tolerance.
c. Reports of potency compared to other strong opioids vary: The Appendix 33 has a cautious conversion, considering fentanyl TD 1.4 times more potent than buprenorphine TD.
d. Available in lower strength doses than fentanyl transdermal patches, so more scope for titration. Patch strengths of 5, 10, 15, or 20 μg/h are available as 7-day patches; 33, 52.5, and 70 μg/h patches can be changed every 3 to 4 days.
e. Starting dose:
1. Opioid naïve patient: start at lowest dose (i.e., 5 μg/h), changed every 7 days.
2. Switching from another strong opioid:
Use cautious conversion ratio based on current opioid dose (see Appendix 32).
Switching from another strong opioid to transdermal buprenorphine may cause opioid withdrawal (gastric flulike symptoms), which can be managed by PRN doses of the previous opioid.

f. Morphine and other mu-receptor agonists at an appropriate dose (buprenorphine TD 5 μg/h is equivalent to approximately 12 mg morphine PO in 24 hours) may be used for breakthrough pain.
g. Titration:
1. If over a period of several days, three or more PRN doses of breakthrough opioid analgesia are being used daily, increase buprenorphine TD patch strength.
2. Increase TD patch dose weekly—this makes it unsuitable for acute pain where rapid titration is necessary.

- Other opioids are encountered less frequently.
  - Fentanyl (immediate release transmucosal)
  a. Indications:
  1. Various preparations of transmucosal fentanyl are now available, including sublingual and buccal tablets, lozenge, and nasal spray.
  2. Transmucosal fentanyl products are designed to provide rapid onset pain relief for a short duration which better fits the profile of breakthrough pain or incident pain.
  b. It is thought best practice to use PO strong opioids first line for breakthrough pain and then switch to transmucosal fentanyl only if the patient experiences prolonged undesirable effects or onset of action is too slow.
  c. Immediate release fentanyl should be prescribed on the recommendation of a specialist in palliative care or MDT. Starting dose/titration:
  1. The manufacturers of the various products publish guidelines on their use and titration.
  2. They should not be used in opioid naïve patients or acute noncancer pain.

  - Fentanyl (SC/CSCI)
  a. Indications:
  1. Pain in severe/end-stage renal failure eGFR less than 30 mL/min
  2. When rapid titration of analgesia is required (often at end of life)
  b. Starting dose:
  1. Opioid naïve: 12.5 to 25 μg 1-hourly PRN SC; 100 μg CSCI/24 h.
  2. Switching from other opioids: see Appendix 33. (Fentanyl is considered approximately 100 times more potent than morphine.)
  c. Titration:
  1. On established fentanyl CSCI dose: use PRN SC dose (1-hourly) equivalent to 1/8 to 1/10 of fentanyl 24-hour CSCI dose.
  2. As with other strong opioids CSCI, if three or more PRN doses are required in 24 h, increase CSCI by the equivalent amount:
  For example, fentanyl 100 μg CSCI/24 h background analgesia plus 4 × 12.5 μg SC PRN in 24 hours: increase CSCI fentanyl to 150 μg CSCI/24 h.

- Alfentanil (SC/CSCI)
  a. Indications:
    1. Pain in severe/end-stage renal failure eGFR less than 30 mL/min
    2. Where morphine neurotoxicity develops
    3. Where volume required prevents use of fentanyl
    4. Note: Alfentanil's duration of action is too short to be useful as a SC PRN analgesic. Use fentanyl for PRN dosing.
  b. Starting dose:
    1. Switching from other opioids: see Appendix 33 (Alfentanil is considered approximately 30 times more potent than oral morphine.)
    2. SC PRN dose of alternative opioid should be available (author recommends fentanyl).
  c. Titration:
    1. As with other strong opioids CSCI, if three or more PRN doses are required in 24 hours, increase CSCI by the equivalent amount.
- Methadone
  a. Methadone is an opioid with mixed properties including mu-opioid receptor agonist and NMDA receptor channel blocker.
  b. It has a highly variable plasma half-life and should only be used under specialist supervision for analgesia.
  c. Indications:
    1. In palliative care, it is most often used when pain fails to respond to more conventional analgesia (i.e., regular opioids and nonopioids) and adjuvant (e.g., severe, mixed nociceptive/neuropathic pain).
    2. It can be used in end-stage renal failure.
  d. Starting dose:
    1. Switching from other opioids: This process is complicated, usually requiring supervision in a hospice inpatient unit.
    2. Ultimately, a regular dose is often administered twice daily.
  e. Titration:
    1. PRN dose is most often 1/6 to 1/10 of the total 24-hour oral methadone dose. This should be given no more frequently than every 3 hours (unlike other opioids).
    2. Patients requiring additional analgesia within 3 hours of a methadone dose may be prescribed the following PRN: nonopioid or previous opioid PRN (at half the previous dose).
    3. Increases in regular dose should be undertaken no more frequently than once a week, due to the accumulation of methadone.

Pain—Neuropathic

Presenting Features

- Neuropathic pain results from a lesion/disease of the sensory nervous system.
- Its character is often described as burning, shooting, pins and needles, or numbness and is usually poorly localized

(although it may be associated with a particular sensory dermatomal distribution).
- Abnormal sensation in the region of a pain is often a good indicator of neuropathic aetiology.
- If it becomes chronic, indicators of chronic regional pain syndrome may develop (e.g., autonomic features with changes in skin/hair/nails, oedema, and motor function).

Management

- Opioids and NSAIDs may sometimes be effective at managing neuropathic pain but specific neuropathic analgesics are often required. These are a diverse group, including:
  - antidepressants;
  - antiepileptics;
  - anaesthetics (local: lidocaine; systemic: ketamine).
- Indications for neuropathic analgesia:
  - Monotherapy for neuropathic pain alone, OR
  - Neuropathic pain unresponsive to opioid plus NSAID
- Choice:
  - The most commonly used for long-term management are amitriptyline, duloxetine, gabapentin, and pregabalin.
  - Both antidepressants and antiepileptics have been shown to have similar tolerability and efficacy in neuropathic pain.
  - Carbamazepine is normally used only for trigeminal neuralgia.
  - Others such as nortriptyline, sodium valproate, and ketamine are usually started by a specialist.
  - Steroids (dexamethasone 8 mg) can be used short term (maximum 2 weeks) for pain due to nerve compression, while waiting for neuropathic analgesia or definitive treatment (e.g., radiotherapy) to have an effect.
  - It is usual practice to start with either an antidepressant or antiepileptic:
    a. If initial drug poorly tolerated/ineffective, switch to a drug from the other category.
    b. If no benefit, try combination of antidepressant and antiepileptic.
- Commonly used neuropathic analgesics:
  - *Amitriptyline* (tricyclic antidepressant—serotonin and norepinephrine reuptake inhibitor [SNRI])
    a. Its sedative side effect can be useful in patients whose pain causes difficulty sleeping.
    b. Benefit in neuropathic pain often seen in subantidepressant doses.
    c. Starting dose: 10 mg PO at night.
    d. Titration: Can be increased weekly, often done stepwise from 10 to 25 mg then by 25 mg weekly if required. Maximum dose 150 mg.

- *Duloxetine* (SNRI)
  a. Similar efficacy and side effect profile to amitriptyline
  b. Starting dose: 30 mg daily
  c. Titration: Increase after 1 week to 60 mg. Can be increased by further 30 mg weekly. Maximum dose 120 mg.
- *Gabapentin*
  a. Generally preferred over pregabalin.
  b. Starting dose: typically 300 mg daily (100 mg three times daily or 300 mg once daily). Requires dose reduction in renal failure.
  c. Titration: Increase by 300 mg daily every 3 to 7 days. Benefit usually experienced by 600 mg three times daily, but maximum recommended dose is 1200 mg three times daily.
- *Pregabalin*
  a. Advantage over gabapentin is twice daily dosing (rather than three times), but no significant analgesic benefit.
  b. Starting dose: 75 mg twice daily; requires dose reduction in renal failure.
  c. Titration: Increase weekly by 150 mg daily in divided doses (i.e., to 150 mg twice daily then 225 mg twice daily, if required). Maximum dose 300 mg twice daily.
- Other neuropathic analgesics (used under specialist guidance)
  - *Steroids*
    a. May be helpful as a short course in managing pain due to metastatic spinal cord compression or nerve root compression while definitive treatment awaited or to manage pain flare following radiotherapy or where no radiotherapy/surgery is possible.
  - *Nortriptyline* (NRI)
    a. Alternative to amitriptyline
  - *Ketamine*
    a. NMDA-receptor channel blocker
    b. Used in neuropathic pain unresponsive to other measures
    c. Potential for urinary tract, hepatobiliary, and neuropsychiatric side effects, so most often given as a short course
    d. May be given as CSCI (100–500 mg CSCI/24 h) or regular oral dose (10–100 mg four times daily).
  - *Methadone*
    a. May be used in complex mixed neuropathic/nociceptive pain (see Pain - Nociceptive > Management - Opioids earlier).
  - *Lidocaine plasters*
    a. Increasingly used to treat localized neuropathic pain, but data on efficacy are poor. Mechanism of effect is unclear and may owe a significant part to placebo.
    b. Consider only if other neuropathic analgesics have failed or are contradicted.
    c. If used, benefit over a 2-week period should be assessed and plasters stopped if no benefit seen.

Pain—Other Types
Malignant Bone Pain

- *Presenting Features*
  - Pain is well localized to bony skeleton in region of known metastatic disease.
- *Management*
  - Radiotherapy: appropriate in patient with prognosis of months as benefit can take 2 to 3 months. Pain flare may occur shortly after treatment and will require additional analgesia. Analgesics may need to be reduced if successful pain relief is achieved by radiotherapy.
  - Intravenous bisphosphonates have a role in treating painful metastatic disease.
  - Surgery: for painful osteolytic metastases at risk of fracture (or following pathological fracture) in patient fit enough to undergo surgical intervention.
  - Analgesia:
    a. NSAIDs and strong opioids are most commonly used (see earlier).
    b. Steroids may provide short-term relief while titrating other analgesia but should not be used for more than 2 weeks.

Smooth Muscle Spasm

- *Presenting features*
  - Spasmodic pain in oesophagus, bowel (including rectum), or bladder
- *Management*
  - Oesophageal spasm: nitrates (glycerol trinitrate [GTN]) or nifedipine 5 mg three times daily PO (titrated to 20 mg TDS);
  - Bowel spasm: hyoscine butylbromide 20 mg PO/SC 4-hourly PRN or QDS
  - Bladder spasm: oxybutynin 5 mg PO twice daily (titrated to 5 mg PO QDS)

Skeletal Muscle Spasm

- *Presenting Features*
  - Painful chronic spasm associated with nerve injury in advanced neurologic disease or malignancy
- *Management (see also "Advanced Neurological Diseases")*
  - Baclofen, tizanidine, dantrolene, and diazepam all have similar efficacy. Start with baclofen and use diazepam only if short course (<1 month).
    a. *Baclofen:* starting dose of 5 mg can be given once, twice or three times daily (maximum starting dose 5 mg three times daily). Titration: increase daily dose by 5 mg to 15 g (in divided doses) every week to maximum 100 mg daily. Withdraw slowly over 2 weeks if discontinuing.
    b. *Tizanidine:* staring dose 2 mg once daily. Titration: increase by 2 mg every 4 days (divided doses). Maximum dose 9 mg four times a day.
    c. *Dantrolene:* starting dose 25 mg once daily. Titration: increase daily dose by 25 mg once a week and give as divided doses. Maximum 100 mg four times a day. Monitor liver function (LFTs).

d. *Diazepam:* dose 2 to 5 mg at night and PRN for maximum 4 weeks.

Tenesmus

- *Presenting Features*
  - Painful sensation of rectal fullness, often due to local tumour.
- *Management*
  - Manage aggravating factors such as constipation.
  - Use NSAIDs, amitriptyline, nifedipine, or antiepileptics (doses as detailed earlier: see Pain - neuropathic and Pain - other types > smooth muscle spasm).

Pain—Total Pain

> **GUIDELINE**
>
> Twycross, R. (2003). *Introducing palliative care* (4th ed.). London: Radcliffe Medical Press.

Definition

- Total pain is the concept that pain includes many contributing factors, notably:
  - biological: disease, treatment, comorbidities, fatigue;
  - psychological: anxiety/depression, fear, experiences, change in body image;
  - social: loss of role, job, change in relationships, isolation;
  - spiritual: faith, loss, search for meaning, fear of unknown.

Presenting Features

- Patients will often identify the factors that contribute to the pain (but not always and may need help exploring these).
- Pain resistant to management with analgesics often has a total component.
- It may manifest as overwhelming pain and/or be disproportionate to the degree of pain expected from known disease.

Management

- Consider holistic, individualized approaches to the management of pain (i.e., choose management options addressing the contributing factors as identified by the patient):
  - Analgesics as for nociceptive/neuropathic pain. But be prepared to reduce/stop analgesics if no benefit experienced.
  - Helping the patient achieve sleep at night can be a particularly helpful initial step.
  - Other approaches: physiotherapy, transcutaneous electrical nerve stimulation (TENS), complimentary therapies, counselling, management of anxiety/depression, addressing social issues, distraction, relaxation.

Pain—Nonpharmacologic Interventions

- Consider nonpharmacologic interventions where possible or when patients are reluctant to try analgesia.

Options

- Radiotherapy for painful metastases
- Splints for fractured bones or braces for spinal stabilization
- TENS: useful for localized neuropathic pain
- Physiotherapy: especially useful for pain associated with immobility or muscle spasm/contractures
- Complimentary therapies: evidence for these is inconsistent, but they may well address components of total pain (see earlier); for example: acupuncture, reflexology, aromatherapy, art and music therapies.

Pain—Interventional Techniques

Presenting Features

- Pain resistant to systemic analgesia or where effectiveness of analgesia limited by side effects.
- Pain limited to one region or clear source (e.g., compression of specific nerve[s] by malignant tumour).

Management

- Consider referring patients for specialist advice if any of the following techniques may be helpful:
  - *Cordotomy:* for pain in one side (hemithorax), such as that caused by mesothelioma.
  - *Neurolysis:* indicated in patients with limited prognosis when pain fails to respond to other measures and a clear cause/pathway is evident. Effectiveness and tolerability are assessed with local anaesthetic before proceeding to neurolytic block. Regions that can be targeted include coeliac plexus (often implicated in pancreatic/upper GI pain); superior hypogastric (pelvic pain); ganglion of Impar (perineal pain).
  - *Neuraxial (intrathecal and epidural):* Indications include intolerable neuropathic pain especially with sympathetically mediated component. When systemic analgesia is ineffective or limited by side effects. The challenge with this technique is provision of ongoing specialist monitoring and management in the community as this needs to be undertaken by experienced specialist teams.

Respiratory

> **PATIENT RESOURCES**
>
> Breathlessness Intervention Service, Cambridge University Hospitals. www.cuh.nhs.uk/breathlessness-intervention-service-bis/resources/patient-information-leaflets.

Breathlessness

- Breathlessness is a very common symptom in palliative care—in patients with malignant, respiratory, and neurological disease.

- Consider if there is a potentially reversible problem with an appropriate treatment acceptable to the patient (Table 26.1). As with all decisions in palliative care, consider options for management in the context of the life-limiting illness and disease trajectory.
- Where the underlying cause of dyspnoea cannot be treated or when patient wishes, prognosis, or performance status make it inappropriate to do so, management should be aimed at palliating symptoms.
- Mainstays of management are nonpharmacological therapies, opioids, and benzodiazepines. Anxiolytic antidepressants may also have a role in patients who have sufficient prognosis to benefit.
- Choice of palliative management option will depend largely on estimated prognosis: Breathlessness in patients expected to live months-years should use predominantly non-harmacological therapies initially, while severe breathlessness in patients with days-weeks will likely rely more on opioids and benzodiazepines (Fig. 26.1).
- Local palliative care centres may have specific breathlessness clinics.
- Management options include:
  a. *Education*
    - Improving patient understanding of the physiology of breathing/breathlessness and providing techniques to optimize breathing can be very helpful. A useful resource is the Breathing, Thinking, Functioning (BTF) approach designed at Cambridge University Hospitals Breathlessness Intervention Service.
    - Focus on improving breathing technique, using positions to ease breathlessness, changing thought

TABLE 26.1 Potentially Reversible Causes of Dyspnoea and Management Options

Cause	Potential Management
Large airway obstruction	Stent, laser/cryotherapy
Small airway obstruction	Optimize bronchodilator dose and delivery: salbutamol and ipratropium nebulizer, oral corticosteroids
Pulmonary embolus	Anticoagulation: low-molecular-weight heparins
Pulmonary oedema	Diuretics
Pulmonary fibrosis	Optimize treatment, oral corticosteroids
Pleural effusion	Pleural drain (temporary or indwelling PleurX drain), pleurodesis
Ascites	Paracentesis
Pain (in chest wall/pleura or elsewhere)	Analgesia
Infection	Antibiotics
Radiation pneumonitis (consequent to radiotherapy)	Dexamethasone (8 mg daily)
Anaemia	Blood transfusion
Anxiety	Beta blocker/lorazepam
Acute Type 2 respiratory failure (in acute exacerbation of COPD)	Non-Invasive Ventilation (NIV) if decompensated respiratory acidosis
Superior vena cava obstruction	Radiotherapy, stent

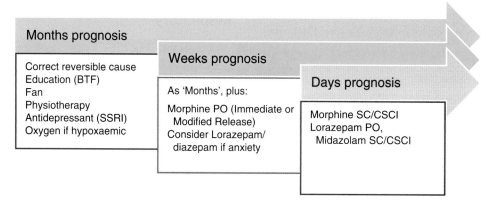

• **Fig. 26.1** Summary: management options for breathlessness according to likely prognosis. *BTF,* Breathing, thinking, functioning; *CSCI,* continuous subcutaneous infusion; *SC,* subcutaneous; *SSRI,* selective serotonin reuptake inhibitor.

processes around breathlessness, and maintaining function and efficient use of energy.
- CBT and relaxation are also helpful.
- Teaching patients simple techniques for recovering control over their breathing when they feel particularly breathlessness is valuable. For example, the use of a fan, sitting forward, and focusing on breathing out (rather than in).

b. *Physiotherapy*
- Maintaining activity helps maintain function, prevent muscle wasting and deconditioning.
- Physiotherapists are also crucial in optimizing efficient breathing technique.

c. *Fan*
- Air flow over the nose and mouth has been shown to be effective in reducing the sensation of breathlessness.
- A handheld fan is a simple, portable, and effective device for easing breathlessness.
- Similarly, air flow through an open window or larger fan is effective.

d. *Antidepressants*
- Selective serotonin reuptake inhibitors (SSRIs) may benefit breathless patients, especially where anxiety is a contributing factor (e.g., sertraline, dosed as for anxiety/depression).

e. *Opioids*
- Reduce sensation of breathlessness and respiratory effort through reducing response to hypercapnia, hypoxia, and exercise.
- Morphine is first choice strong opioid; but if side effects limit dose, oxycodone is an alternative and is titrated in the same way (although twice as potent as morphine).
- Starting dose will depend on whether the patient is already using morphine (for pain or breathlessness) or not (Tables 26.2 and 26.3).

f. *Benzodiazepines*
- Patients with prognosis of months: avoid.
- Prognosis of weeks: use if significant anxiety component to breathlessness. Use oral benzodiazepine with shorter half-life (lorazepam) initially.

TABLE 26.2 Starting Doses & Titration of Morphine for Breathlessness in Opioid Naïve Patients

	Months Prognosis	Weeks-Months Prognosis	Days Prognosis
Morphine PO (immediate release)	1 mg twice daily → 1 mg four times daily → 1 mg every 4 h → 2 mg every 4 h → 3 mg every 4 h → 5 mg every 4 h → further increases by 30%–50% (increase weekly)		2.5–5 mg every 4 h
Morphine PO (modified release)	5 mg twice daily	5 mg twice daily. Titrate total daily dose once a week by 10 mg. I.e. to 10 mg twice daily → 15 mg twice daily. Maximum effective dose usually 30 mg daily	N/A
Morphine SC	N/A	N/A	2.5–5 mg every 4 h
Morphine CSCI/24 h	N/A	N/A	Start with 10 mg CSCI/24 h

Oxycodone is an alternative in patients unable to tolerate morphine. As morphine to oxycodone potency is 1:2, start with half the equivalent morphine dose.
CSCI, Continuous subcutaneous infusion; *SC*, subcutaneous.

TABLE 26.3 Starting Doses & Titration of Morphine for Breathlessness in Patients Already Taking Morphine

	Months Prognosis	Weeks Prognosis	Days Prognosis
Morphine PO PRN (immediate release)	25%–100% of the 4-hourly analgesic dose (e.g., morphine total 60 mg PO in 24 h → 4-hourly analgesia dose = 1/6 of 24-h dose = 10 mg PO → breathlessness dose = 2.5–10 mg PO morphine)		
Morphine PO (modified release)	Titrate pre-existing morphine modified release (MR) dose according to *regular* PRN morphine immediate release (IR) use. (e.g., Morphine MR 30 mg BD but taking 4 doses of morphine IR 5 mg every day for breathlessness → increase Morphine MR to 40 mg twice daily).		N/A
Morphine SC PRN	N/A	N/A	Half of oral PRN dose (PO:SC 1:2), calculated as above.
Morphine CSCI/24 h	N/A (unless vomiting and needs temporary replacement, then as for Days Prognosis)		Half of current oral 24 h dose

If established on oxycodone, the same principles apply.
CSCI, Continuous subcutaneous infusion; *PRN*, as needed; *SC*, subcutaneous.

TABLE 26.4	Breathlessness: Benzodiazepine Dose and Choice		
	Months Prognosis	**Weeks Prognosis**	**Days Prognosis**
Lorazepam	Avoid	If significant anxiety 500 µg every 4 h	If significant anxiety 500 µg–1 mg every 4 h
Diazepam	Avoid	Avoid unless significant anxiety. Minimal effective dose (e.g. 2 mg twice daily, titrated slowly)	N/A
Midazolam SC	N/A	N/A	2.5–5 mg every one hour
Midazolam CSCI	N/A	N/A	Minimum 10 mg CSCI/24 h

CSCI, Continuous subcutaneous infusion; *SC*, subcutaneous.

- Prognosis of days: benzodiazepines often used parenterally in combination with opioid. Intent of benzodiazepine use is to relieve distress. Sedation may be a consequence, but is likely anyway due to exhausting effect of dyspnoea and deteriorating condition.
- Doses as in Table 26.4

g. *Oxygen*
- Long-term therapy for patients who are hypoxaemic due to life-limiting illness (e.g., COPD, interstitial lung disease, cardiac failure, cystic fibrosis, neuromuscular disorders, obstructive sleep apnoea [OSA], pulmonary hypertension).
- Ambulatory oxygen should be supplied to patients qualifying for long-term oxygen therapy who are mobile and wish to leave the home OR patients who desaturate on exercise.
- Nocturnal oxygen can be used for patients with nocturnal hypoxaemia.
- Oxygen's potential for psychological dependence and associated complications (drying/bleeding of nasal mucosa, hazards of equipment/tubing, risks in hypercapnic respiratory failure) means it should only be started if absolutely necessary.

Cough
- Management is guided by whether the cough is productive or not, and whether the patient is able to expectorate.

Productive, Able to Expectorate
- Treat cause/infection: antibiotics
- Loosen secretions: 0.9% saline nebulizers 2.5 to 5 mL four times daily; carbocisteine 375 to 750 mg three times daily
- Physiotherapy
- Bronchospasm: salbutamol

Productive, Unable to Expectorate
- Antimuscarinics (e.g., glycopyrronium; see section on end-of-life symptom control); hyoscine transdermal patches may be helpful if prognosis of weeks
- Cough suppressants (see upcoming discussion)

Nonproductive
- If irreversible cause, a dry cough should be suppressed.
  a. Peripheral suppressants: simple linctus may help pharyngeal irritation
  b. Central suppressants:
  - Opioid naïve patients: pholcodine 10 mL three times daily; codeine 30 to 60 mg four times daily or morphine 2.5 to 5 mg PO every 4 hours. Titrate morphine as for pain.
  - Patients established on strong opioid: dose equivalent to PRN analgesic dose can be tried.
  - Diazepam 5 mg PO daily if other measures ineffective.

Other Symptoms

Bronchorrhoea
- Bronchorrhoea is large volume mucous production which is seen most often in alveolar cell (and other) lung cancers.
- Radiotherapy should be considered, but if this is not possible, the following can be tried:
  - Antimuscarinics: glycopyrronium (SC and CSCI), hyoscine (transdermal, SC, and CSCI)
  - Corticosteroids PO: dexamethasone 4 to 8 mg PO daily
  - Octreotide CSCI 300 µg CSCI/24 h

Haemoptysis
- Consider using antibiotics (if due to infection); low-molecular-weight heparin (if due to pulmonary embolism); radiotherapy (for bleeding tumour).
- Tranexamic acid 1 g PO three times daily can be used to improve coagulation; reduce dose to 500 mg three times daily 1 week after bleeding stops. Alternatively, can be stopped 1 week after bleeding ceases, but resume if bleeding recurs.
- Minor/moderate haemoptysis may herald a massive haemorrhage. For management of massive haemoptysis see "Emergencies—Haemorrhage (Massive)"

Lymphangitis Carcinomatosis
- Corticosteroids (dexamethasone 8 mg PO daily) may improve symptoms.

- Diuretics may have some benefit (furosemide 40 mg + daily)

Gastrointestinal Symptoms

GUIDELINES

Watson, M., Lucas, C., Hoy, A., et al. (2009). *Oxford handbook of palliative care.* Oxford: Oxford University Press. NHS Scotland. *Scottish palliative care guidelines.* www .palliativecareguidelines.scot.nhs.uk/.

Nausea, Vomiting, and Regurgitation

- Nausea and vomiting should be assessed separately: They can occur independently or together.
- When considering vomiting, it is important to distinguish this from expectoration and true regurgitation.
  - Expectoration: should be managed as for cough
  - Regurgitation: often due to intrinsic or extrinsic compression of oesophagus by tumour. If due to oesophageal mass, it may be amenable to stenting/balloon dilatation (if patient can tolerate procedure)

Potential Causes

- Drugs: opioids, NSAIDs, antibiotics, iron supplements
- Metabolic: hypercalcaemia, uraemia
- Treatments: radiotherapy, chemotherapy
- Intracerebral malignancy (primary or secondary)
- Gastrointestinal stasis, constipation

- Bowel obstruction
- Vestibular dysfunction
- Psychological factors: anxiety, fear
- Paraneoplastic
- Infection

Potentially Reversible Causes

- Constipation, pain, infection, hypercalcaemia, ascites, raised intracranial pressure, medications

Management

Based on the following principles:
1. Identify underlying cause
2. Treat/manage cause if reversible
3. Have a clear rationale for pharmalogical management: Choose antiemetic or antinausea medication based on likely cause
4. Administer antiemetic:
   a. regularly: give a stat dose before starting regular antiemetic;
   b. by appropriate route (often parenteral, especially if vomiting);
   c. be prepared to titrate regular dose after 24 hours; and/ or
   d. rotate antiemetics if initial choice is ineffective after 24 to 48 hours.

Table 26.5 summarizes antiemetic choice by underlying aetiology.
- Specific considerations:
  - Some nausea/vomiting may require combinations of antiemetics. When choosing combinations, use

TABLE 26.5 Antiemetic Choice According to Underlying Aetiology/Cause

Stimulus/Cause of Nausea or Vomiting	Central Receptor	Antagonist—Appropriate Antiemetic Choice	Peripheral Action
Drugs (morphine), metabolites, toxins, uraemia, hypercalcaemia	D2 (CTZ)	Haloperidol	None
Gastric stasis	D2 (CTZ)	Metoclopramide	Cholinergic/blocks dopamine brake in gut; prokinetic effect
Raised intracranial pressure	H1 (VC)	Cyclizine	Antimuscarinic (slows bowel)
Motion	Achm (VC)	Hyoscine *Hydro*bromide	Anticholinergic; reduces secretions and spasm
Vestibular	D2, 5HT2, H1	Prochlorperazine	
Various	D2, 5HT2, Achm, H1 (VC and CTZ)	Levomepromazine	
Cytotoxic chemo, Radiotherapy (RT)	5HT3	Ondansetron (metoclopramide)	5HT3 receptors in bowel; ondansetron is very constipating
Anxiety, fear	GABA mimetic (cerebral cortex)	Lorazepam	

Receptors: *5HT2/3*, serotonin; *Achm*, acetylcholine; *D2*, dopamine; *H1*, histamine.
Location of receptors (VC), vomiting centre; (CTZ), chemoreceptor trigger zone.

antiemetics with different (complimentary) central actions. Be aware that some combinations will be antagonistic (e.g., cyclizine + metoclopramide antagonize one another's actions peripherally).

- Ondansetron is very specific in its mode of action and very constipating. Aside from its use in cytotoxic chemotherapy and radiotherapy, the only other main indication is disseminated abdominal/gastrointestinal (GI) malignancy (which can release large amounts of serotonin).
- Route of administration and dosing:
  - Antiemetics should be given parenterally if vomiting is persistent or severe as this will impair absorption of oral medications.
  - If antiemetic is given CSCI, regular opioid dose can also be replaced in this way until nausea/vomiting is controlled.
  - Once nausea/vomiting is settled for over 48 hours on CSCI medication, switch to the equivalent oral antiemetic dose.
  - Unless underlying cause resolves, antiemetics will likely be required long term. The exception is when starting an opioid, as tolerance to nausea may develop in a week or so.
- Table 26.6 summarizes dosing and route of administration.

Constipation

- Constipation is a common problem in patients with life-limiting illness.

- Patients may experience infrequent/irregular bowel evacuations and difficulty in defecating. Stool may be hard.
- Causes include debility, diet (reduced intake/low residue), poor fluid intake, medications (opioids, antimuscarinics, diuretics, 5HT3 receptor antagonists), and biochemical abnormalities (hypercalcaemia, hypokalaemia).
- Consequences include pain, urinary retention, confusion, overflow diarrhoea.
- Many laxatives are available, and often classified by action although there is much overlap.
- Laxative choice should be based upon patient preference/ability—almost all will work if given in sufficient dose.

Management

- Anticipate constipation (e.g., when starting an opioid prescribe prophylactic laxatives).
- Encourage general measures to aid regular bowel habit (e.g., fluid intake, fibre in diet, mobility, good access to toilet).
- Use oral laxative first (rather than rectal):
  - Combination of stimulant and softener/osmotic is usual.
  - Titrate dose until desired consistency and frequency are achieved.
- Patients with spinal cord compression/cauda equina/neurological disease may need a bowel regime to aid defecation. This often consists of senna tablets 3 nights

TABLE 26.6	**Antiemetics: Dosing by Route of Administration**			
	Dose and Frequency			
Antiemetic	**PO**	**SC**	**CSCI**	**Notes**
Haloperidol*	500 µg–1.5 mg at night and every 4 hr PRN		2–5 mg/24 h	Good at End of Life (EoL), when anxiolytic / anti-psychotic properties may also be beneficial
Metoclopramide*	10 mg three times daily to 20 mg four times daily (10 mg every 4 hr PRN with maximum 24-hr dose of 100 mg)		30–100 mg/24 h	Good prokinetic, comparatively large volume for SC injection
Cyclizine	50 mg twice/thrice daily or every 8 hr PRN		100–150 mg/24 h	Can cause cutaneous irritation
Levomepromazine*	6.25 mg at night and every 4 hr PRN (up to 25 mg in 24 h)		12.5–25 mg/24 h	Broad-spectrum, second line antiemetic. Useful PRN in addition to another regular antiemetic
Ondansetron	4–8 mg twice/thrice daily		8–16 mg/24 h	Very constipating
Domperidone	10 mg three times daily	Unavailable	Unavailable	Good prokinetic which does not cross blood-brain barrier (no antidopaminergic effects), but only available PO and PR
Lorazepam	500 µg–1 mg once daily and every 4 hr PRN	N/A		Useful for anticipatory nausea/vomiting

*Avoid in Parkinson disease and Lewy body dementia.
CSCI, Continuous subcutaneous infusion; *PRN*, as needed; *SC*, subcutaneous.

TABLE 26.7	**Laxatives Classified by Mode of Action and Dose**	
Stimulants	• Senna 15 mg at night (prophylaxis); 15–30 mg twice daily (established constipation) • Sodium picosulphate 5–10 mL twice daily • Bisacodyl 5–10 mg at night (prophylactic); 20 mg at night to 20 mg twice daily (established constipation)	Avoid in bowel obstruction
Softeners	• Docusate 100–200 mg twice daily	May be useful in partial bowel obstruction
Osmotic	• Macrogols	Avoid lactulose unless indicated in hepatic impairment (requires large volume of fluid, causes bloating/flatus and abdominal cramps)
Bulk forming	• Ispaghula husk, methylcellulose	Generally avoided as may worsen constipation if patient unable to take sufficient fluids
Rectal agents	• Glycerol suppository (lubricates/softens stool) • Bisacodyl suppository (stimulates rectal mucosa) • Microenema • Phosphate enema	Avoid in patients at risk of bleeding (e.g., thrombocytopenia) or infection (neutropenia)
Peripheral opioid antagonists	• Methylnaltrexone bromide (injection) • Naloxegol (oral)	For opioid-induced constipation where other measures have failed

per week, with glycerol/bisacodyl suppository given the following morning to empty rectum and sigmoid colon.
• Table 26.7 classifies laxatives by mode of action and dose.

Diarrhoea

• Ensure adequate fluid intake while managing the cause.
• Causes include:
  • laxatives;
  • other medications (e.g., antibiotics);
  • infection;
  • faecal impaction: sudden onset diarrhoea after period of constipation;
  • radiotherapy (colitis);
  • malabsorption:
    a. Pancreatic insufficiency (cystic fibrosis [CF], pancreatic cancer, pancreatectomy): steatorrhoea (i.e., pale, fatty stools with offensive odour)
    b. Gastrectomy: steatorrhoea
    c. Colectomy: profuse, watery stools
  • carcinoid tumour: profuse diarrhoea.

Management

• Laxatives: stop and review doses
• Antibiotics: check for/treat *Clostridium difficile*
• Faecal impaction: appropriate laxatives, often macrogols
• Radiotherapy (colitis): steroids (dexamethasone 8 mg daily for 1–2 weeks)
• Malabsorption—steatorrhoea: replace pancreatic enzymes with every meal/snack/drink that is not clear fluid; PPI
• Carcinoid tumour: 5HT3 receptor antagonist (ondansetron), octreotide
• Nonspecific: loperamide or opioids (e.g., codeine, morphine)

Acid Reflux, Gastritis, Oesophagitis

• Can be a problem in tumours affecting the stomach and oesophagus.

Management

• Proton pump inhibitors can be used at up to double dose (e.g., lansoprazole 30 mg twice a day, omeprazole 40 mg daily).
• The H_2-antagonist ranitidine can be used in doses up to 600 mg daily (in divided doses twice daily or four times daily). It can also be given CSCI (150–300 mg CSCI/24 h).

Hiccup

• Diaphragmatic spasms, often caused by irritation from gastric distension or hepatomegaly. Renal failure and steroids are other potential causes in patients with LLI.

Management

• Antiflatulent/prokinetic/PPI, for example:
  • peppermint water 10 mL PRN; or
  • metoclopramide 10 mg three times daily PO; or
  • lansoprazole 30 mg daily.
• Smooth muscle relaxant (e.g., nifedipine 5 mg three times daily)
• Suppression of central hiccup reflex, for example:
  • baclofen 5 to 10 mg three times daily PO;
  • haloperidol 1 to 3 mg twice daily;
  • midazolam 10 mg + CSCI/24 h for severe hiccup in patients in last days of life.

Ascites

- May be due to malignant or nonmalignant aetiology.
- If patient is too frail for either diuretics or invasive procedures, symptom management with analgesia and antiemetics should be maximized.

Causes

- *Nonmalignant:* advanced hepatic disease with portal hypertension, cardiac failure
- *Malignant:* tumours of ovary/endometrium, bowel, liver (primary or secondary), peritoneal metastases from other tumours (e.g., breast)

Management

- *Nonmalignant:* diuretics (spironolactone and furosemide) are especially valuable in portal hypertension. Expect 0.5 to 1 kg/24 h weight loss; may take 2 to 4 weeks to achieve significant reduction in ascites:
  a. Monitor for electrolyte disturbance, hypotension, and renal function. Monitor U&Es weekly or before changing dose.
  b. Dose/titration:
     - Start spironolactone 100 to 200 mg every morning. Increase by 100 mg every 3 to 7 days (maximum response after 2–3 days). Usual maintenance 300 mg every morning. Maximum 400 mg every morning or 200 mg every morning in patients who are frail/elderly/renally impaired.
     - If no change after 2 weeks, consider adding furosemide 40 mg for a few days. This can be increased by 40 mg every 3 to 7 days to a maximum of 160 mg/day.
  c. Stop diuretics if not tolerated, ascites unchanged, or renal function impaired.
- *Malignant:*
  a. Diuretics can be tried, but likely to be less successful than in nonmalignant ascites, as ascites is often due to factors other than portal hypertension alone.
  b. Paracentesis provides effective relief of symptoms, but fluid may reaccumulate within weeks and require repeat drainage.
  c. Indwelling, tunneled ascitic drains (PleurX peritoneal catheter drainage system) are recommended for patients with recurrent ascites resistant to treatment. Patients can empty these themselves every few days as needed.

Anorexia, Cachexia, Dysphagia

- All three can cause significant distress to the patient and those important to them. Managing these symptoms is important, but consideration needs to be given to the fact that they are often an inevitable consequence of advanced disease in the final days of life.

Anorexia

- There is a loss of appetite for food.
- Manage underlying/contributing factors if possible (e.g., nausea, constipation, oral problems, ascites).

- Encourage patients to eat what they like rather than specific foods or supplements.
- Steroids (e.g., dexamethasone 2–4 mg daily PO) may help improve appetite but effects are often short lasting.
- Megestrol acetate 80 to 160 mg daily may be better for longer term appetite stimulation but there is a risk of thromboembolism.
- Both steroids and progestogens increase catabolism of skeletal muscle.
- Prokinetics may improve early satiety.

Cachexia

- This is a common but complex problem seen in advanced LLI including heart failure, respiratory disease, and cancer.
- Likely related to factors such as development of chronic inflammatory state (due to cytokine production), abnormal metabolism, and anorexia.
- The consequence is loss of fat and skeletal muscle which is not improved by increasing nutritional intake alone.
- Management: manage anorexia, optimize nutrition.

Dysphagia

- Look for reversible cause (e.g., oesophageal tumour) amenable to stent/balloon dilatation.
- Prokinetics may be helpful.

Malignant Bowel Obstruction

- Most often associated with cancer of bowel or ovary. Intrinsic or extrinsic compression of the bowel by tumour (e.g., peritoneal metastases) can cause obstruction in multiple sites.
- Often a clinical diagnosis: Investigations may show site of obstruction, but not always (i.e., functional obstruction).
- Symptoms may wax and wane for many months before complete obstruction develops.
- Symptoms depend on site of obstruction:
  - High obstruction of gastric outlet and small bowel—large-volume vomiting is predominant feature, often faeculent once established.
  - Low obstruction of colon—constipation is predominant feature with vomiting coming later.
  - Both can cause colicky abdominal pain and vomiting with or without nausea.

Management

- Consider surgical/interventional options.
  - In advanced malignancy with peritoneal disease, obstruction is likely to be at several sites and patients are likely to be unfit for surgery. But suspected obstruction at a single site may be amenable to surgery (e.g., colostomy for obstructing rectal mass); stent to gastric outlet or duodenum.
  - Parenteral fluid and nutritional support may be an appropriate temporary measure for patients in whom there is potential for intervention by surgery or stent.
- Symptomatic treatment for patients unsuitable for surgery:
  - On initial presentation, management is aimed at encouraging peristalsis (prokinetic [e.g., metoclopramide

30–120 mg daily CSCI]—stop if causes colic), reducing peritumour oedema and compression (dexamethasone 8 mg daily PO/SC), and softening stool (docusate 100–200 mg twice daily).

- If symptoms do not resolve in 2 to 3 days or obstruction is thought to be complete, treat nausea (cyclizine 150 mg CSCI/24 h), colic (hyoscine butylbromide 60–120 mg CSCI/24 h), and pain (CSCI opioids). In complete bowel obstruction, the aim is to reduce the volume and frequency of vomits and associated symptoms.
- If high-volume vomiting, consider Ryle tube for drainage or pharmacological management (hyoscine butylbromide as above, octreotide 300 μg CSCI/24 h, or ranitidine 150 mg CSCI/24 h).

Oral Symptoms
Oral Candidiasis

- Typical presentation is with altered taste and adherent white candida plaques but may present with redness/soreness.
- When diagnosing oral candidiasis, consider if oesophageal extension is likely.

Management
- Good denture hygiene and mouth care
- Oropharyngeal: nystatin 100,000 units/mL (1 mL four times daily for 7 days) or miconazole gel (5–10 mL four times daily for 7 days) for mild infections; fluconazole (50 mg once daily for 7 days) for moderate-severe infections
- Oesophageal candidiasis: fluconazole 50 mg daily for 7 to 14 days
- In immunocompromised: longer courses of fluconazole may be necessary

Mouth Ulcers and Oral Stomatitis
Mouth Ulcers—Treatment
- Corticosteroids (e.g., hydrocortisone oromucosal tablets 2.5 mg four times daily)

Oral Inflammation/Stomatitis—Treatment
- Correct reversible causes such as badly fitting dentures.
- Maintain oral hygiene with mouthwashes if brushing too painful (e.g., sodium chloride, sodium bicarbonate, or chlorhexidine [alcohol free]).
- Coating agents can help in oral mucositis due to chemo/radiotherapy (e.g., GelClair® and Orabase®).
- Local anaesthetics may help (e.g., lidocaine ointment 5%, cocaine hydrochloride 2%).
- NSAIDs may help (e.g., benzydamine 0.15% mouthwash).
- Systemic analgesics (opioids and nonopioids) may be helpful but may need to be given parenterally (CSCI).
- Treat any secondary infection.

Xerostomia
- Often the consequence of medications (e.g., morphine, antimuscarinics) or treatment for cancer (e.g., radiotherapy).

Management
- Stimulate natural saliva (e.g., using sugar-free chewing gum).
- Use artificial saliva (e.g., Biotene Oral Balance gel®, AS Saliva Orthana®)
- Pilocarpine:
  - Particularly useful after radiotherapy for head/neck cancer
  - Dose 5 to 10 mg PO four times daily (pilocarpine 4% eyedrop solution is an alternative; use 3 drops PO four times daily)

Sialorrhoea
- Seen most often in patients with advanced neurological disease

Management
- Tricyclic antidepressants (e.g., amitriptyline 10 mg at night)
- Hyoscine hydrobromide transdermal patch 1 mg/72 h; up to two patches can be applied at one time
- Propantheline 15 mg three times daily
- Atropine (1% eye drops) 2 to 3 drops three times daily

Neurological Symptoms (See Also "Advanced Neurological Diseases")
Seizures

- Seizures may be due to pre-existing epilepsy or a presenting or later feature of intracerebral malignancy or neurodegenerative disease.

Management
- For acute management see "Emergencies - seizures."
- If known epileptic on established therapy:
  - consider increase in current antiepileptic dose (AED);
  - consider addition of levetiracetam.
- If initiating AED for new seizure in patients with irreversible intracerebral lesion/malignancy:
  a. in patient with intracerebral mass/metastases with peri-tumour oedema, consider dexamethasone 16 mg daily PO (temporary measure); will require titration downwards to lowest tolerated dose;
  b. Antiepileptics:
     - Sodium valproate 200 mg PO twice daily (modified release); titrate by 200 mg twice daily every 3 days, maximum 2.5 g daily; OR
     - Levetiracetam 250 mg PO twice daily; titrate by 250 mg twice daily every 2 weeks, maximum 3 g daily.
- Second line (e.g., uncontrolled seizures currently taking an oral antiepileptic or when other antiepileptic contraindicated/not tolerated); levetiracetam, dose as above.

Intracerebral Malignancy
- Intracerebral malignancy may cause a variety of symptoms, but most usually:
  - weakness, incoordination, dysphasia;
  - headache;

- seizures;
- nausea/vomiting;
- reduced consciousness.
- Radiotherapy may exacerbate symptoms.
- Dexamethasone may reduce any symptoms related to intracerebral oedema.

Management With Steroids

- Consider high-dose dexamethasone trial (e.g., 8 to 16 mg PO daily).
- Symptomatic improvement should be seen in 2 to 3 days.
- Monitor for hyperglycaemia, measuring Capillary Blood Glucose (CBG) minimum twice weekly in patients with no known diabetes or daily in patient with diabetes.
- If unable to swallow, dexamethasone can be given subcutaneously (best given once/twice daily in doses before lunchtime to reduce risk of insomnia).
- Discontinue dexamethasone if:
  - no improvement after 1 week;
  - side effects result from steroids (e.g., uncontrolled hyperglycaemia, restlessness).
- If improvement in symptoms after 1 week, titrate dose down to lowest tolerated. Typical reduction of daily dose by 2 to 4 mg, reduced weekly. See Table 26.10.
- Following cerebral radiotherapy, steroid dose should not be reduced until 1 week after radiotherapy is completed. Reduce as above.

Fatigue

- Fatigue is a common symptom in patients with advanced LLI, especially cancer and its treatment.
- It is often related to cachexia (see GI symptoms management).

Management

- Check for symptomatic anaemia.
- Perform thyroid function tests.
- Manage other symptoms (e.g., uncontrolled pain, insomnia, mood disturbance).
- Review concurrent medications.
- Recommend:
  - regular exercise;
  - sleep hygiene;
  - pacing/prioritization of activities.
- For fatigue refractory to these measures consider a psychostimulant (e.g., methylphenidate or modafinil).

Delirium

GUIDELINES

National Institute for Health and Care Excellence. (2013). *Delirium: Diagnosis, prevention and management. NICE clinical guideline 103.* www.nice.org.uk/guidance/cg103.
Inouye, S.K., et al. (1990). Clarifying confusion: The confusion assessment method. A new method for detection of delirium. *Annals of Internal Medicine, 113,* 941–948.

• BOX 26.1 Confusion Assessment Method, Four Item

1. Acute onset and fluctuating course
   a. Is there evidence of an acute change in mental status from the patient's baseline?
   b. Did the abnormal behaviours fluctuate during the day or change in severity?
2. Inattention
   a. Did the patient have difficulty focusing attention (e.g., being easily distractible) or have difficulty keeping track of what was being said?
3. Disorganized thinking
   a. Rambling or irrelevant conversation, unclear/illogical flow of ideas, unpredictable switching from one subject to another
4. Altered level of consciousness
   a. Vigilant (hyperalert), lethargic (drowsy, easily roused), stupor (difficult to rouse), unrousable

If YES to 1+2+3 or 4, a diagnosis of delirium is suggested.

Diagnosis/Presenting Features

- Onset typically acute (within hours or days) and fluctuates hourly/daily.
- Cognitive function impaired (e.g., worsened concentration, slow responses, and disorientation).
- Perception altered (e.g., visual or auditory hallucinations).
- Physical function impaired (e.g., reduced mobility, reduced movement, restlessness, agitation, changes in appetite, sleep disturbance).
- Social behaviour (e.g., lack of cooperation with reasonable requests, withdrawal, or alterations in communication, mood, and/or attitude).
- Be particularly vigilant for signs of hypoactive delirium.
- Several tools for identifying/diagnosing delirium are available. The key is to suspect delirium, especially in patients who may present with hypoactive type. Consider use of the Confusion Assessment Method (Box 26.1).

Management

1. Identify/treat reversible causes (if appropriate), for example:
   - infection (e.g., urinary tract infection [UTI], lower respiratory tract infection [LRTI]);
   - medications: morphine, sedatives, steroids, anticholinergics, tricyclics, neuroleptics, dopaminergics;
   - metabolic: hyperosmolar hyperglycaemic state (HHS)/hypoglycaemia, hepatic failure, hypercalcaemia, uraemia, hyponatraemia;
   - hypoxia;
   - dehydration;
   - urinary retention, constipation;
   - drug/alcohol withdrawal, including withdrawal of nicotine, antidepressants;
   - psychological distress.

2. Provide constant environment:
   - Quiet room, subdued lighting
   - Ensure access to sensory aids (i.e., glasses, hearing aids)
   - Clock, calendar, routine should be on clear display to patient in room
   - Familiar objects and people (involve family, friends, carers)
   - Few interruptions
   - Repeated reassurance and explanation (use lucid intervals)
   - Simple, respectful communication (use short sentences, calm manner; allow thinking time for patient)
   - Avoid moving patient between rooms
3. Ensure safety of patient and others.
4. Medications:
   - Chronic/mild delirium:
     i. Haloperidol only (benzodiazepines do not improve cognition; may worsen it). Dose 1 to 5 mg SC or 500 µg to 5 mg PO stat and PRN, with typical maintenance dose 2.5 to 10 mg CSCI/24 h or 0.5 to 3 mg twice daily PO
   - Acute/severe delirium (+/– agitation):
     i. First line: haloperidol only. Dose 2.5 to 5 mg PO/SC/IM hourly; max 20 mg/24 h, with maintenance dose typically half of the first 24-hour dose OR based on stat doses used
     ii. Second line: add benzodiazepines—only if sedation is needed and/or alcohol or benzodiazepine withdrawal is a factor

Note: Chronic confusion, dementia (behaviour that challenges), and other symptoms specific to neurodegenerative disease are included in additional sections.

Chronic Confusion

- Presenting features:
  - Onset/course typically chronic (days to weeks)
  - Pattern is constant: little/no fluctuation, may be progressive
  - Cognitive function may be normal or impaired (disorientated) BUT consciousness not altered
  - Hallucinations unusual
  - Physical impairment rare; health generally good
  - Memory loss prominent in confusion caused by dementia, mood may be depressed
  - Confusion due to dementia will gradually worsen over months

Management

1. Exclude depression.
2. General measures as for delirium (see Delirium).
3. Medication:
   - Chronic confusion: risperidone 0.25 to 1 mg at night (gradual increase to 1 mg twice daily)
   - Acute on chronic confusion with delirium: haloperidol as for delirium (see Delirium)
   - Insomnia: trazodone 50 to 100 mg at night

Skin Symptoms

> ### GUIDELINES
>
> International Lymphoedema Framework and Canadian Lymphedema Framework. (2010). *International Lymphoedema Framework position document: The management of lymphoedema in advanced cancer and oedema at the end of life.* www.lympho.org.
> British Lymphology Society and Lymphoedema Support Network. (2016). *Consensus document on the management of cellulitis in lymphoedema.* www.lymphoedema.org/images/pdf/CellulitisConsensus.pdf.

Lymphoedema and Oedema

Classification of Oedema in Patients With Life-Limiting Illness

- Oedema in advanced disease is common and often multifactorial in nature, occurring when net capillary filtration exceeds lymphatic drainage. It may or may not have impaired lymphatic drainage (lymphoedema) as a component.
  - *Causes of impaired lymphatic drainage (lymphoedema):* metastatic lymphadenopathy, surgery (especially when lymph nodes removed), radiotherapy, immobility, longstanding increased flow
  - *Causes of increased capillary filtration:* hypoalbuminaemia, venous hypertension (cardiac failure, extrinsic compression from tumour, inferior vena cava obstruction/superior vena cava obstruction (SVCO), venous thrombosis), medications (e.g., corticosteroids, NSAIDs, hormones, chemotherapy)
- Oedema and lymphoedema may present therefore in patients with advanced cancer, heart failure, respiratory disease, renal failure, neurological disease, or liver disease. As oedema becomes chronic, inflammatory and fibrotic changes develop.
- Lymphoedema services are often part of local palliative care provision and will normally manage patients with primary (congenital) lymphoedema and secondary lymphoedema due to the effects of disease or its treatment. They are also a useful source of reference for patients with more general oedema at the end of life.

Signs and Symptoms

- Oedema may be a well-recognized complication of the underlying diagnosis (e.g., in cardiac or hepatic failure).
- Consider underlying venous thrombosis if asymmetric oedema develops acutely in a limb.
- Lymphoedema classically presents as follows:
  - In a discrete anatomic location, due to underlying cause (e.g., arm lymphoedema following axillary node clearance).
  - Skin will indurate or pit when pressure is applied.
  - Skin becomes thickened and changes become chronic: Hyperkeratosis, papillomata, and lymphangiectasia develop.

- Cellulitis and lymphorrhoea (leakage of lymph fluid due to breaks in skin) are recognized complications.

Management

- *Of lymphoedema:* Management is aimed at reducing swelling and thereby restoring function and reducing discomfort. It is tailored to the individual and their stage of underlying illness; early intervention is important to prevent chronic changes. Contraindications are unusual but include uncontrolled cardiac failure. Patients diagnosed with acute deep vein thrombosis (DVT) must wait 8 weeks before receiving intensive lymphoedema intervention and those with arterial insufficiency (ABPI <0.5) should not have compression.
- Consider investigation/treatment for underlying or exacerbating causes (e.g., for malignancy, venous thrombosis, cardiac failure, anaemia, or management of medications exacerbating oedema).
- Complete/complex decongestive therapy (CDT) is the mainstay of management. Management is initiated by specialist lymphoedema practitioners and where possible, self-care is taught to the patient/family. CDT involves:
  - manual lymphatic drainage (MLD). This stimulates lymphatic tissues, decongesting deep lymphatics and increasing drainage of lymph from the affected site. MLD is undertaken by specialized professionals who can teach a simplified version (simple lymphatic drainage) to patients or carers;
  - compression bandaging, hosiery, or Velcro compression devices. These increase tissue pressure to reduce oedema and promote drainage of lymph (when used with MLD) while preventing backflow evacuated lymph. Multi-layered compression can contain dressings to absorb lymphorrhoea;
  - skin care and infection prevention. Skin care with the intent of avoiding infection/cellulitis includes maintaining skin hydration (using emollients daily), careful hygiene, and avoidance of skin trauma;
  - exercise. Undertaken under compression to improve venous drainage, uptake of lymph, and to soften fibrosis. It may be active or passive;
  - elevation of the affected limb (to a level above the heart) can be helpful in patients with advanced disease who are unable to exercise.
- *Of cellulitis associated with lymphoedema:*
  - First line:
    a. Oral amoxicillin 500 mg 8-hourly is treatment of choice
    b. If evidence of *Staphylococcus aureus* infection: flucloxacillin 500 mg four times daily in addition to or as alternative to amoxicillin
    c. In patients with confirmed penicillin allergy: erythromycin 500 mg four times daily or clarithromycin 500 mg twice daily
    d. If complicating factors (e.g., animal scratch/bite) then discuss with microbiologist

- Second line (if poor response to amoxicillin/flucloxacillin after 48 hours):
  a. Clindamycin 300 mg four times daily
- *Duration of antibiotics.* Continue antibiotics until all signs of acute infection have resolved. This often means treatment for a minimum of 2 weeks but may be as long as 1 to 2 months. Note that skin changes/discoloration may persist after infection resolves.
- *Other measures.* Do not use compression garments in the acute attack but replace as soon as the affected area is able to tolerate them. Elevation of affected limb and bed rest is important. Exercise can be resumed once inflammation subsides.

Sweating (Paraneoplastic)

Presenting Features

- Uncontrolled sweating is often associated with malignancy.
- It may be associated with paraneoplastic pyrexia (i.e., pyrexia in absence of infective cause).
- Sweating may affect one specific part of the body or be more generalized.

Management

- Antipyretics:
  - Paracetamol 500 mg to 1 g four times daily
  - Naproxen 250 to 500 mg twice daily (or alternative NSAID)
- Antimuscarinics:
  - Amitriptyline 10 to 50 mg at night
  - Propantheline 15 to 30 mg twice daily
  - Hyoscine hydrobromide or glycopyrronium
- Other:
  - Propranolol 10 to 20 mg twice daily, gabapentin

Pruritus

Causes

- A relatively common symptom in advanced LLI, pruritus may have a wide variety of causes.

Management

1. *General:*
   - Establish, treat, and remove any causes (e.g., skin infection, medication).
   - Keep skin moisturized: Use emollient daily, use aqueous cream instead of soap, avoid hot baths, dry skin by patting.
   - Avoid sweating (see section on managing sweating) and keep skin cool.
   - Macerated skin should be dried and hydrocortisone 1% used if localized inflammation (dermatitis) present.
   - Topical antipruritics include menthol 0.5% to 2%, phenol 0.5% to 3%, and camphor 0.5% to 3%.
   - Use sedative antihistamines at bedtime or regularly (e.g., chlorphenamine 4 mg three times daily).
2. *Cause specific:*
   - Rashes: antihistamines (topical cream or systemic); menthol in aqueous cream; hydrocortisone 1% cream

- Opioids: chlorphenamine 4 mg three times daily or cetirizine 10 mg daily; switch to alternative opioid; ondansetron (4–8 mg twice daily)
- Cholestasis: measures to resolve cholestasis if appropriate (e.g., biliary stent); cholestyramine (often poorly tolerated), sertraline 50 to 100 mg once daily, rifampicin 150 to 600 mg once daily, naltrexone 12.5 to 25 mg once daily (if not taking opioid analgesia)
- Uraemia: localized itch can respond to topical capsaicin cream; ultraviolet B (UVB) phototherapy, gabapentin 100 mg after haemodialysis or doxepin 10 mg twice daily
- Hodgkin lymphoma: prednisolone 10 to 20 mg three times daily
- Paraneoplastic/other causes: paroxetine 5 to 20 mg once daily or sertraline 50 to 100 mg once daily, mirtazapine 15 mg daily

Malignant Wound Management (Bleeding From Wounds, Odour and Infection, Fistulae)

- Wounds due to cancer can cause a variety of problems.
- Ideally, palliative radiotherapy, surgery, or even chemotherapy may help their management, but in advanced disease these are not always possible.
- In all cases, aim to make dressings as unobtrusive and comfortable as possible, change dressings as infrequently as possible, and protect surrounding healthy tissues.
- Pain should be managed using approaches as outlined in "Symptom Management—Pain." If wounds are significantly painful, systemic analgesia will often be required:
  - It is advisable to make PRN analgesia available which can be given prior to changing dressings on malignant wounds.
  - If changing of dressings causes significant distress, lorazepam 500 µg to 1 mg PO can also be given prior to dressing change.
  - An increase in pain in a wound may be a sign of infection (see upcoming discussion).

Bleeding (for Other Sources of Bleeding, See "Bleeding")

- Haemostatic can be used topically or systemically:
  - Topical: Tranexamic acid 10% (500 mg/5 mL ampoule) applied to gauze and held against bleeding surface of wound.
  - Systemic: Tranexamic acid 1 g PO three times daily. Due to potential side effects, halve dose or stop 1 week after bleeding is stopped. Resume if bleeding recurs.
- Other options:
  - Gauze soaked in adrenaline 1:1000 solution (1 mg in 1 mL) and applied to areas of bleeding (note prolonged/repeated use may cause further ischaemia and further bleeding)
  - Alginate dressings

Odour and Infection

- Tumours breaching the skin surface (whether primary or metastatic) are liable to ischaemia, necrosis, and anaerobic infection.

- Infection may be acute or chronic. If evidence of infection develops, treat as for cellulitis (e.g., flucloxacillin or erythromycin).
- Odour is often due to the presence of anaerobic bacteria. Options for managing odour include metronidazole topical gel 0.75% applied to the wound or dressing daily OR metronidazole PO 400 mg three times daily for 1 week. If odour improves, metronidazole may be reduced to 200 mg once daily (indefinite).

Exudate and Enterocutaneous Fistulae

- Exudate requires containment with highly absorbent dressings. Undamaged skin around the wound should be protected with a barrier cream such as Cavilon™.
- When fistulae develop, management should include:
  - protecting surrounding skin (see earlier);
  - containing any effluent—using ostomy collection bags if necessary;
  - reducing fistula output. Octreotide may be given subcutaneously (e.g., 100 µg SC twice or thrice daily).

Depression and Anxiety

Depression

- Depression is a significant problem in patients with LLI of all types.
- Its presence should be actively sought, and it should not be assumed that low mood or depression in patients with LLI is inevitable.

Diagnosis

- Many physical symptoms of depression are common in LLI, such as loss of appetite, disturbed sleep, fatigue, psychomotor slowing.
- In palliative care patients, withdrawal, anhedonia, feelings of guilt, hopelessness, or wishes for death/suicide may suggest depression.
- The simple question "Are you feeling depressed?" can be helpful in identifying depression.
- A variety of screening tools are available—those that have fewer questions are often more appropriate for the palliative population (e.g., Edinburgh Depression Scale).
- Use of the Distress Thermometer can assist in identification of factors contributing to distress.

Management

- Assess for medications that may affect mood, delirium, hypothyroidism, and dementia.
- Ensure good palliative care is provided, including adequate management of any physical symptoms, spiritual needs, and social support needs. Review depressive symptoms once these have been addressed.
- As for any depressive episode, mild-moderate depression may be managed with psychological support and cognitive behavioural therapy.
- If an antidepressant is indicated (moderate-severe depression) and anticipated prognosis long enough to benefit

(i.e., >1 month) then choice can be based upon side effects/safety profile and patient comorbidities:

- First choice is usually an SSRI. If partially effective, titrate dose. If ineffective switch to alternative SSRI or mirtazapine.
- Sertraline (SSRI, 50-mg starting dose in depression; 25 mg starting dose if anxiety). Safer in chronic renal failure and after myocardial infarction (MI).
- Citalopram (SSRI, 10-mg starting dose). Good in anxiety, safer in patients with seizures. Oral suspension available.
- Mirtazapine (15-mg starting dose). Possibly faster mode of action than other antidepressants. Sedative effect and appetite stimulation may be helpful. Safe in cardiac failure and diabetes.
- Amitriptyline. Useful if concurrent pain or insomnia. Avoid if significant cardiac disease/after MI, in hepatic failure, in patients with glaucoma. Greater risk in overdose.
- Duloxetine (serotonin norepinephrine reuptake inhibitor [SNRI]). May be useful when patients have concurrent neuropathic pain.
- Methylphenidate. May be used in patients whose prognosis is thought to be weeks at most, when time is insufficient for conventional antidepressant. May have onset of action within days. Dose 5 mg PO twice daily (maximum 40 mg daily).

Anxiety

- May present with depression, or alone.
- In patients with days to live, manage with benzodiazepines.
- For patients with longer prognosis:
  - Venlafaxine (SNRI) can be helpful. Start with 37.5 mg PO twice daily.
  - Sertraline (start with 25 mg daily PO) and citalopram are alternatives.
  - Pregabalin is useful in patients with concurrent neuropathic pain.
  - Benzodiazepine may also be required.

Bleeding

- For massive haemorrhage, see "Emergencies."
- For haemoptysis, see "Symptom Management—Respiratory."
- For bleeding wounds, see "Symptom Management—Skin."
- Bleeding can occur from a number of anatomic sites; management may be directed at the bleeding site or via systemic therapy.
- Ensure that any medications that may encourage bleeding have been reviewed and stopped if necessary (e.g., LMWH, warfarin, aspirin, clopidogrel, NSAIDs).
- Treat for any infection which may exacerbate bleeding (e.g., UTI, chest infection).
- Consider referring for radiotherapy (e.g., to bladder, lung), local coagulation (e.g., cryotherapy or diathermy) if appropriate.
- *Systemic treatment* (for any bleeding site):
  - Tranexamic acid PO. Give 1 g three times daily initially. One week after bleeding stops, this may be stopped completely or reduced to 500 mg three times daily. If bleeding recurs, resume 1 g three times daily and continue indefinitely.
  - Note: There is risk of clot retention if used for haematuria.
- *Local treatment:*
  - Topical tranexamic acid: 10% solution (500 mg/5 mL applied on gauze) for cutaneous bleeding or epistaxis;

TABLE 26.8 Dexamethasone Starting Doses (PO)

Indication	Daily Dose (Daily Dose >4 mg Usually Given in Two Divided Doses, Before Lunchtime)
Appetite (anorexia)	4 mg
Liver capsule pain	4–8 mg
Pain due to nerve compression	4–8 mg
Bowel obstruction	8 mg Note: Often given as a trial SC. Ensure steroid reviewed daily as may stimulate appetite which can cause significant distress in patient with irreversible obstruction.
Intracerebral oedema/raised ICP, nausea and vomiting due to raised ICP	8–16 mg Note: If for nausea/vomiting in ICP give in combination with antiemetic SC/CSCI.
Superior vena cava obstruction	16 mg
Metastatic spinal cord compression	16 mg

Subcutaneous Dexamethasone:
Dexamethasone can be given by SC injection. The injectable formulation varies, most often either 3.3 mg/mL or 3.8 mg/mL. For practical purposes, consider dexamethasone 4 mg PO equivalent to either 3.3 mg or 3.8 mg SC.

CSCI, Continuous subcutaneous infusion; *ICP*, intracranial pressure; *SC*, subcutaneous.

Steroid	Dexamethasone		Prednisolone	Hydrocortisone
Equivalent anti-inflammatory dose	1 mg		7.5 mg	25 mg
Relative glucocorticoid activity	30		4	1
Relative mineralocorticoid activity	Minimal mineralocorticoid action		0.8	1

TABLE 26.9 Steroids: Approximate Equivalent Anti-Inflammatory, Glucocorticoid and Mineralocorticoid Properties

5% solution (500 mg/10 mL) as mouthwash or for rectal bleeding
- Silver nitrate stick applied to bleeding points
- Sucralfate paste or suspension

Special Notes on Steroids

GUIDELINE

Diabetes UK. (2018). *End of life diabetes care.* https://www.diabetes.org.uk/resources-s3/2018-03/EoL_Guidance_2018_Final.pdf.
National Institute of Clinical Excellence. *Clinical Knowledge Summary 'Corticosteroids - oral'.* https://cks.nice.org.uk/corticosteroids-oral#!scenario.

Indications for and Use of Steroids (Dexamethasone)

- Steroids are indicated in the palliative management of various conditions. The most commonly used in palliative care is dexamethasone—dose varies depending on condition/symptom being managed (Table 26.8).
- When used, consideration should be given to their side effects, notably hyperglycaemia, muscle wasting (proximal myopathy), mood disturbance, osteoporosis, and adrenal suppression.
- Corticosteroids vary in their ratio of mineralocorticoid to glucocorticoid properties. See Table 26.9. This determines their therapeutic action - glucocorticoid properties being used in palliative care for anti-inflammatory action. High mineraolcorticoid action is generally undesirable (due to resulting water retention), but useful in adrenal replacement.
- Generally, just one corticosteroid should be prescribed. See Table 26.9 for equivalent anti-inflammatory doses.
- Dexamethasone should be started at an appropriate dose (see Table 26.8), and reduction in dose attempted once symptoms improved (or after 2 weeks at most).
- Gastric protection in the form of lansoprazole (or similar) should be given, especially to patients also taking NSAIDs.
- Check capillary blood glucose (CBG) in all patients prior to commencing corticosteroids.
- To avoid insomnia, steroids should be given in divided doses with the latest dose at lunchtime.
- Steroids may be given by SC injection. This may be helpful as a temporary measure in a patient with dysphagia or

Starting Dose	Weekly Reduction in Daily Dose by	If Recurrent Symptoms
>8 mg daily	4 mg then once <8 mg daily as below	Increase back to lowest effective dose, then try more cautious reduction (e.g., 1–2 mg weekly)
<8 mg daily	2 mg	

TABLE 26.10 Tapering Dexamethasone Dose

vomiting (e.g., due to intracerebral mass/oedema), but steroids should not be routinely continued when a patient is in the last days of life (discussion to come).

Monitoring Patients Taking Corticosteroids

- CBG should be monitored in all patients: daily in patients with known diabetes (to enable titration of oral hypoglycaemic medications/insulin) and twice weekly in those not known to have diabetes.
- Monitor symptom benefit and reassess after 1 week.
- See management of steroid-induced diabetes (below).

Stopping/Withdrawing Steroids

- At the time of starting steroids, a plan should be made for review and reducing the dose.
- Monitor patients for signs of hypoadrenal crisis when steroids withdrawn.
- Stop steroids abruptly if:
  - steroids bring no symptomatic benefit after 1 week;
  - unacceptable side effects occur less than 1 week after starting;
  - a patient enters the last days of life (stop steroids when patient is dying and no longer responsive). In this situation, steroids can be stopped abruptly, however long the duration. But if steroids are potentially managing significant symptoms (e.g., raised ICP or SVCO), consider alternative symptom management options (e.g., prophylactic midazolam CSCI) to prevent seizures.
- Taper steroids gradually when:
  - patient has been taking more than 4 mg dexamethasone for over 1 week or a lower dose for over 2 weeks in total (as this may have suppressed endogenous production);
  - risk of rebound symptoms exists (e.g., significant cerebral oedema);

- The aim is to stop all courses of steroids completely, unless the patient suffers significant recurrence of symptoms. In this case, maintain on minimal effective dose.
- Table 26.10 provides guidance on how to taper the steroid dose.

Management of New Onset Steroid-Induced Diabetes

- Steroid-induced diabetes can occur in patients previously not known to have diabetes. It can occur with any corticosteroid taken for more than a few days.
- Steroids taken in the morning tend to cause a rise in blood glucose around late afternoon/early evening. This can be managed by giving gliclazide or isophane insulin in the morning.
- CBG should be checked before starting steroids in all patients. If CBG is above 8 mmol/L, check with a venous sample and manage accordingly before starting steroids.
- In patient with LLI, aim for CBG in the range of 6 to 15 mmol/L to minimize symptoms of hyperglycaemia.
- When discontinuing steroids, reduce hypoglycaemic medications.
- Patients already known to have diabetes should have their medication titrated according to any changes in CBG exacerbated by steroids.
- *Management of new steroid-induced diabetes when steroids given once daily* (mornings):
  - Check CBG before evening meal.
  - If CBG consistently above 15 mmol/L, start gliclazide 40 mg with breakfast.
  - Titrate gliclazide by increments of 40 mg daily until CBG 6 to 15 mmol/L. Maximum morning dose 240 mg daily. If still high, add gliclazide 40 to 80 mg in evening.
  - If gliclazide ineffective, switch to morning insulin and seek specialist advice.

Care in the Last Days of Life

Prognostication

> **GUIDELINES**
>
> National Institute for Health and Care Excellence. (2015). *Care of dying adults in the last days of life. NICE clinical guideline 31.* www.nice.org.uk.
> Thomas, K., Wilson, J.A. and GSF Team. (Dec 2016). *GSF PIG 6th Edition. National Gold Standards Framework Centre in End of Life Care.* http://www. goldstandardsframework.org.uk.
> Leadership Alliance for the Care of Dying People. (2014). *One chance to get it right: Improving people's experience of care in the last few days and hours of life.* www.gov.uk/ government/uploads/system/uploads/attachment_data/ file/323188/One_chance_to_get_it_right.pdf.

- Judging whether a person is entering the last few days of life can be challenging.

- Regardless of how much experience a professional has, there always remains some uncertainty. It is important to openly acknowledge this, especially to the patient and those caring for him/her.
- The following clinical signs may suggest a person is dying:
  - Global clinical deterioration despite optimal management of underlying life-limiting illness or concurrent problems
  - Daily deterioration in performance status
  - Profound fatigue, minimal oral intake (sips of fluid only), and difficulty swallowing oral medications
  - Signs such as agitation, Cheyne–Stokes breathing, significant deterioration in level of consciousness, mottled skin, noisy respiratory secretions
- In this situation, ensure that a person's symptomatic and physical care needs are anticipated, and that measures are put in place to address their holistic care.
- Involve the patient as much as they are able or desire. When no longer able to contribute, consider any advance decisions they had made and recorded.
- Attending to the understanding, wishes, and needs of those important to them—especially any carers—will be crucial in providing successful care in the last days of life.

Stopping Treatments

> **GUIDELINES**
>
> National Institute for Health and Care Excellence. (2017). *Nutrition support for adults: Oral nutrition support, enteral tube feeding and parenteral nutrition. NICE clinical guideline 32.* www.nice.org.uk/.
> General Medical Council. (2010). *Treatment and care towards the end of life: Good practice in decision making.* www.gmc-uk.org.

- As death approaches, it is appropriate to rationalize and consider stopping treatment and medications.
- Making an informed decision to stop any treatment can be made by any patient with capacity.
- If a medication or treatment is stopped either intentionally or because it is no longer possible to administer it, thought should be given to ensure ongoing symptom control is unaffected. Alternative means of providing medications for symptom control should be used whenever possible.

Medications

- Medications that can be stopped:
  - Oral medications for which there is no parenteral replacement once a patient loses the ability to swallow
  - Oral medications not contributing to symptom control (e.g., prophylactic medications such as statins)
- Medications that should be continued/alternative found:
  - Medications required for symptom control (e.g., long-term opioids for pain)
  - Medications whose withdrawal may cause severe symptoms (e.g., long-term antiepileptic medications)

- Means of continuing medications:
  - When the oral route is no longer viable, consider liquid formulation that can be given via percutaneous endoscopic gastrostomy (PEG)/radiologically inserted gastrostomy (RIG) (if available). Only continue medications considered necessary for ongoing symptom relief.
  - Most medications for symptom control at end of life can be given CSCI via a syringe driver (see "Syringe Drivers").

Nutrition and Hydration

- A patient with capacity to do so may choose to stop clinically assisted nutrition and hydration at any point.
- Consider the benefits, burdens, and risks of nutrition and hydration separately.
- For a person in the last hours to days of life, the burdens and risk of clinically assisted nutrition and hydration usually outweigh the benefits. Guidance from the General Medical Council (GMC) and Department of Health is available to assist decision making.
- Both should be reviewed regularly, particularly if the patient exceeds his or her anticipated prognosis.
- Nutrition:
  - Most people in the last days to week of life will gradually stop eating.
  - Clinically assisted (parenteral or enteral) nutrition may be stopped by any patient with capacity to make this decision or in the patient's best interests if he or she is not competent to give consent (if those responsible for a best interests decision conclude that the burdens and risks outweigh benefits).
- Hydration:
  - In most circumstances, the dying process entails a person gradually ceasing to take oral fluids and when in the last hours to days of life, parenteral replacement is unlikely to be appropriate.
  - A person's hydration status and needs should be assessed as he or she enters the last few days of life.
  - Clinically assisted fluids can be stopped by any patient with capacity to do so or in the patient's best interests if not competent to consent (if those responsible for a best interests decision conclude that the burdens and risks outweigh benefits).
  - Regular mouth care should be provided to patients in the final days to week of life.

Noninvasive Ventilation

- As with other treatments, noninvasive ventilation (NIV) can be stopped at any time by a patient competent to make the decision to do so.
- Specialist support from palliative care teams/professionals with working knowledge of the legal and ethical guidelines and practicalities around stopping NIV should be available to healthcare professionals and patients in this situation.
- When stopping, medication may be given to alleviate any symptoms experienced, particularly for patients requiring NIV 24 hours a day:

- For example, SC/CSCI opioids for breathlessness, with SC/CSCI benzodiazepines for breathlessness and anxiety. See "Symptom Control—Breathlessness," "Care in the last days of life - anticipatory medications," and "Syringe Driver" for doses/guidance.

Anticipatory Medications and Care

For guidance on doses of CSCI medications at end of life, see "Syringe Driver."
- Everything possible should be done to anticipate symptom, care, and support needs for people in the last days of life and those important to them.
- Equipment needed to manage a patient at home (e.g., hospital bed, commode, hoist) should be anticipated wherever possible and adequate support by professional carers arranged.
- Anticipatory medications should be readily available for subcutaneous administration:
  - Medications should have appropriate community administration instructions/record.
  - A minimal number of medications should be available to avoid confusion (for more options, see relevant symptom control sections).
- Commonly used anticipatory medications are listed in Tables 26.11 and 26.12, along with appropriate indications for their use and doses. All injections should be administered subcutaneously. There may be variation to this in local guidance: local guidance should be followed wherever possible.
- If patients regularly require PRN doses (e.g., three or more PRN doses of analgesia daily), their regular (CSCI) dose should be increased accordingly.
- Note: Guidance around opioid use in renal failure will vary according to local policy. See "End-Stage Renal Failure" for guidance.

Syringe Driver

GUIDELINES

MIMS Online. (2016). *Syringe driver compatibility*. www.mims.co.uk.

Palliativedrugs.com. *Syringe driver compatibilities*. https://palliativedrugs.com.

Indications and Practicalities

- Syringe drivers are used to enable delivery of symptom-control medications when an alternative to the oral route is required, for example:
  - at end of life when the patient is no longer able to swallow;
  - as a temporary measure in a patient with vomiting or dysphagia.
- They are battery-powered devices that enable the administration of medications by CSCI. The most common in current use is the CME McKinley T34.

TABLE 26.11 Anticipatory PRN Medications For Symptom Control (Opioid Naïve Patients)

Symptom/Indication	Medication	PRN Dose (SC Unless Stated Otherwise)
Pain	Morphine (opioid naïve patient)	2.5–5 mg 1-hourly
	Diamorphine (opioid naïve patient)	2.5–5 mg 1-hourly
Nausea/vomiting	Haloperidol	1–2 mg 4-hourly
	Levomepromazine	6.25–12.5 mg 4-hourly
Secretions	Glycopyrronium	200–400 µg 4-hourly
	Hyoscine butylbromide	20 mg 4-hourly
Delirium	Haloperidol	1–5 mg SC 4-hourly (see also section on delirium)
Agitation	Midazolam	2.5–5 mg 1-hourly
Seizures	Midazolam OR	10 mg for prolonged/distressing seizures (may also be given via buccal route; see also section on seizures)
	Diazepam	10 mg PR
Risk of distressing life-threatening event (e.g., massive haemorrhage, airway obstruction)	Midazolam	10 mg IM (if haemorrhage)

IM, Intramuscular; *PRN*, as needed; *SC*, subcutaneous.

TABLE 26.12 Anticipatory PRN Opioid Analgesia: Patients on Regular/Established Opioids

Regular Opioid	PRN SC Opioid	Additional Information
Morphine or oxycodone—ORAL	1/12 of patient's current daily (24 h) oral dose	Replace regular oral opioid with CSCI dose when patient is unable to swallow
Morphine or oxycodone—CSCI	1/6 of total daily CSCI dose	
Diamorphine—CSCI	1/6 of patient's current CSCI dose	
TD opioid patch (e.g., buprenorphine or fentanyl)	Provide PRN medication at appropriate dose (see approximate equivalences in "Pain" or Appendix 33 and/or seek specialist advice)	Continue TD opioid patch until death; titrate analgesia by adding in regular CSCI opioid if indicated
Methadone	Seek specialist guidance	

Ensure patient has anticipatory medications for other symptoms also - see Table 26.11
CSCI, Continuous subcutaneous infusion; *PRN*, as needed; *TD*, transdermal.

- Infusion through the skin is achieved by plastic/Teflon cannula:
  - The best sites for these are upper arms and anterior chest wall and suprascapular region, but abdominal wall and thighs can also be used.
  - Sites should be inspected regularly for signs of reaction/irritation. They should be rotated every 3 to 5 days.
- CSCI administration is off label use for most medications.
- The conventional infusion period is 24 hours, which helps ensure contents remain stable and sterile and achieves more even plasma concentration of medication than repeated SC injections:
  - Contents are changed (and adjusted as necessary) once daily.

- Combinations of medications (e.g., analgesia plus antiemetic) can be used. When using combinations of medications:
  - check compatibility data as some will not mix and may precipitate, affecting symptom control (see Appendix 31);
  - water for injection is the normal diluent, with a few exceptions;
  - dilute contents to the maximum volume possible to reduce risk of skin reactions at the infusion site;
  - usually up to three drugs are combined;
  - combination and dosing is limited by volume: The maximum fill volume of a McKinley T34 is 34 mL in a 50-mL syringe, although 22 mL in a 30-mL syringe is more commonly used.

- It is good practice to ensure patients have additional PRN medications available for symptom control. It can take hours to appreciate the benefit of starting CSCI medications and SC alternatives should be available for symptoms such as breakthrough pain or nausea.

Starting Doses

See also "Symptom Management Specific to Advanced Chronic Kidney Disease/End-Stage Renal Failure" for patients with known renal impairment.

- Syringe driver starting doses:
  - Table 26.13 gives common staring doses for CSCI medications.
  - See section on symptom control of nausea and vomiting for CSCI doses of antiemetics (Table 26.6).
- *Patients on established medications.* Remember to stop the equivalent oral medications (e.g., modified release opioid), if switching to CSCI delivery (Table 26.14):
  - Converting from PO to CSCI and vice versa:
    a. Medications are normally more potent SC (CSCI) than PO, and as such a dose reduction is usual.
    b. Refer to local guidelines on dose conversion, seek specialist advice (and refer to opioid equivalence

tables (Appendix 33)/antiemetic dosing table in symptom control section (Table 26.6)).
c. If symptoms controlled and a switchback from CSCI to PO is indicated, remember to increase doses where necessary. CSCI is usually stopped when the first PO dose is given.

TABLE 26.13 Starting Doses for CSCI Medications in the Last Days to Week of Life

Symptom/ Medication	CSCI/24 h
Pain (opioid naïve)	Morphine 10 mg CSCI/24 h OR Oxycodone 5–10 mg CSCI/24 h OR Diamorphine 10 mg CSCI/24 h
Agitation	Midazolam 10–20 mg CSCI/24 h
Nausea/ vomiting	Haloperidol 3–5 mg/24 h OR CSCI equivalent of alternative antiemetic
Secretions	Glycopyrronium 600 µg–1.2 mg/24 h
Risk of seizures	Midazolam 20 mg+/24 h

CSCI, Continuous subcutaneous infusion.

TABLE 26.14 Guidance on Switching From Established PO and Transdermal to Continuous Subcutaneous Infusion Medications

Symptom/Medication	CSCI/24 h
Pain: Morphine or oxycodone PO regular dose (immediate or modified release) continuing as CSCI equivalent	PO:SC potency ratio for both morphine and oxycodone is approximately 1:2, so HALVE the total oral 24-h dose and administer CSCI For example, morphine 100 mg total PO/24 h = morphine 50 mg CSCI/24 h For example, oxycodone 40 mg total PO/24 h = oxycodone 20 mg CSCI/24 h
Pain: Morphine PO regular dose switching to equivalent CSCI diamorphine (see "Symptom Control—Pain" and Appendix 33 for guidance)	PO morphine: SC diamorphine potency ratio is approximately 1:3 For example, morphine 30 mg total PO/24 h = diamorphine 10 mg CSCI/24 h
Pain: Transdermal buprenorphine or fentanyl patches	Continue transdermal patch and supplement with SC PRN strong opioid (morphine, diamorphine, or oxycodone if no renal impairment) If requiring three or more PRN SC opioid doses daily, supplement with CSCI opioid For example, additional three doses of morphine 5 mg SC in 24 h Start morphine 15 mg CSCI/24 h in addition to transdermal patch Seek specialist advice on dosing.
If nausea/vomiting:	CSCI equivalent of previous antiemetic See Table 26.6 in "Symptom Management Guidelines; Gastrointestinal Symptoms"
Established antiepileptic medication	Midazolam 20 mg+/24 h Levetiracetam and sodium valproate are used CSCI in some regions: seek specialist advice.

For renal failure, seek specialist advice and refer to "End-Stage Renal Failure."

CSCI, Continuous subcutaneous infusion; *PRN,* as needed; *SC,* subcutaneous.

- Converting from transdermal to CSCI:
  a. When a patient is in the last days to week of life, transdermal opioids should be continued. Any additional analgesic requirements are supplemented by PRN SC and CSCI strong opioid.

Advanced Neurological Disease

- See also sections:
  - "Symptom Management Guidelines; Pain—Other Types; Skeletal Muscle Spasm"
  - "Symptom Management Guidelines; Neurological Symptoms—Seizures, Fatigue, Delirium"

General Problems

> **GUIDELINE**
>
> NG 97. *Dementia: assessment, management and support for people living with dementia and their carers.* https://www.nice.org.uk/guidance/ng97.

- Most symptoms can be managed successfully, using the general guidelines above (see section on symptom control).
- Needs can change rapidly and so require ongoing assessment and specialist input.
- In addition to local palliative care services, local specialist services for people with advanced neurological diseases often exist. (e.g., specialist nurses/teams to support people with Motor Neurone Disease, Multiple Sclerosis, Parkinson's Disease).
- There are a few specific considerations/medications outlined in this section.

Communication

- Patients should be reviewed by a speech and language therapist.
- They should have access to both low-level (e.g., alphabet board) and high-level (e.g., eye-gaze computer systems) augmentive and alternative communication (AAC) technologies.
- Deteriorating communication ability should be a trigger for advance care planning (see "Basics Principles" i.e., initial section of chapter).

Nutrition, Hydration, and Poor Swallow

- Management of reduced oral intake should be considered early in the course of disease. If appropriate and desired, procedures to provide long-term enteral access (e.g., PEG) should be planned and undertaken while a patient remains well enough to undergo the procedure.
- Poor nutrition, anorexia/cachexia and aspiration may be inevitable consequences of the end stage of advanced neurological disease; and where reversal of underlying cause is not possible, symptomatic treatment should be provided (see "Care in the Last Days of Life").

- Similarly, hydration needs must be assessed in context and managed according to individual risk/benefit.
- A decision may be reached to continue feeding/fluids orally at risk, and manage complications symptomatically should they occur.
- Mouth care should always be provided to patients when they are no longer able to swallow.

Recurrent Infection

- Infections such as UTI or chest infection/aspiration are seen in advanced respiratory disease due to the consequences of the disease itself (recurrent aspiration from impaired swallow or interventions to manage symptoms—e.g., UTI associated with catheterization).
- When treating infection, consider general principles (see "Basic Principles"), routes available to administer medication (PO, PEG, RIG), and likelihood of treatment success (may be reduced if multiple-drug-resistant infection or irreversible underlying aetiology such as aspiration from at-risk feeding).
- If treatment of underlying infection is not desired or indicated, symptoms should be managed.

Muscle Spasms/Spasticity (See Also Section on Pain)

- Further to pain-relieving measures as described previously, the following may be considered in people with neurodegenerative disease causing painful muscle spasm:
  - Gabapentin and clonazepam may also be used if other medications are poorly tolerated.
  - Botulinum toxin injections can be used for isolated muscle spasm.
  - Physiotherapy input and specialist spasticity services are usually available locally.
  - Midazolam CSCI may be required as the end of life approaches.

Activities of Daily Living

- Equipment is available (usually via physiotherapy/occupational therapy services and/or specialist services for people with advanced neurological disease) and should be provided to aid activities of daily living and mobility.

Dementia

- Dementia may be the primary diagnosis or comorbidity in a patient with life-limiting illness.
- As with all illnesses, medications to address the underlying pathology are the mainstays of management.
- Advanced dementia may have associated complications, including:
  - reduced nutritional intake and weight loss (forgetting to eat or poor swallowing);
  - recurrent infections (aspiration, debility, reduced fluid intake);
  - behaviour that challenges and makes the patient at risk to self or others.

Management of Behaviour That Challenges

- Drug treatments for the control of violence, aggression, and extreme agitation should be used to calm the person with dementia and reduce the risk of violence and harm, rather than treat any underlying psychiatric condition. Aim to reduce agitation or aggression without causing unnecessary sedation.
- If required give medications for behaviour that challenges orally first line, SC second line. However, IM injections may be used if required.
- If SC/IM preparations are needed, lorazepam, haloperidol, or olanzapine should be used. Wherever possible, a single agent should be used in preference to a combination.
- If a patient exhibiting agitation/delirium is at the end of life, manage as for agitation (see "Emergencies").
- People with Alzheimer's disease, vascular dementia, mixed dementias, or dementia with Lewy bodies with severe non-cognitive symptoms (psychosis and/or agitated behaviour causing significant distress) may be offered treatment with an antipsychotic drug. (See also "Parkinson's Disease and Parkinson Plus Syndromes."):
  - Target symptoms for treatment should be identified and individual risk/benefit considered. Treatment should be discussed with patients and/or those important to them.
  - The antipsychotic should be commenced at low dose and reviewed regularly (monthly). Monitor for neuroleptic sensitivity (i.e., changes in cognition and physical function).

Management of Reduced Oral Intake and Infection (See Earlier Discussion - 'Nutrition, Hydration & Poor swallow')

- Managing these complications of advanced dementia should always be undertaken in context (i.e., with involvement of the patient, those important to the patient, and with due consideration to the stage of underlying disease) (see "Basic Principles").

Parkinson's Disease and Parkinson Plus Syndromes

> **GUIDELINES**
>
> National Institute for Health and Care Excellence. (2006). *Parkinson's disease: Diagnosis and management in primary and secondary care. NICE clinical guideline 35.* www.nice.org.uk.
>   NICE Pathway. (2014). *Managing Parkinson's disease.* http://pathways.nice.org.uk/pathways.

- Advanced end-stage Parkinson disease may cause specific symptomatic problems: Bradykinesia, rigidity, tremor, and pain are possible.
- Goal of management is to optimize dopamine treatment/administration, while avoiding dopamine antagonists.

- Worsening of symptoms may be due to loss of dopaminergic response. Optimize administration and regular dosing of dopaminergic medications but consider stopping these at end of life/when of no benefit.
- Difficulty with swallowing may cause problems with administration of oral dopaminergic medications:
  - Madopar is available in dispersible formulations and/or other dopaminergic medications can be given via PEG if present.
  - Rotigotine transdermal patches are available and can be used under specialist guidance.
- Pain: optimize analgesia (see "Symptom Control—Pain"). Skeletal muscle relaxants (e.g., midazolam CSCI) may be necessary, especially where dopaminergic medications can no longer be taken or are of little benefit.
- Nausea and vomiting. Domperidone and cyclizine are preferred antiemetics (see section on symptom control related to nausea and vomiting).
- Hallucinations/delirium:
  - Exclude any potentially reversible causes.
  - Dopaminergic drugs are a potential cause.
  - Quetiapine (minimum 12.5 mg at night) is the only recommended antipsychotic.
  - In advanced disease, where a parenteral route is required, levomepromazine +/- midazolam may be more appropriate (see "Emergencies—Agitation").

Motor Neurone Disease (MND)/Amyotrophic Lateral Sclerosis (ALS)

> **GUIDELINE**
>
> National Institute for Health and Care Excellence. (2016). *Motor neurone disease—assessment & management. NICE clinical guideline 42.* www.nice.org.uk.

- Many principles of symptom management in MND are common to other advanced life-limiting illness, as above, but those in this section pertain specifically to motor neurone disease.

Ventilatory Support

- *NIV.* Patients can be offered NIV if they develop signs and symptoms of respiratory impairment (e.g., breathlessness, weak cough/sniff, disturbed/nonrefreshing sleep, nightmares, daytime drowsiness, morning headache, fatigue, shallow breathing, recurrent chest infection, accessory muscle use, abdominal paradox, orthopnoea, increased respiratory rate).
- This is set up and monitored according to patient wishes with the local specialist multidisciplinary team (MDT)/respiratory ventilation service. It can be stopped by a patient with capacity at any time (see "Care in the Last Days of Life").

Cough

- Breath stacking (manual or assisted) and mechanical cough assist devices can be used to improve effectiveness of cough. This may be particularly helpful in clearing secretions associated with infection.

End-Stage Renal Failure

> **GUIDELINE**
>
> Scottish Palliative Care Guidelines. (2015). *Renal disease in the last days of life*. www.palliativecareguidelines.scot.nhs.uk/.

- Renal failure is considered end stage when estimated glomerular filtration rate (eGFR) falls to below 15 mL/min/1.73m^2 (chronic kidney disease [CKD] Stage 5).
- However, symptoms are common in patients with CKD4 (eGFR 15–29 mL/min/1.73m^2) and symptom control/pharmacological considerations mentioned later are appropriate for all patients with eGFR below 30 mL/min.
- Note on eGFR and creatinine clearance. Most pharmacokinetic studies used an estimate of creatinine clearance based on Coackroft-Gault equation. Dose adjustments of drugs were therefore based upon this. Estimated GFR (eGFR)—most often based on MDRD calculation—is not the same as creatinine clearance, but an acceptable substitute when considering whether adjustments need to be made in the dosing of medications. eGFR is adjusted to body surface area and as such should be used with caution if body size is unusually low or high. eGFR should be taken as an indication of the need to modify drug doses.
- Chronic kidney disease may be the underlying LLI or a comorbidity. It is most often due to:
  - diabetes;
  - hypertension, cardiovascular disease;
  - renal disease (e.g., glomerulonephritis, polycystic kidney disease [PKD]), infection, or obstructive uropathy;
  - malignancy (e.g., myeloma, tumour causing obstructive uropathy, effects of chemotherapy);
  - medications (e.g., lithium, long-term NSAIDs).
- Patients with end-stage renal failure may be managed in a variety of ways: either conservatively or with a form of renal replacement therapy (peritoneal dialysis or haemodialysis).

Symptoms

- Patients with end-stage renal failure have at least as many symptoms as patients with advanced disease, cancer, possibly more.

- Many similarities exist between symptoms experienced in end-stage renal failure (ESRF) and other LLI toward the end of life (e.g., pain, fatigue/lethargy, nausea/vomiting, anorexia).
- However, there are some symptoms specific to ESRF, which are often a consequence of uraemia or drug toxicity. For example:
  - pain due to renal disease, renal osteodystrophy, carpal tunnel syndrome, osteoporosis, osteomyelitis, renal neuropathy;
  - calciphylaxis (painful tissue ischaemia due to calcification of small blood vessels);
  - itch;
  - fluid overload;
  - restless legs, muscle cramps.
  - In addition to symptoms due to disease, the demands of treatment can be a significant source of distress for patients with advanced renal disease; these can be a significant factor in patients choosing to withdraw from dialysis.

Indicators of Poor Prognosis (Being in the Final Months to Year of Life) in Advanced and End-Stage Renal Failure (Chronic Kidney Disease 4 or 5)

- Symptomatic renal failure (e.g., nausea/vomiting, fluid overload, anorexia, pruritus, declining performance status) in patients having conservative management
- Patients choosing conservative management
- Poor tolerance of dialysis (e.g., hypotension preventing haemodialysis)
- Progressive cachexia and decline in performance status and increasing symptom burden despite dialysis
- Patients declining or withdrawing from dialysis (Note: Average survival for patients discontinuing haemodialysis varies but is likely in the range of several days to 2 weeks.)

Pharmacological Considerations in Chronic Kidney Disease 4 and 5

NB: Modifications to medications are appropriate in any patient with established acute kidney injury (eGFR <30) as well as those with CKD.

General Considerations

- Renal failure can reduce the oral absorption, alter the distribution, and reduce the excretion of many different drugs (and/or their metabolites):
  - Where possible, use medications that do not rely on renal excretion.
  - Nephrotoxic medications should be avoided if there is some residual renal function.
  - Medications that rely on renal excretion should be reduced in dose.
- Some medications will be removed by dialysis. In patients having dialysis, seek advice on medications from specialist teams.

- Detailed guidance on dose adjustment of medications in renal failure can be found in the British National Formulary (BNF), Palliative Care Formulary, or Summary of Product Characteristics (available online).
- *In patients with end-stage renal disease estimated to be in their final hours to days of life:*
  - Side effects from potential accumulation of medications and/or their metabolites need to be weighed carefully against the need to achieve timely symptom control, comfort, and dignity.
  - If there is a delay/difficulty in sourcing preferred 'renally safe' medications, and patients are experiencing uncontrolled symptoms/distress, then the priority should be to provide symptom control with the medications available.
  - In this situation smaller doses of less ideal mediation (e.g., morphine/diamorphine) can be given less frequently.
  - Note: Patients with a previously normal renal function dying from any cause may well develop renal failure/acute kidney injury (AKI) due to the physiologic processes that occur as death approaches (e.g., reduced fluid intake). In this patient group, modifications to well-tolerated, established medications for symptom control (e.g., morphine) are generally not needed. It is not appropriate to monitor renal function in the final days of life.

Symptom Management Specific to Advanced Chronic Kidney Disease/End-Stage Renal Failure

- As with most advanced LLI, maximizing therapy aimed at managing the disease and its complications is an important part of symptom management.
- As disease progresses and prognosis deteriorates it is important to review these medications and discontinue them where possible.

Medications Used to Manage Advanced Chronic Kidney Disease/End-Stage Renal Failure (and Its Complications)

- Calcium, vitamin D
- Phosphate binders
- Diuretics
- Iron, erythropoietin: for anaemia
- Antihypertensives
- Secondary prevention of cardiovascular disease (e.g., statins, antiplatelet therapy)
- Fluid restrictions

Managing Medications Used in Advanced Chronic Kidney Disease/ End-Stage Renal Failure

- Medications for advanced CKD and its complications should be reviewed when it becomes clear that a patient is deteriorating.
- Table 26.15 provides a guide as to when it may be appropriate to discontinue these medications.

Management of Symptoms Specific to Advanced Chronic Kidney Disease/ End-Stage Renal Failure

- The following guidance is appropriate for all patients with eGFR below 30 mL/min/1.73m^2 (CKD 4 or 5). It suggests alternative medications for symptom management in advanced renal disease. The general principles guiding use of these medications are mostly described under the general symptom control section. Please also refer to this section.
- Local practice may vary: Seek advice of local specialist palliative care team.
- Patients undergoing dialysis: Seek specialist advice for these patients as some medications (e.g., gabapentin and pregabalin) are cleared by dialysis.
- Table 26.16 summarises the medications most appropriate to use, and those best avoided.

TABLE 26.15	Management of Medications in Advanced Chronic Kidney Disease/End-Stage Renal Failure
Medication	**When to Consider Stopping**
Medications for anaemia: iron, erythropoietin	Stop in final weeks of life
Medications to maintain dialysis access (e.g., warfarin)	Stop when dialysis stops
Medications to reduce cardiovascular risk (e.g., statin, aspirin)	Stop when dialysis stops, or tablet burden felt to be too great
Calcium, vitamin D	Stop when dialysis stops or when patient is no longer swallowing
Phosphate binders	Stop when patient is no longer eating
Diuretics	Continue for as long as possible
Medications for symptom control (e.g., long-term analgesia, antiemetics)	Continue while patient is able to swallow and replace where possible with equivalent continuous subcutaneous infusion medication until death

TABLE 26.16	Summary of Medications for Symptom Control When Estimated Glomerular Filtration Rate Is Below 30 mL/min/1.73m²	
Symptom	Avoid	Manage With
1. Pain	Codeine, tramadol, NSAIDs (if any remaining renal function), morphine, diamorphine, oxycodone (used in some centres; use with caution)	Paracetamol, buprenorphine TD, fentanyl TD, fentanyl SC/CSCI, alfentanil CSCI, methadone, amitriptyline (titrate slowly), gabapentin (reduce dose), pregabalin (reduce dose), ketamine (specialist use)
2. Anxiety, depression	Venlafaxine, mirtazapine, duloxetine	Sertraline, lorazepam/diazepam (reduced dose)
3. Nausea/vomiting	Metoclopramide (long term)	Domperidone, haloperidol (reduce dose), cyclizine (reduce dose), ondansetron, levomepromazine (reduce dose)
4. Restless legs	—	Clonazepam, gabapentin (reduced dose)
5. Muscle jerks (myoclonic)	Diazepam (if possible)	Lorazepam, clonazepam
6. Breathlessness	Diazepam (if possible)	Fentanyl SC PRN/CSCI, alfentanil CSCI, lorazepam, midazolam PRN (reduced dose)
7. Delirium	—	Olanzapine, haloperidol (reduce dose)
8. Agitation	—	Midazolam (reduce doses), levomepromazine (reduce doses)
9. Respiratory secretions	Hyoscine hydrobromide	Glycopyrronium, hyoscine butylbromide
10. Pruritus	—	Capsaicin, gabapentin
11. Seizures	Phenobarbital	Sodium valproate, midazolam CSCI

For doses of medications in the table above, please see the main text.
CSCI, Continuous subcutaneous infusion; *NSAID,* nonsteroidal antiinflammatory drugs; *PRN,* as needed; *SC,* subcutaneous.

Pain

- Paracetamol: 500 mg to 1 g four times daily
- NSAIDs: ONLY for use in patients undergoing dialysis if they have no residual renal function
- Opioids:
  - Buprenorphine transdermal (TD) patches: no dose reduction required. Useful for chronic, stable pain. Consider the time taken to titrate dose—use in patients with weeks to months to live to give time for titration.
  - Fentanyl TD patches: may require dose reduction: titrate slowly. Useful for chronic, stable pain. Consider the time taken to titrate dose—use in patients with weeks to months to live to give time for titration.
  - Fentanyl injection SC PRN or CSCI: useful for opioid naïve patients with severe renal failure in the last days to week of life requiring rapid titration. Starting doses typically 12.5 to 25 μg SC 1-hourly PRN and 100 μg CSCI/24 h.
  - Alfentanil injection CSCI: useful for replacing other opioids via CSCI at end of life, and those requiring rapid opioid titration. Alfentanil SC is 10 times as potent as diamorphine SC (i.e., 10 mg diamorphine SC is approximately equivalent to 1 mg SC alfentanil). It is too short acting to use as SC PRN.
  - Methadone: specialist use. May be used orally or converted to CSCI at end of life (halve oral dose if

starting CSCI as considered twice as potent SC, compared to PO); may require dose reduction in severe renal failure.
- Others:
  - Amitriptyline: start with low dose (10 mg at night) and titrate slowly.
  - Gabapentin: requires dose reduction. Creatinine clearance (mL/min) 15 to 29 ml/min: 100 to 600 mg daily, titrated slowly. Creatinine clearance below 15 ml/min: 100 mg alternate days to 300 mg daily. (See manufacturer's summary of product characteristics for guidance; these doses are both lower than manufacturer's guidance.)
  - Pregabalin: requires dose reduction. Creatinine clearance 15 to 29 ml/min: 25 to 150 mg once daily. Creatinine clearance below 15 ml/min: 25 to 75 mg once daily.
  - Clonazepam: specialist use. May be helpful for nerve pain. Dose 500 μg to 2 mg at night.
  - Ketamine: specialist use. Typical starting dose 5 to 10 mg PO four times daily.

Anxiety, Depression

- Sertraline: no dose reduction required
- Lorazepam (severe anxiety): 500 μg 6-hourly
- Diazepam (severe anxiety): avoid if possible. If necessary, start with reduced dose (e.g., 2.5 to 5 mg at night, titrate slowly.

Nausea/Vomiting

- Manage according to likely cause (see section Symptom Management Guidelines > GI—nausea etc...)
- Ondansetron: no dose reduction required (i.e., 4–8 mg PO/SC twice daily
- Cyclizine: no dose reduction required but may exacerbate dry mouth, therefore start with 25 to 50 mg PO/SC thrice daily
- Haloperidol: reduce dose by 50%—start with 500 μg at night
- Metoclopramide: reduce dose by 50%—start with 5 mg PO/SC thrice daily
- Domperidone: start with low dose (e.g., 10 mg PO once or twice daily)
- Levomepromazine: start with low dose (i.e., 6.25 mg PO/SC at night and/or 6-hourly PRN)

Restless Legs

- Clonazepam: 500 μg PO at night, titrate slowly
- Gabapentin: dose reduced according to renal function as mentioned above under 'pain'.

Muscle Jerks (Myoclonic)

- Lorazepam or clonazepam (doses as mentioned above)

Breathlessness

- Opioids: fentanyl or alfentanil (doses as mentioned above under 'Pain')
- Benzodiazepines: lorazepam (doses as mentioned above) or midazolam starting at 2.5 mg SC 1-hourly PRN (at end of life)

Delirium

- See section on symptom management of neurological symptoms, delirium.
- Olanzapine is an alternative, starting at 5 mg daily.

Agitation

- See section on "Emergencies—agitation".
- Lower doses of midazolam (starting at 2.5 mg SC 1-hourly) and levomepromazine (6.25 mg SC 4-hourly) may be effective.

Respiratory Secretions

- Glycopyrronium 200 μg SC 4-hourly or hyoscine butylbromide 20 mg SC 4-hourly

Pruritus

- See section on symptom management—skin, pruritus.

Seizures at End of Life

- See section on emergencies—seizures.
- If CSCI required, midazolam is preferred. Phenobarbital should be avoided unless intractable seizures in last hours to days of life.
- Sodium valproate preferred if oral antiepileptic is appropriate; dose unchanged.

End-Stage Respiratory Disease

> ### GUIDELINES
>
> National Institute for Health and Care Excellence. (2010). *Chronic obstructive pulmonary disease in over 16s: Diagnosis and management. NICE clinical guideline 101.* www.nice.org.uk.
>   National Institute for Health and Care Excellence. (2011, updated March 2017). *End of life care for adults. NICE quality standard 13.* www.nice.org.uk.
>   Royal College of General Practitioners. (2016). Gold standards framework proactive identification guidance. https://www.goldstandardsframework.org.uk/cd-content/uploads/files/PIG/NEW%20PIG%20-%20%20%2020.1.17%20KT%20vs17.pdf

- The end stage of respiratory disease is not clearly defined.
- However, when the underlying disease becomes unresponsive to usual medical treatment (resulting in persistent or worsening symptoms) and estimated prognosis is less than 1 year, these factors suggest that the patient is in the 'end stages and approaching the end of life'.

Indicators of Poor Prognosis (Being in the Final Months to Year of Life) in Advanced Respiratory Disease

- Frequent exacerbations and hospital admissions
- Patients too unwell for pulmonary rehabilitation
- Patients who qualify for long-term oxygen therapy (LTOT)
- COPD with forced expiratory volume 1 (FEV1) less than 30% predicted
- Medical Research Council Dyspnoea Scale grade 4/5 (i.e., breathless on walking 100 yards or on minimal exertion)
- Cachexia, weight loss, low body mass index (BMI)
- Comorbidities such as heart failure

Symptom Management Specific to End-Stage Respiratory Disease

- Many symptoms experienced in end-stage respiratory disease can be managed according to general symptom management guidelines for pain, breathlessness, cough, secretions, anxiety, and depression (as detailed above).
- It is important always to consider whether symptoms in end-stage respiratory disease are reversible, for example:
  - treating infection with antibiotics;
  - treating inflammation with steroids;
  - managing bronchospasm with salbutamol and ipratropium.
- Management options specific to the underlying cause of the respiratory disease should always be optimized (e.g., beta-2 agonists and muscarinic antagonists, corticosteroids).
- When symptoms are no longer controlled by optimal medical treatment, palliative approaches should be employed. It is appropriate to manage uncontrolled symptoms with opioids or benzodiazepines. Anxiety about

casing respiratory depression should not prevent use of these medications where needed.

- Local specialist teams (Respiratory, Palliative Care) should remain involved in supporting patients and their needs.

Oxygen in End-Stage Respiratory Disease

- Oxygen may be helpful in the palliation of breathlessness due to hypoxia (see section on Symptom Management Guidelines > Respiratory—breathlessness).
- Appropriate use of oxygen:
  - Many patients will be on LTOT (PaO_2 <7.3 kPa).
  - If not, short-burst oxygen therapy (oxygen given intermittently for 10–20 minutes at a time) can be considered for breathlessness not responding to other measures.
  - Use a 24% or 28% Venturi mask at a flow rate of 2 to 4 L/min.
  - Use oxygen with caution if symptoms of CO_2 retention such as headache, lethargy, hand flap, and confusion.
- As disease progresses, routine measurement of oxygen saturations becomes less appropriate. In fact, it may cause undue concern to patients for whom no remedial measures are possible.
- Focus should be switched to managing symptoms of breathlessness regardless of measured oxygen saturations.

Anticipating Care Needs and Management

- Patients will often have extensive experience of hospitalization for management of exacerbations with their condition and may well have strong opinions on the treatment they would or would not want.
- If so, they should be encouraged to record an advance care plan or advance decision to refuse treatment.
- For patients with respiratory disease, opportunity should be created to discuss considerations such as whether they want further hospital admission, antibiotics (at home/in hospital or not at all), and ventilation (were this to be considered appropriate).
- Clinical condition and symptom burden can deteriorate rapidly in patients with advanced respiratory disease. For those patients who choose to have symptoms managed in the community, arrangements should be made to ensure anticipatory medication for symptom control/end-of-life care is readily available to them at home.

End-Stage Heart Failure

GUIDELINES

National Institute for Health and Care Excellence. (2010). *Chronic heart failure in adults. NICE clinical guideline 108.* www.nice.org.uk/.

CIED Working Group. (2016). Cardiovascular implanted electronic devices in people towards the end of life, during CPR and after death: Guidance from the Resuscitation Council (UK), British Cardiovascular Society and National Council for Palliative Care. *Heart.* doi:10.1136/heartjnl-2016-309721.

- Heart failure may be the sole underlying life-limiting illness, but is often encountered as a comorbidity or consequence of another condition (e.g., cardiomyopathy secondary to effects of chemotherapy or cor pulmonale).
- All management options for heart failure are designed to improve symptoms; some will improve survival, none cure the disease.
- Severity of heart failure is classified according to the New York Heart Association (NYHA) functional system:
  - Class I (no limitation of physical activity or symptoms, but heart failure symptoms in the past) to class IV (symptomatic at rest and discomfort from any physical activity).
  - NYHA grading allows assessment of symptomatic response to treatment.
- Further classification can be based upon which side of the heart is predominantly affected. Treatment is based on whether left ventricular systolic dysfunction (reduced LVEF) is present or not.

Symptoms

- Many patients with heart failure experience similar symptoms to those with advanced malignant disease, such as breathlessness, pain, fatigue, and depression.
- However, there are some symptoms of heart failure (such as fluid retention) that require disease-specific management. Disease-specific treatments are the mainstay of symptom control.
- Consequently, some modifications to general palliative symptom management are required to address the differing aetiology of symptoms in heart failure (described below).
- The risk of sudden death in patients with heart failure has declined, but this potential may still cause anxiety and underlines the need for advance care planning.
- Patients should be screened for depression.
- Initial management is pharmacological. However, cardiac resynchronization therapy pacing (CRT-P) or defibrillator (CRT-D) devices may improve cardiac function and symptoms.

Indicators of Poor Prognosis (Being in the Final Months to Year of Life) in Advanced Heart Failure

- NYHA grade III/IV with symptoms becoming resistant to maximum tolerated medications
- Increasing frequency of episodes of decompensation/hospitalization
- No further possible interventions
- Complications of heart failure or medications used to manage it (e.g., renal failure, hypotension at rest, hyponatraemia)
- Anaemia
- Life-limiting comorbidity
- Factors common to other LLI (i.e., cachexia, declining performance status)

Symptom Management Specific to End-Stage Heart Failure

- Medications designed to manage disease should be continued for as long as possible as they all have symptomatic benefit.

Medications Used to Manage Heart Failure (and Its Symptoms)

- *In patients with left ventricular systolic dysfunction:*
  - First line: ACE inhibitors and beta blockers
  - Second line (if symptoms despite first line medications): an aldosterone antagonist or an angiotensin II receptor antagonist
  - Digoxin if worsening heart failure despite first and second line treatment
  - Sacubitril valsartan (Entresto)
- *In all types of heart failure:*
  - Diuretics for relief of fluid retention/congestive symptoms
  - Amlodipine for hypertension and/or angina
  - Aspirin in atherosclerotic disease
  - Amiodarone, anticoagulants may be used

Managing Cardiac Medications to Improve Symptoms in Advanced End-Stage Heart Failure (Table 26.17)

- *Medications that improve survival and symptoms:*
  - Aldosterone antagonists, ACE inhibitors, angiotensin receptor blockers, beta blockers
  - Continue these for as long as possible
  - Consider dose reduction if symptomatic hypotension, worsening renal impairment, or tablet burden
- *Medications that improve symptoms:*
  - Loop diuretics: Continue unless patients become clinically hypovolaemic or anuric. To symptomatically manage fluid overload at the end of life. Furosemide may be given by CSCI, starting at a CSCI dose over 24 hours identical to their previous oral dose.

TABLE 26.17 Management of Medications in Advanced Cardiac Failure

Medications That Can Be Stopped Early	Medications to Continue as Long as Possible
Cholesterol-lowering drugs	Loop diuretics Note: Furosemide can be continued continuous subcutaneous infusion if required (see text)
Antihypertensives	ACE inhibitors
Digoxin (if in sinus rhythm or renal failure)	Beta blockers
Antiarrhythmic (if no symptomatic arrhythmia)	Angiotensin receptor blockers
	Aldosterone antagonists

- Antiarrhythmic: Continue if symptomatic tachycardia present. Otherwise, these can be discontinued relatively early.
- Antianginals. Can be stopped if no angina.
- Antihypertensives become less important in advanced cardiac failure. Stop if symptomatic hypotension.
- Digoxin should be stopped in renal failure, and in patients with sinus rhythm.

Secondary Prevention

- Cholesterol-lowering drugs can be discontinued early.

Pharmacological Considerations in End-Stage Heart Failure
Medications to Avoid

- Some medications may worsen symptoms and are best avoided; but a pragmatic approach must also be applied to symptom control—particularly for patients believed to be in the last days to week(s) of life.
- Concurrent renal failure may necessitate careful consideration of medications used to control symptoms, such as opioids (see section on renal failure).
- Medications to avoid where possible:
  - NSAIDs and cyclooxygenase 2 (COX-2) inhibitors: can exacerbate heart failure and fluid retention and may cause renal toxicity
  - Antimuscarinic medications, including cyclizine
  - Tricyclics: may exacerbate arrhythmias
  - Corticosteroids, progestogens
  - Medications that prolong the QT interval

Managing Cardiac Devices
Types of Implantable Cardiovascular Implanted Electronic Devices

- Patients with heart disease/failure may have one of several implantable devices. It is important to consider which type of device a patient has, as they are managed differently at end of life.
- Commonly encountered devices can be categorized as follows:
  - Pacemakers for bradycardia
  - Cardiac resynchronization therapy devices: These are biventricular pacemakers, used primarily for managing cardiac failure. If purely for pacing this is termed CRT-P. If it includes additional defibrillator component for patients at risk of ventricular arrhythmia causing sudden death this is termed CRT-D.
  - Implantable cardioverter defibrillator (ICD): for treatment of ventricular arrhythmia
- Patients with cardiac failure may have either CRT-P, CRT-D, or ICD.
- Note: More unusually, other devices with external components such as a left ventricular assist device (LVAD) may be present. Specialist advice should be sought on the management of these in patients at the end of life.

Deactivation of Defibrillator Component of Devices at End of Life

- The aim of deactivating the defibrillator function is to prevent inappropriate shocks at the end of life.
- Defibrillation shocks may be delivered by ICD or CRT-D devices.
- When the defibrillator function is deactivated, any pacing function is normally left unchanged.
- Deactivation of a defibrillator is not the same as a Do Not Attempt Cardiopulmonary Resuscitation (DNACPR) decision. Both require full discussion when possible.
- Discussion about the circumstances in which the defibrillator function of a device may be turned off should be started prior to implantation:
  - This should be revisited as a patient's condition deteriorates.
  - A competent patient can make a decision for deactivation at any stage.
  - It may be recorded in an advance care plan.
  - It should be explained to patients that deactivation is not painful, death is not likely to be immediate, and the pacemaker function will not be deactivated.

Practicalities of Defibrillator Deactivation

- *Planned deactivation (in the community):*
  - This should come as a shared, informed decision, often after several discussions with the patient, those important to the patient, and multidisciplinary teams involved in care.
  - The patient's informed consent should be recorded (or—if made in the person's best interests—appropriate people involved, and documentation completed).
  - The general practitioner, specialist nurse, or palliative care team should liaise with local cardiac services to arrange deactivation.

- Deactivation itself is undertaken by a cardiac physiologist who should be able to see the patient in his or her own home if necessary.
- *Emergency deactivation:*
  - Where there is no time to arrange a cardiac physiologist, temporary defibrillator deactivation can be achieved by placing a doughnut-shaped magnet over the device and taping it securely in place.
  - This should only be used only as a temporary measure while full deactivation is being arranged.
  - The magnet will not deactivate the pacemaker function.

Deactivation of Other Pacemaker Function at End of Life

- *Pacemakers for bradycardia:* These are not normally deactivated (as they aid symptom control), unless specifically requested by a patient.
- *CRT-P:* Not normally deactivated as beneficial in symptom control.
- In rare circumstances, patient may request deactivation of his or her pacemaker. This should be a shared, informed decision and deactivation undertaken by a cardiac physiologist as for a defibrillator.
- Note: CRT-P and pacemakers are not deactivated by magnets.

After Death

- An active pacemaker (including CRT-P) needs no immediate management.
- If still active, an ICD/CRT-D should be fully deactivated by a cardiac physiologist as soon as possible after death and before attempts are made to remove the device.
- All cardiovascular implanted electronic devices should be explanted prior to cremation. They are usually then returned to local device services for disposal.

Appendix 1

Routine Schedule of Immunizations

Age	Immunization
2 months	DTaP/IPV/Hib and PCV and MenB and Hep B Rotavirus (oral drops)
3 months	DTaP/IPV/Hib/Hep B Rotavirus (oral drops)
4 months	DTaP/IPV/Hib/Hep B and MenB and PCV
12–13 months	Hib/MenC and MMR and PCV and MenB
2–8 (up to 18 for children in clinical risk groups) years annually. Given at school to children from reception to year 4.	Nasal flu spray
3 years 4 months–5 years (preschool)	DTaP/IPV, or dTaP/IPV, and MMR
12–13 years (girls only)	HPV (2 doses given 6–24 months apart)
14 years (school year 9)	Td/IPV and MenACWY. Check MMR status and vaccinate if necessary.
65 onwards	Flu annually and PCV once
70 years	Shingles

aP, Acellular pertussis; *D,* diphtheria; *d,* low-dose diphtheria; *flu,* influenza; *Hep B,* hepatitis B; *Hib, Haemophilus influenzae* b; *HPV,* human papillomavirus; *IPV,* inactivated polio vaccine; *MenACWY,* meningitis A,C,W,Y; *MenB,* meningitis B; *MenC,* meningococcal C; *MMR,* mumps, measles, rubella; *PCV,* pneumococcal vaccine; *T,* tetanus.

Incubation Period and Infectivity of Common Diseases

Disease	Incubation Period	Period of Infectivity	Exclusion From School or Nursery
Bacillary dysentery (shigellosis)	1–7 days	Mean 7 days	For 48 hours after last diarrhoea
Campylobacter	1–10 days	1–3 weeks	For 48 hours after last diarrhoea
Cryptosporidiosis	1–14 days	2–4 weeks	For 48 hours after last diarrhoea
Enteroviral infection	2–3 days	1–2 weeks	None
Escherichia. coli enteritis	2–48 hours or longer	12 days or longer	For 48 hours after last diarrhoea
Gastroenteritis (rotaviral)	2–4 days	6–10 days	48 hours from last diarrhoea or vomiting
Gastroenteritis (adenoviral)	8–10 days	7–14 days	48 hours from last diarrhoea or vomiting
Gastroenteritis (Norwalk virus)	4–77 hours	0–3 days	3 days after onset
Gastroenteritis (unidentified)	N/A	N/A	48 hours from last diarrhoea or vomiting
Giardiasis	5–20 days	2 weeks	24 hours from last diarrhoea
Salmonellosis	4 hours to 5 days	Adults 4 weeks (median)	For 24 hours after last diarrhoea
Typhoid and paratyphoid	3–56 days	2 weeks to indefinite	Until 24 hours after last diarrhoea
Other Diseases			
Chickenpox	11–20 days	–4 to +5 days	5 days from start of rash
Conjunctivitis	3–29 days	2 weeks	None
Haemophilus influenzae	4–5 days	Indefinite (untreated)	24 hours from start of antibiotics
Head lice	N/A	Indefinite (untreated)	None
Hand, foot, and mouth disease	3–5 days	7 days	None
Hepatitis A	2–6 weeks	–17 days to +2 weeks	Exclude until 7 days after onset of jaundice or symptom onset if there is no jaundice
Hepatitis B	6 weeks to 6 months or longer		None (although may be too ill to attend during acute infection)
Hepatitis C	2 weeks to 6 months		None
Herpes simplex	1–6 days	1–8 weeks (primary infection)	None
		1–3 days (recurrence)	
Impetigo	N/A	N/A	Until lesions crusted or 48 hours after starting antibiotics
Infectious mononucleosis	33–49 days	At least 2 months	None
Influenza	1–3 days	3–7 days	None

Disease	Incubation Period	Period of Infectivity	Exclusion From School or Nursery
Measles	9–18 days	–2 to +3 days	From prodromal symptoms to 4 days after the onset of the rash
Meningococcal disease	N/A	Indefinite (untreated) <2 days (treated)	For the duration of the illness
Meningococcal infection	2–10 days		Until 48 hours after starting treatment
Mumps	15–24 days	Days –6 to +4	3 days before to 5 days after the start of the swelling
Pertussis	5–21 days	≥6 weeks, or 1 week if given a macrolide	48 hours after starting antibiotic treatment if they feel well enough to attend, or 21 days after onset of illness if no antibiotics given
Rabies	9 days to 9 weeks (possibly up to 2 years)	Until death	N/A
Rubella	15–20 days	Day 1–6	1 week before the rash appears to 6 days after
Scabies	7–27 days	Indefinite until treated	Until after first treatment
Scarlet fever	½–5 days	3 days if treated	24 hours after starting antibiotics
Slapped cheek disease	13–18 days	–6 to –3 (i.e., prodrome only)	None
Streptococcal pharyngitis	½–5 days	Indefinite (untreated)	None
Tetanus	4–21 days	Not contagious	None
Threadworms	2–4 weeks	Indefinite	None
Tinea	2–4 weeks	Indefinite	None
Tuberculosis	4 weeks to years	Smear positive: until 2 weeks after starting treatment	Until 2 weeks after starting treatment. No exlusion necessary for nonpulmonary Tb
Warts	1–24 months	While present	None

A Suggested Table of Immunizations for Travel

This schedule is for an adult who has been fully immunized as a child according to the UK recommendations. Few travellers will need all the immunizations below; they should only be given if appropriate to the travel planned. Individual health problems and exposure risks should always be taken into account. Other vaccines such as tuberculosis (TB) and chickenpox may be needed.

Day 0	Rabies, Japanese encephalitis, tickborne encephalitis, hepatitis B
Day 7	Rabies, Japanese encephalitis
Day 14	Tickborne encephalitis
Day 28	Rabies, Japanese encephalitis, hepatitis B
At some point in the above schedule (either together or spread out over the month). Immunization early in the month (at least 1 week before departure) will allow time for immunity to develop.	BCG, cholera, hepatitis A, meningococcal ACWY, polio, tetanus, and diphtheria (as Td), typhoid, yellow fever

If exposure to risk continues, further immunizations against hepatitis B will be needed at 2 months and at 1 year from the first dose, and against tickborne encephalitis at 9 months to 1 year after the last dose.

Appendix 4

Notification of Infectious Diseases

The notification of the following diseases is required by law in the United Kingdom, and the doctor is not excused from notification by considerations of confidentiality. The following list applies to England and Wales, with variations for Scotland and Northern Ireland indicated.

Acute Encephalitis	Malaria*
Acute Infectious Hepatitis*	Measles
Acute Meningitis	Meningococcal Septicaemia
Acute Poliomyelitis	Mumps
Anthrax	Plague
Botulism[†]	Rabies
Brucellosis[†]	Rubella
Cholera	Scarlet Fever*
Diphtheria	Severe Acute Respiratory Syndrome (SARS)[†]
Enteric Fever (typhoid or paratyphoid fever)	Smallpox
Food Poisoning*	Tetanus
Haemolytic Uraemic Syndrome[†]	Tuberculosis
Infectious Bloody Diarrhoea*,[†]	Typhus*
Invasive Group A Streptococcal Disease*,[†]	Viral Haemorrhagic Fever (VHF)
Legionnaires Disease*	Whooping Cough
Leprosy*,[†]	Yellow Fever

*Not in Scotland
[†]Not in Northern Ireland
Also notifiable in Scotland: Clinical syndrome due to *E. coli 0157* infection. Haemophilus influenza b. Necrotizing fasciitis. Tularaemia. West Nile Fever.
Also notifiable in Northern Ireland: Chickenpox. Dysentery. Gastroenteritis <2 years. Leptospirosis. Relapsing Fever.

Appendix 5

Child Health Promotion

History and Examination	Health Education
Neonatal Examination	
a. Elicit and consider concerns expressed by the parents	a. Feeding and nutrition b. Sleeping position
b. Review family history, pregnancy, and birth	c. Baby care
c. Assess risk of hearing defect and refer accordingly	d. Sibling management e. Crying and sleep problems
d. Full physical examination, including weight and head circumference	f. Transport in a car g. Advice on reducing risk of SIDS
e. Check for CDH and testicular descent	
f. Inspect eyes, check red reflex	
g. Check PKU, thyroid tests, cystic fibrosis, medium chain acyl-CoA deficiency have been done/are organized	
h. Screen for haemoglobinopathy, if relevant i. Vitamin K according to protocol j. Consider need for BCG and Hep B vac	
First 2 Weeks	
In addition to the neonatal examination:	
a. Assess the level of support and assistance that each new parent is likely to require b. Newborn hearing test	a. Nutrition b. The effects of passive smoking c. Accident prevention—bathing, scalding by feeds, fires d. Immunization
6–8 Weeks	
a. Check history, review growth and development, and ask about parental concerns	a. Immunization b. Nutrition c. Dangers of fires/falls/overheating/scalds
b. Physical examination, weight, head circumference (and length, if indicated); testes in boys	d. Recognition of illness and what to do
c. Check for CDH	
d. Enquire about concerns regarding vision, squint, and hearing	
e. Check whether the baby is in the high-risk category for hearing loss and refer if necessary	
f. Discuss and perform immunizations	
2, 3, and 4 Months and 13 Months	
a. Primary immunizations	

History and Examination	Health Education
6–9 Months	
a. Enquire about parental concerns regarding health and development, vision, and hearing	a. Accident prevention—choking, scalds, and burns (including sunburn), falls
b. Look for evidence of CDH c. Check for testicular descent	b. Anticipate increased mobility (eg, safety gates, guards)
d. Observe visual behaviour and look for squint	c. Nutrition d. Dental prophylaxis
e. Distraction test for hearing (HV) f. Infant feeding and obesity risk	e. Reinforce advice about safety in cars and passive smoking f. Developmental needs
18–24 Months	
a. Enquire about parental concerns particularly regarding behaviour, vision, and hearing	a. Accident prevention—falls from heights, drowning, poisoning, road safety
b. Confirm that the child is walking with a normal gait, and that speech and comprehension are appropriate for age c. Arrange detailed vision, hearing, or language assessment if indicated d. Remember the prevalence of iron deficiency anemia	b. Nutrition c. Developmental needs—language and play d. Need to mix with other children—playgroup, etc. e. Avoidance and management of behaviour problems
e. Measure height	

Note: Inform the community paediatric services if there is any anxiety about a child's educational potential.

36–54 Months	
a. Enquiry and discussion about vision, squint, hearing, behaviour, language acquisition, and development	a. Accidents—fires, roads, drowning b. Road safety
b. Discuss, if appropriate, whether the child is likely to have special educational problems and refer as appropriate	c. Preparation for school d. Nutrition and dental care
c. Measure the height and chart it	
d. Refer for hearing test if concerned	

Department of Health. (2004). *National service framework for children, young people, and maternity services*. London: DoH.

Appendix 6

Stages of Child Development

Summary of Development: Birth to 16 Weeks

	0–4 Weeks	6–8 Weeks	12–16 Weeks
Social	Watches mother and may smile	Responsive smile by 6 weeks and vocalizes	Recognizes family, shows pleasure
Motor			
Ventral suspension	Head hangs down until 3–4 weeks then up momentarily	Head held in horizontal plane, and briefly up by 8 weeks	Head maintained well above plane of body by 12 weeks
Prone	Head to side, pelvis high, knees drawn up under abdomen	Chin up intermittently at 6 weeks, well up at 8 weeks Pelvis flat	Head and shoulders up, and chest by 16 weeks Weight on forearms
Supine	Head to side, limbs flexed or ATNR posture	ATNR posture common but head to midline by 8 weeks	ATNR declining Head and hands now to midline
Pull-to-sit	Complete head lag	Less head lag	Slight head lag
Held sitting	Very round back Head drops forward	Back rounded Head briefly up	Back straighter and head up
Held standing	Walking and placing reflexes present until 6 weeks	Sags at hips and knees, getting head up by 8 weeks	Increasingly bears weight on legs
Hands	Strong grasp reflex Hands often closed	Grasp reflex present but slight by 8 weeks Fingers extend more often	Grasp reflex fades between 12 and 16 weeks Can hold rattle briefly
Vision	Blink and pupil reflexes Eye righting reflex Random movements but can fixate	Smoother conjugate eye movements Fixates on face/objects and follows through 45–90 degrees	Follows through 130 degrees Hand regard common (12–20 weeks)
Vocalization/hearing	Cries, stills, or startles to sounds	Eyes turn to sounds Starts vocalizing	Varied coos, squeals, and laughs Turns to sounds

ATNR, Asymmetric tonic neck reflex.

Summary of Development: 4–10 Months

	4–6 Months	6–8 Months	8–10 Months
Personal and social behaviour	Responsive to all comers Smiles at self in mirror Excited at approach of food	Discriminates between family and strangers Attracts attention Hand feeds biscuit	Wary of strangers Waves bye-bye Attempts to use spoon
Gross motor	No head lag in traction Rolls prone to supine Back straight in supported sitting	Lifts head up in supine Rolls supine to prone/creeps Sits without lateral support Bears weight on feet (5–8 months)	Sits steadily, pivots, and leans Can get from prone to sitting Pulls self to stand and crawls
Fine motor and vision	Reaches and grasps toys (4–6 months) Plays with toes Very alert visually	Transfers cube hand to hand (5–7 months) Can hold two cubes Any squint reported after 6 months is abnormal	Pincer grasp of pellet (8–12 months) Releases object and looks for it (7–11 months) Points at 1 mm sweet
Language and hearing	Varied sounds and squeals Consonants such as *ba* or *da*	Starts to babble *da-da* Turns to sounds (4–8 months)	Varied babble *ma-ma, ba-ba, da-da* Indicates and understands "no" Locates sounds well

Summary of Development: 12–24 Months

	12–15 Months	18–24 Months
Personal and social behaviour	Shows affection and may be shy Indicates wants, points, claps hands (10–18 months)	Becoming egocentric, clinging, and resistant Loves domestic mimicry
	Mouthing stops (12–15 months) Enjoys casting (12–15 months)	Definitely stopped mouthing and casting (by 18 months)
	May manage cup and spoon with spills (10–17 months)	Helps undress Independent with cup and spoon (15–24 months)
Gross motor	Walks holding on (8–12 months)	Walks well (12–18 months)
	Walks alone (11–15 months)	Climbs stairs, kneels (14–22 months)
Fine motor and vision	Fine pincer grasp Bangs bricks together (8–14 months) Holds two cubes Scribbles (12–18 months)	May show hand preference (after 15 months) Builds 2 to 3 cubes Turns pages (15–24 months)
Language and hearing	*Mama, Dada,* with meaning (9–15 months) Three to four clear words (12–18 months)	Can point to three parts of body, has 6–20 words and jargon (15–24 months)

Summary of Development: 2–5 Years

	2–3 Years	3–4 Years	5 Years Old
Personal and social skills	Enjoys solitary play, alongside peers, not sharing Possessive: tantrums if thwarted Feeds quite neatly, using spoon and fork or fingers May be clean and dry by day, with supervision, or may refuse to cooperate	Plays with peers, sharing toys Enjoys make-believe play Shows concern and sympathy for others, and able to take turns by 4 years Easily manages spoon and fork and then knife Mostly dry day and night Can wash hands, dress and undress by 4 years, except fastenings	Plays complicated cooperative games Makes friends Comforts playmates and siblings in distress Almost completely independent in self-help skills now Can carry out simple domestic tasks and run errands
Gross motor	Now very mobile Runs, kicks ball, tries to throw Walks up and down stairs two feet to a step Propels tricycle by pushing with feet on floor	Up stairs one foot per step at 3, and down by 4 years Can walk, then run on tip-toe, and hop, by 4 years Enjoys climbing, pedals a tricycle skillfully	Enjoys running, jumping, climbing, swings and slides, and starting to play ball games Can stand on one leg, hop 10 times, and heel-toe walk a narrow line
Fine motor and vision	Neat prehension, and controlled release Tower of 6–8 bricks Holds pencil in fist Circular scribble (24 months) copies vertical line, imitates circle (30 months) Simple puzzles and can thread large beads Difficult age to test vision Recognizes two-dimensional symbols and may match letters at 30 months	Tower of 9–10 and imitates 3 cube bridge at 3 years, steps or gate by 4 years Awkward tripod grasp of pencil at 3 years—copies circle and imitates cross Dynamic tripod after 4 years; draws man with head, trunk, and legs Can do letter-matching vision tests, using linear charts, each eye separately, by 3½ to 4 years	Can write name, copy a square and a triangle Draws man with detailed features and limbs Can fold paper and use scissors to cut out shapes Performs Snellen chart type of vision test
Language and hearing	Listens to simple stories and understands two-part instructions Can say 50–100 single words and join two to three ("Daddy gone car") Many questions: what? and who? Long monologues, still some jargon, enjoys nursery rhymes and jingles Toy tests of hearing or may point to named pictures	Intelligible but immature speech, 3–5 word sentences, knows name and sex, at 3 years Long stories, constant more abstract questions, grammar mostly correct, and speech clear, by 4 years Knows age and address, 6+ colours and can count to 4+ Can do cooperative (conditioned) hearing tests	Enjoys riddles and jokes Understands negatives and complex questions and instructions Gives long descriptions and explanations Speech easily intelligible with few errors Manages full audiometry and speech discrimination now

Stages of Puberty

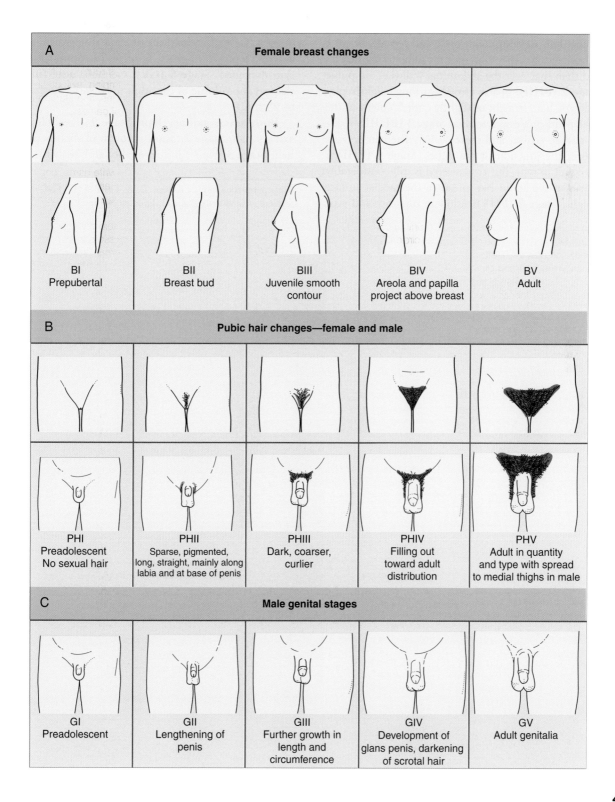

A   **Female breast changes**

BI
Prepubertal

BII
Breast bud

BIII
Juvenile smooth
contour

BIV
Areola and papilla
project above breast

BV
Adult

B   **Pubic hair changes—female and male**

PHI
Preadolescent
No sexual hair

PHII
Sparse, pigmented,
long, straight, mainly along
labia and at base of penis

PHIII
Dark, coarser,
curlier

PHIV
Filling out
toward adult
distribution

PHV
Adult in quantity
and type with spread
to medial thighs in male

C   **Male genital stages**

GI
Preadolescent

GII
Lengthening of
penis

GIII
Further growth in
length and
circumference

GIV
Development of
glans penis, darkening
of scrotal hair

GV
Adult genitalia

(A) The stages of breast development in a female. Stage 1 (BI): Preadolescent: elevation in papilla only. **Stage 2 (BII):** Breast bud stage: elevation of breast and papilla as a small mound. Enlargement of areolar diameter. **Stage 3 (BIII):** Further enlargement and elevation of breast and areola, with no separation of their contours. **Stage 4 (BIV):** Projection of areola and papilla to form a secondary mound above the level of the breast. **Stage 5 (BV):** Mature stage; projection of papilla only, due to recession of the areola to the general contour of the breast. (This last stage may not be reached in women until after their first pregnancy.)

(B) Pubic hair development: male and female. Stage 1 (PHI): Preadolescent. The vellus over the pubes is not further developed than that over the abdominal wall (i.e., no pubic hair). **Stage 2 (PHII):** Sparse growth of long, slightly pigmented downy hair, straight or slightly curled, chiefly at the base of the penis or along the labia. **Stage 3 (PHIII):** Considerably darker, coarser and more curled. The hair spreads sparsely over the junction of the pubes. **Stage 4 (PHIV):** Hair now adult in type, but area covered is still considerably smaller than in the adult. No spread to the medial surface of the thighs. **Stage 5 (PHV):** Adult in quantity and type with distribution of the horizontal (or classically feminine) pattern. Spread to medial surface of thighs but not up linea alba or elsewhere above the base of the inverse triangle (spread up linea alba occurs later and is rated Stage 6).

(C) Male genital development. Stage 1 (GI): Preadolescent: testes, scrotum, and penis are of about the same size and proportion as in early childhood. **Stage 2 (GII):** Enlargement of scrotum, and testes. Skin of scrotum reddens and changes in texture. Little or no enlargement of penis at this stage. **Stage 3 (GIII):** Enlargement of penis, which occurs at first mainly in length. Further growth of testes and scrotum. **Stage 4 (GIV):** Increased size of penis with growth in breadth and development of glans. Testes and scrotum larger; scrotal skin darkened. **Stage 5 (GV):** Genitalia adult in size and shape. (The volume of the adult testis varies in size from 12 to 25 mL.)

Both sexes: axillary hair. Stage 1: Preadolescent. No axillary hair. **Stage 2:** Scanty growth of slightly pigmented hair. **Stage 3:** Hair adult in quality and quantity.

With permission from Lissauer, T., & Clayden, G. (2005). *Illustrated textbook of paediatrics* (3rd ed.). London: Mosby.

Appendix 8

Predicted Normal Peak Flow Values in Children (Under 15 Years of Age)

Height		Peak Flows (L/min)
(cm)	(ft–in)	
91	3–0	100
99	3–3	120
107	3–6	140
114	3–9	170
122	4–0	210
130	4–3	250
137	4–6	285
145	4–9	325
152	5–0	360
160	5–3	400
168	5–6	440
175	5–9	480

Appendix 9

Peak Expiratory Flow in Normal Subjects

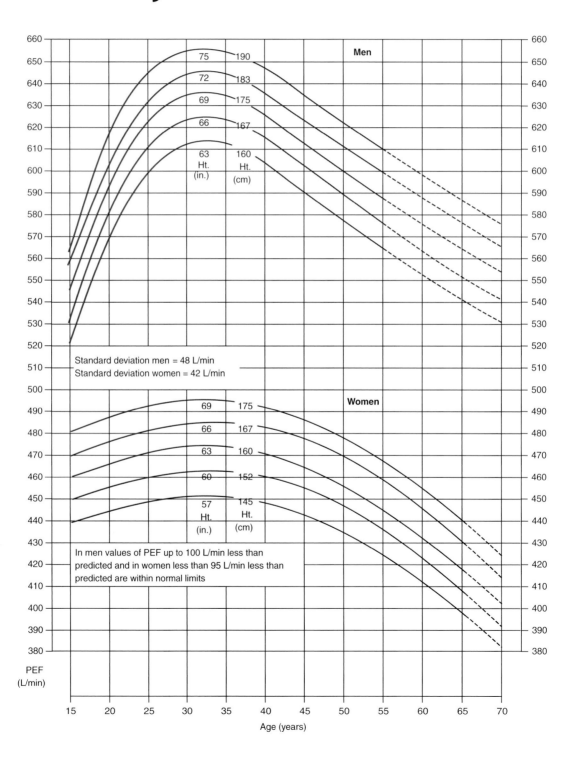

Standard deviation men = 48 L/min
Standard deviation women = 42 L/min

In men values of PEF up to 100 L/min less than predicted and in women less than 95 L/min less than predicted are within normal limits

PEF (L/min)

Age (years)

Appendix 10

FEV$_1$/FVC Charts

Females

Age (Years)		Height (m)							
		1.45	1.50	1.55	1.60	1.65	1.70	1.75	1.80
25	FEV$_1$	2.5	2.7	2.9	3.1	3.4	3.6	3.8	4.0
	FVC	2.9	3.1	3.3	3.6	3.8	4.0	4.2	4.4
30	FEV$_1$	2.4	2.6	2.8	3.0	3.2	3.4	3.7	3.9
	FVC	2.8	3.0	3.2	3.4	3.6	3.9	4.1	4.3
35	FEV$_1$	2.3	2.5	2.7	2.9	3.1	3.3	3.5	3.7
	FVC	2.6	2.9	3.1	3.3	3.5	3.7	4.0	4.2
40	FEV$_1$	2.1	2.3	2.6	2.8	3.0	3.2	3.4	3.6
	FVC	2.5	2.7	2.9	3.2	3.4	3.6	3.8	4.0
45	FEV$_1$	2.0	2.2	2.4	2.6	2.9	3.1	3.3	3.5
	FVC	2.4	2.6	2.8	3.0	3.3	3.5	3.7	3.9
50	FEV$_1$	1.9	2.1	2.3	2.5	2.7	2.9	3.2	3.4
	FVC	2.2	2.5	2.7	2.9	3.1	3.3	3.6	3.8
55	FEV$_1$	1.8	2.0	2.2	2.4	2.6	2.8	3.0	3.2
	FVC	2.1	2.3	2.6	2.8	3.0	3.2	3.4	3.7
60	FEV$_1$	1.6	1.8	2.1	2.3	2.5	2.7	2.9	3.1
	FVC	2.0	2.2	2.4	2.6	2.9	3.1	3.3	3.5
65	FEV$_1$	1.5	1.7	1.9	2.1	2.4	2.6	2.8	3.0
	FVC	1.8	2.1	2.3	2.5	2.7	3.0	3.2	3.4
70	FEV$_1$	1.4	1.6	1.8	2.0	2.2	2.4	2.7	2.9
	FVC	1.7	1.9	2.2	2.4	2.6	2.8	3.0	3.3

Males

Age (Years)		Height (m)							
		1.55	1.60	1.65	1.70	1.75	1.80	1.85	1.90
25	FEV$_1$	3.4	3.6	3.8	4.1	4.3	4.5	4.7	5.0
	FVC	3.9	4.2	4.5	4.8	5.1	5.4	5.7	6.0
30	FEV$_1$	3.3	3.5	3.7	3.9	4.2	4.4	4.6	4.8
	FVC	3.8	4.1	4.4	4.7	5.0	5.3	5.5	5.8
35	FEV$_1$	3.1	3.3	3.6	3.8	4.0	4.2	4.5	4.7
	FVC	3.7	4.0	4.3	4.5	4.8	5.1	5.4	5.7
40	FEV$_1$	3.0	3.2	3.4	3.6	3.9	4.1	4.3	4.5
	FVC	3.6	3.8	4.1	4.4	4.7	5.0	5.3	5.6
45	FEV$_1$	2.8	3.0	3.3	3.5	3.7	3.9	4.2	4.4
	FVC	3.4	3.7	4.0	4.3	4.6	4.9	5.2	5.4
50	FEV$_1$	2.7	2.9	3.1	3.3	3.6	3.8	4.0	4.2
	FVC	3.3	3.6	3.9	4.2	4.4	4.7	5.0	5.3
55	FEV$_1$	2.5	2.8	3.0	3.2	3.4	3.7	3.9	4.1
	FVC	3.2	3.5	3.7	4.0	4.3	4.6	4.9	5.2
60	FEV$_1$	2.4	2.6	2.8	3.1	3.3	3.5	3.7	4.0
	FVC	3.0	3.3	3.6	3.9	4.2	4.5	4.8	5.0
65	FEV$_1$	2.2	2.5	2.7	2.9	3.1	3.4	3.6	3.8
	FVC	2.9	3.2	3.5	3.8	4.1	4.3	4.6	4.9
70	FEV$_1$	2.1	2.3	2.5	2.8	3.0	3.2	3.4	3.7
	FVC	2.8	3.1	3.3	3.6	3.9	4.2	4.4	4.8

Girls

Height		FEV$_1$	FVC
Metres	Inches		
0.80	32	0.41	0.46
0.90	35	0.56	0.64
1.00	39	0.75	0.86
1.10	43	0.98	1.11
1.20	47	1.24	1.43
1.30	51	1.55	1.79
1.40	55	1.90	2.20
1.50	59	2.29	2.68
1.60	63	2.73	3.22
1.70	67	3.23	3.82
1.80	71	3.77	4.48

Boys

Height		FEV$_1$	FVC
Metres	Inches		
0.80	32	0.40	0.46
0.90	35	0.56	0.65
1.00	39	0.76	0.89
1.10	43	1.00	1.17
1.20	47	1.28	1.52
1.30	51	1.61	1.92
1.40	55	2.00	2.38
1.50	59	2.43	2.92
1.60	63	2.93	3.53
1.70	67	3.49	4.22
1.80	71	4.11	4.99

Summary of Management of Asthma in Adults

Reproduced from Scottish Intercollegiate Guidelines Network and British Thoracic Society. (2016). *British guideline on the management of asthma.*

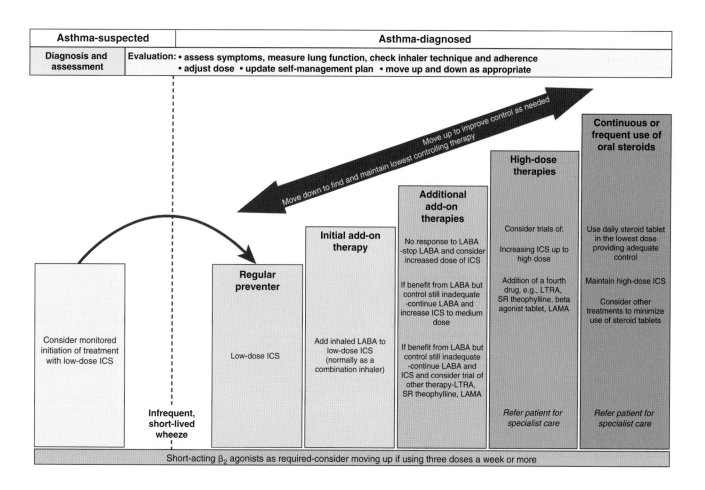

Summary of Management of Asthma in Children

Reproduced from Scottish Intercollegiate Guidelines Network and British Thoracic Society. (2016). *British guideline on the management of asthma.*

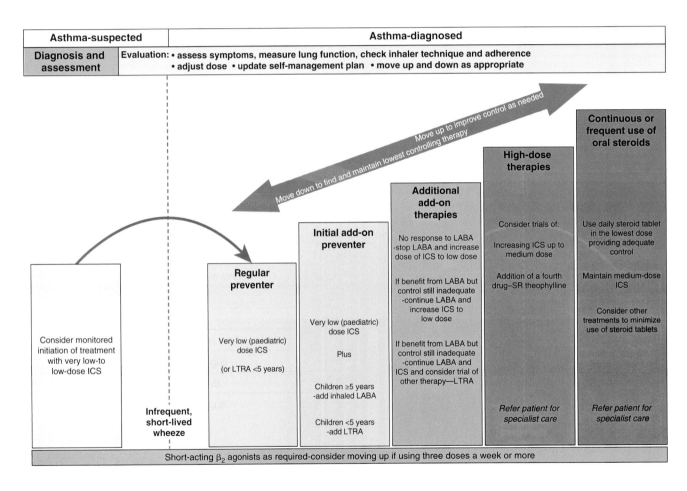

Appendix 11C

Management of Acute Severe Asthma in Adults in General Practice

Reproduced from Scottish Intercollegiate Guidelines Network and British Thoracic Society. (2016). *British guideline on the management of asthma.*

Management of acute severe asthma in adults in general practice

Many deaths from asthma are preventable. Delay can be fatal. Factors leading to poor outcome include:

- Clinical staff failing to assess severity by objective measurement
- Patients or relatives failing to appreciate severity
- Underuse of corticosteroids

Regard each emergency asthma consultation as for acute severe asthma until shown otherwise.

Assess and record:

- Peak expiratory flow (PEF)
- Symptoms and response to self treatment
- Heart and respiratory rates
- Oxygen saturation (by pulse oximetry)

Caution: Patients with severe or life-threatening attacks may not be distressed and may not have all the abnormalities listed below. The presence of any should alert the doctor.

Moderate asthma	Acute severe asthma	Life-threatening asthma

INITIAL ASSESSMENT

PEF >50%–75% best or predicted	PEF 33%–50% best or predicted	PEF <33% best or predicted

FURTHER ASSESSMENT

• SpO$_2$ ≥92% • Speech normal • Respiration <25 breaths/min • Pulse <110 beats/min	• SpO$_2$ ≥92% • Can't complete sentences • Respiration ≥25 breaths/min • Pulse ≥110 beats/min	• SpO$_2$ <92% • Silent chest, cyanosis or poor respiratory effort • Arrhythmia or hypotension • Exhaustion, altered consciousness

MANAGEMENT

Treat at home or in surgery and ASSESS RESPONSE TO TREATMENT	**Consider admission**	**Arrange immediate ADMISSION**

TREATMENT

• β$_2$ Bronchodilator:
  – via spacer (give 4 puffs initially and give a further 2 puffs every 2 minutes according to response up to maximum of 10 puffs)
 	
If PEF >50%–75% predicted/best:
• Nebulizer (preferably oxygen driven) (salbutamol 5 mg)
• Give prednisolone 40–50 mg
• Continue or increase usual treatment
 	
If good response to first treatment (symptoms improved, respiration and pulse settling and PEF >50%) continue or increase usual treatment and continue prednisolone
	• Oxygen to maintain SpO$_2$ 94%–98% if available
	• β$_2$ Bronchodilator:
	  – nebulizer (preferably oxygen driven) (salbutamol 5 mg)
	  – or via spacer (give 4 puffs initially and give a further 2 puffs every 2 minutes according to response up to maximum of 10 puffs)
	• Prednisolone 40–50 mg or IV hydrocortisone 100 mg
	• **If no response in acute severe asthma: ADMIT**
		• Oxygen to maintain SpO$_2$ 94%–98%
		• β$_2$ Bronchodilator and ipratropium:
		  – nebulizer (preferably oxygen driven) (salbutamol 5 mg and ipratropium 0.5 mg)
		  – or via spacer (give 4 puffs initially and give a further 2 puffs every 2 minutes according to response up to maximum of 10 puffs)
		• Prednisolone 40–50 mg or IV hydrocortisone 100 mg immediately

Admit to hospital if any: • Life-threatening features • Features of acute severe asthma present after initial treatment • Previous near-fatal asthma Lower threshold for admission if afternoon or evening attack, recent nocturnal symptoms or hospital admission, previous severe attacks, patient unable to assess own condition, or concern over social circumstances	**If admitting the patient to hospital:** • Stay with patient until ambulance arrives • Send written assessment and referral details to hospital • β$_2$ bronchodilator via oxygen-driven **nebulizer in ambulance**	**Follow up after treatment or discharge from hospital:** • **GP review within 2 working days** • Monitor symptoms and PEF • Check inhaler technique • **Written asthma action plan** • Modify treatment according to guidelines for chronic persistent asthma • Address potentially preventable contributors to admission

Management of Acute Severe Asthma in Children in General Practice

Reproduced from Scottish Intercollegiate Guidelines Network and British Thoracic Society. (2016). *British guideline on the management of asthma.*

Management of acute asthma in children in general practice

Age 2–5 years

ASSESS AND RECORD ASTHMA SEVERITY

Moderate asthma
- SpO_2 ≥92%
- Able to talk
- Heart rate ≤140/min
- Respiratory rate ≤40/min

Acute severe asthma
- SpO_2 <92%
- Too breathless to talk
- Heart rate >140/min
- Respiratory rate >40/min
- Use of accessory neck muscles

Life-threatening asthma
SpO_2 <92% plus any of:
- Silent chest
- Poor respiratory effort
- Agitation
- Confusion
- Cyanosis

Moderate asthma path:
- $β_2$ agonist 2–10 puffs via spacer and facemask (given one puff at a time inhaled separately using tidal breathing)
- Give one puff of $β_2$ agonist every 30–60 seconds up to 10 puffs according to response
- Consider oral prednisolone 20 mg

Acute severe asthma path:
- Oxygen via face mask
- 10 puffs of $β_2$ agonist or nebulized salbutamol 2.5 mg
- Oral prednisolone 20 mg

Life-threatening asthma path:
- Oxygen via face mask
- Nebulize every 20 minutes with:
  - salbutamol 2.5 mg
  +
  - ipratropium 0.25 mg
- Oral prednisolone 20 mg
  or
- IV hydrocortisone 50 mg if vomiting

Assess response to treatment 15 mins after $β_2$ agonist

IF POOR RESPONSE ARRANGE ADMISSION

IF POOR RESPONSE REPEAT $β_2$ AGONIST AND ARRANGE ADMISSION

REPEAT $β_2$ AGONIST VIA OXYGEN-DRIVEN NEBULIZER WHILST ARRANGING IMMEDIATE HOSPITAL ADMISSION

GOOD RESPONSE
- Continue $β_2$ agonist via spacer or nebulizer, as needed but not exceeding 4 hourly
- **If symptoms are not controlled repeat $β_2$ agonist and refer to hospital**
- Continue prednisolone for up to 3 days
- Arrange follow-up clinic visit within 48 hours
- Consider referral to secondary care asthma clinic if 2nd attack within 12 months

POOR RESPONSE
- Stay with patient until ambulance arrives
- Send written assessment and referral details
- Repeat $β_2$ agonist via oxygen-driven nebulizer in ambulance

---

LOWER THRESHOLD FOR ADMISSION IF:
- Attack in late afternoon or at night
- Recent hospital admission or previous severe attack
- Concern over social circumstances or ability to cope at home

NB: If a patient has signs and symptoms across categories, always treat according to their most severe features

Age >5 years

ASSESS AND RECORD ASTHMA SEVERITY

Moderate asthma
- SpO_2 ≥92%
- Able to talk
- Heart rate ≤125/min
- Respiratory rate ≤30/min
- PEF ≥50% best or predicted

Acute severe asthma
- SpO_2 <92%
- Too breathless to talk
- Heart rate >125/min
- Respiratory rate >30/min
- Use of accessory neck muscles
- PEF 33%–50% best or predicted

Life-threatening asthma
SpO_2 <92% plus any of:
- Silent chest
- Poor respiratory effort
- Agitation
- Confusion
- Cyanosis
- PEF <33% best or predicted

Moderate asthma path:
- $β_2$ agonist 2–10 puffs via spacer and mouthpiece (given one puff at a time inhaled separately using tidal breathing)
- Give one puff of $β_2$ agonist every 30–60 seconds up to 10 puffs according to response
- Consider oral prednisolone 30–40 mg

Acute severe asthma path:
- Oxygen via face mask
- 10 puffs of $β_2$ agonist or nebulized salbutamol 5 mg
- Oral prednisolone 30–40 mg

Life-threatening asthma path:
- Oxygen via face mask
- Nebulize every 20 minutes with:
  - salbutamol 5 mg
  +
  - ipratropium 0.25 mg
- Oral prednisolone 30–40 mg
  or
- IV hydrocortisone 100 mg if vomiting

Assess response to treatment 15 mins after $β_2$ agonist

IF POOR RESPONSE ARRANGE ADMISSION

IF POOR RESPONSE REPEAT $β_2$ AGONIST AND ARRANGE ADMISSION

REPEAT $β_2$ AGONIST VIA OXYGEN-DRIVEN NEBULIZER WHILST ARRANGING IMMEDIATE HOSPITAL ADMISSION

GOOD RESPONSE
- Continue $β_2$ agonist via spacer or nebulizer, as needed but not exceeding 4 hourly
- **If symptoms are not controlled repeat $β_2$ agonist and refer to hospital**
- Continue prednisolone for up to 3 days
- Arrange follow-up clinic visit within 48 hours
- Consider referral to secondary care asthma clinic if 2nd attack within 12 months

POOR RESPONSE
- Stay with patient until ambulance arrives
- Send written assessment and referral details
- Repeat $β_2$ agonist via oxygen-driven nebulizer in ambulance

---

LOWER THRESHOLD FOR ADMISSION IF:
- Attack in late afternoon or at night
- Recent hospital admission or previous severe attack
- Concern over social circumstances or ability to cope at home

NB: If a patient has signs and symptoms across categories, always treat according to their most severe features

Appendix 12

Care Pathway for Respiratory Tract Infections

Care pathway for respiratory tract infections (RTIs)

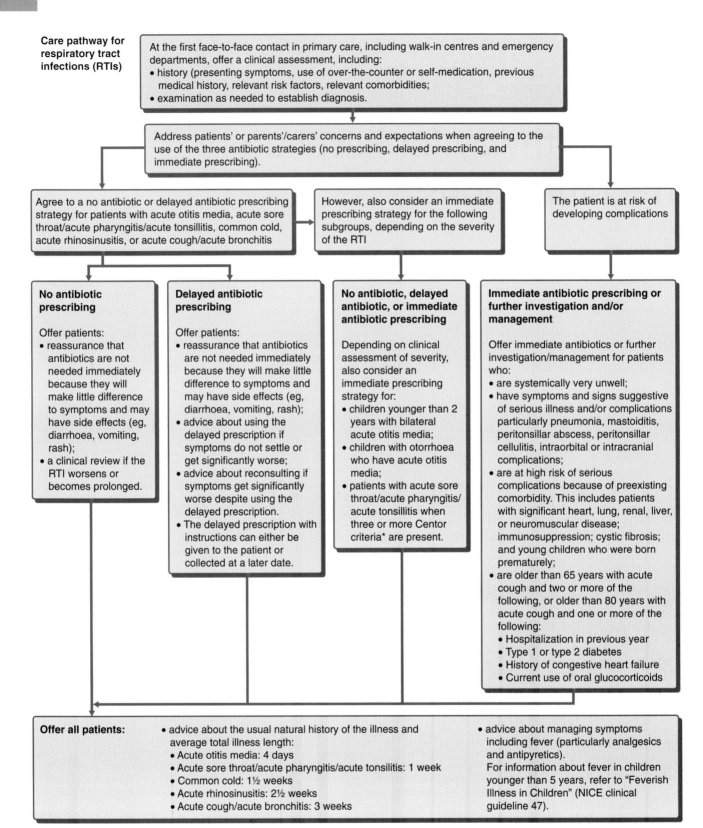

At the first face-to-face contact in primary care, including walk-in centres and emergency departments, offer a clinical assessment, including:
- history (presenting symptoms, use of over-the-counter or self-medication, previous medical history, relevant risk factors, relevant comorbidities;
- examination as needed to establish diagnosis.

Address patients' or parents'/carers' concerns and expectations when agreeing to the use of the three antibiotic strategies (no prescribing, delayed prescribing, and immediate prescribing).

Agree to a no antibiotic or delayed antibiotic prescribing strategy for patients with acute otitis media, acute sore throat/acute pharyngitis/acute tonsillitis, common cold, acute rhinosinusitis, or acute cough/acute bronchitis

However, also consider an immediate prescribing strategy for the following subgroups, depending on the severity of the RTI

The patient is at risk of developing complications

No antibiotic prescribing

Offer patients:
- reassurance that antibiotics are not needed immediately because they will make little difference to symptoms and may have side effects (eg, diarrhoea, vomiting, rash);
- a clinical review if the RTI worsens or becomes prolonged.

Delayed antibiotic prescribing

Offer patients:
- reassurance that antibiotics are not needed immediately because they will make little difference to symptoms and may have side effects (eg, diarrhoea, vomiting, rash);
- advice about using the delayed prescription if symptoms do not settle or get significantly worse;
- advice about reconsulting if symptoms get significantly worse despite using the delayed prescription.
- The delayed prescription with instructions can either be given to the patient or collected at a later date.

No antibiotic, delayed antibiotic, or immediate antibiotic prescribing

Depending on clinical assessment of severity, also consider an immediate prescribing strategy for:
- children younger than 2 years with bilateral acute otitis media;
- children with otorrhoea who have acute otitis media;
- patients with acute sore throat/acute pharyngitis/acute tonsillitis when three or more Centor criteria* are present.

Immediate antibiotic prescribing or further investigation and/or management

Offer immediate antibiotics or further investigation/management for patients who:
- are systemically very unwell;
- have symptoms and signs suggestive of serious illness and/or complications particularly pneumonia, mastoiditis, peritonsillar abscess, peritonsillar cellulitis, intraorbital or intracranial complications;
- are at high risk of serious complications because of preexisting comorbidity. This includes patients with significant heart, lung, renal, liver, or neuromuscular disease; immunosuppression; cystic fibrosis; and young children who were born prematurely;
- are older than 65 years with acute cough and two or more of the following, or older than 80 years with acute cough and one or more of the following:
  - Hospitalization in previous year
  - Type 1 or type 2 diabetes
  - History of congestive heart failure
  - Current use of oral glucocorticoids

Offer all patients:
- advice about the usual natural history of the illness and average total illness length:
  - Acute otitis media: 4 days
  - Acute sore throat/acute pharyngitis/acute tonsilitis: 1 week
  - Common cold: 1½ weeks
  - Acute rhinosinusitis: 2½ weeks
  - Acute cough/acute bronchitis: 3 weeks
- advice about managing symptoms including fever (particularly analgesics and antipyretics).

For information about fever in children younger than 5 years, refer to "Feverish Illness in Children" (NICE clinical guideline 47).

*Centor criteria are presence of tonsillar exudate, tender anterior lymphadenopathy or lymphadenitis, history of fever, and an absence of cough.
Reproduced with permission from National Insititute for Health and Care Excellence. (2008). *Respiratory tract infections—antibiotic prescribing. NICE clinical guideline 69.* www.nice.org.uk.

Guidance for DMARD Prescribing

GUIDELINE

British Society of Rheumatology. (2017). BSR and BHPR guideline for the prescription and monitoring of non-biologic disease-modifying anti-rheumatic drugs. *Rheumatology*, *56*(6), 865–868.

Generic Recommendations Before Commencing Any DMARD

a. The decision to initiate DMARDs should be made in conjunction with the patient/carer and be supervised by an expert in the management of rheumatic diseases.
b. Patients should be provided with education about their treatment to promote self-management.
c. When appropriate, patients should be advised about the impact of DMARD therapy upon fertility, pregnancy, and breastfeeding.
d. Baseline assessment should include height, weight, blood pressure, and laboratory evaluation: FBC, eGFR, ALT, and/or AST, albumin.
e. Patients should be assessed for comorbidities because these may influence DMARD choice, including evaluation for respiratory disease and screening for occult viral infection.
f. Vaccinations against pneumococcus and influenza are recommended.

Drug-Specific Recommendations

- *Methotrexate*: All patients should be co-prescribed folic acid supplementation at a minimal dose of 5 mg once weekly to be taken on a different day than the methotrexate.
- *Azathioprine*: Patients should have baseline thiopurine methyltransferase (TPMT) status assessed.
- *Hydroxychloroquine*: Patients should have baseline formal ophthalmic examination, ideally including objective retinal assessment (e.g., using optical coherence tomography) within 1 year of commencing an antimalarial drug.

Prescribing DMARDS in Patients With Comorbidities

- Pre-existing lung disease is not a specific contraindication to DMARD therapy; however, caution is advised when using drugs associated with pneumonitis in patients with poor respiratory reserve.
- In patients with deranged liver biochemistry, hepatotoxic DMARDs should be used with caution, with careful attention to trends in test results.
- In patients with impaired liver synthetic function (e.g., cirrhosis), DMARD therapy should be used with extreme caution.
- Patients with chronic viral hepatitis infection should be considered for antiviral treatment prior to immunosuppressive DMARD initiation.
- DMARDs must be used with caution in chronic kidney disease, with appropriate dose reduction and increased frequency of monitoring.
- Cardiovascular disease and prior malignancy are not considered contraindications to DMARD therapy.

Drug Monitoring

Recommended DMARD Blood Monitoring Schedule When Starting or Adding a New DMARD

- Check FBC, creatinine/calculated GFR, ALT and/or AST, and albumin every 2 weeks until on stable dose for 6 weeks; then once on stable dose, monthly FBC, creatinine/calculated GFR, ALT and/or AST, and albumin for 3 months; thereafter, FBC, creatinine/calculated GFR, ALT and/or AST, and albumin at least every 12 weeks. More frequent monitoring is appropriate in patients at higher risk of toxicity.
- Dose increases should be monitored by FBC, creatinine/calculated GFR, ALT and/or AST, and albumin every 2 weeks until on stable dose for 6 weeks then revert to previous schedule.

Drug Specific Monitoring Recommendations

Summary of Monitoring Requirements

Drug	Laboratory Monitoring	Other Monitoring
Apremilast	No routine laboratory monitoring	None
Azathioprine	Standard monitoring schedule[a]	None
Ciclosporin	Extend monthly monitoring longer term	BP and glucose at each monitoring visit
Gold	Standard monitoring schedule[a]	Urinalysis for blood and protein prior to each dose
Hydroxychloroquine	No routine laboratory monitoring	Annual eye assessment (ideally including optical coherence tomography) if continued for >5 years
Leflunomide	Standard monitoring schedule[a]	BP and weight at each monitoring visit
Mepacrine	No routine laboratory monitoring	None
Methotrexate	Standard monitoring schedule	None
Methotrexate and leflunomide combined	Extend monthly monitoring longer term	None
Minocycline	No routine laboratory monitoring	None
Mycophenolate	Standard monitoring schedule	None
Sulfasalazine	Standard monitoring schedule for 12 months then no routine monitoring needed	None
Tacrolimus	Extend monthly monitoring longer term	BP and glucose at each monitoring visit

BP, Blood pressure.
[a]Standard monitoring schedule as per the guidance in 'Drug Monitoring'

Perioperative DMARD Management

- Steroid exposure should be minimized prior to surgical procedures; and increases in steroid dose to prevent adrenal insufficiency are not routinely required.
- DMARD therapy should not routinely be stopped in the perioperative period, although individualized decisions should be made for high-risk procedures.

Intercurrent Infections

- During a serious infection, methotrexate, leflunomide, sulfasalazine, azathioprine, apremilast, mycophenolate mofetil, ciclosporin, and tacrolimus should be temporarily discontinued until the patient has recovered from the infection.

Recommendations for Shared Care Agreements

- The prescriber has responsibility for ensuring patients are adhering to monitoring guidance.

- When prescribing takes place in primary care, it should be supported by local written shared care agreements, highlighting responsibilities of each party (patient, secondary care, primary care).
- Contact rheumatology team urgently and consider interruption in treatment if any of the following develop: white cell count $<3.5 \times 10^9$/L; mean cell volume >105 fL; neutrophils $<1.6 \times 10^9$/L; creatinine increase >30% over 12 months and/or calculated GFR <60 mL/min; unexplained eosinophilia $>0.5 \times 10^9$/L; ALT and/or AST >100 units/L; platelet count $<140 \times 10^9$/L; unexplained reduction in albumin <30 g/L.
- As well as responding to absolute values in laboratory tests, it is also relevant to observe trends in results (e.g., gradual decreases in white blood cells or albumin, or increasing liver enzymes).
- For clinically urgent abnormalities, emergency access to specialist rheumatology advice, with response within one working day, should be available as per National Institute for Health and Care Excellence guidelines.

Dermatomes and Myotomes

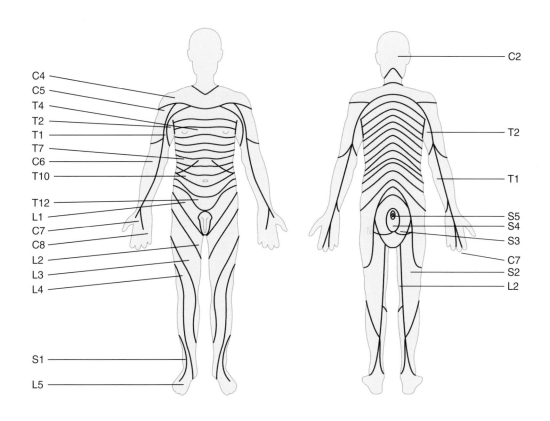

Muscle group	Nerve supply	Reflexes
Diaphragm	C(3), 4, (5)	
Shoulder abductors	C5	
Elbow flexors	C5, 6	Biceps jerk C5, 6
Supinators/pronators	C6	Supinator jerk C6
Wrist extensors	C6	
Wrist flexors	C7	
Elbow extensors	C7	Triceps jerk C7
Finger extensors	C7	
Finger flexors	C8	
Intrinsic hand muscles	T1	Abdominal reflex T8–12
Hip flexors	L1, 2	
Hip adductors	L2, 3	
Knee extensors	L3, 4	Knee jerk L3, 4
Ankle dorsiflexors	L4, 5	
Toe extensors	L5	
Knee flexors	L4, 5 S1	
Ankle plantar flexors	S1, 2	Ankle jerk S1, 2
Toe flexors	S1, 2	
Anal sphincter	S2, 3, 4	Bulbocavernosus reflex S3, 4
		Anal reflex S5
		Plantar reflex

Appendix 15

Testing Peripheral Nerves

Nerve Root	Muscle	Test—By Asking the Patient to
C3, 4	Trapezius	Shrug shoulder, adduct scapula
C4, 5	Rhomboids	Brace shoulder back
C5, 6, 7	Serratus anterior	Push forward against resistance
C5, 6, 7, 8	Pectoralis major (clavicular head)	Adduct arm from above horizontal and forward
C6, 7, 8, T1	Pectoralis major (sternocostal head)	Adduct arm below horizontal
C5	Supraspinatus	Abduct arm the first 15 degrees
C5, 6	Infraspinatus	Externally rotate arm, elbow at side
C6, 7, 8	Latissimus dorsi	Adduct horizontal and lateral arm
C5, 6	Biceps	Flex supinated forearm
C5, 6	Deltoid	Abduct arm between 15 and 90 degrees
Radial Nerve		
C7, 8	Triceps	Extend elbow against resistance
C5, 6	Brachioradialis	Flex elbow with forearm halfway between pronation and supination
C6, 7	Extensor carpi radialis longus	Extend wrist to radial side with fingers extended
C5, 6	Supinator	Arm by side, resist hand pronation
C7, 8	Extensor digitorum	Keep fingers extended at MCP joint
C7, 8	Extensor carpi ulnaris	Extend wrist to ulnar side
C7, 8	Abductor pollicis longus	Abduct thumb at 90 degrees to palm
C7, 8	Extensor pollicis brevis	Extend thumb at MCP joint
C7, 8	Extensor pollicis longus	Resist thumb flexion at IP joint
Median Nerve		
C6, 7	Pronator teres	Keep arm pronated against resistance
C6, 7, 8	Flexor carpi radialis	Flex wrist towards radial side
C7, 8, T1	Flexor digitorum sublimis	Resist extension at PIP joint (while you fix the proximal phalanx)
C8, T1	Flexor digitorum profundus I and II	Resist extension at the DIP joint
C8, T1	Flexor pollicis longus	Resist thumb extension at interphalangeal joint (fix proximal phalanx)
C8, T1	Abductor pollicis brevis	Abduct thumb (nail at 90 degrees to palm)
C8, T1	Opponens pollicis	Thumb touches fifth fingertip (nail parallel to palm)
C8, T1	First and second lumbricals	Extend PIP joint against resistance with MCP joint held hyperextended

Nerve Root	Muscle	Test—By Asking the Patient to
Ulnar Nerve		
C7, 8	Flexor carpi ulnaris	Abducting little finger, see tendon when all fingers extended
C8, T1	Flexor digitorum profundus III and IV	Fix middle phalanx of little finger, resisting extension of distal phalanx
C8, T1	Dorsal interossei	Abduct fingers (use index finger)
C8, T1	Palmar interossei	Adduct fingers (use index finger)
C8, T1	Adductor pollicis	Adduct thumb (nail at 90 degrees to palm)
C8, T1	Abductor digiti minimi	Abduct little finger
C8, T1	Opponens digiti minimi	With fingers extended, carry little finger in front of other fingers
Nerve Root		
L4, 5, S1	Gluteus medius and minimus (superior gluteal nerve)	Internal rotation at hip, hip abduction
L5, S1, 2	Gluteus maximus (inferior gluteal nerve)	Extension at hip (lie prone)
L2, 3, 4	Adductors (obturator nerve)	Adduct leg against resistance
Femoral Nerve		
L1, 2, 3	Iliopsoas	Flex hip with knee flexed and lower leg supported (patient lies on back)
L2, 3	Sartorius	Flex knee with hip externally rotated
L2, 3, 4	Quadriceps femoris	Extend knee against resistance
Sciatic Nerve		
L4, 5, S1, 2	Hamstrings	Flex knee against resistance
L4, 5	Tibialis posterior	Invert plantarflexed foot
L4, 5	Tibialis anterior	Dorsiflex ankle
L5, S1	Extensor digitorum longus	Dorsiflex toes against resistance
L5, S1	Extensor hallucis longus	Dorsiflex hallux against resistance
L5, S1	Peroneus longus and brevis	Exert foot against resistance
S1	Extensor digitorum brevis	Dorsiflex hallux (muscle of foot)
S1, 2	Gastrocnemius	Plantarflex ankle joint
S1, 2	Flexor digitorum longus	Flex terminal joints of toes
S1, 2	Small muscles of foot	Make sole of foot into a cup

Source: Medical Research Council. (1976). *Aids to the examination of the peripheral nervous system*. London: HMSO. Crown copyright material is reproduced with the permission of the Controller of HMSO and the Queen's Perrinter for Scotland.

Appendix 16

Drug Levels

Drug	Therapeutic Range
For the following drugs, blood should be taken predose:	
Carbamazepine	4–12 mg/L
Ethosuximide	40–100 mg/L
Phenobarbital	20–40 mg/L
Phenytoin	10–20 mg/L (child: 6–14 mg/L)
Primidone	As for phenobarbital
Theophylline	10–20 mg/L
For the following drugs, blood should be taken at the times indicated:	
Digoxin (8–12 hours after last dose)	0.6–2.0 µg/L toxicity 1.8–3.0 µg/L
Lithium (12 hours after last dose)	0.4–1.0 mmol/L
Valproate (2 hours after last dose)	50–100 mg/L

Checklist to Guide the Review of a Patient With Multiple Sclerosis

This is not a list of questions to be asked of every person with MS on every occasion. It is a list to remind clinicians of the wide range of potential problems that people with MS may face, and which should be actively considered as appropriate. A positive answer should lead to more detailed assessment and management.

INITIAL QUESTION

It is best to start by asking an open-ended question such as:
"Since you were last seen or assessed has any activity you used to undertake been limited, stopped, or affected?"

Activity Domains

Then, especially if nothing has been identified, it is worth asking questions directly, choosing from the list below those appropriate to the situation based on your knowledge of the person with MS:
"Are you still able to undertake, as far as you wish, the following?"
- Vocational activities (work, education, other occupation)
- Leisure activities
- Family roles
- Shopping and other community activities
- Household and domestic activities
- Washing, dressing, using toilet
- Getting about (either by walking or in other ways) and getting in and out of your house
- Controlling your environment (opening doors, switching things on and off, using the phone)

If restrictions are identified, then the reasons for these should be identified as far as possible considering impairments (see below), and social and physical factors (contexts).

Common Impairments

It is worth asking about specific impairments from the list below, again adapting to the situation and what you already know:
"Since you were last seen have you developed any new problems with the following?"
- Fatigue, endurance, being overtired
- Speech and communication
- Balance and falling
- Chewing and swallowing food and drink
- Unintended change in weight
- Pain or painful abnormal sensations
- Control over your bladder or bowels
- Control over your movement
- Vision and your eyes
- Thinking, remembering
- Your mood
- Your sexual function or partnership relations
- How you get on in social situations

Final Question

Finally, it is always worth finishing with a further open-ended question:
"Are there any other new problems that you think might be due to MS that concern you?"

Reference

National Institute of Health and Care Excellence. (2014). *Multiple sclerosis in adults: Management.* NICE clinical guideline 186. www.nice.org.uk.

Medical Management of Obesity

Pharmacological Management

Consider pharmacological management with orlistat if:

1. adequate weight loss has not been achieved with appropriate lifestyle measures; and
2. the patient has been appropriately counselled about adverse effects; and
3. the patient has a body mass index (BMI) >28 with associated risk factors or >30.

Continue pharmacological management:

1. beyond 3 months only if 5% of their initial body weight has been lost (although allow for less ambitious targets in people with type 2 diabetes in whom rate of weight loss might be slower);
2. beyond 12 months after discussing the benefits and limitations of treatment with the patient.

Surgical Management

Consider referral for bariatric surgery if:

1. BMI ≥40 or BMI 35–40 with a comorbidity that would be improved with weight loss (e.g., type 2 diabetes, hypertension); and
2. all nonsurgical options have been tried and clinically beneficial weight loss has not been achieved/maintained; and
3. the patient is receiving or will receive intensive treatment in a specialist service; and
4. the patient is fit for anaesthesia; and
5. the patient commits to long-term follow-up.

National Institute of Health and Care Excellence. (2014). *Obesity: Identification, assessment and management. NICE clinical guideline 189.* www.nice.org.uk.

Immunizations in Pregnancy

Immunizations Contraindicated in Pregnancy

Vaccine	Comments
BCG	Live mycobacterium
Cholera (oral)	No evidence of safety; benefit unlikely to outweigh theoretical risk
Measles	Live virus. Avoid pregnancy for 3 months after vaccination
Mumps	Live virus. Avoid pregnancy for 3 months after vaccination
Rubella	Live virus. Avoid pregnancy for 3 months after vaccination
Typhoid	Live bacterium
Ty21a	
Varicella	Live virus. Consider giving VZIG if exposed to chickenpox in pregnancy
Yellow fever	Live virus. Give patient a written waiver if travelling to a country requiring a certificate. If risk of contracting the disease is high the patient may choose to have the immunization.

Immunizations which may be given in pregnancy if patient and physician judge that the potential benefit outweighs the risk

That risk is theoretical. In almost all of these immunizations there is no evidence either way. If deciding to give the immunization, it may be thought prudent to wait until the second or third trimester in case a reaction to the vaccine were to trigger a first-trimester miscarriage.

Vaccine	Comments
Diphtheria/tetanus	
Hepatitis A	The patient may choose immunoglobulin as a safer alternative.
Hepatitis B	
Immunoglobulin	
Influenza	The vaccine is positively indicated in pregnant women. They are more prone to pulmonary complications than nonpregnant women.
Japanese encephalitis	Inactivated virus but there is no consensus on its safety.
Meningococcus	
Pneumococcus	
Pertussis	The vaccine is positively indicated in pregnancy (ideally between 16 and 32 weeks) to protect newborn babies via passive immunity.
Polio (oral)	Paralysis seems more likely in pregnancy than in the non-pregnant woman. Neonatal infection carries a high mortality rate.
Rabies	
Typhoid (Vi capsular polysaccharide)	

Adapted from Centers for Disease Control and Prevention. (2008). *CDC Health Information for International Travel*. Atlanta, GA: Mosby; National Institute for Health and Care Excellence. (2008). *Antenatal care: Routine care for the healthy pregnant woman*. National Collaborating Centre for Women's and Children's Health. Commissioned by the National Institute for Health and Clinical Excellence. NICE clinical guideline 62. www.nice. org.uk; Martinez, L. (Ed.). (2002). *International travel and health*. Geneva: World Health Organization.

Edinburgh Postnatal Depression Scale

Instructions for Users

1. The mother is asked to underline the response which comes closest to how she has been feeling in the previous 7 days.
2. All 10 items must be completed.
3. Care should be taken to avoid the possibility of the mother discussing her answers with others.
4. The mother should complete the scale herself, unless she has limited English or has difficulty with reading.
5. The EPDS may be used at 6–8 weeks to screen postnatal women. The child health clinic, postnatal checkup, or a home visit may provide suitable opportunities for its completion.

Scoring the EPDS

- Response categories are scored 0, 1, 2, and 3 according to increased severity of the symptom.
- Items marked with an asterisk are reverse scored (i.e., 3, 2, 1, and 0). The total score is calculated by adding together the scores for each of the 10 items.
- Mothers who score above a threshold 12/13 are likely to be suffering from a depressive illness of varying severity. Nevertheless, the EPDS score should not override clinical judgment. A careful clinical assessment should be carried out to confirm the diagnosis. The scale indicates how the mother has felt during the previous week, and in doubtful cases it may be usefully repeated after 2 weeks. The scale will not detect mothers with anxiety neuroses, phobias, or personality disorders.

As you have recently had a baby, we would like to know how you are feeling. Please UNDERLINE the answer which comes closest to how you have felt IN THE PAST 7 DAYS, not just how you feel today. Here is an example, already completed.

1. I have felt happy:
   Yes, all the time
   <u>Yes, most of the time</u>
   No, not very often
   No, not at all

This would mean: "I have felt happy most of the time" during the past week. Please complete the other questions in the same way.

In the Past 7 Days:

1. I have been able to laugh and see the funny side of things:
   As much as I always could
   Not quite so much now
   Definitely not so much now
   Not at all
2. I have looked forward with enjoyment to things:
   As much as I ever did
   Rather less than I used to
   Definitely less than I used to
   Hardly at all
3. *I have blamed myself unnecessarily when things went wrong:
   Yes, most of the time
   Yes, some of the time
   Not very often
   No, never
4. *I have been anxious or worried for no good reason:
   No, not at all
   Hardly ever
   Yes, sometimes
   Yes, very often

5. *I have felt scared or panicky for no very good reason:
   Yes, quite a lot
   Yes, sometimes
   No, not much
   No, not at all
6. *Things have been getting on top of me:
   Yes, most of the time I haven't been able to cope at all
   Yes, sometimes I haven't been coping as well as usual
   No, most of the time I have coped quite well
   No, I have been coping as well as ever
7. *I have been so unhappy that I have had difficulty sleeping:
   Yes, most of the time
   Yes, sometimes
   Not very often
   No, not at all
8. *I have felt sad or miserable:
   Yes, most of the time
   Yes, quite often
   Not very often
   No, not at all
9. *I have been so unhappy that I have been crying:
   Yes, most of the time
   Yes, quite often
   Only occasionally
   No, never
10. *The thought of harming myself has occurred to me:
    Yes, quite often
    Sometimes
    Hardly ever
    Never

Admission Procedures for Patients With Mental Health Problems

Compulsory Admission

The team needed to complete a Section 2 or Section 3 consists of:

a) the general practitioner (GP) (or an independent section 12–approved doctor if the GP is not available);
b) an approved mental health professional (AMHP);
c) an approved psychiatrist (duty consultant or specialist registrar).

The procedure to follow between 9 am and 5 pm for assessment of a patient who may need to be sectioned from home might be as follows:

- Obtain relevant information from a partner who may know the patient better.
- Review the records to assess:
  - risk of violence;
  - past history of outcomes of previous sections;
  - previous responses to treatment.
- Phone the family or carer to obtain their assessment of the:
  - current situation and urgency;
  - need for police support;
  - risk of violence, access to weapons.
- Ensure the patient is at home and someone is in to allow access.
- Explain the procedure and arrange a time to visit.
- Contact the duty AMHP and duty psychiatrist:
  - Provide basic information: name, date of birth, address, past history, current problem, reason for assessment, phone number of patient, name of carer or relative at home, how to contact you in the next few hours, name of key worker, any known risk of violence or self-harm.
  - Decide on the need for police support.
  - Arrange a time to meet together at the home.
- If a joint visit is not possible decide:
  - when each will visit;
  - how to discuss assessments and decide on need for sectioning;
  - where to leave the section form for GP to sign (e.g., will it be left with relative or brought to surgery?).
- If the GP visits first, take the section forms and complete, if appropriate.
- Avoid sedating the patient as this makes subsequent assessment difficult.
- Avoid asking the relative to sign Section 2 or 4, as this increases guilt and may disrupt future relationships.
- If the two doctors cannot do a joint assessment, they must examine the patient within 5 days of each other.
- Organize a hospital bed (the AMHP is responsible for arranging transport).
- If the GP and AMHP disagree on the need for sectioning:
  - record the basis of each decision in writing;
  - identify a home care plan;
  - decide who will reassess and when;
  - instruct the carer in what to do if the situation changes.
- Ask family or carer to make a GP follow-up appointment to find out how they are coping and what has happened to the patient, and future plans.
- Complete item of service claim form.

Voluntary Admission

- If patient is known to hospital staff and a bed is available and the patient accepts admission: arrange admission, write a letter, organize transport.
- If patient is known to hospital staff but there are no beds available: contact the bed manager or psychiatric nurse manager.
  1. If a bed is found, arrange admission as above.
  2. If a bed is not immediately available and a 2-hour delay is acceptable, if supported by CPN or crisis team:
     a) arrange for the hospital to phone you and family when bed available;
     b) write letter and give to patient or relative;
     c) ask the family to phone the GP if they have not heard from hospital in 2 hours.
  3. If a bed is not immediately available and a delay is not acceptable:
     a) phone the A&E psychiatric registrar or A&E mental health nurse;
     b) consider referral to A&E;
     c) other options according to local guidance.
- If the patient is not known to hospital staff: if Monday to Friday, 9 am to 5 pm then:
  a) check catchment area and relevant consultant;
  b) phone the consultant on pager or mobile or contact his or her secretary to ask the psychiatrist to phone you ASAP:
     - if the consultant is available arrange for domiciliary visit or admission;
     - if consultant is not available, phone the SHO or registrar and proceed as above;
     - if out of hours, follow the local protocol for voluntary admission if available.

Note: The out of hours service should ensure that the protocol is in the doctor's bag.

Appendix 22

The Early Warning Form for Use in Psychotic Illness

EARLY WARNING SIGNS

Name: ....

I am at risk of developing episodes of: ....
....

My early warning signs are (e.g., changes in sleep, eating/drinking or mood, becoming quiet or loud or more withdrawn):

1. ....
2. ....
3. ....

Whenever I have any of these signs I will respond by: ....
....
....

My health worker is: ....   Phone ....

My home contact is: ....   Phone ....

My advocacy contact is: ....   Phone ....

If I have any concerns about my illness I will contact: ....
.... immediately.

Reproduced with permission from Falloon, I.R.H., et al. (1993). *Managing stress in families: Cognitive and behavioural strategies for enhancing coping skills.* London: Routledge.

Appendix 23

AUDIT

The Alcohol Use Disorders Identification Test: Interview Version

Initially give an explanation of the content and purpose of the questions and the need for accurate answers. Read questions as written. Record answers carefully. Begin the AUDIT by saying, "Now I am going to ask you some questions about your use of alcoholic beverages during this past year." Explain what is meant by "alcoholic beverages" by using local examples of beer, wine, vodka, etc. Code answers in terms of "standard drinks." Place the correct answer number in the box at the right.

1. How often do you have a drink containing alcohol? ☐
   (0) Never [Skip to Questions 9–10]
   (1) Monthly or less
   (2) 2 to 4 times a month
   (3) 2 to 3 times a week
   (4) 4 or more times a week

2. How many drinks containing alcohol do you have on a typical day when you are drinking? ☐
   (0) 1 or 2
   (1) 3 or 4
   (2) 5 or 6
   (3) 7, 8, or 9
   (4) 10 or more

3. How often do you have six or more drinks on one occasion? ☐
   (0) Never
   (1) Less than monthly
   (2) Monthly
   (3) Weekly
   (4) Daily or almost daily

   Skip to Questions 9 and 10 if Total Score for Questions 2 and 3 = 0

4. How often during the last year have you found that you were not able to stop drinking once you had started? ☐
   (0) Never
   (1) Less than monthly
   (2) Monthly
   (3) Weekly
   (4) Daily or almost daily

Continued

5. How often during the last year have you failed to do what was normally expected from you because of drinking? ☐
   (0) Never
   (1) Less than monthly
   (2) Monthly
   (3) Weekly
   (4) Daily or almost daily

6. How often during the last year have you needed a first drink in the morning to get yourself going after a heavy drinking session? ☐
   (0) Never
   (1) Less than monthly
   (2) Monthly
   (3) Weekly
   (4) Daily or almost daily

7. How often during the last year have you had a feeling of guilt or remorse after drinking? ☐
   (0) Never
   (1) Less than monthly
   (2) Monthly
   (3) Weekly
   (4) Daily or almost daily

8. How often during the last year have you been unable to remember what happened the night before because you had been drinking? ☐
   (0) Never
   (1) Less than monthly
   (2) Monthly
   (3) Weekly
   (4) Daily or almost daily

9. Have you or someone else been injured as a result of your drinking? ☐
   (0) No
   (2) Yes, but not in the last year
   (4) Yes, during the last year

10. Has a relative or friend or a doctor or another health worker been concerned about your drinking or suggested you cut down? ☐
    (0) No
    (2) Yes, but not in the last year
    (4) Yes, during the last year

Record total of specific items here: ☐
An AUDIT score in the range of 8–15 represents a medium level of alcohol problems where brief interventions would be appropriate. Scores of ≥16 represent a high level of alcohol problems with higher levels of intervention and monitoring recommended. Scores of ≥20 suggest dependent drinking and merits further assessment.[1]
AUDIT-C uses the first three questions only. If the score is ≥3 then complete the full questionnaire.

[1]Babor, T. F., Higgins-Biddle, J. C., Saunders, J. B., et al. (2001). *Audit, the alcohol use disorders identification test: World Health Organization (WHO)*. www.who.int/Alcohol_AUDIT.

International Prostate Symptom Score (IPSS)

	Not at All	Less Than One Time in Five	Less Than Half the Time	About Half the Time	More Than Half the Time	Almost Always
1. Incomplete emptying Over the past month, how often have you had a sensation of not emptying your bladder completely after you have finished urinating?	0	1	2	3	4	5
2. Frequency Over the past month, how often have you had to urinate again less than 2 hours after you finished urinating?	0	1	2	3	4	5
3. Intermittency Over the past month, how often have you found you stopped and started again several times when you urinated?	0	1	2	3	4	5
4. Urgency Over the past month, how often have you found it difficult to postpone urination or felt sudden urges to urinate?	0	1	2	3	4	5
5. Weak stream Over the past month, how often have you had a weak urinary stream?	0	1	2	3	4	5
6. Straining Over the past month, how often have you had to push or strain to begin urination?	0	1	2	3	4	5

	None	Once	Twice	Three Times	Four Times	Five Times or More
7. Nocturia Over the past month, how many times did you typically get up to urinate from the time you went to bed at night to the time you got up in the morning?	0	1	2	3	4	5

(Scoring items 1–7: 0–7 = mild; 8–19 = moderate; 20–35 = severe)

Continued

Quality of Life	Delighted	Pleased	Mostly Satisfied	No Strong Feelings Either Way	Mostly Dissatisfied	Unhappy	Terrible
If you were to spend the rest of your life with urinary conditions just the way they are now, how would you feel about it?	0	1	2	3	4	5	6

Appendix 25

Body Mass Index

Body mass index $= W/H^2$

Women

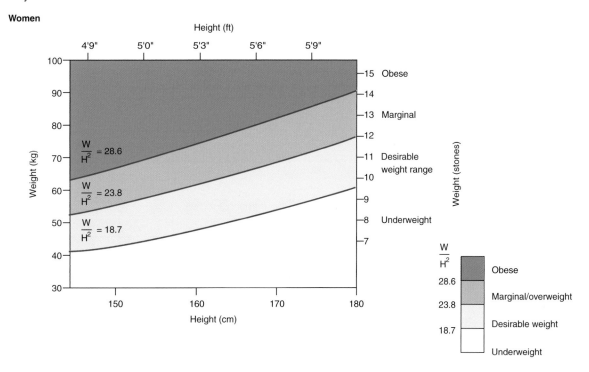

Men

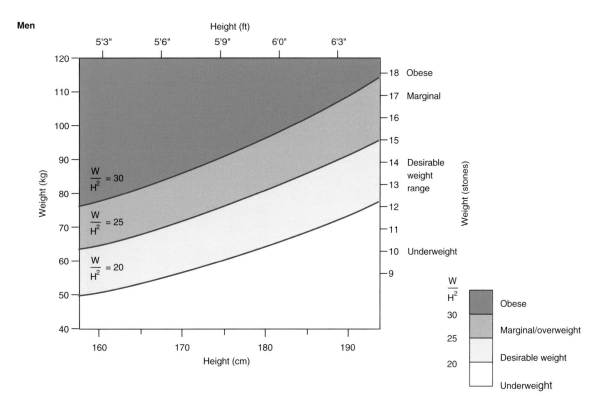

Appendix 26

Reference Ranges for Young Adults

Reference ranges vary according to laboratory and test method. The following are given as typical ranges but if the laboratory performing the test gives a range that differs from these it should be used instead. The range will also vary according to age and gender.

Blood

Biochemistry and Immunology

Serum or plasma		Immunoglobulins:	
Acid phosphatase:		IgG	6–13 g/L
total	1–5 IU/L	IgM	0.5–2.0 g/L
prostatic	0–1 IU/L	IgA	1.0–4.0 g/L
ACTH	10–80 ng/L	Lactate dehydrogenase	70–250 IU/L
Alkaline phosphatase	30–300 IU/L	Magnesium	0.7–1.0 mmol/L
Alanine aminotransferase	5–35 IU/L	Osmolality	280–295 mosmol/kg
Amylase	<120 IU/L	Phosphate (inorganic)	0.8–1.4 mmol/L
Asparate aminotransferase	5–35 IU/L	Potassium	3.4–5.2 mmol/L
Bicarbonate	21–26 mmol/L	Prolactin	Male: 80–400 mu/L
Bilirubin	<17 mmol/L		Female: 90–520 mu/L
Calcium	2.26–2.60 mmol/L		Postmenopausal female: 80–280 mu/L
Chloride	95–105 mmol/L	Protein:	
Cholesterol	<5.5 mmol/L	total	60–80 g/L
Complement:		albumin	35–50 g/L
C3	0.69–1.5 mg/L	PSA	0–4 ng/mL
C4	0.12–0.27 mg/L	Sodium	133–145 mmol/L
		Total thyroxine	70–140 nmol/L
Cortisol:		Free T4	10–26 pmol/L
9:00 am	130–690 nmol/L	Free T3	3–9 pmol/L
midnight	Half the am value	Triiodothyronine	1.2–3.0 nmol/L
Creatinine	70–130 mol/L	TSH	0.3–3.8 mu/L
Creatine kinase	<200 IU/L	Triglycerides**	<0.55–1.90 mmol/L
α-Fetoprotein	<10 ku/L	Urea	2.5–6.7 mmol/L

γ-Glutamyl transferase:		Uric acid:	
men	11–51 IU/L	men	0.15–0.42 mmol/L
women	7–33 IU/L	women	0.10–0.36 mmol/L
Glucose (fasting)	3.4–5.5 mmol/L		
Growth hormone	<5.5 mu/L	*Arterial blood gases*	
		pH	7.35–7.45
		PaO$_2$	12–14 kPa
		PaCO$_2$	4.6–6.0 kPa

*To convert cholesterol from mmol/L into mg/dL multiply by 39.
**To convert triglycerides from mmol/L into mg/dL multiply by 89.

Haematology

Haemoglobin	13.5–18.0 g/dL (men)
	11.5–16.0 g/dL (women)
MCV	82–98 fL
MCH	26.7–33.0 pg
MCHC	31.4–35.0 g/dL
WBC	3.2–11.0×10^9/L
Neutrophils	1.9–7.7×10^9/L
Monocytes	0.1–0.9×10^9/L
Eosinophils	0.0–0.4×10^9/L
Basophils	0.2–0.8×10^9/L
Platelets	120–400×10^9/L
Reticulocytes	25–100×10^9/L (or <2%)
Ferritin	30–230 µg/L (male)
	6–80 µg/L (female)
	14–180 µg/L
	(postmenopausal female)

Urine

Sodium	100–250 mmol/24 h
Potassium	14–120 mmol/24 h
Albumin:	
– microalbuminuria	20–200 mg/L
– proteinuria	>200 mg/L
Albumin/creatinine ratio:	
– microalbuminuria	2.5 mg/mmol (men) or 3.5 mg/mmol (women) to 30 mg/mmol
– proteinuria	>30 mg/mmol
Creatinine clearance	85–125 mL/min (men); 75–115 mL/min (women)
Osmolality	350–1000 mosmol/kg

Appendix 27

Anaphylaxis Algorithm

Reproduced from Working Group of the Resuscitation Council (UK). (2008). *Emergency treatment of anaphylactic reactions. Guidelines for healthcare providers.* London: Resuscitation Council (UK), by permission of the Resuscitation Council.

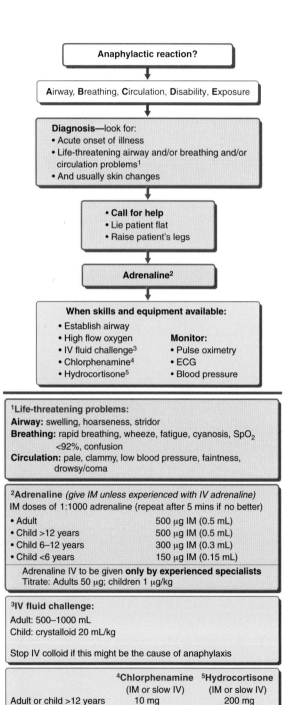

Appendix 28

Problems Associated With Specific Causes of Disability

	Audiovisual	Endocrine	Psychiatric/ Psycologic	CNS	Cardiovascular	Muscular/ Skeletal and Skin	Other	Inheritance
Cerebral palsy 1:500	Visual impairment Hearing impairment		Depression Variable intellectual capacity	Epilepsy		Orthopaedic problems Neuromuscular problems	Genitourinary problems Incontinence Constipation Dental problems Recurrent aspiration Oesophagitis, gastrooesophageal reflux ± bleeding/ anaemia Swallowing/eating difficulties	
Down syndrome 1:700	Visual impairment (multifactorial), cataracts Hearing impairment (multifactorial) Annual assessments recommended	Hypothyroidism Annual TFT recommended	Depression Alzheimer type dementia (clinical onset uncommon before 40 years)	Epilepsy usually clonic/tonic	Congenital heart defects (present in 40%–50%)	Atlantoaxial instability Skin disorders, alopecia, eczema	Blood dyscrasias Childhood leukaemia Sleep apnoea Increased susceptibility to infections Coeliac disease	Most cases are sporadic; 4% due to translocation involving chromosome 21 or rarely parental mosaicism
Prader-Willi 1:10,000– 25,000	Strabismus myopia	NIDDM (secondary to obesity) Hypogonadism Delayed puberty	Hyperphagia impulse control difficulties Self-injury			Scoliosis, kyphosis Hypotonia Skin picking	Infantile failure to thrive, then hyperphagia and severe obesity High tolerance to pain Decreased ability to vomit Sleep apnoea Osteoporosis Undescended testes Dental abnormalities	Atypical. Most cases are sporadic

Condition							
Fragile X 1:6000	Visual impairment (multifactorial) Hearing impairment Recurrent ear infections	Attention deficit/ hyperactivity Variable intellectual capacity Disabled in social functioning	Epilepsy Usually clonic/ tonic, complex partial	Aortic dilatation, mitral valve prolapse (related to connective tissue dysplasia)	Connective tissue dysplasia Scoliosis Congenital hip dislocation	Hernias (CT related) Abnormalities of speech and language	X-linked
Phenylketonuria 1:10,000– 20,000		Variable intellectual capacity Phobic anxiety Disabled in social functioning	Epilepsy Hyperactivity Tremor and pyramidal tract signs Extrapyramidal syndromes			Eczema	Autosomal recessive
Angelmann syndrome 1:10,000	Glaucoma	Easily excitable Hyperactive	Severe developmental delay Epilepsy		Joint contractures and scoliosis (in adults)	Speech impairment Movement and balance disorder Characteristic EEG changes	Variety of genetic mechanisms on chromosome 15
Williams <1:20,000	Hyperacusis Strabismus	Variable intellectual capacity Attention deficit problems in childhood	Perceptual and motor function reduced	Cardiac abnormalities Hypertension CVAs Chronic hemiparesis	Joint contractures Scoliosis Hypotonia	Renal abnormalities	Microdeletion on chromosome 7
Rett 1:14,000 Females	Refractory errors	Severe intellectual disability	Epilepsy Vasomotor instability	Prolonged QT interval	Osteopenia Fractures Scoliosis	Hyperventilation Apnoea Reflux Feeding difficulties Growth failure	Usually sporadic X-linked

Continued

	Audiovisual	Endocrine	Psychiatric/ Psycologic	CNS	Cardiovascular	Muscular/ Skeletal and Skin	Other	Inheritance
Noonan <1:10,000	Strabismus Refractive errors Vision/hearing impairments		Mild intellectual disability	Epilepsy	Pulmonary valvular stenosis ASD, VSD, PDA	Scoliosis Talipes equinovarus Pectus carinatum/ excavatum	Abnormal clotting factors, platelet dysfunction Undescended tests, deficient spermatogenesis Lymphangiectasia Hepatosplenomegaly Cubitus valgus, hand abnormalities	Autosomal dominant, may be sporadic
Tuberous sclerosis 1:6000– 17,000	Retinal tumours Eye rhabdomyomatas		Variable intellectual capacity Behavioural difficulties Sleep problems	Cerebral astrocytomas Epilepsy	Rhabdomyomatas Hypertension	Bone Rhabdomyomata	Kidney and lung hamartomata Polycystic kidneys Liver rhabdomyomata Dental abnormalities Skin lesions	Autosomal dominant
Neurofibromatosis 1:300	Hearing impairment (glioma affecting auditory nerve)	Various endocrine abnormalities	Variable intellectual capacity	Variable clinical phenomena depending on site of the tumours Epilepsy		Skeletal abnormalities especially kyphoscoliosis	Variable clinical phenomena depending on the location of the neurofibroma Tumours are susceptible to malignant change Other varieties of tumours may be associated	Autosomal dominant

The Community Dependency Index

Score the patient under the following nine headings. A score <75 suggests moderate disability; <50 suggests severe disability.

Personal Toilet

5 = Client can wash hands and face, comb hair, clean teeth and shave. Must be able to get to water, brushes, without help and operate them independently.

0 = Any help or supervision needed or difficulty with personal toilet.

Feeding

10 = Independent. The client can feed himself a meal from a tray or table when someone puts the food within reach. He must put on his own assistive device if this is needed, cut up food, spread butter and so on. He must accomplish this in a reasonable time (that is acceptable to the client).

5 = Food must be cut for the client or some help is necessary with the items above. Unreasonable time or effort required if feeds independently.

0 = Client unable to feed himself.

Moving From (Wheel) Chair to Bed and Return

15 = Independent in all phases of this activity.

Chair: client can safely stand up from sitting in his chair (high chair allowed) without help from another person, and sit down again. Client must be able to get in/out bed without help, and, once in bed be able to turn and move up and down in the bed as necessary.

Or wheelchair: client can safely approach the bed in his wheelchair, lock brakes, lift footrests, transfer safely to the bed and lie down. Once in bed he must be able to turn and move up and down the bed as necessary. Client must be able to transfer back into the wheelchair safely including changing the position of the wheelchair for the return transfer.

10 = Client can independently sit down and stand up from chair, or transfer in and out of a wheelchair, but still has difficulty or needs help in bed.

5 = Help or supervision needed to ensure client's safety in all parts of this activity; or client performs all or parts of this activity with difficulty.

0 = Client unable to perform this activity.

Getting On and Off the Toilet or Commode (During Day and Night)

10 = Client is able to reach the toilet/commode area unassisted. He is able to transfer on and off the commode,

fasten and unfasten clothes, prevent spoiling of clothes, use toilet paper without help. He may use equipment or stable fittings for support if needed (e.g., rail, raised toilet seat or side of bath). If he uses a commode he must be able to position it for use, empty it and clean it out.

5 = Client has difficulty with part of this activity or client needs help because of imbalance or in handling clothes or in using toilet paper or in flushing the toilet.

0 = Client needs help to empty the commode or is not able to transfer.

Note: If the client can use the toilet independently during the day but has the commode at night, which someone else empties, then score = 5.

Walking 50 Yards Outside the House or Using a Wheelchair

Walking

15 = Client gets in/out of the house unassisted. He can walk at least 50 yards without help or supervision outside his home. He may wear braces and prostheses and use walking aids. He must be able to reach and operate aids without help.

10 = Client has difficulty or needs minimal help or supervision in any of the above but can walk at least 50 yards.

Wheelchair

5 = Client cannot walk but can propel a wheelchair independently. He must be able to go round corners and turn around. He must be able to get in and out of the house independently (access). He must be able to push the wheelchair at least 50 yards. If the wheelchair is used indoors he must be able to manoeuvre himself to a table, bed or toilet. Do not score for wheelchair use if the client gets a score for walking.

0 = Client unable to walk or propel a wheelchair for 50 yards.

Dressing and Undressing

10 = Client is able to put on and remove and fasten all clothing and tie shoelaces (adaptations/aids allowed). This activity includes putting on and removing prostheses, braces and corsets where these are prescribed. Special clothing, such as slip-on shoes or dresses that open down the front, may be used where necessary.

5 = Client has difficulty or needs help in putting on and removing or fastening any clothing. Where helped he must do at least half the work himself. He must accomplish this in a reasonable time.

0 = Client needs help with all or most of dressing.

Continued

Bathing Self

5 = Client can use a bath or shower. He must be able to do all the steps involved in whichever method is employed without another person helping him. Verbal supervision is allowed.

0 = Client has difficulty or needs help.

Note: Where the client's home does not have bathing/shower facilities, score 5 for using a bath/shower in another facility or having an all-over wash if independent. Where client has an all-over wash because he is unable to use the bath/shower then score = 0.

Ascending and Descending Stairs

10 = Client is able to get up and down stairs safely, without help or supervision. He may and should use the handrails and walking aids when needed. He must be able to carry walking aids up and down the stairs if needed. If a stair lift or vertical lift is used, the client must be able to use it without help or supervision (including transfers).

5 = Client has difficulty, needs help or supervision in any one of the above items.

0 = Client unable to climb the stairs.

Note: If the client does not have stairs in the house, count as 10 because they are not an obstacle to independence in the home, even if they are obstacles in the community.

Continence of Bowels

10 = Client is able to control bowels and has no accidents. He can use a suppository or take an enema when necessary (e.g. spinal cord injury). He can manage external devices (e.g. colostomy).

5 = Client needs help with any of the above.

0 = Client does not have bowel control.

Continence of Bladder

10 = Client able to control his bladder day and night. Clients who wear external device and leg bag must put them on independently, clean and empty the bag and stay dry day and night.

5 = Client has control of bladder, but cannot get to the toilet or commode in time (e.g. due to poor mobility) or needs help with an external device.

0 = Client does not have bladder control.

Appendix 30

Nottingham Extended Activities of Daily Living Questionnaire (EADL)

Score the patient on each item on a scale of 0 to 3 where "3" represents independent function, "2" represents alone with difficulty, "1" represents alone with help, and "0" represents unable.

Subscale	Item
Mobility	1. Do you walk around outside?
	2. Do you climb stairs?
	3. Do you get in and out of the car?
	4. Do you walk over uneven ground?
	5. Do you cross roads?
	6. Do you travel on public transport?
Kitchen	7. Do you manage to feed yourself?
	8. Do you manage to make yourself a hot snack?
	9. Do you take hot drinks from one room to another?
	10. Do you do the washing up?
	11. Do you make yourself a hot drink?
Domestic	12. Do you manage your own money when you are out?
	13. Do you wash small items of clothing?
	14. Do you do your own housework?
	15. Do you do your own shopping?
	16. Do you do a full clothes wash?
Leisure	17. Do you read newspapers or books?
	18. Do you use the telephone?
	19. Do you write letters?
	20. Do you go out socially?
	21. Do you manage your own garden?
	22. Do you drive a car?
	Total (0–66)

Drug Stabilities in Syringe Drivers

Notes on using tables of drug mixture stabilities
- The following tables are separated into mixtures containing two or three drugs, ordered by diamorphine first, then the other drugs in alphabetical order.
- The maximum dose for each drug in each syringe size is given. Provided the doses for every drug in the combination is less than or equal to these maximum values, then the mixture is stable for 24 hours. Above the maximum doses stated the solution is either unstable or has not been tested and it is not possible to say whether it is stable or not.
- All drug mixtures should be protected from light where possible.

- It is considered best practice to give dexamethasone as a bolus dose as it has a long duration of action and frequently causes compatability problems in mixture.
- The following combinations are not stable:
  - diamorphine, dexamethasone, and levomepromazine
  - diamorphine, dexamethasone, and midazolam
  - diamorphine, cyclizine, and metoclopramide
  - octreotide and levomepromazine
  - octreotide and cyclizine
  - octreotide and dexamethasone
  - diamorphine, metoclopramide, and ondansetron

Drug Combination	8 mL in a 10-mL Syringe		14 mL in a 20-mL Syringe		17 mL in a 30-mL Syringe		Comments
Maximum Dose (mg) Known to be Stable in:							
Two drug combinations for subcutaneous infusion which are stable for 24 h							
Diluent: Water for Injections BP							
Diamorphine and cyclizine	160 160*	If diamorphine dose >160, cyclizine dose must be no more than 80	280 280*	If diamorphine dose >280, cyclizine dose must be no more than 140	340 340*	If diamorphine dose >340, cyclizine dose must be no more than 170	If exceed these doses then likely to get precipitate *Maximum recommended daily dose 150
Diamorphine and haloperidol	800 24	400 32	–		–		If exceed these doses then likely to get precipitate
Diamorphine and hyoscine HBr	1200 3.2		–		–		–
Diamorphine and hyoscine butylbromide (Buscopan)	1200 160		–		–		–
Diamorphine and ketorolac	47 40		82 74		90 90		–
Diamorphine and levomepromazine (Nozinan)	400 80		700 140		850 170		Mixture can be irritant, dilute to largest possible volume

Drug Combination	Maximum Dose (mg) Known to be Stable in:			Comments
	8 mL in a 10-mL Syringe	14 mL in a 20-mL Syringe	17 mL in a 30-mL Syringe	
Diamorphine and metoclopramide	1200 40	2100 70	2550 85	Mixture can be irritant, dilute to largest possible volume
Diamorphine and midazolam	400 16	700 28	850 34	—
Diamorphine and octreotide	200 0.9	350 1.6	425 1.9	—
Diamorphine and ondansetron	40 5	70 9	85 11	

Three drug combinations for subcutaneous infusion which are stable for 24 h

Diluent: Water for Injections BP

Drug Combination	8 mL in a 10-mL Syringe	14 mL in a 20-mL Syringe	17 mL in a 30-mL Syringe	Comments
Diamorphine and cyclizine and haloperidol	160 160 16	280 280 28	340 340 34	Above these doses the mixture is likely to precipitate. Only stable if diamorphine and haloperidol are well diluted before dexamethasone is added. Use only if no other options
Diamorphine and haloperidol and midazolam	560 4 32	980 7 56	1190 8.5 68	—
Diamorphine and levomepromazine and metoclopramide	400 80 24	700 140 42	850 170 51	—

Appendix 32

Guidelines for the Urgent Referral of Patients With Suspected Cancer

Cancer Type	Referral Guidelines

Lung cancer	*Urgent referral for chest x-ray*
	• Haemoptysis
	• *Unexplained* or persistent (>3 weeks):
	  – Cough
	  – Chest/shoulder pain
	  – Dyspnoea
	  – Weight loss
	  – Chest signs
	  – Hoarseness
	  – Finger clubbing
	  – Features suggestive of metastasis from a lung cancer (e.g., brain, bone, liver, or skin)
	  – Cervical/supraclavicular lymphadenopathy
	  – Unexplained change in symptoms in someone with underlying chronic respiratory disease
	Urgent referral to a chest physician
	Any of the following:
	• Chest x-ray suggestive/suspicious of lung cancer (including pleural effusion and slowly resolving consolidation)
	• Persistent haemoptysis in smokers/ex-smokers >40 years of age
	• High suspicion of lung cancer despite normal chest x-ray
	• History of asbestos exposure and recent onset of chest pain, shortness of breath, or unexplained systemic symptoms where a chest x-ray indicates pleural effusion, pleural mass, or any suspicious lung pathology
	• Signs of superior vena cava obstruction (swelling of face/neck with fixed elevation of jugular venous pressure) (consider immediate referral)
	• Stridor (consider immediate referral)

Upper GI cancer	*Urgent referral*
	• Dysphagia: food sticking on swallowing (any age)
	• Dyspepsia at any age combined with one or more of the following:
	  – Chronic GI bleeding
	  – Progressive unintentional weight loss
	  – Iron deficiency anaemia
	  – Persistent vomiting
	  – Suspicious barium meal result
	• Unexplained upper abdominal pain and weight loss, with or without back pain
	• Upper abdominal mass
	• Obstructive jaundice (depending on clinical state)
	• Consider urgent referral for those with unexplained worsening of dyspepsia combined with at least one of the following:
	  – Barrett oesophagus
	  – Peptic ulcer surgery >20 years ago
	  – Known dysplasia, atrophic gastritis, intestinal metaplasia
	• Consider urgent referral for those without dyspepsia who have:
	  – persistent vomiting and weight loss
	  – unexplained weight loss and iron deficiency anaemia
	• Refer urgently for endoscopy patients age ≥55 years with unexplained and persistent recent-onset dyspepsia alone

Cancer Type	Referral Guidelines
Lower GI cancer	*Urgent referral* All ages • A definite palpable right-sided abdominal mass consistent with involvement of the large bowel • A definite palpable rectal (not pelvic) mass • Men with unexplained iron deficiency anaemia and an Hb of ≤11 g/100 mL • Women who are not menstruating with unexplained iron deficiency anaemia and an Hb of ≤10 g/100 mL ≥40 years old • Rectal bleeding *with* a change in bowel habit to looser stools and/or increased frequency of defecation persistent for 6 weeks ≥60 years old • Rectal bleeding for at least 6 weeks *without a* change in bowel habit and *without anal* symptoms • Change of bowel habit to looser stools and/or increased frequency of defecation, *without* rectal bleeding and persistent for 6 weeks
Breast cancer	*Urgent referral* • Patients with a discrete hard lump with fixation • Women aged ≥30 with a discrete lump that persists after their next period, or presents after the menopause • Women aged <30 with a lump that enlarges, or is fixed and hard, or in whom there are other reasons for concern (eg, family history) • Those with a lump or with suspicious symptoms and a past history of breast cancer • Those with unilateral eczematous skin or nipple change that does not respond to topical treatment • Those with nipple distortion of recent onset • Those with spontaneous unilateral bloody nipple discharge • Men aged ≥50 with a unilateral, firm subareolar mass *Conditions that require referral—but not necessarily urgently* • Discrete lump in younger women (age <30 years) • Breast pain not responding to initial treatment and/or with unexplained persistent symptoms
Gynaecologic cancer	*Urgent referral* • Clinical features suggestive of cervical cancer on examination • Unexplained vulval lump • Vulval bleeding due to ulceration • Postmenopausal bleeding (PMB) in women not on HRT • On tamoxifen with PMB • On HRT: persistent or unexplained bleeding for >6 weeks after stopping HRT *Consider urgent referral* • Persistent intermenstrual bleeding and negative pelvic examination *Urgent ultrasound scan (USS)* • Palpable abdominal or pelvic mass that is not obviously uterine fibroids or gastrointestinal or urologic. If the scan suggests cancer, or if urgent USS is not available, urgent referral should be made
Urologic cancers	*Urgent referral* Prostate: – Hard irregular prostate typical of carcinoma – Normal prostate but rising or raised age-specific PSA, with or without lower urinary tract symptoms Bladder and kidney: – Painless macroscopic haematuria – Age ≥40 with recurrent or persistent urinary tract infection associated with haematuria – Unexplained microscopic haematuria in adults aged ≥50 years – Abdominal mass identified clinically or on imaging thought to arise from the urinary tract Testis: – Swelling or mass in the body of the testis Penis: – Any suspected penile cancer *Non-urgent referral of microscopic haematuria in a patient aged <50 years* – To a renal physician if there is proteinuria or a raised serum creatinine – To a urologist if there is no proteinuria and serum creatinine is normal
Haematologic cancers	*Urgent referral* • Blood count/film reported as suggestive of acute leukaemia (immediate referral) • Spinal cord compression or renal failure suspected of being due to myeloma (immediate referral) • Persistent unexplained splenomegaly

Continued

Cancer Type	Referral Guidelines

Skin cancers	*Urgent referral*
	• A lesion suspected to be melanoma
	• Suspicion of squamous cell carcinoma:
	  – Non-healing keratinizing or crusted tumours >1 cm with significant induration on palpation
	  – Patients in whom squamous cell carcinoma has been diagnosed from a biopsy undertaken in general practice
	  – After an organ transplant with new or growing cutaneous lesions

Head and neck cancer	*Urgent referral*
	• Unexplained lump in the neck that is of recent onset or a previously undiagnosed lump that has changed over 3–6 weeks
	• Unexplained persistent swelling in the parotid or submandibular gland
	• Unexplained persistent sore or painful throat
	• Unexplained persistent pain in the head or neck for >4 weeks associated with otalgia (earache) but a normal otoscopy
	• Unexplained ulceration of oral mucosa or mass persisting for >3 weeks
	• Unexplained red and white patches of the oral mucosa (including suspected lichen planus) that are painful or swollen or bleeding
	• Any other patients with persistent symptoms or signs (>6 weeks) related to the oral cavity in whom a definitive diagnosis of a benign lesion cannot be made
	• Unexplained tooth mobility lasting >3 weeks (to a dentist)
	• Hoarseness for >3 weeks. Order urgent chest x-ray. If positive, refer to a team specializing in the management of lung cancer. If negative, refer urgently to a team specializing in head and neck cancer
	Thyroid cancer
	• Tracheal compression due to thyroid swelling (immediate referral)
	• Solitary nodule increasing in size
	• Thyroid swelling associated with:
	  – history of neck irradiation
	  – family history of an endocrine tumour
	  – unexplained hoarseness or voice changes
	  – cervical lymphadenopathy
	  – prepubertal patient or patient aged 65 or older

Brain tumours	*Urgent referral:* when a brain tumour is suspected in a patient with:
	  – progressive neurologic deficit
	  – new onset seizures
	  – headaches
	  – mental changes
	  – cranial nerve palsy
	  – unilateral sensorineural deafness
	• Headaches of recent onset with features suggestive of raised intracranial pressure (eg, vomiting, drowsiness, posture-related headache, pulse-synchronous tinnitus, or other focal or non-focal neurologic symptoms)
	• A new, qualitatively different, unexplained headache that becomes progressively severe
	• Suspected recent-onset seizures (refer to neurologist)
	Consider urgent referral when there is rapid progression of:
	• subacute focal neurologic deficit
	• unexplained cognitive impairment, and/or behavioural disturbance
	• personality change

Sarcoma	*Urgent referral*
	Suspected spontaneous fracture needs immediate x-ray. Refer if it suggests possible cancer. A palpable lump with one or more of the following characteristics:
	  – Size >5 cm
	  – Painful
	  – Increasing in size
	  – Deep to fascia, fixed or immobile
	  – Recurrence after previous excision
	• Suspected Kaposi sarcoma in a patient who has HIV
	• Increasing, unexplained, or persistent bone pain or tenderness, particularly pain at rest (especially if not in the joint) or an unexplained limp
	Investigate urgently first

Children's Cancers	Referral Guidelines
General	*Urgent referral* • When a child presents three or more times with the same problem and investigation reveals no clear diagnosis • Persistent back pain after investigation and taking parental anxiety into account

Leukaemia	• Unexplained petechiae (refer immediately)
	• Hepatosplenomegaly (refer immediately)
	• Take blood for FBC and film (and refer urgently if positive) if any of the following is present:
	  – Fatigue
	  – Pallor
	  – Unexplained irritability
	  – Unexplained fever
	  – Persistent or recurrent upper respiratory tract infections
	  – Generalized lymphadenopathy
	  – Persistent or unexplained bone pain
	  – Unexplained bruising

Lymphoma	• Hepatosplenomegaly (immediate referral)
	• Mediastinal or hilar mass on chest x-ray (immediate referral)
	• Lymphadenopathy (particularly if there is no evidence of previous local infection) with at least one of the following:
	  – Nodes >2 cm in size
	  – Nontender, firm/hard nodes
	  – Progressively enlarging
	  – Associated with other signs of general ill health, fever, and/or weight loss
	  – Involves axillary nodes (in the absence of any local infection or dermatitis) or supraclavicular nodes
	• Shortness of breath and unexplained petechiae or hepatosplenomegaly

Brain and CNS tumours	*Urgent referral*
	Altered level of consciousness (immediate referral)
	• Headache and vomiting that cause early morning waking or occur on waking (immediate referral)
	• Children aged <2 years with any of the following (immediate referral):
	  – Bulging fontanelle
	  – Extensor attacks
	  – Persistent vomiting
	  – New onset seizures
	• Children of any age with any of the following (immediate or urgent referral):
	  – New onset seizures
	  – Cranial nerve abnormalities
	  – Visual disturbance
	  – Gait abnormality
	  – Motor or sensory signs
	  – Unexplained deteriorating school performance or developmental milestones
	  – Unexplained behavioural and/or mood changes
	• Children age ≥2 years, and young people, with persistent headache where you cannot carry out an adequate neurologic examination
	• Children <2 years old with any of the following:
	  – Abnormal increase in head size
	  – Arrest or regression of motor development
	  – Altered behaviour
	  – Abnormal eye movements
	  – Lack of visual following
	  – Poor feeding or failure to thrive
	  – Squint (where the urgency will depend on other factors)

Neuroblastoma	*Refer urgently children with:*
	  – proptosis
	  – unexplained back pain, leg weakness
	  – unexplained urinary retention

Continued

Children's Cancers	Referral Guidelines
Wilms tumour Soft tissue sarcoma	*Refer urgently* children with haematuria *Refer urgently* children with an unexplained mass if associated with one or more of the following characteristics: – Nontender – Progressively enlarging – Size >2 cm in maximum diameter or deep to fascia – Associated with enlarging regional lymph node
Bone sarcoma	*Refer* children or young people with rest pain, back pain, or unexplained limp (discuss with paeditrician). Refer urgently if there is persistent localized bone pain and/or swelling and x-ray suggests cancer
Retinoblastoma	*Refer urgently* children with a white pupillary reflex, a new squint, or change in visual acuity suggestive of cancer, or any visual problems and a family history of retinoblastoma

Opioid Dose Conversion Chart

(all doses in milligrams (mg) unless otherwise stated)

Oral Opioid (24 h)		CSCI Opioid (24 h)					Subcutaneous PRN Opioid q4h				Opioid Transdermal Patch	
Morphine	Oxycodone	Morphine	Oxycodone	Diamorphine	Alfentanil	Fentanyl	Morphine	Oxycodone	Diamorphine	Fentanyl	Fentanyl	Buprenorphine
20	10	10	5	5	500 µg	100 µg	2	1	1	12.5 µg	–	10 µg/h
30	15	15	7.5	10	1 mg	200 µg	2.5	1.5	2	25 µg	–	15 µg/h
45	20	20	10	15	1.5	300 µg	4	2	2.5	37.5 µg	12 µg/h	20 µg/h
90	45	45	20	30	3	600 µg	8	4	5	75 µg	25 µg/h	35 µg/h
140	70	70	35	45	4.5	900 µg	12	6	8	100 µg	37 µg/h	52.5 µg/h
180	90	90	45	60	6	Max. CSCI 900 µg as limited by volume (50 µg/mL)	15	8	10	Max. PRN 100 µg as limited by volume (50 µg/mL)	50 µg/h	70 µg/h
230	115	115	60	75	7.5		20	10	12.5		62 µg/h	105 µg/h
270	135	135	70	90	9		25	12	15		75 µg/h	122.5 µg/h
360	180	180	90	120	12		30	15	20		100 µg/h	140 µg/h
450	225	225	110	150	15		35	18	25		125 µg/h	(Manufacturer's recommended maximum is 140 µg/h)
540	270	270	135	180	18		45	20	30		150 µg/h	
630	315	315	160	210	21		50	25	35		175 µg/h	
720	360	360	180	240	24		60	30	40		200 µg/h	

Notes:
- The conversions stated here are only approximate, and are based upon manufacturers' and other sources of data. There may be local guidelines stating different conversion ratios: these should be followed where they exist.
- When switching between opioids, it is recommended that the calculated equivalent dose of the new opioid is reduced by 25–50%.
- Alfentanil: Fentanyl based on 5:1 (this is the modal average taken from several different data sources; range 3.3–6:1)
- Fentanyl PRN dose is calculated as 1/8th of 24 h dose (mean average taken from different sources; range 1/10th to 1/6th)

Index

Page numbers followed by "*f*" indicate figures, "*t*" indicate tables, and "*b*" indicate boxes.